ENDOVASCULAR SURGERY

FOURTH EDITION

ENDOVASCULAR SURGERY

FOURTH EDITION

Wesley S. Moore, MD

Professor and Chief Emeritus
Division of Vascular Surgery
University of California Medical Center
Los Angeles, California

Samuel S. Ahn, MD, FACS

University Vascular Associates
Los Angeles, California
DFW Vascular Group
Dallas, Texas

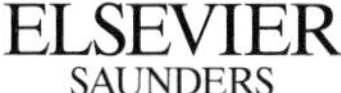
SAUNDERS

ELSEVIER
SAUNDERS

1600 John F. Kennedy Bovlevard
Suite 1800
Philadelphia, Pennsylvania 19103-2899

ENDOVASCULAR SURGERY **ISBN: 978-1-4160-6208-0**

Library of Congress Cataloging-in-Publication Data
Endovascular surgery / [edited by] Wesley S. Moore, Samuel S. Ahn. --
4th ed.
p.; cm
Includes bibliographical references and index.
ISBN 978-1-4160-6208-0 (hardcover : alk. paper)
1. Blood-vessels--Endoscopic surgery. 2. Angioscopy. 3. Angioplasty
I. Moore, Wesley S. II. Ahn, Samuel S.
[DNLM: 1. Vascular Surgical Procedures--methods. 2. Angioplasty, Balloon--methods. 3. Endoscopy--methods. WG 170]
RD598.5.E53 2011
617.4'130597--dc22 2010039799

Acquisitions Editor: Judith Fletcher
Developmental Editor: Rachel Yard
Publishing Services Manager: Anne Altepeter
Senior Project Manager: Beth Hayes
Marketing Manager: Cara Jespersen
Design Direction: Lou Forgione

Printed in the United States of America

Last digit is the print number: 9 8 7 6 5 4 3 2 1

Contributors

Justin S. Ahn, BS
Medical Student
University of Texas Southwestern
Dallas, Texas
Axillosubclavian Vein Thrombectomy, Thrombolysis, and Angioplasty

Samuel S. Ahn, MD, FACS
President
University Vascular Associates
Los Angeles, California
DFW Vascular Group
Dallas, Texas
Laser Atherectomy
Femoral-Popliteal-Tibial Graft Occlusion: Thrombolysis, Angioplasty, Atherectomy, and Stent
Endovascular Treatment of Visceral Artery Aneurysms
Axillosubclavian Vein Thrombectomy, Thrombolysis, and Angioplasty
Thoracoscopic Dorsal Sympathectomy

Paul M. Anain, MD, FACS
Vascular & Endovascular Center
Endovascular Center West New York
Buffalo, New York
Femoral-Popliteal-Tibial Graft Occlusion: Thrombolysis, Angioplasty, Atherectomy, and Stent

George Andros, MD
Medical Director
Amputation Prevention Center
Valley Presbyterian Hospital
Los Angeles, California
Arterial Access

Enrico Ascher, MD, FACS
Director
Vascular and Endovascular Surgery
Maimonides Medical Center
Professor of Surgery
Mount Sinai School of Medicine
New York, New York
Duplex-Guided Infrainguinal Interventions
Inferior Vena Cava Filter Placement

Martin R. Back, MD
Professor of Surgery
Division of Vascular and Endovascular Surgery
University of South Florida
Tampa, Florida
Duplex Ultrasound Surveillance of Dialysis Access Function

J. Dennis Baker, MD
Professor of Surgery
Division of Vascular Surgery
University of California – Los Angeles
Gonda Vascular Center
Los Angeles, California
Duplex Ultrasonography

Dennis F. Bandyk, MD
Professor of Surgery
Division of Vascular and Endovascular Surgery
University of South Florida College of Medicine
Tampa, Florida
Vascular Laboratory Surveillance After Arterial Intervention
Duplex Ultrasound Surveillance of Dialysis Access Function

Joel E. Barbato, MD
Assistant Professor of Surgery
Division of Vascular Surgery
University of Minnesota
Saint Paul, Minnesota
Endovascular Repair of Thoracic Aortic Aneurysms

Donald T. Baril, MD
Assistant Professor
Division of Vascular Surgery
Department of Surgery
University of Pittsburgh Medical Center
Pittsburgh, Pennsylvania
Peripheral Atherectomy

Marc Bosiers, MD
Vascular Surgeon
Department of Vascular Surgery
AZ Sint-Blasius Hospital
East Flanders
Belgium
Subclavian and Vertebral Arteries: Angioplasty and Stents

Jacob Buth, MD, PhD, FRCS
Consulting Vascular Surgeon
Department of Surgery
Eindhoven, The Netherlands
Peripheral Arterial Atherectomy for Infrainguinal Arterial Occlusive Disease

James Caridi, MD, FSIR
Associate Professor and Chair
Vascular and Interventional Radiology
University of Florida
Gainesville, Forida
Angiography

Jeffrey P. Carpenter, MD
Professor and Chief of Surgery
Department of Surgery
Robert Wood Johnson Medical School
Camden, New Jersey
Magnetic Resonance Imaging and Angiography

Neal S. Cayne, MD
Director of Endovascular Surgery
Division of Vascular Surgery
New York University School of Medicine
New York, New York
Endovascular Repair of Ruptured Abdominal Aortic Aneurysms

Rabih A. Chaer, MD
Assistant Professor of Surgery
Division of Vascular Surgery
University of Pittsburgh School of Medicine
Pittsburgh, Pennsylvania
Peripheral Atherectomy

Elliot L. Chaikof, MD, PhD
Professor of Surgery
Chief
Division of Vascular Surgery
Department of Surgery, Emory University School of Medicine
Atlanta, Georgia
Percutaneous Thrombectomy and Mechanical Thrombolysis Catheters

Kristofer M. Charlton-Ouw, MD
Assistant Professor
Department of Cardiothoracic and Vascular Surgery
University of Texas Medical School – Houston
Houston, Texas
Balloon Angioplasty in Aortoiliac Arterial Occlusive Disease
Intravascular Stenting in Aortoiliac Arterial Occlusive Disease

Joe P. Chauvapun, MD
Assistant Professor
Department of Surgery
Division of Vascular Surgery
Harbor–UCLA Medical Center
David Geffen School of Medicine
University of California – Los Angeles
Los Angeles, California
Duplex Ultrasound Surveillance of Dialysis Access Function

Julia F. Chen
Research Associate
DFW Vascular Group
Dallas, Texas
Laser Atherectomy

Charlie Cheng, MD
Assistant Professor
Vascular and Endovascular Surgery
Department of Surgery
University of Texas Medical Branch
Galveston, Texas
Guidewires, Catheters, and Sheaths

Jae S. Cho, MD
Associate Professor of Surgery
Division of Vascular Surgery
Department of Surgery
University of Pittsburgh School of Medicine
Pittsburgh, Pennsylvania
Endovascular Repair of Thoracic Aortic Aneurysms

Timothy A. M. Chuter, BM, BS, DM
Professor of Surgery
Department of Vascular Surgery
University of California – San Francisco
San Francisco, California
Repair of Thoracoabdominal Aortic Aneurysms Using Branched Endografts

Daniel Clair, MD
Professor of Surgery
Department of Vascular Surgery
Cleveland Clinic
Lerner College of Medicine
Cleveland, Ohio
Mesenteric Syndromes

Anthony J. Comerota, MD, FACS, RVT
Director
Jobst Vascular Center
Toledo, Ohio
Catheter-Directed Thrombolysis for Lower Extremity Acute Deep Venous Thrombosis
Pulmonary Thrombolysis

Milton Conley, MD
Fellow
University of California – Los Angeles
Oroville, California
Axillosubclavian Vein Thrombectomy, Thrombolysis, and Angioplasty

Richard Brad Cook, MD
Fellow
University Medical Center
University of California – Los Angeles
Endovascular Ablation of Veins

Hans Coveliers, MD
Vascular Surgeon
VU Medical Center
Amsterdam, The Netherlands
Laparoscopic Aortic Surgery

Miguel Cuesta, MD
Vascular Surgeon
VU Medical Center
Amsterdam, The Netherlands
Laparoscopic Aortic Surgery

Mark G. Davies, PhD, MBA, FACS, FRCS, FRCSI
Professor of Cardiovascular Surgery
Vice Chair
Research and Education
Vice Chair
Finance and Administration
Program Director
Vascular Surgery

Department of Cardiovascular Surgery
The Methodist Hospital
Methodist DeBakey Heart and Vascular Center
Weill-Cornell Medical School
New York, New York
The Methodist Hospital
Houston, Texas
Balloon Angioplasty in Aortoiliac Arterial Occlusive Disease
Intravascular Stenting in Aortoiliac Arterial Occlusive Disease

Luis R. Davila-Santini, MD
Vascular Fellow
North Shore Long Island Jewish Health System
MMC Eastern Vascular Associates
Bronx, New York
Radiation Physics and Radiation Safety

Koen Deloose, MD
Vascular Surgeon
Department of Vascular Surgery
AZ Sint-Blasius Hospital
East Flanders, Belgium
Subclavian and Vertebral Arteries: Angioplasty and Stents

Brian G. DeRubertis, MD
Assistant Professor of Surgery
Division of Vascular Surgery
Department of Surgery
David Geffen School of Medicine
University of California – Los Angeles
Los Angeles, California
Balloon Angioplasty and Stenting for Femoral-Popliteal Occlusive Disease
Stent-Grafting for Infrainguinal Arterial Occlusive Disease
Innominate and Common Carotid Arteries: Angioplasty and Stents
The Use of Embolization Techniques in Endovascular Surgery

Jean-Paul de Vries, MD, PhD
Head
Department of Vascular Surgery
St. Antonius Hospital
Nieuwegein, The Netherlands
Endarterectomy in Infrainguinal Arterial Occlusive Disease

Edward B. Diethrich, MD
Arizona Heart Institute
Hospital and Translational Research Center
Phoenix, Arizona
Thrombolysis in Aortoiliac Arterial Occlusive Disease
Endovascular Repair of Aortic Arch Aneurysm Using Supra-Aortic Trunk Debranching

Jeroen Diks, PhD
Resident
Department of Surgery
Albert Schweitzer Hospital
Dordrecht, The Netherlands
Laparoscopic Aortic Surgery

Sharif Ellozy, MD
Assistant Professor of Surgery and Radiology
Department of Surgery
Mount Sinai School of Medicine
New York, New York
Management of Complications After Endovascular Abdominal Aortic Aneurysm Repair

Darwin Eton, MD, FACS
Professor of Surgery
University of Chicago
Chicago, Illinois
Stem Cell Infusion for Development of Collateral Circulation

Robert J. Feezor, MD
Assistant Professor of Vascular Surgery and Endovascular Therapy
Department of Surgery
University of Florida
Gainesville, Florida
Angiography

Mark F. Fillinger, MD
Professor of Surgery
Department of Vascular Surgery
Dartmouth-Hitchcock Medical Center
Lebanon, New Hampshire
Computed Tomographic Scanning

Nicholas J. Gargiulio, III, MD, FACS
Associate Professor of Clinical Surgery
Albert Einstein College of Medicine
Montefiore Medical Center
Division of Vascular Surgery
Department of Surgery
Bronx, New York
Endovascular Repair of Ruptured Abdominal Aortic Aneurysms

Hugh A. Gelabert, MD
Professor of Surgery
Division of Vascular Surgery
University of California – Los Angeles
Gonda Vascular Center
Los Angeles, California
Clinical Decision Making and Hemodialysis Graft Thrombosis
Central Venous Catheter Malfunction

Alexander Gevorgyan, MD
Oral Maxillofacial Surgeon
Clinic of Oral, Maxillofacial, and Plastic Surgery
Yerevan, Armenia
Endovascular Treatment of Visceral Artery Aneurysms

Ramyar Gilani, MD
Assistant Professor
Department of Vascular Surgery
Baylor College of Medicine
Houston, Texas
Aortoiliac Graft Limb Occlusion: Thrombolysis, Mechanical Thrombectomy

Suzanne S. Gisbertz, MD, PhD
Department of Surgery
VU Medical Center
Amsterdam, The Netherlands
Endarterectomy in Infrainguinal Arterial Occlusive Disease

Peter Gloviczki, MD
Joe M. and Ruth Roberts Professor of Surgery
Division of Vascular Surgery
Mayo Clinic
Rochester, Minnesota
Endoscopic and Percutaneous Techniques for Treatment of Incompetent Perforators

Roy K. Greenberg, MD
Director
Endovascular Research and Peripheral Vascular Core Laboratory
Associate Professor of Surgery
Department of Vascular Surgery
Cleveland Clinic Lerner College of Medicine
Case School of Medicine
Associate Professor of Biomedical Engineering
Case School of Biomedical Engineering
Case Western Reserve University
Cleveland, Ohio
Endovascular Repair of Abdominal Aortic Aneurysm Using Fenestrated Grafts

Irvin Hawkins, MD
(Retired) Cardiovascular Radiology Fellow
Shands Hospital
Department of Radiology
University of Florida
Gainesville, Florida
Angiography

Anil P. Hingorani, MD
Associate Professor
Division of Vascular Surgery
Mount Sinai Medical Center
Brooklyn, New York
Duplex-Guided Infrainguinal Interventions
Inferior Vena Cava Filter Placement

Kim J. Hodgson, MD
Professor and Chair
Division of Vascular Surgery
Department of Vascular Surgery
Southern Illinois University School of Medicine
Springfield, Illinois
Preparing the Endovascular Operating Room Suite
Endovascular Treatment of Renovascular Disease

Douglas B. Hood, MD
Associate Professor of Vascular Surgery
Southern Illinois University School of Medicine
Springfield, Illinois
Endovascular Treatment of Renovascular Disease

L. Nelson Hopkins, MD
Professor and Chair of Neurosurgery
Professor of Radiology
Director
Toshiba Stroke Research Center
State University of New York – Buffalo
Buffalo, New York
Complication Management in Carotid Stenting

Daniel M. Ihnat, MD, FACS
Associate Professor of Clinical Surgery
Division of Vascular Surgery
University of Utah
Salt Lake City, Utah
Endovascular Management of Infrapopliteal Occlusive Disease

Khalid Irshad, FRCS
Associate Surgical Specialist
Wishaw Hospital
Wishaw, Scotland
United Kingdom
Endovascular Repair of Aortic Arch Aneurysm Using Supra-Aortic Trunk Debranching

Reda Jamjoom, MD, Med, FRCS(C)
Vascular Surgery Fellow
McGill University
Montreal, Quebec, Canada
Thrombolysis in Dialysis Access Salvage

Colleen L. Jay, MD
Surgical Resident
Post-Doctoral Research Fellow
Department of Surgery
Feinberg School of Medicine
Northwestern University
Chicago, Illinois
Brachiocephalic Graft Occlusion
Endovascular Repair of Abdominal Aortic Aneurysm: Comparative Technique and Results of Currently Available Devices

Jeffrey Jim, MD, MS
Assistant Professor of Surgery
Section of Vascular Surgery
Washington University School of Medicine
St. Louis, Missouri
The Transjugular Intrahepatic Portosystemic Shunt Procedure for Portal Hypertension

Juan Carlos Jimenez, MD
Assistant Professor
Gonda Vascular Center
University of California – Los Angeles
Los Angeles, California
Complications Associated With Endovascular Management of Aortoiliac Arterial Occlusive Disease
Endovascular Treatment of Visceral Artery Aneurysms
Endoscopic Vein Harvest

Colleen M. Johnson, MD
Assistant Professor
Division of Vascular Surgery
Southern Illinois University School of Medicine
Springfield, Illinois
Preparing the Endovascular Operating Room Suite

Jagajan Karmacharya, MBBS, FRCS, FACS
Assistant Professor
Division of Vascular and Endovascular Surgery
Department of Surgery
Miller School of Medicine
University of Miami
Miami, Florida
Endovascular Treatment of Vascular Injuries

Vikram S. Kashyap, MD, FACS
Department of Vascular Surgery
The Cleveland Clinic Foundation
Cleveland, Ohio
Principles of Thrombolysis
Aortoiliac Graft Limb Occlusion: Thrombolysis, Mechanical Thrombectomy
Catheter-Directed Therapy of Superior Vena Cava Syndrome

Karthikeshwar Kasirajan, MD
Professor of Surgery
Associate Department of Surgery
Emory University School of Medicine
Atlanta Veterans Administration Medical Center
Atlanta, Georgia
Carotid Bifurcation Stented Balloon Angioplasty With Cerebral Protection
Endovascular Management of Anastomotic Aneurysms
Endovascular Repair of Acute and Chronic Thoracic Aortic Dissections

Arash Keyhani, DO
Vascular Surgeon
Department of Surgery
Harbor–UCLA Medical Center
Long Beach Memorial Medical Center
Long Beach, California
Intravascular Ultrasound

Ali Khoynezhad, MD, PhD
Director
Department of Thoracic Aortic Surgery
Associate Professor of Surgery
Division of Cardiothoracic Surgery
Cedars-Sinai Medical Center
Los Angeles, California
Training and Credentialing

Brian N. King, MD
Fellow in Vascular Surgery
Montefiore Medical Center
Albert Einsein College of Medicine
Bronx, New York
Complications and Their Management After Endovascular Intervention in Infrainguinal Arterial Occlusive Disease

Kenneth R. Kollmeyer, MD, PhD
Endovascular Surgeon
DFW Vascular Group
Clinical Assistant Professor of Surgery
University of Texas Southwestern Medical School
Dallas, Texas
Laser Atherectomy

George Kopchock, MD
Division of Vascular Surgery
Harbor–UCLA Medical Center
Torrance, California
Intravascular Ultrasound

Kenneth Kuchta, MD
Associate Clinical Professor
Anesthesiology
David Geffen School of Medicine
University of California – Los Angeles
Los Angeles, California
Anesthetic Management for Endovascular Procedures

Gregory J. Landry, MD, MCR
Associate Professor of Surgery
Department of Surgery
Oregon Health and Science University
Portland, Oregon
Endovascular Management of Popliteal Aneurysms

Peter F. Lawrence, MD
Bergman Professor of Vascular Research
Wiley Barker Chief of Vascular Surgery
Director of the Gonda Vascular Center
David Geffen School of Medicine
University of California – Los Angeles
Los Angeles, California
Pharmacologic Adjuncts in Endovascular Surgery

W. Anthony Lee, MD
Associate Professor of Surgery
Division of Vascular Surgery and Endovascular Therapy
University of Florida College of Medicine
Gainesville, Florida
Arterial Closure Devices

Elad I. Levy, MD, FACS, FAHA
Professor of Neurosurgery
Professor of Radiology
Director
Endovascular Fellowship and Stroke Service
Department of Neurosurgery
School of Medicine and Biomedical Sciences
State University of New York – Buffalo
Buffalo, New York
Complication Management in Carotid Stenting

Timothy K. Liem, MD
Associate Professor of Surgery
Adjunct Associate Professor of Radiology
Division of Vascular Surgery
Oregon Health Sciences University
Portland, Oregon
Endovascular Management of Popliteal Aneurysms

Evan C. Lipsitz, MD
Interim Chief
Division of Vascular Surgery
Department of Surgery
Montefiore Medical Center
Albert Einstein College of Medicine
Bronx, New York
Reducing Radiation Exposure During Endovascular Procedures
Complications and Their Management Following Endovascular Intervention in Infrainguinal Arterial Occlusive Disease

Harold Litt, MD, PhD
Assistant Professor of Radiology and Medicine
Chief
Cardiovascular Imaging
Department of Radiology
University of Pennsylvania School of Medicine
Philadelphia, Pennsylvania
Magnetic Resonance Imaging and Angiography

Alan B. Lumsden, MD
Medical Director
Methodist DeBakey Heart & Vascular Center
Professor and Chair
Department of Cardiovascular Surgery
The Methodist Hospital
Houston, Texas
Balloon Angioplasty in Aortoiliac Arterial Occlusive Disease
Intravascular Stenting in Aortoiliac Arterial Occlusive Disease

Michel S. Makaroun, MD
Professor of Surgery
Chair
Division of Vascular Surgery
University of Pittsburgh
Pittsburgh, Pennsylvania
Endovascular Repair of Thoracic Aortic Aneurysms

Michael L. Marin, MD
Department of Surgery
Mount Sinai Medical Center
New York, New York
Endovascular Grafting in Aortoiliac Arterial Occlusive Disease

Natalie Marks, MD, RVT
Vascular Laboratory Technical Director
Department of Vascular Surgery Division
Maimonides Medical Center
Brooklyn, New York
Duplex-Guided Infrainguinal Interventions

Tara M. Mastracci, MD, FRCSC, MSc
Assistant Professor of Surgery
Department of Vascular Surgery
Cleveland Clinic Foundation
Cleveland, Ohio
Endovascular Repair of Abdominal Aortic Aneurysm Using Fenestrated Grafts

Jon S. Matsumura, MD
Division of Vascular Surgery
Department of Surgery
University of Wisconsin School of Medicine and Public Health
Madison, Wisconsin
Brachiocephalic Graft Occlusion
Endovascular Repair of Abdominal Aortic Aneurysm: Comparative Technique and Results of Currently Available Devices

Jordan D. Miller, MD
Associate Professor
Department of Anesthesia
David Geffen School of Medicine
University of California – Los Angeles
Los Angeles, California
Anesthetic Management for Endovascular Procedures

Joseph L. Mills, Sr., MD
Professor of Surgery
Chief
Division of Vascular and Endovascular Surgery
Division of Vascular Surgery
Department of Surgery
University of Arizona Health Sciences Center
Tucson, Arizona
Endovascular Management of Infrapopliteal Occlusive Disease

Frans L. Moll, MD, PhD
Professor and Head
Department of Vascular Surgery
University Medical Center Utrecht
Utrecht, The Netherlands
Endarterectomy in Infrainguinal Arterial Occlusive Disease

Wesley S. Moore, MD
Professor and Chief Emeritus
Division of Vascular Surgery
University of California Medical Center
Los Angeles, California
The Concept of Endovascular Surgery

Sabareesh K. Natarajan, MD, MS
Clinical Assistant Instructor
Health Sciences
Department of Neurosurgery
School of Medicine and Biomedical Sciences
State University of New York – Buffalo
Buffalo, New York
Complication Management in Carotid Stenting

Peter Neglen, MD, PhD
Vascular Surgery
Flowood, Mississippi
Iliofemoral and Inferior Vena Cava Stenting in Chronic Venous Insufficiency

Nicolas A. Nelken, MD, FACS
Vascular Surgeon
Kaiser Hawaii
Assistant Clinical Professor of Surgery
University of California – San Francisco
Kaiser Permanente
Honolulu, Hiawai
Computed Tomographic Angiography in Peripheral Arterial Occlusive Disease
Percutaneous Thrombectomy Devices in Thrombosed Dialysis Access

Daniel I. Obrand, MD, FRCSC
Assistant Professor of Surgery
Department of Vascular Surgery
McGill University
Montreal, Quebec, Canada
Thrombolysis in Dialysis Access Salvage

Takao Ohki, MD
Chairman and Professor
Department of Surgery
Jikei University School of Medicine
Minato-ku, Tokyo
Reducing Radiation Exposure During Endovascular Procedures

Dawn Olsen, PA
Vascular PA-C
Arizona Heart Institute
Phoenix, Arizona
Endovascular Repair of Aortic Arch Aneurysm Using Supra-Aortic Trunk Debranching

Arthur Olson, MD
Clinical Assistant Professor
Radiation Safety Officer and Director of Medicophysics
State University of New York
Downstate Medical Center
Brooklyn, New York
Radiation Physics and Radiation Safety

Kenneth Ouriel, MD
Columbia University
New York, New York
Principles of Thrombolysis

Thomas F. Panetta, MD
Medical Director
Axcess, Inc.
Great Neck, New York
Radiation Physics and Radiation Safety
Vascular Stents

Juan C. Parodi, MD
(Retired)
University of Miami Miller School of Medicine
Miami, Florida
Endovascular Treatment of Vascular Injuries

Nirav Patel, MD
Southland Neurologic Associates
Los Alamitos, California
Inferior Vena Cava Filter Placement

Sheela T. Patel, MD
Assistant Professor of Surgery
Department of Surgery
University of Miami Miller School of Medicine
Miami, Florida
Endovascular Treatment of Vascular Injuries

Patrick Peeters, MD
Vascular Surgery
Department of Cardiovascular and Thoracic Surgery
Imelda Hospital
Bonheiden, Antwerp, Belgium
Subclavian and Vertebral Arteries: Angioplasty and Stents

Gregory Pierce, MD
Staff Interventional Radiology
Section of Vascular and Interventional Radiology
Imaging Institute
Cleveland Clinic
Cleveland, Ohio
Catheter-Directed Therapy of Superior Vena Cava Syndrome

Alessandra Puggioni, MD
Vascular Surgeon
Department of Surgery
Scottsdale Vascular Services
Scottsdale, Arizona
Endoscopic and Percutaneous Techniques for Treatment of Incompetent Perforators

Feng Qin, MD
Attending, Vascular Surgery
Lenox Hill Heart and Vascular Institute
New York, New York
Vascular Stents

William J. Quinones-Baldrich, MD
Professor of Surgery
Director of Endovascular Service
Department of Vascular Surgery
David Geffen School of Medicine
University of California – Los Angeles
Los Angeles, California
Combined Endovascular and Surgical Approach to Thoracoabdominal Aortic Pathology

Seshadri Raju, MD, FACS
Vascular Surgery
The Rane Center for Veinous and Lymphatic Disease
Flowood, Mississippi
Iliofemoral and Inferior Vena Cava Stenting in Chronic Venous Insufficiency

Venkatesh J. Ramiah, MD
Internal Medicine
Troy, Michigan
Endovascular Repair of Aortic Arch Aneurysm Using Supra-Aortic Trunk Debranching

Donald B. Reid, MD, FRCS
Wishaw Hospital
Wishaw, Scotland, United Kingdom
Thrombolysis in Aortoiliac Arterial Occlusive Disease
Endovascular Repair of Aortic Arch Aneurysm Using Supra-Aortic Trunk Debranching

Todd D. Reil, MD, FACS
Associate Professor of Surgery
Director of Endovascular Surgery
Department of Vascular Surgery
Department of Surgery
University of Minnesota Minneapolis, Minnesota
Endovascular Treatment of Visceral Artery Aneurysms

Linda M. Reilly, MD
Professor of Surgery
Director
General Surgery Residency Program
Division of Vascular Surgery
University of California – San Francisco
San Francisco, California
Repair of Thoracoabdominal Aortic Aneurysms Using Branched Endografts

David A. Rigberg, MD
Associate Professor of Vascular Surgery
Department of Surgery
University of California – Los Angeles
Los Angeles, California
Endovascular Ablation of Veins
The Transjugular Intrahepatic Portosystemic Shunt Procedure for Portal Hypertension

Kyung M. Ro, MD
Department of Radiology
The Permanente Medical Group
Redwood City Medical Center
Redwood City, California
Thoracoscopic Dorsal Sympathectomy

Sean P. Roddy, MD
Associate Professor of Surgery
Department of Surgery
Albany Medical College
Albany, New York
Billing and Coding in an Endovascular Practice

Julio A. Rodriguez-Lopez, MD
Assistant Program Director
Vascular Surgery Program
Medical Director
Wound Healing Center
Arizona Heart Hospital
Department of Vascular and Endovascular Surgery
Arizona Heart Institute Midwestern University
Glendale, Arizona
Endovascular Repair of Aortic Arch Aneurysm Using Supra-Aortic Trunk Debranching

Luis Sanchez, MD
Professor of Surgery and Radiology
Section of Vascular Surgery
Department of Surgery
Washington University St. Louis School of Medicine
St. Louis, Missouri
Iliac Artery Aneurysms

Peter A. Schneider, MD
Vascular and Endovascular Surgeon
Chief of Vascular Therapy
Hawaii Permanente Medical Group
Kasier Foundation Hospital
Honolulu, Hawaii
Balloon Angioplasty Catheters
Carotid Bifurcation Stented Balloon Angioplasty With Cerebral Protection

[†]James M. Seeger, MD
Devoted Chief of Vascular Surgery
Division of Vascular Surgery
University of Florida – Gainesville
College of Medicine
Gainesville, Florida
Angiography

Adnan H. Siddiqui, MD, PhD
Assistant Professor
Director of Neurosurgical Research
Director of Neuroendovascular Critical Care
Department of Neurosurgery and Radiology
School of Medicine and Biomedical Sciences
State University of New York – Buffalo
Buffalo, New York
Complication Management in Carotid Stenting

Michael B. Silva, Jr., MD
The Fred J. and Dorothy E. Wolma Professor of Vascular Surgery
Professor of Radiology
Director
Texas Vascular Center
University of Texas Medical Branch
Galveston, Texas
Guidewires, Catheters, and Sheaths

Daniel Silverberg, MD
Attending Vascular Surgeon
Department of Vascular Surgery
The Chain Sheba Medical Center
Tel Hashomer, Israel
Tel-Aviv University
Sackler School of Medicine
Ramat Gan, Israel
Endovascular Grafting in Aortoiliac Arterial Occlusive Disease
Management of Complications After Endovascular Abdominal Aortic Aneurysm Repair

[†]Deceased.

Niten H. Singh, MD
Assistant Professor
Surgery
Uniformed Services
University of the Health Sciences
Bethesda, Maryland
Department of Vascular Surgery
Madigan Army Medical Center
Tacoma, Washington
Balloon Angioplasty Catheters

Joshua C. Smith
Class of 2012
Lake Erie College of Osteopathic Medicine
Erie, Pennsylvania
Endoscopic Vein Harvest

Kenneth V. Snyder, MD, PhD
Assistant Professor
Department of Neurosurgery
School of Medicine and Biomedical Sciences
State University of New York – Buffalo
Buffalo, New York
Complication Management in Carotid Stenting

Subhash Thakur, MD
Vascular Surgeon
Jobst Vascular Center
Toledo, Ohio
Pulmonary Thrombolysis

Alexander V. Tielbeek, MD, PhD
Consulting Radiologist
Head of Training Program
Department of Radiology
Catharina Hospital
Eindhoven, The Netherlands
Peripheral Arterial Atherectomy for Infrainguinal Arterial Occlusive Disease

Frank J. Veith, MD
Professor of Surgery
New York University
New York, New York
Professor of Surgery
William J. von Liebig Chair in Vascular Surgery
The Cleveland Clinic
Cleveland, Ohio
Reducing Radiation Exposure During Endovascular Procedures
Endovascular Repair of Ruptured Abdominal Aortic Aneurysms

Omaida Velazquez, MD
Professor of Surgery
Department of Surgery
University of Miami Miller School of Medicine
Miami, Florida
Endovascular Treatment of Vascular Injuries

Jürgen Verbist, MD
Vascular Surgery
Department of Cardiovascular and Thoracic Surgery
Imelda Hospital
Bonheiden, Antwerp, Belgium
Subclavian and Vertebral Arteries: Angioplasty and Stents

Grace J. Wang, MD
Assistant Professor of Surgery
Department of Vascular Surgery
Hospital of the University of Pennsylvania
Philadelphia, Pennsylvania
Magnetic Resonance Imaging and Angiography

Jeffrey Wang, MD
Chief
Orthopaedic Spine Service
UCLA Comprehensive Spine Center
Santa Monica, California
Percutaneous Thrombectomy and Mechanical Thrombolysis Catheters

Grayson H. Wheatley, MD
Department of Cardiovascular Surgery
Arizona Heart Institute
Phoenix, Arizona
Endovascular Repair of Aortic Arch Aneurysm Using Supra-Aortic Trunk Debranching

Rodney A. White, MD
Chief
Vascular Surgery
Associate Chair
Department of Surgery
Harbor–UCLA Medical Center
Professor of Surgery
School of Medicine
University of California – Los Angeles
Torrance, California
Training and Credentialing
Intravascular Ultrasound

Cecilia K. Wieslander, MD
Dallas, Texas
Thoracoscopic Dorsal Sympathectomy

Michael Wilderman, MD
Vascular Surgery Fellow
Department of Surgery
Washington University
St. Louis, Missouri
Iliac Artery Aneurysms

Willem Wisselink, MD, FACS
Professor of Surgery
Chief
Division of Vascular Surgery
VU University Medical Center
Amsterdam, The Netherlands
Laparoscopic Aortic Surgery

Preface

Endovascular surgery and other catheter-based interventions are taking on an increasingly important role in the management of patients with vascular disease. Vascular surgeons and interventionalists alike are recognizing the importance of this therapeutic modality and are constantly seeking training and updates to fully make use of these treatment options in their daily practice. When the first two editions of this book were prepared, there were a limited number of vascular surgeons with sufficient experience to contribute chapters. Since then, the situation has changed considerably. In the third edition, as well as the current fourth edition, every chapter has been written by a vascular surgeon, thus emphasizing the emerging role of the vascular surgeon in this important and expanding field. Currently, it is estimated that endovascular surgery represents 50% to 70% of the average vascular surgeon's practice.

The field of endovascular surgery has progressed significantly since the third edition. The fourth edition reflects this progress and maturation. For example, the promising laser angioplasty and atherectomy technology that was discussed in the second edition was dropped in the third edition because of disappointing results; however, it is reintroduced in the fourth edition to reflect recent clinically relevant developments. Aortic stent grafting has taken on an even more important position, particularly concerning fenestrated endografts and the combined open and endovascular hybrid techniques for thoracic and abdominal aneurysms and dissections. In addition to complete updates of prior chapters, interventional management of superficial and deep venous disease has been greatly expanded.

The book has kept its major sections, which include general principles, imaging, and the various therapeutic modalities. Sections are also broken out anatomically to address the variety of endovascular techniques appropriate for each anatomic location (such as the aortoiliac system, the infrainguinal arteries, the visceral arteries, and the supra-aortic trunks). The management of specific problems (such as vascular graft thrombosis, endografting for aneurysms and traumatic injuries, dialysis access salvage, and venous surgery) are updated with real and promising developments. We have also added a new section of representative instructional case presentations, featuring integrated clinical and angiographic data. These case presentations reinforce the thinking process that go into clinical decision-making. *Color versions of many of the illustrations can be found at http:www.expertconsult.com.*

This book is designed to meet the needs of those who are first entering the field as well as experienced endovascular surgeons who wish to update their skills and have access to a current database of results. To accomplish these objectives, the text covers the basic technical aspects of a variety of procedures in all anatomic locations, except for of heart and intracranial circulation. Individual chapters are prepared to stand alone so that the text can be used as a data resource. When several interventional options are available for a given lesion, the immediate and long-term results are compared and the advantages and disadvantages of each technique are discussed. Finally, pharmacologic adjuncts and methods to prevent intimal hyperplasia and late failure are addressed.

It is the editors' expectation that this book will be comprehensive and up-to-date and will serve the needs of the vascular specialist for several years to come.

Wesley S. Moore
Samuel S. Ahn

Contents

†Deceased.

X

VENOUS DISEASE

XI

ENDOSCOPIC VASCULAR SURGERY

XII

MISCELLANEOUS ENDOVASCULAR TECHNIQUES

SECTION I

GENERAL PRINCIPLES

CHAPTER

1

The Concept of Endovascular Surgery

Wesley S. Moore

The care of patients with vascular disease, including the direct repair of lesions of the vascular tree, was previously the uncontested province of the vascular surgeon. Resection of aneurysms, endarterectomy for carotid bifurcation disease, and bypass creation for aortoiliac or infrainguinal occlusive disease continued to improve and develop as a function of technical and technologic refinement. With an increase in the population threatened with vascular disorders, many surgeons limited their practice to vascular surgery, and younger generations sought additional residency training in this rapidly expanding specialty. As a result of many factors, the field of vascular surgery experienced accelerated growth for more than 40 years. Improvements in training, operative experience, and technologic improvement in grafts, instruments, and suture materials took place during this time. The growth in the specialty combined with an increased operative experience led to a better long-term treatment outcome for patients with vascular disorders. In spite of these advances, most vascular operations continue to be quite invasive, carry a significant risk of morbidity and mortality, and frequently require a long recovery period before patients can return to their premorbid level of activity.

In the late 1960s, Charles Dotter, a radiologist, pioneered the concept of intravascular intervention, so-called endovascular therapy.[1] The concept evolved from experience with catheter-based angiography. The development of guidewire-directed catheter technology permitted selective catheterization of virtually any branch of the aorta from a percutaneous femoral arterial approach. Dotter conceived of the idea of using a series of coaxial catheters of increasing diameter to dilate stenotic atherosclerotic lesions of the iliac arteries. This technique was limited by the size of the hole that could be safely made in the femoral artery. With the introduction of the balloon angioplasty catheter by Grüntzig, a revolution in catheter-based therapy took place.[2] Thus, through a small femoral artery puncture, a balloon catheter expandable to the size necessary to treat a remote lesion could be introduced. Although the immediate results of this technique were quite good, use of the technology was limited in a small percentage of patients owing to elastic recoil of the atherosclerotic plaque or the development of intimal hyperplasia with recurrent stenosis at the site of dilatation. To address these problems, metallic stents, initially balloon expandable (as developed by Palmaz et al.[3]) and subsequently self-expanding, were introduced. Catheter-based therapy also permitted the development of intra-arterial thrombolysis directed at the site of thrombosis, which could be used rather than large intravenous systemic doses to effect clot dissolution in a localized area. Other adjunctive techniques, such as atherectomy or the partial removal of a plaque using a catheter, have some limited long-term benefit. There were also several misadventures along this fascinating road of investigation and development. Perhaps the best example of such a misadventure was the attempt to use laser technology as an adjunct to balloon angioplasty. Although this appeared to be very promising at first, it quickly fell victim to a high incidence of intermediate-term failure.

The most recent development has been a hybrid of a limited surgical exposure and the catheter-based introduction of a stent graft to treat aneurysmal disease. There have also been some attempts to use stent grafts after angioplasty to manage occlusive disease better with placement of a new vascular lining. Thus the field of endovascular therapy can be defined as any catheter-based intervention, introduced at an easily accessible remote site, to treat occlusive or aneurysmal disease in either the arterial or the venous system.

As endovascular therapy became competitive with and, in many cases, more desirable than direct vascular repair, the traditional role of the vascular surgeon was challenged. The vascular surgeons argued that their specialty training and practice provided a better clinical background and a better understanding of patients with vascular disease than did the background of interventional specialists. Because of the vascular surgeons' experience, they were better able to judge whether patients with vascular disorders needed intervention and, if so, what procedure would be most likely to strike a balance between the best result and the lowest risk. Although these were cogent arguments, the number of referrals to vascular surgeons began to erode because primary care physicians, who believed that they were capable of making diagnostic and therapeutic judgments, were more naturally attracted to less-invasive procedures for their patients. As interventional cardiologists expanded their domain to the peripheral vascular system, the threat to vascular surgeons became even better defined because the cardiologists also had clinical management skills and could serve as both physician and interventionist.

As the threat to the specialty and to the traditional acceptance of vascular surgeons as vascular disease specialists became apparent, some vascular surgeons began to seek interventional training to remain competitive. Interventional radiologists and cardiologists were reluctant to offer training to a competing specialty, however, particularly when they had an obligation to train their own residents. We recognized this problem and, in 1989, offered the first national postgraduate course at the University of California, Los Angeles, Medical Center to provide both didactic and practical training for surgeons wishing to acquire interventional skills. To emphasize the fact that intra-arterial intervention was another form of surgery and, hence, should be included in the vascular surgeons' repertoire, we decided to use the term "endovascular surgery" as an alternative to the term "endovascular therapy," which was used by interventional radiologists. The term endovascular surgery was quickly accepted by the vascular surgery community and served to emphasize the fact that vascular surgeons can and should add interventional skills to their training and subsequent practice. By doing so, vascular surgeons will be able to maintain a leadership position as the specialists who are best equipped to care for patients with vascular disease. When faced with a patient with a vascular problem, vascular surgeons can draw from extensive training, background, and experience. They understand how to use the vascular diagnostic laboratory in a carefully directed, cost-effective manner. They can determine whether invasive diagnostic studies are indicated or can be effectively replaced with noninvasive alternatives. Because vascular surgeons have the best perspective of the natural history of vascular disease, they can choose medical management when it is a reasonable alternative. When intervention is indicated, the vascular surgeon who has skill in both open and endovascular surgery can make a choice based on a balance among risk, the need for rapid patient recovery, and long-term outcome. In contrast, the specialist whose only interventional skills are catheter based can select only one alternative, which may or may not be the best for a specific patient.

References

1. Dotter CT, Judkins MP: Transluminal treatment of arteriosclerotic obstruction: description of a new technique and preliminary report of its application, *Circulation* 30:645–670, 1969.
2. Grüntzig A, Hopff H: Perkutane rekanalisation chronischer arterieller Verschlüsse mit einen neuen Dilatationskatheter: Modifikation der Dotter-technik, *Dtsch Med Wochenschr* 99:2502–2551, 1974.
3. Palmaz JC, Siggitt RR, Reuter SR, et al: Expandable intraluminal graft: preliminary study, *Radiology* 156:73–77, 1985.

CHAPTER

2

Preparing the Endovascular Operating Room Suite

Colleen M. Johnson, Kim J. Hodgson

The 1990s ushered in the era of endovascular surgery and saw it develop from the rudimentary balloon angioplasty to highly complex and sophisticated endoluminal graft placement. In the latest decade this evolution has continued, and now highly complex hybrid procedures combining both open and endovascular techniques are allowing interventionists to treat an even broader range of vascular maladies. This evolution has been fueled by continued developments in catheter-based technology, which have led to an exponential increase in the number of conditions now suitable for endoluminal therapy.[1] Endovascular interventions have evolved to the extent that the majority of open surgical revascularization procedures now have a completely percutaneous alternative, or one that significantly minimizes the surgical dissection once required. The advances that have led to a paradigm shift in the treatment of abdominal aortic aneurysms, from a purely open operation to the endovascular procedure commonly performed today, are now being applied to the treatment of thoracic and thoracoabdominal aneurysms.[2]

The ability to safely deliver and precisely place these endoluminal devices is paramount to the overall success of these minimally invasive procedures and maintenance of a low complication rate. Not surprisingly, one of the most crucial requirements for procedural success is the ability to adequately visualize the target anatomy and interventional instrumentation, best found in a contemporary well-equipped endovascular suite.[3-5] Early endoluminal interventions were performed on easily visualized 0.035-inch systems, without complicated delivery systems or embolic filters, using radiopaque balloon-deployed stents, none of which place significant demands on an imaging system. The imaging requirements of those days, however, are long behind us, at least for those who desire to practice the full spectrum of endovascular interventions. Although many of the basic endovascular procedures can be performed in existing suites, whether they are located in radiology, the cardiac catheterization laboratory, or the operating room, an environment of proper sterility and equipped as an operating room is necessary to perform the evolving combined, or hybrid, open and endovascular procedures.[6-8] In this chapter, an overview of basic equipment, adjunctive hardware and software, and appropriate personnel required in a contemporary endovascular operating suite capable of handling the needs of the vascular interventionist is presented.

THE ENDOVASCULAR OPERATING ROOM

Design and Infrastructure

The modern endovascular operating room has to fulfill the dual role of providing state-of-the-art imaging capabilities in a fully equipped operating room. The basic structure of the operating room must conform to all state and federal regulations. Typically there are requirements for installation of lead lining in the wall and lead shields around equipment and personnel to minimize radiation exposure to patients and operating room personnel. Provisions must be made for adequate overhead operative lighting, and electric, anesthetic gases, and vacuum outlets must be available.[9,10] Adequate space must also be allotted for an anesthesia machine and the appropriate physiologic monitors. Storage space for all associated equipment is mandatory. Many suites have a combination of cabinetry and drawers in conjunction with rolling wire racks that can hold a variety of catheters and make them easily accessible and visible to the operating surgeon. The storage systems must also be appropriate to hold sutures and other commonly used surgical instruments. Ideally, additional space for a control booth should be incorporated into the floor plan for a new endovascular operating room suite, though this may be a dispensable luxury. Scrub sinks with appropriate soap dispensers must be available. Furthermore, a substerile area with an autoclave may be useful if surgical instruments have to be sterilized rapidly for immediate use. Although no standards for minimum surface area have been set, it is hard to imagine an endovascular operating room that was too large. Consider when designing, not just the space required for the radiographic equipment, but a minimum of 500 to 600 square feet of additional space to accommodate adjunctive instrumentation and equipment such as intravascular ultrasound (IVUS) and portable power injection devices.

The ventilation system in the operating room should be designed to provide clean air and to reduce the possibility of contamination. This is achieved by maintaining positive pressure ventilation, which prevents air flow from less clean areas into the cleaner endovascular operating suite. Furthermore, two filter beds are installed in series in the air conditioning system, which is designed to perform 15 air exchanges of filtered air per hour. Clean air enters the room from the ceiling and exhausts through exits near the floor. It is desirable to have a laminar air-flow system, with recirculated air being passed through a high-efficiency particulate filter.[11]

Choosing the Venue

Determining whether to locate an endovascular operating room within the confines of an existing operating room, in a catheterization laboratory, or in the radiology department has much to do with institutional infrastructure, material resources, personnel, and, perhaps most important, politics. The various venues are often viewed as "home turf" for their respective primary users, which explains why most surgeons want the facility located in the operating room.[10] Despite many of these territorial notions, any of these areas can be suitably adapted to accommodate the required standards of sterility and functionality, and, in fact, it is not unheard of for a hospital to have several endovascular operating rooms in several different locations, providing unfettered access to a range of disciplines and specialties, albeit at increased cost. Considering that surgical access is presently required for most aortic endografting (EVAR) and that the use of iliac conduits and hybrid procedures requiring sternotomy or abdominal reconstructions is on the rise, as is the incorporation of fluoroscopy into many standard vascular surgical procedures, it makes a lot of sense to have at least one endovascular operating room located within the operating room area.[6-8]

After a decade with their heads in the sand, vascular surgeons were finally awakened by EVAR to the need to incorporate interventional procedures into their practices and into vascular fellowship training programs. With 75% of abdominal aortic aneurysms having suitable anatomy for EVAR and even ruptured aneurysms showing benefit from the endovascular approach,[12-14] vascular surgeons could no longer afford to marginalize the endovascular therapies. Having far from embraced endovascular therapy over the years, vascular surgeons owe their continued involvement with EVAR to the need for their services to provide vascular access, which bought them precious time to play catch-up in the game of endovascular skills acquisition. Not surprisingly, after having acquired an endovascular skill set, most vascular surgeons have gone out on their own, working completely independently of interventional radiology. Because the operating room is their traditional place of work, most surgeons choose it as their preferred venue for endografting despite the cumbersome and inferior imaging often available there. Although some advocate that the superior sterility of the operating room environment is indispensible for even standard EVAR cases because of the requisite surgical vascular access, most with experience working in the catheter laboratory environment are comfortable with femoral cutdowns and even iliac conduits in a standard angiographic room. Most, however, prefer an angiographic operating room environment for cases requiring abdominal or thoracic debranching.

The potential for conversion to open repair is another often-cited argument for EVAR being performed in an operating room rather than an angiographic suite. Although compelling in concept, the reality is that emergency surgical conversions are extremely rare, and most emergency remedies can be effected endovascularly, or problems at least temporized endovascularly pending definitive surgical repair. In fact, the most frequent EVAR complications relate to access artery or pathway trauma, the majority of which can be readily addressed in an angiographic suite environment. Because they are a consequence of relatively large and stiff delivery systems, the hope was that technologic advances would reduce delivery system size and thereby these complications. Unfortunately, these smaller endoluminal delivery systems have not been developed, and the need for open femoral artery access and occasional iliac conduits persists. Therefore, although both venues, the operating room and the angiographic suite, can be made to work for standard EVAR cases, combining the advantages of each into an endovascular operating room will continue to offer benefits when combined surgical and endovascular procedures are being performed.

The most common approach to building an endovascular operating room entails a variable degree of "conversion" of an existing operating room into one more suitable for radiographic imaging. Therefore one is starting with a fully equipped operating room with adequate lighting, sterile instruments, and adequate space for anesthesia machines and monitors, lacking only imaging capabilities. The complete package of fluoroscopic imaging equipment consists of three basic components: a fluoroscopic operating table, a radiographic unit, and a postprocessing/hard copy storage and output device. The least expensive operating room conversion is simply to add a portable fluoroscopy unit with a standard radiolucent table.[15] Although this may provide adequate imaging for some procedures in some patients, the field of endovascular therapy has moved beyond the stage where adequate is desirable. At the bare minimum, upgrading to a floating tabletop radiographic table with an operator-controlled portable C-arm adds functionality and fluidity to endovascular procedures. The current state-of-the-art endovascular operating suite, however, incorporates the further addition of fixed overhead-mounted x-ray tube and image intensifier, which dramatically improves both the image quality and ease of image acquisition[9,10] but typically requires both a spacious operating room and available adjacent space for the associated advanced radiographic necessities such as power generators and postprocessing and archival computers. The differences between these levels of conversion are addressed more thoroughly later in this chapter.

Radiographic Imaging Equipment

Vascular surgeons commonly perform angiography in the operating room to assess intraoperative conditions or on completion of a bypass procedure to assess the results of revascularization. These are often single-shot angiograms requiring little operator skill and nothing more sophisticated than a portable radiographic unit. On the contrary, endoluminal interventions require real-time imaging, most commonly provided through fluoroscopy, which may be available in the operating room as either a portable C-arm unit or a C-arm unit affixed to either the ceiling or the floor.[9,10] The inherent advantages and disadvantages of each system are highlighted in Table 2-1. Although there have been significant improvements in portable fluoroscopic equipment over the past decade, portable units remain inferior to fixed-based imaging with regard to power, resolution, flexibility, fluidity of image acquisition, and postprocessing capabilities that can elucidate pathology obscured by motion or radiologic artifact. As endovascular interventions have become increasingly complex and instrumentation progressively smaller, portable imaging systems simply do not allow for adequate visualization of the pathology, catheters, and guidewires. In addition, endoluminal grafts cannot be deployed with optimal precision to achieve maximal aortic neck coverage without encroachment on the renal artery orifices unless imaging is of adequate quality (Figure 2-1).

TABLE 2-1 Comparison of Mobile and Fixed Ceiling-Mounted C-arm

	Mobile Unit	Fix-Mounted Unit
Image quality	Inferior	Superior
Reliability	Less reliable	Very reliable
Radiation exposure	More	Less
Availability	Portable and able to be used in multiple venues	Restricted to a single room
Special construction	None needed	Required
Rotational imaging	Not available	Available

Radiographic resolution is dependent on the focal spot size of the x-ray tube, with smaller being better. Although portable fluoroscopy units can have comparably small focal spot sizes with those of fixed units, and the improved resolution that results, they achieve this by trading off both power output and available frame rates. Commonly used portable C-arm units have focal spot sizes ranging from 0.30 to 0.14 mm in diameter. In contrast, fixed units routinely have focal spot sizes of 0.15 mm or less in diameter, thus providing markedly improved image resolution.[12]

Another inherent limitation of portable C-arm units is the fixed distance between the x-ray tube and the image intensifier. In contrast, the image intensifier on fixed units can be positioned either closer to or farther away from the x-ray tube, effectively "closing the C" and thereby allowing positioning of the image intensifier closer to the patient. The ability to adjust the distance between the image intensifier and x-ray tube reduces x-ray scatter, thereby reducing radiation exposure to everyone in the operating room.[9,10] Portable C-arm units use a smaller power generator for greater maneuverability and portability of the entire unit. This is in stark contrast to the fixed units that have a larger, remote power generator with increased power capability, resulting in improved tissue penetration, which can be important in the imaging of larger patients or in lateral projections. Newer portable units have incorporated the use of collimation and filtering that was previously seen only in fixed units. The former constrains the x-ray beam to penetrate only the area of interest, reducing radiation exposure to the patient and staff, whereas the latter evens out the image exposure by interposing partially radiodense filters in areas of the field that are relatively radiolucent.

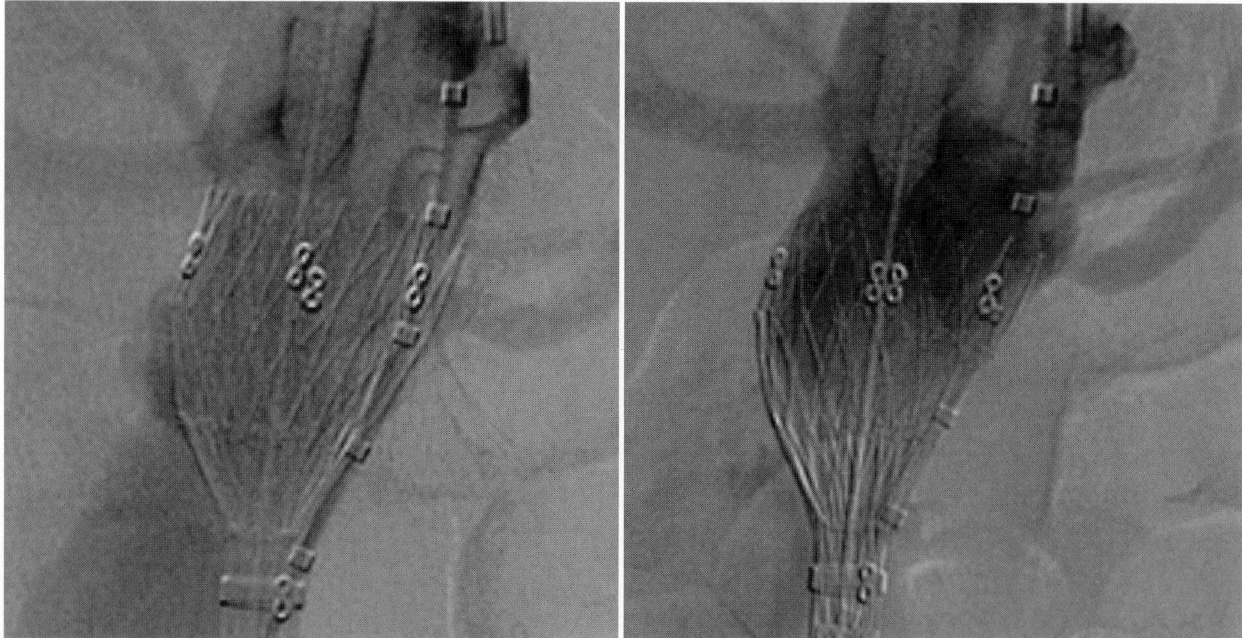

FIGURE 2-1 Image quality is important for the precise deployment of intravascular devices. The stent graft seen in the image on the *left* is just above the renal arteries. The image quality facilitates a slight caudad repositioning of the device inferior to the renal arteries as seen in the image on the *right*.

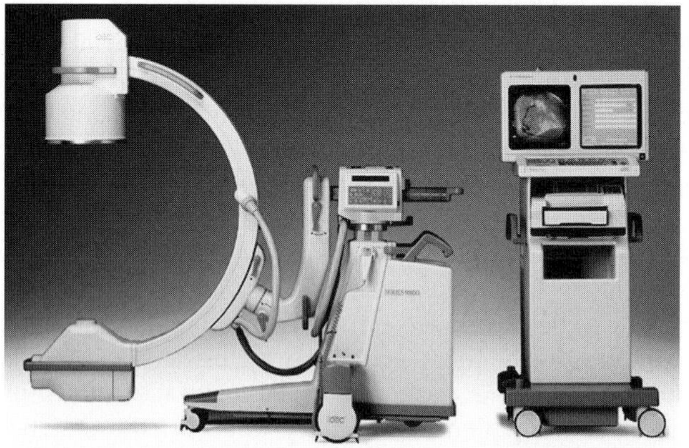

FIGURE 2-2 Portable fluoroscopy units can be used in any operating room and can be positioned within the confines of operating tables and instrument setups. However, the limitations of a smaller field of view and the fixed distance between the tube and image intensifier can make these less desirable for procedures that require more precise imaging.

Additional advantages of fixed imaging units relate to their maximum available image intensifier size. Portable C-arm units are usually equipped with a 9-inch image intensifier; however, some newer models have image intensifiers as large as 12 inches (Figure 2-2). Fixed units can be installed with much larger image intensifiers, up to 17 inches (Figure 2-3), which allow for a wider anatomic area, such as from the renal arteries to the common femoral arteries, to be seen in the same image. The latest and greatest endovascular suites incorporate flat-panel radiographic detectors that are physically smaller and therefore less obtrusive and encumbering, despite their ability to provide an even larger field of view. Rectangular rather than circular like standard image intensifiers, flat-panel detectors can be rotated into landscape or portrait orientations to optimize the visualized field for the anatomic area of interest. In landscape orientation the field is wide enough to image both lower extremities simultaneously, enabling digital subtraction bolus chase angiography.

Although the smaller image intensifier sizes typically found in portable units may be adequate for endovascular interventions in focal fields, such as renal or iliac angioplasty, larger fluoroscopic fields make aortic endografting easier and safer as there is less repositioning of the imaging unit or patient required for passage of devices and to ensure accurate endograft placement. Not only do radiographic reference points maintain their apparent position (because parallax is not an issue so long as the field has not been shifted), but also larger image intensifiers further obviate the need for constant fluoroscopic panning to visualize the vessels and catheters during complex interventions. A final concern about portable digital C-arm units, especially older models, is their propensity to overheat with prolonged use. If this occurs, the unit shuts down and cannot be restarted until the unit has cooled sufficiently. This may take upwards of 15 to 20 minutes, during which time an alternate C-arm must be brought in or there is a break in the

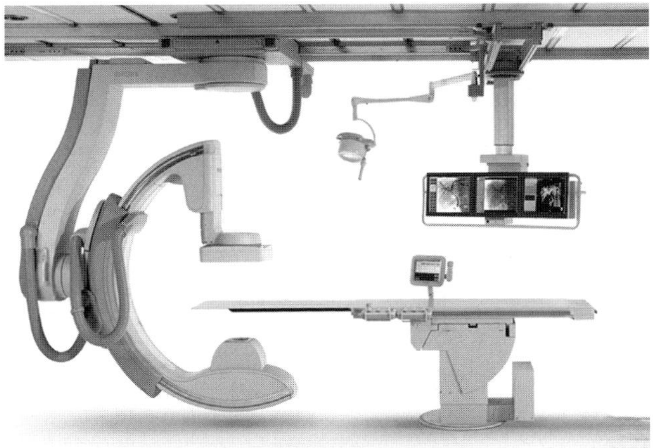

FIGURE 2-3 The fixed-mounted suite as seen in this image provides the opportunity to adjust the distance between the tube and the image intensifier allowing for the operator to view any anatomic field. The image intensifier is small and less obtrusive. The table moves to provide images at different anatomic levels and does not require repositioning of the fluoroscopy tube as with portable units.

middle of the procedure during which no imaging can be obtained. Although this may not be an issue of great concern for a patient undergoing placement of a tunneled dialysis catheter, it can have disastrous consequences during complex EVAR procedures.

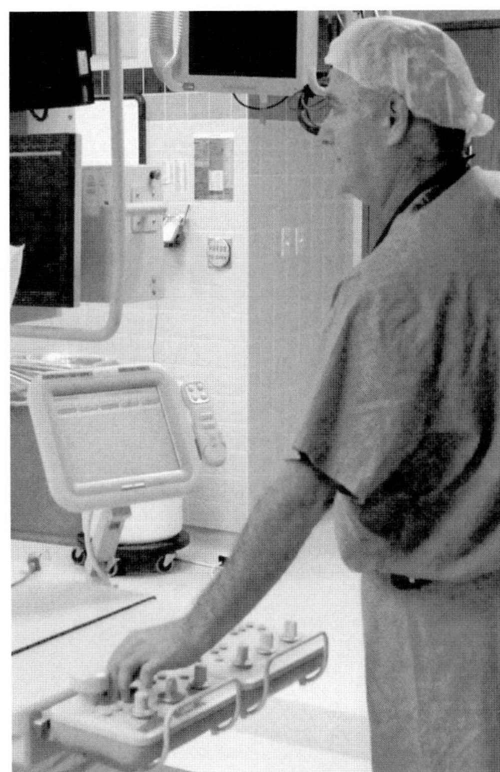

FIGURE 2-4 Table-mounted controls can be draped sterilely and adjusted by the operating surgeon or placed outside the operative field to be used by a technician allowing for maximal versatility and control by the operating team.

The Operating Table

Operating suites are generally equipped with versatile operating tables that permit a myriad of positions suitable for use by multiple surgeons of varying specialties.[9,10] For endovascular procedures, however, the primary requirement for the table is that it be radiolucent. Radiolucent tables used for vascular imaging can be portable or fixed, similar to the imaging units. The ideal fixed-type table is normally constructed of a nonmetallic carbon-fiber tabletop supported at a single end, usually the head. It can be rotated from side to side and tilted for Trendelenburg and reverse Trendelenburg positioning. This type of table provides unobstructed access for the C-arm from head to toe because there are no structural elements to obstruct the course of the C-arm. Because it is constructed of radiolucent material, imaging is not obstructed by structural elements of the table, and visualization is excellent. In the past, the fragile construction of these tables limited their use in obese patients. Currently available tables have improved construction and can support patients up to 500 pounds while offering superior imaging quality.

In the typical operating room portable fluoroscopy scenario the C-arm is panned over the field of interest to evaluate various areas of the vascular tree and observe passage of endovascular instrumentation. Changing fields of view by moving the C-arm, however, is far less fluid and convenient than sliding the table beneath the image intensifier, a simple maneuver that can be performed by the operator rather than a cumbersome one that requires an intermediary to perform. Movable tables provide for fluid positioning of the patient in the horizontal plane using controls mounted on the table. In addition, the table-mounted controls allow for selection of multiple radiographic settings including radiographic gantry rotation, image intensifier size, collimation, table height, and others (Figure 2-4). The controls are readily accessible to the endovascular surgeon because they are covered by a clear plastic window incorporated into the drapes covering the patient.

Tableside controls allow the surgeon greater autonomy to maneuver the patient and do away with the need to communicate the necessary table or C-arm movements to ancillary operating room personnel. This is the type of table most commonly found in radiologic and cardiac catheterization suites and is floor mounted. In the model shown in Figure 2-3, which is equipped with a fixed-mount radiographic unit and a movable table, the x-ray tube and the image intensifier remain stable while the table moves freely with the patient in the horizontal plane. When using moving tables care must be taken to

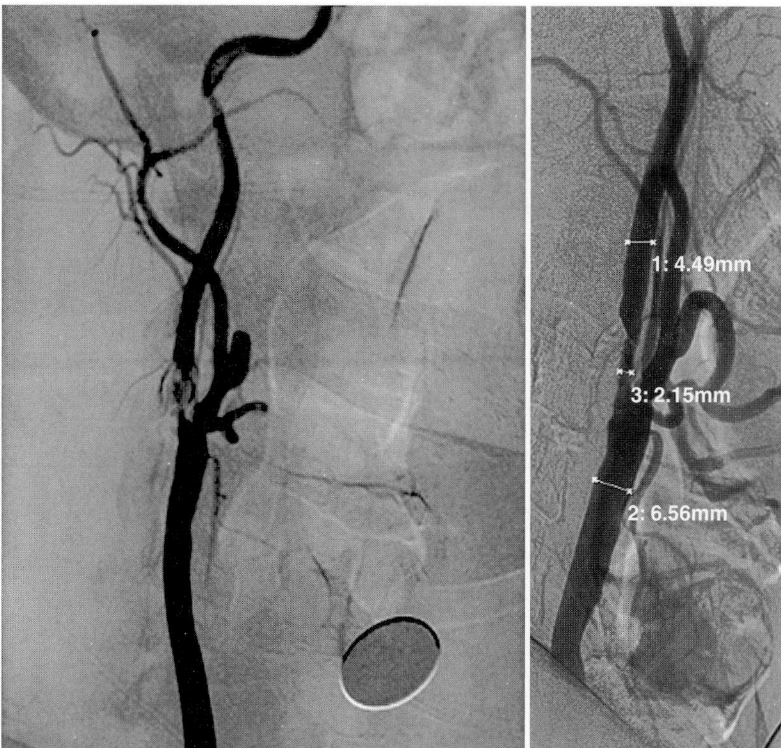

FIGURE 2-5 Measurements for exact sizing of stent and other endoluminal devices is facilitated by the ability to increase the magnification of images as seen here. The image on the *left* was taken to identify the area of carotid artery stenosis; however the magnified image on the *right* provides a large image that makes caliper placement more precise.

provide an adequate length of intravenous tubing, electrocardiographic lead wires, pulse oximetry, and any other necessary monitoring lines to allow the patient to travel under the image intensifier. This may be cumbersome, especially if the patient is under general anesthesia. Another advantage to this setup is the ability to install a long leg exchanger if traditional cut-film runoff imaging is desired. Several manufacturers offer radiolucent tables suitable for an endovascular suite, which vary in price and features, as well as weight tolerances.[16]

IMAGE ACQUISITION AND DISPLAY

Cut-film radiographic imaging has largely fallen by the wayside and is presently regarded as both tedious and wasteful of resources because of the silver salts utilized in the emulsions of standard x-ray film. The state of the art in vascular radiographic imaging is digital subtraction angiography. This technique has many advantages over cut-film radiography, including a reduction in the amount of iodinated contrast agent required for diagnostic imaging and the ability to postprocess images to reduce motion artifacts or other radiographic flaws that can degrade the images. The images can also be magnified, which allows for calibration and accurate measurement of vessel diameters and stenoses (Figure 2-5), and electronically merged to show an image with contrast opacification throughout the field of view even when proximal and distal vessels were best opacified on different frames of the angiographic run because of delayed transit time of the contrast agent.

Modern imaging systems have many additional features that facilitate the performance of more complex endovascular procedures. A large bank of monitors allows the operating surgeon to observe the patient's electrocardiographic and hemodynamic data in real time alongside reference radiographic images from prior angiographic runs, all while following live fluoroscopy. Additional monitors in the bank permit display of computed tomographic (CT) or magnetic resonance scans, three-dimensional reconstructions thereof, and duplex or IVUS imaging. Variable-size image intensifiers provide the versatility and the flexibility to view a variety of anatomic regions. Finer details can be examined with magnification and increased image resolution in a small field (e.g., carotid arteries), or, conversely, a wide field of view can be included on one screen (e.g., aortoiliac arteries). Road mapping can be another helpful feature when tortuous, stenotic, or occluded vessels are being traversed with guidewires. This technique allows for the live fluoroscopic image to be superimposed on a reference angiographic image, allowing the operating surgeon to easily monitor the advancement of the guidewire through the vessel as it negotiates turns or traverses stenoses, facilitating safe guidewire passage while minimizing the risk of dissections and perforations. This is, however, contingent on there having been no movement of the area being imaged since the time of acquisition of the reference image, a situation that compromises the accuracy of the road map because the real-time location of the vascular anatomy is no longer where the road map portrays it. Even if the movement does not shift the vascular anatomy of interest, shifted adjacent areas can induce distracting radiographic noise into the live fluoroscopic image. It is for this reason that road mapping of the abdominal or thoracic regions can be challenging because of ever-present intestinal and pulmonary movement.

As mentioned earlier, current angiographic systems use rectangular flat-panel detectors rather than the older circular image intensifiers. These can be rotated into "portrait" or "landscape" orientations, the former having the larger of the rectangular dimensions oriented vertically while in the latter case it is oriented horizontally. This capability allows the operator to orient the flat-panel detector whichever way optimizes the area of desired imaging. Flat-panel detectors are also significantly less bulky than the older image intensifiers, rendering their gantries more easily rotated, which has facilitated the incorporation of rotational angiography yielding three-dimensional angiograms, as well as limited CT scans, termed flat-panel CT. Rotational angiography provides more complete imaging of a vessel with a single angiographic run and can assist in identifying the optimal projection for further imaging or intervention, which otherwise might have required a series of trial-and-error single injections in selected projections. Both rotational angiography and flat-panel CT scanning can assist in the translumbar treatment of type 2 endoleaks following endovascular repair of abdominal aortic aneurysms by allowing three-dimensional assessment of the location of the translumbar needle that otherwise would have required repetitive back-and-forth anteroposterior and lateral gantry positioning.

A variety of other image acquisition settings can be used to optimize angiographic evaluations. Variable frame rates can be used to acquire radiographic images, from 0.5 to 30 frames per second. Typically, most examinations are performed at 2 to 3 frames per second. Slower frame rates reduce radiation exposure but may compromise the evaluation if optimal opacification of the area of interest occurs in the now longer time period between exposures. Collimation is a technique that allows one to focus on a particular anatomic area while cropping unwanted regions. For example, in a lower-extremity angiogram, the field can be focused on the course of the superficial femoral artery, excluding the lateral thigh. This technique improves image quality and reduces radiation exposure. In the same manner, filters can be used to partially shield areas of relative radiolucency that otherwise tend to have increased brightness on the angiogram, rendering the image more evenly exposed.[9] Bolus "chasing" is another feature that may be useful when performing a lower-extremity runoff examination. In this feature, available only with fix-mounted imagers, a single bolus of iodinated contrast material is administered in the infrarenal aorta, and imaging is performed as the table steps under the image intensifier or vice versa. As the contrast media pass through the arterial system, the relative positions of the patient and the image intensifier are changed to "chase" the contrast down the legs. With a 15-inch or larger image intensifier, or a peripheral-size flat-panel detector, the pelvis and both lower extremities can be visualized with a single bolus of contrast from the aorta to the feet.

Image storage and reproduction are other important features of modern radiographic equipment. Instant review of both fluoroscopic and radiographic images is possible and is becoming the standard by which most surgeons operate. Most radiographic "runs" are currently being stored on magnetic or optical disks. Angiographic images can be postprocessed to optimize the image and annotate it, if so desired, at the end of the procedure. For example, patient motion or heavy breathing at the beginning of an angiographic run will offset the mask image from later images with contrast in the field of view, causing degradation of the image. By selecting a new digital mask frame just before arrival of the contrast media, these motion artifacts can often be minimized or even eliminated.[17]

ANCILLARY EQUIPMENT

Duplex Ultrasonography

Duplex ultrasonography is another imaging modality used in conjunction with fluoroscopy that can facilitate initial access to the vascular system. In addition, some centers are performing many endovascular interventions under duplex imaging alone.[18-20] Although this has been reported, it will not entirely replace angiography in the endovascular operating room. Therefore it may be hard to justify the cost of a dedicated duplex scanner in the operating room when most of its functions can be performed angiographically. Both the ultrasound base units and their scanheads have become more diminutive over the past decade, despite significant improvements in both B-mode image quality and complementary Doppler information. Smaller scanheads are less likely to impede access to target vessels when used to assist in vascular access. Although all

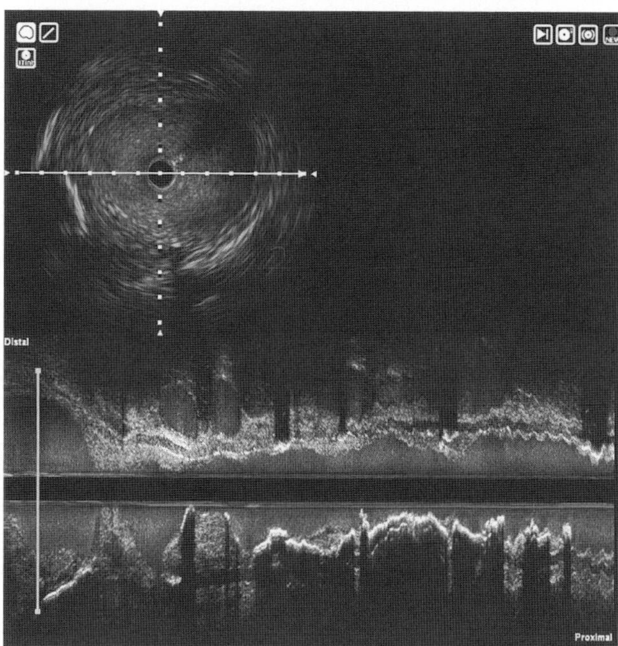

FIGURE 2-6 IVUS imaging can provide real-time ultrasound images in a transverse orientation. The images can be reconstructed to provide a longitudinal vessel view that can provide an additional modality to assess plaque morphology, degree of stenosis, or vessel diameter.

duplex scanheads can be placed in sterile covers to allow their use within the sterile field, traditional stand-alone duplex scanners require operating room personnel to control duplex settings and functions. Newer integrated units, however, allow the surgeon to perform the study and adjust the controls simultaneously, by virtue of tableside control panels. The duplex scanner may also be useful for obtaining vascular access when pulses are not readily palpable, such as in a scarred groin or a patent femoral artery distal to an iliac occlusion. Similarly, duplex scanning has proved useful for ultrasound-guided puncture of the popliteal or posterior tibial veins for venography.[10]

Intravascular Ultrasonography

In contrast to duplex ultrasonography, IVUS was developed to interrogate vessels from within.[18] Although not essential, many surgeons have found that IVUS provides a more accurate assessment of vessel diameter and degree of stenosis. IVUS allows for real-time cross-sectional imaging to be reconstructed into a longitudinal vessel view (Figure 2-6). This imaging modality is useful for arterial imaging after angioplasty to assess for the presence of a dissection and determine the need for placement of a stent. For endoluminal aortic grafts, IVUS can be used to confirm diameter measurements of the aortic and iliac landing zones to help select the correct size endograft, as well as being helpful in evaluating attachment site apposition. In situations where iodinated contrast administration must be minimized, placement of an endoprosthesis is possible by using solely IVUS, and once the deployment is complete 20 mL of iodinated contrast can be used to assess for endoleaks. This renders patients with chronic renal insufficiency eligible for endovascular repair of abdominal aortic aneurysms with a much reduced risk of further renal function compromise.

IVUS imaging is used more frequently in venous imaging. It allows the operator to see the vein in a more natural state when not distended by a large contrast injection. It allows for visualization of venous webs and synechiae that previously went undetected. Newer catheters with lower crossing profiles are making the technology easier to use, with smaller sheath sizes and improved imaging quality. Previously, IVUS required a large portable cart with a drive unit, processor, and monitor, similar to that seen with duplex ultrasonography. Newer units, however, can be integrated into the angiographic system itself, with table-mounted controls and image display on a dedicated larger monitor within the bank of monitors, allowing easy comparison between IVUS imaging, angiographic images, and even previously obtained CT scans, all on separate monitors. Despite these assets for IVUS, however, in the "real world" the majority of endovascular procedures of all kinds are routinely performed without any type of ultrasonographic guidance or evaluation. Therefore both duplex ultrasound and IVUS capabilities would be considered optional for an endovascular operating room.

Thrombolytic Catheters and Wires

Intravascular thrombosis can occur spontaneously or concomitantly with an endovascular intervention. In either scenario, it is a situation that all endovascular surgeons should be equipped for and adept at treating. Treatment modalities in this arena have expanded significantly in recent years. Previously, the mainstay of therapy has been via the use of multi–side-hole infusion catheters and wires positioned within the clot to passively infuse thrombolytic agents into the thrombus, a technique termed pharmacologic thrombolysis. A syringe setup can be used to facilitate a forceful, pulsed infusion of small aliquots of the lytic agent into the clot, termed "pulse spray" thrombolysis. Some believe that this technique enhances the speed and extent of clot lysis, either by delivering the lytic agent deep into the clot where it might not otherwise be able to penetrate, by the mechanical disruptive effect of the spray itself, or through a combination of both of these mechanisms. None of these postulates, however, have ever been proved.

BOX 2-1

BASIC TOOLS FOR ENDOVASCULAR DIAGNOSIS OR INTERVENTION

Diagnostic Angiography

Puncture needle and J-wire
Sheath (4F or 5F)
Multipurpose catheter (straight and pigtail)
Soft-tip or J guidewire
Nonionic contrast
Power injector (for aortograms and vena cavograms)

Angioplasty

Preformed catheter in at least two different shapes
Guidewires
Hydrophilic, angled and steerable
0.035-inch and 0.014-inch diameter wires
Long sheaths (various lengths and diameters)
Guiding catheters
Balloons in a variety of lengths and diameters
Inflation gauge

Thrombolysis

Multihole infusion catheter or infusion wire
Percutaneous mechanical thrombectomy device

In the pursuit of faster clot lysis, most practitioners have taken up the use of at least one of the various types of mechanical thrombectomy devices, a term used to describe a device that physically disrupts clot. These devices work under one of three principles: rheolytic thrombectomy (Possis Medical, Minneapolis, MN), fragmentational thrombectomy (Bacchus Vascular, Santa Clara, CA), and ultrasonic lytic enhancement (EKOS, Bothell, WA). Rheolytic and fragmentational devices can be used independently or in conjunction with pharmacologic agents, which offer an endovascular solution to patients who have a contraindication to the use of lytic agents. The EKOS device uses ultrasonic energy to open up the fibrin network, allowing deeper penetration of the lytic agent into the clot, enhancing the speed and extent of clot lysis. As is often the case when many devices employing different strategies are available, none has been shown to be inherently superior to the others, at least not yet, and current use is largely based on operator experience and preference. Given the need to be able to address intravascular thrombosis, however, at least one type of mechanical thrombectomy device should be stocked in the modern endovascular operating suite.

STOCKING THE ENDOVASCULAR OPERATING ROOM

A variety of equipment and supplies not seen in the standard vascular operating suite will be needed to properly equip a modern endovascular operating room (Box 2-1). Unfortunately, the requisite inventory, let alone additional desirable equipment, can be voluminous and expensive and hospitals are often reluctant to stock a new endovascular operating room when similar supplies are often stocked in existing imaging venues such as interventional radiology and the cardiac catheterization laboratory. This can be problematic for surgeons initiating an endovascular program because it is simply not possible to offer comprehensive endovascular care without instant access to the requisite tools of the trade. Querying off-site stores and waiting for supplies to be brought in not only is wasteful of time but also can affect the quality of patient care and be potentially injurious to patients. Consequently, pressure needs to be brought to bear on those in charge to ensure that the endovascular operating room is adequately stocked. Bear in mind that many vendors are willing to stock balloons, stents, and other basic supplies on consignment, whereby the hospital does not actually pay for the products until they are used. This arrangement can substantially lessen the financial outlay necessary to stock an endovascular operating room, at least partially circumventing this hurdle. If this cannot be accomplished, as is often the case with devices for which there are few or no competitive products, vascular surgeons should strongly consider gaining access to other facilities so the appropriate equipment is on hand. Although more specific details about endovascular equipment and its proper use are given in later chapters specifically dedicated to these procedures, this chapter provides an overview of equipment that needs to be readily available to the endovascular surgeon to provide comprehensive endovascular care.

Angiographic Sheaths, Catheters, and Guidewires

Because storage space in the endovascular suite is always at a premium, acquiring the optimal mix of angiographic guidewires and catheters can be a challenging task. For percutaneous access using the Seldinger technique, puncture needles and "entry" guidewires (those without hydrophilic coatings) are required. The use of hydrophilic guidewires as initial "entry" wires during cannulation of the access vessel is not recommended because of the risk of shearing of the hydrophilic polymeric coating by the bevel of the needle with resultant systemic embolization.[9,19] Usually, a 16-gauge beveled needle with a short J-tipped 0.035-inch guidewire is adequate for gaining vascular access. A variety of sizes of sheaths should be on hand, through which are passed guidewires, balloons, and other endoluminal devices. For a simple diagnostic angiogram, a 5F sheath is adequate. Depending on the size and the type of balloon or stent to be used for intervention, as well as whether or not a guiding catheter is to be used, a 7F or 8F sheath may be needed. Aortic endografting often requires sheaths in the 16F to 24F range, depending on the specific device being used. Femoral arteries with minimal disease can generally tolerate percutaneous introduction of a sheath up to 10F without excessive risk of complications, obviating the need for a surgical cutdown.[20]

For abdominal or thoracic aortic endografting, sheaths in the 16F to 24F range are placed into the femoral artery via open surgical cutdowns, although some authors have described placing large sheaths percutaneously with the aid of puncture-sealing (closure) devices. Several percutaneous closure devices are commercially available, incorporating a collagen plug, suture-mediated closure, or a small staple placed on the outside of the artery to tamponade or coagulate the puncture site in an effort to reduce access site complications and the requisite period of bed rest. These devices are designed to occlude an 8F or smaller puncture site. For larger-size sheaths, a Perclose ProGlide (Abbott Vascular, Abbott Park, IL) device can be used.[21] The Perclose device uses a sheathed needle and a surgical suture to engage the edges of the femoral artery, after which a knot is tied extracorporeally and is slipped down through a special guide to achieve hemostasis.

The Perclose ProGlide has been used in the "Preclose" technique to close arteriotomies up to 24F. To perform a percutaneous aneurysm repair using this technique the femoral artery is cannulated with use of a micropuncture kit. The puncture must be on the anterior surface of the common femoral artery at least 1 cm proximal to the femoral bifurcation. After confirmation of a satisfactory cannulation a 0.035-inch guidewire is advanced into the artery. The first Perclose ProGlide is then advanced into the artery, rotated 30 degrees medially, and deployed. The sutures are left extracorporeally and clamped. A second Perclose ProGlide is then placed in the same femoral artery, rotated 30 degrees laterally, and deployed. The sutures are clamped. The procedure then proceeds in the normal fashion. At the conclusion of the procedure the 0.035-inch guidewire is left in place while the two previously placed sutures are secured. If hemostasis is adequate, the 0.035-inch guidewire can be removed. If the technique fails, the 0.035-inch guidewire can be used to deploy a third device or to facilitate sheath placement until open surgical repair of the artery can be accomplished.[22]

Catheters can be classified by any of a number of characteristics. A common distinction is whether they have only one hole at the end (an end-hole catheter) or multiple side holes in addition to an end hole to provide better dispersion of contrast into the vessel flow stream. For nonselective or "flush" aortograms, a multi–side-hole pigtail, tennis racquet, or Omni Flush (AngioDynamics, Queensbury, NY) catheter is usually recommended. When used with a power injector, these catheters provide a sufficient bolus of contrast material for imaging in these high-flow areas.[9,10,19] In addition to the diagnostic multi–side-hole catheters previously described, there are other multi–side-hole catheters that are straight in configuration with side holes distributed over a length of 10 to 60 cm, for use in infusing thrombolytic agents into thrombosed segments of the vascular system. Some angiographic catheters are used to perform selective catheterization of branch vessels for enhanced visualization of the vessel and its nutrient bed. These catheters are designed with various tip shapes and forms to facilitate catheterization of branch vessels, either singly or in conjunction with guidewires (Figure 2-7). They are commonly used for selective subclavian, mesenteric, or renal imaging, as well as to cross over the aortic bifurcation.

Although these diagnostic catheters are often used to "guide" a guidewire into a branch vessel, they are technically not "guiding catheters," which is a term applied to oversized catheters through which balloons, stents, and other devices are deployed. Guiding catheters can be thought of as sheaths with preformed curves at their tips, except that, unlike sheaths, guiding catheters do not have hemostatic valves at their hubs. Therefore they require a Touhy-Borst adapter to be attached to their hubs to maintain hemostasis, as the luminal diameter of guiding catheters is in the 0.072- to 0.089-inch range, far larger than the 0.014- to 0.035-inch guidewires commonly used through them. Guiding catheters are especially helpful in delivering balloons and stents across difficult or unusual angles (e.g., renal, mesenteric, or proximal brachiocephalic arteries) because they provide external support for passage of the device to supplement the internal support of the guidewire along which the device is tracking. They also help negate the frictional effects of iliac tortuosity and stenoses, rendering catheters and guidewires more steerable and responsive. Furthermore, the use of guiding catheters permits contrast agent injection immediately before stent deployment to ensure precise positioning of the stent (Figure 2-8).

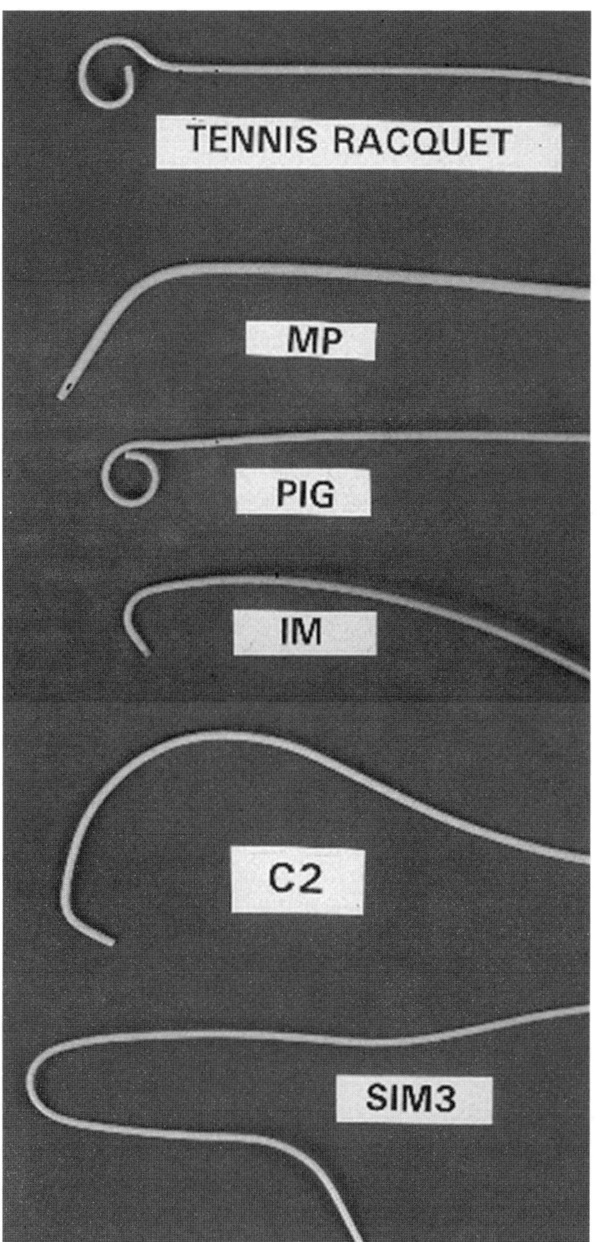

FIGURE 2-7 Angiographic catheters come in a variety of shapes and sizes. Various catheter tip configurations are depicted here. *(Courtesy AngioDynamics, Inc., Queensbury, NY.)*

Guidewires play a prominent role in obtaining access to and navigating through the vascular system. Several guidewire features have to be taken into consideration for appropriate selection, including diameter, overall length, tip shape, tip flexibility, antifriction coatings, and overall stiffness. Initial access is usually best established with a soft-tipped J-wire because initial guidewire passage is usually blind and this tip configuration is least likely to dissect plaque. When there are stenotic lesions or bifurcations close to the site of puncture, however, a steerable (i.e., angled tipped) guidewire may be desirable. As mentioned previously, care must be taken not to use a hydrophilic-coated guidewire as the initial access wire because its hydrophilic coating can be scraped off by contact with the bevel of the entry needle. Stiff wires, such as Amplatz (Boston Scientific, Natick, MA) and Lunderquist (Cook Medical, Bloomington, IN) wires, are typically required for the delivery of endoluminal grafts to straighten out naturally occurring curves in the iliac system and to provide maximal internal support for the passage of the endograft delivery system. The extreme stiffness of the body of these guidewires and the relatively abrupt transition from their floppy tips to their stiff bodies renders these guidewires ill-suited for passage through the vascular system on their own, so they are generally delivered into the desired location through a catheter that has already been placed there over a softer guidewire. Special infusion wires have been designed to deliver thrombolytic agents into occluded vessels or grafts, either independently or in concert with a coaxial infusion catheter. In contradistinction to the stiff guidewires, these hollow-core infusion wires are often too floppy throughout their length to negotiate significant turns in the vascular system so they too are usually delivered to their desired location through a previously placed catheter.

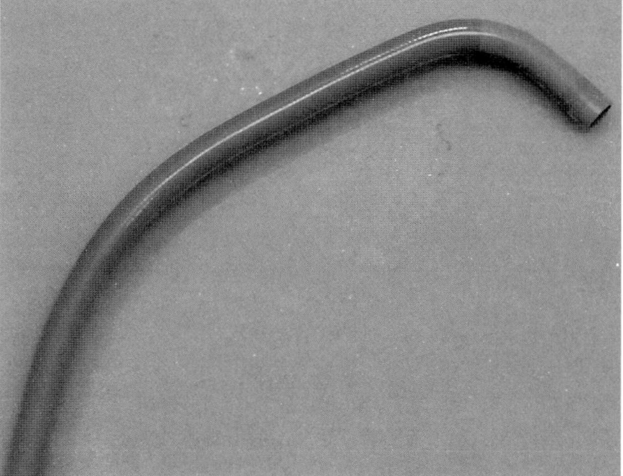

FIGURE 2-8 Guiding catheters are braided and stiffer than angiographic catheters. These are designed to be placed in the orifices of vessels and facilitate precise placement of intravascular devices as contrast can be injected around the device directly to the area of interest. When selecting a guiding catheter it is important to consider how the vessel will constrain the catheter and reshape it.

Angiographic Contrast Agents and Their Administration

The radiopacity of angiographic contrast agents is derived from the iodine content of the agent and varies widely among different preparations, as does the osmolality of the agent. Contrast agents with higher osmolality can induce significant discomfort when injected into the patient. This can be particularly problematic when evaluating patients with ischemic rest pain because these patients are likely to develop muscle spasms when exposed to the increased osmolality of any contrast agent. The resulting involuntary patient movement can severely compromise the image quality obtained. Traditional ionic contrast agents dissociate in blood, effectively doubling their osmolality, whereas newer nonionic agents are lower in osmolality and maintain that characteristic when injected, minimizing contrast-associated patient discomfort. For this reason they are generally preferred but can cost considerably more than ionic agents of similar iodine content. Though often alleged, there is no convincing evidence that nonionic contrast agents are associated with reduced rates of nephrotoxicity or other complications in euvolemic patients without hypercoagulable states.

Contrast agent infusion can be accomplished via hand injection with a syringe or power injection of precise amounts of contrast material at set flow rates and pressure limits. Although hand injection is suitable for most types of lower extremity angiography and selective angiography of mesenteric and brachiocephalic vessels, power injection is an absolute necessity for imaging in high-flow vessels such as the aorta and vena cava where larger contrast boluses must be delivered quickly for adequate vessel opacification. Care should be taken to avoid power injection through end-hole–only catheters unless the flow rate is set sufficiently low, lest a potentially injurious "jet effect" of contrast material be produced from the end of the catheter. An added advantage of power injection is that there is the option to step back or even leave the room so as to minimize radiation exposure to the operator during the angiographic runs because the power injector can be controlled from a remote site, typically the lead-lined and glassed control room.

Balloons and Stents

Percutaneous balloon angioplasty, with or without stents, has been performed with varying success rates in virtually every vascular bed in the body, from intracranial branch vessels to distal tibial arteries.[23-25] Therefore a broad range of balloon lengths and diameters is available to meet the wide variations seen in vascular anatomy. For iliac angioplasty, use of balloons with diameters in the 7- to 12-mm range and with lengths of 2 to 4 cm would cover the majority of lesions commonly encountered. Smaller-size balloons (4 to 8 mm) are used for femoropopliteal, renal, and subclavian artery angioplasty. Although angioplasty is typically performed in the latter two vessels with relatively short (2 to 4 cm) balloons, lengths of up to 10 cm are commonly employed in the superficial femoral artery. Special high-pressure angioplasty balloons are available for severely calcified lesions, whereas low-pressure "elastomeric" balloons expand and conform to the vessel wall making them suitable for occluding blood flow in emergency situations and for "modeling" endovascular grafts to the underlying vessel's contours. The well-stocked endovascular operating room therefore will have balloons ranging in size from 2 to 12 mm in diameter and 2 to 10 cm in length, with catheter shaft or working lengths of 75 to 120 cm.

In an attempt to limit the amount of restenosis caused by elastic recoil of the vessel wall after angioplasty, intravascular stents that scaffold the plaque were developed (Figure 2-9). Stents can be categorized by a number of characteristics, including their metal of composition (e.g., stainless steel or nitinol), flexibility, mechanism of deployment (e.g., balloon deployed or self-expanding), radiopacity, and metallic surface area.[20] All of the nitinol stents make use of the thermal memory properties of this metallic alloy and deploy via self-expansion, which is instantaneous at body temperature once the restraining cover is retracted. Nitinol stents typically deploy without significant foreshortening, but their precision of deployment is less than that of balloon-deployed stents, so care must be taken when they are deployed. Stainless-steel stents can be self-expanding (e.g., Wallstent, Boston Scientific) or balloon expandable. Although the Wallstent is considerably more flexible and available

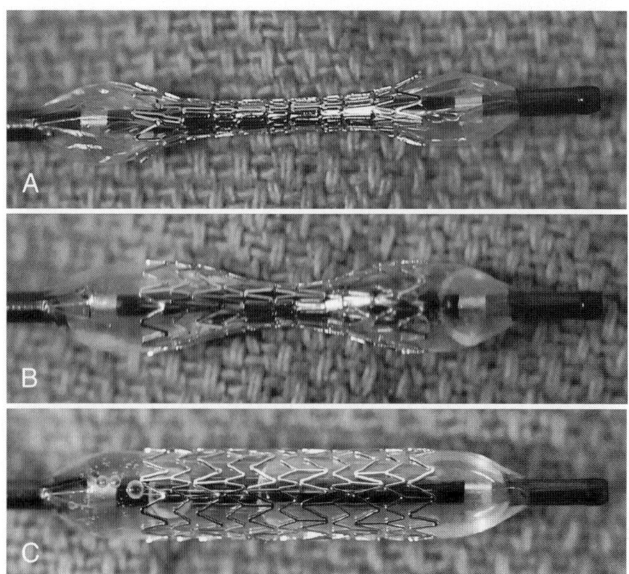

FIGURE 2-9 Stents can be balloon expandable or self-expanding. The balloon-expandable stents can be more precisely placed, have more radial force, and are less flexible than self-expanding stents. The images demonstrate how a balloon-expandable stent deploys from the edges toward the middle.

in substantially longer lengths than most balloon-deployed stents, it has less radial expansion force, particularly at its ends, rendering the Wallstent an ill-advised choice for orificial lesions such as the typical renal artery stenosis. Furthermore, the Wallstent foreshortens considerably during deployment, and the extent of foreshortening is not always predictable, making it difficult to use these stents near vessel origins lest they are inadvertently covered, or "jailed," by the stent or in orificial stenoses of aortic branch vessels where the stent may be left hanging into the aorta. Many of the commercially available stents have been designed and approved for use in the biliary system, but not-so-subtly marketed for use in the vascular system, a practice currently being scrutinized more closely by the Food and Drug Administration. Although the specific handling characteristics of a specific stent may have an impact on its suitability for use in a specific situation, there are no compelling data available to conclude that one stent is superior to another in any respect. Stents covering the applicable range of diameters and lengths should be readily available but represent a significant inventory to store and purchase, unless a consignment arrangement can be fostered.

Balloon-deployed stents are generally more precise in their deployment and have significantly greater radial expansion force than self-expanding stents. They are also much easier to visualize than self-expanding stents, before, during, and after deployment. For these reasons they are the generally preferred type of stent for orificial stenoses where both precise deployment location and enhanced radial expansion force are critical. Their only limitations pertain to their crushability, rendering them ill-suited for use in areas subject to extrinsic compression (such as in the superficial femoral or carotid arteries) or flexion (such as in the common femoral or popliteal arteries). Last, balloon-deployed stents are generally not available in lengths of more than 60 to 80 mm, whereas self-expanding stents can be found in much longer lengths.

Covered Stents or Stent Grafts

Stimulated by efforts to develop an endovascular treatment for abdominal aortic aneurysms, covered stents or "stent grafts" have been designed that function as internal bypass grafts within an aneurysm. In this application, the stents serve to anchor the graft, replacing the sutures used during open repair, and to provide column strength to resist distal endograft migration. The same technology has been extrapolated to the treatment of peripheral arterial occlusive and aneurysmal disease, effectively "relining" an artery after its balloon dilatation or recanalization. This strategy has been most commonly applied to the superficial femoral artery. As with bare metal stents, the metal used in stent grafts is either stainless steel or nitinol, and the fabric covering can be either Dacron or polytetrafluoroethylene. Covered stents have also proved useful in the treatment of traumatic arteriovenous fistulas, pseudoaneurysms, and peripheral aneurysms. The durability of these devices and their associated repairs remains unknown, though it continues to be the subject of ongoing investigations.

At this time, aortic endografts are approved for the treatment of nonruptured abdominal and thoracic aortic aneurysms, both of which are elective procedures. Therefore maintaining a significant inventory of these costly devices is necessary only if "off-label" use for the treatment of ruptured aneurysms, dissections, or traumatic disruptions is desired. In contradistinction to balloons and stents, these more expensive endoprostheses are rarely consigned, which severely limits their availability for emergency procedures in hospitals not otherwise performing a sufficiently high volume of aortic endografting that would justify the maintenance of a good breadth of sizes of these devices. Similarly, peripheral endografts are less likely to be consigned than their bare metal brethren, but because they are considerably less expensive than aortic endografts, maintaining an inventory of them is less cost prohibitive.

Ancillary Equipment

When stocking a modern endovascular suite it is important to prepare for the breadth of elective procedures that may be performed, as well as the emergency situations that may be encountered. The development of retrievable inferior vena cava (IVC) filters has resulted in an increase in the numbers of IVC filters that are placed. There are a host of filters available for use, each with its own unique design and suggested retrieval times and mechanisms. Although many can be initially deployed from either the internal jugular (IJ) vein or the common femoral vein approach, most are retrieved via an IJ approach. Most presently available IVC filters are suitable for use only with IVC diameters of 28 mm or less and are reasonably equally efficacious. Consequently, most institutions only stock one type, and most operators become familiar with the deployment and retrieval of only one or two types.

Snares are another type of adjunctive endovascular device that should be readily available in the endovascular operating suite. Snares are routinely used to retrieve hooked IVC filters, to strip fibrin sheaths off of hemodialysis catheters, and to facilitate cannulation of the contralateral limb in endovascular aneurysm repair. Although the most commonly used snare is of the single-loop variety, basket snares and multilooped snares are also available. Loop snares come in multiple sizes and function as lassos within the vessel to capture the ends of devices, which are then typically retracted out of the body through the sheath. Basket snares, on the contrary, capture objects from their side without requiring access to the end of an object.

Vascular surgeons are increasingly becoming the go-to interventionists for procedures requiring coil, particulate, or liquid agent embolization. These procedures are performed for a variety of pathologies including gastrointestinal or traumatic bleeding, embolization of splenic artery aneurysms, uterine fibroid embolization, and endoleak embolization. Each of these may best be accomplished with different embolic materials, the details of which are beyond the scope of this chapter. Particulate embolization microspheres are available in a variety of sizes, depending on the diameter of the vessel the surgeon is trying to occlude. They can also be impregnated with chemotherapeutic agents for use in catheter-directed chemotherapy of neoplasms. Liquid and particulate embolization agents are typically carried to their target vessels by blood flow once infused through a selectively placed catheter. In contrast, embolization coils, which range in postrelease diameters from 2 to 12 mm, are typically deposited at or just beyond the end of the selectively positioned catheter. They are used to occlude flow through larger vessels and assume a predetermined shape and size once advanced out the end of the catheter. They are coated or intertwined with thrombogenic material to help induce intravascular thrombosis and are available in standard 0.035-inch wire diameter or micro 0.014-inch diameter sizes. Although vessel occlusion with embolization coils often requires the use of multiple coils to achieve the desired occlusion, endovascularly placed plugs are now available that can often achieve the desired vessel occlusion with a single plug. Their size and predeployment stiffness, however, render them unsuitable for use to occlude vessels any farther out than one could place a 6F sheath. Liquid agents often used to induce thrombosis or occlude flow through a vessel include cyanoacrylate or thrombin glues, sclerosing agents such as sodium tetradecyl sulfate or ethanol, and macerated thrombin-soaked topical hemostatic agents.

ENDOVASCULAR SUITE PERSONNEL

In the traditional operating room, support staff is composed of a scrub nurse or a surgical technologist, who passes instruments to the surgeon, and a circulating nurse, who brings supplies and instruments that are needed. In an endovascular operating room, a radiologic technologist is mandatory to assist in the operation of the imaging equipment, whether it is a portable C-arm or a fixed-mounted unit. Dedicated angiographic rooms typically have a lead-lined and glassed control room from which the majority of radiographic acquisition and playback selections can be made, along with a duplicate set of controls mounted tableside. Personnel with special training on the use of the equipment and the subtleties of image manipulation are needed to provide additional support during the procedure. Ideally, a team of dedicated radiologic technologists familiar with the nuances of the complex equipment, as well as the various catheters, guidewires, and other endoluminal instrumentation and devices, should be assigned to the endovascular operating suite.

In contrast to the operating room, where the patient is monitored and drugs are administered by anesthesia personnel, most endovascular diagnostic and therapeutic procedures are performed with the patient under local anesthesia with supplemental intravenous sedation. Although the vascular surgeon is ultimately responsible for the care and well-being of the patient, a nurse is typically present to assist in this regard, administering drugs under the direction of the vascular surgeon and monitoring the patient's vital signs and oxygen saturation. This often requires additional training regarding sedation protocols and pharmacology. Although most diagnostic and therapeutic endovascular procedures can be performed by using local anesthesia provided by the nurse, the services of anesthesia personnel should be employed if deeper sedation is required or if a more complex procedure is anticipated.[2] Adequate monitoring of the patient's airway and cardiopulmonary status while he or she is under heavy sedation is simply too distracting to the operating surgeon and beyond the scope of training of a typical nurse. Although aortic endografting is most commonly performed, at least in our practice, with the patient under local anesthesia (for the femoral cutdowns) and anesthesia-provided deep intravenous sedation, many vascular surgeons prefer epidural or general anesthesia for these procedures. The only benefit we can see for these latter forms of anesthesia would be the ability to suspend respiration during angiographic runs to improve image clarity by elimination of respiratory motion artifacts, something that is rarely necessary and does not, in our opinion, justify these more invasive forms of anesthesia.

COST CONSIDERATIONS

Some institutions have the luxury of designing and building an endovascular suite from the ground up, but most hospitals opt for reconfiguring an existing suite. There are significant cost considerations in planning a dedicated endovascular suite, and this becomes a major financial issue if the hospital does not have the patient volume to support such a facility. Hospital administrators will favor portable units because they are inherently more versatile and cost-efficient. Although most endovascular surgeons, given the option, would chose to work with a fixed-mount unit for deployment of endoluminal aortic grafts, portable C-arm fluoroscopy units are routinely used in practice with acceptable results.[15] In the big picture, however, the improved image quality, ease of image acquisition, and postprocessing capabilities strongly favor a dedicated angiographic operating room with fixed radiographic imaging.

Fix-mounted units are inherently more expensive than portable C-arm units related to the infrastructure modifications necessary to meet state and local regulations, such as the installation of lead lining in the walls of the room. This provision may not apply to rooms in which only portable fluoroscopy units are to be used. Other structural modifications may be required, such as supporting I-beams and embedded electrical conduits, all of which increase the overall price of construction or remodeling. Additional funds need to be budgeted for fluoroscopic tables, protective shields, and surgical lighting fixtures required to make a functional endovascular operating suite.

Although small in comparison with the initial outlay required to construct an endovascular operating room, the recurring cost of endovascular supplies and devices quickly adds up to an imposing sum. Savings can often be realized through aggressive negotiation with manufacturers to obtain competitive pricing and, in many cases, to procure products on consignment. There are numerous purveyors of aortic endografts, guidewires, catheters, balloons, and stents, most of which perform similarly, giving the purchaser ample competitive options.

A final consideration regarding the design of an endovascular operating room that has significant impact on cumulative long-term costs is the overall efficiency of the entire operation, beginning with the preadmission planning and extending through the discharge of the patient. The overwhelming majority of endovascular procedures can now safely be performed on an outpatient or observational basis, meaning efficient patient flow can translate into significant savings for the hospital. Therefore the design of the endovascular operating room needs to take into account operational considerations relating to location, space, and personnel requirements. The close proximity of a multipurpose "admission-recovery-discharge" ward to the endovascular suite is desirable because this allows for smooth patient flow into and out of the endovascular suite, and ultimately to home or a hospital room. Costs can also be pared by having a dedicated area outside the endovascular suite for monitoring of the patient after removal of all catheters because it frees up the endovascular suite, which is more costly, for use by other patients. Immediately after a procedure, the patient is simply transported to the recovery area where the introducer sheath is removed and pressure is applied to the site if a percutaneous closure device is not used. Routine use of closure devices speeds this process along and allows the suite to be turned over faster. This time-saving maneuver improves turnover time and maximizes the use of the endovascular operating room.

CONCLUSION

Setting up an endovascular operating suite can follow a variety of models ranging from the inexpensive portable fluoroscopy in the operating room model to the full-fledged angiographic operating room. The choice of approach largely depends on the available budget and space, with the latter model being the most desirable, but clearly the largest and most expensive. The range of procedures that can be performed in the dedicated angiographic operating room, however, by virtue of its superior imaging, will be significantly greater. Regardless of the model chosen, the cost does not end with the room and imaging equipment, as stocking the variety of endovascular devices necessary to provide the full spectrum of endovascular care can add substantial extra expense. Furthermore, staffing the facility with qualified personnel can prove problematic, particularly if endovascular procedure volumes are low, as they often are in start-up operations. Nonetheless, the vascular surgeon should strive for access to the best available imaging environment possible, as imaging is paramount for the successful performance of endovascular procedures.

References

1. Green RM, Chuter TAM: Evolution of technologies in endovascular grafting, *Cardiovasc Surg* 3:101–107, 1995.
2. Henretta JP, Hodgson KJ, Mattos MA, et al: Feasibility of endovascular repair of abdominal aortic aneurysms with local anesthesia with intravenous sedation, *J Vasc Surg* 29:793–798, 1999.
3. Calligaro KD, Dougherty MJ, Patterson DE, et al: Value of an endovascular suite in the operating room, *Ann Vasc Surg* 12:296–298, 1998.
4. Criado FJ: On becoming an endovascular surgeon, *J Endovasc Surg* 3:140–145, 1996.
5. Haji-Aghii M, Fogarty TJ: Balloon angioplasty, stenting, and role of atherectomy, *Surg Clin North Am* 78:593–616, 1998.
6. Brueck M, Heidt MC, Szente-Varga M, et al: Hybrid treatment for complex aortic problems combining surgery and stenting in the integrated operating theater, *J Interv Cardiol* 19:539–543, 2006.
7. Fulton JJ, Farber MA, Marston WA, et al: Endovascular stent-graft repair of pararenal and type IV thoracoabdominal aneurysms with adjunctive visceral reconstruction, *J Vasc Surg* 41:191–198, 2005.

8. Zhou W, Reardon ME, Peden EK, et al: Endovascular repair of a supra-aortic debranching with antegrade endograft deployment via an anterior thoracotomy approach, *J Vasc Surg* 43:1045–1048, 2006.
9. Hodgson KJ, Mattos MA, Sumner DS: Angiography in the operating room: equipment, catheter skills and safety issues. In: Yao JST, Pearce WH, editors: *Techniques in Vascular Surgery*, Stamford, CT, 1997, Appleton & Lange.
10. Mansour MA: The new operating room environment, *Surg Clin North Am* 79:477–487, 1999.
11. Mangram AJ, Horan TC, Pearson ML, et al: Guideline for prevention of surgical site infection, *J Surg Outcomes* 2:61–103, 1999.
12. Lombardi JV, Fairman RM, Golden MA, Carpenter JP, Mitchell M, Barker C, et al: The utility of commercially available endografts in the treatment of contained ruptured abdominal aortic aneurysm with hemodynamic stability, *J Vasc Surg* 40:154–160, 2004.
13. Peppelenbosch N, Geelkerken RH, Soong C, Cao P, Steinmetz OK, Teijink JA, et al: Endograft treatment of ruptured abdominal aortic aneurysms using the Talent aortouniiliac system: an international multicenter study, *J Vasc Surg* 43:1111–1123, 2006.
14. May J, White GH, Stephen MS, Harris JP: Rupture of abdominal aortic aneurysm: concurrent comparison of outcome of those occurring after endovascular repair versus those occurring without previous treatment in an 11-year single-center experience, *J Vasc Surg* 40:860–866, 2004.
15. Makaroun M, Zajko A, Orons P, et al: The experience of an academic medical center with endovascular treatment of abdominal aortic aneurysms, *Am J Surg* 176:198–202, 1998.
16. Dietrich EB: Endovascular intervention suite design. In: White RA, Fogarty TJ, editors: *Peripheral Endovascular Interventions*, St. Louis, 1996, Mosby.
17. Slonim SM, Wexler L: Image production and visualization systems: angiography, US, CT and MRI. In: White RA, Fogarty TJ, editors: *Peripheral Endovascular Interventions*, St. Louis, 1996, Mosby.
18. Wilson EP, White RA: Intravascular ultrasound, *Surg Clin North Am* 27:614–623, 1998.
19. Hodgson KJ, Mattos MA, Sumner DS: Access to the vascular system for endovascular procedures: techniques and indications for percutaneous and open arteriotomy approaches, *Semin Vasc Surg* 10:206–211, 1997.
20. Duda SH, Wiskirchen J, Erb M, et al: Suture-mediated percutaneous closure of antegrade femoral arterial access sites in patients who have received full anticoagulation therapy, *Radiology* 210:47–52, 1999.
21. Jean-Baptiste E, Hassen-Khodja R, Haudebourg P, et al: Percutaneous closure devices for endovascular repair of infrarenal abdominal aortic aneurysms: a prospective, non-randomized comparative study, *Eur J Vasc Endovasc Surg* 35:422–428, 2008.
22. Lee WA, Brown MP, Nelson PR, Hubu TS: Total percutaneous access for endovascular aortic aneurysm repair. ("Preclose" technique), *J Vasc Surg* 45:1095–1101, 2007.
23. Mazighi M, Yadav JS, Abou-Chebl A: Durability of endovascular therapy for symptomatic intracranial atherosclerosis, *Stroke* 39:1766–1769, 2008.
24. Wojak JC, Dunlap DC, Hargrave KR: Intracranial angioplasty and stenting: long-term results from a single center, *AJNR Am J Neuroradiol* 27:1882–1892, 2006.
25. Clair DG, Dayal R, Faries PL, et al: Tibial angioplasty as an alternative strategy in patients with limb threatening ischemia, *Ann Vasc Surg* 19:63–68, 2005.

CHAPTER

3

Training and Credentialing

Ali Khoynezhad, Rodney A. White

Training and credentialing for endovascular procedures have evolved as the technology has matured and various interventional subspecialties adapt training programs to address pertinent issues. Although the ideal would be for institutions to form endovascular services with significant forethought and planning, in most cases these services evolved on the basis of the expertise of individual clinicians who had an interest in adapting newer treatment methods for specific illnesses. In many cases, this may have occurred as interventional radiologists applied their diagnostic imaging and catheter-based skills to the percutaneous treatment of vascular lesions. In addition, peripheral endovascular methods have been used by surgeons who maintained their diagnostic radiographic skills and began to use endovascular methods as techniques evolved. There are also a number of cardiac surgeons who are actively involved in treating patients with open and endovascular peripheral operations. Some are trained in both vascular and cardiac surgery. More commonly, they are simultaneously trained and board certified by the traditional cardiovascular training programs in cardiac and vascular surgery. Cardiologists also treated peripheral vascular lesions, either as a means to improve peripheral vessel access for cardiac interventions or as part of a combined peripheral and coronary interventional service.

Each subspecialty has specialized skills that influence the efficacy and safety of endovascular methods, with the ideal endovascular specialist being an individual who has extensive knowledge of both catheter-based interventions and surgical techniques. The future vascular specialist may be trained in all these areas. Many institutions are assessing the need for endovascular training and are evaluating the optimal way to accomplish this goal. In the interim, practicing physicians in various subspecialties will be modifying their practice to accommodate the use of endovascular surgical methods. This entails the establishment of ways to provide training and facilities for application of these methods in an environment that maximizes involvement of appropriate subspecialties. The role of individuals will vary from institution to institution depending on the expertise of those involved and the institution's capability to accommodate the new methods.

ENDOVASCULAR PHYSICIANS

Although the organization of the endovascular team will be determined by the expertise and interest of various subspecialists and by the quality of interventional facilities, two types of clinical skills are required to be a member of this team. Interventional catheter-based manipulation and imaging skills are needed for both diagnostic and therapeutic interventions, whereas surgical skills are required to determine the indications for endovascular therapy versus conventional surgical treatment. Surgical expertise is also needed to treat possible complications of endovascular mishaps that may require either emergent or elective surgical conversion or correction. A combination of interventional catheter-based and diagnostic skills might be found in an appropriately trained vascular or cardiac surgeon, although usually in most settings the endovascular team consists of both interventional radiologists or cardiologists and vascular or cardiac surgeons. This collaborative approach may be necessary in many hospitals to complement the catheter-based and vascular surgical skills of the involved physicians. Although some institutions have been unable to address the development of a service because of either facility constraints or political controversy among the subspecialties, many hospitals are developing congenial arrangements that fulfill the needs of all involved parties.

Several guidelines have been proposed to address the credentialing and training of various subspecialists, and there are many points of agreement regarding the essentials for safe application of endovascular technology.[1-12] Although there are points of disagreement in earlier versions of these documents, ongoing conversations among the involved groups are resolving the remaining issues and are delineating mechanisms for addressing controversial areas and establishing an endovascular service in various types of institutional environments. Essential to an effective environment are the establishment of training, credentialing, and practice guidelines for the vascular specialist of the future and the provision of facilities that accommodate the needs of the endovascular team.

NATIONAL GUIDELINES FOR PHYSICIAN CREDENTIALING

The Joint Commission requires that specific privileges be delineated for each hospital staff member. Each hospital is required to monitor the appropriateness of care provided by its physicians and to establish mechanisms to assess new technologies before they can be used clinically. These directives have been accommodated in most instances by establishing departmental guidelines for new physicians or for physicians using techniques or methods that they have not used previously. For interventional and surgical procedures, this usually entails observation of a specified number of procedures by a proctor. Reporting procedural outcomes, both initially and after long-term follow-up, is optional if considered appropriate by the hospital's credentialing body.

Qualifications to perform a particular procedure are based on skills acquired by the physician during residency or fellowship training, a supervised preceptorship, or approved courses when appropriate. Frequently, expertise in new technology is developed during initial experimental trials of devices under the auspices of institutional review boards and Food and Drug Administration investigational programs. Thus physicians can obtain appropriate training to use new techniques via a number of means, from formal training to acquisition of skills during initial animal evaluations and clinical trials.

SPECIALTY GUIDELINES FOR PHYSICIAN CREDENTIALING

Endovascular device development and application have been influenced by various specialists, primarily surgeons, radiologists, and cardiologists, in the context of the effect these methods have on each group's primary patient population. Each specialty has independently arrived-at training, credentialing, quality assurance, and educational guidelines for applications solely within its discipline (such as coronary catheterization, cerebral angiography). Controversy and uncertainty have arisen when guidelines are developed for areas of mutual interest. In addition, because different patient groups may be treated, different criteria of success may be employed; each specialty emphasizes credentialing criteria based on its tradition and the evolution of endovascular techniques within its domain. Patients with minimal disease (no symptoms), moderate disease (intermittent claudication), or severe disease (limb-threatening ischemia) can be treated by identical techniques. The short- and long-term success in each of these groups is different. Furthermore, although some measure immediate hemodynamic or angiographic success, others emphasize long-term clinical evaluation, maintenance of patency (as documented by duplex scanning), or hemodynamic success (as measured in a noninvasive vascular laboratory). Both these points have been just recently incorporated in the most recent multisocietal consensus statement on peripheral arterial disease (TASC II).[13] This document is a result of cooperation among 14 medical and surgical vascular, cardiovascular, radiology, and cardiology societies in Europe and North America,[13] and it is based on recommended reporting standards of peripheral and endovascular procedures.[14-17]

Each specialty had established preliminary criteria for application of general endovascular interventions based on interest, the ability to treat a particular segment of the patient population, and the tradition of equating expertise with completion of a large number of procedures.[1-11] The emphasis in several of the earlier documents was on establishment of credentials for performance of percutaneous transluminal angioplasty, whereas the perspective of the vascular surgeon has been to address more broadly a large number of methods and techniques being developed. Guidelines for other procedures in addition to percutaneous transluminal angioplasty and stent placement have evolved with advances in the technology and proved safety and effectiveness. Table 3-1 summarizes the number of previously recommended interventions for credentialing of various groups. In 2004, the American College of Cardiology, American College of Physicians, Society for Vascular Surgery, Society for Cardiovascular Angiography and Interventions, and Society for Vascular Medicine Task Force on Clinical Competence published their consensus statement.[12] The following presents an overview of the content of this document and outlines various recommendations made for a particular specialty or intervention.

TABLE 3-1 Required Number of Catheterizations and Interventions

	SCVIR*	SCAI	ACC†	AHA†	SVS/ISCVS (1993)†	SVS/ISCVS (1998)†
Catheterizations/ angiograms	200	100 (50‡)	100	100	50‡	100 (50‡) Catheterizations
Interventions	25	50 (25‡)	50 (25‡)	5 (25‡)	10 (15‡)	50 (25‡) Procedures
Live demonstration	Yes	Yes	Yes	Yes	Yes	Yes

Reprinted with permission from White RA, Hodgson K, Ahn S, et al. Endovascular interventions training and credentialing for vascular surgeons, *J Vasc Surg* 1999, 29:177-186.
* *SCVIR*, Society of Cardiovascular and Interventional Radiology; *SCAI*, Society for Cardiac Angiography and Interventions; *ACC*, American College of Cardiology; *AHA*, American Heart Association; *SVS/ISCVS*, Society for Vascular Surgery/International Society for Cardiovascular Surgery.
†Includes knowledge of thrombolysis or thrombolytic therapy.
‡As primary interventionist.

CREDENTIALING DOCUMENTS FOR GENERAL PERIPHERAL INTERVENTIONS

Several articles addressed the performance of peripheral endovascular procedures, with most addressing the needs of a particular subspecialty rather than the requirements for an endovascular specialist.[1-12] This has occurred because each subspecialty has a dramatically different background and different training requirements for current interventional practice. Interventional cardiologists and radiologists have viewed endovascular surgery from their perspective (i.e., delivery systems and diagnostic modalities that are important in performing current procedures in their fields). Vascular and cardiac surgeons have viewed endovascular technology as an ancillary or a complementary technique to current open surgical methods. With the evolution of endovascular technologies, the surgical training base has expanded, with many of the current investigational studies of large-vessel endovascular prostheses being heavily dependent on surgical skills for the selection and treatment of patients undergoing vessel access for device delivery, as well as for the treatment of complications.

The consensus statement published by the American College of Cardiology, American College of Physicians, Society for Vascular Surgery, Society for Cardiovascular Angiography and Interventions, and Society for Vascular Medicine represents one of the few multidisciplinary guidelines for endovascular training, and offers training algorithms for various specialists.[12] The authors distinguish between expertise in vascular medicine and catheter-based peripheral interventions.[12] The former includes comprehensive knowledge of vascular disease, diagnostic tools, and therapeutic options. The writing committee recommends formal training in vascular medicine after 3 years of internal medicine to achieve competence. This additional year of training would entail training into various rotations including vascular surgery for 1 to 2 months and noninvasive vascular laboratory for 3 to 4 months to interpret at least 100 duplex ultrasonographies, and physiologic vascular testing.[12] These recommendations are derived from guidelines of the American College of Cardiology for training in vascular medicine and are crucial for any physician treating patients with peripheral vascular disease.[18] Although these cognitive skills are part of the training for surgeons treating patients with peripheral arterial disease, they have not been traditionally part of the residencies and fellowships in cardiology or radiology.

The concerning issue arises as the eligibility requirements for the board examination in general vascular medicine include only the American Board of Internal Medicine.[19] This has been an issue of controversy and criticism from radiologists and surgeons, who are effectively excluded from obtaining the vascular medicine "board certification." This exclusion criterion has no other functional basis than to fulfill the internal agenda of American College of Cardiology; this board certification is currently promoted to be a "benchmark of expertise in the field of vascular medicine" in hospitals[19] and may be enforced in the near future for hospital credentialing and public-relation purposes.

The second area of expertise in this consensus statement is less controversial, as it outlines a true multispecialty solution for ensuring adequate training and competency in catheter-based peripheral interventions. The eligibility requirements include board certification in the American Board of Surgery, American Board of Radiology, or American Board of Internal Medicine.[12] Furthermore, 12 months of experience in peripheral interventions is necessary that would include 100 diagnostic peripheral angiograms (50 as primary operator) and 50 peripheral interventions (25 as primary operator).[12,19] The writing committee describes the necessity of proficiency in peripheral (noncoronary) endovascular interventions, not limited to balloon angioplasty stents, stent grafts, and thrombolysis.[12] It is recommended to have a case mix distributed among various vascular beds and to include thrombus management and catheter-guided thrombolysis of arterial limb ischemia or venous thrombosis. The number of required procedures and recommendations is derived from the original "Special Writing Group of the Councils on Cardiovascular Radiology, Cardio-Thoracic and Vascular Surgery, and Clinical Cardiology, the American Heart Association."[4] For established physicians, there is an alternative training route that includes achieving the aforementioned procedural requirements in a 2-year period. For maintenance of competency, a "minimum of 25 peripheral vascular interventions per year along with documented favorable outcomes and minimal complications" is recommended.[12,19] This is an encouraging change from outdated documents from the American Heart Association, in which the authors limited the maintenance of privileges unless physicians acquire the level of training suggested in the paper within 3 years of publication of the document.[4]

CREDENTIALING DOCUMENTS FOR SPECIFIC PERIPHERAL INTERVENTIONS

In addition to consensus statements and documents elaborating on general requirements for peripheral (noncardiac) interventions, there have been guidelines specific to carotid artery stenting and thoracic endovascular aortic repair (TEVAR).[9-11] A similar writing committee that processed the aforementioned consensus statement for peripheral endovascular interventions has convened to publish a multidisciplinary recommendation on carotid artery stenting and TEVAR.[9,10] Both procedures are gaining popularity and require more rigid training algorithms and competency criteria, because the procedures can be more technically demanding and associated with significantly more morbidity and mortality than other peripheral interventions.

Competency guidelines on (extracranial) carotid artery stenting were written by a multispecialty group consisting of members of the Society for Cardiovascular Angiography and Interventions, the Society for Vascular Medicine, and the Society for Vascular Surgery.[9] The group distinguishes three elements of competency, namely, cognitive, technical, and clinical components. The cognitive requirements include pathophysiology, clinical manifestation, natural history, diagnosis, and treatment options for carotid artery disease. The technical component entails a minimum of 30 cervicocerebral angiograms and 25 carotid artery stentings (with half as primary operator), familiarity with advanced wire skills, and management of procedural complications of carotid artery stenting.[9] Finally, clinical requirements for performing carotid artery stenting involve the ability to weigh risks and benefits of stenting versus open carotid endarterectomy, periprocedural management of patients, as well as competency in outpatient surveillance. As with the consensus statement for peripheral interventions, there is a residency/fellowship and a practice pathway, both of which would lead into competency in all three aforementioned elements. The members of the writing committee do not require a minimum of carotid artery stents per year. However, maintenance of competency in noncarotid interventional work along with courses in continuing medical education is essential.[9]

TEVAR remains a true hybrid procedure. Although an endovascular procedure, the performance without surgical expertise is not possible, as typically a 24F to 29F (outer diameter) sheath is used to deliver the stent graft. An injury to the iliac artery injury is not uncommon and may need surgical attention in case of "iliac on the stick." An iliac conduit is used in approximately 10% to 15% of the patients who will require an open operation.[20] Not infrequently extra-anatomic bypasses to brachiocephalic vessels are warranted to allow for adequate proximal landing zone. In addition, approximately 2% of the patients will need either emergent or urgent open thoracic aortic repair within the first 2 months after TEVAR.[21] Therefore open surgical expertise remains one of the key competencies for performing TEVAR. This is in contrast to all previously discussed peripheral interventions, thereby excluding cardiologists or radiologists as independent operators. Furthermore, there is a compendium of endovascular skill sets that is needed to deal with a host of intraprocedural issues, such as inadvertent coverage of critical brachiocephalic or mesenteric vessels, selective catheterization and potential stenting of these vessels, requirement for advanced imaging including intravascular ultrasound, balloon angioplasty, and stenting of iliac vessels. Furthermore, a thorough knowledge of the natural history of various aortic pathologies, follow-up and treatment of patients with aortic disease, and sound risk and benefit analysis of open versus endovascular repair are a necessity for the treating surgeon (or team of physicians).

There are two recent documents entailing competency guidelines for performing TEVAR.[10,11] The first is derived from a writing committee with members of the Society for Vascular Surgery, Society of Interventional Radiology, Society for Cardiovascular Angiography and Interventions, and Society for Vascular Medicine.[10] The eligibility requirements include the highest level of certification in each specialty: American Board of Thoracic Surgery, American Board of Vascular Surgery, American Board of Radiology with added certification in interventional radiology, and American Board of Internal Medicine with added certification through interventional cardiology, or endovascular certification of the American Board of Vascular Medicine.[19] Furthermore, the following elements of competency are required: catheter-based peripheral interventional requirements as outlined by consensus statement of the American College of Cardiology, American College of Physicians, Society for Vascular Surgery, Society for Cardiovascular Angiography and Interventions, and Society for Vascular Medicine; performance of 25 abdominal endovascular repairs or 10 TEVAR in the past 2 years; knowledge of natural history and management options of thoracic pathologies by taking 20 hours of devoted continued medical education; and surgical expertise by involvement of a board-certified cardiac or vascular surgeon. The authors convey the idea that the majority of physicians interested in TEVAR will not have all four aforementioned requirements and will need to collaborate with other physicians who would complement the elements of competency. Furthermore, the writing committee recommends a minimum of 10 hours of continued medical education and 10 TEVAR procedures on a biannual basis to maintain the competency.[10]

The second guideline for competency and credentialing for TEVAR is written by the Taskforce for Endovascular Surgery of the Society of Thoracic Surgeons and American Association for Thoracic Surgery.[11] The authors are concerned about "rapid adoption" of the technology and deviation from standards of physician education and indications without long-term proved benefit for quality and safety of the patient. The writing committee suggests the following competencies in a 2-year period: longitudinal clinical experience with 20 patients, including 10 patients undergoing open repair; a minimum of 25 wire or catheter placements; performance of 10 abdominal endovascular repairs or five TEVARs, experience with large-bore sheaths in iliac and femoral arteries; and experience with iliac conduit along with open repair, as well as angioplasty and stenting of iliac arteries. In addition to the five core competencies, the authors recommend attending a TEVAR course offered by the Society for Vascular Surgery or Society of Thoracic Surgeons/American Association for Thoracic Surgery. They stress again the need for a collaborative team approach when offering TEVAR to patients with various aortic pathologies.

Both credentialing and competency guidelines were published in 2006, and one would have hoped to have a unified version among all specialties treating patients requiring TEVAR. Although both stress the necessity of cardiac or vascular surgical expertise and the importance of multidisciplinary collaboration, the first document is requesting more rigid requirements for peripheral interventions, whereas the second document from cardiac surgeons is requesting performance of 10 open thoracic aortic operations thereby excluding many surgeons (and obviously all nonsurgical colleagues). Despite advances in endoluminal treatment of thoracic aortic pathologies, cardiac surgeons were (initially) slow in adapting to the new "disruptive" technology: few have undergone dedicated endovascular training and acquired comprehensive peripheral endovascular skills, although many thoracic surgery training programs have now incorporated such training in the curriculum. The concern in lack of adequate number of peripheral interventional cases among cardiothoracic surgeons is projected in the consensus document by the Society of Thoracic Surgeons and American Association for Thoracic Surgery: 25 peripheral interventions may not be adequate training to deal with unexpected complications and difficult arterial anatomies.

On the other hand, there are some concerns with the document by the Society for Vascular Surgery, Society of Interventional Radiology, Society for Cardiovascular Angiography and Interventions, and Society for Vascular Medicine. Foremost, it is not truly a consensus statement of all involved physicians; the cardiac surgery community, which has traditionally had (and in many places still has) the majority of referrals for thoracic aortic disease, is not represented. Furthermore, there were no minimum requirements for open aortic operations. Although the need for open conversions is relatively low, they will need prompt and competent "complication rescue."[21] Just having a board-certified vascular or cardiac surgeon as a member of the treating physician team is probably not adequate. The current operative experience of that surgeon is a critical issue. For example, a "noncardiac" thoracic surgeon who is certified by the American Board of Thoracic Surgery would not be able to offer life-saving emergent open aortic repair, which may also require cardiopulmonary bypass and (in case of zone II or higher deployed stent grafts or retrograde aortic dissection) hypothermic circulatory arrest. Similarly, a board-certified vascular surgeon who specialized in venous pathologies and dialysis access would be unable to provide effective open "complication rescue."

A key concept in TEVAR has been part of both credentialing and competency documents: collaboration and a team approach are the most effective and safest way to offer complex hybrid procedures to a morbid patient population. It is clear that both cardiac and vascular surgeons should be leaders in this multidisciplinary model. TEVAR should be a procedure to help cultivate the strong bond between the "brother specialties"; the traditional cardiovascular surgeon had been one specialty until the 1970s treating manifestations of atherosclerosis in various locations in the "circle" first described by William Harvey.[22] Both specialties share a number of "giants": Michael E. DeBakey, the founding editor of the *Journal of Vascular Surgery*, has numerous contributions to various vascular beds. "The cardiac and vascular services are separated in many places. I object to that for the simple reason that I consider the cardiovascular system a unified system," he said in an interview in 1997.[23] Cardiologists have no self-imposed barriers, such as the diaphragm and the clavicle, originally dividing vascular and cardiac surgery. Their realm now is the entire circulatory system. A unifying group of cardiac and vascular surgeons would have the same concept in mind.[24]

References

1. String ST, Brener BJ, Ehrenfeld WK, et al: Interventional procedures for the treatment of vascular disease: recommendations regarding quality assurance, development, credentialing criteria, and education, *J Vasc Surg* 9:736–739, 1989.
2. Spies JB, Bakal CW, Burke DR, et al: Guidelines for percutaneous transluminal angioplasty, *Radiology* 177:619–626, 1990.
3. Wexler L, Dorros G, Levin DC, King SB: Guidelines for performance of peripheral percutaneous transluminal angioplasty, *Catheter Cardiovasc Diagn* 2:128–129, 1990.
4. Levin DC, Becker GJ, Dorros G, et al: Training standards for physicians performing peripheral angioplasty and other percutaneous peripheral vascular interventions, *Circulation* 86:1348–1350, 1992.
5. Spittell JA, Creager AA, Dorros G, et al: Recommendations for peripheral transluminal angioplasty: training and facilities, *J Coll Cardiol* 21:546–548, 1993.
6. White RA, Fogarty TJ, Baker WM, et al: Endovascular surgery credentialing and training for vascular surgeons, *J Vasc Surg* 17:1095–1102, 1993.
7. White RA, Hodgson K, Ahn S, et al: Endovascular interventions training and credentialing for vascular surgeons, *J Vasc Surg* 29:177–186, 1999.
8. Babb J, Collins TJ, Cowley MJ, et al: Revised guidelines for the performance of peripheral vascular interventions, *Catheter Cardiovasc Interv* 46:21–23, 1999.
9. Rosenfield K, Cowley MJ, Jaff MR, et al: SCAI/SVMB/SVS clinical competence statement on carotid stenting: training and credentialing for carotid stenting—multispecialty consensus recommendations, a report of the SCAI/SVMB/SVS writing committee to develop a clinical competence statement on carotid interventions, *J Vasc Surg* 41(1):160–168, 2005.
10. Hodgson KJ, Matsumura JS, Ascher E, et al: SVS/SIR/SCAI/SVMB clinical competence statement on thoracic endovascular aortic repair (TEVAR)—multispecialty consensus recommendations, a report of the SVS/SIR/SCAI/SVMB Writing Committee to develop a clinical competence standard for TEVAR, *J Vasc Surg* 43:858–862, 2006.
11. Kouchoukos NT, Bavaria JE, Coselli JS, et al: Guidelines for credentialing of practitioners to perform endovascular stent-grafting of the thoracic aorta, *J Thorac Cardiovasc Surg* 131(3): 530–532, 2006.
12. Creager MA, Goldstone J, Hirshfeld JW Jr, et al: ACC/ACP/SCAI/SVMB/SVS clinical competence statement on vascular medicine and catheter-based peripheral vascular interventions, *J Am Coll Cardiol* 44(4):941–957, 2004.
13. Norgren L, Hiatt WR, Dormandy JA, et al: Inter-Society Consensus for the Management of Peripheral Arterial Disease (TASC II), *J Vasc Surg* 45(Suppl. S):S5–S67, 2007.
14. Rutherford RB, Flanigan DP, Gupta SK, et al: Suggested standards for reports dealing with lower extremity ischemia, *J Vasc Surg* 4:80–94, 1986.
15. Ahn S, Rutherford R, Becker G, et al: Reporting standards for endovascular procedures, *J Vasc Surg* 17:1103–1107, 1993.
16. Chaikof EL, Blankensteijn JD, Harris PL, et al: Reporting standards for endovascular aortic aneurysm repair, *J Vasc Surg* 35(5):1048–1060, 2002.
17. Ahn S, Rutherford R, Johnston KW, et al: Reporting standards for infrarenal endovascular abdominal aortic aneurysm repair, *J Vasc Surg* 25:405–410, 1997.
18. Spittell JA Jr, Nanda NC, Creager MA, et al: Recommendations for training in vascular medicine. American College of Cardiology Peripheral Vascular Disease Committee, *J Am Coll Cardiol* 22:626–628, 1993.
19. American Board of Vascular Medicine requirements. http://www.vascularboard.org/cert_reqs.cfm. Accessed on October 4, 2008.
20. Khoynezhad A, Donayre CE, Bui H, et al: Risk factors of neurologic deficit after thoracic aortic endografting, *Ann Thorac Surg* 83:S882–S889, 2007.
21. Khoynezhad A, Donayre CE, Smith J, et al: Risk factors for early and late mortality following thoracic endovascular aortic repair, *J Thoracic Cardiovasc Surg* 135(5):1103–1109. 1109e1-e4, 2008.
22. Harvey W: *Exercitatio anatomica de motu cordis et sanguinis in animalibus*. ed 4 (Translated by Chauncey D. Leake), Springfield [IL], 1958, Charles C Thomas Publisher.
23. DeBakey MD, Roberts WC: Michael Ellis DeBakey: a conversation with the editor, *Am J Cardiol* 79:929–950, 1997.
24. Roberts CS: Cardiovascular surgery as a single specialty: The case to unify cardiac and vascular surgery, *J Thorac Cardiovasc Surg* 136:267–270, 2008.

CHAPTER

4

Radiation Physics and Radiation Safety

Thomas F. Panetta, Luis R. Davila-Santini, Arthur Olson

There are two types of radiation. *Nonionizing radiation* includes radio waves, microwaves, and lasers. *Ionizing radiation* includes cosmic rays, x-rays, gamma rays, and charged particles. In radiology, ionizing radiation including x-rays and gamma rays is most commonly used. Magnetic resonance imaging uses radio waves. Charged particles are emitted only by various isotopes and by high-energy accelerators. X-rays are electromagnetic radiation emitted from outside the nucleus, and gamma rays, emitted from isotopes such as technetium, come directly from the nucleus. The way they interact with tissue and the biologic damage they produce are identical.

Several different units are used to describe radiation exposure: *roentgens, rad,* and *rem. Roentgens* are the amount of ionization produced in a specific volume of air. One roentgen equals 2.58×10^4 coulomb/kg of air or 1.61×10^{12} ion pairs/cc of air. A *rad* is the amount of energy absorbed by material (100 erg/g = 1 rad). Recently, the Système International has been adopted in which the rad has been replaced by the gray. One *gray* (Gy) equals 100 rad. *Rem* (roentgen equivalent mammal) is a measure of biologic effectiveness of irradiation. Rem = rad × quality factor. The quality factors for neutrons, alphas, and protons are greater than one. For x-rays, gamma rays, and electrons the quality factor equals one. In diagnostic radiology, where x-rays and gamma rays are the primary source of exposure, the conversion factors for converting roentgens to rad to rems are approximately one. Therefore roentgens ≅ rad ≅ rem ≅ 0.01 Gy.

Mechanisms of Interaction

Ionizing radiations are photon and particulate radiations whose principal mode of interaction with molecules is the ejection of electrons from bound orbitals. This results in ionization. Neutrally charged particles such as x-rays and gamma rays cause ionization through the photoelectric or Compton effect. Neutrons cause it by collisions with protons. This is a billiard ball—type of interaction that ejects protons from hydrogen atoms.

As charged particles, such as electrons, positrons, protons, and alpha particles, penetrate tissues they push or pull on the bound electrons of tissue molecules through their electrostatic forces of attraction and repulsion. This takes place as the particles hurtle through tissue. Their initial kinetic energy is given up rapidly in the process, and the charged particles quickly come to a halt. For electrons released by x-ray interactions, the distances traversed are typically much less than a millimeter. For beta rays (electrons) released by radionuclides this distance is more or less on the order of a millimeter. The energy released per unit length of distance traversed is the linear energy transfer (LET) of the particle. For an uncharged radiation, the LET is that of the initially released charged particle. The LET of diagnostic ionizing radiation is typically on the order of 1 keV/μm. For neutrons and alpha particles the LET is typically 10 to 100 times greater.

CELLULAR EFFECTS

The effect of radiation on humans can also be grouped into two general areas. *Somatic effects* are those effects occurring to the tissue of the person being irradiated. *Genetic effects* are those that will affect reproductive cells and therefore future generations.

Direct and Indirect Effect

Injury to macromolecules of tissue might take place directly from interaction with ionizing particles or indirectly by chemical interaction with the by-products of the ionization (Table 4-1). This is the initial stage of biologic effect that might result in cellular dysfunction.

The primary action of the radiation is to cause ionization. The indirect effect would be ionization of water to form an OH radical and H^+ ion. These can go through various interactions forming different radicals that can eventually combine with DNA to produce damage. These reactions are in competition with recombination whereby the radicals may combine to form water. Chemical sensitizers and protectors either enhance or reduce the indirect effect. The direct effect produces damage to the DNA by ionizing DNA atoms directly.

For low LET radiation (x-rays), the indirect effect accounts for about two thirds of damage—only one third is produced by direct effect, whereas the direct effect accounts for the majority of damage for high LET radiation. The DNA and RNA may be damaged in at least three different ways: (1) base damage, which is mainly to the pyrimidine bases, cytosine, thymine, and uracil; (2) single chain breaks; and (3) double chain breaks.

The effect of the ionization results in single and double strand breaks in DNA resulting in chromosome aberrations. Doses of 25 to 50 rad and greater can be estimated on the basis of the amount of aberrations. The translocations of DNA in chromosomes may lead to cancer and genetic mutations.

Cell Survival

Information about the effects of radiation can also be obtained by observing cell life after irradiation. One method used to study the effects of ionizing radiation on cells is to plot the replicative response of cells as a function of the absorbed dose. If we define response as the ability to produce colonies in a culture medium, then we can determine the fractional number of cells "surviving" after any given radiation dose and plot the relationship. Such a relationship is called a "survival curve."

Typically, such a curve will show a slow response to radiation at low doses as indicated by the initially gradually decreasing survival with increasing doses. Ultimately, the decrease in the fraction of surviving cells becomes linear on the semilogarithmic plot as dose increases. The shoulder of the survival curve indicates that damage to the cell must accumulate from multiple interactions in the cell before replicative death is likely. The likelihood of accumulating sufficient damage to any one particular cell depends on how much radiation is given to the culture. If too little radiation is given, no one cell will have accumulated enough damage, and the replicative capacity of all cells will remain intact. This is true for the initial low-dose parts of the curve. As the damage to cells accumulates, some cells will accumulate slightly more damage than other cells and therefore their replicative capacity will be more likely to be impaired. The gradual drop-off in survival before the shoulder is indicative of this accumulation of damage. After a dose of significant magnitude, almost all cells have accumulated barely sublethal damage and any more injury will result in replicative dysfunction. Under such a condition, the semilogarithmic survival curve is expected to be a straight line. The straight-line portion of the curve is indicative of this situation.

There are a number of factors that influence the fractional survival of cells including the type of ionizing radiation, the dose, the dose rate, the target cell type, and the situation of the target cells. The fractional survival of cells differs depending on the type of radiation used. There is an increasingly lethal effect as the LET of the ionizing irradiation increases. Alpha rays are potentially more harmful per dose than are fast neutrons or x-rays. Particles with higher LET are expected to produce a greater relative biologic effect than are particles with lower LET.

Relative biological effectiveness (RBE) is a term that describes the response of tissues for any given radiation relative to the response that one would obtain for 250-kVp x-rays. A comparison of radiations and their LETs and RBEs is given in Table 4-2. For a given dose, the rate at which the dose is delivered is a significant factor in determining the impairment to the replicative mechanism. If the doses are given in bursts that are separated by a significant interval of time (fractionated) then there is a transient flattening of the otherwise steep decline in the survival curve. Spreading out the absorbed dose to cells over time is less effective biologically than if the dose is given acutely. The reason for this phenomenon is that at low dose rates or between dose fractions cells

TABLE 4-1 Source of Ionizing Particles

A. $H_2O + hv$	→	$H_2O^+ + e^-$	Lifetime about 100 μs
H_2O^+	→	$OH + H^+$	Lifetime about 1 μs
$H_2O^+ + H_2O$	→	$OH + H_3O$	
B. $H_2O + hv$	→	H_2O^*	
H_2O^*	→	$H + OH$	Lifetime about 1 μs

* Excited water molecule.
hv, High voltage.

TABLE 4-2 Comparison of Radiations and Their LET and RBE

Ionizing Radiation	LET (keV/μm)	RBE
Gamma rays	0.3-10	1.0
Beta rays	0.5-15	1-2
Neutrons	20-50	2-5
Alphas	80-250	5-10

LET, Linear energy transfer; *RBE,* Relative biological effectiveness.

can repair sublethal damage before too much damage accumulates, and therefore more dose will be required to make up for the repair.

If the cells are irradiated during their late S-phase, they are least sensitive to radiation-induced impairment of their replicative capacity. During mitosis, the cells are most sensitive to radiation-induced impairment of the replicative capacity.

For this reason, those cells that actively proliferate are expected to be more sensitive to radiation. Immature undifferentiated cells tend to have a greater radiosensitivity than well-differentiated, mature cells. The greater length of time that cells spend in mitotic and developmental activity will increase their sensitivity. These observations are known as the Bergonié-Tribondeau law, a generalized principle for which major exceptions exist.

Cells that are hypoxic are less radiosensitive than those that are not. The presence of oxygen enhances the effect of the radiation. The oxygen enhancement ratio (OER) is the ratio of the dose required to produce an effect in hypoxic cells to that required in aerated cells. For x-rays, the OER is typically around 2.5 to 3.0. For higher LET radiations, the OER is less, typically less than 2.0. Many substances exist that can change and alter the radiosensitivity of cells to radiation.

Chromosomal Aberrations

Another way to examine the sensitivity of cells to radiation is to examine cells for chromosomal aberrations and to score the number of aberrations observed for a given dose against the normal incidence of such aberrations. This can then be plotted as a function of dose. In particular, examination of dicentric chromosomal aberrations in T-lymphocytes can be used to estimate whole body exposures to individuals accidentally exposed to doses in excess of approximately 25 rad. To date, biologic research seems to agree with the long-held theory that the "target" of the radiation in the cell is the DNA, which is contained primarily in the chromosomes. There are 23 pairs of chromosomes, which contain approximately 6×10^9 pairs of DNA bases. Most mutations occur during cell replication. Mutations occur in both germ cells and somatic cells although they are much less apparent in somatic cells unless tissue proliferation is promoted (as with cancer and some congenital birth defects). Most mutations in germ cells are lethal. Exposure to ionizing radiation may produce breaks in the DNA chain (which can be repaired by enzymatic excision and reconstruction). DNA is a double-stranded helix—shaped group of acids and bases and is capable of repair (one side of the chain is capable of replicating the proper base on the other side). The common belief that radiation damage is irreparable and cumulative is not completely true. If only one side of the chain is damaged it can be referred to as a sublethal damage and may be repairable. If both sides of the chain are damaged, there is usually no repair and the cell will die or mutate.

In a great majority of cells, structural changes of the chromosomes arise as a result of radiation damage inflicted during the interphase period of the cell cycle. At this time, the chromosomes are not organized; the altered structures arise through a breakage of the component strands of the chromosomes followed by the rejoining of broken ends to form configurations different from the original ones. Mutations result from the damage to chromosomes. Two general classes of mutations are seen. One is due to visible changes in the chromosome structure, probably because of chain breaks that are incorrectly repaired. The other type is due to invisible alterations in the chromosomes because of base damage. Equal doses of radiation given over a longer period of time are less damaging than if it is given as an instantaneous shot. Cells having a high mitotic rate are more sensitive to radiation than those reproducing slowly. A high mitotic rate allows the cell less time to repair the damage. Once the cell tries to reproduce with a damaged DNA, it will either die or produce two mutant cells. This is called the *law of Bergonié and Tribondeau.*

Cells and tissue types fall into four groups of radiosensitivity. The *most sensitive* generally include stem cells of the classic self-renewing systems. These include lymphocytes, precursor erythroblasts, and the primitive cells of the spermatogenic series and the lens of the eye. *Sensitive* cells divide regularly but mature and differentiate between divisions. These include cells of the gastrointestinal tract, hematopoietic cells, and more differentiated spermatogonia and spermatocytes. *Insensitive* cells are generally postmitotic cells with a relatively long life. These include cells of the liver, kidney, pancreas, and thyroid. The *most insensitive* cells are those fixed postmitotic cells that are highly differentiated and do not divide including those in brain, nerve, and fat.

SOMATIC EFFECTS

Short-Term and Long-Term Effects

Generally, large doses of radiation are required for short-term effects to be demonstrated; however, doses of 10 rad have been shown to decrease the lymphocyte count. A dose of 15 rad will reduce sperm counts, detectable approximately 8 weeks later. Whole-body doses on the order of 25 rad can be detected as chromosomal aberrations in T-lymphocytes; however, such individuals would not exhibit the characteristic signatures such as anorexia, nausea, and vomiting. The threshold whole-body dose required to elicit signs and symptoms of radiation exposure in only a small percentage of exposed individuals is 40 to 60 rad delivered acutely. Such signs occur in 50% of individuals exposed acutely to 120 to 200 rad (Table 4-3).

If large doses of radiation are given to the total body at one time, the individual can die as a result of the radiation-induced damages. There is a significant dose-rate effect for low LET radiation. At low dose rates the effect of radiation is significantly reduced. Most human and animal data are obtained from high dose rate studies. The lethal dose when 50% of the exposed population die is usually referred to as LD50. The LD50/60 (the dose at which 50% of the people would die within 60 days) for humans is approximately 350 rad. This is for total body irradiation. Death of acute radiation exposure is a threshold effect and would occur in only a small number of individuals exposed to 200 rad. After a dose of approximately 700 rad, virtually all individuals would die within 30 to 60 days after exposure.

In this range, the common cause of death is hematopoietic system failure because the bone marrow is no longer able to produce future blood cells. At higher acute doses, other organ systems show severe responses earlier than the hematopoietic system and are usually the cause of death. These include the gastrointestinal system, which responds in the dose range of 700 to 5000 rad, and the central nervous system, which responds to doses in excess of 5000 rad. The individual can die as a result of major complications to three general areas.

Fortunately, doses of this magnitude are rarely used in diagnostic examinations. Careful technologists and radiologists will always limit the area of the patient being exposed to the smallest area yielding the necessary clinical information.

TABLE 4-3 Response to Radiation Exposure

Dose	Response
0-200 rad	None. Very unlikely anyone would die. About 50% of the population would exhibit some signs of anorexia, nausea, and vomiting when exposed to 120-200 rad.
200-500 rad	Hematopoietic: Death occurs in several weeks usually as a result of infections.
500-5000 rad	Gastrointestinal: Death in days resulting from starvation.
5000 rad	Central nervous system: Death in minutes to hours; brain stops functioning.

To demonstrate the importance of shielding, a whole-body dose of 800 rad to mice would yield no survivors. If only one leg of each mouse is not exposed, a significant number of mice survive even at doses up to 1000 rad. Protecting the intestines also increases the survival. Useless exposure of uninvolved patient parts will directly increase the risk of the examination. In addition, the amount of scatter is proportional to the field size, so using the smallest possible field size also reduces exposure to everyone else.

Fertility and Sterility

Radiation damage to the testis or ovary can impair fertility. If the dose is high enough sterility may result; however, this requires depletion of the majority of the reproductive cells. Thus the effect is dose dependent and there is a threshold. The germ cells of the human testis may be highly radiosensitive depending on their degree of maturation. The spermatogonia is the most sensitive cell stage whereas the later stages of spermiogenesis are highly resistant. A dose of 150 to 200 rad is sufficient to kill enough young sperm cells that temporary sterility occurs. A dose of 300 to 500 rad (delivered instantaneously or within a few days) is required to cause permanent sterility. A dose of 100 to 200 mrad/day in dogs has been tolerated indefinitely without detectable effects on their sperm count.

The female ovum follows a different course. Three days postpartum, there are no stem (oogonial) cells, only oocytes. There are three types of follicles: (1) immature, (2) nearly mature, and (3) mature. A dose of 50 rad will cause temporary sterility, probably damaging the cells in the mature follicle stage. A dose of 400 rad would produce permanent sterility; however, a dose of 600 to 2000 rad is tolerated if given over a period of weeks. The threshold for permanent sterility in females decreases with age.

Long-Term Effects

The principal long-term somatic effect of concern to the medical community is cancer. The radiation-induced cancers of principal importance include leukemia, thyroid cancer, and breast cancer. Others of importance include skin and lung cancer. Risks depend on age at exposure; time since exposure; type of cancer; dose received; tissue exposed; protraction of dose; sex; and a host of other factors that might include genetic characteristics, living environment, smoking habits, and other factors that are not well understood. In general, children, women, and smokers are more sensitive to radiation-induced cancers than adults, men, and nonsmokers. Human data, however, are minimal, and most risk estimates are based on a combination of human and animal data.

The mechanism by which radiation may produce carcinogenic changes is thought to be the induction of mutations in the structure of single genes, changes in gene expression without mutation, or oncogenic viruses, which, in turn, cause cancer. The effects of radiation that lead to cancer are generally dose dependent and irreversible. Radiation has been shown to activate proto-oncogenes that give rise to oncogenes. Radiation itself has been shown to enhance tumor promotion, tumor progression, and the conversion of benign to malignant growths. Many promoting agents, such as chemicals, induce free radicals in cells (as does radiation), and these free radicals can damage DNA. There are several chemical/biological agents that have been shown to modify radiation-induced genetic transformation in the laboratory. If the tumor-promoting agent 12-0-tetradecanoyl-phorbol-acetate is present when irradiation is given, the genetic transformation rate is increased 10-fold when compared with radiation alone. High levels of vitamins A and E repress the effect of radiation. High levels of T_3 hormone increase the number of genetic transformations, whereas low levels of T_3 decrease the number of transformations.

Dose-Response Model

Because there is no adequate knowledge of the effects at low doses, the estimate for dose effect depends on the shape of the dose versus effect curve. There are two dose-response models of importance for radiation-induced cancer: (1) a linear no-threshold model and (2) the linear-quadratic model. The linear no-threshold model assumes all doses increase risk in proportion to the dose received. The linear-quadratic model has a linear response in the low-dose range with an increasing response incidence as dose increases. In this model low doses are less potent carcinogens on a risk per rad basis than are higher doses.

Risk Versus Dose

Most radiation safety workers will use the linear model. The linear-quadratic model results in lower estimates at lower dose levels. The linear-quadratic model is supported by data from Nagasaki and Hiroshima. The linear model is a more realistic estimate of high LET radiation.

Types of Risks

There are principally two types of risks that are used to describe radiation-induced cancer. *Absolute risk* examines the incidence of cancer in excess of the natural incidence of cancer in a population. Risks of this type are often expressed in terms of incidence per million people per year per rem. To interpret this risk, let us say the risk is 2 per million persons per year per rem (PYR = persons per year per rem). In this case, the risk would begin after a minimum latent period and continue at that rate until the risk expires. For example, the risk of cancer developing within the next 32 years after an initial exposure of 10 rem and a minimum latent period of 2 years might be 30 years × 10 rem × 2 per million PYR = 600 per million or 0.06%. Stated another way, if 1 million people are exposed to 2 rem, 600 additional cancers might be expected in the following 32 years. It is not clear, however, that absolute risk is an accurate descriptor of the way radiation-induced cancers develop.

Many data indicate that the *relative risk* is a more appropriate descriptor. For relative risk, the likelihood of the development of radiation-induced cancer within any period of time after the latent period is expressed as a multiple of the natural age-specific risk of the development of a cancer within that period of time. For example, if an exposure to radiation increases the risk of development of cancer by a factor of 1.01 (1%), then, after an initial latent period, the risk of cancer developing in a person during any year is 1% greater than the person's natural risk of having that cancer develop within that year. Because natural risk increases with age a person's risk for the development of radiation-induced cancer always remains 1% that of the current natural risk.

Human data are drawn from very small numbers. The largest sources of human data are listed in Table 4-4. Of all the human data published, the majority applies to A-bomb survivors. There were about 280,000 of whom only 41,719 received doses greater than 0.5 rad. Of these 3435 died of some form of cancer between 1950 and 1985. Another 34,272 survivors were used as the control group, and 2501 have died of cancer. In general, there were approximately 400 to 600 extra cancers produced in the exposed over what would be expected.

Another study, which followed 82,000 exposed survivors of the atomic bomb, recorded approximately 250 radiation-induced cancers. The average exposure to these survivors was 14 rem. The next largest human study is of 14,500 people who received x-ray treatments (1935 to 1954) to the spine for a form of arthritis (ankylosing spondylitis) with doses of 500 to 3000 rem. These patients showed an increase (140) of cancer and leukemia. A group of 2652 children were treated by x-rays to reduce the thymus gland. The thymus doses ranged from 200 to 600 rad. The thyroid doses ranged from 5 to 1100 rem. Thyroid cancer developed in 37 of the children. Large doses of radiation can produce cancer and leukemia. There is a time period that elapses before this effect is evident; this latent period will vary depending on, for example, the rate of growth of the tumor, interval of clinical testing, dose level, and age of patient. The latest estimates for overall cancer-induced death are that a whole-body exposure of 10

TABLE 4-4 Largest Sources of Human Data

Skin cancer	Early x-ray workers.
Bone tumors	Radium watch dial painters. Thoratrast injections.
Leukemia	Japanese A-bomb survivors. Early radiologists (lifetime doses of 200-2000 rad). Ankylosing spondylitis (14,106 patients received radiation therapy treatments).
Thyroid cancer	Patients irradiated for tinea capitis: 10,834 patients aged 0-15 years resulted in 39 thyroid cancers, whereas the control group yielded 16.
Thymus	Thymus irradiation: 2652 patients younger than 1 year old were given radiation therapy for thymus reduction. Thirty-seven cancers were recorded vs. one in the control group.
Breast cancer	Fluoroscopic examination of chest (31,710 women examined by multiple fluoroscopic examinations from 1930-1952). By 1980 a total of 482 cancer deaths had been observed. Japanese A-bomb survivors.
Lung cancer	Underground miners exposed to radon. Patients with cervical cancer: 82,000 women treated for cervical cancer by radiation, lung received 10-60 rad.

TABLE 4-5 Cancer Risks From Radiation Exposure

	Risk	
Malignancy	**Extra cases per 100,000 exposed to 10 rem**	**Cases per 100,000 unexposed people**
Leukemia mortality	110	900
Thyroid induction	300—Children	30 M, 100 F
Thyroid induction	150—Adult	
Breast mortality	70—All ages	3600
Breast mortality	295—Age 15 yr	
Lung mortality	190	7800 M, 3400 F
Digestive mortality	170	1300
Skin induction	20 doses of 100 rad generally required	
All other organs	Low risk	
All cancer deaths	800	22,000

F, Female; *M*, male.

rad given to 100,000 persons of all ages would yield an extra 800 cancer deaths (all types including leukemia) in addition to the 20,000 that would have occurred without any radiation exposure. In other words, this would be an excess 3.7% of the normal expectation. On the basis of recent studies, the risks and mean latency periods for several types of cancers are discussed below and summarized in Table 4-5.

Leukemia

The principal radiation-induced leukemias include chronic granulocytic leukemia and acute leukemias. Human data do not suggest that chronic lymphocytic leukemia is radiation induced. The minimum latent period for radiation-induced leukemia is approximately 2 years, and, depending on the age at exposure, the risk period tends to peak at 5 to 10 years after exposure. The relative risk then declines to essentially no excess risk after 20 years following the initial exposure. The mortality rate is significantly elevated at 0.4 Gy (40 rad) and above but not at lesser doses. The number of excess deaths resulting from leukemia was approximately 110 per 100,000 persons per 10 rad. This is approximately the same number of extra cases that would result from a continuous exposure of 0.1 rem/yr. If the dose rate is increased to 1 rem/yr, the number of extra leukemias would jump to 400 per 100,000 people exposed. The effect is very age dependent. For example, the excess relative risk due to a 10-rad exposure for people under the age of 15 years is approximately 3.6% whereas for people 16 to 25 years it is approximately 0.3%, and for people over 26 years it drops to 0.03%. The dose-response function for radiation-induced leukemia seems to best be described by a linear-quadratic function.

Thyroid Cancer

Radiation-induced thyroid cancers are typically of the well-differentiated papillary type; few are of the follicular type. As such, they tend to be easily treated; the cure rate for such cancers is approximately 90%. Women are more susceptible to radiation-induced thyroid cancer than are men (3:1); however, they are also three times as likely to have thyroid cancer develop even if unirradiated. Hence, the relative risks are the same, but the absolute risk is three times higher in females. The latent period for such cancers is at minimum 5 to 10 years with a mean of about 20 years. At present, there is no evidence for a maximum limit on the latent period.

The absolute risk for radiation-induced thyroid cancer is approximately six cases per million PYR for women and two per million PYR for men. This applies only to externally administered radiation. Children are the most sensitive; the relative risk for children is twice as great as the risk for adults. The best estimate for children over age 5 years yields a relative risk of 8.3% excess cancers per 100 rad. For children under age 5 years the risk goes up to 23% excess cancers per 100 rad. The excessive risk estimate for children over age 5 years is 300 extra cases per 10 rem exposure. For uptake of iodine-131 the cancer incidence is apparently much less. The risk for thyroid adenoma is 12 cases per million PYR. The linear no-threshold risk model is the most appropriate for this cancer. Doses of 6 to 30 rad in children have shown a statistical increase in thyroid cancer.

Breast Cancer

The minimum latent period for radiation-induced breast cancer varies with age. Independent of the age at exposure, the pattern for increased incidence of radiation-induced breast cancer follows the same age characteristic patterns of the spontaneous natural incidence of breast cancer. In general, however, the minimum latent period for women exposed after age 25 years is 5 years with a mean of 20 to 25 years. Data do not indicate any increased risk in breast cancer for men. The risk for radiation-induced breast cancer death is approximately 70 extra cancers per 100,000 people exposed to a dose of 10 rem. The risk of breast cancer is also very age dependent with the highest risk at age 15 years: 295 per 100,000 women exposed to 10 rem; this drops to 52 at age 25 years; to 43 at age 35 years; to 20 at age 45 years; and to 6 at age 55 years. Another way to look at the data is by using the excessive relative risk method. In other words, what is the percent increase above the normal incidence rate? A woman exposed at age 15 years to a dose of 10 rem would have an additional 1.2% risk of breast cancer death, almost the same as the incidence of the development of breast cancer. A 45-year-old woman would have a 0.03% risk of cancer death resulting from a 10-rem dose. The linear no-threshold risk model is the most appropriate model for this cancer.

Lung Cancer

Data on radiation-induced lung cancer are confounded by two important factors: (1) exposure of some of the study groups to inhaled radon, which produces a high LET alpha particle, and (2) the variable smoking habits among members of the study groups. The extra cancer mortality due to a 10-rem exposure to 100,000 people is 190. Children seem to have a lower risk (at age 5 years the number of extra deaths is only 17; at age 15 years it rises to 54). The excess incidence is approximately four cases per million PYR with use of a linear no-threshold risk model. The minimum latent period is approximately 10 years for individuals 25 years or older with a mean of approximately 25 years. For individuals less than 25 years old, risk does not increase until they reach about age 35 years. The linear-quadratic risk estimate may be more appropriate for this cancer; this estimate is about three times less than the linear one.

Skin Cancer

Compared with the previously mentioned cancers, skin cancer does not appear to be a significant concern after exposure to low doses of ionizing radiation. The tumors most commonly found after exposure to ionizing radiation include squamous cell and basal cell carcinomas. Perhaps the most extensive study of radiation-induced skin cancer is that in 2226 children who were irradiated with epilating doses of 100-kVp x-rays to the scalp for tinea capitis. The doses were approximately 450 rad. Of the 1680 white members of the group, 80 basal cell carcinomas were produced, whereas only 3 were found in the control group. No skin cancers were found in the nonwhite group. The risk of the development of skin cancer is about 20 per 100,000 persons exposed to 10 rem. Melanomas do not appear to be induced by ionizing radiation. Radiation-induced skin cancer is a concern to radiologists receiving substantial radiation doses (hundreds of rad) to their hands during fluoroscopy.

Radiation-Induced Mortality From Cancer

For a variety of reasons, not all people die of the radiation-induced cancers. As such, the death rate is lower. The national death rate from individual cancers is 5 to 200 per 100,000 persons per 10 rem. Risks are sometimes given in terms of increased risk and sometimes in terms of mortality risk. For example, the absolute risk of a radiation-induced thyroid cancer is about 6 per million PYR. Mortality risk from radiation-induced thyroid cancer is 1 million PYR or less. It is important to keep these differences in mind. Benign thyroid tumors are also induced by radiation but are not accounted for in cancer risk estimates. The lifetime mortality risk from an acute whole-body dose of 10 rem is 800 per 100,000 exposed individuals. These risks are almost the same if population is exposed to 0.1 rem/yr continuous radiation.

OTHER SOMATIC EFFECTS

Cataracts

Cataract is another radiation-induced effect with a threshold. The effective threshold for cataract is approximately 200 rad dose to the lens of the eye. If the dose is protracted, threshold increases. The cataracts may not appear for 35 years and may show up as early as 6 months from the date of exposure. A typical time frame is within 2 to 3 years. It is important to note that studies investigating radiation-induced cataracts include lens opacities that do not interfere clinically with vision. Doses required to produce cataracts that interfere with vision would be higher. One study indicates the average latent period to be about 8 years for persons receiving 200 to 600 rad. This is lowered to 4 years for doses of 650 to 1100 rad. NOTE: There have been no cases in persons receiving less than 200 rad.

Nonspecific Life-Shortening

In laboratory animals, mammals exposed to whole-body radiation died earlier than the unirradiated controls. This effect increased with increased dose. From these experiments, it was concluded that there is a life-shortening effect from radiation. Most of the cause of accelerated death was the onset of cancer. Mortality from other diseases has not been significantly increased by radiation in human populations.

GENETIC EFFECTS

Approximately 10% of all live births in the United States have some form of genetic mutation, one third of which are serious. The development of a mature sperm cell (spermatozoa) takes approximately 10 weeks. Cells in order of increasing maturity are spermatogoniums (stem cells), primary spermatocytes, secondary spermatocytes, spermatids, and spermatozoa.

The sensitivity of the cell decreases as it matures. Postspermatogonial cells are rather resistant to radiation. After a moderate exposure (200 rad) there is a period of fertility followed by a period of infertility (temporary sterility) when the last spermatogonial cells have been used. There are no significant hormonal changes in the male. The mature spermatozoa are much more likely to produce genetic mutation. This is why conception should be postponed after a large exposure to radiation. A dose of 250 rad will produce temporary sterility in the male for 1 to 2 years, and an exposure of 600 rad will cause permanent sterility. In males, a dose of 15 rad may reduce sperm count and may cause temporary sterility. There is a dose-rate effect, that is, the higher the dose rate the higher the mutational frequency. The spermatogonia are more dose-rate sensitive. This is attributable to some type of repair process.

At low dose rates, the male is much more sensitive than the female in producing mutations. The genetic effect can be reduced if a time period between irradiation and conception is permitted; 6 months is usually recommended. The reason for this is understood in males. The same effect is noted in females; however, the mechanism is not understood. In addition, there does not seem to be a lower threshold dose below which no mutations are produced; a linear extrapolation from high-dose data appears valid.

Doses in the range of 300 to 400 rad to the ovaries of women approaching menopause may cause long-term impairment of fertility or permanent sterility. In younger women, the impairment to fertility is temporary. Gonadal irradiation may cause genetic defects in progeny of the irradiated persons. Investigations in animals, particularly mice, have led the Biologic Effects of Ionizing Radiation (BEIR) Committee to suggest that a dose of 1 rad delivered to the entire population might cause a 0.1% incidence of genetically affected offspring. This should be compared with the normal incidence of 11%. Sometimes a doubling dose is quoted to indicate risk. This is the dose that must be given to all adults for many generations to double the current incidence of genetically affected offspring. The doubling dose for humans is thought to be between 50 and 250 rem. The estimates for doubling dose (dose required to double mutation rate) are listed in Table 4-6.

Recent data indicate that if more than 7 weeks intervened between irradiation and conception (in female mice) the number of mutations drops to zero implying complete repair of genetic damage. This probably relates to about 6 months in humans. This effect (decrease in mutation rate with increased interval between irradiation and conception) exists for both males and females. The mechanism for females is not understood. It is estimated that a continuous dose of 1 rem per generation will increase the natural incident rate of mutation by approximately 1%.

OTHER SOURCES OF RADIATION

Humans are exposed to radiation from different sources from conception to death. The most common is external background radiation. It is estimated that the average exposure to a person at sea level is approximately 26 mrem/yr. At higher altitudes, there is less air to absorb this radiation, resulting in higher radiation levels. Without the layer of air to protect us, we would receive about 1000 times more radiation exposure. In addition, there exist in the atmosphere natural radioactive

TABLE 4-6 Dose Required to Double Mutation Rate

Double dose	Supporting data
3 rem	This is the average dose a person will receive over a 30-year period (reproductive lifetime). All mutations are produced by background radiation.
20-200 rem	Based on animal data
100 rem	Hiroshima and Nagasaki

materials that were present in or on the earth when it was formed. There are also radionuclides, which are produced by the interaction of cosmic radiation and matter. The incident cosmic ray knocks out a nucleon producing a radionuclide and possible neutron activation. The most common radionuclides produced this way are ^{14}C, ^{3}H, ^{22}Na, and ^{7}Be. Carbon-14 and tritium contribute the most to the background dose to humans.

Humans also increase the amount of radionuclides in the atmosphere because of nuclear reactors, as well as nuclear weapons. A nuclear reactor produces ^{14}C, most of which will be released into the atmosphere; however, the dose to humans from this is 100 times less than that which is produced naturally.

Humans also receive a radiation dose because of radionuclides present in the earth or transferred from the atmosphere to the earth. Most of the exposure comes from primordial radionuclides. Thorium and uranium undergo radioactive decay through complex decay schemes that have half-lives of thousands and millions of years. Some of the uranium and thorium isotopes also decay by fission, which produces additional isotopes. Radon, a gas, is the daughter of radium, a solid; as radium decays, radon is emitted (radium—1,600-year half-life). When possible, the radon gas will escape into the atmosphere and will expose the population (approximately 2×10^9 Ci of radon enters the atmosphere each year). There are other naturally occurring radioisotopes that can end up in, for example, building materials, granite, concrete, and marble, which will also expose the population. The average whole-body dose from external terrestrial radiation is about 30 mrem. Typical exposures for background and man-made radiation are listed in Table 4-7.

Of the total 360 mrem/yr received by the U.S. population, 18% comes from medical examinations and 66% from radon. No change in cancer rates have been identified in areas of high natural background; however, increase in chromosome aberrations has been reported.

TABLE 4-7 Typical Exposures for Background and Human-Made Radiation

NATURAL BACKGROUND	*EXPOSURE*	*HUMAN-MADE*	*EXPOSURE*
External (cosmic rays)		Medical	53 mrem/yr
New York City	27 mrem/yr	Occupational	20 mrem/yr
Denver	50 mrem/yr	Average to U.S. population	1 mrem/yr
Internal		Other (weapons testing)	5 mrem/yr
Radioactive potassium, calcium, etc.	39 mrem/yr	Nuclear industry	0.1 mrem/yr
Inhaled (radon)		Coal burning	0.2 mrem/yr
Effective total body	200 mrem/yr	Consumer products	10 mrem/yr
Bronchial epithelium	2400 mrem/yr	Typical exposures from specific human-made radiation	
Can be as great as	20,000 mrem/yr	Color TV	0.5 mR/hr
Terrestrial radionuclide exposure		Mammography	1000 mR/exposure
New York City	28 mrem/yr	Dental	500 mR/film
Denver	90 mrem/yr	CT scanner	2000 mR/slice
Guarapari, Brazil	640 mrem/yr	Airport, x-ray unit	0.2 mR
Madras states in India	1300 mrem/yr	Transatlantic flight	0.5 mR
Niue Island in Pacific	1000 mrem/yr	Airline crew members	160 mR/yr
Average noncoastal United States	46 mrem/yr	Three Mile Island	10 mrem (<50 miles)
Guangdong, China	400 mrem/yr	Three Mile Island	80 mrem (<1 mile)
Reading Prong (radon)	150 mrem/yr	Chernobyl	200 deaths resulting from acute radiation syndrome
Radon emitted from soil	2,000,000,000 curies/yr	Tobacco (1 pack/day) to small regions in bronchial epithelium	16,000 mrem/yr

MEDICAL USE OF RADIATION

Without question, the use of radiation in the medical field has provided large benefits to society. It is important to realize, however, that medical radiation accounts for 90% of the man-made radiation exposure to the U.S. population. The amount of radiation used in the medical community must be kept as low as reasonably achievable. There are three major sources of unnecessary exposure to medical radiation: (1) poor equipment and sloppy techniques by practitioners or radiologic technologists; (2) malpractice: practitioners using x-rays for purposes of defending themselves in possible malpractice suits; and (3) poor judgment on the part of the practitioner, employers, and/or patients. Significant injury to patients can occur with improper exposure to radiation (Figure 4-1).

Real Effect

Approximately 80% of medical attention is given within 3 years of a patient's death. The true effect of medical radiation may be much less than other types of exposure. The total number of extra leukemias produced by the medical radiation (if the patients live another 20 years) is about 300 to 600 in United States. The total number of solid tumors is approximately 100 to 2000; the number of genetic mutations is estimated at 100 to 2000, of which one third are serious.

RECOMMENDATIONS

X-ray equipment should meet the Federal Diagnostic X-ray Equipment Performance Standard or, as a minimum for equipment manufactured before August 1, 1974, the Suggested State Regulations for Control of Radiation (40 FR 29749). General-purpose fluoroscopy units should provide image intensification; fluoroscopy units for nonradiology specialty use should have electronic image-holding features unless such use is demonstrated to be impracticable for the clinical use involved. Photofluorographic x-ray equipment should not be used for chest radiography.

X-ray facilities should have quality assurance programs designed to produce radiographs that satisfy

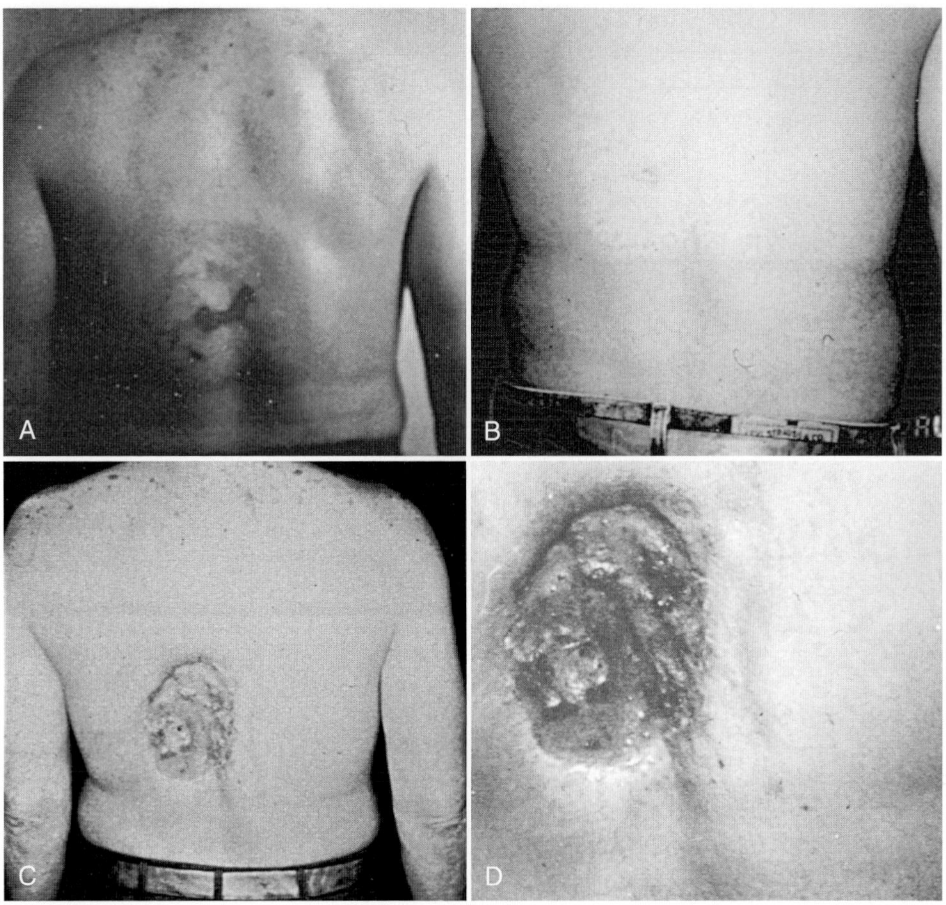

FIGURE 4-1 **A,** Radiation injury to back after prolonged C-arm exposure. Patient is 7 weeks after radiation exposure. **B,** Same patient 18 weeks after injury. **C,** Delayed necrosis is apparent. Patient is 18 months after injury. **D,** Closeup view of injury at 18 months.

diagnostic requirements with minimal patient exposure. Such programs should contain material and equipment specifications, equipment calibration and preventive maintenance requirements, quality control of image processing, and operational procedures to reduce retake and duplicate examinations.

Proper collimation should be used to restrict the x-ray beam as much as practicable to the clinical area of interest and within the dimensions of the image receptor. Shielding should be used to further limit the exposure of the fetus, and the gonads of patients with reproductive potential, when such exclusion does not interfere with the examination being conducted.

Technique appropriate to the equipment and materials available should be used to maintain exposure as low as is reasonably achievable without loss of requisite diagnostic information. Measures should be undertaken to evaluate and reduce, where practicable, exposures for routine nonspecialty exams that exceed the Entrance Skin Exposure Guides, as listed in Table 4-8.

TABLE 4-8 Entrance Skin Exposure Guides

Examination (projection)	Entrance Skin Exposure: FDA* Guidelines	HSCB
Chest (P/A)	17 mR	10 mR
Skull (lateral)	154 mR	125 mR
Abdomen (A/P)	485 mR	338 mR
Cervical spine (A/P)		125 mR
Thoracic spine (A/P)	405 mR	310 mR
L/S spine (A/P)	622 mR	520 mR
Retrograde pyelogram	638 mR	364 mR
Feet (D/P)	106 mR	140 mR
Dental	289 mR	170 mR
CT body		5,000 mR
Mammography		450 mR
Fluoroscopy		3000 mR/min
105-mm spot film		100 mR
Barium enema		12,000 mR
GI series		8000 mR
Ovarian dose from		
Abdomen x-ray		75 mR
Chest x-ray (P/A)		1 mR
Barium enema		3000 mR

* *A/P,* anterior-posterior; *CT,* Computed tomography; *D/P,* dorsal-plantar; *FDA,* Food and Drug Administration; *GI,* gastrointestinal; *HSCB,* Health Science Center at Brooklyn; *L/S,* lumbo-sacral; *P/A,* posterior-anterior.

RADIATION SAFETY LIMITS

The population is divided into two general classes. *Occupational exposure* (e.g., x-ray technologist, nuclear power plant operator) means the radiation dose is received by an individual in a controlled area or in the course of such individual's employment in which the individual's duty involves exposure to radiation. It does not include any dose received for the purpose of medical diagnosis or therapy. *Nonoccupational exposure* is in those people who may get exposed to radiation but who do not directly work with sources of radiation.

Controlled Versus Noncontrolled Area

A *controlled* area is any area where access is controlled for the purpose of protecting individuals from exposure to radiation and radioactive material. It does not include any area used as a residence. A *noncontrolled* area is any area where access is not controlled; virtually anyone may enter. The *maximum permissible dose* to an individual must be no greater than 0.5 rem in 52 consecutive weeks; the exposure level must be less than 2 mrem in any 1 hour or 100 mrem in 7 consecutive days.

DOSE LIMITS

There are no dose limits to the patient at this time for medical procedures. There are limits to those individuals who may get exposed as a result of their employment and to those individuals who may get exposed because they are in the area where radiation is used. No individual in a controlled area shall receive doses in excess of (1) 5 rem/yr to total body, bone marrow, lens of eyes, and gonads; (2) 75 rem/yr to hands; (3) 30 rem/yr to forearms; and (4) 15 rem/yr to all other organs. No individual shall receive a nonoccupation exposure in excess of (1) 0.5 rem/yr to any organ and (2) 2.0 mrem/h to any organ. A fetus shall not receive exposure in excess of 0.5 rem per gestation. *Note:* this does not include medical exposure the fetus may receive as a result of the mother undergoing diagnostic examination or therapy.

In addition to these specific limits, the federal government has adopted the "as low as reasonably achievable" (ALARA) principle. Simply put, ALARA means that all unnecessary exposure should be eliminated when financially and technically feasible.

Maximum Permissible Body Burdens

Maximum permissible body burdens (MPBB) state the limit on internally absorbed radioactive materials that would yield 5 rems/yr. In turn the maximum permissible concentration (MPC) is that amount in air (or water) that would result in the person receiving the MPBB.

PERSONNEL MONITORING

Film Badges

A small piece of dental film in a light-tight paper container is inserted into a specially designed holder. The individual generally wears this for a period of 1 to 3 months, after which the badge is returned to a company for processing. By measuring the optical density and the pattern on the film, the company can estimate the amount and the type of radiation. The holder has different filter materials: none, thin aluminum, heavy copper, and cadmium, which attenuate the radiation to different degrees. High energy betas may penetrate the zero filter and the aluminum but not the copper and cadmium, whereas a high energy x-ray beam would penetrate all three. In either case, a different density pattern would result. Badges do not offer protection from radiation; they supply information about previous exposure only. Reports can be 2 months delayed for monthly badges.

LIMITS FOR X-RAY EQUIPMENT

Fluoroscopic Output

The entrance exposure to the patient shall be measured 1 cm above the tabletop for under-table tube configurations; 30 cm above the tabletop for above-table tube configurations; and 30 cm from the input surface of the image intensifier for C-arm units. For fluoroscopic equipment with automatic brightness control, the maximum permissible exposure to the patient is 10 R/min except (1) during recording of the fluoroscopic image and (2) when an optional high R mode is provided; then the limit shall be 5 R/min unless the high R mode is activated. There is no limit for the high R mode.

For fluoroscopic equipment without automatic brightness control the maximum permissible exposure to the patient is 5 R/min except (1) during the recording of the fluoroscopic image and (2) when an optional high R mode is provided; then there is no limit for the high R mode.

X-Ray Field Size

The fluoroscopic and radiographic x-ray field shall not exceed the visible field size by more than 3% of the source image-receptor distance (SID) along any edge.

Half Value Layer

To reduce entrance patient exposure, the primary x-ray beam must be filtered to remove the low-energy photons. There must be enough added filtration to result in the x-ray beam having a half rvalue layer of no less than (1) 2.3 mm Al at 80 kVp for general x-ray and (2) 0.3 mm Al at 30 kVp for mammography.

Scatter Radiation

There is no limit for the amount of scatter from a radiographic exam. However, for fluoroscopy, the x-ray unit shall have some type of shielding to limit the exposure to the operator, or other personnel, to 100 mR/hr at the point of closest approach.

The amount of scatter radiation depends on the kVp (higher kVp results in proportionally more Compton scatter), field size (increased field size increases the amount of scatter), and patient thickness (thicker patient, more scatter). One rule of thumb is that at 1 m the amount of scatter is approximately 0.1% of the entrance patient exposure. The average energy of the scattered beam is about the same as the primary beam. This is due to the fact that low-energy photons of the primary beam are absorbed, not scattered; the higher-energy photons, when scattered, have reduced energy.

SHIELDING DESIGNS

To ensure that exposure levels are within acceptable amounts, a shielding design is generally performed before an x-ray installation is started. Lead is generally used in diagnostic installations, concrete in many high-energy therapy installations. Lead is very effective at absorbing low-energy x-rays because of its high Z. At higher energies, where Compton is the major interaction, electron density is more important. Most materials have similar electron densities; therefore a pound of concrete would attenuate about the same amount as a pound of lead. Because a pound of concrete is much less expensive than a pound of lead, it is generally used in radiation therapy installations. Even in diagnostic installation, concrete may be substituted for lead; however, it must be much thicker—$^1/_{16}$ inch of lead is equivalent to about 3.5 inches of concrete.

PRACTICAL ISSUES IN RADIATION SAFETY

Optimal protection for all personnel involved in fluoroscopic procedures is of utmost importance. The physician performing the procedure is responsible for the safety of himself or herself and those around himself or herself. A radiation safety educational program will help reduce exposure, improve the working environment, and limit radiation exposure risks. As discussed earlier in this chapter, federal regulations require providers and institutions to comply with the ALARA principle. Physicians should be aware of the principle and strive to attain radiation doses *a*s *l*ow *a*s *r*easonably *a*chievable. The U.S. guidelines and regulations for radiation safety are dictated by the state. Every institution then establishes its own policy and procedures governing all aspects of radiation safety based on state regulations. Every fluoroscopist should be aware of the institutional guidelines for protective wear and monitoring of exposure. There have been multiple articles published in the literature that attempt to assess the radiation exposure to physicians and/or technologists performing fluoroscopic procedures such as cardiac catheterization and orthopedic procedures by recreating the same conditions in the laboratory. There are many variables that alter the exposure doses (angle of beam or image intensifier, time of exposure, distance from beam, background scatter, amount of protective garments, just to name a few). The most practical knowledge for the physician, however, is that there are three main factors that limit the dose of exposure: distance, time, and protective garments.

Distance

The closer the physician needs to stand to the radiation beam, the more protected he or she should be. Most institutional guidelines recommend a thyroid collar in addition to a lead apron for all personnel standing less than 3 feet away from the tube. The effective dose rate to personnel is reduced by approximately a factor of two every time the distance from the patient is increased by 40 cm. As standard practice, it is advisable to step away from the image intensifier as much as possible without compromising one's ability to perform the procedure.

Time

The amount of time of exposure to radiation is also an important factor contributing to overall dose exposure. The new technologies provide for last-image-hold ability, as well as low dose settings that are designed to reduce radiation times. It is important to remember that the effective dose of exposure is accumulated over days, weeks, months, and years as sequential fluoroscopic procedures are performed. Therefore all providers should have monitoring devices to quantify exposure over time. Limiting the amount of exposure in every procedure, even in small amounts, over time will decrease the effective dose rate and limit the lifetime exposure risk.

Protective Garments

Lead protective garments are standard required protection to anyone being exposed to radiation. Lead aprons and/or skirt and vest garments need to be between 0.35 and 0.5 mm thick, properly stored, and inspected every 6 months to a year for cracks, creases, or rupture to ensure adequate protection. The garments not only protect the covered organs but also reduce the total body effective dose of exposure as much as 16-fold. The use of a thyroid collar protects the thyroid from the minimal exposure risk and also reduces the total effective dose by a factor between 1.7 and 3. Protective 0.15-mm lead–equivalent glasses or goggles limit the eye lens dose and provide about 70% attenuation even in high energy (kVp) beams. The angle and distance of the beam to the patient will determine the amount of scatter. Increased exposure dose results from oblique or lateral views and higher image intensifier distance from the patient and table. These factors should be considered while acquiring the images. Shields attached to the ceiling and screens that move in and out of the procedure room also provide increased protection from radiation.

An underestimated occupational hazard associated with the use of lead gowns, aprons, and vests is cervical and lumbar spine injuries. The rationale for a skirt and vest in contrast to a full lead apron is to split the weight of the lead between the shoulders and the hips, thus distributing the weight between the upper cervical/thoracic spine and the lumbar spine. Using lighter lead is an obvious approach within the limits of lead thickness and safety requirements. However, in those who have symptoms of cervical disk disease, a single-piece lead gown with a tight belt around the waist is effective in transmitting all the weight to the hips, thus relieving all the weight from the cervical spine. For those who have symptoms, early diagnosis with magnetic resonance imaging and a physical therapy program can frequently reduce symptoms and control the risk of more serious injury.

CONCLUSION

The implementation of safety guidelines and the use of the spectrum of protection devices reduce the lifetime exposure risk to radiation. However, with increased use of endovascular techniques in vascular surgery, the risks are substantial and not necessarily negligible. All physicians involved in performing fluoroscopic procedures should be aware of the risk and take responsibility in protecting and educating themselves and their staff.

CHAPTER

5

Reducing Radiation Exposure During Endovascular Procedures

Evan C. Lipsitz, Frank J. Veith, Takao Ohki

Endovascular aortoiliac aneurysm repair has recently been approved by the U.S. Food and Drug Administration. Other endovascular procedures for the treatment of such entities as aortoiliac occlusive disease and renal artery stenosis are also being employed more frequently. It has been estimated that up to 80% of all abdominal aortic aneurysms are amenable to treatment with endovascular grafting and that in the near future at least 40% to 70% of all vascular interventions will be performed by using an endovascular method.[1] These procedures require the use of digital cinefluoroscopy, which exposes both the patient and the staff to ionizing radiation.

BIOLOGIC EFFECTS OF RADIATION

The biologic effects of radiation can be divided into two types, deterministic and stochastic.[2] *Deterministic* effects are observed only when many cells in an organ or a tissue are killed by a dose above a given threshold. *Stochastic* effects are due to radiation-induced injury to the DNA of a single cell, and there is no threshold below which the risk is eliminated. The probability of an effect is small, however. Stochastic effects may be somatic, affecting somatic cells, or hereditary, affecting germ cells. It is these stochastic effects that are of concern because there is no low threshold.

Radiation exposure is cumulative, and effects are permanent. The total exposure for an individual performing fluoroscopic procedures is the sum of his or her exposure during these procedures, the background exposure, and any incidental instances of medical exposure (e.g., diagnostic chest x-ray examinations). In the United States, the average person receives approximately 3.5 millisieverts per year of background exposure.[3] This dose increases with altitude, doubling at every 2000 m. Other local effects, such as those caused by radionuclides in the soil, can significantly affect the amount of background radiation. Table 5-1 highlights the current recommended dose limits for both occupational and civilian settings.

UNITS OF MEASUREMENT

There are several different measures of radiation exposure. *Absorbed* dose is the energy delivered to an organ divided by the mass of the organ, expressed in grays. *Equivalent* dose is the average absorbed dose in an organ or tissue multiplied by a radiation weighting factor, expressed in sieverts. In general, radiation used in medicine has a weighting factor of one, so that the absorbed dose and the equivalent dose are considered equal. Total effective dose is the sum of the equivalent doses in all tissues and organs multiplied by a tissue weighting factor for each organ or tissue used to evaluate total body exposure.[2]

ROLE OF EXPERIENCE

Some endovascular procedures can be quite complex and may require lengthy fluoroscopic times, especially at tertiary referral centers, which generally have affiliated training programs. In a study of radiation exposure during cardiology fellowship training, Watson and colleagues[4] found a statistically significant increase in exposure for cases done in the first versus the second year of fellowship. This difference was largely accounted for by an increase in fluoroscopy time but not cine time, reflecting the fact that less-experienced operators take longer to position the catheters. These

TABLE 5-1 Yearly Recommended Dose Limits

	Dose limit (mSv/yr)*	
Application	**Occupational**	**Public**
Effective dose	20	1
Equivalent dose in lens of eye	150	15
Skin	500	50
Hands and feet	500	—

From Radiological protection and safety in medicine. A report of the International Commission on Radiological Protection. *Ann ICRP* 1996, 26:1-47.
**mSv*, millisievert.

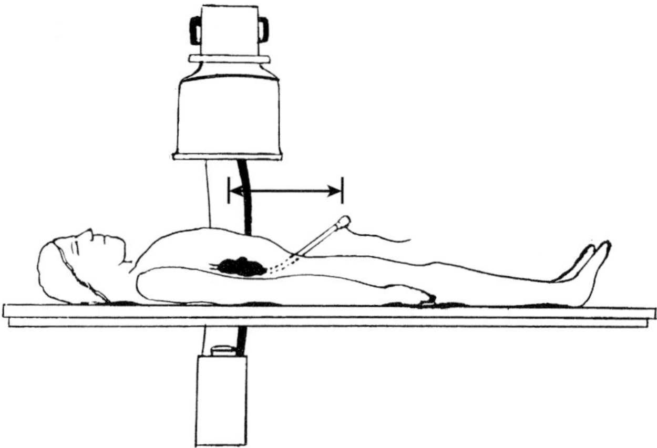

FIGURE 5-1 There is a fixed working distance from the sheath to the area of interest, in this case the abdominal aorta.

results have implications for fellowship training programs, in which the teaching of less-experienced operators results in increased radiation exposure for patients and staff alike. The needs of training must be balanced against increased fluoroscopy times and resulting exposure.

SPECIFIC RECOMMENDATIONS

General Principles

Radiation exposure is proportional to total fluoroscopy time. Therefore the most effective way to reduce exposure to both the patient and the staff is to reduce the total fluoroscopy time. Several steps can be taken toward this end. When there is a stable wire position, catheter-guidewire exchanges do not need to be visualized in their entirety. When repositioning the field of interest by moving either the table or the C-arm unit, the desired position should be estimated and then fine-tuned under fluoroscopic guidance rather than imaged along the entire course. This is also true when obtaining oblique or angled projections. When performing cine-acquisition, each screening should be carefully planned and should have a specific objective. Poorly planned runs add no information to the procedure and increase exposure, contrast load, and operative time. For example, a subtraction run over the upper abdomen without breath holding, either in an intubated patient under anesthesia or voluntarily in the awake patient, is likely to produce a useless image. The most important factors are (1) to be constantly aware of when the fluoroscope is on and (2) whether fluoroscopic imaging is required at that moment. Simply measuring the fluoroscopic time may be enough to increase awareness and reduce overall fluoroscopy time. Hough and associates[5] found that the use of audible radiation monitors, which were dose sensitive, led to a significant reduction in exposure to the staff wearing the monitors.

The next most effective way to reduce exposure is to increase the distance from the source. The exposure to the operator caused by scatter decreases with the square of the distance from the source. This is known as the *inverse square law*. There is a substantial drop in the amount of scattered radiation once one moves 30 to 50 cm from the scatter source.[6,7] For most endovascular interventions, the working distance from the source is largely fixed by the distance between the area of interest and the arterial access site (Figure 5-1). The radiation dose to the operator during cardiac interventions has been shown to increase 1.5 to 2.6 times when the operator moves from the femoral to the subclavian position.[8] Kuwayama and coworkers[9] found that radiation to the operator was increased approximately twofold to threefold when a transcarotid versus a transfemoral route was used for neuroradiologic procedures. In this same study, the transcarotid approach led to a 10-fold increase in exposure to the hands.

Endovascular aortoiliac aneurysm repair requires prolonged imaging over the abdomen and the pelvis. Penetration of these tissues requires more energy and results in a significantly higher exposure rate to the patient and staff than imaging the periphery.[10] A recent study of dose levels in interventional and neurointerventional procedures found that renal and visceral artery angioplasty procedures (in addition to transjugular intrahepatic portosystemic shunt and embolization procedures) were associated with a higher likelihood of clinically significant patient radiation dose than other procedures.[11]

Use of the Fluoroscope and Patient Positioning

The radiation exposure of the operator is proportional to that of the patient. Therefore, reducing patient exposure will also reduce operator exposure. Several methods can be used to achieve this. The beam should be positioned under the patient (i.e., posteroanterior

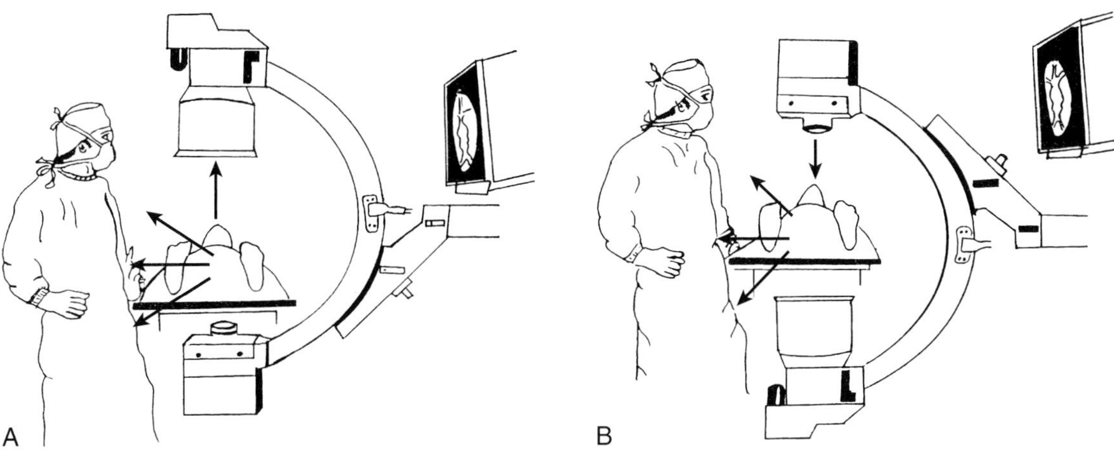

FIGURE 5-2 **A,** In posteroanterior imaging, the majority of scatter is directed at the level of the patient and below. **B,** In anteroposterior imaging, the majority of scatter is directed at the level of the patient and above.

imaging) (Figure 5-2, *A*). This will decrease scatter, as well as the amount of exposure to the operator's hand. Placing the beam in the anteroposterior position (source anterior to patient, image intensifier posterior to patient, patient supine) results in approximately four times more exposure to the operator's head, neck, and upper extremities (Figure 5-2, *B*).[6] Additionally, these areas are far more difficult to shield than the area below the waist. Obtaining oblique views will also have an impact on the scattered radiation dose. The right anterior oblique view will result in significantly more scatter to an operator standing on the patient's left than the left anterior oblique view. The reverse is true when the operator stands on the patient's right.[12]

The image intensifier should be positioned as close as possible to the patient. This reduces the amount of scatter by allowing for lower entrance exposure and also results in a sharper image (Figure 5-3). Pulse mode fluoroscopy at rates of 15 to 30 frames per second or less greatly reduces exposure as compared with continuous mode fluoroscopy.

A larger image-intensifier mode requires less radiation than a smaller one. The radiation dose approximately doubles with each successively smaller image-intensifier setting.[13] Large image-intensifier sizes should be used whenever possible. Avoid excessive use of high-level, or cinefluoroscopy, mode. This mode should be used only for essential acquisitions.

The amount of radiation produced by the fluoroscope is dependent on the amount of energy used to generate the beam. The factors determining this are milliamperes (mA) and kilovolts (kV). The mA setting controls the number of photons produced.[13] Low mA level produces a mottled image, which can be eliminated by increasing the mA at the cost of higher radiation. The kV control determines the penetration of the beam and image contrast. For most fluoroscopic units, mA and kV settings are determined by an automatic brightness control, which sets the values using feedback from the image obtained. If these are not set, however, the use of higher kV and lower mA levels will reduce exposure while not greatly affecting image quality. One study found that increasing the fluoroscopy voltage from 75 to 96 kV decreased the entrance dose by 50%.[14]

There are factors intrinsic to the fluoroscopic unit itself (e.g., design and manufacture of the unit) that affect the radiation dose. Mehlman and DiPasquale,[7] in a study that used both an OEC 9600 and a Philips BV-29, found that the deep and shallow unprotected collar exposure, as well as the eye exposure, was increased by at least 1.5 times when using the OEC 9600. There was a substantial increase in deep and shallow unprotected waist exposure that could not be precisely measured owing to the short exposure times and low readings with the Philips BV-29. These differences may be accounted for by the increased mA generated by the OEC 9600 (3.3 mA/69 kV) as compared with the Philips BV-29 (2.7 mA/72 kV). In another study, Watson and colleagues[4] found a statistically significant difference between two wall-mounted units that used different imaging technologies. A General Electric LU-C MPX/L500 PULSCAN 17178 Video Processor using pulsed progressive fluoroscopy resulted in a 45% higher dose per case than a Philips DCI-S Poly-Diagnostic using digital imaging technology. This difference was largely due to differences in the techniques used for image acquisition, because progressive pulsed fluoroscopy generally reduces radiation exposure. Finally, a heavier patient will require greater radiation energy to penetrate tissues, with a consequent increase in radiation exposure to the patient and the staff. We have found increased doses of radiation in heavier patients, although the amount is difficult to quantify because of differences in the duration of high-level fluoroscopy in each case.

Although the collimation of all fluoroscopic units is regulated by federal law, the ratio of the field of view

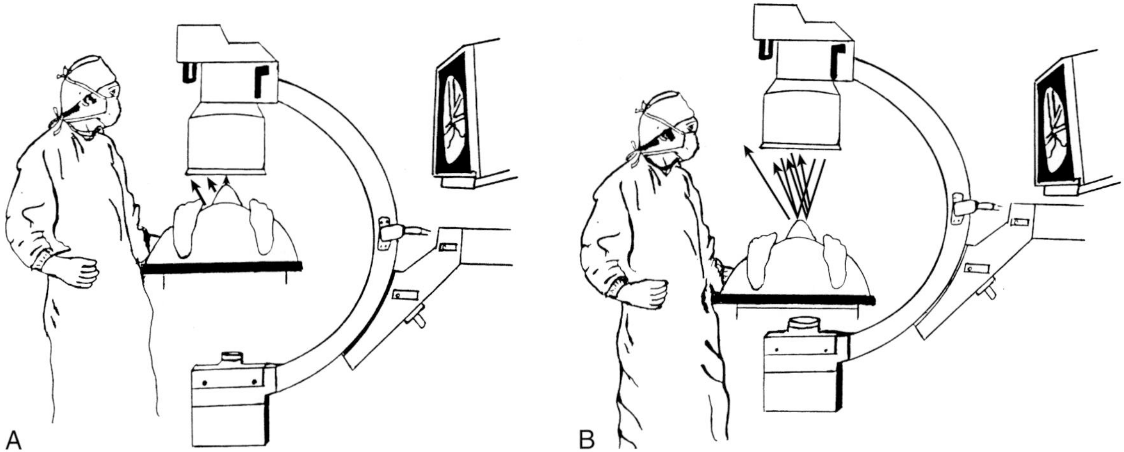

FIGURE 5-3 **A,** Image intensifier is located close to the patient. Less energy is required for tissue penetration, and scatter is reduced, resulting in a clearer image. **B,** Image intensifier is located far away from the patient. More energy is required for tissue penetration, and there is increased scatter, resulting in reduced image quality.

to the total exposed area is not 1:1. In fact, Granger and associates[15] found that the percent difference between the total exposed area and the field of view may be quite significant even though the fluoroscopic unit is in compliance. They evaluated 18 fluoroscopic units from different manufacturers and of different ages and found that only 67% of the units met federal compliance standards. For units not in compliance, the measured difference between the total exposed area and the field of view ranged from 22% to 48%. For units in compliance, the difference ranged from 5% to 32%. This excess exposed area provides no additional clinical information, increases the radiation doses to the patient and the staff, and reduces image contrast and quality. After the units were serviced, a 40% average reduction in beam area was achieved, and 100% of the units met compliance standards.

Although automatic collimation is part of all current systems, reducing the field size by using manual collimation will greatly decrease exposure and has the added benefit of enhancing image quality by reducing the amount of stray radiation. Lindsay and coworkers[8] found that by collimating the field of image during radiofrequency catheter ablation, the radiation dose to the patient and the staff was reduced by 40%.

Antiscatter grids mounted in front of the input screen decrease the amount of scatter reaching the image intensifier and thus improve image quality. They also greatly increase both the amount of radiation required to obtain a satisfactory image and the amount of backscatter reaching the patient and the staff.[16] Removal of these grids can reduce the radiation dose by a factor of two to four but with some loss of resolution. This is not the case during pediatric procedures, in which grids can and should be removed without loss of image quality.[16]

The fluoroscope should undergo at least biannual inspection and calibration as required by law. More frequent quality control checks are probably in order. If the unit requires service and any components are replaced, the fluoroscope should be recalibrated.

Radiologic Protection

Protective barriers should be readily available and should be used liberally. The most important of these is the lead apron. Aprons are generally available in 0.5- and 0.25-mm thicknesses. In optimal circumstances, the 0.5-mm thickness has the ability to attenuate 98% to 99.5% of the radiation dose, whereas the 0.25-mm thickness attenuates approximately 96% of the dose.[13,17] Deterioration of the apron's lead lining occurs with use and is increased by rough handling or improper storage. Aprons should undergo periodic screening and replacement if inadequate protection is found, depending on the location of the defect. It has been recommended that aprons should be replaced if there are defects over noncritical areas for which the sum of all defects exceeds 670 mm^2, or the equivalent of a 29-mm diameter circular hole. If the defects are over critical areas, such as the gonads or thyroid, aprons should be replaced if the sum of the defects exceeds 11 mm^2, or the equivalent of a 3.8-mm diameter circular hole. A thyroid shield with a greater than 11 mm^2 defect should be replaced.[18] Many aprons are not of the wraparound type and therefore do not provide circumferential protection. Scattered radiation from the sides may produce unprotected exposure.

A thyroid collar and protective glasses are essential. These glasses are highly variable in the amount of protection afforded and allow for a low of 3% to a high of 98% transmission of the radioactive beam.[19] The greatest protective effect is obtained with glasses containing lead. Glasses at the lower end of this spectrum may provide protection from ultraviolet rays but not ionizing radiation. Also of note is that a significant amount of the ocular exposure, up to 21%, is the result of scatter from the operator's head.[19] Depending on the head position of the operator during the procedure, side shields or wraparound configurations are necessary to provide adequate protection.

A lead acrylic shield, which can be either ceiling mounted or positioned on a mobile floor stand, should be placed between the operator and the patient to reduce exposure further. Eye radiation can be reduced by a factor of 20 to 35 with the use of a ceiling-suspended lead glass shield.[8,12] Lead-lined gloves also help reduce exposure but can be cumbersome. Because (1) backscattered radiation is more intense than forward scattered radiation[20] and (2) with the C-arm in the posteroanterior orientation, the greatest exposure due to scatter occurs from under the table, we use a lead drape suspended from the operating table on the operator's side to reduce exposure. Using this additional shield eliminates a significant amount of this scatter.[6]

Patient and Staff Monitoring

The use of radiation badges by all persons working with fluoroscopy is mandatory. The position of the badges is important. A badge must be worn at waist level under the lead apron. An additional badge should also be worn on the collar to monitor the head dose and to aid in calculating the total effective dose because there is a large and variable difference between the "over-lead" and "under-lead" doses.[21] Ring badges are also advisable. Waist and collar badges should be worn on the operator's left side when working on the patient's right and on the operator's right side when working on the patient's left (i.e., the badge should face the source directly). Ring badges should be worn on the hand most likely to be exposed. A self-retaining device to stabilize the sheaths may also reduce exposure. Monitoring of all at-risk body positions is essential because dominant-hand finger doses were shown not to correlate with doses estimated by shoulder badges in interventionists performing percutaneous drainage procedures.[22] Although the use of badges is mandated, it is the responsibility of the individual to wear them and of the institution to have a monitoring program that provides feedback to the exposed individuals.

Many patients are exposed to fluoroscopy only once. However, patients undergoing endovascular aneurysm repair require follow-up radiologic studies such as computed tomographic scans, and those having had peripheral or visceral intervention frequently must undergo repeated diagnostic and/or therapeutic studies. Many patients undergoing these procedures are older and are less likely to have potential malignancies. Because of the long screening times, however, patients should be warned about the possible development of transient skin erythema, which may present up to several weeks after the procedure, and other exposure-related skin conditions.

In one large prospective study of interventional radiologists, Marx et al.[21] found that the only variable correlating with over-lead collar dose was number of procedures performed per year, and the only variable correlating with waist under-lead dose was thickness of the lead apron (0.5 mm vs. 1 mm). This study also included a questionnaire on the practice habits of the interventional radiologists involved. Nearly half of the respondents reported wearing their radiation badges rarely or never. One half of the respondents either had exceeded or did not know whether they had exceeded monthly or quarterly occupational dose limits at some time within the past year. With regard to protection habits, 30% rarely or never wore a thyroid shield, 73% rarely or never wore lead glasses, 70% rarely or never used a ceiling-mounted lead shield, and 83% rarely or never wore leaded gloves. In another study a questionnaire was administered to 130 physicians including consultant radiologists in the United Kingdom. Participants were asked to estimate the doses received by patients undergoing various radiologic procedures. The actual exposure was underestimated in 97% of cases. The fact that ionizing radiation is not used in either ultrasound or magnetic resonance imaging was not recognized by 5% and 8% of physicians, respectively.[23] These results indicate that there can be significant misunderstanding and complacency even among the most at-risk population of physicians, who have substantial background and education in radiation safety and physics.

We have previously reviewed our own radiation exposure incurred during 47 endovascular aortic or iliac aneurysm repairs performed over a 1-year period.[24] Other fluoroscopic procedures such as diagnostic angiography, peripheral and visceral artery angioplasty and stenting, fluoroscopically assisted thromboembolectomy, and inferior vena caval filter placement were not included.

Each of three surgeons wore three radiation dosimeters, as follows: (1) on the waist under the lead apron, (2) on the waist outside the lead apron, and (3) on the collar outside the thyroid shield. A ring dosimeter was worn on the ring finger of the left hand of each surgeon. Additional badges were placed around the operating room to estimate the exposure to the scrub and circulating nurses. Patient entrance doses were calculated by using the fluoroscopic energies, and positions were recorded during each case. Total effective doses were calculated and were compared with standards established by the International Commission on Radiological Protection (ICRP).[2]

Yearly total effective doses for the surgeons (underlead) ranged from 5% to 8% of the ICRP occupational exposure limit. Outside-lead doses for all surgeons approximated the recommended occupational limit. Ring and calculated eye doses ranged from 1% to 5% of the ICRP occupational exposure limits. Lead aprons attenuated 85% to 91% of the dose. Patient entrance doses averaged 360 millisieverts per case (range 120 to 860 millisieverts). Outside-lead exposure to the scrub and the circulating nurses was 4% and 2%, respectively, of the ICRP occupational limits.

Our results suggested that a team of surgeons could perform 386 hours of fluoroscopy per year or 587 endovascular aortoiliac aneurysm repairs per year and remain within occupational exposure limits. This does not take into account other endovascular procedures performed by the surgeons, which would reduce these figures accordingly. Other studies have confirmed doses below occupational limits but noted that there can be significant variability depending on the fluoroscopic equipment used and operator technique.[25,26]

Additional Equipment to Help Reduce Exposure

Several available devices are helpful in reducing total radiation exposure. Use of a floating table simplifies positional changes and reduces the need to adjust the fluoroscope constantly. Use of a power injector (ACIST injection system, Eden Prairie, MN) ensures that an adequate volume of contrast material is delivered, which maximizes image quality and reduces the need for multiple screening runs. This is especially important when imaging the thoracic or abdominal aorta and its branches. An equally important benefit is that use of a power injector allows the operator to increase distance from the source. The same effect can be achieved by adding extension tubing to the catheter injection port during manual injection. The tabletop should be maximally radiolucent. The equipment used (stent grafts, guidewires, catheters) should be well marked with radiopaque indicators that are easily visualized so that one does not have to strain or to increase the image intensifier size to see them.

Noninvasive vascular imaging techniques, such as duplex Doppler and intravascular ultrasonography, contribute anatomic information that can aid in the performance planning of endovascular procedures and thereby reduce fluoroscopic time and contrast load. Marking appropriate landmarks on the screen with an erasable pen allows one to work under regular fluoroscopic guidance rather than using road-mapping, which may lead to increased exposure.

SUMMARY

The most important points to remember are that radiation exposure is cumulative and that it is permanent. The major factors increasing exposure are increased fluoroscopy time and the proximity of the surgeon to the operative field.

The maximum allowable occupational and civilian radiation exposure doses have been lowered with time. It is likely that with increasing knowledge about the effects of radiation, this trend will continue. We recommend keeping exposure to less than 10% to 20% of established occupational limits. Each center performing endovascular procedures should actively monitor its effective doses and educate personnel regarding methods to reduce exposure.

References

1. Ohki T, Veith FJ, Sanchez LA, et al: What percentage of abdominal aortic aneurysms can be treated endovascularly? The role of a surgeon-made device. Presented at the 23rd Annual Meeting of the Southern Association for Vascular Surgery. January 28–30, 1999, Naples, FL.
2. Radiological protection and safety in medicine: A report of the International Commission on Radiological Protection, *Ann ICRP* 26:1–47, 1996.
3. National Council on Radiation Protection and Measurements: Ionizing Radiation Exposure of the Population of the United States. Report No. 93. Bethesda, MD, National Council on Radiation Protection and Measurements, 1987.
4. Watson LE, Riggs MW, Bourland PD: Radiation exposure during cardiology fellowship training, *Health Phys* 73:690–693, 1997.
5. Hough DM, Brady A, Stevenson GW: Audible radiation monitors: the value in reducing radiation exposure to fluoroscopy personnel, *AJR Am J Roentgenol* 160:407–408, 1993.
6. Boone JM, Levin DC: Radiation exposure to angiographers under different fluoroscopic imaging conditions, *Radiology* 180:861–865, 1991.
7. Mehlman CT, DiPasquale TG: Radiation exposure to the orthopaedic surgical team during fluoroscopy: "how far away is far enough?" *J Orthop Trauma* 11:392–398, 1997.
8. Lindsay BD, Eichling JO, Ambos HD, Cain ME: Radiation exposure to patients and medical personnel during radiofrequency catheter ablation for supraventricular tachycardia, *Am J Cardiol* 70:218–223, 1992.
9. Kuwayama N, Takaku A, Endo S, et al: Radiation exposure in endovascular surgery of the head and neck, *AJNR Am J Neuroradiol* 15:1801–1808, 1994.
10. Ramalanjaona GR, Pearce WH, Ritenour ER: Radiation exposure risk to the surgeon during operative angiography, *J Vasc Surg* 4:224–228, 1986.
11. Miller DL, Balter S, Cole PE, et al: Radiation Doses in Interventional Radiology Procedures: The RAD-IR Study Part I: Overall Measures of Dose, *J Vasc Interv Radiol* 14:711–727, 2003.
12. Pratt TA, Shaw AJ: Factors affecting the radiation dose to the lens of the eye during cardiac catheterization procedures, *Br J Radiol* 66:346–350, 1993.

13. Aldridge HE, Chisholm RJ, Dragatakis L, Roy L: Radiation safety in the cardiac catheterization laboratory, *Can J Cardiol* 13:459–467, 1997.
14. Heyd RL, Kopecky KK, Sherman S, et al: Radiation exposure to patients and personnel during interventional ERCP at a teaching institution, *Gastrointest Endosc* 44:287–292, 1996.
15. Granger WE, Bednarek DR, Rudin S: Primary beam exposure outside the fluoroscopic field of view, *Med Phys* 24:703–707, 1997.
16. Coakley KS, Ratcliffe J, Masel J: Measurement of radiation dose received by the hands and thyroid of staff performing gridless fluoroscopic procedures in children, *Br J Radiol* 70:933–936, 1997.
17. Kicken PJ, Bos AJJ: Effectiveness of lead aprons in vascular radiology: results of clinical measurements, *Radiology* 197:473–478, 1995.
18. Lambert K, McKeon T: Inspection of lead aprons: criteria for rejection, *Health Phys.* 80:S67–9, 2001.
19. Cousin AJ, Lawdahl RB, Chakraborty DP, Koehler RE: The case for radioprotective eyewear/facewear: practical implications and suggestions, *Invest Radiol* 22:688–692, 1987.
20. Lo NN, Goh SS, Khong KS: Radiation dosage from use of the image intensifier in orthopaedic surgery, *Singapore Med J* 37:69–71, 1996.
21. Marx MV, Niklason L, Mauger EA: Occupational radiation exposure to interventional radiologists: a prospective study, *J Vasc Interv Radiol* 3:597–606, 1992.
22. Vehmas T, Tikkanen H: Measuring radiation exposure during percutaneous drainages: can shoulder dosimeters be used to estimate finger doses? *Br J Radiol* 65:1007–1010, 1992.
23. Shiralkar S, Rennie A, Snow M, Galland RB, Lewis MH, Gower-Thomas K: Doctors' knowledge of radiation exposure: questionnaire study, *BMJ* 327:371–372, 2003.
24. Lipsitz EC, Veith FJ, Ohki T, et al: Does the endovascular repair of aortoiliac aneurysms pose a radiation safety hazard to vascular surgeons? *J Vasc Surg* 32:704–710, 2000.
25. Ho P, Cheng SW, Wu PM, et al: Ionizing radiation absorption of vascular surgeons during endovascular procedures, *J Vasc Surg* 46:455–459, 2007.
26. Geijer H, Larzon T, Popek R, Beckman KW: Radiation exposure in stent-grafting of abdominal aortic aneurysms, *Br J Radiol* 78:906–912, 2005.

CHAPTER

6

Arterial Access

George Andros

Endovascular intervention begins with vascular access. The necessary fundamentals are technical skill and familiarity with the use and the organization of essential tools (e.g., needles, guidewires, catheters, and sheaths) and the sequence of how they fit together. From this beginning, the interventionist learns angiography, both primary and selective, and progresses to more advanced procedures: angioplasty, stenting, and thrombolysis. As the surgeon's experience expands, new procedures with alternative methods and devices are added. The road to proficiency begins with mastery of *percutaneous vascular* access, the subject of this chapter. Access by way of a surgically exposed artery is essentially identical to percutaneous access; for the experienced vascular surgeon, little further elaboration is necessary.

SELECTING THE ACCESS SITE

Selection of the access site is a two-part process. (1) An artery with a secure, direct, and uninterrupted pathway to the target legion or the arterial territory of interest is selected (Figure 6-1). (2) The artery is cannulated on the basis of specific local landmarks (Figures 6-2 and 6-3).

Although there are pros and cons to the use of each of the access sites (Table 6-1), the femoral approach (preferably from the right) is the first choice for angiography and most interventions. By using retrograde femoral puncture, access to the entire thoracoabdominal aorta (and its ramifications) is standard; catheterization of the contralateral iliofemoral tree and runoff is readily performed. With *antegrade* femoral puncture, the interventionist can selectively catheterize vessels as distal as the infrapopliteal arteries and beyond.

Arterial puncture in the upper extremity (usually the left) also provides access to both the thoracic and abdominal aortas and their runoffs. Every interventionist should acquire upper extremity access experience at one or more of the available sites. As a routine, however, the use of upper extremity access is usually limited to those instances in which the common femoral arteries are occluded or otherwise unavailable (e.g., a recently implanted aortofemoral bypass graft).

Cannulation of the artery at the selected site is a standardized procedure irrespective of the artery selected and begins with arterial puncture. There are two methods of achieving intra-arterial access (Figure 6-4, *A*).

- Through-and-through puncture completely across both walls of the artery. The needle is then withdrawn *backward* into the lumen.
- Single-wall entry, in which only the anterior wall is punctured by gentle pressure as the arterial pulsation is "palpated" through the slowly advancing needle. Pulsatile flow signals entry into the arterial lumen.

For each method of entry, there are appropriate types of needles.

- For single-wall entry, a simple disposable needle, preferably with a stabilizing flange, is used. We believe this to be the preferred device for the safest method of accessing arteries and veins. The bevel is placed anteriorly.
- Through-and-through puncture, or double-wall entry, can be performed with a single-wall entry needle, but a multipart needle, of which there are many types, is often used. The multipart needle with its inner core is used to puncture both walls of the artery. The inner needle is then removed, and the outer needle is withdrawn backward into the arterial lumen. The original Seldinger needle comprised four parts, including an obturator.

Puncture of small arteries, such as the brachial artery at the antecubital fossa, is facilitated by the use of a multipart "micropuncture kit," available from several manufacturers. A small-caliber needle is inserted first

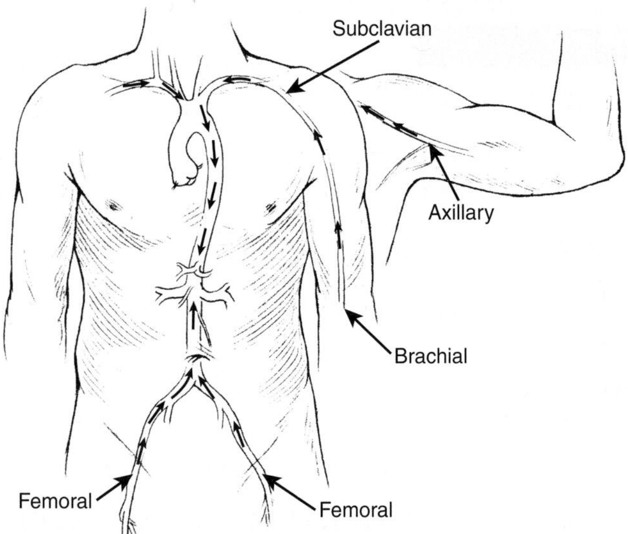

FIGURE 6-1 Sites for arterial access.

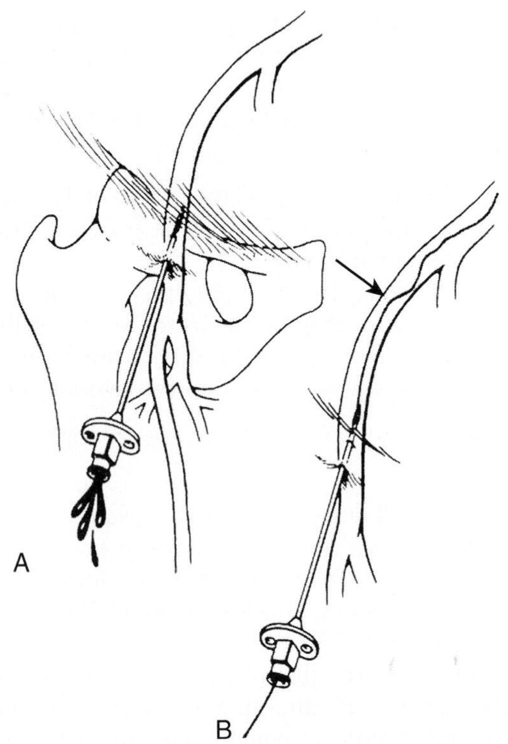

FIGURE 6-2 Common femoral artery puncture. **A,** Entry into common femoral artery. **B,** Guidewire passed with floppy portion well advanced.

followed by a 0.018-inch guidewire. Next, the needle is exchanged for paired coaxial catheters. The smaller inner catheter accommodates the guidewire and permits the larger outer catheter to dilate the subcutaneous track. After both catheters are securely advanced into the artery, the guidewire and the small inner catheter

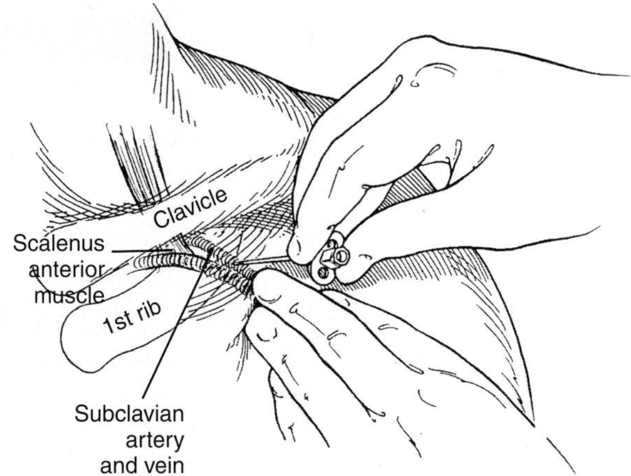

FIGURE 6-3 Left subclavian artery puncture. *a.,* Artery; *ant.,* anterior; *m.,* muscle; *v.,* vein.

are removed; the remaining larger catheter will then accept a 0.035-inch guidewire, which is capable of supporting larger devices.

THE SELDINGER TECHNIQUE

The Seldinger method, first described in 1953, is the fundamental technique for vascular access (Figure 6-5). So widespread is its application for the insertion of catheters that virtually every medical student has some personal hands-on experience with its elegant simplicity. The steps include the following:

- Localization of the entry point by palpation of the appropriate arterial pulse.
- Angulated entry into the vessel lumen (see Figure 6-4, *B*). As previously noted, anterior single-wall entry with the bevel pointed anteriorly is preferred.
- Verification of the intraluminal position by pulsatile flow from the arterial hub. When in doubt, a puff of contrast material is administered under fluoroscopic guidance. A guidewire is passed into the arterial lumen and is advanced so that the stiff portion of the guidewire is securely intraluminal. If the tissues surrounding the punctured artery are fibrotic, as they might be in the case of previous arterial catheterization, or if the artery is calcified and rigid, the needle is exchanged for a dilator or a series of graduated dilators to enlarge the track.
- Finally, exchange of the needle or the dilating catheter for the intended catheter or the appropriate sheath. The guidewire can then be safely removed or exchanged.

TABLE 6-1 Comparison of Sites for Arterial Access

Site	Advantages	Disadvantages	Comment
Femoral	Easily accessed	Possible tortuosity	First choice among the sites
	Large vessel	Long pathway for catheter manipulations to remote targets	Obesity may complicate puncture
	SPR set up for right-handed access	May be compromised by ASO	Left side accessed from the patient's right
	Most devices designed for femoral access		Predictable complications
	Right or left artery available		
	Permits brachiocephalic and aortic/runoff access		
	Easily compressed		
	Puncture complication easily managed		
Brachial	Usually patent and disease free	Prone to thrombosis	Second-choice site
	Either side accessible	Patient comfort compromised by arm or arm board	"Micropuncture" set a useful adjunctive device
	Most target lesions are accessible	Long tortuous route for catheter manipulations	Brachial site best for angiography and some simple interventions
Axillary	Large vessel	Major complication, "short hematoma"	Small catheters in the hands of experienced operator
	Short working distance to the aorta	Brachial plexopathy	Use best limited to angiography
	Access from the left avoids crossing the cerebrovascular orifices	Uncomfortable patient position	
Subclavian	Large vessel	Potential for pneumothorax	Useful for angiography, PTA/stenting, thrombolysis
	Very short working distance to the aorta	Prolonged bimanual compression	Angle of approach desirable for renal angioplasty
	Accessible bilaterally, left side preferred	Increased risk of hematoma with larger catheters	Sheath removed when PTT returns to normal
	Access to arch, thoracic aorta, and entire runoff		Most difficult access—requires experience
	Each leg may be accessed antegradely		
Radial	Ease of access and compression for early patient discharge	Very long working distance	A novelty
	Radial artery may be expandable	Radial artery may thrombose—later unusable for bypass graft	
		Hand ischemia potential	
		Nerve damage potential	

ASO, Arteriosclerosis obliterans; *PTA,* percutaneous transluminal angioplasty; *PTT,* partial thromboplastin time; *SPR,* special procedures room.

GUIDEWIRES AND SHEATHS

Several features distinguish guidewires. Variations in the tip of the catheter include J-shaped tips of various sizes with or without a movable core. Tips can also be flexible or "floppy," such as the Bentson wire; steerable, such as the Wholey wire; platinum tipped for visibility in negotiating tortuous arteries; and so forth. Guidewires are of various lengths and stiffness to (1) permit exchanges over the reinforced portion of the wire and (2) allow devices to be exchanged and deployed. Appropriate guidewire coatings, such as the hydrophilic coating of the Terumo Glidewire (Terumo, Someset, NJ), facilitate wire advancement through torous and irular channels.

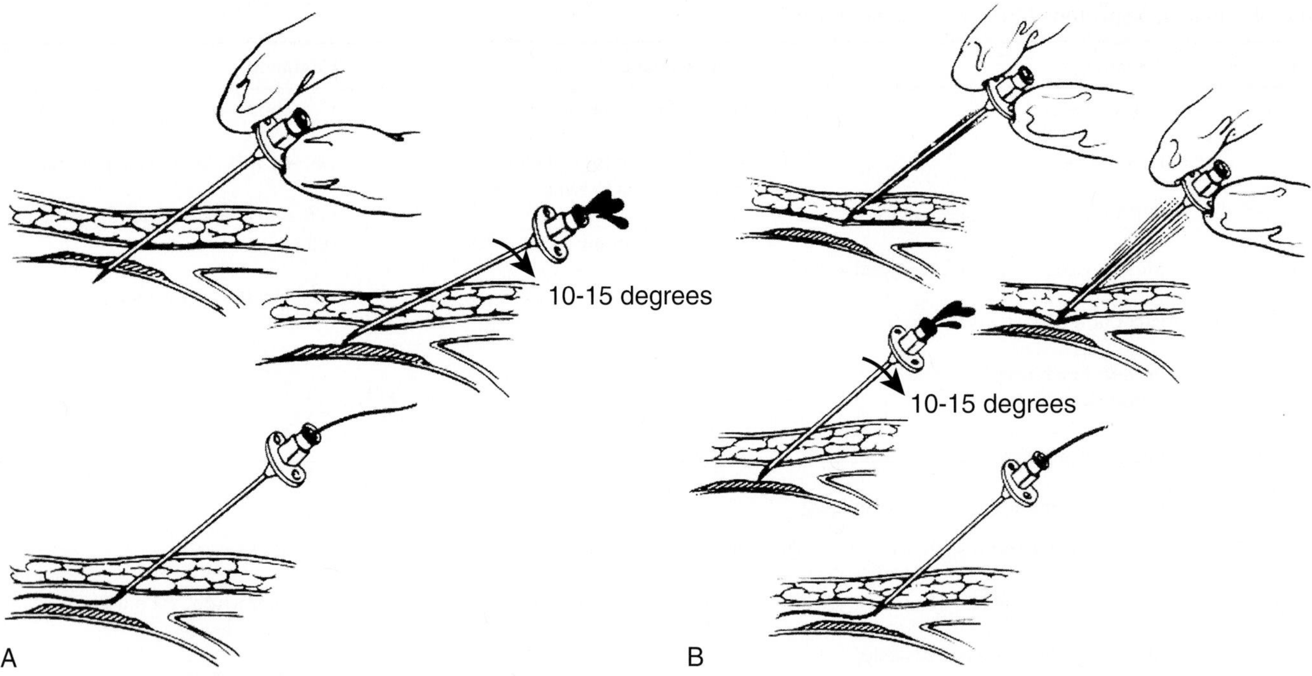

FIGURE 6-4 **A,** Through-and-through (double-wall) puncture. **B,** Single (anterior wall) puncture.

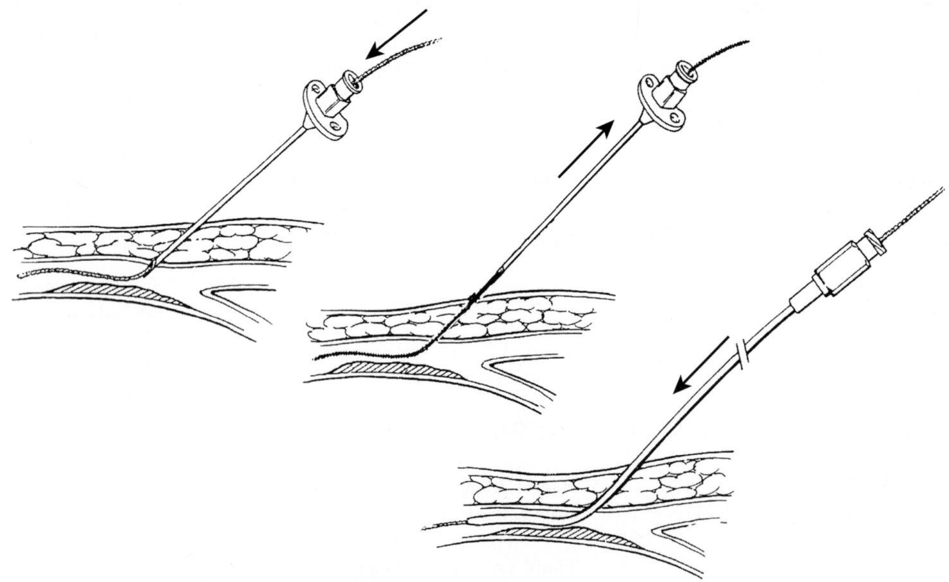

FIGURE 6-5 The Seldinger technique.

Introducing sheaths are composed of (1) a catheter portion with a hydrostatic valve with side arm for fluid injection and (2) an inner dilator. They have multiple purposes, which dictate their diameter, length, and construction.

- Securing access for one or more catheter or guidewire exchanges
- Securing access through fibrotic subcutaneous tissue (such as groin) that has undergone previous intervention, either surgically or with catheter techniques
- Securing smooth access through calcified or sclerotic arteries
- Straightening of tortuous arteries

- Passage and guidance of interventional devices such as balloon angioplasty catheters, stents, selective angiography catheters, thrombolysis and thrombectomy catheters, and other catheters (e.g., "guiding catheters")
- Facilitating intraprocedural angiography to assess the status of an intervention (e.g., angioplasty and stent placement)

FOUR ESSENTIAL TECHNIQUES

After the fundamentals have been learned, there are four essential access techniques that every interventionist must master (and perhaps a fifth if one includes learning to obtain access by way of an upper extremity artery).

Retrograde Femoral Puncture

Puncture of the femoral artery is simplified by knowledge of its position referable to osseous anatomic landmarks. In the majority of cases, there is approximately 3 cm of common femoral artery between the inguinal ligament and the femoral bifurcation suitable for introduction of a needle, a guidewire, and a catheter; it lies over the junction of the medial third and middle third of the femoral head. Importantly, this relationship varies little with the patient's body habitus, age, and so forth (Figure 6-6). This point is commonly designated as lying two fingerbreadths lateral to the pubic symphysis on a line joining the symphysis with the anterior iliac spine. Because increasing numbers of patients undergoing arterial catheterization are obese, it may be difficult to orient the common femoral artery to the standard landmarks. Hence, it is useful to lay the entry needle directly on the patient and to identify its relationship to the femoral head by using fluoroscopy.

Attempts to enter the femoral artery may result in a puncture that is too distal into either the deep or the superficial femoral arteries, especially in the obese patient. Catheterization of either of these vessels carries an increased risk for postprocedural hematoma or pseudoaneurysm development. By establishing the relationship between the skin puncture wound and the femoral head, it is easier to puncture the common femoral artery. If there is any concern regarding the intraluminal passage of guidewire once the needle tip has entered the femoral artery, the guidewire should be advanced under fluoroscopic guidance. Alternatively, a "puff" of contrast material together with road-mapping assists in negotiating passage of a guidewire. Using the standard Bentson guidewire, at least 20 cm of the guidewire is advanced through the needle so that exchanges can be safely achieved. It is usually safe to let the Bentson guidewire tip buckle so that the stiffer portion will be safely within the artery. After the 18F thin-walled needle has punctured the artery and the 0.035-inch guidewire has passed into the artery, a 4F dilator is exchanged for the needle to permit passage of a No. 5 catheter or sheath. If, however, the groin is densely scarred and fibrotic, it may be desirable to pass a No. 6 dilator in anticipation of introducing a 5F sheath. With access established and the sheath in place, the next step, crossing the iliac arteries, can be taken.

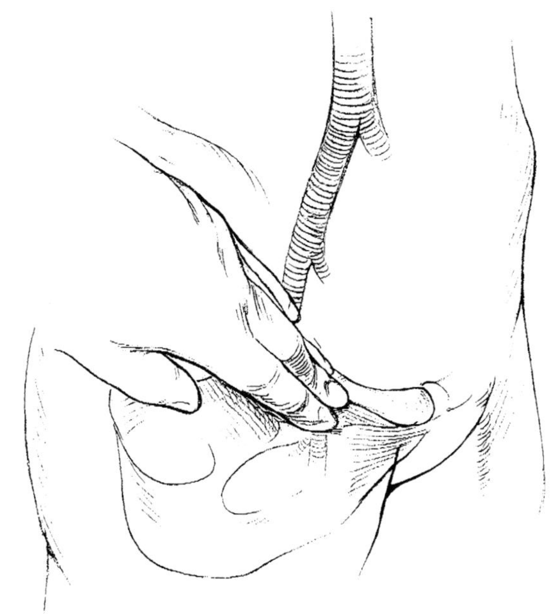

FIGURE 6-6 Retrograde femoral puncture orientation.

ANTEGRADE FEMORAL PUNCTURE

Antegrade femoral puncture is a simple technique of achieving direct access to the common femoral artery and its superficial femoral and popliteal artery runoff (Figure 6-7). It is an optimal technique for selective distal angiography or ipsilateral intervention. The most common error, again often a result of patient obesity, is puncture of the superficial or deep femoral artery. Less commonly, the external iliac artery is punctured; entry into this artery may result in either difficult passage of the guidewire at the beginning of the procedure or a retroperitoneal hematoma at the end (Figure 6-8). A three-dimensional sense of the location of the common femoral artery is invaluable: when in doubt, revert to the "needle on the skin under fluoroscopy" trick.

After preliminary skin infiltration with lidocaine and the establishment of cutaneous access, the needle is inserted in an antegrade direction just distal to the anterior iliac spine and passes through the inguinal ligament to

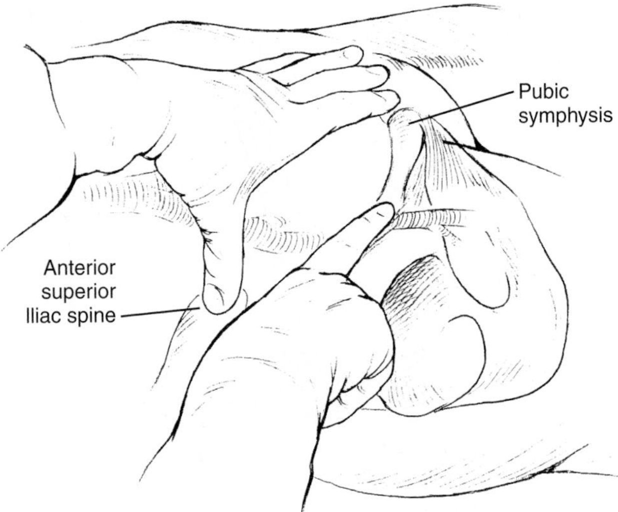

FIGURE 6-7 Antegrade femoral puncture orientation.

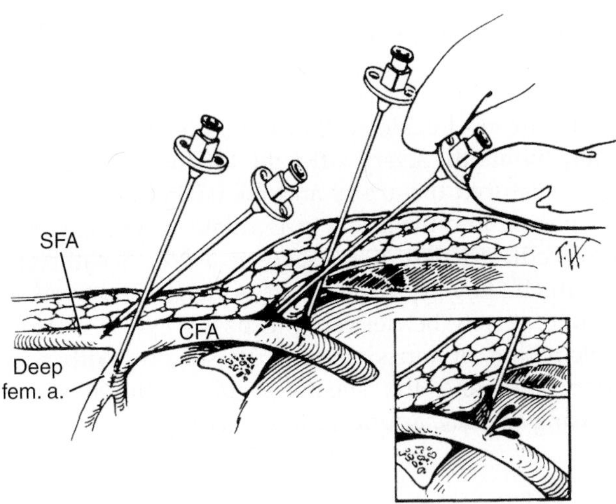

FIGURE 6-8 Antegrade femoral puncture with external iliac puncture and extraperitoneal hemorrhage *(inset)*. *CFA,* Common femoral artery; *fem a.,* femoral artery; *SFA,* superior femoral artery.

engage the common femoral artery. If the patient is very obese, it is often necessary for an assistant to retract the abdominal panniculus in a cephalad direction to allow an appropriate angle of entry. As in the case of retrograde femoral puncture, it is sometimes useful to pass the guidewire under fluoroscopic control, supplemented by contrast agent administration with or without roadmapping. If the guidewire enters the deep femoral artery, the needle tip may be moved either medially or laterally to redirect it into the superficial femoral artery. This may not be possible if the needle has entered the artery too close to the femoral bifurcation. This circumstance should be ascertained by angling the image intensifier into an anterior oblique position and injecting contrast material to localize the entry point of the needle. This will also help in redirecting the guidewire into the superficial femoral artery. In those instances when the guidewire enters the deep femoral artery, it is possible to "bounce" the guidewire tip off the lateral aspect of the femoral artery to redirect it to the more medially placed orifice of the superficial femoral artery; alternatively, the guidewire tip can be steered with a Wholey wire.

The technique of redirecting the guidewire down the superficial femoral artery that we prefer is to exchange the needle for a cobra catheter that is 30 cm in length. This is securely positioned in the deep femoral artery and is slowly withdrawn under fluoroscopic guidance as contrast material is injected with the image intensifier in a right anterior oblique angle, which opens a space between the deep and the superficial femoral arteries. The catheter tip is directed anteromedially as it is withdrawn and will "pop" into the superficial femoral artery orifice. The guidewire is then reinserted, and it advances almost invariably into the superficial femoral artery; the catheter follows (Figure 6-9).

Puncturing the Pulseless Femoral Artery

If no femoral pulse can be palpated to enable retrograde femoral puncture and arterial access, there are eight techniques that can be used to meet this challenge (Figure 6-10).

- Even if the iliac artery is completely occluded, the femoral artery usually has a "soft" compliant spot, as is often noted in patients with complete aortic occlusions who undergo aortofemoral bypass. Similarly, when a patient is sedated on the angiographic table, the pulse that was previously nonpalpable in the office may be detected. The artery *believed* to be pulseless may, in fact, have a sufficient pulse to guide needle placement.
- The arterial fibrosis and calcification associated with arteriosclerosis render the common femoral artery itself palpable. Just as the surgically exposed artery can be felt to be a thickened cord, it can be palpated transcutaneously. It is into this thickened, calcified vessel that a needle can be effectively directed.
- Under magnified fluoroscopy, careful examination of the region of the femoral head can reveal arterial calcification to help localize the common femoral artery.
- When the contralateral iliofemoral system is patent, lumbar aortography is usually performed before intervention. This angiogram visualizes the common femoral artery distal to the iliac occlusive lesion. Using the angiogram and bony references, the needle can be directed to the site of the femoral artery, as visualized on the preintervention lumbar aortogram; a complementary technique is to perform lumbar

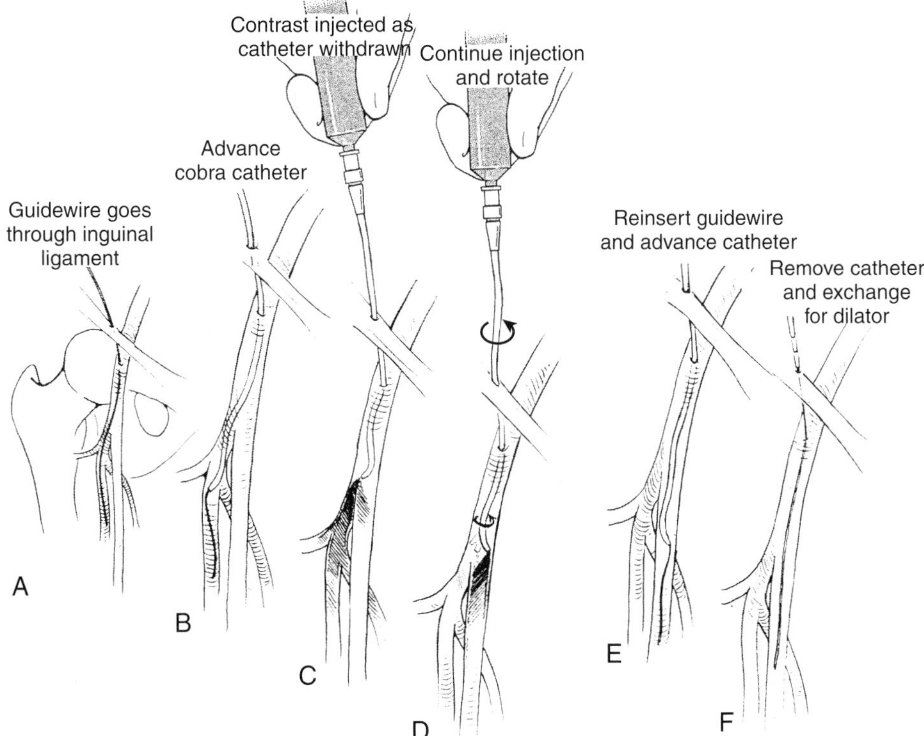

FIGURE 6-9 Redirecting the catheter from the deep to the superficial femoral artery.

aortography and road-mapping. By using the road map and direct fluoroscopy, the needle can be directed within the live image on the screen. Of course, when working with fluoroscopy, lead gloves should be used.

- Two ultrasound techniques have been used to localize the common femoral artery. First an ultrasound probe or a duplex machine can be brought to the special procedures room and can be used to determine the position of the common femoral artery. The position is then marked on the skin to facilitate puncture.
- A second ultrasound technique employs the so-called smart needle, which has an ultrasound probe at its tip. As the needle approaches the artery, the needle emits an ultrasound signal, which identifies proximity to the pulseless vessel.
- Occasional attempts to enter the common femoral artery will result in puncture of the common femoral vein with appearance of dark nonpulsatile venous blood. By noting the exact position of the needle within the common femoral vein, the needle can be withdrawn and then reinserted 1 to 2 cm laterally, the normal distance between the artery and the vein. Bear in mind, however, that the pulseless femoral artery often has low pressure and low pulse pressure so that the arterial blood may be dark and may resemble venous blood; what appears to be a venous puncture may, in fact, be an arterial puncture. If the origin of the dark, minimally pulsatile blood flow is in doubt, the needle should not be withdrawn. A puff of dye is then injected to identify the location of the needle.
- Finally, the junction of the middle third and the medial third of the femoral head is the normal location of the common femoral artery, as visualized fluoroscopically. A needle aimed at this point, especially if it encounters a firm "crunchy" sclerotic structure, will often engage the nonpulsatile artery.

With one of these techniques, percutaneous access can be obtained in virtually every instance. Once access to the lumen has been attained, the Seldinger technique is employed.

Crossing "Over-the-Top"

Gaining access to the iliofemoropopliteal system from the contralateral femoral artery "over the aortic bifurcation" is indispensable. Moreover, it is a technique that is learned with surprising ease. Several maneuvers and devices facilitate the procedure (Figure 6-11).

- The aortic bifurcation can be localized not only by its usual position in relation to L4 but also by its relation to the iliac crests. If there is aortic calcification, this also helps with localization and orientation. It is sometimes helpful to angle the image intensifier obliquely to view the iliac artery orifice. This widens

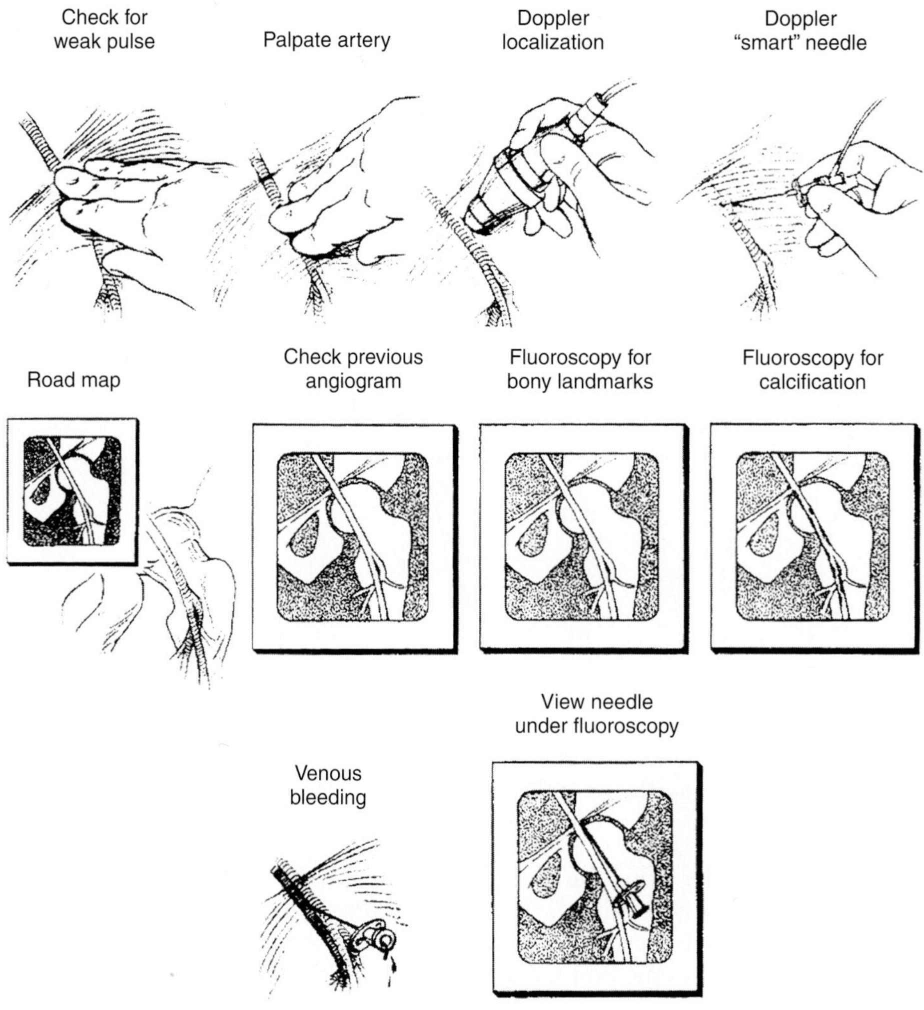

FIGURE 6-10 Adjuncts to puncture of the pulseless femoral artery.

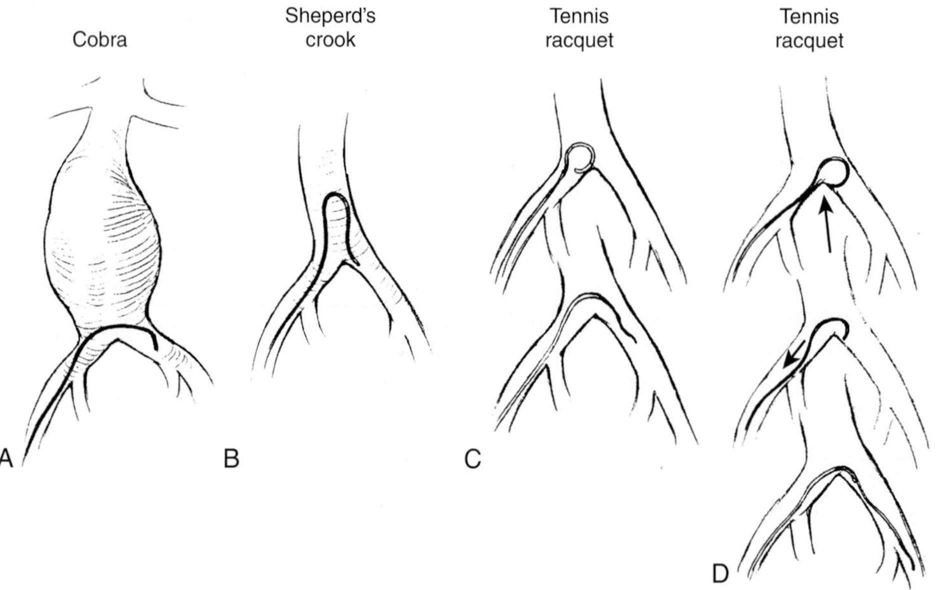

FIGURE 6-11 Directing a catheter and a guidewire over the aortic bifurcation ("over the top").

the apparent angle of entry into the iliac artery and facilitates passage of guidewire down the external iliac artery rather than the internal iliac artery. A preliminary lumbar aortogram with or without road-mapping also helps establish landmarks.

- The choice of catheter to cannulate the contralateral iliac artery is decisive. We generally use a tennis racquet catheter to perform lumbar aortograms. If the aorta is of normal width, the same catheter can be withdrawn under fluoroscopic guidance to the aortic bifurcation; the tip tends to uncoil and usually "hooks" the iliac artery orifice. At least 6 to 8 inches of a soft guidewire, such as a Bentson or Wholey wire, can then be directed into the iliac system; guidewire buckling is permissible. The catheter is then passed over the wire to secure access before catheter and guidewire exchanges are effected.
- For narrower aortas, particularly in women, we find the Sos catheter useful. It is advanced into the distal lumbar aorta and is reconfigured so that the tip points distally. With about 1 cm of guidewire exposed, the catheter tip is then dragged retrogradely into the orifice of the common iliac artery. The guidewire is advanced until it is securely positioned in the iliofemoral system before changes are attempted.
- It is worth noting that, when guided over the aortic bifurcation, the guidewire tends to pass from the external iliac artery through the common femoral artery directly into the superficial femoral artery rather than down the deep femoral artery in almost all cases.

In the case of a wide aortic bifurcation, as in the pressure of an aneurysm, a cobra catheter is effective in directing the guidewire over the aortic bifurcation. Some interventionists have recommended the use of a "Balken" guiding sheath for this purpose; the latter device has the advantage of permitting antegrade angiography to monitor the course of interventions.

Calcification with stenosis and tortuosity often make crossing the aortic bifurcation difficult. The need to traverse extensive iliofemoral occlusive disease is a relative contraindication to gaining access to the contralateral femoropopliteal segment because this may cause damage to the inflow of an outflow artery intended for treatment. In this instance, an alternative approach should be used. Tortuosity is often a problem in torquing and directing catheters and guidewires, particularly when traversing the aortic bifurcation. The effect of tortuosity can be reduced by employing a 15- or 20-cm introducing sheath, which helps straighten the artery.

There are many opportunities to gain skill in the over-the-top technique. We use it often after lumbar aortography to visualize the distal runoff of the contralateral limb by performing selective femoral, popliteal, and tibial angiograms. This selective catheterization technique produces angiograms of startlingly improved quality and permits acquisition of femoral angiograms with multiple projections. By incorporating these techniques into routine angiographic practice, experience can be gained not only in these so-called diagnostic procedures but also in subsequent and concomitant interventions.

COMPLICATIONS

Complications of catheter-based interventions, like all conditions, are better managed with prevention rather than treatment. Damage to the arteries at the puncture site and at remote locations of secondary catheterization is lessened by puncturing the proper artery. Hematomas, pseudoaneurysms, and arteriovenous fistulas in the groin usually result from failure to puncture the common femoral artery or from selecting a very diseased artery to gain access. Technique in handling catheters and guidewires is important. They should be manipulated and advanced in small increments, gently and without force to avoid dissections. The liberal use of sheaths of the smallest appropriate size helps forestall damage to the entry artery. Dye-induced nephropathy, particularly in patients with diabetes, can be virtually eliminated with the use of mannitol and diuretics (to establish diuresis, either by single injection or by infusion) and with dopamine infusion (to enhance renal flow). Direct injection of contrast material into the renal arteries should be avoided, if possible, and the minimal amount of contrast material, diluted if possible, should always be employed, whatever the status of renal function. Carbon dioxide angiography should be considered.

COMMENT

The performance of angiograms provides the best opportunity to gain skill in the use of needles, guidewires, sheaths, and catheters. We believe that vascular surgeons should perform their own angiograms in the special procedures room. It is the vascular surgeon who knows, in intimate detail, the information needed for vascular reconstruction, as well as which lesions are to be treated with endovascular techniques and which are to be treated with open surgery. After gaining expertise in the primary skills of angiography, more advanced techniques, such as antegrade femoral puncture and other techniques mentioned in this chapter, can be attempted. There are, however, hindrances to gaining this skill. Prime among the roadblocks to gaining endovascular skills is interspecialty rivalry with interventional radiologists and, increasingly, invasive cardiologists.

By mastering endovascular techniques and employing them in the special procedures room, the vascular surgeon will seldom find it necessary to combine inflow angioplasty with femorodistal or femorofemoral bypass. He or she would perform angiography and endoluminal intervention as a single procedure and would perform bypass grafting at a later date. By having access to the special procedures room and skill in percutaneous techniques, the surgeon would soon realize that minimally invasive techniques using a cutdown seldom are necessary. Likewise, scheduling of percutaneous procedures in the operating room would become rare. By performing the intervention in the special procedures room those cases that require multiple sites of access—such as bilateral femoral puncture for kissing balloon techniques, the seldom-performed popliteal puncture, and the manipulation of multiple guidewires—could be undertaken far more easily than in the operating room with a mobile C-arm and a radiolucent table.

Gaining percutaneous arterial access for diagnostic and therapeutic procedures is akin to making an incision in open surgery. Just as the position, the size, and the orientation of the incision can optimize visualization of the organs to be examined and treated, so does properly selected and performed arterial access allow remote interrogation and treatment of arterial lesions. Knowledge of when to use forceps, needle holders, and retractors is analogous to expertise in the selection and the use of needles, guidewires, sheaths, and endoluminal devices. No surgeon can progress without skill and experience in the use of the former, and no endovascular surgeon can gain technical mastery without training and experience in the latter.

CHAPTER

7

Guidewires, Catheters, and Sheaths

Michael B. Silva, Jr., Charlie C. Cheng

Most interventionists gain knowledge of guidewires, catheters, and sheaths through actual handling of the devices, with little thought given to the complex scientific and engineering processes that led to their development. Suppliers of these products are eager to offer a variety of devices that are tailored to specific needs and may have subtly different handling characteristics, making the task of selecting and stocking an inventory difficult for the practitioner.

The maturation of an endovascular practice goes through predictable phases in the buildup and the use of this fundamental inventory. Initially, only a few product choices are available, and the interventionist makes do with what is on hand. With growing experience, more difficult anatomic challenges, and a wider offering of therapeutic endovascular alternatives, the perceived need for additional wire, catheter, and sheath options increases substantially. In this second phase, a variety of competing products are tested, and inventory increases markedly. Ultimately, the interventionist becomes facile with a more moderate selection of devices and is able to adapt catheters with favored shapes and handling characteristics to a wide number of anatomic conditions. In this mature phase, inventory stabilizes, with new products being introduced as new technologies are developed or significant improvements are made.

This chapter does not promote a particular brand or list of products necessary for the successful conduct of an endovascular practice; rather, it offers background and definitions that may be useful in assisting the practitioner in sorting through the myriad of options presented for consideration. The number and the variety of products that are needed will be directly related to the number and the variety of procedures to be performed and the previously mentioned phase of maturation of one's endovascular practice.

GUIDEWIRES

Guidewire Design Characteristics

Guidewires are designed to have the characteristics of *pushability* and *flexibility*. Pushability refers to the characteristics associated with the direct transfer of forces on the wire from manipulations outside the patient's body as they translate to forward advancement of the wire or device inside the patient. Flexibility is a characteristic that usually works in a manner counter to pushability. The more stiff a wire, or the less flexible it is, the more pushable it will be.

Most guidewires have a single steel core called a mandrel surrounded by a coiled wire and coated with a substance to make the guidewire slippery. The tip of the guidewire, always more flexible than the rigid body, is frequently made of a smaller wire that is bonded to the distal tip of the mandrel. These design characteristics—slipperiness and maximal flexibility—allow the tip of the guidewire to be manipulated past tortuous lesions or tight stenoses while limiting the risk of dissection or perforation. (This is why turning the wire around and using the rigid back end to make it more pushable is not recommended.)

Guidewire tips are available in three shapes: straight, angled, or J-shaped. The type of tip chosen imparts variable degrees of *steerability* under fluoroscopic guidance. Steerability refers to the ability to direct the intravascular tip of the guidewire by manipulating the extra-anatomic portion by twisting, pulling, and pushing. Torque devices may be used to assist in wire manipulation (Figure 7-1). These bullet-shaped devices tighten down on the external protruding part of the wire and provide something larger to grip and twist. Alternatively, the use of powder-free or textured gloves can enhance one's ability to manipulate wires—especially the hydrophilic variety.

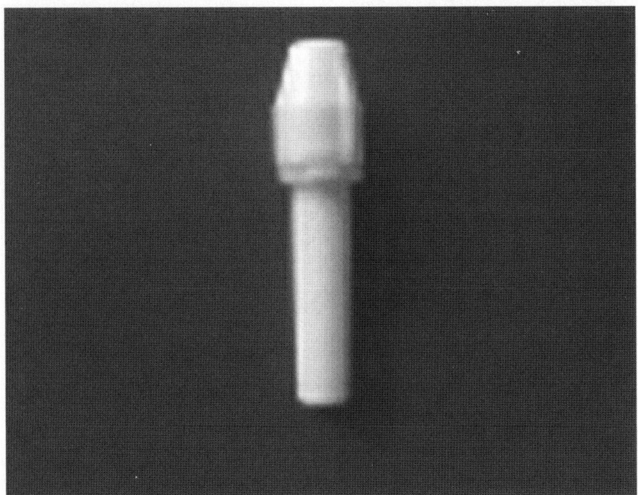

FIGURE 7-1 Wire torque device.

Guidewires are sized by their maximal transverse diameter (in hundredths of inches) and by their length (in centimeters). The guidewires most commonly used in peripheral vascular procedures come in three diameters: 0.035 inch, 0.018 inch, and 0.014 inch. For most angiographic procedures and most aortoiliac interventions, a 0.035-inch guidewire is used. *Trackability* of a wire refers to the ability of a catheter or an endovascular device such as a balloon catheter or stent to pass over the wire through tortuous anatomic configurations. Generally, a larger-diameter wire that is stiffer provides better trackability than one that is smaller and more flexible.

For infrageniculate lesions or tight renal and carotid stenoses, one may use a 0.014-inch or 0.018-inch wire. Use of these smaller wires allows the operator to advance a lower-profile balloon across a tight lesion in a smaller artery. A balloon with a lower profile has a smaller transverse diameter in its folded or deflated state, which allows it to traverse a tighter stenosis than one with a higher profile.

Occasionally, one will need a 0.038-inch wire for passage of a large-diameter sheath or delivery of an endograft through a tortuous iliac artery. Passage of these large devices may be facilitated by the additional trackability provided by a wire of greater diameter and stiffness.

Guidewires come in a variety of lengths. The most commonly used lengths for general-purpose guidewires are 145, 150, or 180 cm. Exchange wires, which allow the exchange of catheters or interventional devices without losing access across a remote lesion, are usually 260 or 300 cm in length. Increasing the length of the wire makes handling and manipulations more difficult and increases the chance of contamination. When performing any intervention, one should try to maintain the wire across the lesion until the completion angiogram has been obtained and is satisfactory. This allows additional interventional procedures such as stent placement to be performed after suboptimal intermediate interventions through a channel that remains constant. A good rule for selecting wire length is as follows:

Total length of wire needed
= Length of wire from insertion site to lesion
+ Length of catheter or interventional device
+ 10 cm

A wire length of less than this may not allow one to remove the catheter while maintaining fixation of the wire across the lesion. Docking devices are available in some wire systems that allow one to extend the length of a wire that is in place by adding a second wire to the end of the first via an attachable dock. These docking systems are of sufficiently low profile that they allow for subsequent passage of catheters and interventional devices over the added wire, over the docking system, and onto the initial wire.

Balloons and other devices equipped with a side-hole exit for the wire rather than the original end-hole configuration are often referred to as rapid-exchange catheters, and they offer some advantages when wire length is a factor (Figure 7-2). By allowing the wire to exit from the side of the catheter—15 to 30 cm from the tip for instance—they eliminate the need for the protruding wire to be longer than the device length. This is particularly useful when performing coronary, carotid, or upper extremity interventions from a retrograde femoral approach.

Quantum Maverick Monorail Catheter Schematic

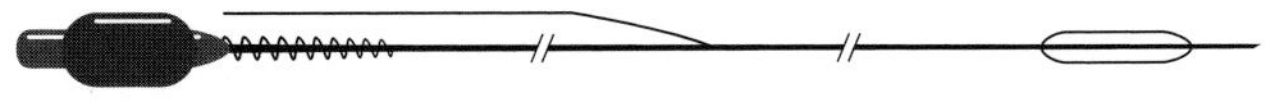

Quantum Maverick Over-the-Wire Catheter Schematic

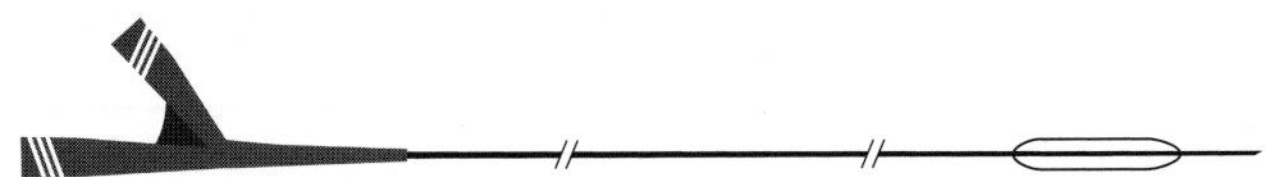

FIGURE 7-2 *(Upper)* Rapid exchange device (monorail) with wire exiting from the side. *(Lower)* Over-the-wire version of the same device.

Guidewire tip shape and coatings facilitate function. Non–hydrophilic-coated J-tip catheters are useful for initial catheter introduction via the Seldinger technique. Although dissection may occur with any type of wire, these wires offer characteristics that may reduce the frequency of this complication compared with use of hydrophilic wires with angled or straight tips. J-tip wires are also useful for passage of a wire through a stent when use of an angled or a straight wire may lead to inadvertent passage through a fenestration in the stent. Angled- or shapable-tip guidewires are steerable and are therefore useful in manipulating the catheter across a tight stenosis or into a specific branch vessel. We limit the use of straight wires to catheter exchanges.

Most guidewires have a hydrophilic coating of either polytetrafluoroethylene or silicone, which decreases the coefficient of friction during catheter exchange or while traversing stenoses or occlusions. The interventionist should be aware of the tactile differences noted with different wires as they are advanced into an artery. Even with a dissection, the passage of a very hydrophilic wire or a reduced-diameter wire in the subintimal plane may offer the technician so little resistance that he or she is unaware of the dissection. The use of fluoroscopy during wire advancement is an important adjunct to the tactile information one feels with wire advancement. A visibly spinning and freely advancing wire suggests that it is in the vessel lumen. A wire that will not spin and turns back on itself, or consistently tracks to the other iliac artery as it is advanced through the aortic bifurcation, may suggest it is in a subintimal plane.

In contrast, attempted passage of a standard J-tip wire through an introducer needle and into an artery in an extraluminal plane will offer resistance alerting the operator to stop and confirm location with a handheld injection of contrast agent—a quick and easy way to reduce significant complications. For the beginning interventionist, a nonhydrophilic J-tip wire is our recommended starting wire. A good practice is to wipe the guidewire with a sponge soaked in heparin and saline solution frequently and routinely between each catheter manipulation. This minimizes the amount of thrombotic debris that accumulates on the wire and decreases friction during subsequent catheter or wire exchanges. Care must be taken when wiping a wire not to remove any length of the wire from its implanted and intended position. The practice of wiping toward the body reduces the possibility of inadvertent wire removal.

Guidewire Selection

Paradoxically, as one gains experience with catheter-based therapy, the number of guidewires and catheters needed to complete complex interventions becomes fewer. Our recommendations should serve as a reference for the reader but are by no means comprehensive (Table 7-1). For initial entry into the artery, we recommend a J-tip wire, which is associated with the lowest risk of dissection. J-tip wires come in a wide variety. Some have a movable core that can convert the distal end of the wire from a flexible state to a rigid one. For initial introduction, one should be chosen that is not hydrophilic and has medium rigidity. The Bentson wire has a floppy tip, is of medium to firm rigidity, and, although straight in its packaged state, forms a functional large J-tip when being advanced through an artery or a vein.

Glidewires (Terumo, Somerset, NJ) can be either straight or angled and are hydrophilic. Angled Glidewires are steerable and may be manipulated with torque at the skin level with or without an external torquing device. We do not recommend the use of straight Glidewires during initial access because they are associated with the greatest chance of dissection. If dissection is suspected but not confirmed, the interventionist can perform a few simple tests. First, if a J-wire is used, one can attempt to spin the wire under fluoroscopy. The curved J-tip will not move freely in a subintimal plane. One can also perform handheld contrast agent injection.

Smaller-diameter wires include 0.018-inch and 0.014-inch wires. These may be useful in renal, carotid, or infrageniculate manipulations. Use of these wires is accompanied by use of appropriately sized catheters, balloon angioplasty catheters, and stents. Their use necessitates an expanded inventory and some redundancy (e.g., one may carry 4-mm balloon angioplasty catheters for use with a 0.018-inch or 0.014-inch system and different 4-mm balloon catheters for use with a 0.035-inch system). The smaller-diameter systems are necessary in many instances when introduction of the lowest-profile balloon catheters is needed. Recent advances in design have improved the 0.014-inch wires so that they are more rigid throughout their body, allowing for improved trackability. The 0.014-inch system is currently our preferred system for angioplasty and stenting of the carotid, visceral, and tibial vascular beds.

Infusion wires have been designed for use during thrombolytic infusion therapy. These wires have a proximal infusion port and a lumen that allows one to infuse through the distal aspect of the wire. Typically, these wires are passed through a multi–side-hole infusion catheter (Figure 7-3). Using a coaxial system and a Tuohy-Borst adapter (Cook, Bloomington, IN) (Figure 7-4), one may infuse thrombolytic agents through the infusion catheter directly into the clot while simultaneously infusing either additional thrombolytic agent or heparin into the distal circulation via the infusion wire.

EMBOLIC PROTECTION WIRES

A new class of wires has been developed to provide embolic protection during balloon angioplasty and stenting procedures. Initially conceived as an integral adjunct to carotid angioplasty and stenting, these

TABLE 7-1 Types of Guidewires and Catheters

Guidewire	Diameter (0.001 × inches)	Length (cm)	Features	Function
GENERAL				
J tip (Cook, Bloomington, IN)	18, 21, 25, 28, 32, 35, 38	80, 100, 125, 145	Variable tip curve 1.5, 3, 7.5, 15 TFE* coated	Catheter introduction Passage through stents or tortuous vessels
Bentsen (Cook, Bloomington, IN)	18, 21, 25, 28, 32, 35, 38	145, 180	15-cm flexible tip with distal 5 cm soft	Atraumatic negotiation of tortuous or strictured vessel
Glidewire (Terumo Medical, Ann Arbor, MI)	18, 25, 32, 35	120, 150, 180, 260	Hydrophilic, angled, or shapable tip	Crossing difficult lesions
EXCHANGE				
Amplatz Super Stiff (Cook, Bloomington, IN)	35, 38	80, 145, 180, 260	Stiff mandrel with flexible tip	Catheter exchange, good trackability Straightens acute aortoiliac bifurcation
Rosen (Boston Scientific, Quincy, MA)	35	150, 180, 260	1.5-mm J-tip	Good trackability Supports advancing catheter
Wholey (Mallinckrodt, St. Louis, MO)	35	145, 190, 300	17-cm floppy tip	Steerable tip, stiff core catheterization
Lunderquist-Ring (Cook, Bloomington, IN)	38	125	Very stiff	Used through a catheter, flossing, straightening tortuous iliac arteries for endograft delivery
Renal				
TAD (Mallinckrodt, St. Louis, MO)	35 tapers to 18 tip	145, 200	36-cm tapered tip Guidewire extension available	Good for crossing a stenosis with little trauma Good trackability with little trauma
TAD II	Same as TAD		20-cm tapered tip	Short renal arteries
Spartacore (Guidant, Santa Clara, CA)	14	145, 180	Atraumatic tip, 1:1 torquing	Rigid support Low-profile 14 system

*TFE, Tetrafluoroethyl.

devices are likely to assume an expanded role in those peripheral interventions where embolic debris is expected or needs to be avoided. The devices are based on a 0.014-inch wire platform and are therefore compatible with all current carotid stenting systems. The EZ filter wire (Boston Scientific, Natick, MA) (Figure 7-5) comes in one size and has a flexible "wind-sock"–type filter system. It is constrained in an outer sheath as it crosses the lesion and is then deployed passively as the sheath is removed. Passing a constraining catheter over the wire and collapsing the filter basket accomplish retrieval. The Emboshield (Abbott Vascular Devices, Abbott Park, IL) (Figure 7-6) is a device that is advanced over a wire, once the wire has crossed the lesion to be angioplastied. It is not attached to the wire but is constrained from distal migration by a specialized wire tip. Because the filter is free—like a cable car—on the wire it has the benefit of not responding directly to small inadvertent wire movements that are sometimes encountered with balloon and stent exchanges.

One of the more novel embolic protection systems conceived is the Flow Reversal System (W. L. Gore & Associates, Flagstaff, AZ) (Figure 7-7). This system consists of a sheath placed in the common carotid artery that has an inflatable cuff. Once it is positioned in the carotid and the cuff is inflated, prograde flow into the common carotid is stopped. A wire with a balloon occluder is advanced into the external carotid and

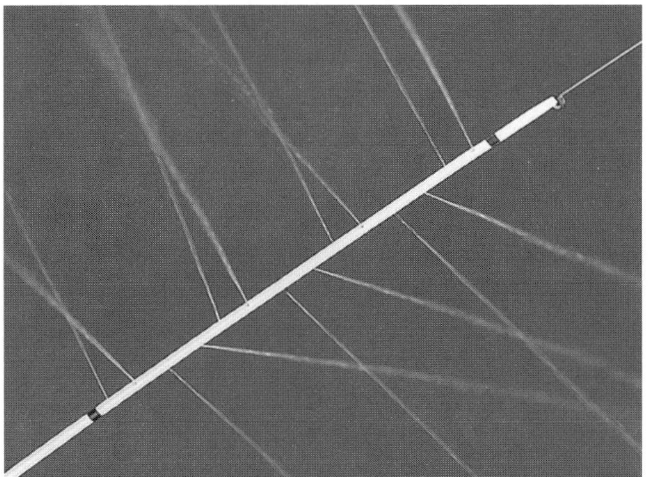

FIGURE 7-3 Cook Infusion catheter.

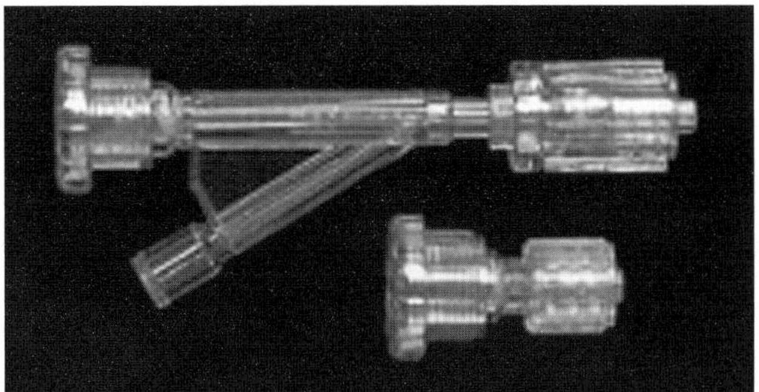

FIGURE 7-4 Cook Touhy-Borst valve adapter.

inflated, preventing retrograde flow from the external carotid artery into the common or internal carotid. The side port of the femoral access sheath is then connected to the venous circulation of the contralateral femoral vein via tubing with a filter device in line. These separate components create a negative pressure gradient from the internal carotid back down the sheath, through the filter, and into the contralateral femoral venous system. This system has the practical advantage of not requiring the embolic protection device to be passed across the internal carotid lesion—a source of potentially unprotected embolization with other device designs.

CATHETERS

Catheter Design

Catheters may be made from polyurethane, polyethylene, polypropylene, Teflon, or nylon, with polyurethane catheters having the highest coefficient of friction and Teflon having the lowest. Catheters are sized according to their outer diameter (in French units) and their length

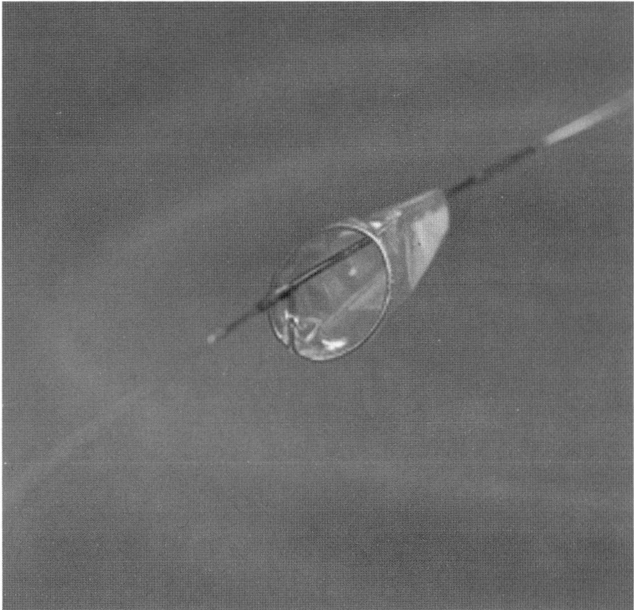

FIGURE 7-5 Boston Scientific EZ Filter Wire for Embolic Protection.

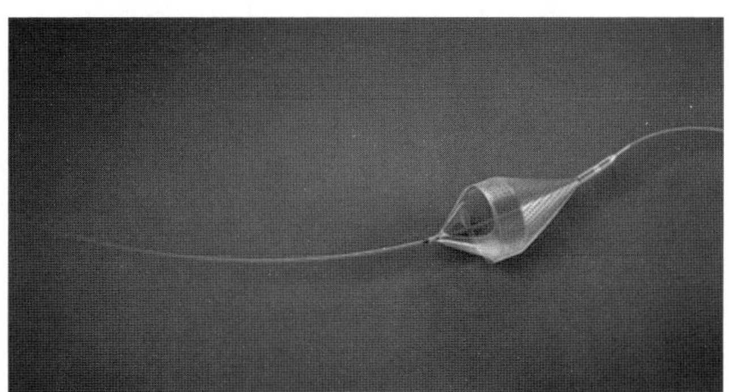

FIGURE 7-6 Abbott Emboshield.

(in centimeters). To convert French sizes to metric sizes one divides by pi—3.14. A 6F catheter therefore will be slightly less than 2 mm in diameter. Although catheters that have smaller internal diameters are available, most catheters used in angiography will accommodate a 0.035-inch guidewire. We stock and use mostly 5F catheters, but 4F and 6F catheters are occasionally used. These are matched with their appropriately sized sheaths. The most commonly used catheter lengths are 65 and 100 cm.

Functionally, catheters may be either selective or nonselective. Nonselective or flush catheters, which have multiple side and end holes that allow a large cloud of contrast agent to be infused over a short period of time, are used for large-vessel opacification and in high-flow systems (Figure 7-8). These nonselective catheters may be straight, or they may have shaped ends

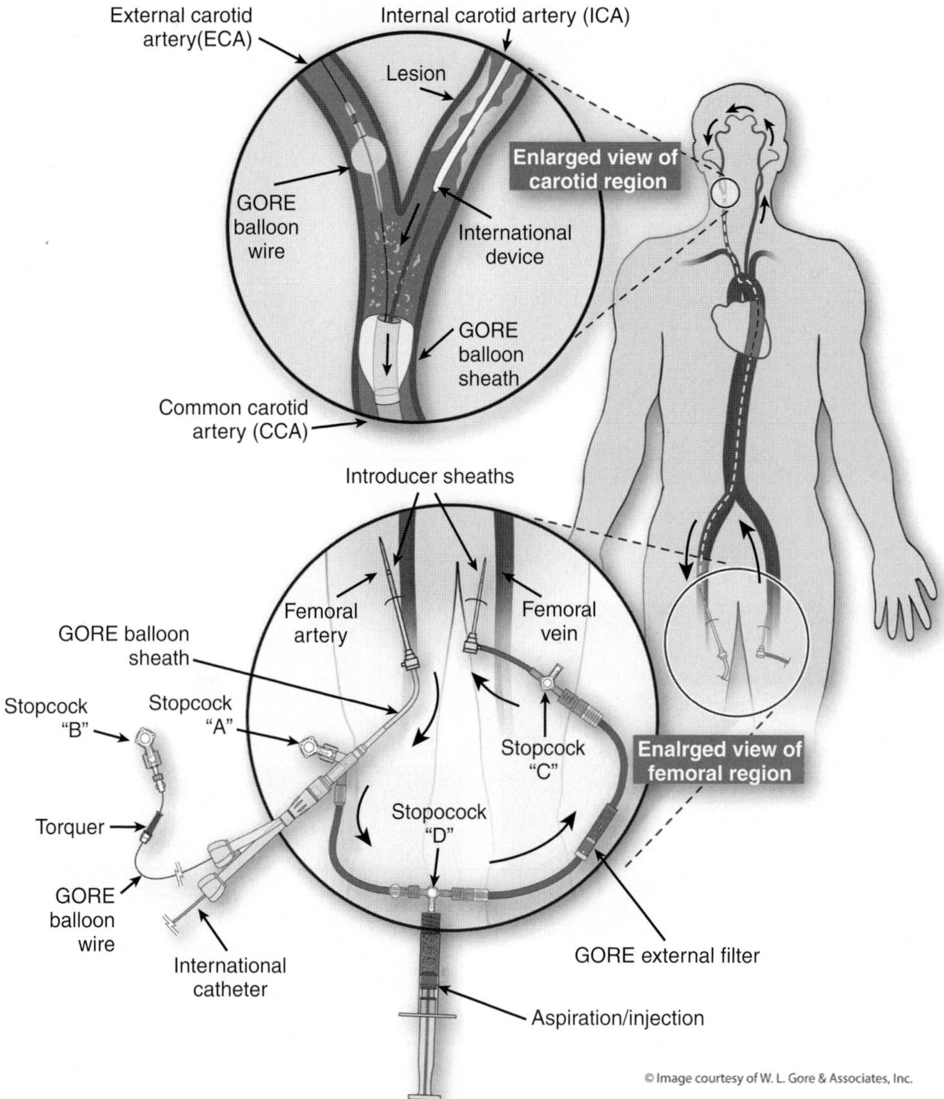

FIGURE 7-7 Gore reversal-of-flow embolic protection system.

(e.g., tennis racquet or pigtail catheters). There are numerous variations of the curled pigtail shape with subtle modifications of the tightness of the curls. We have found them interchangeable.

Selective catheters have only a single hole at their tip and are used to intubate vascular families (branches off the aorta) before advancement of the wire. They are available in many shapes and lengths that are designed to facilitate intubation of branch vasculature (Figure 7-9). With angiography that includes selective catheterization, one uses smaller amounts of contrast material at lower injection rates to obtain adequate arterial opacification. When using selective catheters, care must be taken to avoid intimal injury or dissection of the artery from either direct catheter tip advancement or the forceful injection of contrast material. Additionally, a "jet effect" can occur when forceful injection of contrast material pushes the catheter out of the vessel of interest and back into the aorta. Lengthening the "rise of rate" of injection on the power injector control panel can limit these negative effects.

Catheter information, such as maximal flow rate, bursting pressure, inner diameter, outer diameter, and length, is detailed on the package label. We routinely review the catheter package before opening it. This allows us to reaffirm compatibility of the catheter with the wire and the introducer sheath while visually assessing the shape of the tip as it relates to the anatomic angles we are attempting to navigate.

Flow rate (Q) through a catheter varies with its internal radius and is inversely proportional to the catheter length. Poiseuille's equation can be used to describe the factors associated with flow through a catheter. The equation can be written:

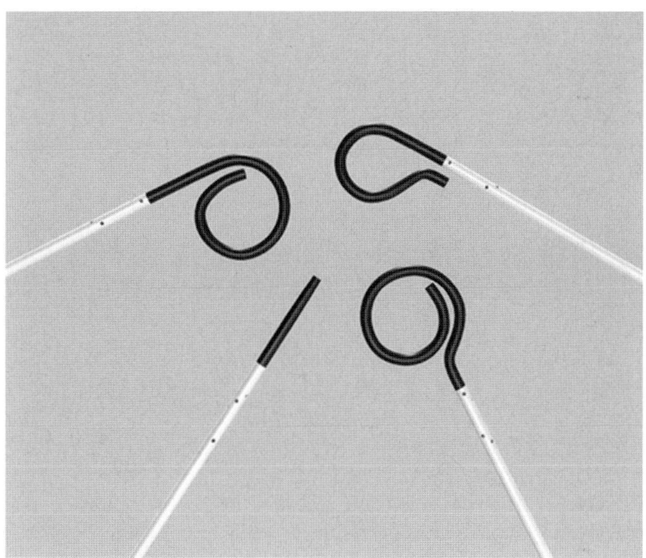

FIGURE 7-8 A variety of nonselective flush catheters.

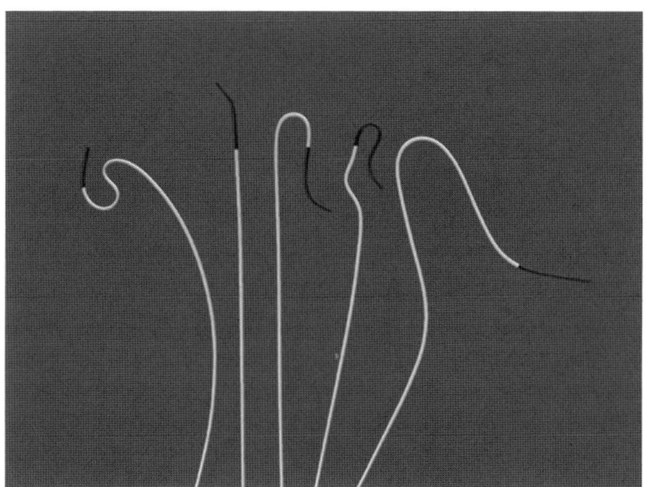

FIGURE 7-9 A variety of selective shaped catheters.

$$Q = \frac{P\pi R^4}{8\eta\ L}$$

In this equation: Q is flow, P is the pressure drop over the length of the catheter, R is the internal radius raised to the fourth power, L is the length of the catheter, and η is the viscosity of the fluid. Table 7-2 shows the effect of altering radius and length on flow rates for several commonly used catheters.

Catheter Selection

Prevention of thrombus formation is desired in any vascular cannulation. There is an increasing likelihood of thrombus formation as catheter size increases with respect to the internal diameter of the vessel lumen. One can minimize this by selecting the smallest catheter that will achieve the intended purpose and removing the catheter as early as possible. Thrombus may also form within a catheter while it is in the lumen of the vessel. We recommend regular aspiration of blood from catheters before planned injection and flushing with heparinized saline solution once the catheter is found to be free of clot.

TABLE 7-2 Catheter Maximal Flow Rate

Size (F)	Length (cm)	Contrast agent used (mL/s)
5	65	15
5	100	11
6	65	21
6	100	17

The head shape of a catheter determines its function. All catheters, regardless of shape, should be advanced over a wire to limit the potential for intimal injury during advancement and positioning. Nonselective catheters, such as the pigtail catheter, are designed to be used in larger-diameter vessels, such as the aorta. Once the wire has been withdrawn and the curl of the pigtail has been formed in the aorta, the leading edge of the catheter curl offers a relatively blunt profile. As such, these catheters can be carefully advanced or repositioned distally without reinserting the wire. We recommend, however, that a wire be reinserted before removing any shaped catheter through the iliac or the brachial artery into which it is introduced. This practice limits the potential for the catheter tip to score and injure the intima as it is removed. Another useful technique is to allow a length of wire to protrude from the end of the catheter during repositioning from one part of the aorta to another. This technique reduces the likelihood that the catheter will lodge inadvertently in the various branches of the aorta before reaching its intended position.

To cannulate the contralateral iliac artery for selective iliac injection, one can often use the nonselective flush catheter used for the initial aortogram. The wire is reinserted and is advanced to the tip of the catheter orifice to open the angle of the curl. The catheter is withdrawn to the bifurcation so that the tip engages the orifice of the contralateral common iliac artery. The wire is then advanced distally, and the catheter is advanced over the wire. To minimize arterial injury, care should be taken not to advance or withdraw the unfurled pigtail catheter without reintroducing the wire.

For selective cannulation of branches of the aorta, one should choose a catheter with a head shape that corresponds to the anatomic angle of the branch to be entered. In selective catheterization, the catheter tip itself is manipulated into the orifice of the branch vessel. Injections at lower pressures may be performed after this step; however, for higher-pressure injections, the catheter will need to be advanced farther into the branch to prevent losing access as a result of catheter whip and recoil. First passing the wire more distally and then advancing the catheter into the target vessel will accomplish this with the least likelihood of injury.

For arch vessels, we recommend starting with a vertebral catheter. This catheter has perhaps the most minimally selective design, with a 1-cm tip angled at approximately 30 degrees to the straight access. With practice, however, it is possible to use this catheter for each of the thoracic arch vessels. Alternatively, a number of elaborately designed catheters have been developed to facilitate cannulation of arch vessels. The Headhunter or the Simmons may be appropriate for this. If unsuccessful with one of the aforementioned catheters, one may try the Mani, the Vitek, or the HN4.

Most of the more elaborately shaped selective catheters must be reformed in the aortic arch or the abdominal aorta proximal to the vessel that one is attempting to intubate. Once the catheter is reformed into its planned shape, the operator withdraws and rotates the catheter under fluoroscopic guidance until it engages the orifice of the desired branch vessel.

For renal and visceral arteries, we recommend a Cobra catheter or a Shepherd's hook. The catheter should be advanced above the intended artery and rotated as it is gently pulled inferiorly. This manipulation will result in intubation of the renal or the visceral orifice; position can be confirmed with a puff of contrast material. Once the orifice of the intended artery has been intubated, a guidewire with a floppy tip is advanced into it distally so that the catheter may then be advanced over the stiffer portion of the wire.

In arteries of the lower extremity, we use a simple selective straight catheter over a guidewire for selective arteriography. Occasionally, one cannot manipulate a guidewire across a tight stenosis. In this case, the catheter may be advanced to the area of stenosis to support the wire as an additional attempt to cross the lesion is made.

A number of catheters have been designed for specific functions or unusual situations. Catheters with a hydrophilic coating, called Glidecaths (Terumo Medical) or Slip-Caths (Cook), may be helpful in crossing tight stenoses (Figure 7-10). For thrombolytic therapy, the Mewissen Infusion Catheter is used in conjunction with Cragg or Katzen (Boston Scientific) wires. When assessing a patient with an aneurysm for the potential use of an aortic endograft, aortography is performed with a 5F pigtail catheter that is marked with radiopaque markers at 1-cm increments. This allows for the measurement of aortic and iliac segments and aids in selection of appropriately tailored limbs for the endoprosthesis. Additionally, a catheter with radiopaque markings spaced 2.8 cm apart is available. This catheter is useful in performing an inferior venacavogram before vena cava filter placement. The 2.8-cm measurement can then be used to determine easily the transverse diameter of the vena cava and to identify those venae cavae that are too large for standard filter placement.

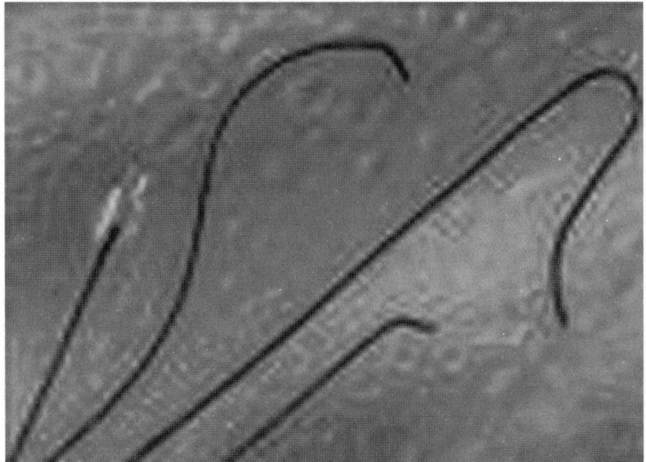

FIGURE 7-10 Terumo Glide catheters. The bottom catheter with the slightly angled head is routinely used to intubate most arch branches.

With the proliferation of accurate noninvasive imaging techniques and the growing acceptance of the appropriateness of endovascular therapeutic intervention for treatment of atherosclerotic disease, purely diagnostic angiography is performed infrequently in our practice. More commonly, our patients undergoing catheterization are candidates for potential intervention in addition to angiographic inspection. As such, we routinely perform catheterizations through introducer sheaths with hemostatic valves. This facilitates introduction of various endovascular devices while minimizing blood loss and trauma to the artery at the insertion site.

SHEATHS

Introducer Sheaths

Once percutaneous access has been obtained and wire access to the blood vessel has been established, we prefer to dilate the track gradually with progressively enlarging dilators. Dilators, like catheters, are sized according to their outer diameter in French units (F). Sheaths, in contradistinction, are sized according

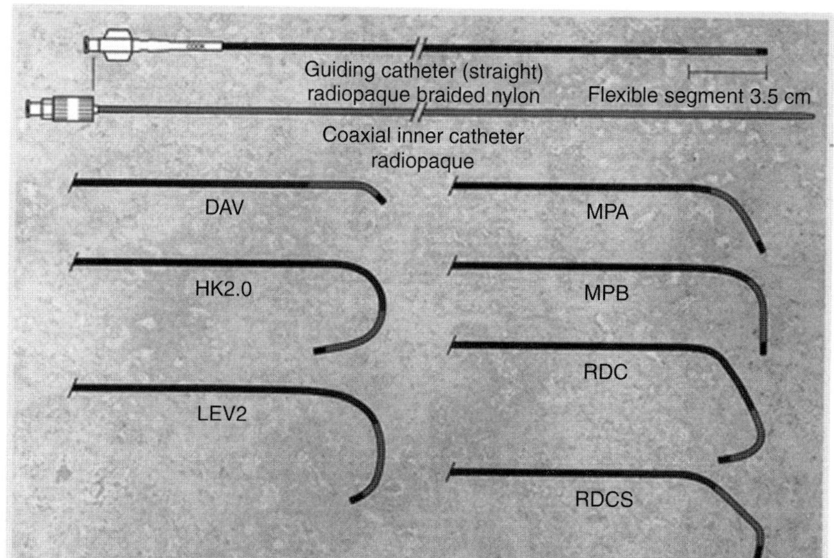

FIGURE 7-11 Guide catheters. Some come with an obturator, sized by outer diameter in French units and length in centimeters do not have a side infusion port. Use of a Tuohy-Borst radiopaque tips preferred.

to their inner diameter also in French units. Consequently, if we are planning to use a 5F sheath, we sequentially pass 4F, 5F, and 6F dilators. The final size of the hole in the artery will be determined by the outer size of the 5F sheath, which is just over 6F. Progressive dilatation, although taking a few extra seconds, may cause less trauma to the common femoral artery, reducing the potential for iatrogenic injury.

Introducer sheaths all have hemostatic valves and side infusion ports. The side port may be used to monitor pressures or, in some cases, to inject contrast agent and to eliminate the need for a catheter. Sheaths come in multiple lengths (measured in centimeters). Most commonly, we use 15- or 25-cm lengths. A shorter 6-cm sheath is ideally suited for working on arteriovenous grafts or fistulas. These shorter sheaths are adapted for high-volume infusion and may be left in the graft for dialysis after the procedure if the patient requires same-day dialysis. Occasionally, we will use a long 5F sheath to assist with passage of a catheter through a tortuous iliac artery. When one is planning to perform angioplasty or stenting, the initial 5F sheath placed for diagnostic angiography is exchanged for a larger-diameter sheath, usually 6F or 7F, through which the interventional devices can be passed. We use the smallest size sheath required for the planned intervention.

Guiding Catheters and Guiding Sheaths

Guiding catheters and guiding sheaths are both used to facilitate passage of a smaller catheter or an endovascular device through a tortuous area to a desired treatment location. The larger size of the guiding catheter or the guiding sheath may allow contrast agent injection around the smaller endovascular treatment device in place. For visceral, renal, and carotid artery angioplasty and stenting, use of a guiding catheter or a guiding sheath is preferred. In addition to facilitating passage of the endovascular device, they promote precise positioning by allowing contrast agent injections around the device with concomitant maintenance of wire access across the lesion.

Although the terms "guiding catheter" and "guiding sheath" are sometimes used interchangeably, there are differences between them. Guiding catheters (Figure 7-11) are designed with a stronger external reinforcement material, which aids in supporting balloon or catheter passage through long distances in the aorta to branch vessels. Unlike guiding sheaths, guiding catheters have no hemostatic valve and require the use of a Tuohy-Borst side-arm adapter. Another important distinction between sheaths and catheters is that guiding sheaths are sized according to their internal diameter, whereas guiding catheters are sized according to their outer diameter (both in French units).

Guide sheaths (Figure 7-12) are packaged with a tapered internal obturator for introduction and advancement into an artery. Not all guiding catheters come with internal obturators. The size discrepancy between the internal diameter of the guiding catheter and the wire is usually significant. Advancement of a guiding catheter that is much larger than its wire can be associated with injury to the intima of the artery and an unintentional endarterectomy. To reduce the size mismatch, one may advance a selective catheter over the wire to just beyond the tip of the guiding catheter and then advance both as a unit. We prefer, however, to use only guiding sheaths and guiding

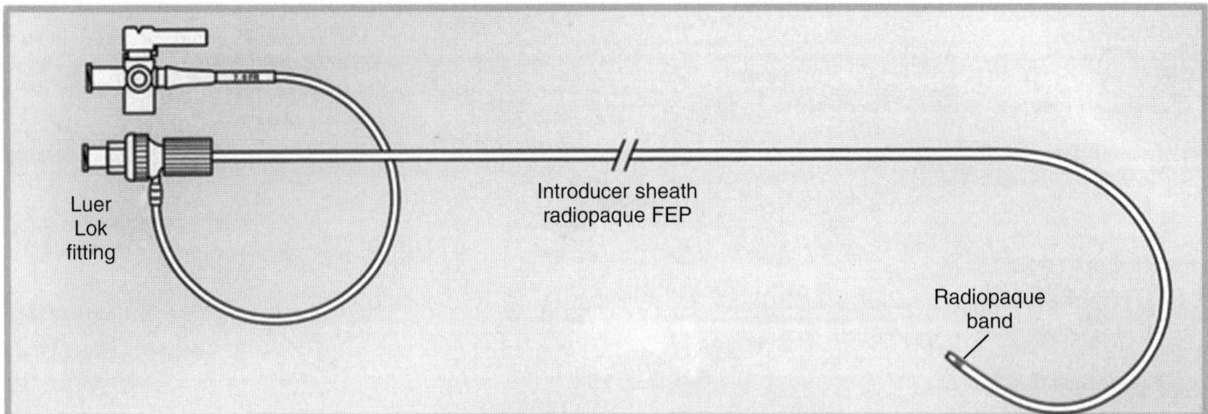

FIGURE 7-12 Guide sheaths. All come with an obturator, sized by inner diameter in French and length in centimeters. Sheaths have an integrated side infusion port.

catheters supplied with internal obturators. Both sheaths and catheters are available with radiopaque tips. These are preferred because they allow for accurate identification of the end of the guide in relation to the endovascular device and the lesion being treated.

Guides are available with preformed distal shapes for use in many anatomic scenarios. Use of a hockey stick–shaped catheter that forms an angle of 90 degrees is useful in the deployment of a renal artery stent. When using a guide to facilitate delivery of a balloon-expandable stent, we attempt to advance the guide past the lesion to be stented. If successful, this allows delivery of the stent through a protected sleeve, limiting the potential for dislodging the stent from its delivery balloon as it traverses the atherosclerotic lesion. The guide is then withdrawn to the orifice of the involved artery, and contrast material is injected for accurate positioning just before deployment.

We initially used an externally supported long sheath with a straight but malleable tip for angioplasty and stenting of the brachiocephalic vessels. Continued improvements in device profile have allowed for the reduction in size of sheaths necessary for the delivery of carotid stents. Long, flexible 6F guide sheaths have greatly simplified the procedure and allow for carotid stent delivery in patients with complex arch anatomy. The Shuttle Select System (Cook) is specifically designed for streamlined carotid access. Long catheters (135 cm) with 6F diameters and a variety of shaped tips specifically designed for accessing the arch vessels allow for advancement of the sheath over the slightly larger diameter catheters (eliminating any step-off) directly into the common carotid arteries, eliminating the need for exchanging an initially placed short sheath for the longer carotid sheath.

Guiding sheaths are particularly useful when performing interventions in the contralateral iliac system. In addition to facilitating passage of stents up and over the bifurcation, they protect the ipsilateral iliac artery from the repetitive passage of balloon catheters, diagnostic catheters, and stents. Most important, they allow for intermediate assessment of the results of preliminary angioplasty with pericatheter puff angiography while maintaining wire access across the lesion. If angioplasty of a contralateral iliac artery is performed without a guide sheath, assessment of the results of angioplasty requires removing the balloon catheter and advancing a diagnostic catheter over the wire. The wire must then be removed and the catheter must be pulled back above the lesion undergoing angioplasty to perform angiography. If one determines that a stent is required owing to suboptimal angioplasty results, one is then forced to recross the freshly treated lesion. If the wire does not pass through the center of the lumen but rather tracks through a portion of the fractured plaque, subsequent stenting may prove catastrophic. We recommend use of a guide sheath for contralateral iliac endovascular interventions. The Shuttle Select system, originally developed for carotid intervention, is now available in a 4F size that allows contralateral tibial interventions with a significant reduction in entry hole diameter.

When using guiding catheters or guiding sheaths, the operator should note that the diameter of these devices is much larger than in those used in simple angiographic procedures. With a larger-diameter introducer one may see a higher rate of access-related complications in the iliac and the femoral systems. In a smaller patient, the catheter may be of sufficient size to occlude the artery or significantly diminish flow distal to the insertion site, subjecting the ipsilateral extremity to some degree of ischemia and predisposing to thrombosis. We administer anticoagulation therapy to the patient once these large-diameter devices are in place. Use of these catheters should be limited, and their removal from a vessel should be prompt.

SUMMARY

In our endovascular training program, we teach three rules of endovascular surgery. Rule number one (we call this "The Inviolate Rule of Endovascular Surgery" for emphasis): "Once across a lesion with a wire, don't remove it until the case is finished." Wires still get pulled out inadvertently, suggesting that the emphasis needs to be stronger.

Rule number two: "Read the package." As we have described in this chapter, sizing methodology for wires, catheters, and sheaths was clearly an afterthought. Wire diameters are in hundredths of an inch and their lengths are in centimeters; dilators and catheters are described in French units by their outer diameters; and sheaths are described in French units by their inner diameters with their lengths in centimeters. For guiding sheaths, the inner diameter is in French units; for guiding catheters, the outer diameter is in French units. Balloon catheters and stents are described by their outer diameter in French units in the undeployed state and in millimeters once they are inflated or deployed. The challenge is putting pieces together that fit. Mercifully, all the information that one needs is included on the front of the package for each of these devices. The corollary to rule number two is that the package will be found in the trash can.

Rule number three: "Everything falls on the floor." This is both self-explanatory and prophetic. We recommend having at least two of everything.

Online References

We have found the following websites useful in exploring the various product offerings in wires, catheters, and sheaths. In addition to detailing available products and specifications, many offer free downloadable images and animations in a variety of formats.

http://www.abbottvascular.com/av_dotcom/url/home/en_US
http://www.bardpv.com/
http://www.bostonscientific.com/home.bsci
http://www.cookmedical.com/home.do
http://www.cordis.com/
http://www.edwards.com/products/productshome.htm
http://www.ev3.net/peripheral/us/
http://www.gore.com/
http://www.medtronic.com/for-physicians/
http://www.possis.com/
http://www.terumomedical.com/

Bibliography

Moore W, editor: *Vascular and Endovascular Surgery: A Comprehensive Review,* ed 7, Philadelphia, 2005, Saunder, p 9,92.

Schneider P, editor: *Endovascular Skills*, ed 2, London, 2004, Taylor & Francis, Inc, p 376.

CHAPTER

8

Balloon Angioplasty Catheters

Niten H. Singh, Peter A. Schneider

Endoluminal blood vessel manipulation by means of balloon angioplasty has become a cornerstone of contemporary vascular therapy. The usefulness of balloon angioplasty has increased steadily since 1980, and at present balloon angioplasty contributes significantly to the management of occlusive disease in most vascular beds. Improving technology and catheter-based techniques have broadened the spectrum of lesions that are amenable to percutaneous transluminal angioplasty (PTA). The development of vascular stents (see Chapter 10, Vascular Stents) has further increased the number of applications for balloon angioplasty.

PTA (with stent placement as needed) is an essential option in the management of aortoiliac and femoropopliteal occlusive disease.[1-6] In other arterial segments, such as renal artery orifice and carotid bifurcation, where primary stent placement is commonly employed, balloon angioplasty is an essential adjunct used to create a pathway in the lesion for stent placement and then to perform poststent angioplasty. Significant advances have been made in the treatment of carotid artery lesions over the last 5 years, and along with this progress some studies have shown that carotid artery stenting is not inferior to carotid endarterectomy in high-risk patients.[7-9] Other aortic branch arteries such as subclavian or innominate arteries are also commonly treated with catheter-based techniques, including balloon angioplasty. Lower-profile systems are facilitating tibial and pedal angioplasty.[10-12] Balloon angioplasty may be used to treat some lesions within bypass grafts and dialysis grafts.[13] PTA shows promise in the central venous system and represents a potentially significant advance in venous reconstruction.

This chapter presents the concepts, the equipment, and the techniques that make balloon angioplasty an integral part of contemporary vascular practice.

STRUCTURE OF BALLOON ANGIOPLASTY CATHETERS

Balloon angioplasty is performed by using a disposable coaxial or monorail platform catheter selected from among many sizes and types to meet the demands posed by the particular lesion being treated. The function of a balloon angioplasty catheter is to exert a dilating force on the endoluminal surface of a blood vessel at a desired location. Although a balloon angioplasty catheter is a relatively simple tool, there are multiple variables that must be considered in choosing a catheter for a given situation. These features include balloon diameter and length, catheter size and length, balloon type, and catheter profile (Figure 8-1).

The angioplasty catheter has two lumens: one that permits the catheter to pass over a guidewire during placement and one to inflate the balloon once it is appropriately placed. Balloon diameters range from 1.5 to 24 mm and are selected with the intent to overdilate slightly the artery being treated (Table 8-1). Balloon length ranges from 1.5 to 22 cm and should be sufficient to dilate the lesion with a slight overhang into the adjacent artery. When balloon angioplasty is performed after stent placement, it is not necessary to overdilate and it is usually not necessary to have the balloon extend into the artery beyond the end of the stent. Radiopaque markers on the catheter at each end of the balloon permit the operator to place the catheter precisely. The shoulder is the tapered balloon end that extends beyond the radiopaque marker. Because the body of the balloon is cylindrical, the taper of the shoulder helps define the balloon's overall shape when it is fully inflated. A short shoulder is desirable when angioplasty is performed adjacent to an area where dilatation is contraindicated, such as a smaller-diameter branch vessel or an ulcerated or an aneurysmal segment. The tip of the catheter, which

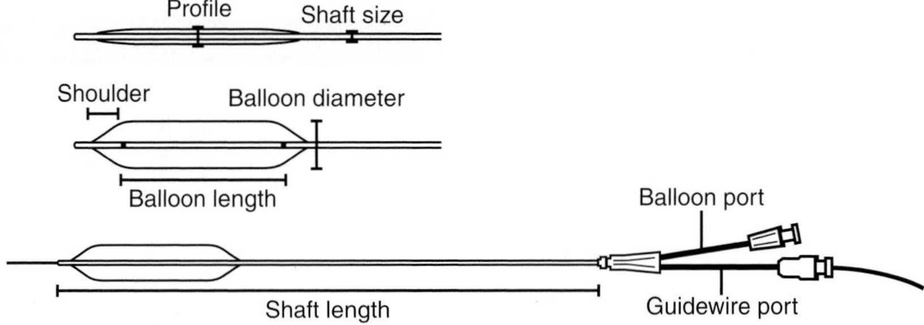

FIGURE 8-1 Balloon angioplasty catheter. It is a simple disposable tool with applications in multiple vascular beds. *(Reproduced with permission from Schneider PA: Endovascular Skills, 2nd ed. New York, Marcel Dekker, 2003.*

TABLE 8-1 Structure and Function of Balloon Angioplasty Catheters

Structure	Function
Balloon diameter	Exert dilating pressure to appropriate diameter on endoluminal surface of blood vessel
Balloon length	Dilate entire length of lesion with slight overhang of balloon onto adjacent artery
Catheter size	Deliver appropriate balloon to lesion on smallest possible catheter
Catheter length	Reach lesion through chosen access site without excessive catheter length
Balloon type	Promote use for high-pressure inflation, low-profile catheter passage, stent placement, or scratch resistance based on various materials
Catheter profile	Determine the size of the access sheath required
Shoulder	Taper balloon to the catheter shaft and determine inflated shape of balloon
Balloon port	Provide a lumen along the catheter shaft and into the balloon used for inflation
Guidewire port	Provide a guidewire lumen for delivery of the catheter to its intended site
Radiopaque markers	Mark end of balloon for correct placement

is the segment that extends beyond the end of the balloon, may also vary in length.

The shaft length may vary from 40 to 150 cm. The shaft must be long enough to reach from the remote access site to the lesion. In general, the shortest catheter that is able to reach the target site is desirable because it is less cumbersome and more responsive to manipulation, requires shorter guidewires, and makes exchanges simpler. Angioplasty catheters that pass over a 0.035-inch guidewire are available over a broad range of balloon sizes (3 mm to more than 2 cm). Catheter shaft sizes range from 3F to 7F and are determined by the balloon type and diameter. Standard angioplasty in its most common working range (diameters from 3 to 8 mm) may be performed with use of 5F catheters. Larger-diameter balloons or heavy-duty (high-pressure) balloons require larger catheter shafts (5.8F to 7F) and larger sheaths. Smaller-diameter balloons (1.5 to 4 mm) are available on 3F shafts, which pass over 0.018-inch and 0.014-inch guidewires. These may be on either coaxial or monorail catheters.

FUNCTION OF BALLOON ANGIOPLASTY CATHETERS

The type of balloon is determined by its material. Standard, noncompliant, 0.035-inch–compatible angioplasty catheters have balloons that are constructed of polyethylene, polyethylene terephthalate, or other low-compliance plastic polymers. Burst pressures range from 8 to 15 atm. At higher pressures, low-compliance balloons will exert force without an increase in diameter or the risk of vessel rupture. Reinforced high-pressure polymer balloons, such as the Blue Max (Boston Scientific, Natick, MA) have burst pressures that exceed 17 atm and may be pressurized to more than 20 atm. These have larger shafts (usually by approximately 1F) than standard balloons. These thick-walled balloons are useful for treating heavily calcified or sharp lesions and recalcitrant lesions, such as those caused by intimal hyperplasia. Recently, newer low-profile noncompliant balloons such as the Dorado (Bard Peripheral Vascular, Tempe, AZ), which range in diameter from 3 to 10 mm, can be placed through a 5F and 6F sheath.

Thinner-walled, compliant balloons are available, which permit a lower profile. Compliance is a highly desirable feature in smaller-artery angioplasty. Slight changes in diameter can be made with adjustments in inflated pressure, rather than changing for a different balloon catheter. These lower-profile catheters are more easily passed through a preocclusive or tortuous lesion, but they are less puncture resistant and are not useful for heavily calcified lesions or stent placement.

The performance of the catheter may be enhanced by a hydrophilic coating, which may be applied by the manufacturer to the balloon surface to permit the balloon to track and cross easily. There are multiple potential applications of this concept of modifying the balloon surface (e.g., antithrombotic therapy and brachytherapy).

The profile of the catheter is the overall diameter of the catheter shaft with the balloon wrapped around it. After a balloon has been inflated, its profile increases in size because the balloon does not wrap as neatly around the catheter once it has been used. The used balloon material forms wings, which may be manually rewrapped around the catheter if necessary. The profile of the balloon affects its ability to pass through a lesion. In general, preinflation of the balloon is not performed because this may make it more difficult to pass it across the lesion. Catheter profile is the main factor limiting the size of the percutaneous access site and is an important consideration in every angioplasty.

MECHANISM OF REVASCULARIZATION WITH BALLOON ANGIOPLASTY

Balloon angioplasty has been the basis of most endovascular procedures. However, the unpredictability of the results of balloon angioplasty makes stent usage necessary on a frequent basis. In some cases, selective stent placement is practiced. Stents are reserved for cases in which there is an inadequate result with balloon angioplasty. In other settings, such as coronary stenosis and renal artery orifice lesions, primary stenting is performed with balloon angioplasty as a complementary technique.

Balloon angioplasty causes desquamation of endothelial cells and histologic damage proportional to the diameter of the balloon and the duration of inflation. Longitudinal fracture of the atherosclerotic plaque and stretching of the media and adventitia increase the cross-sectional area of the diseased vessel.[14,15] Plaque compression does not add appreciably to the newly restored luminal diameter.[16] Postangioplasty arteriography almost always reveals areas of dissection and plaque separation caused by PTA. Areas of dissection are seen more frequently with dilatation of calcified lesions and with dilatation of circumferential lesions. The plaque may become partially separated from the artery wall at the angioplasty site and may remain attached to the proximal and the distal arterial walls. Medial dissection occurs at plaque edges or at plaque rupture sites and tends to be somewhat unpredictable.[13,15] The media opposite the plaque becomes thinner. Because most fractures in the plaque are oriented in the direction of flow, there is a relatively low incidence of acute occlusion at the angioplasty site (due to dissection) or distally (due to atheroembolization).[14-17] Platelets and fibrin cover the damaged surface, and some endothelialization and surface remodeling soon follow. Follow-up angiography shows that most dissection planes have healed within 1 month.[18]

MECHANISM OF BALLOON DILATATION

The dilating force generated by the balloon is proportional to the balloon diameter, the balloon pressure, and the surface over which the balloon material is applied.[19,20] The dilating force is a result of the hydrostatic pressure within the balloon, the wall tension generated by balloon expansion, and the force vector that results from deformation of the balloon by the lesion.

Hydrostatic pressure is proportional to both the inflation pressure and the endoluminal surface area of the lesion that is dilated by the balloon. At any established level of hydrostatic pressure, wall tension is dependent on Laplace's law and is therefore proportional to the radius of the balloon. This explains why larger balloons are more likely to rupture at a given pressure: the larger radius results in increased wall tension.

Most atherosclerotic lesions require 8 atm of pressure or less for dilatation. When the balloon is inflated, the proximal and the distal ends fill first, and the middle section or the body of the balloon, which is usually located at the segment of most severe stenosis, forms a waist (Figure 8-2). This waistlike shape also contributes to the dilating force of the balloon. As the balloon waist is expanded by increasing wall tension, a radial vector force is generated, which is greatest when the waist is tightest. Once the balloon is fully inflated, further inflation to treat a small area of residual stenosis will not contribute to the dilating force but will increase the likelihood of rupture of the balloon. For a given stenosis for which there is a choice of possible balloon diameters, the larger balloon will generate a much higher dilating force. The larger diameter increases the wall tension, and the larger balloon size results in a tighter waist at the point of maximal stenosis and a higher radial force vector.

THE PERFECT ANGIOPLASTY CATHETER

Balloon angioplasty catheters, like all other catheters, must be "pushable" and trackable. The balloon material must be durable and resistant to rupture and must permit very high pressures (20 atm or more). The balloon must be scratch resistant, puncture resistant, and reusable and must collapse to the lowest possible profile. The lumen filling the balloon must be large enough to inflate and deflate the balloon in a short period of time. The catheter must be small enough in caliber to be used safely via standard percutaneous approaches.[19,21]

Present technology does not permit the optimization of all these factors in a single catheter; however, most balloon angioplasty catheters are designed to feature

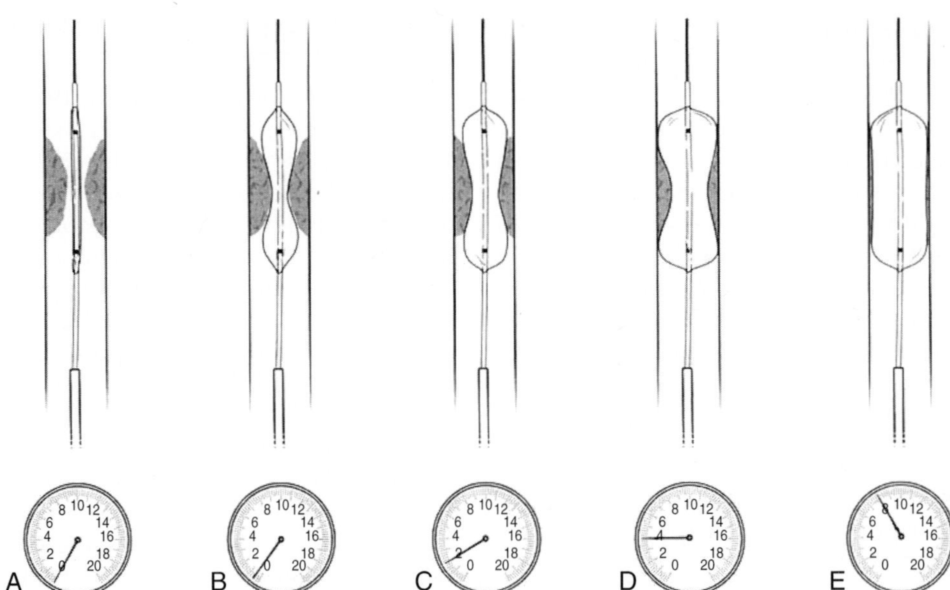

FIGURE 8-2 Dilatation of the atherosclerotic waist. **A,** The balloon catheter is advanced through the lesion. **B,** The proximal and distal ends of the balloon begin to fill at very low pressure. **C,** At 2 atm of pressure, a waist develops where the stenosis caused by the plaque is most severe. **D,** Stenosis remains at 4 atm of pressure as the waist persists. **E,** The waist has been fully dilated. *(Reproduced with permission from Schneider PA:* Endovascular skills, *ed 2, New York, 2003, Marcel Dekker.)*

one or more of these strengths. Basic categories of balloons follow.

1. A wide variety of lesions that require pressures of 2 to 10 atm and intended diameters of 4 to 10 mm may be treated by using standard polyethylene balloons through 5F or 6F sheaths placed over 0.035-inch guidewires.
2. Small-caliber balloons are available (1.5 to 4 mm in diameter), which may be placed through 4F sheaths over 0.014-inch or 0.018-inch guidewires. These catheters confer advantages in specific situations that require small-caliber balloons. Trackability and pushability are poor, however, especially from a very remote puncture site. These features may be improved by placing the sheath as close as possible to the target lesion. Balloon material is less durable and does not permit higher pressures.
3. With their success in coronary procedures, monorail or rapid-exchange systems have been employed in the peripheral vascular system as well. The advantage of this system is the lower profile and routine use of a 0.014-inch guidewire. The guidewire exits 20 to 25 cm from the tip through a side hole thus making it less cumbersome for the operator. The operator can control the guidewire and the catheter together. The disadvantage is that some stability and maneuverability are lost with the smaller platform system.
4. High-pressure balloons are made of more durable polymer material and may be inflated to pressures in excess of 20 atm. The shaft size is larger (5.8F or more), and the profile of the thicker balloon material is higher because the wings of the previously expanded balloon material are not completely collapsible. This requires use of a 7F or larger sheath. However, as stated previously, newer low-profile systems are now available, making this a more desirable option for lesions such as in-stent restenosis.
5. Larger-diameter balloons (>10 mm) are available for aortic or central venous angioplasty. Balloon diameters exceeding 20 mm in diameter are available on 5.8F shafts; however, the profile of these balloons is high, they require more time to inflate and deflate, and they are often more compliant than is desired.

CURRENT PRACTICE OF BALLOON ANGIOPLASTY

Indications for balloon angioplasty vary significantly from one vascular bed to another.[22,23] Balloon angioplasty plays a role, however, in the management of most vascular occlusive problems. Balloon angioplasty is also a useful tool during stent-graft placement for the management of aneurysm disease. In general, the best patients for balloon angioplasty are those with less extensive disease or those with medical comorbidities that contraindicate open surgery.[21,23] The best lesions for balloon angioplasty are focal stenoses and are located in large vessels with good runoff.[2,22] Stents have influenced this equation significantly, making it possible to treat more extensive lesions with angioplasty.[24,25]

The advantage of balloon angioplasty is that it permits mechanical intervention with less associated morbidity than most open surgical options and results in autologous revascularization; however, its use is limited by several factors. Many patients who present with threatening clinical problems have disease that is too extensive to be treated with angioplasty. Applications of balloon angioplasty have expanded dramatically since the development of stents. Balloon angioplasty offers limited long-term success in many settings; the patency and the durability are less than with surgery. Applications of angioplasty and short- and long-term success are limited in smaller-diameter arteries, especially those less than 5 mm in diameter.

ADDITIONAL BALLOON ANGIOPLASTY MODALITIES

Cryoplasty

The PolarCath (Boston Scientific) is a balloon angioplasty catheter that employs cold therapy via the use of nitrous oxide as the inflation material rather than the usual saline and contrast mix placed in an inflation device. The concept of inducing apoptosis via freezing is perceived to reduce the intimal hyperplastic response in the treated segment.[26] The device uses a battery-operated inflation device into which nitrous oxide cylinders are placed. The device then inflates in 2-atm increments to a nominal pressure of 8 atm. The controlled inflation is the other benefit of this balloon angioplasty catheter with reported low incidence of dissection. The registry data from the use of the PolarCath in the femoropopliteal segments have been favorable.[27,28]

Cutting Balloon

The cutting balloon (Boston Scientific) has been used in the coronary system for a number of years. It has been approved for use in the peripheral vascular system and is now available in larger sizes. The device has four longitudinal microsurgical blades (atherotomes) attached to the balloon. These atherotomes allow for the perceived benefit of a more controlled fracture and dilatation of the vessel. It ranges in balloon diameters from 2 to 8 mm but is only available in short lengths (1.5-2.0 cm). It is particularly useful in focal, fibrotic lesions such as vein graft stenosis.[29]

Scoring Balloon

The AngioSculpt (AngioScore, Fremont, CA) is similar to the cutting balloon, but instead of atherotomes it uses a flexible, nitinol scoring element with three rectangular spiral struts that score the target lesion. It is a low-profile system that is 0.018 inch or 0.014 inch, has balloon diameters of 2 to 5 mm, and is available in longer lengths.[30]

TECHNIQUE OF BALLOON ANGIOPLASTY

Equipment for Balloon Angioplasty

A wide selection of balloon angioplasty catheters should be readily available to the operator. A facility with trained support staff, an inventory of other endovascular supplies, and satisfactory radiographic imaging capabilities is essential (see Chapter 2, Preparing the Endovascular Operating Room Suite). Supplies that should be opened and should be placed on the sterile field are listed in Box 8-1.[31-33]

Approach to the Lesion

Before balloon angioplasty, the approach must be planned on the basis of the location of the lesion, its suitability for angioplasty, and the timing of proceeding with PTA. If the location and the appearance of the lesion are known as a result of a prior imaging study (e.g., duplex mapping, magnetic resonance angiography, computed tomographic angiography, or standard arteriography) and it is deemed suitable for angioplasty, the puncture site for remote access may be chosen accordingly. When arteriography is performed initially and PTA is added to the same procedure, the access site chosen for arteriography may be converted to use for a therapeutic procedure, or a new access site may be selected. The shortest distance that provides adequate working room is usually best. The operator should work forehand for best catheter control (Figure 8-3).

After the lesion has been identified, it is marked with external markers placed on the field, by observation of bony landmarks, or by using road-mapping. Heparin is administered. When stent placement is also anticipated, antibiotics are administered. The lesion is crossed with an appropriate guidewire before placing a sheath or opening angioplasty catheters. If the guidewire does not pass easily, the operator may decide on a different approach. If the lesion is preocclusive, the guidewire alone may inhibit flow. In that situation, the patient should be adequately heparinized, and the operator should proceed directly with PTA.

When an arteriographic procedure is converted to an angioplasty procedure, an appropriately sized sheath is placed to minimize injury to the access vessel and simplify access. The smallest-size sheath adequate for the intended balloon catheter is best because complications increase with increasing French size. Sheath changes in the middle of the procedure are awkward and inconvenient; therefore the operator should attempt to place the correct sheath when the decision is made to proceed with PTA. Guidelines for sheath sizing are presented in Table 8-2. The required sheath is selected on the basis of the desired type and diameter of the balloon, the size of the catheter, and the need for a stent.

BOX 8-1

SUPPLIES FOR BALLOON ANGIOPLASTY

Endovascular Inventory

- Balloon angioplasty catheters
- Stents
- Access sheaths
- Guidewires
- Angiographic catheters

Supplies for the Sterile Field

- 4 × 4 gauze
- Entry needle
- No. 11 scalpel
- Mosquito clamp
- Iodinated contrast agent
- Lidocaine local anesthetic agent
- 10-mL syringe
- 20-mL syringe or larger
- 25-gauge needle
- Inflation device
- Gown
- Gloves, drapes

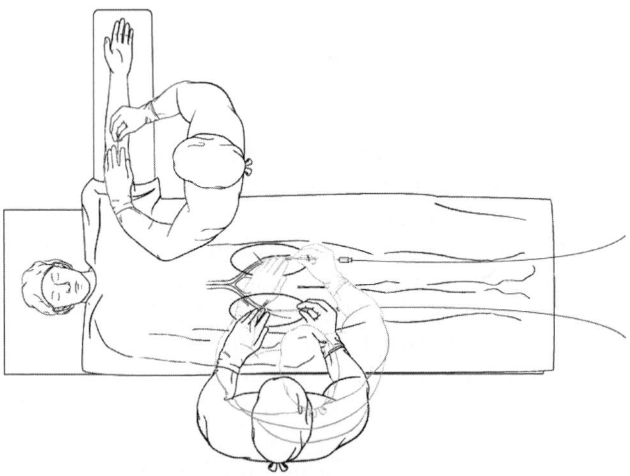

FIGURE 8-3 Working forehand. In this case, the right-handed operator works forehand to manipulate catheters and guidewires. The assistant stands to the side. The fluoroscopic image is observed on the monitor placed on the opposite side of the table. *(Reproduced with permission from Schneider PA:* Endovascular skills, *ed 2, New York, 2003, Marcel Dekker.)*

Selection of a Balloon Catheter

A slight overdilatation at the angioplasty site is generally recommended during standard angioplasty. Ranges of balloon sizes for specific PTA sites are listed in Table 8-3. The diameter of the normal vessel just distal to the lesion is measured to help assess the required balloon diameter (Figure 8-4). Digital subtraction filming requires the use of software measuring packages or the use of catheters with graduated measurement markers for size comparisons. In general, if there is uncertainty about the final desired diameter, it is best to begin with a smaller-diameter balloon and to upsize as needed to avoid overdilatation.

The balloon should be long enough so that there is a short distance of overhang into the adjacent artery. If

TABLE 8-2 Sheath Sizing Guidelines for Balloon Angioplasty

Sheath (F)	Balloon diameter (mm)	Balloon shaft (F)	Anticipated procedure
4	1.5-4	3.8	Small-vessel PTA* (0.014-inch or 0.018-inch guidewire)
5	3-6	5	Infrainguinal, or dialysis graft PTA without stent (0.035-inch guidewire)
6	Up to 8	5	Standard PTA—aortoiliac, infrainguinal, renal, or subclavian
6	Up to 9	5	Placement of balloon-expandable stent (4-9 mm)
6			Placement of self-expanding stent (≤10 mm)
7	Up to 8	5.8	PTA with high-pressure balloon
8	Up to 18	5.8	Aortic PTA
	6-8	5	Placement of 8F guiding catheter for renal, subclavian, or carotid PTA/stent
	8-12	5.8	Placement of balloon-expandable stent (up to 12 mm)
			Placement of self-expanding stent (≥12 mm)

**PTA,* Percutaneous transluminal angioplasty.

the lesion is lengthy or is juxtaposed to an area where dilatation is contraindicated, it is best to choose a shorter balloon and to dilate the lesion with several sequential balloon inflations. The length of the catheter shaft must be adequate to cover the distance from the access site to the lesion.

Balloon Catheter Placement

The selected balloon catheter is wiped and is flushed with heparinized saline solution but is not preinflated. When small-caliber balloon catheters are used, the inflation lumen is primed with dilute contrast to

TABLE 8-3 Selection of Balloon Angioplasty Catheters

			Shaft length (cm)	
Lesion site	**Balloon diameter (mm)**	**Balloon length (cm)**	**Femoral access**	**Brachial access**
Common carotid artery	6-8	2 or 4	120	—
Subclavian artery	6-8	2 or 4	120	75
Axillary artery	5-7	2 or 4	120	30
Renal artery	5-7	2 or 2 or 4	75	120
Aorta	8-18	4	75	—
Common iliac artery	6-10	2, 4, or 6	75*	120
External iliac artery	6-8	2, 4, or 6	75*	120
Superficial femoral artery	4-7	2, 4, 6, or 10	75†	120
Popliteal artery	3-6	2, 4, or 6	75†	120‡
Infrageniculate artery	2-4	2 or 4	75†	—

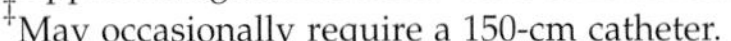

*Approaching these lesions via a contralateral femoral access site usually requires a 75-cm catheter.
†Approaching these lesions via a contralateral femoral access site usually requires a 120-cm catheter and occasionally may require a 150-cm catheter.
‡May occasionally require a 150-cm catheter.

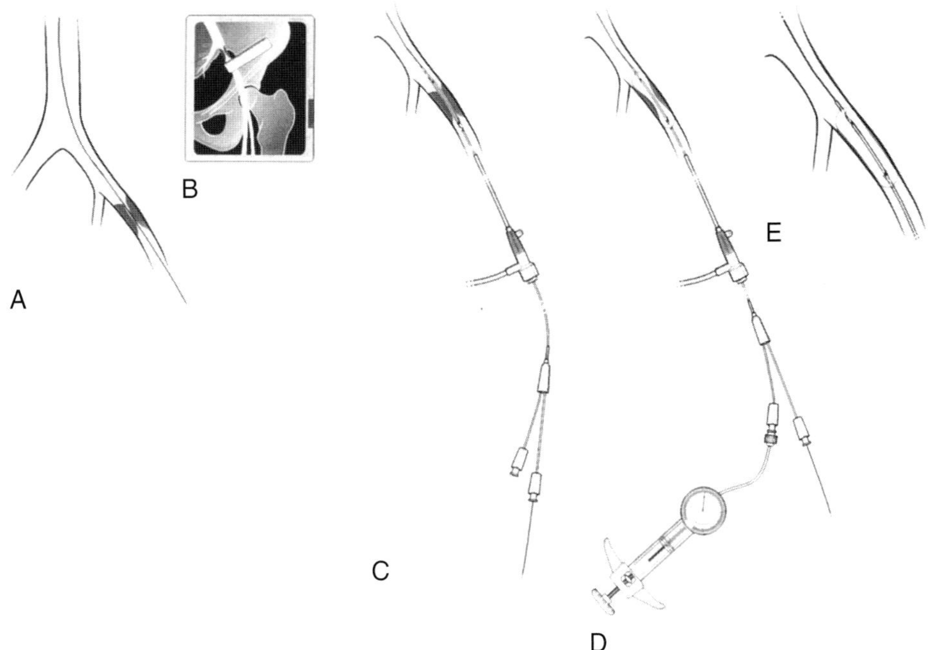

FIGURE 8-4 Balloon angioplasty. **A,** In this case, left external iliac artery stenosis is treated. A guidewire is placed across the lesion. **B,** The diameter of the balloon is selected. The diameter may be determined by measuring the diameter of the adjacent uninvolved artery, either by measuring cut film images directly or, if using digital subtraction imaging, by comparing with a known standard such as a catheter with graduated markers. **C,** The angioplasty catheter is passed over the guidewire, through the access sheath, and across the stenosis. **D,** The balloon is inflated by using the inflation device. **E,** The fully dilated shape of the balloon is confirmed by using fluoroscopy. *(Reproduced with permission from Schneider PA:* Endovascular skills, *ed 2, New York, 2003, Marcel Dekker.)*

help minimize retained air. After placement of the correctly sized sheath, the angioplasty catheter is passed over the guidewire, through the sheath, and into the lesion. The catheter should pass easily through the sheath because the balloon has not yet been inflated. The balloon catheter should track along the guidewire and should advance across the lesion using predetermined markers of the lesion's location. The balloon is centered so that its body dilates the portion of the lesion with the most critical stenosis. This is where the force vector will contribute substantially to the dilating force.

The balloon material may break by snagging on a protruding calcific lesion or a previously placed stent. If this is a concern, a longer sheath may be used to deliver the balloon to the lesion. If the balloon catheter will not track along the guidewire, this may be due to distance, lack of shaft strength, tortuosity, or even subintimal guidewire positioning. If this occurs, consider a stiffer guidewire or a longer sheath.

Occasionally, the lesion itself may be so tight that the balloon catheter cannot be advanced across it. If the balloon will cross the lesion only partially, do not start angioplasty. Withdraw the PTA catheter, and confirm guidewire positioning. Consider (1) adequate anticoagulation, (2) Dottering the lesion by advancing a straight 5F angiographic catheter across the lesion, (3) predilatation with a smaller-diameter (lower-profile) balloon, or (4) a balloon with a hydrophilic coating.

Balloon Inflation

After catheter placement, the balloon is inflated without delay to avoid thrombus formation. The balloon is inflated with use of a 50% contrast agent solution so that the outline of the balloon is visible under fluoroscopy. This permits the operator to observe the location and the severity of the atherosclerotic waist as it is being dilated. Solution is forced into the balloon with use of an inflation device, which also measures the pressure required to dilate the lesion.

The balloon is usually inflated slowly to the minimum pressure that allows the balloon to reach its full profile. Inflation is maintained for a minimum of 30 to 60 seconds and often longer. A spot film of the inflated balloon is often obtained to document its full expansion. After complete deflation of the balloon but before moving the catheter, fluoroscopy is used to visualize the balloon and to ensure that it is fully deflated. Partially flared balloon wings may disrupt fractured atherosclerotic plaque or may damage the tip of the access sheath on withdrawal. During removal of the balloon catheter, the guidewire must be maintained in place across the lesion.

TABLE 8-4 Assessing the Results of Balloon Angioplasty

Method	Comments
Completion arteriography	Only method required in most cases; usually performed in the projection used for PTA* (anteroposterior)
Oblique views	Useful in assessing posterior wall residual stenosis or postangioplasty dissection
Magnified views	Evaluation for dissection flaps or contrast trapping in arterial wall
Pressure measurement	Only quantitative hemodynamic assessment available; time-consuming; results variable; catheter placement across lesion may affect pressure in small-diameter artery
Vasodilator use	An adjunct to pressure measurement when there is no gradient despite the appearance of a substantial lesion
Intravascular ultrasonography	Expensive; particularly effective in finding and measuring diameter of residual stenosis

* *PTA,* Percutaneous transluminal angioplasty.

Completion Arteriography

After the balloon catheter is removed, completion arteriography is performed to evaluate the results of PTA. Completion arteriography is usually performed through the same access site used for balloon angioplasty. The guidewire may be exchanged for an angiographic catheter, which is placed upstream from the lesion. If the tip of the sheath is in proximity to the lesion, contrast material may be injected through the side arm of the sheath to obtain an arteriogram.

Assessment of Angioplasty Results

The most commonly used and readily available method of assessing angioplasty results is completion arteriography. When completion arteriography shows a widely patent PTA site without residual stenosis or significant dissection, the procedure is complete. When residual stenosis or dissection is present, its significance may be evaluated by using adjunctive means of assessment (Table 8-4). Inadequate angioplasty results may be treated with stent placement.[24,25] Stents and their indications are detailed in Chapter 10, Vascular Stents.

Handling of Balloon Catheters

The balloon angioplasty procedure is simpler and is less likely to result in complications when the catheters are handled with excellent technique. Advice about the use of balloon catheters is presented in Box 8-2.

BOX 8-2

HANDLING BALLOON CATHETERS

- Pick catheters before the case to save time and to be sure you have what you need.
- Flush and wipe catheter with heparinized saline solution to decrease thrombogenicity.
- Keep profile of catheter low by avoiding preinflation.
- Check the size of the catheter before placement to avoid unintended overdilatation.
- When correct catheter shaft length is unclear, measure outside the body with angiographic catheter of known length for a quick estimation.
- When best arterial diameter is unclear, underestimate to avoid overdilatation.
- Be sure guidewire is intraluminal before advancing and inflating balloon catheter.
- Push catheter from the tip when entering the hub of the access sheath to avoid kinking the guidewire and the catheter.
- Have some options when the catheter will not advance along the guidewire (see text discussion, Technique of Balloon Angioplasty).
- Be ready to inflate as soon as the balloon crosses the lesion.
- Magnify field of view at the PTA site if needed to ensure correct balloon position.
- Know what to do next when catheter will not advance through lesion (see text discussion, Technique of Balloon Angioplasty).
- Deflate the balloon by aspirating with a large syringe before withdrawal of catheter.
- Rotate the catheter to fold its wings before pulling it into the sheath.
- Employ fluoroscopy during inflation to confirm the location and the severity of the lesion.
- Take a spot film of expanded balloon after complete inflation for documentation and size comparisons.
- Maintain guidewire across the lesion until completion study is satisfactory.
- If balloon bursts, inflate rapidly until it will no longer hold pressure, then exchange it for a new balloon.
- If there is evidence of arterial rupture, reinflate balloon at same location to tamponade.

PTA, Percutaneous transluminal angioplasty.

TABLE 8.5 Complications of Balloon Angioplasty

Systemic	Puncture site	PTA* site	Runoff
Renal failure	Hemorrhage	Dissection	Embolization
Fluid overload	AV fistula	Residual stenosis	Thrombosis
Contrast agent allergy	Hematoma	Thrombosis	Spasm
	Ecchymosis	Rupture	
	Pseudoaneurysm		
	Thrombosis		

* *PTA,* Percutaneous transluminal angioplasty; *AV,* arteriovenous.

Complications of Balloon Angioplasty

The tremendous advantage of PTA is that the incidence and the severity of complications are generally low. Because the durability is not as good as with surgical reconstruction, PTA is useful only when complication rates are acceptable. Patients with very extensive disease are poor candidates for endovascular intervention and have a high chance of experiencing complications if it is attempted.[22] Complications may occur at the access site, at the PTA site, in the runoff, or systemically. Systemic complications and some access site complications may occur with arteriography alone. The total complication rate should be less than 10%, and the rate of serious complications (or those requiring operative intervention) should be less than 5% (Table 8-5).[2,22,23]

References

1. Becker GJ, Katzen BT, Dake MD: Noncoronary angioplasty, *Radiology* 170:921–946, 1989.
2. Johnston KW: Iliac arteries: reanalysis of results of balloon angioplasty, *Radiology* 186:207–212, 1993.
3. O'Donovan RM, Gutierrez OH, Izzo JL: Preservation of renal function by percutaneous renal angioplasty in high-risk elderly patients: short-term outcome, *Nephron* 60:187–192, 1992.
4. Englund R, Brown MA: Renal angioplasty for renovascular disease: a reappraisal, *J Cardiovasc Surg* 32:76–80, 1991.
5. Krepel VM, van Andel GJ, van Erp WFM, et al: Percutaneous transluminal angioplasty of the femoropopliteal artery: initial and long-term results, *Radiology* 156:325–328, 1985.
6. Becker GJ: Intravascular stents. General principles and status of lower extremity arterial applications, *Circulation* 83(suppl):I122–I136, 1991.

7. Gurm HS, Yadav JS, Fayad P, et al: Long-term results of carotid artery stenting versus endarterectomy in high risk patients, *N Engl J Med* 358:1572–1579, 2008.
8. van der Vaart MG, Meerwaldt R, et al: Endarterectomy or carotid stenting: the quest continues, *Am J Surg* 195:259–269, 2008.
9. Ringleb PA, Allenberg J, Bruckmann H, et al: Thirty-day results from the SPACE trial of stent-protected angioplasty versus carotid endarterectomy in symptomatic patients: a randomized non-inferiority trial, *Lancet* 368:1239–1247, 2006.
10. Hynes N, Mahendran B, Manning B, et al: The influence of subintimal angioplasty on level of amputation and limb salvage rates in lower limb critical limb ischemia, *Eur J Vasc Endovasc Surg* 30:291–299, 2005.
11. BASIL Trial participants: Bypass versus angioplasty in severe ischemia of the leg (BASIL): multicentre randomized controlled trial, *Lancet* 366:1925–1934, 2005.
12. Dosluoglu HH, Attuwayaybi B, Cherr GS, Harris LM, Dryjski ML: The management of ischemic heel ulcers and gangrene in the endovascular era, *Am J Surg* 194:600–605, 2007.
13. Kasirajan K, Schneider PA: Early outcome of "cutting" balloon angioplasty for infrainguinal vein graft stenosis, *J Vasc Surg* 39:702–708, 2004.
14. Castaneda-Zuniga WR, Formanek A, Tadavarthy M, et al: The mechanism of balloon angioplasty, *Radiology* 135:565, 1980.
15. Block PC, Baughman KL, Pasternak RC, et al: Transluminal angioplasty: correlation of morphologic and angiographic findings in an experimental model, *Circulation* 61:778, 1980.
16. Szlavy L, Taveras JM: Pathomechanism of percutaneous transluminal angioplasty. In: Szlavy L, Taveras JM, editors: *Noncoronary Angioplasty and Interventional Radiologic Treatment of Vascular Malformations*, Baltimore, 1995, William & Wilkins, pp 21–26.
17. Jain A, Demer LL: In vivo assessment of vascular dilatation during percutaneous transluminal coronary angioplasty, *Am J Cardiol* 60:988–992, 1987.
18. Zarins CK, Lu CT, Gewertz BL, et al: Arterial disruption and remodeling following balloon dilatation, *Surgery* 92:1086–1095, 1982.
19. Abele JE: Balloon catheters and transluminal dilatation: technical considerations, *AJR Am J Roentgenol* 135:901–906, 1980.
20. Orron DE, Kim D: Percutaneous transluminal angioplasty. In: Orron DE, Kim D, editors: *Peripheral Vascular Imaging and Intervention*, St. Louis, 1992, Mosby–Year Book, pp 380–383.
21. Gerlock AJ, Regen DM, Shaff MI: An examination of the physical characteristics leading to angioplasty balloon rupture, *Radiology* 144:421–422, 1982.
22. Pentecost MJ, Criqui MH, Dorros G, et al: Guidelines for peripheral percutaneous transluminal angioplasty of the abdominal aorta and lower extremity arteries, *Circulation* 89:511–531, 1994.
23. Schneider PA, Rutherford RB: Endovascular interventions in the management of chronic lower extremity ischemia. In: Rutherford RB, editor: *Vascular Surgery*, ed 5, Philadelphia, 2000, Saunders, pp 1035–1069.
24. Katzen BT, Becker GJ: Intravascular stents: status and development of clinical applications, *Surg Clin North Am* 72:941–957, 1992.
25. Sapoval MR, Chatellier G, Long AR, et al: Self-expandable stents for the treatment of iliac artery obstructive lesions: long-term success and prognostic factors, *AJR Am J Roentgenol* 166:1173–1179, 1996.
26. Yiu WK, Cheng SW, Sumpio BE: Vascular smooth muscle cell apoptosis induced by "supercooling" and rewarming, *J Interv Radiol* 16:1067–1073, 2005.
27. Laird JR, Jaff MR, Biamino G, McNamara T, Schneinert D, Zetterlund P, et al: Cryoplasty for the treatment of femoropopliteal arterial disease: results of a multicenter prospective registry, *J Vasc Interv Radiol* 16:1067–1073, 2005.
28. Laird JR, Jaff MR, Biamino G, et al: Cryoplasty for the treatment of femoropopliteal arterial disease: extended follow-up results, *J Endovasc Ther* 13:II-52–II-59, 2006.
29. Schneider PA, Caps MT, Nelken N: Infrainguinal vein graft stenosis: cutting balloon angioplasty as the first-line treatment of choice, *J Vasc Surg* 47:960–966, 2008.
30. Scheinert D, Peeters P, Bosiers M, et al: Results of Multicenter first-in-man study of a novel scoring balloon catheter for the treatment of infra-popliteal peripheral arterial disease, *Cath Cardiovasc Interv* 70:1034–1039, 2007.
31. Hinink MGM, Kandarpa K: Extremity balloon angioplasty. In: Kandarpa K, Aruny JE, editors: *Handbook of Interventional Radiologic Procedures*, Boston, Little, 1996, Brown, pp 69–80.
32. Schneider PA: Balloon angioplasty: minimally invasive autologous revascularization. In: Schneider PA, editor: *Endovascular Skills*, St. Louis, 1998, Quality Medical Publishing, pp 107–117.
33. Ahn SS, Obrand DI: Percutaneous transluminal angioplasty. In: *Handbook of Endovascular Surgery*, Georgetown, TX, 1997, Karger-Landes, pp 59–74.

CHAPTER

9

Peripheral Atherectomy

Donald T. Baril, Rabih A. Chaer

Peripheral atherectomy provides an alternative approach to the treatment of atherosclerotic occlusive disease beyond angioplasty and stenting. Atherectomy works via debulking atherosclerotic lesions (including heavily calcified lesions and those with large quantities of thrombus), which has been postulated to lower restenosis rates by removing the offending plaque rather than simply dilating the existing lumen and leaving disease in situ. Furthermore, atherectomy may be used to treat lesions involving a joint space that are under continuous dynamic stress forces, areas where stents may be at increased risk of fracture and subsequent failure. At present, there are three U.S. Food and Drug Administration (FDA)–approved atherectomy devices, the SilverHawk Plaque Excision System (FoxHollow Technologies, Redwood City, CA) (Figure 9-1), the Diamondback 360 Orbital Atherectomy System (Cardiovascular Systems, St. Paul, MN) (Figure 9-2), and the CVX-300 Excimer Laser (Spectranetics, Colorado Springs, CO) (Figure 9-3). There is one additional device, the Pathway PV Atherectomy System (Pathway Medical Technologies Inc., Kirkland, WA), which is currently under clinical trial (Figure 9-4).

HISTORY

Percutaneous atherectomy as an endovascular modality was initially applied in the coronary bed. However, despite the theoretic advantages, several studies showed unfavorable long-term results compared with angioplasty.[1,2] Other studies demonstrated the efficacy of atherectomy when used to treat select lesions with aggressive plaque removal and balloon postdilatation.[3,4] This same technology was subsequently applied to the first generation of peripheral atherectomy devices, including the Simpson AeroCath (Guidant, Santa Clara, CA) and the Auth Rotablator (Boston Scientific, Natick, MA). Despite high initial technical success rates, these devices were associated with poor intermediate and long-term patency rates. Subsequent advances have led to the current generation of atherectomy devices, which are now being applied to treat lesions in both the femoropopliteal and infrapopliteal segments.

ATHERECTOMY DEVICES

Atherectomy devices work via varying mechanisms to remove the offending lesions. Both the SilverHawk Plaque Excision System and the Pathway PV Atherectomy System use a rotational blade to excise plaque. The Diamondback 360 Orbital Atherectomy System relies on the principle of centrifugal force, using an eccentrically mounted diamond-coated crown that rotates at high speed to sand away plaque. The CVX-300 Excimer Laser uses ultraviolet light delivered in short, controlled energy pulses to dissolve arterial plaque (Table 9-1).

INDICATIONS

All the current atherectomy devices are indicated for the treatment of lower-extremity arterial atherosclerotic lesions and symptoms ranging from disabling claudication to critical limb ischemia, including tissue loss and gangrene. These devices are useful to treat areas of high-stress and repetitive motion, where a stent may be prone to fracture or kinking. Furthermore, they may be used to treat lesions at arterial bifurcations or trifurcations in the lower extremities, where angioplasty and/or stenting may jeopardize the artery adjacent to the target vessel.

The SilverHawk Plaque Excision System may be used throughout the infrainguinal arterial system, including the femoropopliteal and infrapopliteal segments. The Diamondback 360 Orbital Atherectomy System may be

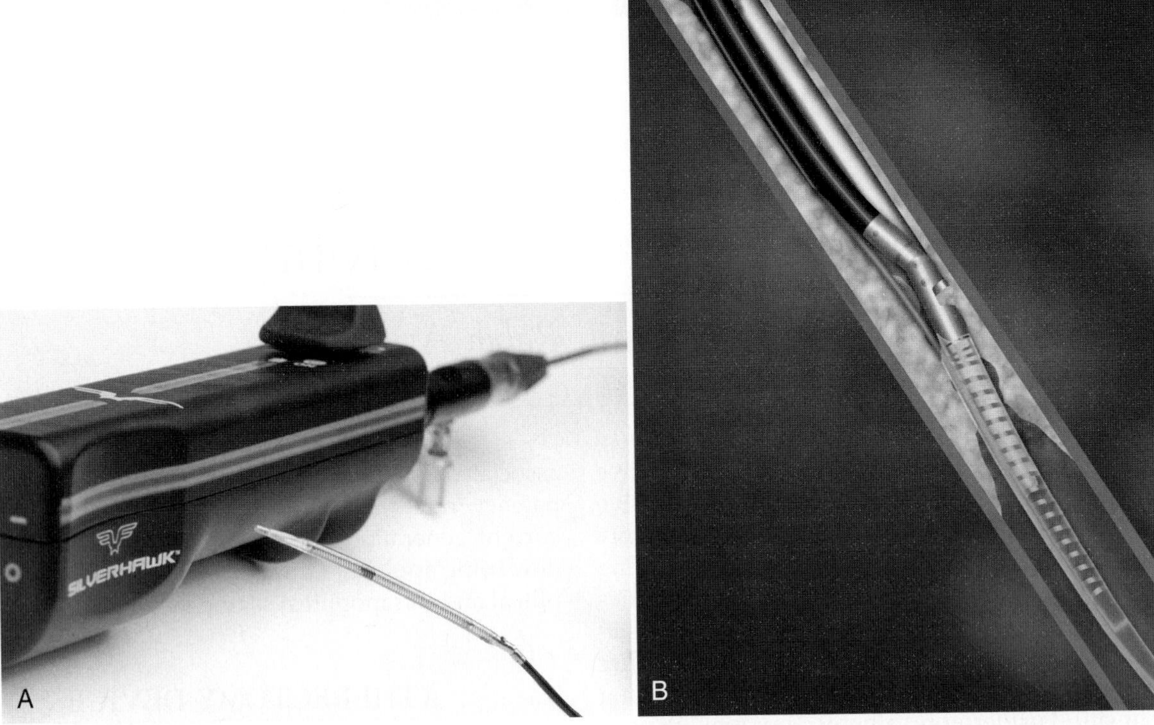

FIGURE 9-1 SilverHawk atherectomy catheter. **A,** Battery-powered motor and atherectomy catheter. **B,** Cutting blade engaging plaque.

used in both the femoropopliteal and infrapopliteal segments as well. The Pathway PV Atherectomy System has been applied in both the femoropopliteal and infrapopliteal segments in clinical trials. Finally, the CVX-300 Excimer Laser may also be used in the femoropopliteal and infrapopliteal segments. However, adjunctive angioplasty is typically necessary when this device is used in the femoropopliteal segment.

SILVERHAWK PLAQUE EXCISION SYSTEM

The SilverHawk atherectomy catheter was approved for peripheral arterial use in 2003 by the FDA. The SilverHawk catheter debulks lesions without the use of a balloon and instead relies on self-apposition against plaque through a hinged system at the distal end of the catheter. The device consists of a detachable, battery-powered motor that attaches to a 0.014-inch monorail atherectomy catheter. The tip of the catheter contains a rotating blade and a plaque collection chamber. The carbide cutting blade rotates at 8000 rpm when activated. This blade has a concave design that is designed to shave the plaque and then pack it into the nose cone storage compartment. The operator places the tip of the catheter just proximal to the target lesion, activates the blade, and then slowly advances the tip of the catheter through the entire length of the lesion, periodically emptying the nose cone. This process is repeated until an adequate flow channel is achieved. The tip of the catheter may be rotated 360 degrees, and thus plaque excision may be carried out in all four quadrants of the lumen. Once the nose cone collection unit is full, the entire catheter must be removed before reinsertion and additional passages.

There are a number of different size catheters available that may treat target vessel sizes ranging from 2 to 7 mm. All of these require a sheath ranging in size from 5F to 8F, are introduced over a 0.014-inch guidewire, and have a crossing profile of 1.9 to 2.7 mm. Access may be achieved via either a contralateral common femoral arterial puncture or an antegrade approach. The use of a filter to protect against distal embolization is optional. The catheter may be used in the flow channel or in a subintimal plane. An additional catheter, the RockHawk (ev3 Endovascular, Plymouth, MN) system, has incorporated changes in the geometry and the material of the cutter structure of the other available catheters to facilitate the breakdown of hard, calcified lesions. A second additional system, the NightHawk (FoxHollow Technologies, Redwood City, CA), which is in clinical trial, uses optical coherence tomography imaging technology embedded in the catheter in conjunction with

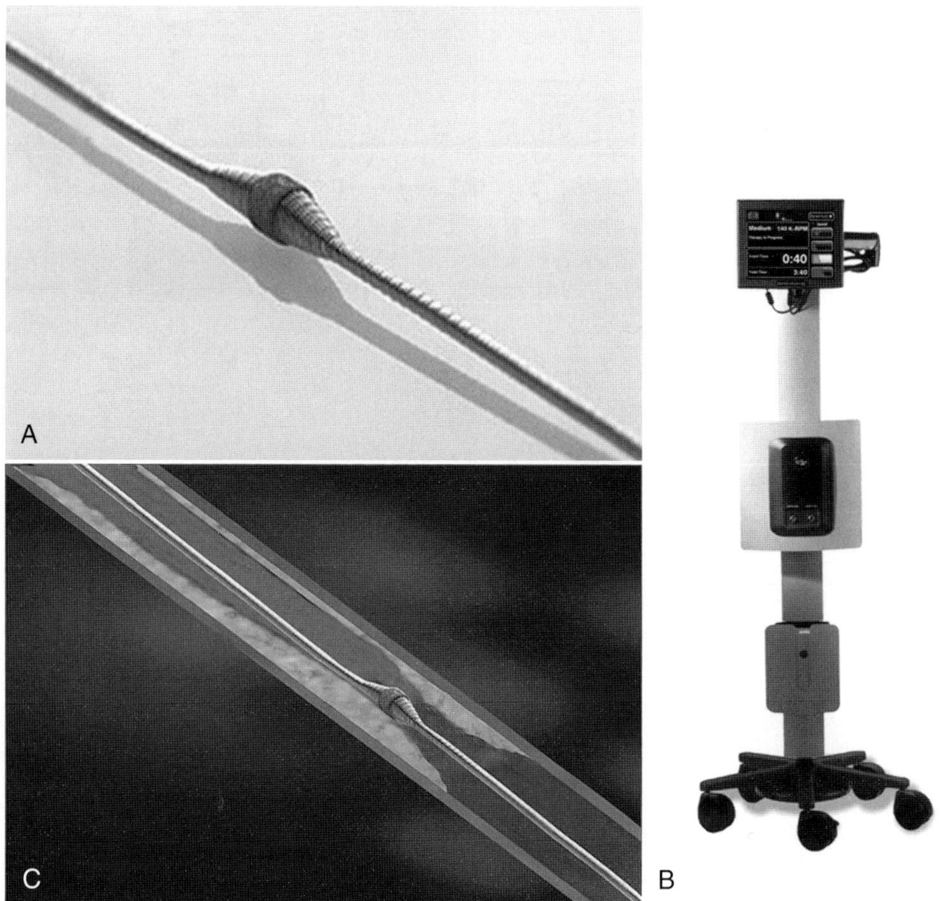

FIGURE 9-2 Diamondback 360 Orbital Atherectomy System. **A,** Diamond grit–coated device. **B,** System base with touch-screen operation panel. **C,** Device engaged in sanding atherosclerotic lesion.

the SilverHawk plaque excision mechanism. The NightHawk device allows for precise visualization of the vascular wall, which provides adjunctive data to conventional angiography during plaque excision.

Results

Although there are no randomized data with regard to the SilverHawk atherectomy catheter, there have been several reports demonstrating its efficacy for the treatment of atherosclerotic lesions in both the femoropopliteal and the infrapopliteal segments. Zeller et al.[5] reported 71 lesions treated in 52 patients with an average lesion length of 48 ± 64 mm. Forty-two percent of these were primary stenoses, 38% were native vessel restenoses, and 20% were in-stent restenoses (which were performed outside of the manufacturer's instructions for use). Adjunctive angioplasty was used in 58% of these procedures, whereas stenting was used in 6%. Primary patency rates at 6 months were 80% for primary lesions, 63% for postangioplasty lesions, and 71% for in-stent restenoses. Zeller et al.[6] subsequently reported longer-term data of 131 lesions in 84 patients with 12-month primary patency rates (as defined by <50% restenoses on ultrasound) of 84% for de novo lesions, 54% for native vessel restenoses, and 54% for in-stent restenoses. At 18 months, these fell to 73%, 42%, and 49% respectively; however, secondary patency rates were 89%, 67%, and 79%.

The largest outcome data of the SilverHawk atherectomy catheter are the nonrandomized, manufacturer-sponsored TALON registry (Treating Peripherals With SilverHawk: Outcomes Collection), which involved 19 centers in the United States and collected data on 1,258 lesions treated in 601 patients.[7] Mean lesion length was 62.5 ± 68.5 mm above the knee and 33.4 ± 42.7 mm below the knee. Procedural success was 97.6% with less than 50% residual stenosis achieved in 94.7% of lesions. Adjunctive angioplasty was used in 21.7% of cases and stenting in 6.3% of cases. Six-month and 12-month freedoms from target lesion revascularization were 90% and 80%. Predictors of target lesion revascularization included a history of myocardial infarction or coronary revascularization and increasing Rutherford classification.

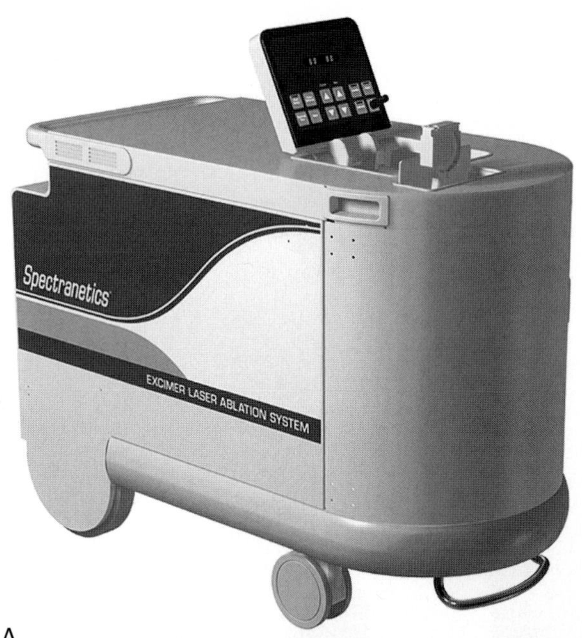

A

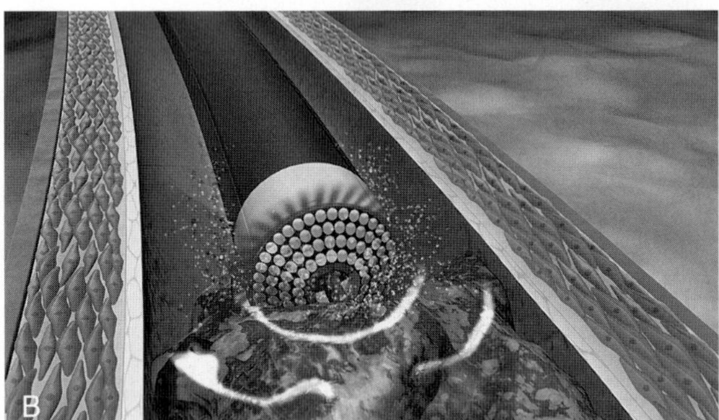

B

FIGURE 9-3 CVX-300 Excimer Laser. **A,** CVX-300 Excimer Laser system base unit. **B,** Plaque photoablation by the Turbo Elite catheter.

Recent data from a prospectively maintained database of 559 lesions treated in 255 patients included 228 in the superficial femoral artery (106 occlusions), 176 in the popliteal artery (84 occlusions), and 229 in the infrapopliteal arteries (130 occlusions).[8] Eighteen-month primary and secondary patency rates for all lesions were 45.9% ± 3.4% and 80.3% ± 2.5%, respectively, with reported 18-month primary and secondary patency rates for claudicants of 59.2% ± 4.9% and 88.1% ± 3.3% and for patients with critical limb ischemia of 34.3% ± 4.5% and 73.6% ± 3.6%. Overall limb salvage was 93.1%.

The use of the SilverHawk atherectomy catheter specifically for the treatment of critical limb ischemia has also been reported. Kandzari et al.[9] reported the results of 160 lesions in 74 limbs ranging from the external iliac to the dorsalis pedis in patients with Rutherford class 5 and 6 disease. Mean above-knee lesion length was 74 ± 88 mm. Technical success was achieved in 99% of patients, with 17% requiring adjunctive angioplasty and/or stenting. The primary end point evaluated was a major event (death, myocardial infarction, unplanned amputation, or repeat target vessel revascularization). At 6 months, 23% of patients met this end point. Amputations that were less extensive than initially planned or avoided completely occurred in 93% of patients at 30 days and 82% at 6 months. Keeling et al.[10] also reported on the use of the SilverHawk atherectomy catheter for the treatment of both claudicants and patients with critical limb ischemia. The technical success was 87.1% with a 1-year primary patency rate of 61.7%. Restenosis was higher in patients with Transatlantic Intersociety Consensus (TASC) C or D lesions compared with those with TASC A or B lesions.

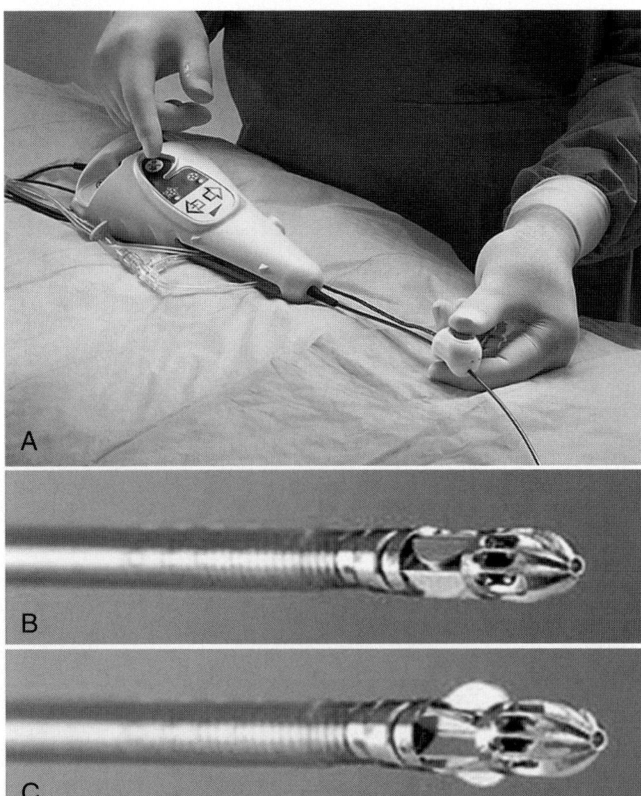

A

B

C

FIGURE 9-4 Pathway PV Atherectomy System. **A,** Control pod, which provides rotational drive to the catheter and allows for control of device rotational speed and tip size. **B,** Catheter tip shown when spinning in a clockwise direction at a set diameter of 2.1 mm. **C,** Catheter tip shown when spinning in a counterclockwise direction at a diameter of 3.0 mm.

Zeller et al.[11] reported additional data on the use of the SilverHawk atherectomy catheter for infrapopliteal lesions alone on 52 lesions in 33 patients. Atherectomy was used alone in 71%. Restenosis (>70% on ultrasound examination) was observed in 14% of lesions at 3 months and 22% at 6 months; however, the cumulative patency rate was 94.1% at 6 months.

TABLE 9-1 Atherectomy Devices

	SilverHawk Plaque Excision System	CVX-300 Excimer Laser	Diamondback 360 Orbital Atherectomy System	Pathway PV Atherectomy System
Manufacturer	FoxHollow Technologies (Redwood City, CA)	Spectranetics (Colorado Springs, CO)	Cardiovascular Systems Inc. (St. Paul, MN)	Pathway Medical Technologies Inc. (Kirkland, WA)
FDA approved	Yes	Yes	Yes	No
Mechanism	Rotational blade plaque excision	Ultraviolet light plaque dissolution	Centrifugal force plaque sanding	Rotational blade plaque excision
Catheter tip size (mm)	1.9-2.7	0.9-2.5	1.25-2.25	2.1
Sheath size (F)	5-8	4-8	6-7	8
Guidewire (in.)	0.014	0.014 or 0.018	0.014	0.014

Complications

The primary complications associated with this device include perforation and distal embolization. Using the first-generation device, Suri et al.[12] reported a 100% rate of embolic debris in 13 lesions treated with the SilverHawk atherectomy catheter with the concomitant use of a FilterWire (Boston Scientific, Natick, MA). This embolic debris ranged in size from 0.5 to 10 mm and, in one patient, led to vessel occlusion that resolved with removal of the filter. Lam et al.[13] also detected emboli during use of the SilverHawk atherectomy catheter using simultaneous Doppler monitoring. Of note, in this study, emboli were detected during the period between passes of the catheter, indicating that debris may shower from the disrupted intimal surface. However, no patient had any clinically significant sequelae from these emboli.

DIAMONDBACK 360 ORBITAL ATHERECTOMY SYSTEM

The Diamondback 360 Orbital Atherectomy System device differs from other atherectomy technologies in that it uses orbiting action to remove plaque and increases lumen diameter by increasing the orbital speed (80,000 to 200,000 rpm). An eccentrically mounted diamond-coated crown rotates at high speed at the end of the catheter to sand away plaque as the crown is slowly advanced through the target lesion. As crown rotation increases, centrifugal force presses the crown against the lesion to effect plaque removal, while the less diseased, more elastic arterial wall flexes away from the crown, minimizing the risk of vessel trauma.[14] As with the other atherectomy devices, the crown is positioned at the proximal portion of the target lesion and slowly advanced. This crown is manufactured in sizes of 1.25 mm, 1.50 mm, 1.75 mm, 2.00 mm, and 2.25 mm to allow for final lumen diameters ranging from 1.25 mm to 3.50 mm based on the rotational speed. This device is placed over a 0.014-inch guidewire and requires a 6F or 7F sheath for access depending on the device size.

Results

The only reported data on outcomes using the Diamondback 360 Orbital Atherectomy System are from the Orbital Atherectomy System Investigational Study (OASIS) trial, a prospective, multicenter, clinical study that enrolled 124 patients with 201 lesions.[15] Fifty-one percent of these lesions were reported to be noncalcified, and 85% were infrapopliteal. This study demonstrated an acute debulking rate, as measured angiographically, of 62%. Device success, as defined by less than 30% residual stenosis on angiography after orbital atherectomy alone, was 78%. The use of adjunctive angioplasty and/or stenting for 84 lesions (42%) increased this to 93%. Ankle-brachial indices were 0.68 at baseline, 0.90 at 30 days, and 0.82 at 6 months. Additionally, the 6-month target lesion revascularization rate was 0.9%.

Complications

In the OASIS trial, there was a serious adverse event rate of 8%, although only 3.2% of these were directly device related. These device-related complications consisted of thrombus formation at the site of the treated lesion, perforations (at the site of the target lesion and distal to the lesion), and embolization.

CVX-300 EXCIMER LASER

The CVX-300 Excimer Laser is used in conjunction with the Turbo-Booster or the Turbo Elite catheter. The laser removes plaque through photoablation, using light to vaporize and ablate tissue. The CVX-300 uses exact energy control with shallow tissue penetration to decrease the thermal injury to the native artery. The energy is released in short pulses rather than in continuous fashion, as was used in previous devices. These short pulses reduce tissue that is within 50 μm of the laser tip to molecular particles through the breaking of molecular bonds, through molecular vibration with resultant heat production, and through the expansion and collapse of vapor bubbles at the laser tip. Plaque is broken down into particles less than 10 μm in size.

The CVX-300 Excimer Laser in combination with the Turbo-Booster or the Turbo Elite catheter may be used for stenoses or complete occlusions. The laser can be used to cross chronic total occlusions by using the "step-by-step" technique whereby the catheter tip is placed in direct contact with the proximal portion of the lesion. The laser is then activated for 5 to 10 seconds and is advanced through the plaque with or without the support of a guidewire. For stenoses, the guidewire is passed beyond the lesion, and the catheter is slowly advanced though the lesion at a rate of 0.5 to 1 mm/s. This is typically not a standalone device because the lumen size obtained is generally 1.5 times the size of the probe, thereby almost always requiring adjunctive balloon angioplasty.

The Turbo-Booster and the Turbo Elite catheters range in working length from 110 to 150 cm with diameters from 0.9 to 2.5 mm. These are introduced over either 0.014-inch or 0.018-inch guidewires through 4F to 8F sheaths depending on the catheter size. The Turbo-Booster allows for directional atherectomy, therefore resulting in a large flow channel in the femoropopliteal segment. This modality may therefore prove to be the preferred method for the treatment of in-stent restenosis.

Results

There have been a number of reports demonstrating the safety and efficacy of the excimer laser for the treatment of infrainguinal occlusive disease. The Peripheral Excimer Laser Angioplasty (PELA) study was a multicenter, prospective, randomized trial comparing laser atherectomy with angioplasty versus angioplasty alone for long superficial femoral artery occlusions.[16] Procedural success was 85% in the laser group and 91% in the angioplasty-alone group. Complication rates were similar, and 12-month primary patency rates were the same for both groups (49%). However, the laser group required less stent implantation compared with the angioplasty group (42% vs. 59%).

Scheinert et al.[17] reported 411 lesions in 318 patients treated with laser-assisted recanalization of chronic superficial femoral artery occlusions with a 90.5% technical success rate. Stent usage was required in 7.3% of cases. At 1 year, primary patency, assisted primary patency, and secondary patency rates were 20.1%, 64.6%, and 75.1%, respectively.

The Laser Angioplasty for Critical Limb Ischemia (LACI) trial was a multicenter trial that enrolled 145 patients who were deemed poor surgical candidates.[18] A total of 423 lesions were treated in 155 limbs. Adjunctive angioplasty was used in 96% of cases and stenting in 45%. Ankle–brachial indices (ABIs) improved from 0.54 ± 0.21 to 0.84 ± 0.20. Six-month limb salvage was 92.5%.

Stoner et al.[19] reported midterm results of 40 patients treated with laser atherectomy with an average follow-up of 461 ± 49 days. Forty-seven lesions were treated, and adjunctive angioplasty was used in 75% of cases. The overall technical success rate (<50% residual stenosis) was 88%. The overall 12-month primary patency was 44%, and the 12-month limb salvage rate in 26 patients with critical limb ischemia was 55%. Chronic renal failure, diabetes mellitus, and poor tibial runoff were all associated with worse outcomes.

Complications

As with the other atherectomy devices, laser atherectomy has a risk of perforation, dissection, thrombosis at the site of atherectomy, and distal embolization. Scheniert et al.[17] reported a perforation rate of 2.2% and a distal embolization and thrombosis rate of 3.9% in their series. The overall procedural complication rate reported from the LACI trial was 12% and included major dissection (4%), thrombosis (3%), distal embolization (3%), and perforation (2%).

PATHWAY PV ATHERECTOMY SYSTEM

The Pathway PV Atherectomy System, which is not yet FDA approved and remains in trial phase, is a rotating, aspirating, expandable catheter that actively removes atherosclerotic debris and thrombus. The Pathway PV System uses a cutting catheter tip that is designed to preferentially remove diseased tissue with minimal damage to the arterial wall. The catheter tip remains at a set diameter of 2.1 mm when spinning in a clockwise direction but expands up to a maximum diameter of 3.0 mm when rotating in a counterclockwise direction. There is an attached control pod that provides rotational drive to the catheter and allows for control of both the device rotational speed and the tip size. Saline solution is delivered to the proximal end of the catheter with use of two separate lines; one of these flushes the motor assembly, while the other infuses saline solution to the treatment area to maximize the catheter's debulking and aspiration capabilities. Excised material is aspirated via ports in the tip into the catheter lumen and transported to a collection bag. This device requires an 0.014-inch guidewire and an 8F sheath. Once introduced to the segment of the target lesion, the catheter tip is placed just proximal to the lesion and then advanced at a maximum rate of 1 mm/s once engaged.

Results

Zeller et al.[20] reported the initial use of the Pathway PV Atherectomy System in 15 patients with a mean lesion length of 61 ± 62 mm. Initial technical success was 100%. Atherectomy alone was performed in 6 (40%) patients, adjunctive balloon angioplasty in 7 (47%), and stenting/endografting in 2 (13%). Primary patency rates, measured by duplex ultrasound scan, at 1 and 6 months were 100% and 73%. Furthermore, the target lesion revascularization rate was 0% at 6 months. ABIs increased significantly from 0.54 ± 0.3 at baseline to 0.89 ± 0.16, 0.88 ± 0.19, and 0.81 ± 0.20 at discharge, 1 month, and 6 months, respectively. Additionally, mean Rutherford categories were 2.92 ± 1.19, 0.64 ± 1.12, and 0.83 ± 1.33 at discharge, 1 month, and 6 months.

Since the initial report, Zeller[21] has presented additional data from a 172-patient multicenter registry. Initial technical success was 99%. Fifty-seven percent of patients required adjuvant angioplasty, and 7% required adjuvant stenting. Target lesion revascularization was 13.8% at 6 months. Mean ABIs were 0.60 ± 0.21 at baseline, 0.91 ± 0.25 at 30 days, and 0.76 ± 0.24 at 6 months. Preliminary data collected from 37 patients using the second-generation device have also been presented. Mean ABIs increased from 0.60 ± 0.28 at baseline to 0.85 ± 0.15 at 30 days. Additionally, Rutherford class decreased from 3.03 ± 0.87 at baseline to 0.90 ± 1.11 at 30 days.

Complications

In the initial report of outcomes in 15 patients, Zeller[21] reported a serious adverse event rate at 30 days of 20%, including one perforation, one pseudoaneurysm at the puncture site, and one dissection in conjunction with a distal embolism. From the subsequent registry data, a major adverse event rate of only 2.9% was reported in 172 patients, consisting primarily of dissection, embolization, and target vessel revascularization.

CONCLUSION

Peripheral atherectomy has continued to evolve since its adaptation from the coronary technology, with a new generation of devices providing an additional means of treating infrainguinal atherosclerotic disease. Atherectomy provides several theoretic advantages compared with angioplasty and stenting including debulking of lesions, minimizing barotrauma by obviating the need for high-pressure angioplasty, and avoidance of the placement of a permanent prosthesis within the treated artery. Furthermore, for anatomic locations that are subject to repetitive force and stress, atherectomy offers an alternative to stenting in such segments, which may place a stent at high risk of fracture and kinking. Additionally, ostial lesions can be treated by atherectomy with less concern of proximal dissection or stent impingement into normal-flow lumens.

Immediate procedural success of these devices has been excellent, but longer-term data are limited. Moreover, the midterm data that have been reported have shown relatively high rates of restenosis. At present, the high restenosis rates reported in most series may not justify the cost and widespread use of the current atherectomy devices. Although it is evident that there are certain clinical scenarios where peripheral atherectomy may be the best therapeutic option, longer-term, randomized data are necessary to better determine the efficacy of these devices and their role in the treatment of infrainguinal atherosclerotic disease.

References

1. Mauri L, Reisman M, Buchbinder M, et al: Comparison of rotational atherectomy with conventional balloon angioplasty in the prevention of restenosis of small coronary arteries: results of the Dilatation vs Ablation Revascularization Trial Targeting Restenosis (DART), *Am Heart J* 145(5):847–854, 2003.
2. vom Dahl J, Dietz U, Haager PK, et al: Rotational atherectomy does not reduce recurrent in-stent restenosis: results of the Angioplasty Versus Rotational atherectomy for Treatment of Diffuse In-stent Restenosis Trial (ARTIST), *Circulation* 105(5):583–588, 2002.
3. Simonton CA, Leon MB, Baim DS, et al: 'Optimal' directional coronary atherectomy: final results of the Optimal Atherectomy Restenosis Study (OARS), *Circulation* 97(4):332–339, 1998.
4. Suzuki T, Hosokawa H, Katoh O, et al: Effects of adjunctive balloon angioplasty after intravascular ultrasound-guided optimal directional coronary atherectomy: the result of Adjunctive Balloon Angioplasty After Coronary Atherectomy Study (ABACAS), *J Am Coll Cardiol* 34(4):1028–1035, 1999.
5. Zeller T, Rastan A, Schwarzwälder U, et al: Percutaneous peripheral atherectomy of femoropopliteal stenoses using a new-generation device: six-month results from a single-center experience, *J Endovasc Ther* 11(6):676–685, 2004.
6. Zeller T, Rastan A, Sixt S, et al: Long-term results after directional atherectomy of femoro-popliteal lesions, *J Am Coll Cardiol* 48(8): 1573–1578, 2006.
7. Ramaiah V, Gammon R, Kiesz S, et al: Midterm outcomes from the TALON Registry: treating peripherals with SilverHawk: outcomes collection, *J Endovasc Ther* 13(5):592–602, 2006.
8. McKinsey J. Novel Treatment of patients with lower extremity ischemia: use of percutaneous atherectomy in 559 lesions. Presented at the American Surgical Association. April 24, 2008, New York, NY.
9. Kandzari DE, Kiesz RS, Allie D, et al: Procedural and clinical outcomes with catheter-based plaque excision in critical limb ischemia, *J Endovasc Ther* 13(1):12–22, 2006.

10. Keeling WB, Shames ML, Stone PA, et al: Plaque excision with the Silverhawk catheter: early results in patients with claudication or critical limb ischemia, *J Vasc Surg* 45(1):25–31, 2007.
11. Zeller T, Sixt S, Schwarzwälder U, et al: Two-year results after directional atherectomy of infrapopliteal arteries with the SilverHawk device, *J Endovasc Ther* 14(2):232–240, 2007.
12. Suri R, Wholey MH, Postoak D, et al: Distal embolic protection during femoropopliteal atherectomy, *Catheter Cardiovasc Interv* 67(3):417–422, 2006.
13. Lam RC, Shah S, Faries PL, et al: Incidence and clinical significance of distal embolization during percutaneous interventions involving the superficial femoral artery, *J Vasc Surg* 46(6): 1155–1159, 2007.
14. Heuser RR: Treatment of lower extremity vascular disease: the Diamondback 360 Degrees Orbital Atherectomy System, *Expert Rev Med Devices* 5(3):279–286, 2008.
15. Dave R. Orbital atherectomy in infrainguinal disease. Presented at Capital Cardiovascular Conference. September 9-12, 2007, Harrisburg, PA.
16. Laird JR. Peripheral Excimer Laser Angioplasty (PELA) trial results. Presented at Transcatheter Cardiovascular Therapeutics. September 24-28, 2002, Washington, D.C.
17. Scheinert D, Laird JR Jr, Schröder M, et al: Excimer laser-assisted recanalization of long, chronic superficial femoral artery occlusions, *J Endovasc Ther* 8(2):156–166, 2001.
18. Laird JR, Zeller T, Gray BH, et al: Limb salvage following laser-assisted angioplasty for critical limb ischemia: results of the LACI multicenter trial, *J Endovasc Ther* 13(1):1–11, 2006.
19. Stoner MC, deFreitas DJ, Phade SV, et al: Mid-term results with laser atherectomy in the treatment of infrainguinal occlusive disease, *J Vasc Surg* 46(2):289–295, 2007.
20. Zeller T, Krankenberg H, Rastan A, et al: Percutaneous rotational and aspiration atherectomy in infrainguinal peripheral arterial occlusive disease: a multicenter pilot study, *J Endovasc Ther* 14(3): 357–364, 2007.
21. Zeller T. The Pathway Medical Device: 6-month results from the European Gen-1 Registry and preliminary results with the Gen-2 Device. Presented at Transcatheter Cardiovascular Therapeutics October 20-25, 2007, Washington, D.C.

CHAPTER

10

Vascular Stents

Feng Qin, Thomas F. Panetta

The use of stents in vascular surgery is a rapidly growing field. Although the clinical use of stents has expanded tremendously, approval by the Food and Drug Administration (FDA) for peripheral vascular use is variable. This has resulted in continued "off-label use" of many stents for vascular applications. Although the FDA does not prevent the utilization of stents for clinical indications, it does regulate inappropriate marketing by industry for off-label use. With the advent of new stent technologies, endovascular treatment of many vascular diseases has become the mainstream therapy. More recently, novel covered stents, heparin bonded stents, drug-eluting stents, and biodegradable stents are evolving for use in the peripheral circulation.[1]

The concept of vascular stents was first described in 1912 by Alexis Carrel.[2] However, it was not until 1964 that the concept was revisited by Charles Dotter, who described the need for an endoluminal "splint" after angioplasty to prevent early failure due to recoil and dissection.[3] In 1969, Dotter[4] described the percutaneous transluminal insertion of coil-spring, stainless-steel, wire stents in the popliteal arteries of dogs. Along with the observations of Julio Palmaz, his work inspired the development of the modern-day stents, as well as the variety of stents that are currently being developed.

STENT CLASSIFICATION

The metals used for stents include stainless steel, nitinol, tantalum, platinum, and various other metal alloys. Construction of stents is quite variable and includes laser-cut, etched, woven, knitted, coiled, or welded constructions. Stent properties, including flexibility, radial strength, hoop strength, radiopacity, and foreshortening characteristics differ among the stents. In addition, various characteristics of a stent such as metal thickness, surface charge, method of stent cleaning and polishing, source of the metal, corrosion resistance, durability, the amount of open area—to—metal surface ratio, "kinkability," and the sharpness of the ends all impact the biocompatibility of the stent and, ultimately, overall results.

The ideal vascular stent should include the following: high radial force/hoop strength to resist recoil, minimal or no stimulation of intimal hyperplasia or restenosis, longitudinal flexibility to negotiate tortuosity, high radiopacity for visualization, radial elasticity or crush resistance, ability to conform to the vessel, low profile and high expansion ratio, minimal or no foreshortening for precise placement, easy deployment system, maintenance of side branch patency, magnetic resonance (MR) imaging compatibility, durability, and low price.

The evolution of stents has occurred along two fundamental design philosophies: balloon-expanded stents and self-expanding stents. The prototypical self-expanding stent variety is the Wallstent (Boston Scientific Vascular, Natick, MA), and the balloon-expanding stent is the Palmaz stent (Cordis Endovascular, Warren, NJ). There are a myriad of commercially available uncovered and covered stents with varying materials, designs, and mechanical properties. Most self-expanding stents are based on thermomechanical properties of nickel-titanium alloys and a more limited number on purely mechanical stent properties. Table 10-1 is provided as a reference table for currently available stents classified by method of expansion, wire compatibility, metal alloy composition, available diameters and lengths, sheath size, and manufacturer. Off-label use is designated.

Mechanical Self-Expanding Stents

Mechanical self-expanding stents are devices composed of stainless steel, which are compressed within a delivery catheter and rely on a mechanical "springlike" design to achieve expansion. After the delivery system is inserted into the artery or vein, the stents are expanded to their predetermined diameter by withdrawing the sheath

TABLE 10.1 The Practical Classification of Vascular Stents

Classification	Maximum guidewire size (in.)	Device	Materials	Diameter (mm)	Length (mm)	Sheath (F)	Manufacturer
Self-expanding	0.035	Xceed Biliary	Nitinol	5-8	20-120	6	Abbott Vascular
		Absolute Biliary	Nitinol	5-10	20-100	6	Abbott Vascular
		Luminexx	Nitinol	4-14	20-120	6	Bard Peripheral Vascular
		LifeStent FlexStar	Nitinol	6-10	20-80	6	Bard Peripheral Vascular
		LifeStent FlexStar XL	Nitinol	6-7	100-150	6	Bard Peripheral Vascular
		Sentinol	Nitinol	5-10	20-80	6	Boston Scientific
		Wallstent	Elgiloy	5-24	18-94	6-12	Boston Scientific
		Zilver 635 Vascular	Nitinol	6-10	20-80	6	Cook Medical
		Smart Iliac	Nitinol	6-10	20-100	6	Cordis Endovascular
		Protégé EverFlex	Nitinol	6-8	20-150	6	ev3 Endovascular
		Protégé GPS	Nitinol	9-14	20-80	6	ev3 Endovascular
		Aurora	Nitinol	6-10	20-80	6-7	Medtronic Cardiovascular
		Complete SE	Nitinol	4-10	20-150	6	Medtronic Cardiovascular
	0.018	Xpert Biliary	Nitinol	3-8	20-60	4-5	Abbott Vascular
		Dynalink Biliary	Nitinol	5-10	28-100	6	Abbott Vascular
		Zilver 518 Vascular	Nitinol	6-10	20-80	5	Cook Medical
		Protégé GPS	Nitinol	6-10	20-80	6	ev3 Endovascular
		Supera	Nitinol	4-10	20-120	7	Idev Technologies
	0.014	Wallstent Biliary Monorail	Elgiloy	6-10	21-37	5	Boston Scientific Corp.
Balloon-expandable	0.035	Omnilink Biliary	316L stainless steel	5-10	12-58	6-8	Abbott Vascular
		Omniflex Biliary	Platinum	5-7	15	6-7	AngioDynamics
		Vistaflex	Platinum	5-10	35-55	7-9	AngioDynamics
		Valeo Biliary	316L stainless steel	6-10	18-56	6-7	Bard Peripheral Vascular
		Express LD	316L stainless steel	5-10	17-57	6-7	Boston Scientific
		Palmaz	316L stainless steel	4-12	10-30	6-7	Cordis Endovascular
		Genesis	Cobalt	5-10	20-80	6-7	Cordis Endovascular
		Visi-Pro	316L stainless steel	5-10	15-60	6-7	ev3 Endovascular
		Bridge Assurant	316L stainless steel	6-10	20-60	6-7	Medtronic
	0.018	Omnilink Biliary	316L stainless steel	4-7	12-18	5-6	Abbott Vascular
		Express Biliary SD Monorail	316L stainless steel	4-7	14-19	5-6	Boston Scientific
		Formula 418	316L stainless steel	5-8	12-30	5-6	Cook Medical
		Genesis	Cobalt	3-8	12-24	5-6	Cordis
		Palmaz Blue	Cobalt	4-7	12-24	5	Cordis

TABLE 10.1 The Practical Classification of Vascular Stents—cont'd

Classification	Maximum guidewire size (in.)	Device	Materials	Diameter (mm)	Length (mm)	Sheath (F)	Manufacturer
		ParaMount Mini GPS	316L stainless steel	5-7	14-21	5-6	ev3 Endovascular
		Racer	Cobalt (MP35N)	4-7	12-18	5-6	MedTronic Cardiovascular
	0.014	RX Herculink Elite Biliary	Cobalt chromium alloy	4-7	12-18	5	Abbott Vascular
		RX Herculink Plus Biliary	316L stainless steel	4-7	12-18	5-6	Abbott Vascular
		Ultra	316L stainless steel	4.5, 5	13-38	5	Abbott Vascular
		Vision	Cobalt	2.75-4	8-28	5	Abbott Vascular
		Liberté	316L stainless steel	2.75-5	8-32		Boston Scientific
		Genesis	Cobalt	4-7	12-24	4-6	Cordis Endovascular
		Palmaz Blue	Cobalt	5-6	14-17	5	Cordis Endovascular
		ParaMount Mini GPS	316L stainless steel	5-7	14-21	5-6	ev3 Endovascular
		Driver	Cobalt	3-4	9-30	6	Medtronic Cardiovascular
		Racer	Cobalt (MP35N)	4-7	12-18	5-6	Medtronic Cardiovascular
Self-expanding stent grafts	0.035	Fluency Plus	Nitinol/ePTFE	6-10	40-80	8-9	Bard Peripheral Vascular
		Wallgraft	PET/Elgiloy	6-14	27-104	9-12	Boston Scientific
	0.035-0.025	Viabahn	Nitinol/ePTFE	5-13	25-150	7-12	W. L. Gore & Associates
		Viabahn with heparin	Nitinol/ePTFE	5-13	25-150	7-12	W. L. Gore & Associates
	0.038	Viatorr	Nitinol/ePTFE	8-12	40-80	10	W. L. Gore & Associates
	0.018	aSpire	Nitinol/ePTFE	5-9	25-100	7	LeMaitre Vascular
Balloon-expanding stent grafts	0.035	iCast	316L stainless/ePTFE	5-12	16-59	6-7	Atrium Medical

PET, Polyethylene terephthalate.

while the stent is maintained in position by a coaxial inner component of the delivery system. Their design allows for a high degree of flexibility, relative ease of placement, and smaller-diameter delivery systems for large-diameter stents. Smaller profiles reduce the potential for complications attributed to injury at the percutaneous puncture site. In comparison with balloon-expandable stents, self-expanding stents characteristically possess less resistance to radial compressive force, or so-called hoop strength.

The Wallstent Endoprosthesis (Boston Scientific) was FDA approved for iliac artery application in 1996. It is made of Elgiloy, a "superalloy," combining cobalt, chromium, nickel, and other metals. Elgiloy contains a relatively small amount of iron and is therefore negligibly ferromagnetic and MR imaging compatible. A platinum core renders the stent struts radiopaque. The woven mesh design of the struts imparts flexibility, as well as an outward self-expanding force to the stent. The Wallstent is constructed of thin Elgiloy stainless-steel wire, which is woven into a flexible, tubular braid configuration (Figure 10-1). It expands by an intrinsic spring action. The separate wires move freely at their interconnections, resulting in a very flexible tubular structure that can be easily placed via a relatively small introducer system (7F introducer for a 12-mm stent). Its flexibility allows the stent to be placed in tortuous arteries. Wallstent

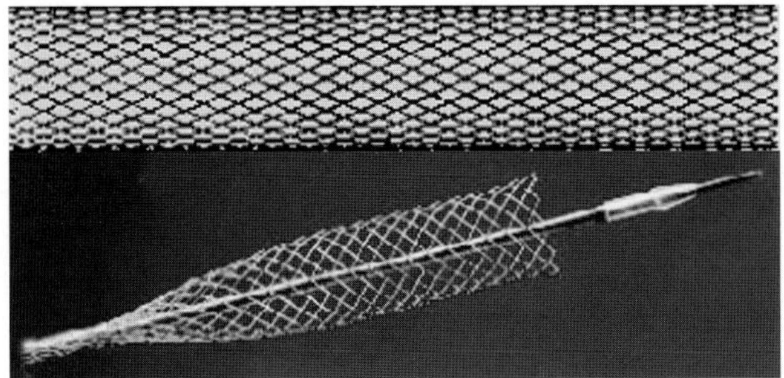

FIGURE 10-1 Wallstent is made of Elgiloy stainless-steel wire woven into a flexible, tubular braid configuration. It expands by an intrinsic spring action with marked shortening.

flexibility facilitates iliac stenting from a contralateral access site across the aortic bifurcation. Intrinsic properties (flexibility, shortening, and column strength) of Wallstents are determined by the thickness of the wires and the braiding angle (the angle between crossing wires at interconnecting points). Potential disadvantages of this design are its tendency for marked shortening during expansion and its low radiopacity. Wallstents are available in diameters of 5 through 24 mm and in lengths of 18 to 94 mm.

When placing a stent in a stenotic vessel, a stent with a diameter approximately 1 mm larger than the desired vessel diameter is selected. Stent length is determined by the vessel diameter, and the length of the lesion is recorded. The Wallstent is packaged constrained into its delivery system consisting in part of two coaxial catheters. The exterior catheter serves to constrain the stent until retracted during deployment. Radiopaque marker bands situated adjacent to the leading and trailing ends of the stent facilitate imaging during deployment. The interior tube serves to hold the stent in place during retraction of the exterior catheter. One must consider marked shortening of the Wallstent that occurs with expansion.[5] The system is then advanced across the lesion such that the leading end of the stent is slightly beyond its desired final position. During deployment, the stent can be pulled back but not advanced because the diverging struts of the partially deployed stent may "catch" the vessel wall. Deployment is initiated by withdrawing the outer catheter while holding the stent in place with the inner plunger. Currently available delivery systems allow recovery and repositioning of up to 75% partially deployed stents.

Thermal Expanding Stents

Although truly a variation or subtype of self-expanding stents, a wide variety of thermal expanding stents are now available for use and, therefore, deserve to be mentioned as a separate class because of their thermomechanical properties. The concept of a thermal expanding stent was first proposed by Dotter's group in 1983.[6] These authors constructed a stent of a nickel-titanium alloy called nitinol (50%-55% nickel, 45%-50% titanium), which possesses the unusual property of thermal memory.[7] Thermal memory is the result of varying crystal lattice structure of the alloy at different temperatures. At high temperatures (approximately 1,000° F) the crystal structure anneals and sets the memory of the alloy's shape. Based on the alloy composition, a transition temperature (usually 90° F for medical-grade nitinol) determines the temperature at which the memory will recover the annealed shape of the nitinol. Cooling below the transition temperature increases the pliability of the nitinol, and increasing the temperature above the transition point recovers the shape determined by the crystal lattice structure predetermined at the annealing temperature.

A variety of thermal expanding stents have been approved for intravascular use in the United States (Table 10-1). These devices will ultimately require clinical evaluation and possibly comparison in randomized trials.

The Xceed Stent (Abbott Vascular, Abbott Park, IL) is a 0.035-inch–compatible, self-expanding, nitinol, biliary stent system. A laser-cut stainless-steel hypotube provides longitudinal strength, and flexibility with advanced electropolish and micropolish results in enhanced durability. Low tip profile facilitates crossing of tight strictures. One-handed ergonomic handle design provides quick, easy, and controlled stent deployment. The triaxial delivery system can be looped during deployment without affecting the accuracy of stent placement. It is available in diameters of 5 to 8 mm and in lengths of 20 to 120 mm.

The Absolute Stent (Abbott Vascular) is a self-expanding, nickel-titanium, biliary stent that is premounted on an over–0.035-inch wire delivery system. Advanced nitinol metallurgy and corrugated ring design provide flexibility and radial strength. Nested ring pattern minimizes stent shortening and enhances stent integrity. Six proprietary radiopaque nitinol markers on the proximal and distal ends of the stent enhance visibility. Absolute stents are available in 20- to 100-mm lengths and 5- to 10-mm diameters. The delivery system is compatible with a 6F sheath or an 8F guiding catheter.

The Xpert Stent (Abbott Vascular) is a 0.018-inch–compatible, self-expanding, nitinol, biliary stent system. Sheath compatibility is 4F for 3- to 5-mm and most 6-mm diameter stents and 5F for some 6-mm (based on length) and all 8-mm diameter stents. Its 0.042-inch tip entry profile provides crossability for tight lesion. Conformable stent design offers low straightening force and excellent kink resistance to ensure wall apposition. Optimized stent architecture enables high radial strength while maintaining a low metal–to–surface area ratio.

It is available in diameters of 3 to 8 mm and in lengths of 20 to 60 mm.

The Dynalink Stent (Abbott Vascular) is a 0.018-inch–compatible, self-expanding, nitinol, biliary stent system. The Dynalink Stent is made of laser-cut nitinol with good flexibility, vessel wall conformability, crush resistance, and minimal foreshortening. It has similar cell geometry to the Multilink coronary stent. This 0.018-inch guidewire–compatible stent system provides 6F sheath/8F guiding catheter compatibility in all diameters (5.0 to 10.0 mm) and in lengths of 28 to 100 mm. The proximal shaft of the delivery system is 4.5F, allowing for contrast injection through a 6F sheath.

The Luminexx Stent (Bard Peripheral Vascular, Tempe, AZ) is a 0.035-inch–compatible, self-expanding, nitinol, biliary stent system. The fundamental design of the stent consists of a zigzag pattern, which has open-cell and flexible mesh design with minimal foreshortening. The stent struts are electropolished to render more rounded edges. A 2-mm flare at the proximal and distal ends of the stent optimizes anchoring of the stent to the vessel wall and minimizes the potential for migration. Four radiopaque tantalum markers at each end of the stent ensure clear visualization to significantly enhance deployment and placement accuracy. The proprietary interlocking "puzzle-marker design" facilitates permanent attachment to reduce potential for migrations. A soft, atraumatic catheter tip formed from the outer sheath retracts over the stent during deployment, rather than through the stent, creating a tipless inner catheter. The 6F-compatible Luminexx stent family ranges from 4- to 14-mm diameters and 20- to 120-mm lengths.

The LifeStent Flexstar Stent (Bard Peripheral Vascular) is a 0.035-inch–compatible, self-expanding, biliary stent system. It has a triple-helix architecture and optimized cell size, which deliver exceptional radial strength and uniform support. The stents can be bent 180 degrees, or even twisted, without kinking. It is available in diameters from 6 to 10 mm and stent lengths from 20 to 80 mm. LifeStent Flexstar XL is a 0.035-inch–compatible, self-expanding, biliary stent system available in stent diameters of 6 and 7 mm and stent lengths of 100 to 150 mm. All diameters and lengths are 6F compatible.

The Sentinol Stent (Boston Scientific Vascular) is a 0.035-inch–compatible, self-expanding, nitinol, biliary stent system. Radial tandem architecture and unique stent-cell geometry are designed for enhanced flexibility and force characteristics. A proprietary manufacturing process was developed to neutralize the stent surface by removing the nickel ions. Stent diameters range from 5 to 10 mm with lengths of 20, 40, 60, and 80 mm and are 6F compatible.

The Zilver Stent (Cook Medical, Bloomington, IN) is an FDA-approved, self-expanding, nitinol stent system for iliac application. Flexible z-cell design provides for excellent wall apposition and conformability. Horizontal tie-bars and z-cell design provide added durability and reduced shortening. Thorough electropolishing on all sides eliminates tiny particles and surface cracks (Figure 10-2). The Zilver 635 series (6F, 0.035 inch) and 518 series (5F, 0.018 inch) are both available in 6- to 10-mm diameter, 20- to 80-mm lengths, and 80- and 125-cm delivery systems. The Zilver PTX Drug-Eluting Stent is coated with paclitaxel. Paclitaxel promotes the assembly of microtubules from tubulin dimers and stabilizes microtubules by preventing depolymerization. This stability results in the inhibition of the normal dynamic reorganization of the microtubule network that is essential for vital interphase and mitotic cellular functions that result in intimal hyperplasia (Figure 10-3). It is currently undergoing pivotal trial evaluation for femoropopliteal applications.

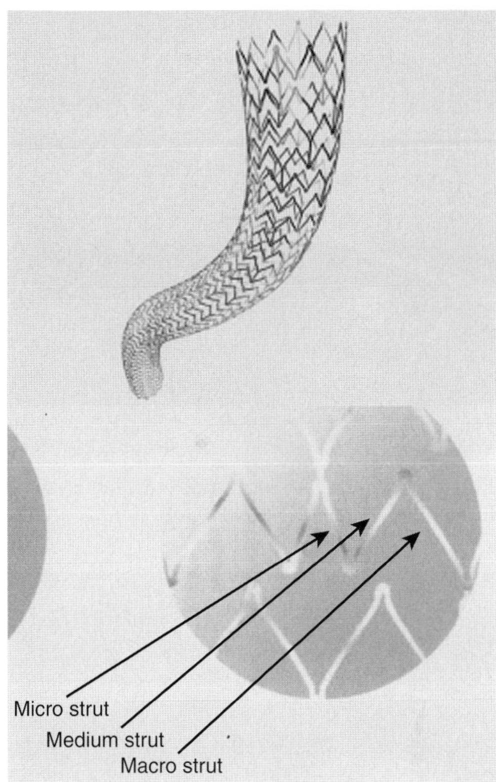

FIGURE 10-2 Zilver Stent has flexible z-cell design, which leads to excellent wall apposition and conformability. Horizontal tie-bars provide added durability with little shortening.

The SMART Stent (Cordis Endovascular) is an FDA-approved, self-expanding, nitinol stent system for iliac applications. The SMART (Shape Memory Alloy Recoverable Technology) stent is a laser-cut, nitinol stent with good flexibility, vessel wall conformability, and crush resistance. Micromesh geometry and segmented stent design provide strong radial strength at increased luminal diameters. The 12 tantalum micromarkers define the ends of the stent for easy visualization and

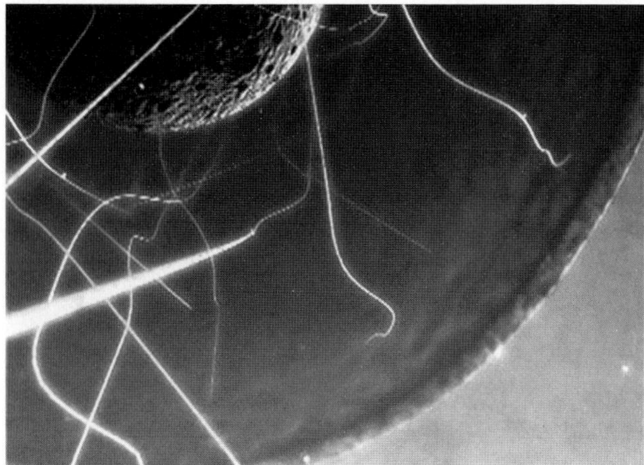

FIGURE 10-3 Paclitaxel stabilizes microtubules, rendering them nonfunctional for vital interphase and mitotic cellular activity.

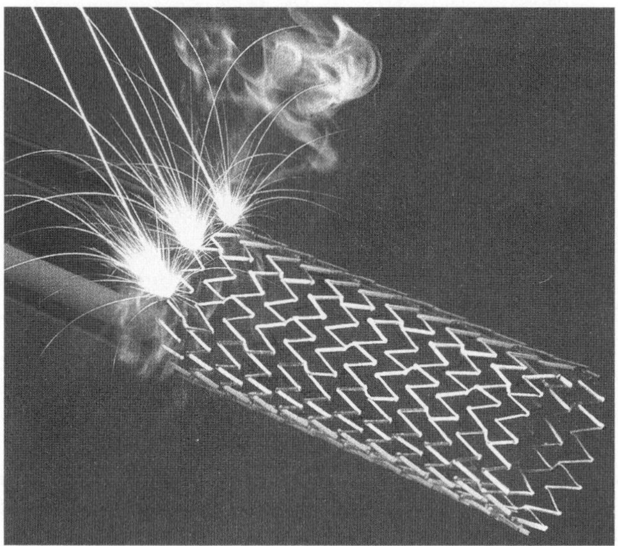

FIGURE 10-4 Micromesh geometry and segmented stent design of SMART stent provides strong radial strength. Flared stent ends with tantalum micromarker offer immediate vessel wall apposition and accurate stent placement.

placement. Flared stent ends offer immediate vessel wall apposition and increase the accuracy of stent placement (Figure 10-4). Its "Control" stent-delivery handle enables incremental deployment and micropositioning of the stent. The stent is available in 6- to 10-mm diameters and lengths from 20 to 100 mm.

The Protégé EverFlex Stent (ev3 Endovascular, Plymouth, MN) is a self-expanding, biliary stent system. It is a flexible, nitinol stent with open lattice design. Its spiral cell connection pattern imparts the stent's flexibility. The three-wave peak design produces expansion force that resists compression while providing excellent wall apposition. The Protégé stent features a retaining ring at the trailing end designed to prevent longitudinal "watermelon seed" forward motion of the stent during its deployment. The delivery catheter also has longitudinal rails to reduce the stored longitudinal forces that may accumulate during the stent deployment process. A side port on the delivery catheter is designed to allow contrast material injection around the stent to check its position before its deployment. The entire product line is 0.035 inch/6F sheath compatible. Stent diameters of 6 and 8 mm are available in lengths from 20 to 150 mm. Protégé GPS Self-Expanding Biliary Stent System is a nitinol stent with the same open lattice design. Tantalum GPS Markers enhance visibility for easier, more precise positioning. Sizes from 9 to 14 mm are 0.035 inch/6F compatible.

The Supera Stent (IDev Technology, Houston, TX) is an interwoven nitinol, self-expanding, biliary stent. The interwoven nitinol design essentially provides both unsurpassed strength and flexibility, which ultimately lead to greater durability. The stent provides exceptional resistance to kinking, crimping, and fracturing. It is available in size ranges from 4 to 10 mm in diameter and 40 to 120 mm in length, mounted on both 90- and 120-cm usable length catheter systems.

The Aurora Stent (Medtronic, Santa Rosa, CA) is a 0.035-inch guidewire/6F to 7F sheath–compatible, self-expanding, nitinol, biliary stent system. Six radiopaque, MR imaging–compatible gold markers provide a clear view of the stent's positioning and placement. It is available in diameters of 6 to 10 mm and in lengths of 20 to 80 mm.

The Complete SE Stent (Medtronic) is another 0.035-inch–compatible, self-expanding, nitinol, biliary stent system. It is available in diameters of 4 to 10 mm with varying lengths from 20 to 150 mm. All sizes are 6F sheath compatible. The system's triaxial design includes an inner shaft, a retractable sheath, and a patented stabilizing sheath that reduces friction during deployment.

Carotid Stents

Carotid stent systems are a special subgroup of self-expanding straight or tapered nitinol stent systems associated with embolic protection devices. Stent-ends are sized with a 1.1:1 to a 1.4:1 stent/artery ratio. Adjacent stents should match the internal diameter as the first stent deployed. If overlap of sequential stents is necessary, the amount of overlap should be kept to a minimum (approximately 5 mm), and no more than two stents should overlap. These stents are included in this chapter focusing more on the stent characteristics. They are not included in Table 10-1 and are discussed in Chapter 38.

The Acculink Carotid Stent System (Abbott Vascular) is a 0.014-inch–compatible, self-expanding, nitinol stent system, which is used with the Abbott Vascular RX Accunet embolic protection system. The self-expanding, crush-resistant nitinol, high-coverage stents are designed

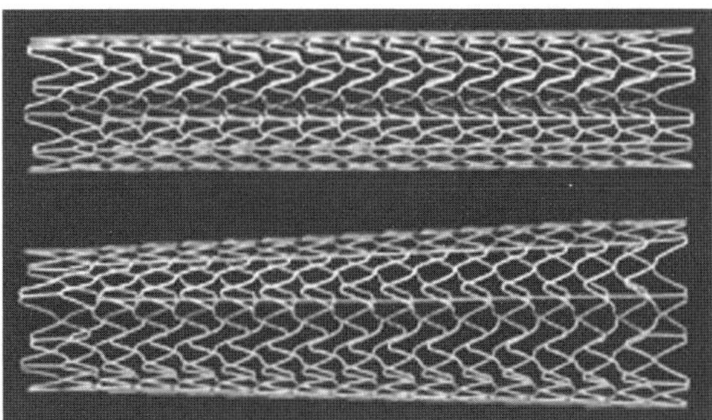

FIGURE 10-5 The self-expanding, crush-resistant Acculink carotid stent has high coverage to reduce embolic risk and three longitudinal spines to reduce stent shortening.

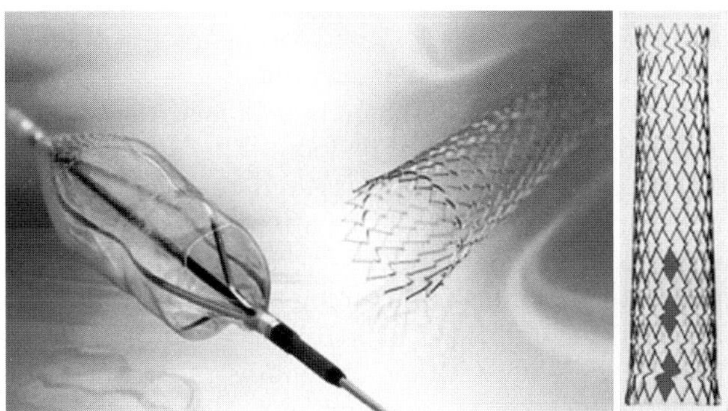

FIGURE 10-6 Xact Carotid Stent has a closed-cell design that creates a tightly knit yet highly flexible mesh, no exposed struts for smooth passage of the retrieval catheter, dense scaffolding to prevent tissue and plaque prolapse, and flared stent ends to facilitate the passage of balloons.

to reduce embolic risk. Three longitudinal spines reduce stent shortening to 1% on the 7.0 × 40 mm stent (Figure 10-5). Straight stents are offered in diameters of 5 to 10 mm and lengths of 20 to 40 mm. Tapered stents (6-8 mm and 7-10 mm tapered diameters) are also available to better match the diameters of both the internal carotid and common carotid arteries. Stents are 6F sheath/8F guide catheter compatible for all available stent sizes. The RX Acculink Carotid Stent System utilizes rapid exchange technology so that a single operator can easily control the embolic protection device and stent delivery system during catheter manipulations.

The Xact Carotid Stent System (Abbott Vascular) is another 0.014-inch—compatible, self-expanding, nitinol stent system. The closed-cell design creates a tight knit yet highly flexible mesh. There are no exposed struts for smooth passage of the retrieval catheter. Dense scaffolding prevents tissue and plaque prolapse, and flared stent ends facilitate the passage of balloons. Targeted radial strength generated by variable cell size offers strength suited to anatomy and lesions of the carotid arteries (Figure 10-6).

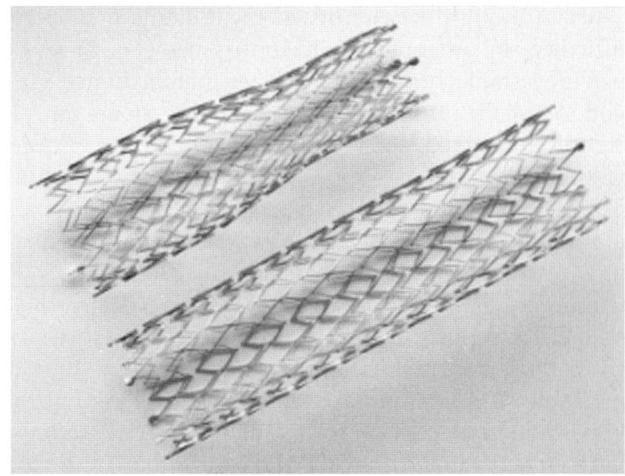

FIGURE 10-7 Protégé carotid stent has open lattice design with tantalum radiopaque markers at the proximal and distal ends of the stent.

The Precise Carotid Stent System (Cordis Endovascular) consists of Precise, over-the-wire, nitinol stent system in conjunction with an Angioguard embolic protection system. The stent has high radial strength, minimal stent shortening, low profile, micromesh geometry, and segmented design to ensure stent conformation to the artery wall. The small-cell geometry maximizes lumen coverage. The stent has a 1-mm flare at each end and will accommodate target vessel diameters between 4 and 9 mm. The Angioguard embolic protection system requires at least 3 to 7.5 mm of normal internal carotid artery distal to the target lesion. The 3.2F low-profile Cordis Angioguard has polyurethane membrane with 100-μm pores to capture clinically significant emboli. The unique umbrella design is able to self-center in the vessel. Eight nitinol struts keep the symmetrical basket in reliable arterial wall apposition.

The Protégé GPS RX Carotid Stent System (ev3 Endovascular) is made of a nitinol stent premounted on a 6F/0.014-inch rapid exchange delivery system used in conjunction with the ev3 embolic protection systems. The stent is cut from a nitinol tube in an open lattice design with tantalum radiopaque markers at the proximal and distal ends (Figure 10-7). Patients must have a vessel diameter of 4.5 to 9.5 mm at the target lesion.

Balloon-Expandable Stents

The majority of balloon-expandable stents are preloaded on an angioplasty balloon catheter before insertion and deployment in the vessel. Once positioned at the appropriate location, the balloon is inflated, expanding the metallic stent. Most balloon-expandable stents possess relatively high radial force but have less longitudinal flexibility when compared with self-expanding stents. Although the rigidity of these stents may cause difficulty in negotiating tortuous vessels, they do provide a stable, nonshifting surface that facilitates early reendothelialization. Balloon-expandable stents can be slightly oversized by being reinflated with a larger balloon if needed, as opposed to the self- and thermal-expandable stents, which can only expand to their nominal diameter predetermined by the nitinol annealing size characteristics.

The Palmaz Stent (Cordis Endovascular) is approved by the FDA for iliac and renal arterial occlusive diseases. It is a rigid stent that is laser cut from a single tube of malleable 316L stainless steel. The stent is configured with staggered rows of rectangular slots circumferentially etched out of its wall[7] (Figure 10-8). These slots allow expansion of the tube to a larger diameter after inflation with a balloon catheter. As with other types of expandable stents, the Palmaz stent will shorten to a certain extent as it is expanded inside a vessel. The medium-sized Palmaz stents are available in diameters ranging from 4 to 9 mm and lengths ranging from 10 to 39 mm. These are mounted on 5F balloon catheters and deployed through 6F or 7F introducer sheaths. The large Palmaz stents have diameters ranging from 8 to 12 mm in lengths as long as 30 mm. These stents

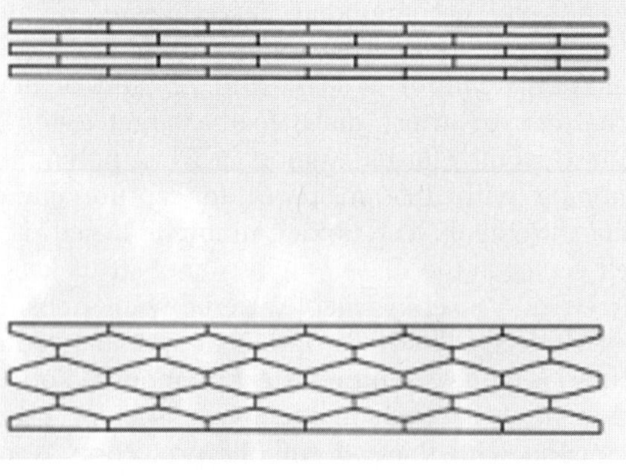

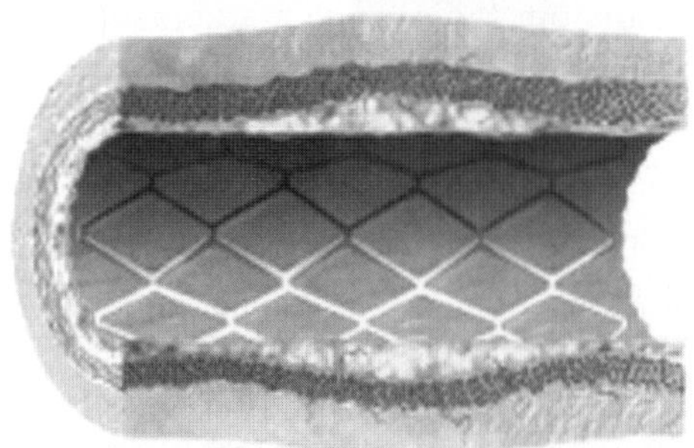

FIGURE 10-8 Palmaz balloon-expandable stent: **A,** unmounted stent; **B,** stent loaded and crimped onto an angioplasty balloon; **C,** fully expanded stent.

require a 5.8F to 7F balloon catheter and a 7F to 10F introducer sheath. The Palmaz-Schatz stents are long, articulated versions of the Palmaz stents, available in diameters ranging from 6 to 10 mm and lengths from 41.8 to 77.8 mm. Palmaz stents can be advanced across the aortic bifurcation for contralateral iliac artery stent placement.

The Palmaz XL Transhepatic Biliary stent is available in 10-mm diameter and lengths of 30, 40, and 50 mm. The stent has the same Palmaz closed-cell design but thicker struts (0.292 mm for Palmaz XL vs. 0.18 mm for Palmaz-Genesis) and much larger cell size. It is able to further expand to 30 mm diameter and maintain strong radial force. It has been used off-label to treat type I endoleaks within the proximal cuff of endovascular aneurysm repairs. The fenestrated Zenith device with Palmaz stents is being designed for the treatment of juxtarenal abdominal aortic aneurysms.

The Palmaz-Genesis Stent is a biliary, L605, cobalt stent premounted on a balloon. The Genesis stent consists of seven rows of staggered cells connected by an S-shaped hinge. This design affords the Genesis stent far greater flexibility and less foreshortening than the Palmaz stent while maintaining good hoop strength. The 0.035-inch series is available in diameters of 5 to 10 mm (6F-7F sheath) and in lengths of 20 to 80 mm. The 0.018-inch series is available in diameters of 3 (5F sheath) to 8 mm (6F sheath) and in lengths of 12 to 24 mm. The 0.014-inch RX (4F-6F sheath) series is available in stent diameters of 4 to 7 mm and stent lengths of 12 to 24 mm.

The Palmaz Blue Stent is another biliary, L605, cobalt stent premounted on a balloon-expandable system. It is designed to provide increased strength, radiopacity, low profile, and superior flexibility and deliverability. The Palmaz Blue, 0.018-inch, over-the-wire (5F sheath) stent series is available in stent diameters of 4 to 7 mm and stent lengths of 12 to 24 mm. The Palmaz Blue, 0.014-inch, RX (5F sheath) series is available in stent diameters of 5 to 6 mm and stent lengths of 14 to 17 mm.

Palmaz stents can be deployed in conjunction with a sheath containing a hemostatic valve, which is used to cross the lesion to be stented. The stent is then inserted through this protective sheath and placed at the deployment site under fluoroscopic guidance. Once in its proper location, the sheath is retracted, and the balloon catheter is inflated. As with arterial angioplasty, diluted contrast placed in the inflation device facilitates visualization during deployment. Once deflated, the balloon is gently rotated counterclockwise, with the stent left in its proper position.

The Omnilink Stent (Abbott Vascular) includes a biliary, balloon-expandable, flexible, 316L stainless-steel stent premounted on a 0.035-inch delivery system.

It has the same multiple linked corrugated ring design (4-4-4 pattern) as the Multilink coronary stent. The linked-ring and open-cell design provide optimum flexibility and conformability. Widened struts throughout the stent provide enhanced radial strength. Two "diameter-specific" Omnilink stent designs were developed—one in 5- to 7-mm diameters and another in 8- to 10-mm diameters. Grip technology helps ensure dependable stent retention, security, and refined balloon pillowing. The 0.035-inch system is available in diameters of 5.0 to 10.0 mm (6F-8F sheath) and in lengths of 12 to 58 mm. The 0.018-inch Omnilink, biliary, balloon-expandable, 316L stainless-steel system is available in diameters of 4.0 to 7.0 mm (6F-8F sheath) and in lengths of 12 to 18 mm.

The Omniflex Stent (AngioDynamics, Inc., Queensbury, NY) is a biliary, balloon-expandable, platinum stent system. It is an alternative stent option for patients allergic to nickel. The stent has virtually no foreshortening on initial deployment and consists of a single wire woven in a sinusoidal fashion, radially coiled, with a longitudinal wire connecting the ends of the stent. The advantages of platinum are essentially the same as those of tantalum, improved radiopacity and MR imaging compatibility, as well as a high degree of flexibility and ability to conform to tortuous anatomy. It is available in diameters of 5 to 8 mm. The Vistaflex Biliary Platinum Stent System is also a balloon-expandable system with a platinum stent. It is available in diameters of 5 to 10 mm and in lengths of 35 and 55 mm.

The Express LD Stent (Boston Scientific Vascular) is a 0.035-inch—compatible, biliary, balloon-expandable, premounted, 316L stainless-steel stent system. Like many balloon-expanded stents, the Express stent is laser cut from a tube of 316L stainless steel. The stent consists of alternating rows of large and small sinusoidal rings with five interconnecting struts between the rings. This cell architecture is designed to provide flexibility and vessel conformability while maintaining hoop strength and radiopacity. It is available in stent diameters of 5 to 10 mm (6F-7F sheath) and stent lengths of 17 to 57 mm. The Express Biliary SD Monorail Premounted Stent System has the same stent design and delivery system but is 0.018-inch compatible. It is available in stent diameters of 4 to 7 mm (5F for 4-6 mm and 6F for 7 mm) and stent lengths of 14 to 19 mm.

The RX Herculink Elite Stent (Abbott Vascular) is a biliary, balloon-expandable, L605 cobalt-chromium alloy stent premounted on the balloon that uses a rapid exchange 0.014-inch/6F delivery system. Ultrastrong cobalt-chromium with thinner struts creates high radial strength, excellent coverage, and enhanced visibility. Its flexible low-profile design provides excellent deliverability and stent conformability. The Xcelon nylon balloon material affords sizing flexibility while providing for 14 atm high-pressure capabilities. Tapered mandrels offer excellent pushability and support. The 4- to 6-mm diameter stent can be overdilated to 7.0 mm, and the 6.5- to 7-mm diameter stent can be overdilated to 8.0 mm. It is available in stent diameters of 4 to 7 mm and stent lengths of 12 to 18 mm.

The RX Herculink Plus Stent (Abbott Vascular) is another 0.014-inch—compatible, biliary, balloon-expandable, 316L stainless-steel stent system. Multiple links connecting rings provide stent flexibility. A robust stent design with nine crests per ring and multiple rings per stent is engineered to increase the stent's coverage and radial strength without compromising flexibility. It is available in stent diameters of 4.0 to 6.5 mm for the 12-mm stent length, and 4.0 to 7.0 mm for the 15- and 18-mm stent lengths. It has small 6F guide catheter compatibility for 4.0 to 6.0 mm and 7F guide catheter compatibility for 6.5 to 7.0 mm.

The Multi-Link Ultra Coronary Stent (Abbott Vascular) is a balloon-expandable, stainless-steel, stent system. Its multilink stent pattern enables high surface coverage for good wall scaffolding and high radial strength for secure lesion stability (Figure 10-9). The flexible delivery system provides smooth tracking and enhanced access to arterial lesions. The GRIP stent-crimping process offers excellent stent retention and smooth surface transitions, protecting stent edges and enhancing passage through tight lesions. The Ultra stent is 0.014 inch compatible and available in stent diameters of 4.5 and 5 mm and stent lengths of 13 to 38 mm.

In this chapter, coronary stents are not discussed. The following coronary stents are included only because they are available as bare metal stents ranging from 4 to 5 mm in diameter and are used in the peripheral

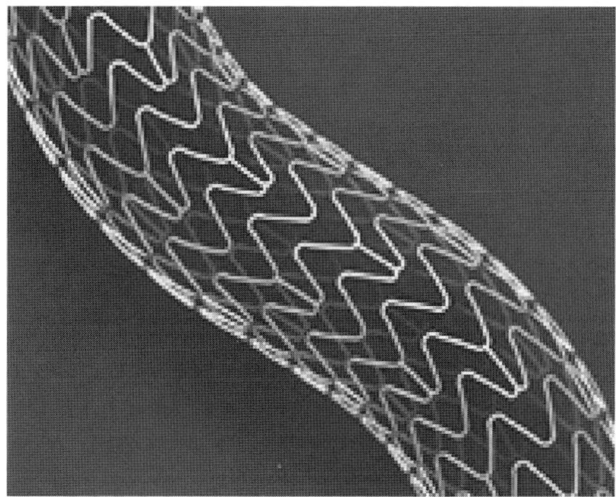

FIGURE 10-9 Multilink pattern of Ultra stent enables high surface coverage for good wall scaffolding and high radial strength for secure lesion stability.

circulation. The Multi-Link Vision Coronary Stent (Abbott Vascular) is a balloon-expandable, cobalt-chromium stent system. Its 0.0032-inch thin struts reduce the stent's profile for easy deliverability and lower restenosis rates. It offers good flexibility and has a low 0.040-inch profile. The Vision stent is 0.014-inch compatible and available in stent diameters of 2.75 and 4 mm and stent lengths of 8 to 28 mm.

The Valeo Stent (Bard Peripheral Vascular) is a biliary, balloon-expandable, 316L stainless-steel stent. The Valeo stent has a triple-helix architecture, which provides flexibility and tracking during delivery and conformability when expanded. The system is premounted on a nylon balloon with a tapered tip and low profile to facilitate crossing tight lesions. It is available in stent diameters of 6 to 10 mm (6F-7F sheath) and stent lengths of 18 to 56 mm.

The Liberté Stent (Boston Scientific) is a coronary, balloon-expandable, 316L stainless-steel stent premounted on an over-the-wire or monorail 0.014-inch balloon catheter system. Uniform cell distribution and small open-cell (2.75 mm^2) area allow for consistent vessel coverage and support (Figure 10-10). Thin struts (0.0038 inch) contribute to exceptional system flexibility and stent conformability. Exceptionally low tip and crossing profiles (0.041 inch) provide enhanced trackability and improved crossability. The Liberté stent is available in diameters from 2.75 to 5 mm and stent lengths of 8 to 32 mm.

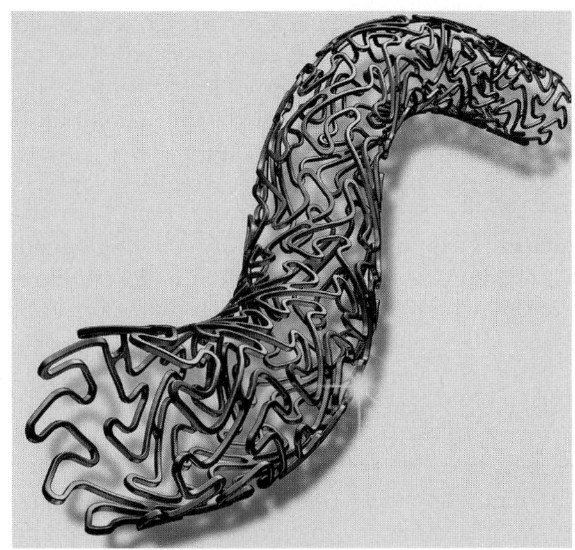

FIGURE 10-10 Liberté Coronary Stent has uniform cell distribution and small open-cell (2.75 mm^2) area allowing for consistent vessel coverage and support.

The Formula 418 Stent (Cook) is a biliary, balloon-expandable, stainless-steel stent that is premounted on the 0.018-inch/4F sheath delivery system. The stent is available in diameters of 3 to 8 mm and lengths of 12 to 30 mm. It has been cleared by the FDA for evaluation of safety and effectiveness for the treatment of renal artery stenosis.

The Visi-Pro Stent (ev3 Endovascular) is another biliary, balloon-expandable, stainless-steel stent that is 0.035 inch compatible with an open lattice design. It is available in stent diameters of 5 to 10 mm and stent lengths of 15 to 60 mm.

The ParaMount Stent (ev3 Endovascular) is a biliary, balloon-expandable, stainless-steel stent system. The GPS, radiopaque, tantalum markers are built into each end of the stent for enhanced procedural accuracy and visibility. Microgrip technology is designed to keep the stent properly centered during expansion. It is available in both 0.014-inch and 0.018-inch guidewire–compatible systems. It is introduced via a 6F guide catheter (5- and 6-mm diameter stents) or a 7F guide catheter for 7-mm stents.

The Bridge Assurant Stent (Medtronic) is a biliary balloon-expandable 316L stainless-steel stent system. The stent has modular design with sinusoidal six-crown architecture to provide strong radial strength. Unlike most balloon-expanded stents, sinusoidal ringed elements of 316L stainless steel with six crowns are laser fused or welded to form a tubular structure with simple rectangular cell geometry. The Bridge stent is characterized by improved hoop strength. Furthermore, the pattern of welding (two of six crowns at opposite sides of the ring) imparts flexibility to the stent in one plane (perpendicular to the plane of the welded crowns). Practically, the stent rotates when negotiating tortuous anatomy. It is 0.035-inch guidewire compatible and available in diameters from 6 to 10 mm and stent lengths of 20 and 60 mm.

The Driver Stent (Medtronic) is a coronary, balloon-expandable, cobalt-chromium bare-metal stent. The modular design with thin, round struts improves stent delivery and achieves optimal vessel wall coverage (Figure 10-11). Its low profile provides good vessel conformability. The small flexible shaft enhances pushability. The Driver Stent is 0.014-inch compatible and available in diameters from 3 to 4 mm and stent lengths from 9 to 30 mm.

The Racer Stent (Medtronic) is the first cobalt-alloy stent approved for peripheral vascular applications. The Racer RX has an exclusive modular design and an advanced cobalt-chromium alloy for stronger radial strength compared with stainless-steel stents but also has thin struts for ease of deliverability. This provides an ideal balance of strength and postdeployment flexibility (Figure 10-12). Racer RX is available in diameters from 4 to 7 mm and stent lengths of 12 and 18 mm. It has a low crossing profile and both 0.014-inch and 0.018-inch guidewire compatibility.

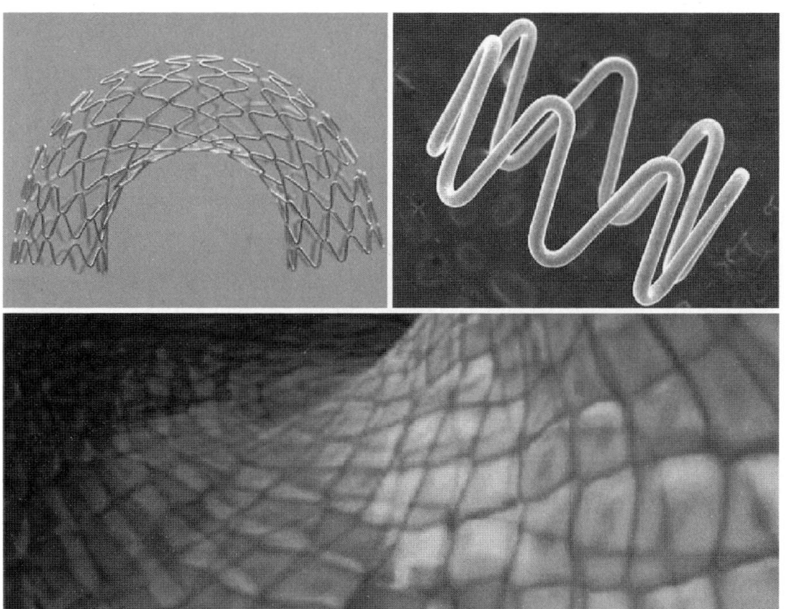

FIGURE 10-11 Cobalt-chromium Driver Stent has a modular design with thin, round struts to help preserve endothelium during stent delivery and achieve optimal vessel wall coverage.

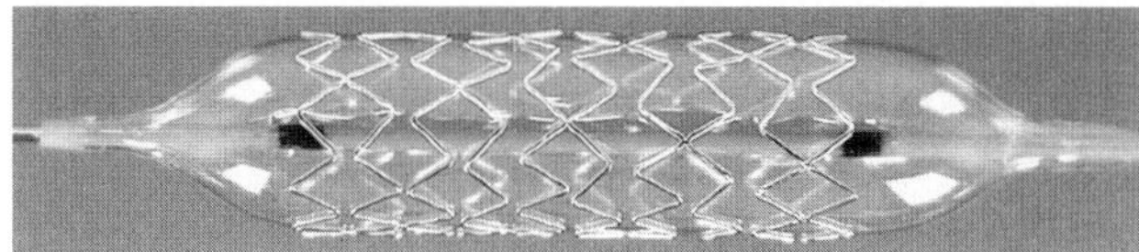

FIGURE 10-12 Racer stent has a modular design.

Stent Grafts

Self-Expanding Stent Grafts

As with other self-expanding stents, thermal expanding stents have been modified and covered with materials such as Dacron and polytetrafluoroethylene (PTFE). These stent grafts are used for the repair of traumatic arterial injuries and aneurysms but are also used in the treatment of arterial occlusive disease.

The Fluency Plus Stent Graft (Bard Peripheral Vascular) is a tracheobronchial, self-expanding, nitinol stent encapsulated within two ultrathin layers of expanded PTFE (ePTFE). Secure adhesive free tip design features optimal balance between shaft pushability and progressive flexibility at the catheter tip, providing excellent trackability to the target lesion site. The luminal surface of the ePTFE is carbon impregnated. Excellent radial expansion force in combination with the 2-mm flared ends minimizes the risk of stent graft dislocation or migration. Minimal stent graft foreshortening during deployment further enhances placement accuracy. The Fluency Plus is available in diameters from 6 to 10 mm (8F-9F sheath) and stent lengths of 40 to 80 mm.

The Wallgraft Endoprosthesis (Boston Scientific) consists of a Wallstent covered with polyethylene terephthalate. The polyethylene terephthalate is attached to the extraluminal surface of the stent with polycarbonate urethane adhesive. A spiral platinum tracer wire enables differentiation of the Wallgraft from the Wallstent fluoroscopically. Otherwise, the only structural difference between the metallic portion of the Wallgraft and the Wallstent is the lack of flaring at the ends of the Wallgraft (Figure 10-13). It is therefore important to oversize the Wallgraft by 1 to 2 mm relative to the diameter of the target vessel. The mechanism of deployment is identical to that of the Wallstent, including the ability to reconstrain the stent when as much as 80% of the stent has been released. The Wallgraft is available in diameters as large as 14 mm and lengths as long as 70 mm. These devices require 9F to 11F introducer sheaths.

The Viabahn Endoprosthesis (W. L. Gore & Associates, Inc., Flagstaff, AZ) is a flexible, self-expanding endoluminal endoprosthesis consisting of an ePTFE lining with an external nitinol stent (exoskeleton). The stent skeleton is constructed from a single strand of nitinol wire formed into a sinusoidal shape and wound in helical fashion around the PTFE tube. The surface of the endoprosthesis is modified with covalently bound, bioactive heparin (Figure 10-14). It is the only covered stent approved for the superficial femoral artery (SFA) application. It is available in diameters from 5 to 13 mm (8F-9F sheath) and stent lengths of 25 and 150 mm. Recommended introducer sheath sizes range from 7F to 14F, and the system is compatible with a 0.025-inch guidewire. To ensure adequate anchoring, the diameter of the endoprosthesis should be 5% to 20% larger than the healthy vessel diameter immediately proximal and distal to the lesion. For occlusive disease, lesions should

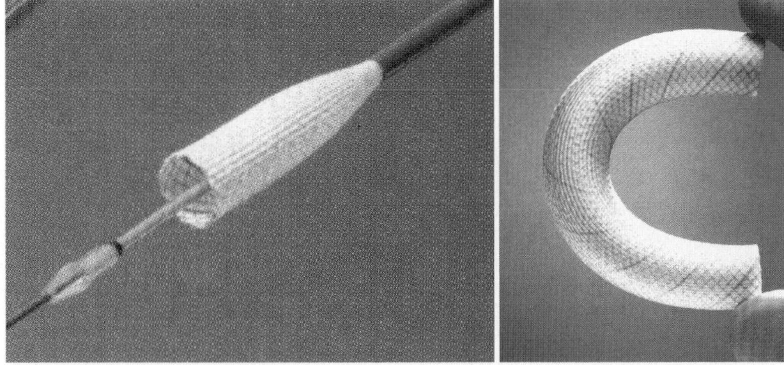

FIGURE 10-13 Wallgraft consists of a Wallstent covered with polyethylene terephthalate. The lack of flaring at the ends of the Wallgraft, as well as a spiral platinum tracer wire, allows differentiation of the Wallgraft from the Wallstent.

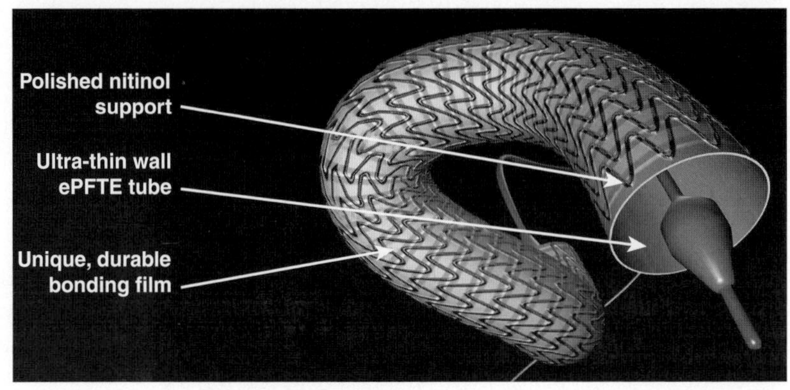

FIGURE 10-14 Viabahn Endoprosthesis consists of an ePTFE lining with an external nitinol stent. The stent skeleton is constructed from a single strand of nitinol wire formed into a sinusoidal shape and wound in helical fashion around the PTFE tube. The surface of the endoprosthesis is modified with covalently bound, bioactive heparin.

be angioplastied to a diameter equal to or greater than the stent graft diameter to allow adequate postballooning of the stent graft. The endoprosthesis should overlap the native vessel at least 1 cm beyond the proximal and distal margins of the lesion. Balloon touch-up (postdilatation) should be performed on the first device before placing the second device. To ensure proper seating, at least 1 cm of overlap between devices is recommended in patients with occlusive disease and longer overlaps for patients with aneurysmal disease. Overlapping devices should not differ by more than 1 mm in diameter. If unequal device diameters are used, the smaller device should be placed first and then the larger device should be placed inside of the smaller device. Balloon dilatation should not be extended beyond the ends of the device and into healthy vessel.

The Viatorr TIPS Endoprosthesis (W. L. Gore & Associates, Inc.) consists of an electropolished nitinol stent that supports a reduced-permeability ePTFE graft. The endoprosthesis is divided into two functional regions: a graft-lined intrahepatic region and an unlined portal region. The interface between the lined and unlined regions is indicated by a circumferential radiopaque gold marker band (Figure 10-15). The delivery catheter is compatible with a 0.038-inch or smaller (0.97 mm)–diameter guidewire and has a working length of 75 cm. It is indicated for the de novo and revision treatment of portal hypertension and its complications such as variceal bleeding, gastropathy, refractory ascites, and/or hepatic hydrothorax.

The aSpire Covered Stent (LeMaitre Vascular, Burlington, MA) is a tracheobronchial device. Its unique design is composed of a double helical nitinol frame molded in a cylindrical coiled fashion and covered with PTFE. The helical turns are 5 mm wide, with 5-mm bare gaps between turns. The stent is not a classic covered stent insofar as it cannot be used to seal aneurysms, arteriovenous fistulas, or vessel ruptures. The goal of this unique construction is to allow for variable vessel wall coverage to promote endothelial ingrowth while potentially maintaining branch or collateral vessel patency. Nitinol scaffold in a double spiral design is engineered to provide radial strength, optimum flexibility, and kink resistance and maintain lumen shape. The ePTFE-covered stent prevents metal-to-tissue inflammatory response. The aSpire stent can be fully apposed to the lumen wall to assess accurate placement and allow repositioning before stent release. It is available in stent diameters of 5 to 9 mm and stent length of 25 to 100 mm.

Balloon-Expanding Stent Grafts

The iCAST Covered Stent (Atrium Medical, Hudson, NH) is a tracheobronchial, balloon-expandable, endoluminal device consisting of a laser-cut 316L stainless-steel

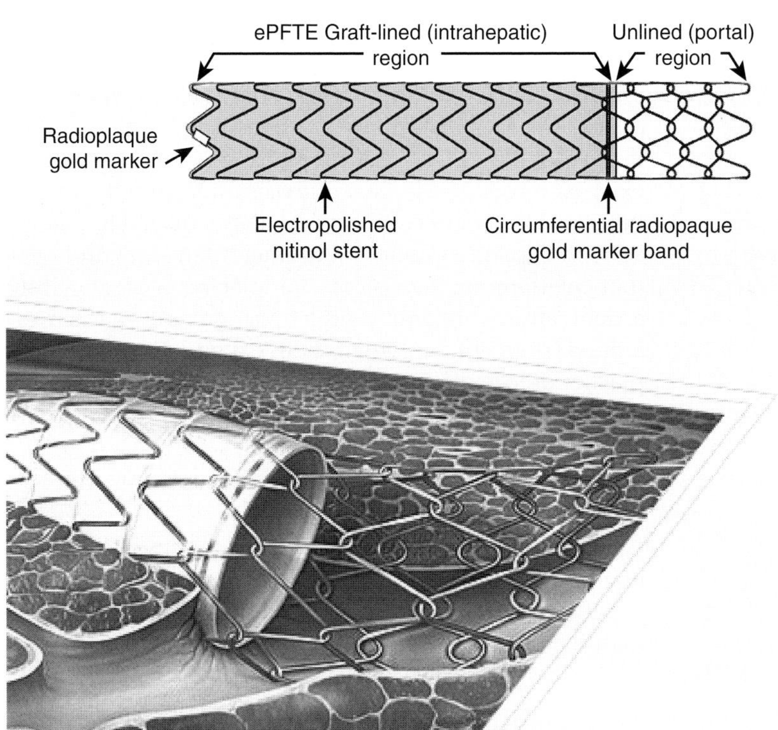

FIGURE 10-15 Viatorr TIPS Endoprosthesis is divided into two functional regions: a PTFE graft-lined 15 intrahepatic region and an unlined portal region.

stent with an encapsulated cover of ePTFE. It is available in stent diameters of 5 to 12 mm and stent lengths of 16 to 59 mm.

INDICATIONS FOR STENTS

As experienced is gained, the indications for stent placement are continuously broadening. The current FDA-approved general indications for intravascular stent placement are as follows:

- Occluded atherosclerotic lesions. Angioplasty alone for occlusions has poor long-term patency, particularly for lesions greater than 2 cm in length.
- Inadequate angiographic and/or hemodynamic angioplasty results. Inadequate results are defined as an intimal dissection and/or residual stenosis of 30% or greater and/or a mean pressure gradient of greater than 5 to 10 mm Hg. Primary stenting of stenotic iliac lesions remains controversial.
- Recurrence. Stenting of recurrent stenosis after balloon angioplasty alone may improve the secondary patency.

The indication for iliac stenting is suboptimal percutaneous transluminal angioplasty (PTA) of common and/or external iliac artery stenotic lesions more than 10 cm in length. A suboptimal PTA is defined as a technically successful dilation but the presence of unfavorable lesion morphology such as:

- An inadequate angiographic and/or hemodynamic result as defined by a 30% or greater residual stenosis after PTA, lesion recoil, or intimal flaps
- Flow-limiting dissections after PTA longer than the initial lesion length
- A 5 mm Hg or greater mean transstenotic pressure gradient after PTA

The indications for innominate and subclavian veins are improving central venous luminal diameter after unsuccessful angioplasty in patients receiving long-term hemodialysis. Indications also include recurrent stenosis or angioplasty failure of the venous outflow tract of a hemodialysis access. Unsuccessful angioplasty is defined as residual stenosis 30% or greater for a vein 10 mm or less in diameter or 50% or greater for a vein more than 10 mm in diameter, a tear that interrupts the integrity of the intima or lumen, abrupt lesion site occlusion, or refractory spasm.

CONTRAINDICATIONS

Stent placement is generally contraindicated:

- In patients who cannot receive antiplatelet and/or anticoagulant therapy.

- With lesions that prevent complete angioplasty balloon inflation or proper placement of the stent or stent delivery system. This includes extravasations at the target site (for bare metal stents), severe vessel tortuosity, or densely calcified lesions.
- With hypersensitivity or contraindication to coating drugs or structurally related compounds including cobalt, chromium, nickel, tungsten, acrylic, and fluoropolymers.

Contraindications for iliac stenting:

- Persistent acute intraluminal thrombus at the proposed stenting site, after thrombolytic therapy
- Arterial perforation or a fusiform or saccular aneurysm during the procedure preceding possible stent implantation

Contraindications for carotid stenting:

- Lesions in the ostium of the common carotid artery
- Patients with total occlusion of the target vessel
- Patients with highly calcified lesions resistant to PTA
- Existence of intraluminal thrombus thought to increase the risk of plaque fragmentation and distal embolization

Contraindications for SFA stenting with Viabahn Endoprosthesis:

- Ostial lesions or lesions involving a major side branch that may be covered by the endoprosthesis
- Less than one distal runoff vessel, which has continuous patency to the ankle

MECHANICAL PROPERTIES OF VASCULAR STENTS

Different mechanical properties of specific vascular stents should be determined when selecting a stent for a particular lesion. Stent properties are crucial for the ultimate site-specific success of endovascular procedures.

Radial Force/Hoop Strength

The radial force of a stent represents its ability to efface the arterial lumen. Radial force is dependent on stent construction, design, material, and size. Hoop strength is the ability of a stent to resist radial compression by external forces. Balloon-expanded stents and self-expanding stents respond in fundamentally different ways to external compression.[8] When an increasing compressive force is applied to a balloon-expanded stent, it initially demonstrates mild elastic deformation. During this phase, the stent will return to its nominal diameter when the external force is removed. However, when the compressive force reaches the yield point, the stent will undergo irreversible plastic deformation and become crushed. Self-expanding stents, conversely, demonstrate a near-linear stress-strain relationship. Therefore they behave in an elastic manner through a large range of external forces. The force required to deform self-expanding stents is generally lower than that required to deform balloon-expanded stents.[8,9] Another interesting finding is that overlapping two stents, or placing a stent within a stent, effectively doubles the hoop strength in the overlapped segment.[8] A stent will experience permanent plastic deformation if the external force exceeds its maximum hoop strength.

Flexibility

The flexibility of various stents is defined by fixing one end of each stent and measuring the force required to bend the stents to a certain degree. The Palmaz stent is the most rigid stent.

Trackability/Pushability

Trackability refers to the ability of a stent with its delivery system to track over a wire. Pushability, although similar, is the force required to push a delivery system over the wire through a tortuous arterial system or lesion. Apart from the flexibility of the stent, this feature is also dependent on the properties of the delivery catheter. Therefore, the trackability of an unmounted balloon-expanded stent can be improved by mounting the stent on a more flexible balloon catheter.

Radiopacity

Radiopacity is measured as the amount of aluminum required to render a stent invisible on fluoroscopy. The stent with the greatest radiopacity is the Palmaz large stent. The Wallstent was slightly less radiopaque.[10]

MR Imaging Compatibility

The ability to assess the patency of metallic stents with MR is becoming increasingly important. Many metallic stents are MR imaging compatible because they are made of inert nonferromagnetic material. These include the nitinol stents, as well as other non–stainless-steel stents such as the Elgiloy, platinum, and tantalum. Because these stents do not experience significant torque when placed in a strong magnetic field, patients can undergo MR imaging examinations in the immediate postimplantation period. MR imaging examinations in recently placed stainless-steel stents that have not undergone endothelialization are generally not recommended because of the risk of stent migration and/or torque. Nonferromagnetic stents cause significantly less artifact on MR angiographic images than stainless-steel stents. The signal loss on MR images of metallic stents is the result of two mechanisms. First, susceptibility artifacts brought about by metal-induced local magnetic field inhomogeneities cause signal loss around the stent struts. Second, radiofrequency artifacts related to the induction of eddy currents in the conductive metallic material cause a reduction of signal within the stent lumen.

With regard to gadolinium-enhanced three-dimensional MR angiography, stainless-steel stents are generally associated with the largest artifacts. Nitinol stents are variable but generally good. Tantalum stents induce minimal artifact.[11]

BIOLOGIC RESPONSE TO INTRAVASCULAR STENT PLACEMENT

The stent size and design itself, as well as the technique of stent deployment, have been shown to influence the intravascular biologic response, which in turn affects the immediate and long-term patency rates.

Most of the currently available stents are made of either stainless steel, tantalum, or nitinol, which on deployment induces an immediate foreign body reaction. The thrombogenicity of the stent is greatly affected by the finishing process during production. Electropolishing, a common finishing process for stainless steels, leads to a more stable and less thrombogenic surface of metal oxides.[12-14]

The electrical charge of most metals and alloys used for intravascular devices is electropositive in electrolytic solutions, whereas all biologic intravascular proteins and cells are negatively charged.[12-14] Palmaz[15] has shown that within seconds after intra-arterial stent deployment, the positive electrical potential of the metallic struts attracts the negatively charged circulating proteins to form a thin layer of randomly oriented fibrinogen strands on the stent surface. This functions to neutralize the stent surface and thereby decreases its thrombogenicity.

Surface tension is another property that influences surface interactions. The critical surface tension of a solid surface must be between 20 and 30 dynes/cm to be thromboresistant. Most metals have a higher critical surface tension and are therefore thrombogenic. The initial layer of proteins covering the metal within seconds after implantation may reduce surface tension and thus decrease thrombogenicity.[13-15]

Additionally, the technique itself of stent implantation may affect thrombogenicity and the rate of endothelialization. At 2 to 15 minutes after implantation, scanning electron microscopy revealed an accumulation of red blood cells and platelets. At 24 hours, this cellular layer is replaced by a layer of fibrin strands oriented in the direction of blood flow. This layer is thought to be conducive to the lateral growth of endothelial cells.[15-17] The ultimate goal of intravascular stenting should be complete endothelial coverage of the stent surface to prevent thrombosis.[18] Ideally, stents should be deployed in such a way that the metal struts are embedded deep enough into the vessel wall to produce troughs where the struts are embedded, surrounded by intima that projects through the meshwork of the stent. The troughs fill with thrombus but the intimal projections are nonthrombogenic and serve as the multicentric source for the endothelialization of the stent. The achievement of this ideal deployment is dependent on multiple factors. These factors include the ratio of the diameter of the stent to the diameter of the blood vessel, the depth of penetration of the struts into the vessel wall, the thickness of the struts, and the composition and integrity of the intimal surface. If the struts are not properly embedded, the entire stented surface becomes covered with thrombus, preventing early endothelialization and thus predisposing to thrombosis and restenosis.[15,16] In general, stent struts will be embedded adequately if the final stent diameter is 10% to 15% larger than the adjacent vessel.

Stent diameter in relation to the vessel diameter plays an important part in determining the final thickness of the neointimal layer. In the third and fourth weeks after insertion, smooth muscle cell proliferation and endothelialization resulted in a neointimal layer of approximately 1 mm in thickness.[16] This relatively uniform thickness represents a greater percentage of luminal narrowing in smaller vessels. This makes it unlikely to achieve long-term patency in vessels smaller than 5 mm in diameter. The diameter of the fully deployed stent should not exceed the diameter of the vessel by more than 20%. Excessive stretching of the vessel wall causes excessive proliferation of the neointima, which may adversely affect the long-term patency.[16,19,20] Optimally, the stent should be deployed so that the struts are embedded in the intimal surface adequately without overstretching the vessel wall, which would stimulate excessive neointimal growth.

Furthermore, the thickness of the stent struts, themselves, can affect the rate at which endothelialization occurs. Thin struts, less than 0.2 mm in thickness, allow for earlier endothelialization than stents with thicker struts.[15] They allow for better intimal embedding and a greater surface area of endothelium exposed to the lumen.

Finally, at several months after stent placement, Palmaz et al.[15,16,21] observed the formation of neointimal vessels and found them to be more abundant around the struts. At 3 to 6 years, the fibromuscular tissue layer covering the stent surface was almost completely replaced by collagen. Of note is that stents placed into the venous system exhibit a faster rate of endothelialization than do intra-arterial stents.[15,16,21]

STENT-RELATED COMPLICATIONS

Stent-related complications include vessel dissection, perforation, or rupture; vessel spasm or recoil; metallic corrosion (interface or fretting corrosion, galvanic corrosion, intergranular corrosion, pitting corrosion); mechanical fatigue; fracture; migration; stenosis; thrombosis; distal embolization; and infection.

Stent thrombosis can cause severe clinical consequences. Carotid stent occlusion can cause a stroke. Coronary drug-eluting stent thrombosis is a low-frequency event but associated with myocardial infarction or death. Drug-eluting stent thrombosis may still occur despite continued dual antiplatelet therapy. Current guidelines recommend that patients receive aspirin indefinitely and that clopidogrel therapy be extended to 12 months in patients at low risk for bleeding.[22]

Stent infection is rare and occurs in 0.45% of cases. *Staphylococcus aureus* is the offending organism in 55% of cases. Overall mortality rate was 27% based on an international inquiry.[23] The mechanisms of this complication include infection at the time of implantation and "seeding" of an implanted graft via bacteremia. Stent infection may lead to thrombosis, pseudoaneurysm, or rupture of an artery. Once a stent is infected, the clinical course progresses rapidly, with conformational changes, sepsis, and arterial rupture. Infected stents should be removed. Arterial resection and reconstruction with autogenous tissue is recommended.

CONCLUSION

The development of endovascular stents has been a major advancement in the treatment of vascular diseases. Although they were primarily designed as adjunctive devices to peripheral angioplasty, modifications in their use have opened the door to even greater applications. Endovascular grafts currently approved for the repair of abdominal aortic aneurysms, and those in clinical trials, would not be available if not for the advancements in the development of intravascular stents. A wide variety of stents with different physical properties are now available, facilitating the technique of minimally invasive vascular surgery. The development of new materials will also make these procedures simpler and safer, as well as broaden their applications. As these devices and techniques evolve, it is imperative for one to be familiar with the different types of stents and their properties to provide optimal therapy for the patient.

References

1. Erbel R, Di Mario C, Bartunek J, et al: Temporary scaffolding of coronary arteries with bioabsorbable magnesium stents: a prospective, non-randomised multicentre trial, *Lancet* 369 (9576):1839–1840, 2007.
2. Carrel A: Results of the permanent intubation of the thoracic aorta, *Surg Gyn Obst* 15:245–248, 1912.
3. Dotter CT, Judkins MP: Transluminal treatment of arteriosclerotic obstruction: description of a new technique and a preliminary report of its application, *Circulation* 30:654–670, 1964.
4. Dotter CT: Transluminally placed coil-spring endarterial tube grafts: long-term patency in canine popliteal artery, *Invest Radiol* 4:320–332, 1969.
5. Hood DB, Hodgson KJ: Percutaneous transluminal angioplasty and stenting for iliac artery occlusive disease. In Pearce WH, Matsumra JS, Yao JST, editors: *Surgical Clinics of North America*, Philadelphia, June 1999, WB Saunders, 79(3): pp 575–596.
6. Becker GJ: Intravascular stents-general principles and status of lower extremity arterial applications, *Circulation* 83(suppl I):1–130, 1991.
7. Black MR, Scoccianti M, White RA: Biomaterial consideration for endovascular devices. In White RA, Fogarty TJ, editors: *Peripheral endovascular interventions*, St. Louis, 1996, Mosby–Year Book, Inc., pp 203–234.
8. Lossef SV, Lutz RJ, Mundorf J, et al: Comparison of mechanical deformation properties of metallic stents with use of stress-strain analysis, *J Vasc Interv Radiol* 5:341–349, 1994.
9. Dyet JF, Watts WG, Ettles DF, et al: Mechanical Properties of metallic stents: how do these properties influence the choice of stent for specific lesions, *Cardiovasc Intervent Radiol* 23:47–54, 2000.
10. Duda SH, Wiskirchen J, Tepe G, et al: Physical properties of endovascular stents: an experimental comparison, *J Vasc Interv Radiol* 11:645–654, 2000.
11. Klemm T, Duda S, Machann J, et al: MR imaging in the presence of vascular stents: a systematic assessment of artifacts for various stent orientations, sequence types, and field strengths, *J Magn Reson Imaging* 12:606–615, 2000.
12. Ratner BD, Johnston AB, Lenk TJ: Biomaterial surfaces, *J Biomed Mater Res* 21:59–89, 1987.
13. Baier RE, Dutton RC: Initial events in interaction of blood with a foreign surface, *J Biomed Mater Res* 3:191–206, 1969.
14. Palmaz JC: Interfacial relationships and future design considerations. In Herman HC, Hirshfield JH, editors: *Clinical use of the Palmaz-Schatz intracoronary stent*, Mt. Kisco, NY, 1993, Futura.
15. Palmaz JC: Intravascular stents: Tissue-stent interactions and design considerations, *AJR* 160:613–618, 1993.
16. Palmaz JC, Tio FO, Alvarado R, et al: Early endothelialization of balloon-expandable stents: experimental observations, *J Intervent Radiol* 3:119–124, 1988.
17. Barth KH, Virmani R, Strecker EP, et al: Flexible tantalum stents implanted in aortas and iliac arteries: effects in normal canines, *Radiology* 175:91–96, 1990.
18. Palmaz JC, Sibbit RR, Reuter SR, et al: Expandable intraluminal graft: a preliminary study, *Radiology* 156:73–77, 1985.
19. Sapoval MR, Long AL, Raynaud AC, et al: Femoralpopliteal stent placement: long-term results, *Radiology* 184:833–839, 1992.
20. Duprat G, Wright KC, Charnsangavej C, et al: Self-expanding metallic stents for small vessels: an experimental evaluation, *Radiology* 162:469–472, 1987.

21. Palmaz JC: Intravascular stents: experimental observations and anatomopathologic correlates. In Castaneda-Zuniga WR, Tadavarthy SM, editors: *New stent developments, interventional radiology,* ed 2, Baltimore, 1992, Williams & Wilkins.
22. ACC/AHA/SCAI Writing Committee: ACC/AHA/SCAI 2005 guideline update for percutaneous coronary intervention: a report of the American College of Cardiology/American Heart Association Task Force on Practice Guidelines, *J Am Coll Cardiol* 47(1):e1–121, 2006.
23. Fiorani P, Speziale F, Calisti A, et al: Endovascular graft infection: Preliminary results of an international inquiry, *J Endovasc Ther* 10:919–927, 2003.

CHAPTER

11

Laser Atherectomy

Julia F. Chen, Kenneth R. Kollmeyer, Samuel S. Ahn

The role of lasers in the treatment of peripheral vascular disease has evolved greatly since the introduction of laser atherectomy in the 1980s. Lasers emit highly amplified, nearly monochromatic, spatially coherent light, which translates to the notion that laser beams can be used to very precisely target small areas of tissue. In peripheral intervention, the laser has become particularly crucial in its ability to vaporize and debulk lesions that would otherwise have been untreatable by balloon angioplasty alone.

Termed "the solution without a problem" when it was first invented in 1960, the laser had already become ubiquitous by the 1980s, with applications in electronics, law enforcement, the military, information technology, and other areas of medicine. Therefore expectations were high for the initial iteration of interventional laser-catheter products. However, complications such as vessel wall dissection and perforation, which ultimately led to thrombosis, restenosis, and failure of revascularization, quickly created a much more pragmatic perspective on the capabilities of existing biomedical laser technologies.

After extensive research and product refinement, the application of lasers in peripheral interventions experienced a resurgence in the 1990s with the discovery of laser-tissue interactions associated with the 308-nm wavelength xenon chloride (XeCl) excimer laser. With decreased complication rates and positive clinical trial outcomes, the excimer laser became the broadly accepted device in both peripheral and coronary interventions.

This chapter reviews the physics and anatomy of lasers and explores the evolution of lasers in peripheral intervention. It continues with a discussion of lasing techniques, lesion selection, and complications, and presents a number of case studies. Last, an overview of current literature is provided, along with comments on future applications of laser technology in the treatment of peripheral vascular disease.

LASER PHYSICS

To develop the laser into what it is in atherectomy today, the fundamental components of a laser had to be considered. The term "laser" is an acronym for *l*ight *a*mplification by *s*timulated *e*mission of *r*adiation in which "light" includes electromagnetic radiation of any frequency, not just the visible spectrum. The principal components of a laser are shown in Figure 11-1.

The *gain medium* can be a solid, liquid, gas, or plasma, with material properties that allow it to amplify light by stimulated emission. It is placed in an *optical cavity,* which is essentially an arrangement of mirrors, allowing light to reflect back and forth. Each pass takes the light through the medium, thus amplifying the light. The mirrors that make up the optical cavity are also called reflectors. Typically, one is a total reflector and the other is a partial reflector. When light comes in contact with the total reflector, 100% of light is deflected through the medium to the other reflector. When light comes in contact with a partial reflector, some light is deflected, whereas some will pass through the partial reflector to generate the laser beam. Light that leaves the system has usually passed through the gain medium numerous times, ensuring that it is an amplified beam.

How does the gain medium amplify the beam? The gain medium absorbs energy through the laser pumping energy source. This energy is usually an electrical current or a light at a different wavelength. As the gain medium absorbs energy, electrons are excited to a high-energy quantum state (Figure 11-2). When electrons are in a high-energy state, they want to return to their lower-energy states, in which case they emit a photon of a specific wavelength. The wavelength of the photon emitted depends on the state of the electron's energy when the photon is released. This emission can be spontaneous or stimulated.

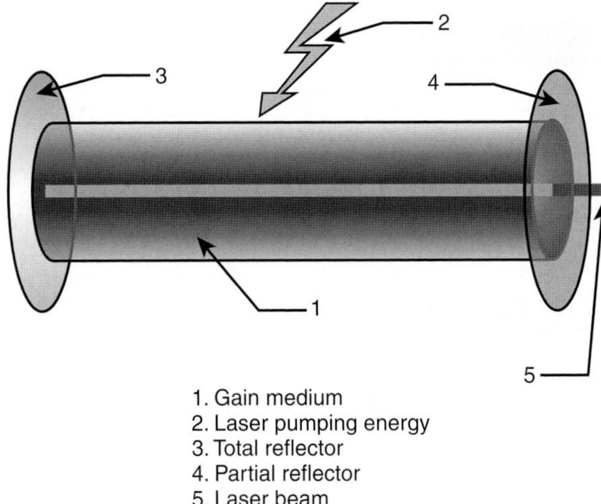

FIGURE 11-1 Principal components of a laser.

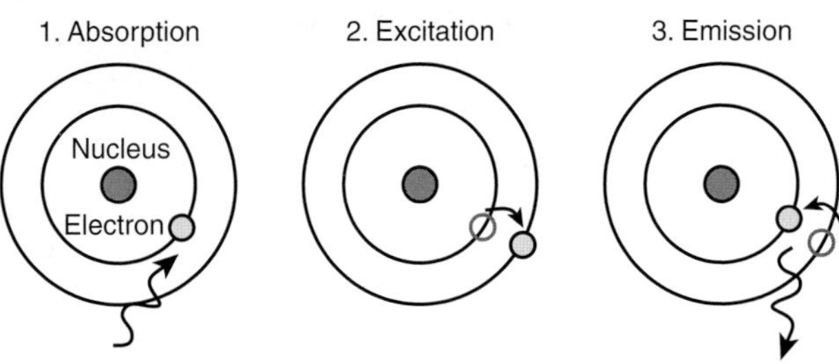

FIGURE 11-2 Photon emission mechanism.

To create monochromatic, coherent, and directional light requires stimulated emission, or a very controlled and organized photon emission. The first photon can stimulate or induce atomic emission such that the subsequent emitted photon (from the second atom) vibrates with the same frequency and direction as the incoming photon, creating coherence.

As these photons pass through the medium, they stimulate emission in additional electrons, all facing in the same direction and frequency. Eventually they hit the reflectors and bounce back, through the medium again, exciting addition emission of the same frequency and direction. This cascade effect creates a *coherent* stream of light that is constantly being *amplified* by additional stimulated emissions. The reflector on the other end is a partial reflecting, reflecting some light and allowing some light to pass through. The light that passes through is the laser beam. This beam is monochromatic, or of one wavelength, and coherent, facing in the same direction. This creates an intense beam of light that can be used to very precisely target anything that will absorb at that wavelength. Depending on the specific gain medium, reflectors, and energy source chosen, a laser of almost any wavelength and intensity can be generated.

In endovascular therapy, the laser beam is subsequently transmitted down fiberoptics that run the length of the catheter. The laser energy is then released at the end of the fiberoptic catheter.

HISTORY OF LASERS IN VASCULAR MEDICINE

Laser applications had already been developed for irradiation of tumors and retinal and skin lesions when the first reported in vitro use of an argon laser to photoablate calcified and noncalcified aortic patches was documented by Marcruz et al.[1] in the early 1980s. Soon after, Lee et al.[2] and Abela et al.[3] reported use of continuous wave argon, neodymium:yttrium aluminum garnet (YAG), and carbon dioxide lasers in atherosclerotic coronary vessels. When Choy et al.[4] reported in vivo transluminal laser recanalization of thrombosed animal arteries using flexible fiberoptics, real interest in the potential role of lasers in vascular medicine began to develop. At that time, the limitations of balloon angioplasty[5,6] had already been explored, leaving a number of difficult lesions uncrossable and thereby untreatable, including 3% to 5% complication rates for distal embolization, thrombosis, and perforation. The hope was that lasers could be used as an adjunctive therapy, facilitate recanalization, and further decrease the need for open surgical bypass and amputation.

Because argon and neodymium:YAG lasers were the only known wavelengths that could be transmitted through fiberoptics, these were the first explored. However, the alarming result of the use of these lasers was that there was a 15% to 20% incidence of perforation with these ridged fiberoptics, creating thrombosis and restenosis and creating very poor long-term patency.[7-9] Necrosis and thermal injury were found in almost all of the reoccluded areas. The two problems that became apparent were that (1) the crude engineering behind the fiberoptic catheter delivery system was traumatic to the vessel and (2) the thermal energy generated by the laser was causing damage to the surrounding tissue around the targeted plaque.

The next iteration of laser atherectomy catheters placed a rounded metal cap at the tip of the catheter.[10] A smooth tip on the fiberoptic catheter would reduce the trauma to vessels caused by the stiff, sharp fibers previously used. In this model, laser energy did not act directly on the tissue but was instead transferred from the laser to the metal tip, which was then heated up, and thermal energy was transferred to the tissue.

Studies with these metal-tipped laser catheters demonstrated an improvement in perforation rate, with the original series exhibiting a perforation rate of less than 2% compared with the original 15% to 20% in the bare fiberoptic fibers.[11,12] This probe became the first Food and Drug Administration (FDA)—approved device for recanalizing peripheral arterial lesions.

Other variations[13,14] of this device were developed subsequently, each with the objective of lowering perforation rates and thermal damage by improving on the design of the fiberoptic catheter or by guiding distribution of laser energy. However, ease of use and questionable efficacy became limitations in their success. Additionally, the attempt to minimize thermal damage of the vessel wall saw a shift from continuous-wave to pulsed-energy lasers,[15,16] a design that sustains in today's laser engineering.

LASER-TISSUE INTERACTIONS AND THE XENON CHLORIDE EXCIMER LASER

In the late 1980s Grundfest et al.[17] proposed the use of ultraviolet (UV) ablation at 308-nm wavelengths via a XeCl excimer laser. This ultimately proved itself to be ideal for plaque photoablation for multiple reasons.

When laser energy is absorbed by tissue, three types of interactions[18] may occur: photothermal, photomechanical, and photochemical. The intensity and nature of each interaction varies depending on the type of laser energy being absorbed and the material absorbing the energy.

Photothermal interactions result from the conversion of laser energy into heat. Excessive heat energy may cause tissue denaturation, coagulation (50°-70° C), tissue water evaporation (>100° C), and carbonization[19] (>350° C). The temperature that is transferred to the tissue depends on the *fluence* (millijoules per square millimeter) and the *penetration depth* of the laser. *Fluence* refers to the energy density of the laser output (higher energy per area = higher fluence). *Penetration depth* refers to the maximum depth at which a material will absorb a specific wavelength of light. Lower penetration depth means higher absorbance (more energy absorbed per area), resulting in lower distribution of laser energy to collateral tissue, allowing for more precise and predictable photoablation.

One of the main problems with early lasers was the rapid build-up of heat in adjacent tissue, resulting from a continuous wave of laser energy. Switching to pulsed ablations dramatically reduced thermal vessel wall damage because a single ablative pulse results in formation of a relatively cool crater wall.[20] However, repeated pulses may still create a temperature buildup (though less rapid than continuous wave) and can still result in damage to surrounding tissue. This further emphasizes the importance of penetration depth in laser-tissue interactions.

TABLE 11-1 Characteristics of Various Lasers

Laser	Mode	Wavelength (nm)	Penetration depth (μm)
XeCl (excimer)	Pulsed	308	30-50
Holmium:YAG	Pulsed	2090	500
Nd:YAG	Continuous	1064	1000
Argon	Continuous	520	400
CO_2	Continuous/ pulsed	10,600	15

What ultimately set the XeCl excimer laser apart[21] was its relatively shallow penetration depth. In the case of the excimer laser, the 308-nm wavelength is absorbed at 30 to 50 μm in tissue. Compare this with the penetration depths of previous iterations of laser atherectomy catheters (Table 11-1), and it becomes clear that the excimer laser has a penetration depth that is significantly lower than that of its predecessors. The reason for this shallow penetration depth is later explained in this section via photochemical interactions.

Quick absorption by plaque also allows less time for scattering of the UV light. This creates small, very precise ablation of targets. A study of lesion ablation via pulse-waved excimer laser found that the action of the XeCl laser radiation revealed channel walls that were flat and uncharred, with close to no damage. Such a channel conspicuously contrasted with channels created by continuous-wave or higher-wavelength laser catheters.

Photomechanical interactions between laser energy and tissue result when laser energy is converted to kinetic energy (typically via tissue heating). The first method by which this may occur is when surrounding tissue expands because of previously described photothermal interactions, causing stress waves to propagate out of the irradiated tissue into adjacent tissue,[22] potentially causing damage to adjacent tissue.

The second method by which photomechanical interactions affect surrounding tissue is via vapor bubble expansion. When tissue water is heated by laser energy, it is converted to water vapor, resulting in fast-expanding and imploding intraluminal vapor bubble that produces microsecond dilation and invagination of the adjacent arterial segment.[23,24] During expansion, the vapor condenses, causing an implosion that creates propagating pressure waves. After collapse, a second, smaller bubble may form and collapse again. The explosive nature of this vapor bubble can result in removal or separation of tissue structures. The size and intensity of this vapor bubble can be significantly reduced by flushing the catheter with saline solution before photoablation (discussed in the Lasing Techniques section of this chapter).

In photoablation using the excimer laser, the key to minimizing surrounding tissue damage is the formation of the *plume*.[25] After vapor bubble expansion and collapse, a plume may be created that carries away the excess heat of the photonic pulse, resulting in a cool, clean crater. Plumes are created when the duration of the laser pulse is much shorter than the time required for heat to diffuse out of the irradiated zone. In general, photonic heating occurs much faster than the time it takes for residual heat to escape into surrounding tissue. With a very short laser pulse, the heat of the irradiated tissue remains confined in the vaporized water and tissue and resulting steam ejects a plume, carrying away the majority of the heat.

Photochemical interactions occur when laser energy is absorbed to excited molecules to higher rotational, vibrational, or electron states, resulting in bond breakage.[26,27] One theory is that this type of interaction is unique to lasers at the UV wavelength because proteins and nucleic acids absorb at 308 nm, resulting in direct breaking of molecular bonds, whereas lasers operating at infrared wavelengths can only indirectly affect organic content via photothermal and photomechanical interactions. Because excimer laser energy is *not* absorbed by water, saline, and other simple liquids, it has a relatively shallow penetration depth. Plaque is composed largely of organic material, which readily absorbs at UV wavelengths. Previous laser catheters operating at higher wavelengths have higher penetration depths in tissue because they rely on absorption by water and subsequent collateral damage to organic material. This can result in absorption to the depth of the tissue wall, increasing the likelihood of thermal damage. Whereas other lasers rely solely on photothermal interactions for ablation, excimer lasers have the distinct advantage of the more direct approach of photochemical interactions as well.

In summary, the relative success of the XeCl excimer laser can be attributed to the following:

- UV light is pulsed, reducing thermal damage to collateral tissue
- UV light breaks molecular bonds, a property unique to UV wavelengths. It does not have to rely exclusively on thermal damage via water absorption.
- UV light has a very shallow penetration depth because of its rapid absorption by organic material.
- At short pulses and at a certain threshold fluence, a plume is formed, carrying away excessive heat, creating a neat, cool crater, leaving little room for thermal damage of surrounding tissue.
- UV ablation combines photothermal, photomechanical, and photochemical effects. Photochemical interactions are the key to reduction of damage typically caused by photothermal and photomechanical effects.

CASE SELECTION

In peripheral endovascular therapy, case selection for uses of laser atherectomy catheters depends entirely on characteristics of the target lesion. Lesions ideal for laser atherectomy intervention include the following: chronic total occlusions, stenotic lesions with suspect significant thrombus (can be detected via intravascular ultrasound [IVUS]), and lesions with large plaque burden (also identifiable via IVUS).[28-31] In particular, patients who are poor candidates for bypass surgery often benefit from intervention via laser atherectomy. With this adjunctive therapy, previously inaccessible lesions via balloon angioplasty become treatable.[32] Patient comorbidities and other patient characteristics have thus far been irrelevant in the decision to intervene via laser atherectomy, though it has been suggested that chronic renal failure and diabetes are risk factors for a negative outcome.[33]

LASING TECHNIQUES

A summary of how to appropriately and effectively operate an excimer laser catheter:

1. Select an appropriately sized catheter.
2. Thread the catheter over the guidewire until the tip of the catheter is in contact with the target plaque or thrombus.
3. Infuse tissue plasminogen activator (t-PA), if desired.
4. Flush the catheter with saline.
5. Apply a few grams of pressure and begin ablation, *slowly* advancing the catheter with each pulse.

1. Select an Appropriate Size and Setting for the Catheter

Currently, the excimer laser catheter system is the Spectranetics CVX-300 Excimer Laser System and Turbo Elite Laser Catheter, manufactured by Spectranetics (Colorado Springs, CO). Catheter selection depends on a combination of the size of the vessel and the nature of the lesion. To debulk the maximum amount of plaque before potential subsequent intervention (angioplasty, stent), typically, the largest possible diameter catheter that will accommodate the vessel is selected. However, heavily calcified, more diseased lesions generally will not yield to larger-diameter catheters. Therefore increasingly severe lesions warrant selection of catheters with decreased diameters. This could result in upsizing and multiple exchanges of laser catheters as ablation of the lesion progresses. Existing excimer lasers for peripheral vascular intervention can be found in Table 11-2. According to Spectranetics guidelines, laser catheter diameter should not exceed two thirds of the reference vessel diameter (Table 11-3).

Smaller catheters have higher fluency and frequency ranges, because there is less risk of perforation. Conversely, larger catheters have lower ranges.[34] Default laser settings are at 45 mJ/mm^2/25 Hz (fluency/frequency), also the recommended start settings. During the procedure, fluency and repetition can be increased as needed to cross the lesion.

2. Thread the Catheter Over the Guidewire Until the Tip of the Catheter Is in Contact With the Target Plaque or Thrombus

As shown in Figure 11-3, the tip of a laser catheter is composed of a bundle of multiple fibers. Each fiber conducts a fraction of the total energy that is ultimately transmitted to its target. To maximize effectiveness of ablation, the tip of the catheter must be in direct physical contact with the targeted lesion. Any fiber that is not in contact with its target will distribute energy to surrounding fluid (saline, blood), resulting in an inadequate amount of pulse energy being transmitted to the tissue, creating a suboptimal result.

3. Infuse t-PA, if Desired

Preliminary data suggest that t-PA infusion before photoablation decreases the risk of distal embolization and facilitates crossing of difficult lesions. t-PA works to lyse any thrombotic components of the lesion throughout the course of ablation. Particles not entirely vaporized that may be carried into the bloodstream (e.g., via the vapor bubble or plume) have already been infused with t-PA and will thus continue to thrombolyse as they travel through the bloodstream, further decreasing the risk of embolization.

4. Flush the Catheter With Saline

Before activation of the laser, the catheter *must* first be generously flushed with saline. Early procedures activated the laser in contrast medium, which created significant pressure on the vessel wall during expansion of the vapor bubble, leading to an unacceptable rate of

TABLE 11-2 Turbo Elite Peripheral Over-the-Wire and Rapid Exchange Catheters

Device	0.9 mm	1.4 mm	1.7 mm	2.0 mm	2.3 mm	2.5 mm
TURBO ELITE PERIPHERAL OVER-THE-WIRE (OTW) CATHETERS						
Model number	410-152	414-151	417-152	420-006	423-001	425-011
Max guidewire compatibility (in.)	0.014	0.014	0.018	0.018	0.018	0.018
Max tip outside diameter (in.)	0.038	0.055	0.068	0.080	0.091	0.101
Max shaft diameter (in.)	0.047	0.056	0.069	0.081	0.091	0.102
Working length (cm)	150	150	150	150	120	110
Sheath compatibility (F)	4	5	5	7	7	8
Fluence (mJ/mm^2)	30-80	30-60	30-60	30-60	30-60	30-45
Repetition rate (Hz)	25-80	25-80	25-80	25-80	25-80	25-80
TURBO ELITE PERIPHERAL RAPID EXCHANGE (RX) CATHETERS						
Model number	410-154	414-149	417-156	420-159		
Max guidewire compatibility (in.)	0.014	0.014	0.014	0.014		
Max tip outside diameter (in.)	0.038	0.057	0.069	0.080		
Max shaft diameter (in.)	0.049	0.062	0.072	0.084		
Working length (cm)	150	150	150	150		
Sheath compatibility (F)	4	5	6	7		
Fluence (mJ/mm^2)	30-80	30-60	30-60	30-60		
Repetition rate (Hz)	25-80	25-80	25-80	25-80		

Max, Maximum.

TABLE 11-3 Catheter Selection

Catheter size (mm)	Proximal vessel diameter (mm)
0.9	≥1.4
1.4	≥2.1
1.7	≥2.6
2.0	≥3.0
2.3	≥3.5
2.5	≥3.8

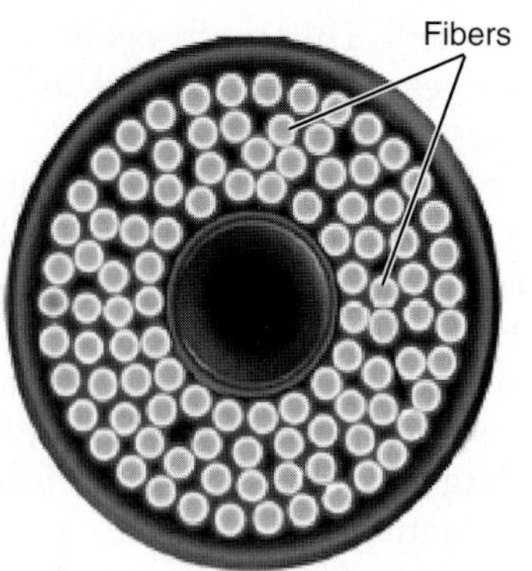

FIGURE 11-3 Cross-section of a laser catheter. The catheter is threaded over a guidewire via the center hole. Fibers must be in continuous contact with the lesion for effective photoablation.

dissection. It turned out that contrast and blood both readily absorb UV light; a large portion of the energy was being absorbed by the medium rather than being transmitted to the lesion.

In the mid-1990s a new technique[35] accurately suggested that replacing blood and contrast with saline would reduce vessel trauma caused by high pressures. UV light is not absorbed by saline, making it an ideal medium for photoablation. Further studies[36] solidified this hypothesis, demonstrating that the immersion medium is crucial in reducing peak pressures on the vessel wall.

5. Apply a Few Grams of Pressure and Begin Ablation, *Slowly* Advancing the Catheter With Each Pulse

A small amount of force must be applied to the catheter to ensure proper ablation.[37] At 0 g of force, ablation occurred with depths linearly correlated to fluency. However, the fiber did not penetrate the tissue. With weight added, the fiber required three or four pulses before penetrating the tissue. To advance the catheter along the lesion, a moderate amount of pressure must be applied to the catheter.

To maximize luminal diameter, the recommended advancement rate is ≤1 mm/s, or ≤6 cm/min (Spectranetics). Excessive weight on the catheter causes rapid advancement, which ultimately results in creation of a less than optimal lumen diameter (Figure 11-4, *A* and *B*).

COMPLICATIONS

The most serious complications resulting from laser intervention are major dissection, thrombosis, and distal embolization. All of these can be prevented with application and adherence to the previously mentioned techniques. Selection of a catheter with too large of a diameter can result in vessel wall perforation. Flushing of saline before use of the laser is crucial to prevention of perforation caused by the low transmission of UV light in contrast and blood. One technique of preventing distal embolization is infusion of t-PA before laser activation. Last, proper handling of the laser during ablation (appropriate advancement rates and pressure application) is necessary to ensure effective photoablation.

CURRENT LITERATURE

Multicenter studies involving peripheral laser atherectomies include the following:

PELA (2001)[38]—Peripheral Excimer Laser Angioplasty: This study randomly assigned 251 patients with claudication and superficial femoral artery (SFA) occlusions ≥10 cm to either laser-assisted angioplasty or balloon angioplasty alone at 13 U.S. and 6 German sites. Stenting was optional for both categories but discouraged. Clinical success was defined as ≥50% patency at 1 year by ultrasound examination, with no serious adverse events. Results for both groups were similar with the exception that the laser group received significantly fewer stents (42% compared with 59% of the angioplasty-only group). Results at 12 months were also similar for both groups. This study showed a trend toward reduced number of stents in the laser group, but the superiority of laser application could not be confirmed.

LACI (2006)[39]—Laser Angioplasty for Critical Ischemia: The purpose of this study was to evaluate the effectiveness of laser angioplasty in patients with critical limb ischemia. Fourteen sites in the United States and Germany enrolled 145 patients with 155 critically ischemic limbs. All were poor candidates for bypass surgery. Treatment included laser atherectomy followed by balloon angioplasty with optional stenting. Stents were implanted in 45% of limbs. At 6-month follow-up, limb salvage was achieved in 110 (92%) of 119

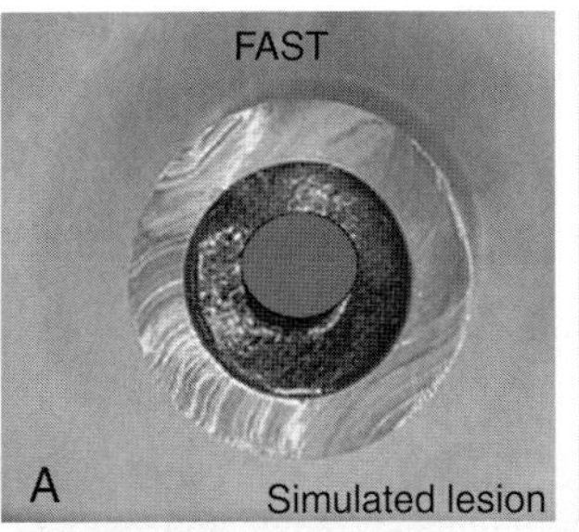

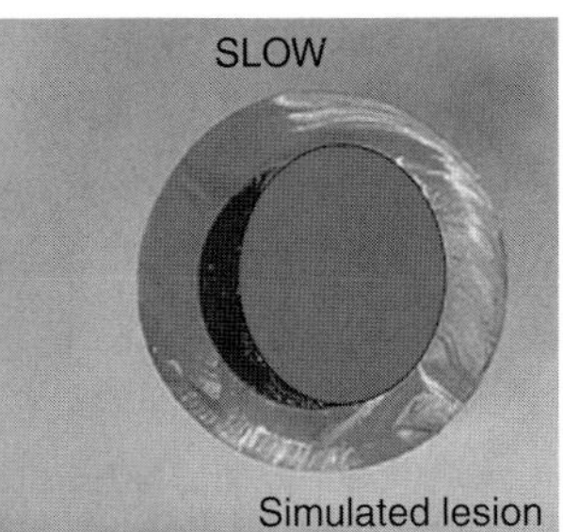

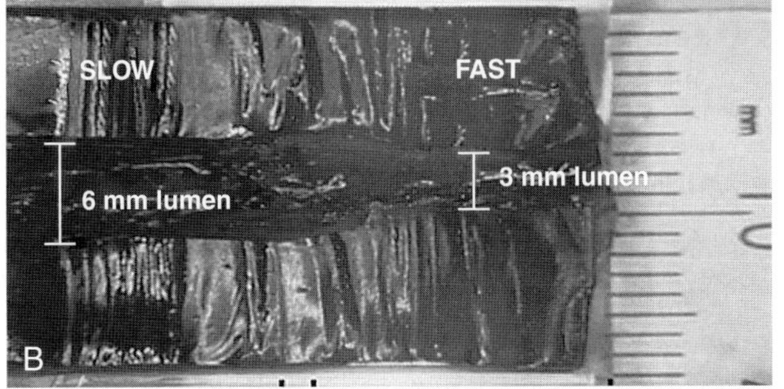

FIGURE 11-4 **A,** Advancement of a Turbo Elite 2.3-mm catheter through a simulated lesion. The *left* image indicates advancement at speed >1 mm/s. The *right* image indicates advancement at a speed <1 mm/s. (*Courtesy Spectranetics Corp.*) **B,** Comparison of multiple catheter advancement rates in a single simulated lesion. (*Courtesy Spectranetics Corp.*)

surviving patients or 93% (118/127) of all limbs. This study concluded that laser-assisted angioplasty was highly effective in limb salvage and revascularization of patients who were unfit for bypass surgery. Other similar studies modeled after the LACI registry include LACI CIS,[40] LACI Belgium,[41] and LACI-RTO (refractory total occlusions), all of which produced excellent limb-salvage rates above 90%.

CELLO (2009)[42]—CliRpath Excimer Laser System to Enlarge Lumen Openings: This most recent study was designed to evaluate the safety and efficacy of the Spectranetics Turbo-Booster addition to the existing Turbo Elite Laser Catheter System. The Turbo-Booster was designed to include lumen diameter during recanalization of lesions. The registry was conducted at 17 sites in the United States, with 65 de novo lesions treated (13 occluded, 52 stenotic). Balloon angioplasty and/or stenting was optional. The primary end point was reduction in lesion diameter measured by Doppler ultrasound after laser ablation before any adjunctive therapy. The primary safety end point was major adverse events at 6 months. Results indicated no major adverse events with a statistically significant improvement in walking impairment and functional status assessments. Lesion diameters were reduced from an average of 77% at baseline to 34%, which was further reduced to 21% after adjunctive therapy. Patency rates were 59% and 54% at 6 and 12 months. Revascularization was not required in 76.9% at 12 months. This study validated the safety and efficacy of the Turbo-Booster laser guide catheter.

In addition to treating infrainguinal disease and critical limb ischemia, more recent single-center studies have demonstrated efficacy of excimer laser ablation in patients with diabetes with critical limb ischemia,[43] recommended the possibility of using embolic filter protection in response to distal embolization during laser photoablation,[44] and experimented with the use of excimer lasers in hemodialysis access intervention.[45] Furthermore, preliminary data from our own retrospective study of more than 450 critically ischemic limbs have shown that the "Lyse and Lase" technique—infusion of thrombolysis before laser ablation—is an effective means of minimizing distal embolization and facilitating crossing of difficult lesions.

CURRENT LIMITATIONS, FUTURE APPLICATIONS

It is apparent that the role of lasers in peripheral intervention continues to evolve. One of the major limitations of the excimer laser today is its ability to create a channel only as wide as the diameter of the catheter itself. The CELLO registry mentioned previously aims to overcome this limitation. Successful application of this technology would mean increased debulking of the target lesion, increased luminal diameter, and possibly decreased restenosis and decreased need for adjunctive therapies such as balloon angioplasty and stenting. The long-term results are yet to be seen. Another possibility for improvement to the existing laser system may be drug delivery to enhance laser ablation and further extend debulking.

Furthermore, so far there have only been published results of applications of the excimer laser in coronary and peripheral vasculature. The decreased use of stents in patients who have received laser treatment, and the success of the excimer laser in otherwise untreatable patients with critical limb ischemia (aside from amputation), suggests that the future of laser may include applications in visceral arteries, renals, or even the carotids.

CONCLUSION

After some initial missteps with the first few iterations of laser photoablation devices, the XeCl excimer laser proved itself to be effective in achieving the originally intended goals for interventional laser photoablation. With appropriate application of lasing techniques, laser atherectomy can open up many possibilities to patients with chronic total occlusions and critical limb ischemia. The exploration of additional potential roles of lasers in vascular medicine continues to be an evolving topic. There are still many improvements to be made and applications to investigate. In the meantime, it seems that lasers have found a niche in peripheral vascular intervention as an effective adjunctive therapy to balloon angioplasty and stenting.

References

1. Marcruz R, Martins JRM, Turpinanba AS, et al: Possibilidades terapeuticas do raio laser em atermas, *Arq Bras Cardio* 34:9–12 (in Portuguese), 1980.
2. Lee G, Ikeda RM, Kozina J, et al: Laser dissolution of coronary atherosclerotic obstruction, *Am Heart J* 102:1074–1075, 1981.
3. Abela GS, Normann S, Cohen D, et al: Effects of carbon dioxide Nd-YAG and argon laser radiation on coronary atheromatous plaque, *Am J Cardiol* 50:1199–1205, 1982.
4. Choy DSJ, Stertzer SH, Rotterdam HZ, et al: Transluminal laser catheter angioplasty, *Am J Cardiol* 50:1206–1208, 1982.
5. Specchia G, Bramucci E, Montemartini C: Indications and limits of transluminal angioplasty, *G Ital Cardiol* 13(4):340–344 (in Italian), 1983.
6. Katzen BT: Percutaneous transluminal angioplasty for arterial disease of the lower extremities, *AJR Am J Roentgenol* 142 (1):23–25, 1984.
7. Ginsburg R, Wexler K, Mitchell RS, et al: Percutaneous transluminal laser angioplasty for treatment of peripheral vascular disease. Clinical experience with 16 patients, *Radiology* 156:619–624, 1985.
8. Geschwind H, Boussignac G, Teisseire B, et al: Percutaneous transluminal laser angioplasty in man, *Lancet* i:844, 1984.
9. Cumberland DC, Tayler DI, Procter AE: Laser-assisted percutaneous angioplasty: initial clinical experience in peripheral arteries, *Clin Radiol* 37:423–428, 1986.
10. Hussein H: A novel fiberoptic laserprobe for treatment of occlusive vessel disease, *Optical Laser Technol Med* 605:59–66, 1986.
11. Cumberland DC, Sanborn TA, Taylor DI, et al: Percutaneous laser thermal angioplasty: initial clinical results with a laserprobe in total periphery artery occlusions, *Lancet* i:1457–1459, 1986.
12. Sanborn TA, Cumberland DC, Greenfield AJ, et al: Peripheral laser-assisted balloon angioplasty: initial multicenter experience in 210 peripheral arteries, *Arch Surg* 124:1099–1103, 1989.
13. Nordstrom LA, Castaneda-Zuniga WR, Von Seggern KB: Peripheral arterial obstructions: analysis of patency 1 year after laser-assisted transluminal angioplasty, *Radiology* 181:515–520, 1991.
14. Spears JR: Percutaneous transluminal coronary angioplasty restenosis: potential prevention with laser balloon angioplasty, *Am J Cardiol* 60:61B–64B, 1987.
15. Deckelbaum LI, Isner JM, Donaldson RF, et al: Reduction of laser-induced pathologic tissue injury using pulsed energy delivery, *Am J Cardiol* 56:662–667, 1985.
16. Isner JM, Clarke RH: The paradox of thermal ablation without thermal injury, *Lasers Med Sci* 2:165–173, 1987.
17. Grundfest WS, Litvack IF, Goldenberg T, et al: Pulsed ultraviolet lasers and the potential for safe laser angioplasty, *Am J Surg* 150:220–226, 1985.
18. Jacques SL: Laser-tissue interactions: photochemical, photothermal and photomechanical, *Surg Clin N Am* 72:531–558, 1992.
19. Thomsen S: Pathologic analysis of photothermal and photomechanical effects of laser-tissue interactions, *Photochem Photobiol* 53:825–835, 1991.
20. Lane RJ, Wynne JJ, Geronemus RG: Ultraviolet laser ablation of skin: healing studies and a thermal model, *Laser Surg Med* 6:504–513, 1987.
21. Nakamura F, Kvasnicka J, Levame M, et al: Acute response of the arterial wall to pulsed laser irradiation, *Lasers Surg Med* 13 (4):412–420, 1993.
22. Vogel A, Schweiger P, Frieser A, et al: Intraocular Nd:YAG laser surgery; light-tissue interaction, damage range, and reduction of collateral effects, *IEEE J Quantum Electron* 26:2240–2260, 1990.
23. Van Leeuwen TG, Meertens JH, Velema E, et al: Intraluminal vapor bubble induced by excimer laser pulse causes microsecond arterial dilation and invagination leading to extensive wall damage in the rabbit, *Circulation* 87(4):1258–1263, 1993.
24. Van Leeuwen TG, van Erven L, Meertens JH, et al: Origin of the arterial wall dissections induced by pulsed excimer and mid-infrared laser ablation in the pig, *J Am Coll Cardiol* 19 (7):1610–1618, 1992.
25. Oraevsky AA, Jacques SL, Pettit GH, et al: XeCl laser ablation of atherosclerotic aorta: luminescence spectroscopy of ablation products, *Lasers Surg Med* 13(2):168–178, 1993.
26. Linsker R, Srinivasan R, Wynne JJ, et al: Far-ultraviolet laser ablation of atherosclerotic lesions, *Lasers Surg Med* 4:201–206, 1984.
27. Cross FW, Bowker TJ: The physical properties of tissue ablation with excimer lasers, *Med Instrum* 21:226–230, 1987.
28. Shrikhande GV, McKinsey JF: Use and abuse of atherectomy: where should it be used? *Semin Vasc Surg* 21(4):204–209, 2008.
29. Das TS: Excimer laser-assisted angioplasty for infrainguinal artery disease, *J Endovasc Ther* 16(2 Suppl. 2):II98–I104, 2009.
30. Tan JW, Yeo KK, Laird JR: Excimer laser-assisted angioplasty for complex infrainguinal disease: a 2008 update, *J Cardiovasc Surg (Torino)* 49(3):329–340, 2008.
31. Topaz O, Ebersole D, Das T, et al: Excimer laser angioplasty in acute myocardial infarction (the CARMEL multicenter trial), *Am J Cardiol* 93:694–701, 2004.
32. Gray BH, Laird JR, Ansel GM, et al: Complex endovascular treatment for critical limb ischemia in poor surgical candidates: a pilot study, *J Endovasc Ther* 9:599–604, 2002.
33. Stoner MC, deFreitas DF, Phade SV, et al: Mid-term results with laser atherectomy in the treatment of infrainguinal occlusive disease, *J Vasc Surg* 46(2):289–295, 2007.
34. Kvasnicka J, Nakamura F, Lange F, et al: Tissue ablation with excimer laser and multiple fiber catheters: effects of optical fiber density and fluence, *J Interven Cardiol* 5(4):263–273, 1992.
35. Tcheng JE, Wells LD, Phillips HR, et al: Development of a new technique for reducing pressure pulse generation during 308-nm excimer laser coronary angioplasty, *Cathet Cardiovasc Diagn* 34 (1):15–22, 1995.
36. Tcheng JE: Saline infusion in excimer laser coronary angioplasty, *Semin Intervent Cardiol* 1:135–141, 1996.
37. Gijsbers GH, van den Broecke DG, Sprangers RL, et al: Effect of force on ablation depth for a XeCl excimer laser beam delivered by an optical fiber in contact with arterial tissue in saline, *Laser Surg Med* 12(6):576–584, 1992.
38. Laird JR. Peripheral Excimer Laser Angioplasty (PELA) trial results. Presented at the Transcatheter Cardiovascular Therapeutics (TCT) Conference; September 24-28, 2002; Washington, DC.
39. Laird JR, Zeller T, Gray BH, et al: LACI Investigators. Limb salvage following laser assisted angioplasty for critical limb ischemia: results of the LACI multicenter trial, *J Endovasc Ther* 13 (1):1–11, 2006.

40. Allie DE, Hebert CJ, Lirtzman CH et al. Infrapopliteal excimer laser-assisted angioplasty in "true limb salvage": a 12-month LACI equivalent study. Poster abstract presented at the Transcatheter Cardiovascular Therapeutics (TCT) Conference, September 15–19, 2003, Washington, DC.
41. Boisers M, Peeters P, Elst FV, et al: Excimer laser-assisted angioplasty for critical limb ischemia: results of the LACI Belgium Study, *Eur J Endovasc Surg* 29(6):613–619, 2005.
42. Dave RM, Patlola R, Kollmeyer K, et al: CELLO Investigators. Excimer laser recanalization of femoropoliteal lesions and 1-year patency: results of the CELLO registry, *J Endovasc Ther* 16 (6):665–675, 2009.
43. Serino F, Cao Y, Renzi C, et al: Excimer laser ablation in the treatment of total chronic occlusions in critical limb ischemia in diabetic patients. Sustained efficacy of plaque recanalisation in mid-term results, *Eur J Endovasc Surg* 39(2):234–238, 2010.
44. Shammas NW, Coiner D, Shammas GA, et al: Distal embolic event protection using the excimer laser ablation in peripheral vascular interventions: results of the DEEP EMBOLI registry, *J Endovasc Ther* 16(2):197–202, 2009.
45. Yevzlin AS, Urbanes A: Excimer laser assisted angioplasty in hemodialysis access intervention, *Semin Dial* 22(5):580–583, 2009.

CHAPTER

12

Percutaneous Thrombectomy and Mechanical Thrombolysis Catheters

Jeffrey Wang, Elliot L. Chaikof

Arterial and venous thromboembolic disease remains a major cause of death and disability despite the discovery of heparin by McLean and Howell in 1916 and its subsequent introduction into clinical practice in 1936.[1] Each year acute limb ischemia affects 14 persons per 100,000 in the U.S. population, with procedures relating to the treatment of acute arterial ischemia comprising 10% to 14% of the annual vascular surgical workload.[2] Venous thromboembolism occurs at a five-fold greater frequency with recent estimates of 77.6 cases per 100,000 person-years.[3] In an effort to reduce the sequelae of postthrombotic syndrome, recent guidelines recommend operative venous thrombectomy or catheter-directed thrombolysis in selected patients with acute iliofemoral deep venous thrombosis (DVT), the latter approach being preferred.[4] Thus the relative number of venous thrombectomy procedures performed over the next decade will likely increase at an even greater pace than those performed for arterial ischemia. These clinical realities will continue to motivate the development of safer and more effective modalities for clot removal.

HISTORY OF THROMBECTOMY DEVICES

Surgical thrombectomy before the 1960s consisted of either direct aspiration through an arteriotomy or flushing of the occluded arterial segment with saline solution through arteriotomies proximal and distal to the site of clot. Alternatively, metal pigtail probes had been described for clot retrieval through an arteriotomy but were often associated with significant vessel wall injury. In 1963 Fogarty and colleagues[5] introduced surgical balloon catheter thrombectomy. Although requiring an arteriotomy, this procedure was less invasive than prior approaches, could be performed with the patient under local anesthesia, facilitated rapid extraction of clot remote from the site of arteriotomy, and was technically simple. Despite the advantages of balloon catheter thrombectomy, acknowledged limitations include the need for surgical arterial exposure; incomplete clot extraction, particularly of clot propagated into smaller branches; potential for vessel injury; and an inability to administer thrombolysis in a sustained manner.

In the 1960s thrombolytic agents were first administered systemically to patients with pulmonary embolism through a peripheral venous route, which evolved during the following decade to catheter-directed therapy to reduce risk of bleeding complications. With growing experience and encouraging results, catheter-directed thrombolysis was subsequently applied to patients presenting with both arterial and venous thromboembolism. There were clear advantages of this technique with respect to balloon thrombectomy. It was less invasive, requiring only percutaneous access; was atraumatic; and facilitated the treatment of difficult-to-access vessels. The ability also existed to eliminate thrombi in smaller branch vessels, inaccessible to balloon catheter thrombectomy. Moreover, in the case of an acute arterial thrombosis, thrombolysis provided a means to define the underlying lesion for optimal planning of subsequent surgical or catheter-based treatment.

Catheter-directed thrombolysis, as a minimally invasive therapy, achieved similar levels of amputation-free survival when compared with surgical intervention in several large randomized trials conducted during the mid-1990s to late 1990s. However, significant limitations of lytic therapy exist, including the inability to safely use this approach in a wide variety of patient populations (Box 12-1). Although relatively simple to initiate,

BOX 12-1

CONTRAINDICATIONS TO LYTIC THERAPY

Absolute
- Active internal bleeding
- Cerebrovascular incident <2 mo
- Pathologic intracranial condition

Major
- Recent major surgery
- Gastrointestinal ulcer or bleeding disorder
- Recent major trauma
- Uncontrolled hypertension

Minor
- Minor surgery
- Recent cardiopulmonary resuscitation
- Bacterial endocarditis
- Liver disease
- Pregnancy
- Left heart thrombus

continuous monitoring in an intensive care unit (ICU) setting with multiple blood draws is required to minimize the risk of bleeding. In addition, patients are often subjected to multiple arteriograms through the course of therapy to monitor the progression of clot lysis. Finally, effective catheter-directed thrombolysis typically entails treatment periods of 24 to 48 hours in duration.

Limitations aside, surgical thrombectomy provides, in an ideal setting, a rapid and complete means for clot extraction, whereas catheter-directed lytic therapy is a minimally invasive, percutaneous treatment. The development of percutaneous mechanical thrombectomy devices was pursued in an attempt to combine the advantages of each of these approaches with direct removal of clot with or without adjunctive thrombolysis. The promise of such a combined strategy would be a reduction in thrombolytic dose, clot lysis time, ICU stay, cost, and total treatment time, with the goal of achieving complete resolution of clot burden in a single setting. By 2000, the U.S. Food and Drug Administration had approved eight mechanical thrombectomy devices for treatment applications, with the majority of these devices initially directed at the treatment of clotted hemodialysis arteriovenous grafts. Current applications have been extended to both venous and arterial beds within all anatomic zones.

CLASSIFICATION OF PERCUTANEOUS MECHANICAL THROMBECTOMY DEVICES

Percutaneous mechanical thrombectomy devices can be classified into five major categories. *Percutaneous aspiration thrombectomy devices* rely on steady suction delivered through a large-lumen aspiration catheter. Many ad hoc strategies and modifications have been developed with use of guide catheters and sheaths. *Pull-back thrombectomy and trapping devices* engage and remove thrombus with a balloon catheter or basket, which retrieves the clot into a trapping device. *Recirculation mechanical thrombectomy devices* use either high-speed rotation (>90,000 rpm) or retrograde fluid jets ranging from 1000 to 10,000 psi to generate hydrodynamic vortexes that ablate the thrombus. *Nonrecirculation mechanical thrombectomy devices* rely on mechanical fragmentation without significant hydrodynamic recirculation and generally function at a relatively low rotational speed (800-5000 rpm). The final category of device uses either direct or indirect ultrasound, laser, or radiofrequency energy to assist thrombolysis.

The first generation of percutaneous mechanical thrombectomy devices exhibited significant limitations. First, clot maceration and aspiration did not occur simultaneously, such that the resulting fragmented thrombus was aspirated through a guide catheter or sheath. This lack of integration reduced the efficiency of thrombus removal and increased the risk of distal embolization. In addition, combined delivery of lytic therapy was cumbersome. The evolution of second-generation devices incorporated concomitant clot fragmentation and aspiration. Moreover, many of these devices had associated infusion ports that facilitated the adjunctive use of catheter-directed lytic therapy. Percutaneous mechanical thrombectomy has emerged as a useful alternative and/or adjunct to both open surgical thrombectomy and pharmacologic thrombolysis.[6-15] The following section is a review of currently available percutaneous mechanical thrombectomy devices.

PULL-BACK THROMBECTOMY AND TRAPPING CATHETERS

Merci Retrieval System

This device consists of a guide catheter with a balloon mounted near the tip along with a microcatheter delivery system and helical clot extraction device (Figure 12-1).

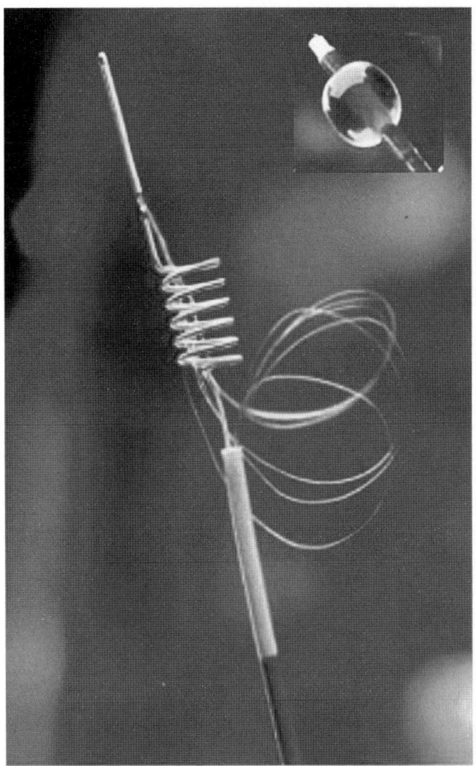

FIGURE 12-1 Merci Retrieval System. *Inset,* The balloon-tipped guide catheter. *(Courtesy Concentric Medical, Inc., Mountain View, CA.)*

The device is primarily intended for clot extraction in the cerebral circulation for treatment of acute stroke.

Mechanism of Action

The guide catheter is placed in the internal carotid artery for anterior circulation strokes or the subclavian artery just proximal to the dominant vertebral artery for posterior circulation strokes. The clot is crossed with a 0.014-inch wire, and the microcatheter delivery system is advanced over the wire beyond the clot. The helical clot extractor is then unsheathed distal to the clot and pulled back to engage the clot. The balloon guide catheter is then inflated to stop the forward flow of blood, and the clot is pulled back toward the guide catheter. During the clot extraction vigorous aspiration through the guide catheter is performed.

Logistical Considerations

The helical extraction coil of the Merci Retrieval System has been fabricated with or without additional capture filaments. It can be delivered through 7F to 9F balloon guide catheters that are 95 cm in length. Microcatheters are 150 cm in length, and retrieval helical clot extractor systems are 180 cm in length with helix diameters of 1.5 to 3 mm. The Merci Retrieval System is relatively simple to use and is minimally traumatic to the native circulation.

There are no published series using the Merci Retrieval Catheter in the peripheral arterial circulation. The MERCI 1 phase 1 trial for clot extraction in the cerebral vasculature showed successful target vessel recanalization in 43% of patients with mechanical embolectomy alone and 64% recanalization with the addition of catheter-directed lytic therapy with tissue plasminogen activator (t-PA).[16]

RECIRCULATION MECHANICAL THROMBECTOMY CATHETERS

Helix Clot Buster

The Helix Clot Buster is a non–wire-guided thrombectomy catheter (Figure 12-2). It uses an impeller, which disrupts and homogenizes the clot to particles less than 10 μm in diameter, which are expelled from side ports. This device is attached to a foot pedal activator with a source of compressed air or nitrogen. The Helix Clot Buster is approved for use in both prosthetic dialysis grafts and native fistulae.

Mechanism of Action

The catheter is placed through a sheath up to the area of treatment. Once the catheter is in place it is actuated by the foot pedal, which will rotate the impeller at the tip of the catheter to speeds greater than 140,000 rpm. The high rotational speed of the impeller causes a recirculation vortex that draws clot material toward the impeller, which aids the removal of thrombus adherent to the wall.[17]

Logistical Considerations

The Helix Clot Buster is delivered through a 7F sheath and comes in 75- and 120-cm working lengths. A guidewire may be used to assist in delivery but is removed during activation. During activation, heparinized saline flush is administered under pressure. The catheter should not be bent within the first 2 cm from the tip or greater than 45 degrees along the shaft. Extensive use of the Helix device can lead to significant hemolysis.[17] The device requires only compressed gas for use.

The Helix device was shown to be equivalent to its predecessor the Amplatz thrombectomy device (ATD) in both efficacy and safety.[18] The Helix device can be placed through a 7F sheath, whereas the ATD required an 8F sheath. The efficacy of the Amplatz thrombectomy device was compared with open surgical thrombectomy for clot extraction from synthetic dialysis grafts in randomized trial.[19] A total of 74 procedures were performed in the open surgical group and 140 procedures in the ATD group. Technical success was defined as greater than 90% thrombus removal and the ability to

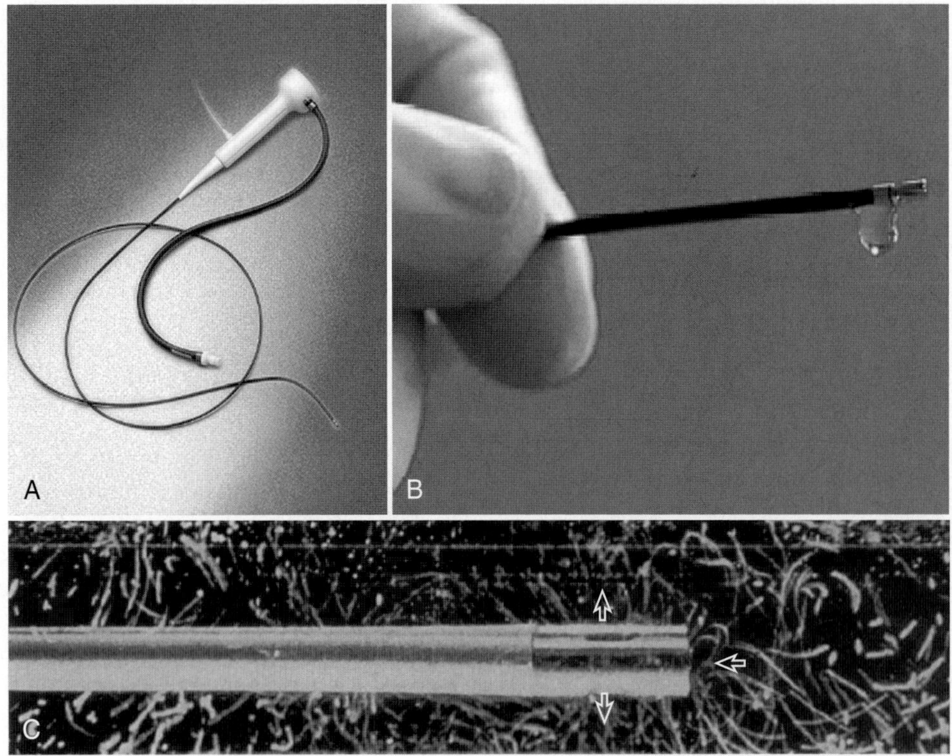

FIGURE 12-2 **A,** Helix Clot Buster device. **B,** Helix Clot Buster device with saline flush through tip. **C,** Illustration of vortex generated by impeller housed in the tip of the device. *(Courtesy eV3, Inc., Plymouth, MN.)*

dialyze after the treatment. Procedural success was achieved in 79% in the ATD group and 73% in the open surgical group (p = not significant [NS]). Patency of the graft at 90 days, as determined by successful dialysis, was 75% and 68% in the ATD and surgical thrombectomy groups, respectively (p = NS).[19]

Delomez et al.[20] reported treatment in 18 patients with either femoral vein, iliac vein, or inferior vena cava (IVC) thrombus with an ATD after placement of a temporary IVC filter. Successful recanalization was achieved in 15 patients (83%). In 8 patients, ATD therapy alone was sufficient for recanalization, whereas additional interventions were required in 7 patients. Görich et al.[21] reported a series of 18 patients with acute occlusions of the femoral artery treated with ATD. Recanalization was achieved in 14 patients with limb salvage of 93% at 8 months. Twelve patients required additional lytic therapy for emboli within tibial vessels.[21]

ThromCat Thrombectomy Catheter

The ThromCat Thrombectomy Catheter is a wire-guided thrombectomy catheter that uses suction, which draws the clot into the catheter, and an impeller, which disrupts and homogenizes the clot into particles (Figure 12-3). The macerated clot is then extracted from the vessel through the catheter into a collection bag. This device consists of the catheter, control unit, and power supply. The ThromCat Thrombectomy Catheter is approved for use in clotted prosthetic dialysis grafts and native fistulae.

Mechanism of Action

The thrombus is first crossed by a guidewire, and the catheter placed proximal to the thrombus. The catheter requires a continuous infusion of sterile saline solution that is injected into the vessel through infusion ports at the tip of the catheter. Once the catheter is activated, it is advanced at 2 mm/s. The control unit generates 700 mm Hg of suction, which draws the clot into the catheter through side extraction ports. The internal helix, which is housed at the catheter tip, rotates at 95,000 rpm and macerates the clot. With each pass of the catheter there is a net loss of blood volume.

Logistical Considerations

The ThromCat Thrombectomy Catheter is delivered through a 6F sheath, uses a 0.014-inch rapid-exchange wire delivery system, and is 150 cm in length. It is designed for use in synthetic dialysis access grafts and native fistulae ranging from 2.5 to 7 mm in diameter. The normal saline infusion occurs at a rate of 15 mL/min, whereas clot extraction occurs at 45 mL/min, so the overall net volume loss is 30 mL/min. Overall, the

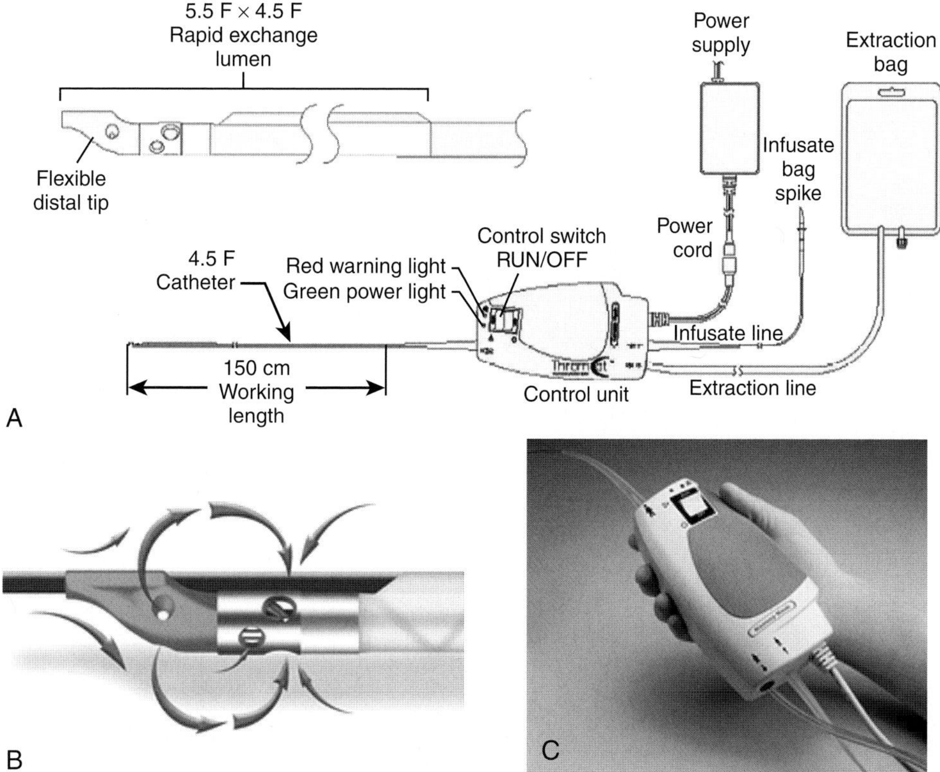

FIGURE 12-3 **A,** Schematic of ThromCat thrombectomy catheter. **B,** Illustration of recirculation vortex generated by the device. **C,** Control unit. *(Courtesy Spectranetics, Colorado Springs, CO.)*

device requires no capital equipment purchases, and the entire system comes in a single package.

AngioJet

The AngioJet is a wire-guided thrombectomy catheter, the mechanism of action of which is based on the Bernoulli principle for direct thrombus fragmentation and subsequent aspiration. If operated in power pulse mode, it can be used for targeted delivery of thrombolytic agents at the affected area. It is approved for use in native peripheral arteries and veins, 3 mm or larger, and in synthetic grafts. The AngioJet is also approved for coronary arteries 2 mm or greater in diameter (Figure 12-4).

Mechanism of Action: Rheolytic Mechanical Thrombectomy

The catheter directs high-speed saline jets in a retrograde direction at 10,000 psi, which produces a Venturi suction gradient. The suction gradient that is generated then fragments and aspirates the thrombus into the device. There are low-speed radial saline jets that maintain isovolumetric balance. The catheter is passed over a wire beyond the distal end of the thrombus before the initiation of treatment. The catheter is then activated and drawn back into the clot at a rate of 1 mm/s.

Mechanism of Action: Power Pulse Spray

Instead of priming the catheter with saline solution, a lytic agent is substituted, and the outflow tract of the AngioJet catheter is occluded with use of a three-way stopcock. The catheter is passed over a wire to the intended area of treatment and advanced into the thrombus with one pedal pump distributing lytic agent at 1-mm intervals. The catheter is then withdrawn with lytic agent infused at 1-mm intervals during the course of withdrawal. The pulsed lytic agent is allowed to dwell in the treated area for 20 to 30 minutes. The outflow tract is opened for drainage, and the catheter primed with saline solution. The catheter is then reintroduced in thrombectomy mode to remove the treated clot.

Logistical Considerations

The AngioJet thrombectomy system is approved for the removal of thrombus in vessels 2 to 12 mm in diameter. The system uses both 0.014- and 0.035-inch guidewires and comes in lengths ranging from 90 to 140 cm. The catheter requires sheaths between 4F and 6F in size. Using the AngioJet system for extensive clot removal can cause hemolysis. The AngioJet thrombectomy system produces a 360-degree suction vortex, which may reduce both the number of passes and the need for rotational positioning. Significantly, it operates

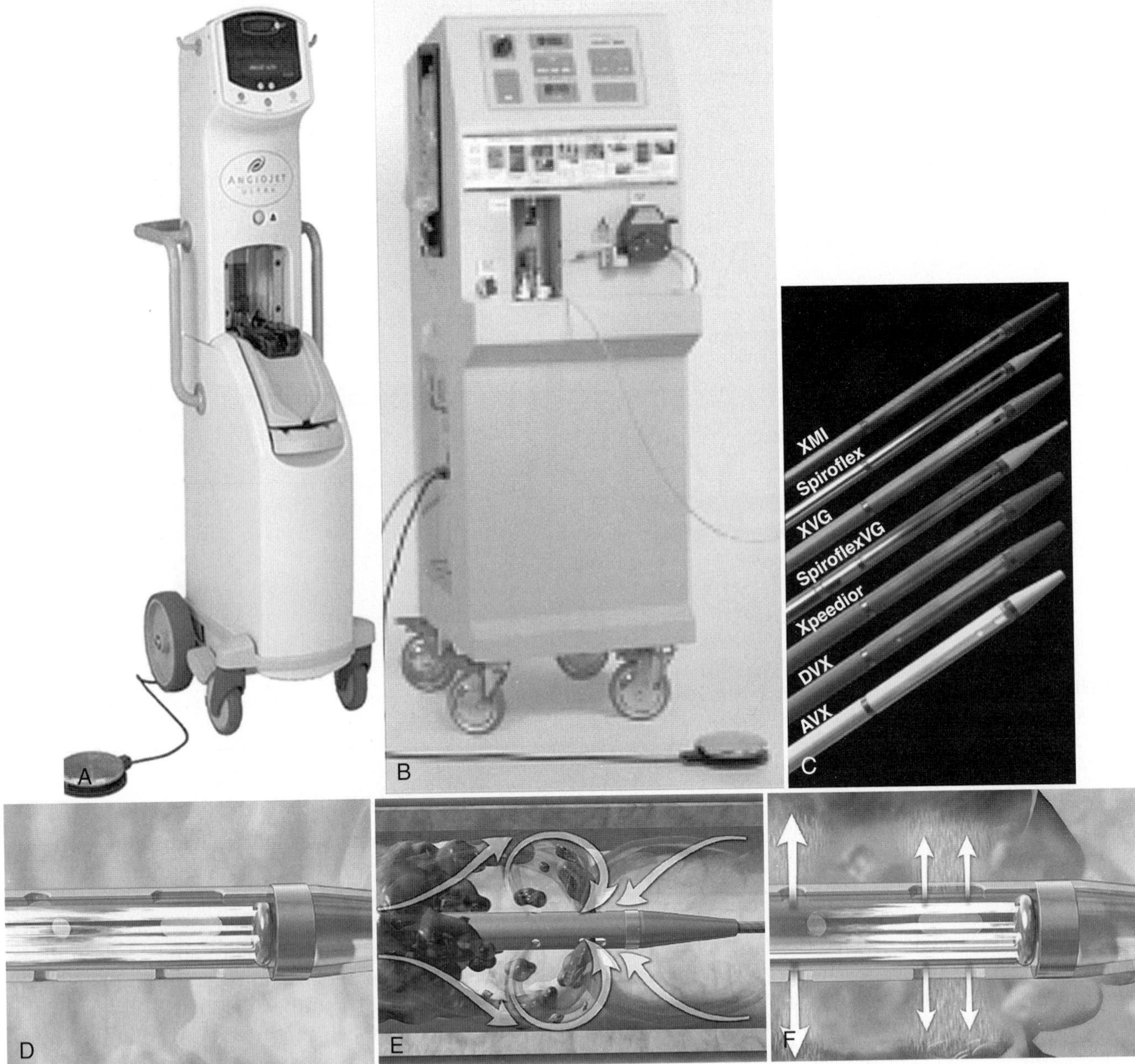

FIGURE 12-4 **A,** AngioJet Ultra base unit. **B,** AngioJet Series 3000 base unit. **C,** Illustration of available catheters. **D,** Catheter tip with retrograde saline jets. **E,** Recirculation vortex produced in thrombectomy mode. **F,** Dispersion of thrombolytic agents in power pulse mode. *(Courtesy Medrad, Inc., Warrendale, Pa.)*

isovolumetrically, which reduces the risk of unintended hypovolemia during clot removal.

The AngioJet thrombectomy system has been compared with open surgical thrombectomy in clotted prosthetic dialysis grafts. A total of 153 patients were enrolled with 82 patients randomly assigned to AngioJet treatment and 71 enrolled in the open surgical group.[22] Technical success, as defined by the ability to undergo dialysis, was achieved in 73% of patients in the AngioJet group and 79% in the open surgical group (p = NS). Three-month patency was 15% for the AngioJet group and 26% for the open surgical group (p = NS).[22]

Kasirajan et al.[23] reported the treatment of 18 patients with extensive DVT using the AngioJet system with nine receiving adjunctive thrombolysis. Ten patients had greater than 50% clot extraction, and 14 reported symptomatic improvement.[23] Recently, Lin et al.[24] reviewed 98 catheter-based interventions for extensive DVT. The AngioJet catheter in power pulse spray mode was used to treat 52 limbs and catheter-directed thrombolysis in 46 limbs. The AngioJet group had complete treatment success in 39 (75%) limbs and partial treatment success in 13 (25%) limbs with immediate clinical improvement noted in 42 (81%) of patients. Catheter-

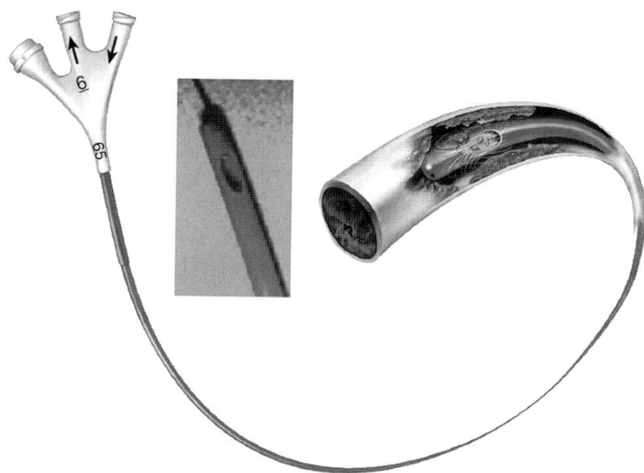

FIGURE 12-5 Hydrolyser percutaneous thrombectomy catheter illustration with picture of catheter tip (*inset*). *(Courtesy Cordis Endovascular, Inc., Warren, NJ.)*

directed thrombolysis was associated with complete treatment success in 32 (70%) limbs with partial treatment success in 14 (30%) limbs with immediate clinical improvement in 33 (72%) patients. Significantly, treatment time, transfusion requirements, ICU stay (2.4 vs. 0.6 days), and total inpatient days (8.4 vs. 4.6 days) were significantly reduced among those treated by AngioJet power pulse spray.[24]

Kasirajan et al.[10] described the treatment of 86 patients presenting with acute and subacute limb-threatening ischemia with the AngioJet device with or without adjunctive catheter-directed thrombolysis. Fifty-one (61.4%) of 83 treated patients had successful recanalization, 19 (22.9%) patients had partial clot removal, and 13 (15.6%) patients did not achieve significant improvement. Additional catheter-directed thrombolysis was used in 50 (58%) patients. However, angiographic improvement was obtained in only 7 (14%) patients. Fifty-six patients were available for follow-up with a patency rate of 79% at 6 months.[10] Silva et al.[9] reported similar results for treatment of 22 vessels in 21 patients with acute ischemia. Initial limb salvage was achieved in 18 of 19 limbs (95%) that was sustained in 89% of limbs at 6 months.

Hydrolyser Percutaneous Thrombectomy Catheter

The Hydrolyser uses a Venturi suction gradient to generate a vortex around the tip of the catheter to fragment and aspirate thrombus (Figure 12-5). The Hydrolyser is indicated for use in dialysis grafts.

Mechanism of Action

The Hydrolyser is placed over a wire and delivered to the area of intended treatment. Once in position, the catheter is connected to a standard power injector, set at 1000 psi, and filled with heparinized saline solution. The saline solution is then injected retrograde through the catheter into the exhaust port. The resultant Venturi gradient causes a surrounding vortex that fragments the clots with removal through an exhaust port.

Logistical Considerations

The Hydrolyser can be introduced through a 6F sheath over a 0.018-inch wire and is available in 65- and 100-cm lengths. As in other rheolytic thrombectomy devices, increased duration of usage is associated with hemolysis. The Hydrolyser does not require an additional drive unit. It functions in an isovolumetric manner.

The Hydrolyser has been used for treatment of pulmonary embolus with promising results.[25,26] In addition, Henry et al.[27] have reported treatment of acute lower limb ischemia in 41 patients in which the device was used in 28 native vessels and 8 bypass grafts. Technical success was achieved in 22 (78%) native arteries and 7 (87%) grafts. This group also reported successful thrombus removal from two patients with IVC thrombosis, as well as from one axillary vein and two pulmonary arteries. At 30 days, 73% of all treated vessels were patent. Rousseau et al.[28] have reported the application of this technology to 25 dialysis access grafts, 14 peripheral bypass grafts, and 15 native arteries. The technical success rates were 82% for fistulas, 100% for synthetic dialysis grafts, 87% for native arteries, and 79% for bypass grafts. The 6-month patency was 56% for fistulas, 62% for dialysis grafts, 78% for native arteries, and 65% for bypass grafts.[28]

NONRECIRCULATION MECHANICAL THROMBECTOMY CATHETERS

Arrow-Trerotola Percutaneous Thrombectomy Device

The Arrow-Trerotola device consists of a catheter-mounted wire basket, which is variable in size, and a rotational drive unit (Figure 12-6). The device comes in both catheter-guided and over-the-wire formats. The catheter can be used for both clot extraction and clot disruption. It is intended for declotting of arteriovenous fistula and synthetic grafts.

Mechanism of Action

The catheter is placed into the clotted graft, and the wire basket is then adjusted to the diameter of the graft up to 9 mm. The catheter is then connected to the rotational drive device to macerate the clot. Aspiration of macerated clot material can be performed by using the large-bore side arm of the provided sheath.

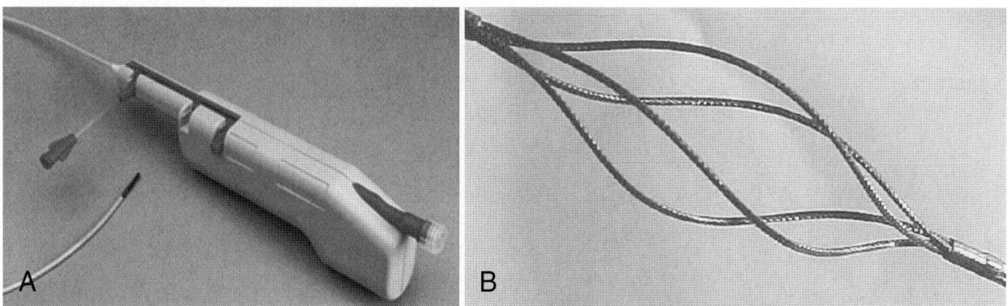

FIGURE 12-6 The Arrow-Trerotola device consists of a rotational drive unit **(A)** and a catheter-mounted wire basket **(B)**, the size of which can be adjusted. *(Courtesy Arrow International, Inc., Redding, PA.)*

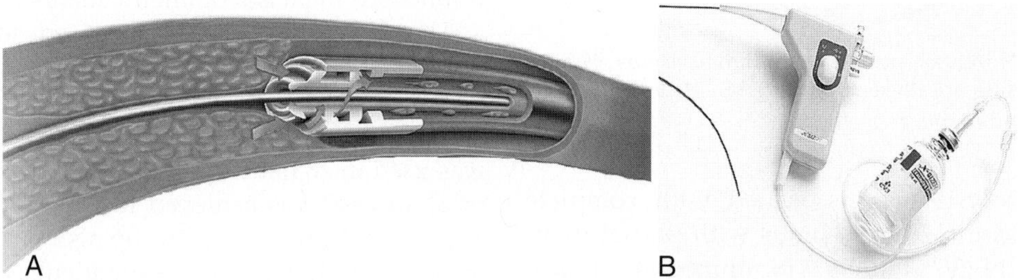

FIGURE 12-7 **A,** Illustration of the X-Sizer thrombectomy catheter within a thrombosed vessel. **B,** Drive unit and connected Vacutainer. *(Courtesy eV3, Endovascular, Plymouth, MN.)*

Logistical Considerations

The catheter-directed version of this device uses a 5F sheath and is available in a 65-cm length. The over-the-wire device uses a 7F sheath and is produced in 65- and 120-cm catheter lengths. The over-the-wire device will accommodate wires of up to 0.025 inch in diameter. The risk of hemolysis is minimal given the low rotational speeds.

The Arrow-Trerotola device has been used in a series of 44 thrombosed arteriovenous dialysis grafts.[29] The initial technical success rate was 79% with 6- and 12-month primary patency of 38% and 18%, respectively. Secondary assisted patency was 74% at 6 months and 69% at 12 months.

X-Sizer Mechanical Thrombectomy Catheter

The X-Sizer thrombectomy catheter is a wire-guided thrombectomy catheter, which uses both mechanical thrombolysis and vacuum aspiration to clear thrombus (Figure 12-7). The device is self-contained and does not require any additional equipment. This device is approved for the removal of clot from synthetic hemodialysis access grafts.

Mechanism of Action

The catheter is first positioned proximal to the intended area of treatment over a guidewire, activated, and slowly advanced through the thrombus. The catheter uses a screw design that rotates at 2100 rpm. The screw both macerates the thrombus and draws it back into the catheter. The removal of the thrombus is performed by vacuum suction, which is provided by the control unit connected to a Vacutainer.

Logistical Considerations

The X-Sizer uses a 0.014-inch wire delivery system. Two cutting diameters are available, 1.5 and 2 mm, both in 135-cm delivery lengths. The X-Sizer requires a 6F or 7F sheath for delivery. There are no capital equipment purchases.

Trellis Infusion System

Trellis device is a wire-guided thrombolysis catheter that is designed for isolated thrombolysis and direct mechanical thrombus fragmentation (Figure 12-8). It is intended for single-setting thrombolysis with targeted delivery of thrombolytic agents.

Mechanism of Action

The catheter is passed to the intended area of treatment over a guidewire. The proximal and distal occlusion balloons are inflated to isolate the area of treatment. The diffusion wire is then activated, and lytic agent is infused into the area between the balloons. Typically, immediately after activating the drive unit 2 mL of lytic agent is

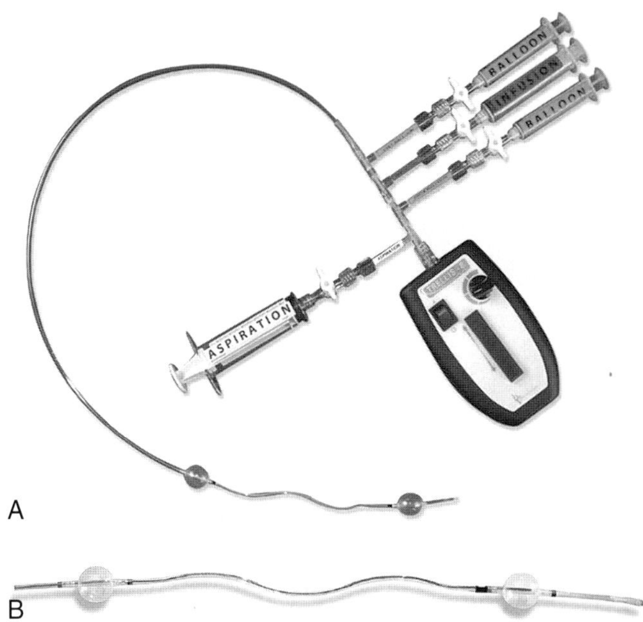

FIGURE 12-8 **A,** The Trellis Infusion System with injection ports and drive unit attached. **B,** Distal portion of catheter with occlusion balloons proximal and distal to treatment area. *(Courtesy Bacchus Vascular, Inc., Santa Clara, CA.)*

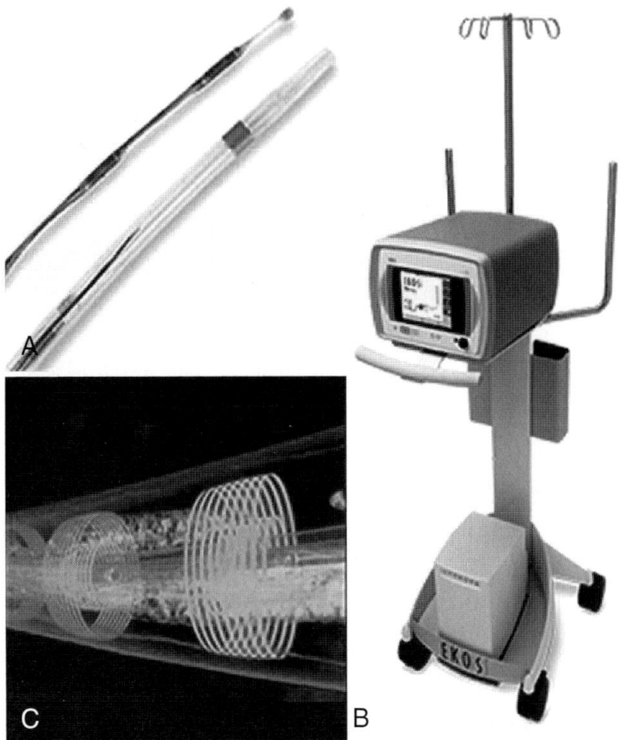

FIGURE 12-9 **A,** Ultrasonic core *(above)* and EKOS lytic catheter *(below)*. **B,** EKOS ultrasound generator unit. **C,** Illustration of ultrasound waves penetrating the clot. *(Courtesy EKOS Corp., Bothell, WA.)*

infused, followed by an additional 2 mL after 1 minute of operation, and thereafter 1 mL/min during an additional 3 minutes of operation. Four minutes after activation the infusion lumen is flushed with 1 mL saline solution. Operation of the diffusion wire should not exceed 30 minutes in a single treatment area or 60 minutes total for multiple areas. After the lytic agent has been diffused by the rotation of the wire, the thrombus is aspirated.

Logistical Considerations

The Trellis-8 infusion system comes in a variety of sizes with occlusion balloon diameters ranging from 5 to 16 mm, catheter lengths of 80 and 120 cm, and treatment zone lengths of 15 and 30 cm. The system is delivered over a 0.035-inch guidewire and requires an 8F sheath. The system is not recommended for situations where the shaft of the device or the treatment area crosses an acute angulation.

Advantages

The Trellis-8 infusion system minimizes the risk of distal embolization; limits the amount of lytic therapy released to the systemic circulation, which reduces the risk of bleeding complications; and minimizes the risk of fluid imbalance.

The use of the Trellis-8 system for DVT was reported by Hilleman and Razavi,[30] who treated DVT in 66 patients with recanalization in 58 (88%) treated patients. The mean lytic infusion time was 18 minutes, and mean total procedure time was 92 minutes. A total of 19% of patients required adjunctive lytic infusion with a mean infusion time of 7 hours. Sarac et al.[31] treated acutely ischemic limbs in 26 consecutive patients with the Trellis system. The technical success rate was 92% with a 30-day amputation-free survival of 96%. The average procedure time was 2.1 hours, and the average infusion time was 0.3 hours. There were no significant bleeding complications reported.

ULTRASONIC ENERGY SYSTEMS

EKOS LYSUS System

The EKOS LYSUS system delivers both lytic agent and ultrasonic energy (Figure 12-9). The catheter delivers standard lytic therapy agents to the clot with local ultrasonic energy used to disrupt the clot and drive the lytic agent into the clot. The EKOS catheter is currently approved for use in the peripheral arterial and venous circulation.

Mechanism of Action

The EKOS system is delivered over a guidewire to the area to be treated, after which the guidewire is removed and replaced with the ultrasonic core. The catheter is connected to the ultrasonic generator, followed by infusion of a lytic agent and normal saline coolant.

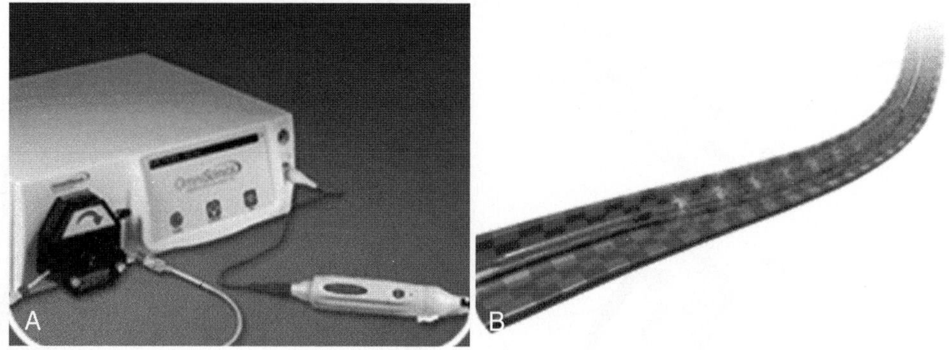

FIGURE 12-10 **A,** OmniWave generator unit. **B,** Illustration of OmniWave catheter delivering ultrasonic energy to the clot. *(Courtesy OmniSonics Medical Technologies, Inc., Wilmington, MA.)*

Logistical Considerations

The EKOS LYSUS system consists of a catheter of 106 or 135 cm in length with treatment lengths ranging between 6 and 50 cm. This system is designed to reduce the time required for lytic therapy, but treatment times typically exceed 2 hours, and the device is not designed for single-setting thrombolysis.

The EKOS LYSUS system was evaluated in the PARES trial for acute limb ischemia.[32] Investigators treated 25 patients with the EKOS LYSUS catheter infusing 1 mg/hr of recombinant t-PA. The technical success rate was 100% with total clot removal achieved in 22 (88%) patients after an average treatment time of 16.9 hours (range: 5-24 hours). There was one bleeding complication resulting from a dislodged introducer sheath. The 30-day patency was 80% without amputation or death at follow-up.

OmniWave Endovascular System

The OmniWave catheter is a thrombectomy system that uses ultrasonic energy, as well as delivery of lytic agent (Figure 12-10). The low-power ultrasonic energy causes cavitation waves that disrupt thrombus without damage to the vessel wall. It is approved for removal of thrombus in the peripheral vasculature.

Mechanism of Action

The thrombus is crossed with a guidewire, and the OmniWave system is then delivered over a guidewire just proximal to the area of intended treatment. The generator is activated. The thrombus is disrupted in particles, 90% of which are less than 10 μm. The catheter is advanced through the thrombus, and multiple passes may be required. Once the treatment is completed the catheter is withdrawn.

Logistical Considerations

The OmniWave Endovascular System has a 100-cm working length, is delivered over a 0.018-inch wire, and requires a 7F sheath for delivery. It requires both the catheter and the generator.

CONCLUSION

Percutaneous thrombectomy and mechanical thrombolytic devices have evolved during the past two decades with significant improvements in the efficiency of clot removal, while limiting distal embolization of the disrupted thrombus. It is anticipated that these results will continue to improve in combination with the introduction of improved locally active thrombolytic agents that can be administered in high dose with limited adverse systemic effects and perhaps growing application of embolic protection devices. Substantial evidence suggests that the incidence of peripheral arterial disease will continue to increase, along with the number of patients with end-stage renal disease receiving hemodialysis. Moreover, opportunities exist for reducing short- and long-term disability from DVT, which occurs in a large number of patients in whom the condition is currently undertreated. Undoubtedly, the potential for rapid thrombus removal at reduced costs will continue to drive the development and application of these devices that will affect the care of an ever-increasing number of our patients.

References

1. Linhardt RJ: Heparin: An important drug enters its seventh decade, *Chem Indust* 2:45–50, 1991.
2. Dormandy J, Heeck L, Vig S: Acute limb ischemia, *Semin Vasc Surg* 12:148–153, 1999.
3. Heit JA: The epidemiology of venous thromboembolism in the community: implications for prevention and management, *J Thromb Thrombolysis* 21:23–29, 2006.
4. Kearon C: Antithrombotic therapy for venous thromboembolic disease, *Chest* 133(6S):454S–545S, 2008.
5. Fogarty TJ, Cranley JJ, Krause RJ, et al: A method for extraction of arterial emboli and thrombi, *Surg Gyn Obst* 116:241–244, 1963.

6. Sharafuddin MJA, Hicks EH: Current status of percutaneous mechanical thrombectomy. Part III. Present and future applications, *J Vasc Interv Radiol* 9:209–224, 1998.
7. Hopfner W, Vicol C, Bohndorf K, et al: Shredding embolectomy thrombectomy catheter for treatment of acute lower-limb ischemia, *Ann Vasc Surg* 13:426–435, 1999.
8. Wagner HJ, Müler-Hülsbeck S, Pitton MB, et al: Rapid thrombectomy with a hydrodynamic catheter: results from a prospective, multicenter trial, *Radiology* 205:675–681, 1997.
9. Silva JA, Ramee SR, Collins TJ, et al: Rheolytic thrombectomy in the treatment of acute limb-threatening ischemia: immediate results and six-month follow-up of the multicenter AngioJet registry, *Cathet Cardiovasc Diagnost* 45:386–393, 1998.
10. Kasirajan K, Beavers FP, Clair DG, et al: Rheolytic thrombectomy in the management of acute and subacute limb threatening ischemia, *J Vasc Interv Radiol* 12:413–420, 2001.
11. Reekers JA, Kromhout JG, Spithoven HG, et al: Arterial thrombosis below the inguinal ligament: percutaneous treatment with a thrombosuction catheter, *Radiology* 198:49–53, 1996.
12. Henry M, Amor M, Henry I, et al: The Hydrolyser thrombectomy catheter: A single-center experience, *J Endovasc Surg* 5:24–31, 1998.
13. Rilinger N, Görich J, Scharrer-Palmer R, et al: Short-term results with use of the Amplatz thrombectomy device in the treatment of acute lower limb occlusion, *J Vasc Interv Radiol* 8:343–348, 1997.
14. Tadavarthy SM, Murray PD, et al: Mechanical thrombectomy with the Amplatz device: human experience, *J Vasc Interv Radiol* 5:715–724, 1994.
15. Varty K, Nydahl S, Butterworth P, et al: Changes in the management of critical limb ischemia, *Br J Surg* 83:954–956, 1996.
16. Gobin YP, Starkman S, Duckwiler GR, et al: MERCI 1: A phase 1 study of Mechanical Embolus Removal in Cerebral Ischemia, *Stroke* 35:2848–2854, 2004.
17. Nazarian GK, Qian Z, Coleman CC, et al: Hemolytic effect of the Amplatz thrombectomy device, *J Vasc Interv Radiol* 5:155–160, 1994.
18. Qian Z, Kvamme P, Raghed D: Comparison of a new recirculation thrombectomy catheter with other devices of the same type: In vitro and in vivo evaluations, *Invest Radiol* 37:503–511, 2002.
19. Uflacker R, Rajagopalan PR, Selby JB, et al: Thrombosed dialysis access grafts: randomized comparison of the Amplatz thrombectomy device and surgical thromboembolectomy, *Eur Radiol* 14:2004–2014, 2009.
20. Delomez M, Beregi JP, Willoteaux S, et al: Mechanical thrombectomy in patients with deep venous thrombosis, *Cardiovasc Intervent Radiol* 24:42–48, 2001.
21. Görich J, Rilinger N, Sokiranski R: Mechanical thrombolysis of acute occlusion of both the superficial and the deep femoral arteries using a thrombectomy device, *AJR Am J Roentgenol* 170:1177–1180, 1998.
22. Vesely TM, Williams D, Weiss M: Comparison of the angiojet rheolytic catheter to surgical thrombectomy for the treatment of thrombosed hemodialysis grafts. Peripheral AngioJet Clinical Trial, *J Vasc Interv Radiol* 10:1195–1205, 1999.
23. Kasirajan K, Gray B, Ouriel K: Percutaneous AngioJet thrombectomy in the management of extensive deep venous thrombosis, *J Vasc Interv Radiol* 12:179–185, 2001.
24. Lin PH, Zhou W, Dardik A, et al: Catheter-direct thrombolysis versus pharmacomechanical thrombectomy for treatment of symptomatic lower extremity deep venous thrombosis, *Am J Surg* 192:345–352, 2006.
25. Skaf E, Beemath A, Siddiqui T, et al: Catheter-tip embolectomy in the management of acute massive pulmonary embolism, *Am J Cardiol* 99:415–420, 2007.
26. Fava M, Loyola S, Huete I: Massive pulmonary embolism: treatment with the hydrolyser thrombectomy catheter, *J Vasc Interv Radiol* 11:1159–1164, 2000.
27. Henry M, Amor M, Henry I, et al: The Hydrolyser thrombectomy catheter: a single-center experience, *J Endovasc Surg* 5:24–31, 1998.
28. Rousseau H, Sapoval M, Ballini P, et al: Percutaneous recanalization of acutely thrombosed vessels by hydrodynamic thrombectomy (Hydrolyser), *Eur Radiol* 7:935–941, 1997.
29. Shatsky JB, Berns JS, Clark TW, et al: Single-center experience with the Arrow-Trerotola percutaneous thrombectomy device in the management of thrombosed native dialysis fistulas, *J Vasc Interv Radiol* 16:1605–1611, 2005.
30. Hilleman DE, Razavi MK: Clinical and economic evaluation of the Trellis-8 infusion catheter for deep vein thrombosis, *J Vasc Interv Radiol* 19:377–383, 2008.
31. Sarac TP, Hilleman D, Arko FR, et al: Clinical and economic evaluation of the trellis thrombectomy device for arterial occlusions: preliminary analysis, *J Vasc Surg* 39:556–559, 2004.
32. Wissgott C, Richter A, Kamusella P, Steinkamp HJ: Treatment of critical limb ischemia using ultrasound-enhanced thrombolysis (PARES Trial): final results, *J Endovasc Therapy* 14:438–443, 2007.

CHAPTER

13

Principles of Thrombolysis

Vikram S. Kashyap, Kenneth Ouriel

Thrombolytic agents are in widespread use for the dissolution of arterial and venous thrombi. Clinical settings in which thrombolysis has played an important role include the acute coronary syndromes, peripheral arterial occlusion, stroke, and deep venous thrombosis. Thrombolytic agents have been employed in each of these areas to achieve dissolution of the occluding thrombus, reconstitution of blood flow, and improvement in the status of the tissue bed supplied or drained by the involved vascular segment. Most commonly, vascular surgeons use thrombolytic therapy in the setting of acute limb ischemia (ALI).

Acute arterial occlusions in the peripheral arteries can be manifested by limb-threatening ischemia. Despite isolated limb ischemia, systemic sequelae from ischemia, comorbidities, and the complications from treatment lead to high mortality rates in the treatment of these patients that may exceed 20%.[1,2] Given the variable presentation of ALI secondary to the extent of the thrombotic process and the abundance of preexisting collateral pathways, a useful stratification is based on the modified Rutherford criteria.[3] In ALI, three broad categories allow stratification of severity of ischemia and also dictate the tempo of management required. The variables that allow stratification include Doppler signals of both pedal arteries and veins, and motor and sensory nerve function of the foot. Grade 1 is a viable foot that is not immediately threatened, and the limb is salvageable with appropriate therapy. There is an audible arterial Doppler signal and no ongoing pain or neurologic deficit. Grade 3 ischemia is severe with irreversible changes. There is profound sensory loss and/or paralysis often with skin marbling. There is neither arterial nor venous Doppler signal, and these patients often require timely amputation to prevent the systemic cardiac, renal, and infectious complications from infarcted limb tissue.

Rutherford grade 2 ischemia requires urgent diagnosis, clinical judgment, and timely intervention to avoid limb loss and minimize the risk of mortality. Patients will not have an arterial Doppler signal but will have venous filling. They will often have minimal sensory loss of the toes (grade 2a) that can progress to sensory loss in the foot and motor dysfunction (grade 2b). The critical differentiation is the subtle sensory deficits in the lower extremity that precede more profound ischemia of the motor nerves and paralysis. These "threatened" limbs require urgent treatment.

On recognition of ALI, treatment begins with anticoagulation, usually with heparin, to limit the propagation of thrombus and perhaps prevent clinical deterioration. After therapeutic anticoagulation is achieved, traditionally, urgent surgical intervention follows using thromboembolectomy, placement of a bypass graft, or other techniques to restore arterial flow to the extremity. Early operative intervention, however, is associated with a significant risk of perioperative mortality. Mortality rates in excess of 25% after open surgical repair for ALI were reported in a classic study by Blaisdell et al. published in the late 1970s.[1] Jivegard and colleagues[2] corroborated these findings a decade later, documenting a 20% mortality rate in patients undergoing operative revascularization for ALI. In spite of advances in surgical technique and perioperative care, the current risk of morbidity and mortality after open surgical intervention continues to be significant.[4-6]

The mortality rate of surgical revascularization performed in the setting of ALI remains high, mostly because many patients poorly tolerate an extensive procedure performed without adequate preoperative preparation.[5,7] Cardiopulmonary complications occur with frequency, accounting for an unacceptably high mortality rate over midterm follow-up. The literature confirms that individuals who present with ALI comprise one of the sickest subgroups of patients that the vascular surgeon is asked to treat.[8] These patients require early intervention to salvage an extremity but are ill-equipped to tolerate an invasive surgical procedure. We think optimizing a combination of endovascular options and reserving open surgical intervention for lesions not amenable to percutaneous intervention may provide the best outcomes for patients presenting with ALI.

THROMBOLYTIC THERAPY

Catheter-directed (regional) thrombolytic therapy offers a less invasive option for patients presenting with peripheral arterial occlusion and acute ischemia. The traditional thrombolytic agents are plasminogen activators converting plasminogen into plasmin. Plasmin is the active molecule that cleaves polymerized fibrin to allow the dissolution of thrombus. Ongoing investigations concentrate on producing agents with a higher affinity for fibrin-bound plasminogen to achieve thrombolysis without systemic thrombolytic activity and the risk of remote bleeding.

In 1933, Tillett and Garner[9] at the Johns Hopkins Medical School discovered that filtrates of broth cultures of certain strains of hemolytic streptococci had fibrinolytic properties. This streptococcal byproduct was originally termed "streptococcal fibrinolysin." The purity of this agent was poor, however. Tillett administered a purified streptokinase (SK) intrapleurally to dissolve loculated hemothoraces in the late 1940s and reported the first intravascular administration of a thrombolytic agent into 11 patients in an article published in 1955.[10]

In 1956, Cliffton, at the Cornell University Medical College in New York, described the first therapeutic administration of thrombolytic agents for vascular thrombotic disease. He later published his results of 40 patients with occlusive thrombi treated with SK and plasminogen in combination.[11] The clinical results were far from exemplary; recanalization was not uniform, bleeding complications were frequent, but this represented the first use of thrombolysis in humans for arterial occlusions. Plasmin is the active molecule that cleaves fibrin polymer to cause the dissolution of thrombus. Early investigators attempted to dissolve occluding thrombi with the direct administration of exogenous plasmin. Free plasmin, however, was ineffective as a thrombolytic agent because it is unstable and autodegrades. Effective thrombolysis was achieved only when *fibrin-bound* plasminogen was converted to its active form, plasmin, at the site of the thrombus.[12]

CLASSIFICATION OF THROMBOLYTIC AGENTS

Several schemes may be used to classify thrombolytic agents. The agents can be grouped by their mechanism of action—those that directly convert plasminogen to plasmin versus those that are inactive zymogens and require transformation to an active form before they can cleave plasminogen. Agents can be classified by their mode of production. Also, thrombolytic agents can be classified by their pharmacologic actions—those that are "fibrin specific" (bind to fibrin but not to fibrinogen) versus those that are nonspecific and those that have a great degree of "fibrin affinity" (bind avidly to fibrin) versus those that do not. We have found it useful to classify thrombolytic agents into groups based on their origin: the SK compounds, the urokinase (UK) compounds, the tissue plasminogen activators (t-PAs), and an additional group consisting of novel agents (Table 13-1).

Streptokinase Compounds

SK is a nonenzymatic protein produced by streptococcus bacteria and was the first thrombolytic agent to be described.[13] SK has a biphasic half-life and initially combines with plasminogen on an equimolar basis. This SK-plasminogen complex converts uncomplexed plasminogen to plasmin leading to thrombolysis with a first half-life of approximately 20 minutes. However, as the process evolves, the SK-plasminogen complex is gradually converted to the SK-plasmin form, which can also convert plasminogen to plasmin with a late half-life of 90 minutes. This mechanism leads to two plasminogen molecules used for SK-mediated plasmin generation. The two half-lives underscore the complexity of SK-mediated reactions and can have a significant impact on the concentration and activity of this drug.

SK is a foreign protein and therefore is antigenic. Most patients have preformed antibodies directed against SK that have developed as a result of prior infections with β-hemolytic streptococci. Thus exogenously administered SK can be inactivated by these neutralizing antibodies and become biochemically inert. These SK antibodies may be overwhelmed through the use of a large initial bolus of drug, which is why a large initial loading dose of SK may be employed.[14] Minor (and occasionally major) allergic reactions to SK have been reported from 1.7% to 18% of cases.[15] These reactions include urticaria, edema, and bronchospasm. Pyrexia may also occur but is usually adequately treated with acetaminophen. However, the major complication of SK is hemorrhage with rates similar to those of other thrombolytic agents. SK-associated hemorrhage may be no different from bleeding associated with any other thrombolytic agent. The primary cause is likely to be the action of the systemic agent on the thrombi, sealing the sites of vascular disintegrity. The generation of free plasmin, however, can contribute to the problem, with degradation of fibrinogen and other serum clotting

TABLE 13-1 Thrombolytic Agents

Agent	Production	Mechanism	Plasma half-life (min)	Fibrin specificity	Fibrin affinity
SK	Bacterial culture	Complex with plasminogen	20/90	+	+
UK (Abbokinase)	Neonatal kidney cell culture	Direct plasminogen activator	14	+	+
Pro-UK (Prolyse)	Prodrug		7	++	+
t-PA (alteplase, Activase)	Recombinant techniques	Direct plasminogen activator	3	++	++
Reteplase (r-PA, Retavase)	rt-PA derivative	Direct plasminogen activator	14	++	+
tNK	Recombinant mutant		15	+++	++
Alfimeprase		Direct fibrinolysis	25		

proteins, as well as the release of fibrin(ogen) degradation products, which are potent anticoagulants themselves and can exacerbate the coagulopathy.

Attempts to produce fibrin-specific agents have led to derivatives of SK that change its biologic activity and the duration of such activity. *p*-Anisoylated human plasminogen SK activator complex (APSAC) is the most studied derivative of SK. It is an acylated complex of SK with human lys-plasminogen. The potency of APSAC has been found to be 10 times that of SK, but it has a longer half-life. Because of this property, it was anticipated that APSAC would be associated with a reduced risk of rethrombosis. Contrary to expectations, APSAC offered little clinical benefit over SK or recombinant t-PA (rt-PA) when studied in the setting of acute coronary occlusion.[16] APSAC shares the same side effect profile of SK because of antistreptococcal antibodies, and therefore retreatment with either drug should not be done within 6 months.

Urokinase Compounds

A trypsin-like serine protease originally isolated from human urine by Macfarlane and Pilling in 1946[17] was found to have fibrinolytic potential in 1947.[18] In the following years, the active molecule was extracted, isolated, and named "urokinase" (UK).[19] The high-molecular-weight form predominates in UK isolated from urine, whereas the low-molecular-weight form is found in UK obtained from tissue culture of kidney cells. Unlike SK, UK activates plasminogen to form plasmin directly without prior binding to plasminogen or plasmin for bioactivity. Plasminogen is the only known protein substrate for UK and is cleaved by first-order reaction kinetics to plasmin. Also in contrast to SK, UK is nonantigenic, and untoward reactions of fever or hypotension are rare. UK requires an initial high loading dose, and like SK it possesses little specific affinity for fibrin and fibrin-bound plasminogen.[20]

Abbokinase

The most commonly used UK in the United States has been of tissue-culture origin, manufactured from human neonatal kidney cells (Abbokinase; Abbott Laboratories, Abbott Park, IL). On intravenous administration, UK is rapidly removed from the circulation via hepatic clearance, and its half-life in humans is estimated to be about 14 minutes. UK has been fully sequenced, and a recombinant form of UK (r-UK) was tested in trials of patients with acute myocardial infarction and in patients with peripheral arterial occlusion.[6,21] r-UK is derived from a murine hybridoma cell line and differs from Abbokinase with a higher molecular weight and a shorter half-life. Despite these differences, the clinical effects of the two agents have been quite similar.

Prourokinase

Husain and colleagues[22] isolated a single-chain form of UK of about 55,000 Da in 1979. This precursor of UK was characterized and subsequently manufactured by recombinant technology. Pro-UK is inert in plasma but can be activated by kallikrein or plasmin to form active two-chain UK. This property accounts for amplification of the fibrinolytic process. As plasmin is generated, more pro-UK is converted to active UK, and the process is repeated. Pro-UK is relatively fibrin specific with preferential activation of fibrin-bound plasminogen. In contrast, SK and UK activate free and bound plasminogen equally and induce systemic plasminemia with resultant fibrinolysis.

A recombinant form of pro-UK has been generated named Prolyse (Abbott Laboratories). This UK compound has the advantage of not originating in a human cell source. Initial clinical data indicate a dose-dependent safety and efficacy profile.[23] Further studies are required to evaluate whether the fibrin specificity of pro-UK translates to a clinical advantage.

Tissue Plasminogen Activators

t-PA is a naturally occurring serine protease produced by endothelial cells. t-PA is involved in the intricate balance between luminal thrombosis and thrombolysis.[24] Natural t-PA is a single-chain (527 amino acid) serine protease with a molecular weight of approximately 65 kDa. t-PA has potential benefits over other thrombolytic agents. The agent exhibits significant fibrin specificity. t-PA is a poor enzyme in the absence of fibrin. However, the presence of fibrin strikingly enhances the activation rate of plasminogen by t-PA. Thus fibrinolysis occurs at the site of thrombus formation without significant conversion of plasminogen in circulating plasma by t-PA.[25] Circulating α_2-antiplasmin is not consumed, fibrinogen is not degraded, and a systemic lytic state is avoided. t-PA also manifests the property of fibrin affinity, that is, it binds strongly to fibrin. Other fibrinolytic agents do not share this property of fibrin affinity.

Alteplase

Although t-PA was identified in the 1940s, its isolation and purification proceeded slowly until the 1980s, when it became possible to extract it from uterine tissue. Wild-type t-PA is a single-chain (527 amino acid) serine protease. Recombinant t-PA was produced in the 1980s by using molecular cloning techniques. Activase (alteplase) (Genentech, South San Francisco, CA), a predominantly single-chain form of t-PA, was approved in the United States for the treatment of acute myocardial infarction and massive pulmonary embolism. This recombinant t-PA has been studied extensively in the setting of coronary occlusion. Results of the limited experience available with the use of t-PA in patients with peripheral vascular occlusions have suggested the occurrence of fewer systemic complications with increased effectiveness of therapy and decreased infusion times. The incidence of intracranial bleeding with t-PA appears to be increased in patients who have been taking oral anticoagulants before therapy, patients weighing less than 70 kg, and patients older than 65 years of age.[26]

Reteplase

In attempting to produce thrombolytic agents that are more effective with a decreased potential for bleeding complications, the native t-PA molecule has been modified. One such modification is reteplase, a third-generation t-PA mutant produced with recombinant technology. Reteplase comprises the kringle 2 and protease domains of t-PA. Reteplase was developed with the goal of avoiding the necessity of a continuous infusion, thereby simplifying ease of administration. Reteplase (Retavase, Centocor, Malvern, PA) is produced in *Escherichia coli* cells and is nonglycosylated, leading to a diminished affinity to hepatocytes. This property accounts for a longer half-life than t-PA, potentially enabling bolus injection versus prolonged infusion. Compared with t-PA, reteplase has improved clot penetration, longer half-life, and a more rapid initiation of thrombolysis, which may account for a decreased risk of hemorrhage.[27] Reteplase has been studied in several small trials, and its safety and efficacy appear to be similar to those of alteplase.[28,29]

Tenecteplase

The novel recombinant plasminogen activator tenecteplase (tNK) was created with three-point mutations of the t-PA molecule. These modifications lead to a greater half-life and fibrin specificity. The longer half-life of tNK allowed successful administration as a single bolus, in contrast to the requirement for an infusion with t-PA. In studies of acute coronary occlusion, tNK performed at least as well as t-PA, with greater ease of administration.[30] Recently, several pilot clinical series have suggested that peripheral arterial thrombolysis with tNK is associated with outcomes similar to those achieved with the older agents.[31]

Other Agents

All commercially available thrombolytic agents act through the activation of plasminogen that is bound to fibrin. The concept of "plasminogen steal" occurs when the substrate is rapidly consumed by thrombolytic agents. Thus the local area of thrombus is rendered devoid of plasminogen and resistant to dissolution. Adding additional thrombolytic agent is not effective. As mentioned, wild-type plasmin was investigated as a fibrinolytic agent early in the history of thrombolysis. Unfortunately, autodigestion of the agent neutralized its activity and rendered the attempts unsuccessful. Recently, however, investigators have successfully developed several novel agents with direct fibrinolytic activity, avoiding the need to activate plasminogen in the process. These agents are plasmin analogues that have fibrinolytic activity but are not autodigested. Plasmin analogues have the potential to achieve more effective thrombolysis than the commercially available thrombolytic agents because they act independent of the endogenous plasminogen supply.

Fibrolase is a direct-acting fibrinolytic enzyme. It is a metalloprotease isolated from the venom of the southern copperhead snake, which dissolves fibrin through rapid hydrolysis.[32] There are some data to suggest that fibrolase dissolves thrombi much quicker than the plasminogen activators.[33] An added advantage of fibrolase is the rapid inactivation by α_2-macroglobulin, which is relatively abundant in the systemic circulation. Presently, Alfimeprase (Nuvelo, San Carlos, Calif), a recombinant variant of fibrolase, is in clinical trials of peripheral arterial occlusion. Also, amediplase (Menarini Group, Florence, Italy) is undergoing evaluation in clinical trials. Amediplase is a chimeric protein that combines part of the t-PA and part of the single-chain UK plasminogen activator (sc-UPA). In animal models, amediplase is a more potent and longer-lasting thrombolytic than alteplase.

Recently, laboratory data indicate that luminal arterial thrombus causes endothelial dysfunction by decreasing nitric oxide (NO) bioactivity.[34,35] Removal of the thrombus by either mechanical means or dissolution with thrombolysis restores blood flow, but endothelial dysfunction persists in multiple animal models. Persistent endothelial dysfunction may be a cause of suboptimal outcomes including rethrombosis after thrombolysis, or angioplasty/stenting. Multiple investigators have recently found that thrombolysis combined with L-arginine supplementation ameliorates thrombus-induced endothelial dysfunction by increasing NO levels.[36,37] The addition of L-arginine to thrombolytic regimens may prove to be an attractive therapeutic adjunct.

CLINICAL TRIAL DATA

Despite results of thrombolytic therapy from a multitude of retrospective studies, a number of questions remained unanswered until the performance of randomized controlled trials in the area of thrombolysis versus surgical revascularization for ALI. The STILE trial compared optimal surgical therapy with intra-arterial catheter-directed thrombolysis for native arterial or bypass graft occlusions.[5] This was a three-armed multicenter comparison of UK (250,000 international units bolus, 4000 international units/min for 4 hr, then 2000 international units/min for up to 36 hr), rt-PA (0.05 to 0.1 mg/kg/hr for up to 12 hr), and primary operation. There was one intracranial hemorrhage in the group receiving UK (0.9%), and there were two in the group receiving rt-PA (1.5%, not significant). Stratification by duration of ischemic symptoms revealed that patients with ischemia of less than 14 days' duration had lower amputation rates with thrombolysis and shorter hospital stays, whereas patients with ischemia for longer than 14 days who had surgical treatment had less ongoing or recurrent ischemia and trends toward lower morbidity. At 6 months, amputation-free survival was improved in patients with acute ischemia treated with thrombolysis, but patients with chronic ischemia had lower amputation rates when treated surgically. Fifty-five percent of patients treated with thrombolysis had a reduction in magnitude of their surgical procedure. Of note, no difference was seen between the use of t-PA and UK.

TOPAS was a multicenter, randomized, prospective trial comparing thrombolysis (r-UK) with surgery for acute lower extremity ischemia of less than 14 days' duration.[6,38] The most effective dose for UK was determined to be 4000 units/min with complete thrombolysis in 71% of patients. After successful thrombolytic therapy, either surgical or endovascular intervention was performed on the lesion responsible for the occlusion. The amputation-free survival for both endovascular and surgical arms was similar at 1 year; however, there was a 43% reduction in open operations in the thrombolytic arm with 30% requiring only endovascular procedures.

Recently, the National Audit of Thrombolysis for Acute Leg Ischemia (NATALI) was published.[39] This represented a 10-year audit of thrombolysis cases performed in the United Kingdom. More than 1100 cases were summarized in this study representing more than 100 cases per year but with significant variation during the decade representing variable enthusiasm for thrombolysis. Overall, there were 75% amputation-free survival, 12% amputation, and 12% death rates in the first 30 days, which compare favorably with historical surgical data. The overall results improved over time, perhaps reflecting improved patient selection and technique. Of note, t-PA was used mostly in the United Kingdom. Distal embolization (2.4%) and reperfusion injury (1.8%) rates were low. Stroke occurred in 26 patients (2.3%) and was thought to be due to hemorrhage or ischemia in equal proportion. The authors concluded that thrombolytic therapy, as an initial management for ALI, was effective in achieving amputation-free survival in the vast majority of patients.

COMPLICATIONS OF REGIONAL LYTIC THERAPY

Complications of local thrombolytic therapy include hemorrhage, distal embolization, pericatheter thrombosis, graft extravasation, fever, and allergic reactions. Distal embolization of clot fragments may cause temporary worsening of symptoms in the treated region. The emboli often disappear with continued thrombolytic therapy; embolectomy is only occasionally required. Pericatheter thrombosis may be avoided by the use of heparin, usually via the sheath side arm in coaxial systems.[40] However, the administration of heparin may lead to a slightly higher remote bleeding rate.

Bleeding, especially intracranial bleeding, is the most feared complication of regional thrombolytic therapy. Bleeding is usually related to systemic effects of the drug, with the most recent experience seeming to indicate that the risk of bleeding correlates more with the duration of therapy than with the actual dose of the agent used. A systemic lytic state is heralded by a 50% drop in fibrinogen from baseline, or an absolute level less than 100 mg/dL. Replacement of fibrinogen with components (e.g., cryoprecipitate or fresh frozen plasma) usually suffices because the half-lives of UK, SK, and t-PA are relatively short. Intracranial bleeding is perhaps the most feared complication of any form of lytic therapy. Any change in the neurologic status of a patient during thrombolytic therapy should be evaluated promptly. The thrombolytic agent should be discontinued till the appropriate evaluation for intracranial bleeding has been performed. In a recent review of 48 studies, rates of major bleeding were 6.2% for UK and 8.4% for t-PA.[41] Intracranial bleeding was infrequent (0.4% UK, 1.1% t-PA). Despite the lack of comparative studies, and the heterogeneity of patients treated, these data suggest a lower complication rate with UK administration.

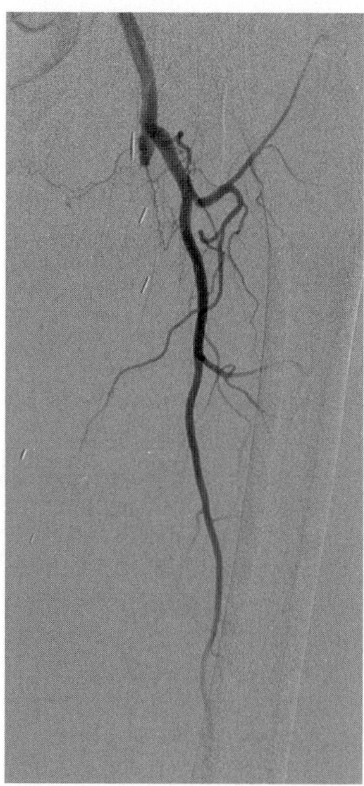

FIGURE 13-1 An 82-year-old woman presented with left leg ALI. A femoral-to-popliteal bypass graft had been performed many years previously. Aortography and selective limb arteriography was performed via a contralateral femoral approach with use of a 5F system. This image reveals patent common femoral and profunda femoris arteries with a stump of the occluded bypass graft.

PATIENT MANAGEMENT AND TECHNICAL CONSIDERATIONS

Intra-arterial thrombolytic therapy has gained prominence as an initial intervention for patients with ALI: infusing thrombolytic agents directly into the occluding thrombus through a catheter-directed approach. Agents such as UK and t-PA can restore adequate arterial perfusion, and subsequent arteriographic studies allow the clinician to identify and address the culprit lesions responsible for the occlusion. Oftentimes, an endovascular procedure can be performed to minimize the risk to the patients. In other cases where open surgical intervention is still necessary, it can be performed on an elective basis in a well-prepared patient.

A plethora of strategies for thrombolysis have been used and are described in a recent consensus document.[42] In this comprehensive review, 33 recommendations were made by a panel of experienced hematologists, radiologists, and vascular surgeons from North America and Europe. The areas covered in this publication are management of patients with lower limb arterial occlusion from presentation to postoperative monitoring. The critical recommendations that deserve emphasis are that thrombolysis for peripheral arterial occlusion should be via a catheter-directed delivery of agent and that systemic thrombolysis should no longer be used. The likelihood of success with thrombolysis is related to the ability to cross the thrombosed region ("guidewire traversal test") and placement of an infusion catheter/wire embedded into the thrombus. Perhaps most important, identifying and treating the "culprit lesion" that led to the thrombotic episode is paramount for a long-term successful outcome. Of note, more than 40 dosage schemes were reviewed and described for thrombolytic infusion. This included strategies of continuous versus stepwise infusion, bolusing or lacing the clot, and intraoperative thrombolysis. The most popular strategies included using UK 4000 units/min for 4 hours, and then decreasing to 2000 units/min for a maximum of 48 hours, t-PA at a dose of 1 mg/hr, and lacing the clot to increase thrombolytic efficiency.

Our preferred current technique is outlined below. First, and of particular importance, thrombolysis should not be attempted in any patient whose ischemia has been of sufficient severity or duration to cause severe motor or sensory impairment or in patients whose ischemia cannot tolerate the anticipated duration of the infusion. Because a systemic lytic state may occur with prolonged regional intravascular thrombolytic therapy, absolute contraindications include active internal bleeding, recent surgery or trauma to the area to be perfused, recent cerebrovascular accident, or

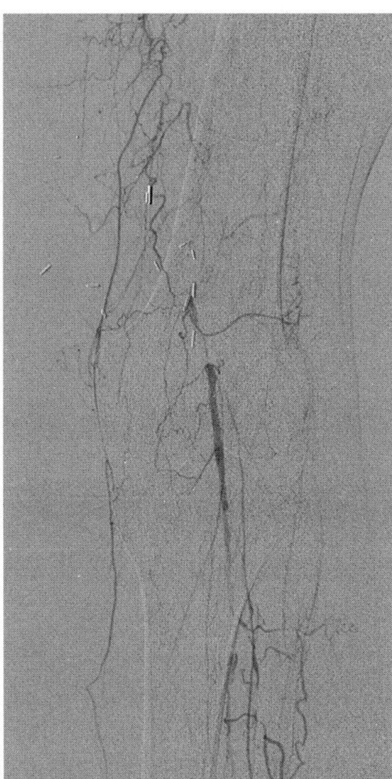

FIGURE 13-2 Delayed imaging reveals faint filling of the popliteal artery via collaterals.

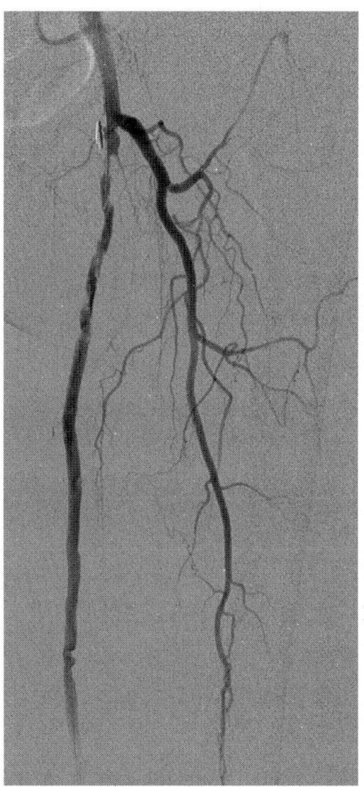

FIGURE 13-3 Power-pulse thrombolysis using the Possis AngioJet system laces the clot with thrombolytic agent, in this case, t-PA. Following a short dwell time, mechanical thrombectomy was performed with use of the same device removing a large fraction of thrombus. Of note, some perfusion to the limb was restored in this case after only 20 minutes with evidence of a Doppler signal in the foot. Catheter-directed thrombolysis was continued to dissolve the remnant thrombus seen in the proximal graft.

documented left heart thrombus. Relative contraindications include gastrointestinal bleeding, severe hypertension, mitral valve disease, endocarditis, hemostatic defects, or pregnancy. After a decision to proceed with thrombolysis, expeditious management in an endovascular suite should ensue.

Access should be chosen carefully and usually is the contralateral femoral artery (Figure 13-1). Multiple puncture attempts can be avoided with the use of duplex ultrasonography in patients with diminished pulses or scarring. Arterial punctures distal to the presumed occlusion should be avoided. Occlusions distal to the mid—superficial femoral artery may be approached with an antegrade ipsilateral puncture, but this information may not be available unless other imaging studies clearly indicate adequate inflow. Multiple-hole catheters are preferred for longer occlusions. If the catheter does not properly penetrate the thrombus, lysis is slowed and inefficient because the lytic agent is "washed out" through collaterals.

Creation of a channel into the thrombus with the angiographic guidewire is of prognostic significance and is technically necessary. Failure to pass the guidewire through the occlusion implies either plaque or a well-organized thrombus, which may be resistant to fibrinolysis. After confirmation of distal arterial patency (Figure 13-2), we power-pulse thrombolysis using the Possis AngioJet system (Figure 13-3). This is performed with a minimal amount of thrombolytic agent (2 mg in 50 mL saline solution) that is laced throughout the clotted region with short bursts of the AngioJet catheter. Of importance, a stopcock is used to turn off the effluent tubing, thus allowing the entire thrombolytic agent to be dispersed into the clot. After 20 minutes, mechanical thrombectomy can be performed without any lytic agent to restore a channel and blood flow into the distal vasculature. We proceed with thrombolysis and have used UK and t-PA preferentially. Bleeding complications appear to correlate most closely with duration of therapy rather than with the total dosage of the agent. Thus we think higher-dose short-term infusions are better tolerated than longer-term low-dose infusions. A higher dose initially (UK 4000 units/min, t-PA 1 mg/hr) appears to be effective in our experience with switching to a lower-dose regimen when there is remnant thrombus on lytic check angiography (UK 1000-2000 units/min, t-PA 0.2-0.5 mg/hr). Valved infusion catheters and infusion wires are used singly or in combination to achieve the appropriate infusion length for intrathrombus infusion. After dissolution of the thrombus, treatment of the "culprit lesion" is critical to durable patency of the thrombolytic procedure (Figures 13-4 through 13-6).

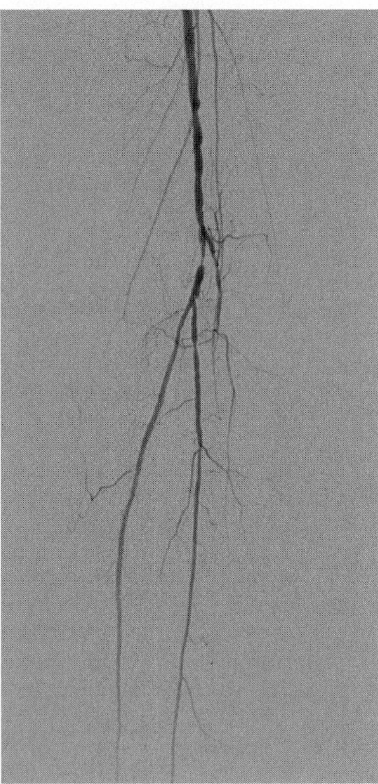

FIGURE 13-4 After resolution of all of the occluding thrombus, the "culprit lesion" was identified as a severe stenosis in the tibioperoneal trunk preventing outflow.

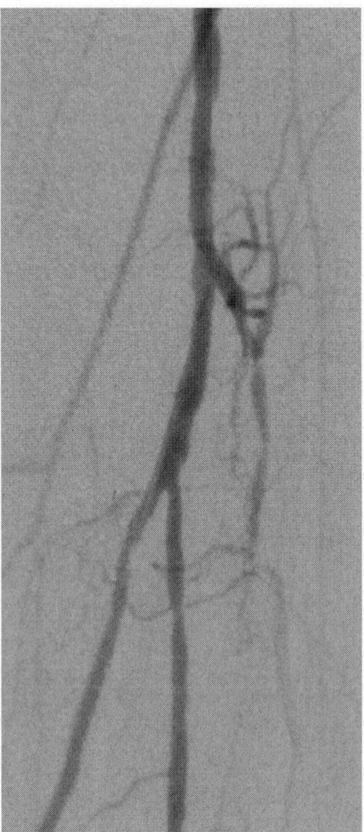

FIGURE 13-5 The tibioperoneal trunk stenosis was treated via percutaneous balloon angioplasty with adequate luminal gain.

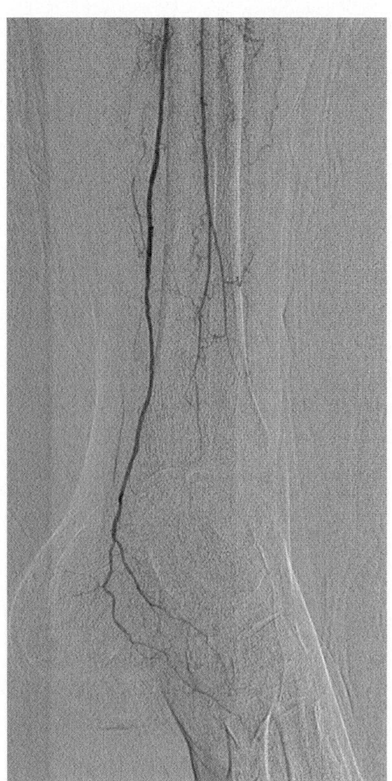

FIGURE 13-6 Endovascular treatment of the occluded graft was successful in returning a posterior tibial pulse in the foot. The patient was discharged without complication and has a patent graft at 6 months of follow-up.

Familiarity with a broad spectrum of novel therapeutic techniques and regimens allows targeted treatment of patients presenting with ALI. A combination of pharmacologic, endovascular, and surgical techniques constitutes the armamentarium of therapeutic strategies that hold the potential to reduce the morbidity and mortality associated with acute vascular occlusion. Considerable judgment must be used in patient selection, and careful planning of the anticipated surgical or endovascular intervention must be done. Thrombolytic therapy appears to be a safe and effective alternative to operation as initial treatment in 70% to 80% of patients presenting with ALI. Although thrombolysis alone can be quite successful in initially restoring patency to a vessel or graft, more often it allows delineation of an underlying arterial stenosis or graft abnormality that then must be treated by operation or angioplasty to maintain patency. Thrombolysis and percutaneous endovascular procedures reduce the need for open operation without increasing the risk of amputation or death.

References

1. Blaisdell FW, Steele M, Allen RE: Management of acute lower extremity arterial ischemia due to embolism and thrombosis, *Surgery* 84(6):822–834, 1978.

2. Jivegard L, Holm J, Schersten T: Acute limb ischemia due to arterial embolism or thrombosis: influence of limb ischemia versus pre-existing cardiac disease on postoperative mortality rate, *J Cardiovasc Surg (Torino)* 29(1):32–36, 1988.
3. Rutherford RB, Baker JD, Ernst C, et al: Recommended standards for reports dealing with lower extremity ischemia: revised version, *J Vasc Surg* 26(3):517–538, 1997.
4. Ouriel K, Shortell CK, DeWeese JA, et al: A comparison of thrombolytic therapy with operative revascularization in the initial treatment of acute peripheral arterial ischemia, *J Vasc Surg* 19(6):1021–1030, 1994.
5. Results of a prospective randomized trial evaluating surgery versus thrombolysis for ischemia of the lower extremity. The STILE trial, *Ann Surg* 220(3):251–266, 1994.
6. Ouriel K, Veith FJ, Sasahara AA: A comparison of recombinant urokinase with vascular surgery as initial treatment for acute arterial occlusion of the legs. Thrombolysis or Peripheral Arterial Surgery (TOPAS) Investigators, *N Engl J Med* 338(16):1105–1111, 1998.
7. Edwards JE, Taylor LM Jr, Porter JM: Treatment of failed lower extremity bypass grafts with new autogenous vein bypass grafting, *J Vasc Surg* 11(1):136–144, 1990.
8. Dormandy JA, Rutherford RB: Management of peripheral arterial disease (PAD). TASC Working Group. TransAtlantic Inter-Society Consensus (TASC), *J Vasc Surg* 31(1 Pt 2):S1–S296, 2000.
9. Tillet WS: The fibrinolytic activity of hemolytic streptococci, *Bacteriol Rev* 2(2):161–216, 1938.
10. Tillett WS, Johnson AJ, McCarty WR: The intravenous infusion of the streptococcal fibrinolytic principle (streptokinase) into patients, *J Clin Invest* 34(2):169–185, 1955.
11. Cliffton EE: The use of plasmin in humans, *Ann N Y Acad Sci* 68 (1):209–229, 1957.
12. Alkjaersig N, Fletcher AP, Sherry S: The mechanism of clot dissolution by plasmin, *J Clin Invest* 38(7):1086–1095, 1959.
13. Tillett WS: The fibrinolytic activity of hemolytic streptococci, *Bacteriol Rev* 2(2):161–216, 1938.
14. Johnson AJ, McCarty WR, Tillett WS: The lysis of artificially induced intravascular clots in man by intravenous infusions of purified streptokinase, *Surg Forum* 9:252–257, 1958.
15. Sharma GV, Cella G, Parisi AF, et al: Thrombolytic therapy, *N Engl J Med* 306(21):1268–1276, 1982.
16. ISIS-3: a randomised comparison of streptokinase vs tissue plasminogen activator vs anistreplase and of aspirin plus heparin vs aspirin alone among 41,299 cases of suspected acute myocardial infarction. ISIS-3 (Third International Study of Infarct Survival) Collaborative Group, *Lancet* 339(8796):753–770, 1992.
17. Macfarlane RG, Pilling J: Observations on fibrinolytic plasminogen, plasmin and antiplasmin content of human blood, *Lancet* 2:562, 1946.
18. Macfarlane RG, Pinot J: Fibrinolytic activity of normal urine, *Nature* 159:779, 1947.
19. Mohler SR, Celander DR, Guest MM: Distribution of urokinase among the common mammals, *Am J Physiol* 192(1):186–190, 1958.
20. Matsuo O, Rijken DC, Collen D: Thrombolysis by human tissue plasminogen activator and urokinase in rabbits with experimental pulmonary embolus, *Nature* 291(5816):590–591, 1981.
21. Teirstein PS, Mann JT III, Cundey PE Jr, et al: Low- versus high-dose recombinant urokinase for the treatment of chronic saphenous vein graft occlusion, *Am J Cardiol* 83(12):1623–1628, 1999.
22. Husain SS, Gurewich V, Lipinski B: Purification and partial characterization of a single-chain high-molecular-weight form of urokinase from human urine, *Arch Biochem Biophys* 220(1):31–38, 1983.
23. Weaver WD, Hartmann JR, Anderson JL, et al: New recombinant glycosylated prourokinase for treatment of patients with acute myocardial infarction. Prourokinase Study Group, *J Am Coll Cardiol* 24(5):1242–1248, 1994.
24. Hoylaerts M, Rijken DC, Lijnen HR, et al: Kinetics of the activation of plasminogen by human tissue plasminogen activator. Role of fibrin, *J Biol Chem* 257(6):2912–2919, 1982.
25. Rijken DC, Hoylaerts M, Collen D: Fibrinolytic properties of one-chain and two-chain human extrinsic (tissue-type) plasminogen activator, *J Biol Chem* 257(6):2920–2925, 1982.
26. De Jaegere PP, Arnold AA, Balk AH, et al: Intracranial hemorrhage in association with thrombolytic therapy: incidence and clinical predictive factors, *J Am Coll Cardiol* 19(2):289–294, 1992.
27. Meierhenrich R, Carlsson J, Seifried E, et al: Effect of reteplase on hemostasis variables: analysis of fibrin specificity, relation to bleeding complications and coronary patency, *Int J Cardiol* 65(1):57–63, 1998.
28. Ouriel K, Castaneda F, McNamara T, et al: Reteplase monotherapy and reteplase/abciximab combination therapy in peripheral arterial occlusive disease: results from the RELAX trial, *J Vasc Interv Radiol* 15(3):229–238, 2004.
29. Valji K: Evolving strategies for thrombolytic therapy of peripheral vascular occlusion, *J Vasc Interv Radiol* 11(4):411–420, 2000.
30. Cannon CP, Gibson CM, McCabe CH, et al: TNK-tissue plasminogen activator compared with front-loaded alteplase in acute myocardial infarction: results of the TIMI 10B trial. Thrombolysis in Myocardial Infarction (TIMI) 10B Investigators, *Circulation* 98(25):2805–2814, 1998.
31. Burkart DJ, Borsa JJ, Anthony JP, et al: Thrombolysis of occluded peripheral arteries and veins with tenecteplase: a pilot study, *J Vasc Interv Radiol* 13(11):1099–1102, 2002.
32. Ahmed NK, Gaddis RR, Tennant KD, et al: Biological and thrombolytic properties of fibrolase: a new fibrinolytic protease from snake venom, *Haemostasis* 20(6):334–340, 1990.
33. Markland FS: Fibrolase, an active thrombolytic enzyme in arterial and venous thrombosis model systems, *Adv Exp Med Biol* 391:427–438, 1996.
34. Kashyap VS, Reil TD, Moore WS, et al: Acute arterial thrombosis causes endothelial dysfunction: a new paradigm for thrombolytic therapy, *J Vasc Surg* 34(2):323–329, 2001.
35. Davis MR, Ortegon DP, Clouse WD, et al: Luminal thrombus disrupts nitric oxide-dependent endothelial physiology, *J Surg Res* 104(2):112–117, 2002.
36. Davis MR, Ortegon DP, Kerby JD: Endothelial dysfunction after arterial thrombosis is ameliorated by L-arginine in combination with thrombolysis, *J Vasc Interv Radiol* 14(2 Pt 1):233–239, 2003.
37. Lin PH, Johnson CK, Pullium JK, et al: L-arginine improves endothelial vasoreactivity and reduces thrombogenicity after thrombolysis in experimental deep venous thrombosis, *J Vasc Surg* 38(6):1396–1403, 2003.
38. Ouriel K, Veith FJ, Sasahara AA: Thrombolysis or peripheral arterial surgery: phase I results. TOPAS Investigators, *J Vasc Surg* 23(1):64–73, 1996.
39. Earnshaw JJ, Whitman B, Foy C: National Audit of Thrombolysis for Acute Leg Ischemia (NATALI): clinical factors associated with early outcome, *J Vasc Surg* 39(5):1018–1025, 2004.
40. Eskridge JM, Becker GJ, Rabe FE, Richmond BD, Holden RW, Yune HY, et al: Catheter-related thrombosis and fibrinolytic therapy, *Radiology* 149(2):429–432, 1983.
41. Ouriel K, Kandarpa K: Safety of thrombolytic therapy with urokinase or recombinant tissue plasminogen activator for peripheral arterial occlusion: a comprehensive compilation of published work, *J Endovasc Ther* 11(4):436–446, 2004.
42. Thrombolysis in the management of lower limb peripheral arterial occlusion—a consensus document, *J Vasc Interv Radiol* 14 (9 Pt 2):S337–S349, 2003.

CHAPTER

14

Arterial Closure Devices

W. Anthony Lee

Successful vessel entry and exit may be arguably two of the most important technical aspects of any percutaneous intervention. It is self-evident that, without proper entry into the vessel, the procedure cannot be performed and, without proper closure of the entry site, a host of complications can ensue that may turn an otherwise successful intervention into a life- or limb-threatening disaster. These two seemingly disparate bookends of the procedure are intimately interrelated, and the success of the back end is critically dependent on the proper execution of the front end[1] (Figure 14-1).

Before the advent of closure devices, the only method of percutaneous hemostasis of the access site was by manual compression. Although mechanical devices (e.g., QuicKlamp, TZ Medical, Portland, OR; FemoStop, Radi Medical Systems, Wilmington, MA) became available that relieved the physical fatigue of those who had to apply the pressure, it did not address the pain and discomfort of having heavy pressure applied on a tender groin and the subsequent need for prolonged bed rest before being allowed to ambulate.

It is important to keep in mind that all of the arterial closure devices have been approved for use only in the common femoral artery. Despite scattered anecdotal experiences of successful closure of other vessels under a variety of unusual circumstances,[2-5] the safety or efficacy of these devices after percutaneous access of prosthetic or autogenous surgical grafts (e.g., vein grafts or aortofemoral limbs) has not been systematically examined.[6] Notably, the small size of the brachial artery and its propensity to spasm make use of a closure device in this location intuitively more risky for injury and ischemic complications.

In this chapter, we will review and compare the different devices that are currently available for closure of arterial access sites and the failure modes unique to each of them. Although the actual instructions for use of the devices are beyond the scope of this chapter, specific technical issues and pitfalls will be discussed as appropriate.

MANUAL COMPRESSION VERSUS ARTERIAL CLOSURE DEVICE

Manual compression is simple, inexpensive, and reliable and does not leave any foreign bodies that may cause an infection or inflammatory reaction or prevent early reintervention through the same site. Despite all of these apparent advantages, manual compression has been far from being an optimal solution to the closure problem. Its disadvantages included (1) the often-overlooked need for proper technique and experience in applying the right amount of pressure at the correct location to prevent bleeding and thrombosis, (2) reduction of blood flow ipsilateral to the side of puncture, (3) operator fatigue caused by the prolonged compression, (4) patient pain and discomfort while pressure is being applied and the obligatory 4 to 6 hours of flat bed rest, and (5) the need for a normal coagulation status.

Arterial closure devices have overcome many of these shortcomings of manual compression with a small but real risk of major complications.[7] In one of the largest comparisons between the two methods involving nearly 13,000 consecutive cardiac catheterizations, the risk of vascular complications after manual compression was over twice that of closure devices for both diagnostic and interventional procedures.[8] These devices principally allow immediate or very rapid (typically <1 minute) closure of the arteriotomy and earlier ambulation[9] by using a variety of mechanisms that include surgical sutures, metallic clips, or bioabsorbable plugs. Because of the mechanical closure of the arteriotomy without reliance on the clotting cascade, hemostasis is largely independent of coagulation status, and the

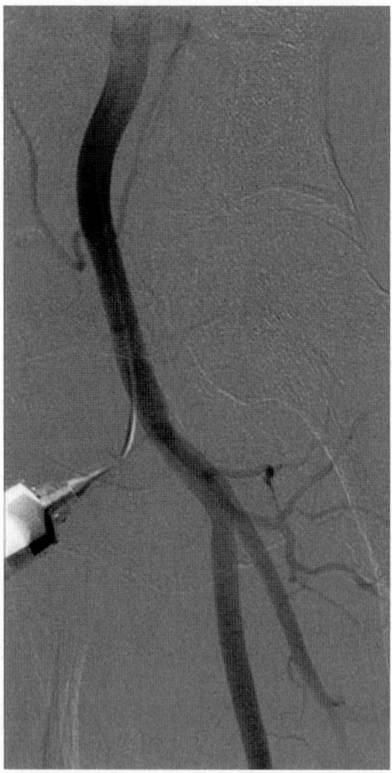

FIGURE 14-1 Femoral arteriogram (30-degree right anterior oblique projection). Ideal femoral access is characterized by (1) an anterior entry, (2) at least 5 to 10 mm proximal to the femoral bifurcation, (3) distal to the inguinal ligament, and (4) single wall puncture.

devices are effective in the fully heparinized patient without the need to wait for the heparin to wear off or be actively reversed with protamine.

Just as with manual compression, there is a learning curve with the initial use of these devices. This learning curve has less to do with the actual steps of the procedure than it has to do with gaining the tactile and visual feedback of the device as it interacts with the artery and its surrounding tissue. It is knowing when to push or pull an extra millimeter, how firmly or gently to actuate a certain lever, when to quit or troubleshoot, and myriad of other unwritten instructions that are never found in a typical Instructions for Use. But most important, it has to do with knowing when and when not to use a closure device. As with all procedures, complications may be overcome with experience, meticulous technique, and careful patient selection. Closure devices are modestly expensive, most are similarly priced at $250 to $300, and neither they nor the procedure is reimbursable. However, the economics of routine use of arterial closure devices must be weighed against the less quantifiable and intangible costs of personnel and fixed resources.[10]

The presence of a permanent foreign body by some of these devices may increase the risk of late arterial stenosis[11-14] or secondary infection, which may lead to a pseudoaneurysm and/or necrotizing arteritis requiring a complex arterial reconstruction.[15] Last, failure of a closure device almost always turns a "simple percutaneous procedure" to a worse problem involving hemorrhage, acute thrombosis, and/or distal embolization with risk to life and limb and necessitating surgical repair.

TABLE 14-1 Hemostasis Pads and Patches

Brand name	Manufacturer
Chito-Seal	Abbott Vascular
Clo-Sur P.A.D.	Scion Cardiovascular
D-Stat Dry	Vascular Solutions
Syvek NT	Marine Polymer Technologies
Neptune Pad	TZ Medical
V+Pad	InterV

ARTERIAL CLOSURE DEVICES

Hemostasis Pads/Patches

A family of vessel closure "aids" described as hemostasis pads/patches has been marketed by a number of manufacturers that purportedly accelerate hemostasis during manual compression. (Table 14-1). These pads (approximately 2-4 cm × 4 cm) are applied directly to the skin puncture site while manual compression is being applied (Figure 14-2). The contact surface of the pads is coated with a variety of "active ingredients" that have included chitosan gel, polyprolate biopolymer, thrombin, and calcium alginate, which in varying degrees are intended to promote the clotting cascade through red blood cell and platelet aggregation within the subcutaneous tract of the catheter/sheath. Ironically, the sheer diversity of active ingredients used by the different pads or patches makes their individual mechanistic claims of action somewhat suspect. The potential benefits of these pads include their lower cost ($30-$80) compared with mechanical closure devices ($200-$300), a shorter compression time compared with the typical 15 to 30 minutes (although without clear reduction in the duration of postcompression bed rest), absence of foreign material near the artery or in the subcutaneous tissues, simplicity, applicability on any site of percutaneous access (e.g., brachial), and ability to reaccess the artery without significant delay.

Despite their plausibility, it has been difficult to convincingly validate the mechanisms of action of these

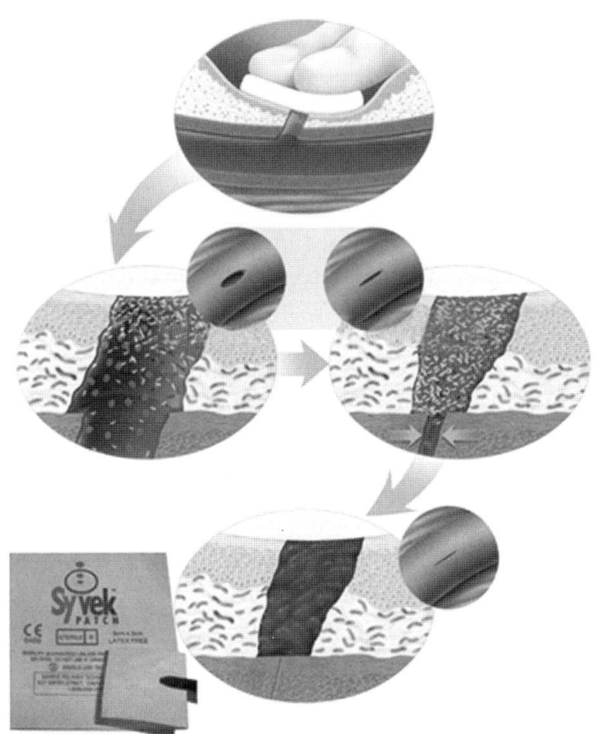

FIGURE 14-2 Syvek NT *(Marine Polymer Technologies, Danvers, MA).*

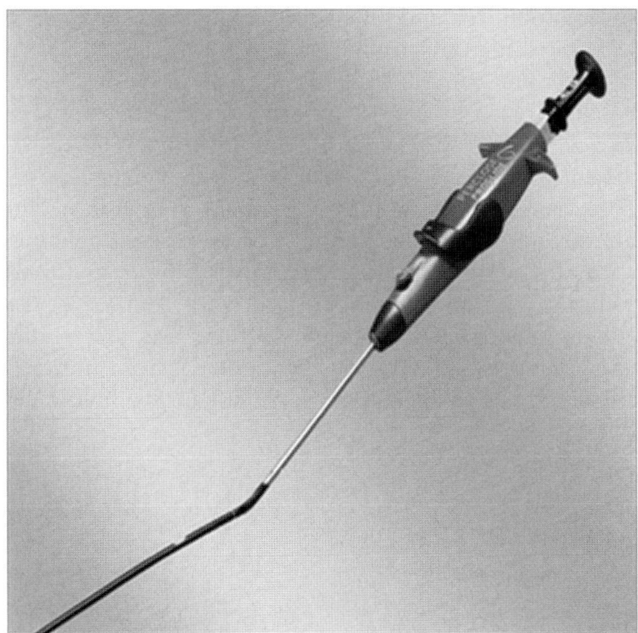

FIGURE 14-3 Perclose Proglide *(Abbott Vascular, Redwood City, CA).*

devices in vivo given the problem of separating the relative contribution of the pad from that of simple compression alone. Indeed, the minimum optimal compression time for hemostasis and duration of bed rest have not been widely studied and are something that may be difficult to study ethically in human subjects. One report involving a large cohort of 5F diagnostic catheterizations showed that ambulation after only 1 hour of bed rest resulted in only a 3% incidence of minor and no major complications.[16] According to the manufacturers, depending on the size of the sheath, hemostasis may be reliably achieved with less than 10 minutes of medium to light compression. These claims notwithstanding, use of hemostasis pads can only be economically justified by virtue of their lower cost over other mechanical arterial closure devices, but as with any other consumer product "you get what you paid for."

Perclose

The Perclose (Abbott Vascular, Redwood City, CA) line of arterial closure devices represents the prototype for suture-mediated closure devices. There are two Perclose devices intended for closure of femoral artery access sites involving 6.5F (Proglide), 8F (Prostar XL 8), and 10F (Prostar XL 10) introducer sheaths.[17] The Prostar XL 8F and 10F versions are similar except for the profile of the delivery systems and will be referred together as the "Prostar" device. The Proglide is the latest iteration of the original Perclose device and has several improvements over its predecessors (Auto-Tie, Closer S) (Figure 14-3). It is a 6F, 0.038-inch–compatible device that deploys a single vertically oriented 3-0 polypropylene suture with use of two nitinol needles, with a preformed slipknot that is tied down by using a combination knot pusher and suture cutter. Although indicated to be used up to 6.5F sheaths, it has been reliably used for 7F sheaths. By comparison, the Prostar is also a 0.038-inch–compatible device, the main shaft of which is 8F/10F with a 20F distal hub that requires a generous blunt subcutaneous dissection to allow the base of the hub to make contact with the surface of the femoral artery (Figure 14-4). It deploys two 3-0 braided polyester sutures in a crossed pattern using four nitinol needles. Slipknots must be tied by the operator (with or without the accompanying knot-tying aid) and cinched down with a knot pusher.

The advantages of suture-mediated devices are the strength of their closure, which resembles a surgical repair, immediate hemostasis even in the setting of full anticoagulation, early ambulation (<60 minutes of bed rest), and early reaccessibility of the artery. The disadvantages of these devices are the cost (Proglide $295, Prostar $495), which as previously mentioned are not reimbursable; permanent foreign material in the artery; risk of infection; device failure leading to early or late bleeding complications (arterial injury from needle deflection or misdeployment and a loose tie from slipknot failure); and a longer learning curve compared with the other devices.

Infectious complications have been associated with Perclose closures almost more than any other closure device.[18,19] Because of the transmural involvement of the suture material with the arterial wall, Perclose infections have almost uniformly resulted in severe necrotizing arteritis and a suppurative soft tissue reaction with an acute pseudoaneurysm that have required complex, femoral reconstruction with use of either autogenous or homograft femoral vein and a sartorius flap[20] (Figure 14-5). This complication has been anecdotally attributed to the higher propensity for seeding of the braided suture in the original versions of this device. Greater awareness of this risk by the interventional community, stricter adherence to aseptic techniques, and introduction of the monofilament suture in the Proglide device should help in this regard.

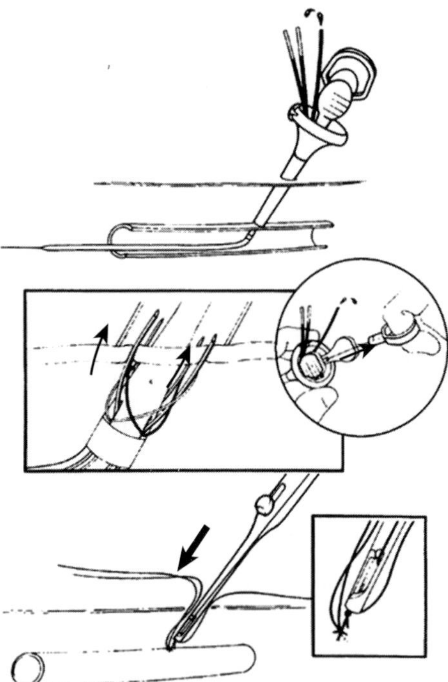

FIGURE 14-4 Perclose Prostar (Abbott Vascular, Redwood City, CA). Note in the *top* illustration how the hub must be inserted deeply through the subcutaneous tissue.

Device-related complications can result in a larger arteriotomy than the original introducer sheath and an increased risk of significant bleeding. If one or more of the needles or sutures fail to deploy correctly, the artery may tear during forcible removal of the misdeployed suture or attempted extrication of the device. Alternatively, the device may cause an intimal dissection with acute occlusion and limb ischemia, which is typically secondary to poor patient selection.[21,22] In either case, surgical repair requires emergent general anesthesia in a poor-risk patient, who may have cardiopulmonary comorbidities, with increased blood loss during the femoral exposure, and arterial repair frequently involving thromboendarterectomy with patch angioplasty.[23] Fortunately, most failures may be managed with manual compression (sometimes longer than what would have been originally necessary) or even a second device. In this latter regard, it is critical to maintain guidewire access until the suture is tied down and removed only after adequate hemostasis is verified. A dilator or sheath may be quickly reinserted to achieve temporary hemostasis while surgical repair or other corrective measures are taken.

The Proglide and Prostar devices have both been used off-label in a technique termed "Preclose" for percutaneous closures of femoral arteries after endovascular aortic repairs.[24,25] Although a detailed description of the technique is beyond the scope of this chapter, in brief, the Perclose sutures are deployed before the insertion of the large-diameter delivery systems and left untied until the end of the procedure. After completion of the endovascular repair, all the catheters and sheaths are removed, and the sutures are tied down over the guidewire. A few minutes of manual pressure are

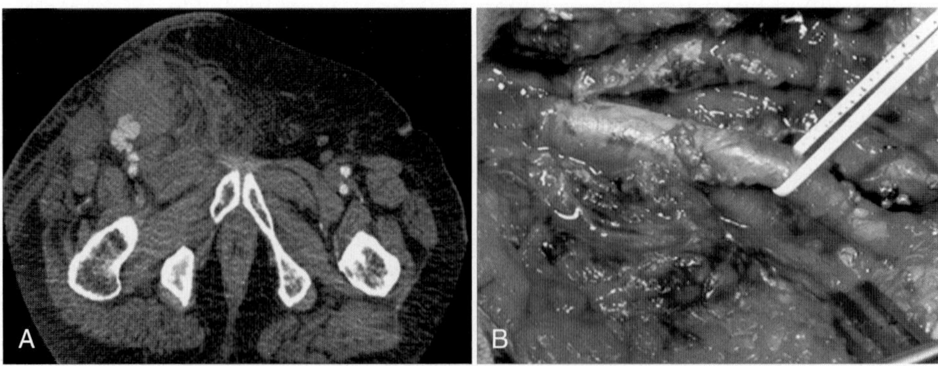

FIGURE 14-5 **A,** Computed tomographic angiogram showing an acute femoral pseudoaneurysm after closure with Perclose device. **B,** Femoral reconstruction with autogenous superficial femoral vein.

usually necessary while the anticoagulation is reversed with protamine sulfate to achieve complete hemostasis. With use of this technique, 18F to 24F sheaths have been closed with success rates of greater than 90%. Indeed, Perclose is the only device that is currently able to be used for percutaneous closure of access sites greater than 12F.

StarClose

The StarClose (Abbott Vascular) is a 6F device that is indicated for closure of femoral access sites after 5F or 6F sheaths. It is composed of a separate 0.035-inch guidewire–compatible introducer sheath and an applicator that deploys a single extravascular nitinol clip (Figure 14-6). The clip is stellate shaped and "grasps" the adventitia around the puncture site and, using the thermal memory property of nitinol, constricts to close the hole. Complete hemostasis requires approximately 15 to 30 seconds after the clip is applied for the nitinol to fully reform on exposure to the body temperature.[26]

StarClose is comparably priced with other devices. Its advantages include relative ease of use (compared with Perclose), absence of any intravascular foreign body (the clip remains completely adventitial), and immediate reaccessibility of the artery with repeat closure with the device. Theoretically, if by sheer chance a repeat puncture were to enter precisely through the center of a previous clip, it would simply expand around the sheath and retract around the site after the sheath is removed, without application of another clip. Successful closures were also reported in stenotic diseased femoral arteries[27] and after antegrade punctures with use of this device.[28] Disadvantages include slightly slower time to complete hemostasis and increased need for additional manual compression[29] compared with other devices, the presence of permanent foreign material, and potential failure of the nitinol clip to actually constrict the arterial wall if it is calcified and rigid. Infrequently the subcutaneous tissue may get entrapped within the clip applicator, and either the clip partially deploys or the applicator cannot be removed,[30] requiring direct surgical extrication and arterial repair.

Angio-Seal

Angio-Seal (St. Jude Medical, St. Paul, MN) uses a dual-layer mechanism comprising a small, low-profile polyglactin footplate that anchors to the luminal side of the artery and is joined by a polyglactin suture to a collagen plug that sits on the outside of the artery (Figure 14-7). A slipknot is used to cinch down the suture, which tightly sandwiches the access site between footplate and the plug to achieve hemostasis (Figure 14-8). The entire mass is fully absorbed in 60 to 90 days. The two versions of the device are indicated for closure of 6F (Angio-Seal VIP) and 8F (Angio-Seal STS Plus) femoral access sites. Anecdotally, however, successful closures of 7F and 9F to 11F sheaths have been performed with use of the VIP and STS devices, respectively. In one study, the device was also used successfully in more than 98% of cases after antegrade femoral punctures.[31] Similarly, single center reports with a combined experience of more than 200 cases of percutaneous brachial punctures have suggested the safety and efficacy of Angio-Seal used in this location with a major complication rate of 0% to 3.1%.[32,33]

The cost of Angio-Seal is comparable with that of the other mechanical closure devices. Its principal advantages include ease of use, reliability, complete

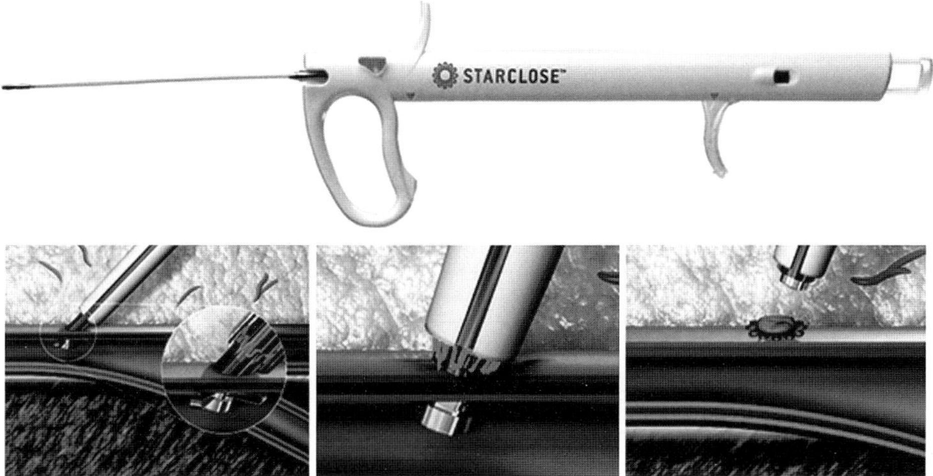

FIGURE 14-6 StarClose (Abbott Vascular, Redwood City, CA). The *bottom panels* illustrate how the clip is applied to the adventitia and constricts to close the arteriotomy.

bioabsorbability, early restickability,[34] extremely low incidence of infection, and overall high rates of success with regard to immediate hemostasis and early ambulation.[35,36] On the other hand, several technical pitfalls deserve mention: (1) In extremely thin patients, because of the lack of sufficient depth of the subcutaneous tissue, the superficial aspect of the collagen plug can actually protrude outside the skin. To remedy this problem, the initial arterial entry should be performed at a relatively shallower angle so that the needle travels within the subcutaneous tissue plane for 1 to 2 cm before arterial entry. Before cutting the suture that is attached to the collagen, a small subcutaneous flap is bluntly raised around the puncture site, used to cover the collagen, and closed with a single subcuticular suture. Another technique that has been described is to use tumescent anesthesia with lidocaine to increase the depth of the subcutaneous layer.[33] (2) Another problem that can occur in thin individuals is that when the connecting suture is cut (typically a few millimeters below the skin) as the last step in the procedure, it is inadvertently cut too close to the slipknot, resulting in unraveling of the knot. In this case, not only will the puncture site start bleeding because of the loss of traction on the collagen plug, but the footplate may become loosened and embolize distally.[37] (3) Although the polyglactin footplate has a low profile, the intravascular location of this component may compromise the lumen in very small (<5 mm) or severely diseased femoral arteries. (4) Occasionally, when the Angio-Seal sheath is inserted too deeply, the collagen plug may actually be deployed intraluminally resulting in immediate or early arterial occlusion.[21,38] There are clear marks on the sheath that indicate the depth of the tip, but careless technique can lead to this avoidable complication. (5) Severe scarring of the subcutaneous tissue from prior surgery or multiple catheterizations can prevent apposition of the plug on the puncture site and result in bleeding through the gap between the arteriotomy and the collagen.

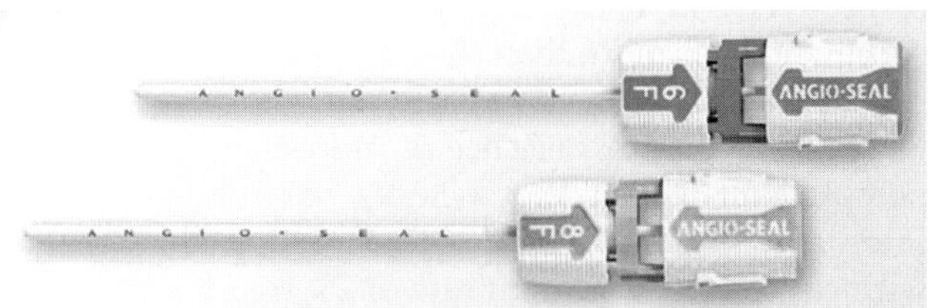

FIGURE 14-7 Angio-Seal VIP (St. Jude Medical, St. Paul, MN). The device is available in 6F and 8F versions.

Boomerang Vascular Closure System

The Boomerang Vascular Closure System (Cardiva Medical, Mountain View, CA) is a hemostasis aid designed to be used as an adjunct to manual compression (Figure 14-9). It is designed to be used for assisted closure after 5F to 7F sheaths. The system is composed of a small nitinol disk (5-6.5 mm diameter) that is attached to a wire (Boomerang Wire, 0.037 inches) and deployed through the existing sheath. As the sheath is removed, the disk is pulled snugly against the inner surface of the arteriotomy, and traction is maintained with the Boomerang Clip applied at the skin level for a minimum of 15 minutes for diagnostic cases and 120 minutes for interventional cases (Figure 14-10). The mechanism of action is purported based on the intrinsic elastic recoil of the artery to reduce the size of the original arteriotomy created by the sheath to the approximate

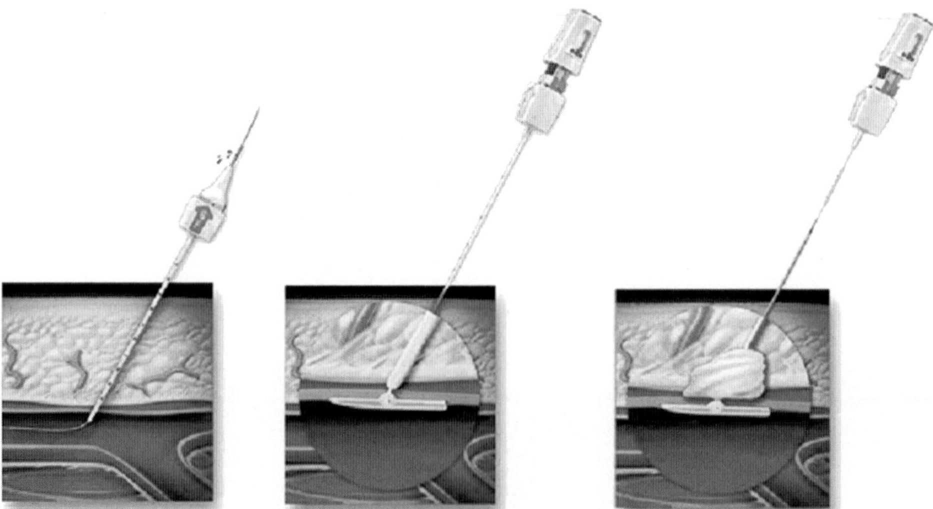

FIGURE 14-8 Steps illustrating the footplate deployed on the luminal side of the arteriotomy and the collagen plug being compacted on the outside of the vessel wall.

equivalent of an 18-gauge needle. Afterward, the nitinol disk is collapsed and pulled through the arteriotomy while manual compression is applied proximally. Compression is applied additionally for 5 to 10 minutes until complete hemostasis is achieved. Recently, the Boomerang Catalyst System II has been introduced, which is coated with a proprietary agent that is intended to shorten the overall time to hemostasis by activating the intrinsic (factor XII mediated) pathway of the coagulation cascade.

The advantages of this system include a simple mechanism of action that is less prone to device failure and absence of any foreign body.[39] Its disadvantages include that (1) manual compression must still be applied and the patient remain in bed rest for a significant duration of time, (2) removal of the collapsed device through the same arteriotomy may reopen the arteriotomy that had just been closed, and (3) elastic recoil may not occur in calcified, heavily diseased arteries. Another potentially problematic issue involves the need to sterilely secure the Boomerang Wire during patient transfer and recovery to avoid contamination and accidental dislodgement, which may result in a larger arteriotomy and significant bleeding. Given these limitations, it is unclear whether even this latest iteration represents

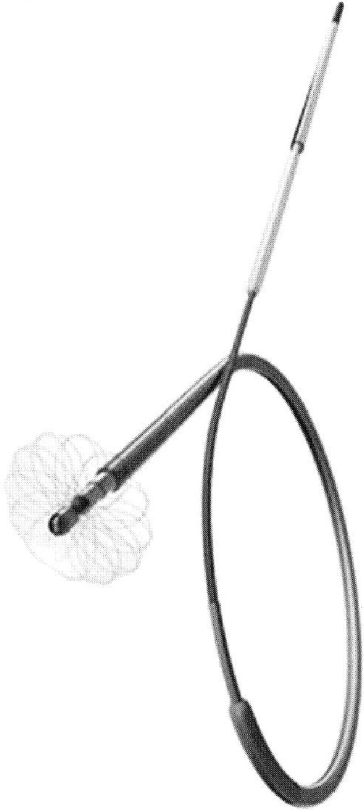

FIGURE 14-9 Boomerang Catalyst Wire (Cardiva Medical, Mountain View, CA).

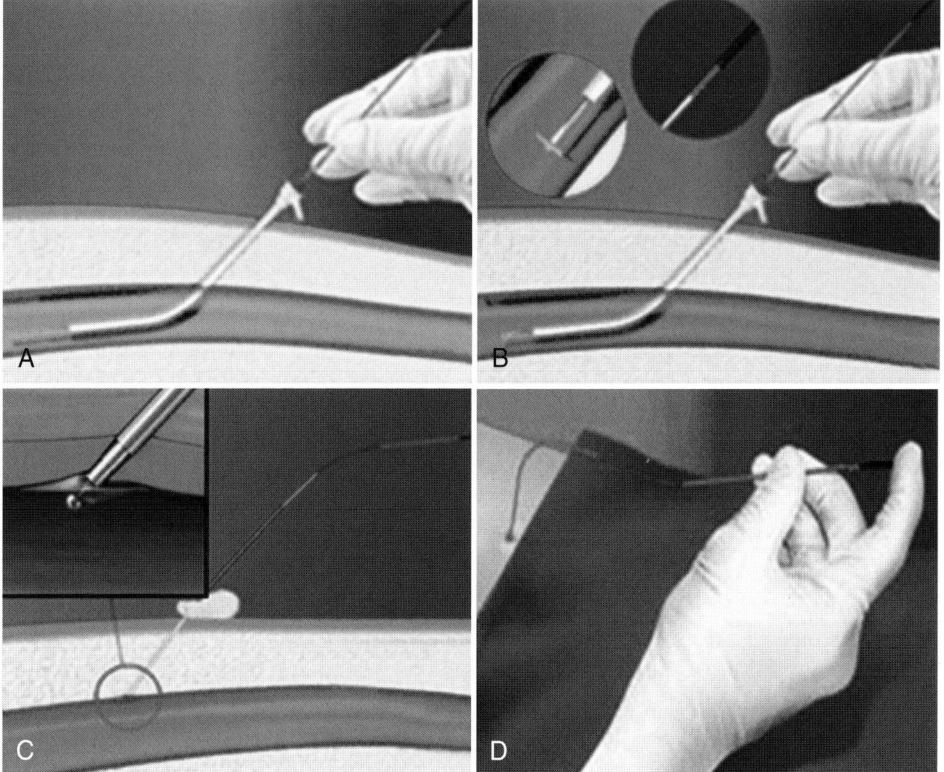

FIGURE 14-10 Deployment of the Boomerang Wire. **A,** Wire is inserted through the existing sheath. **B,** Disk is deployed in the arterial lumen. **C,** Sheath is removed and disk snugged up against arteriotomy. A white clip is attached at skin level to maintain traction. **D,** While manual compression is applied, disk is collapsed and removed.

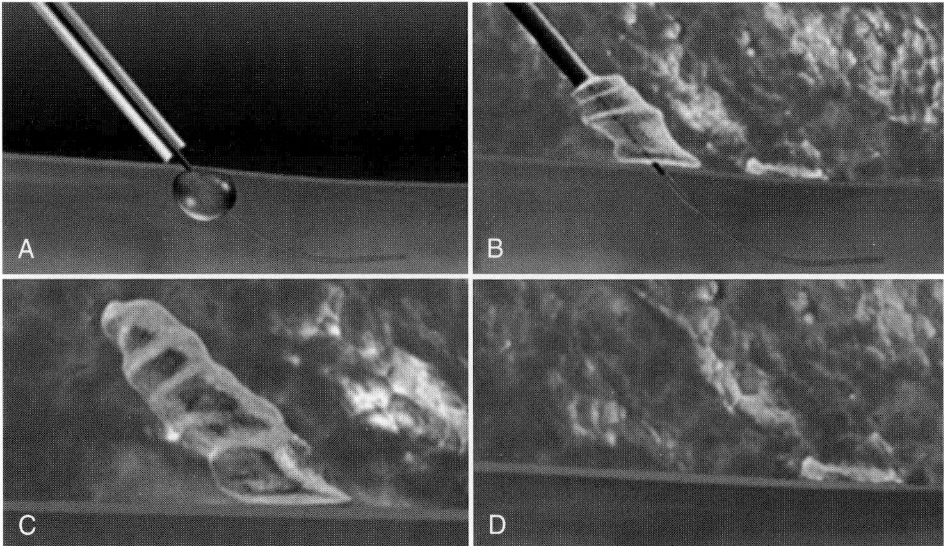

FIGURE 14-11 Mynx (AccessClosure, Mountain View, CA). **A,** Balloon-tipped wire is inserted through existing sheath. **B,** Sealant delivered. **C,** Balloon deflated and removed. **D,** Sealant completely resorbed.

a clear clinical superiority over standard manual compression.

Mynx

The Mynx (AccessClosure, Mountain View, CA) device uses a polyethylene glycol (PEG) sealant delivered through the existing sheath to close the arteriotomy and the sheath tract. A semicompliant balloon-tipped guidewire is inserted through a 6F or 7F sheath, the balloon is temporarily inflated to occlude the arteriotomy, the sealant is delivered to the outside of the arteriotomy and within the tract of the sheath, and the balloon is deflated and removed (Figure 14-11). The PEG sealant is packaged in a dehydrated state and expands by absorption of blood and fluid from the subcutaneous tract. The sealant completely dissolves by hydrolysis within 30 days.

This device shares some of the same advantages as in other closure systems previously mentioned including ease of use, extravascular closure mechanism, early hemostasis (1-2 minutes) and ambulation (2-3 hours) with full anticoagulation,[40] and absence of any permanent foreign body either inside or outside the arteriotomy. Its potential disadvantages include the passive mechanism of the PEG plug to achieve closure versus the active suture-and-anchor mechanism employed by the Angio-Seal device. It is conceivable that, with hypertension, the blood pressure may actually lift the PEG plug away from the arteriotomy, which at best is loosely adherent to the surrounding subcutaneous tissue. In cases of failure of hemostasis and manual compression is required, a portion or the entire plug may be inadvertently extruded intraluminally, risking acute thrombosis and/or distal embolization.

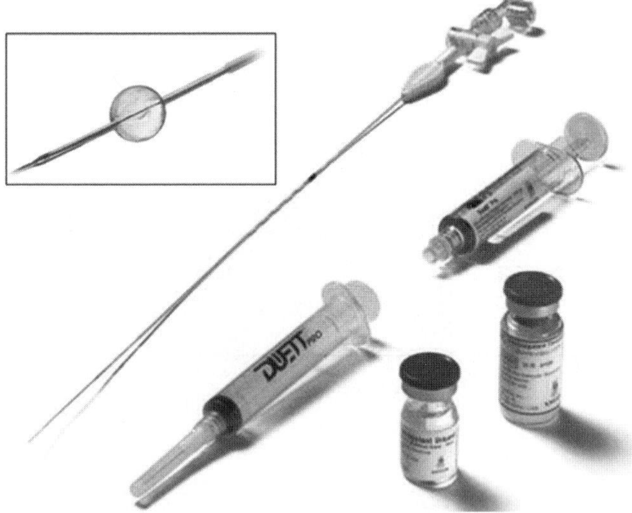

FIGURE 14-12 Duett Pro (Vascular Solutions, Minneapolis, MN). The balloon-tipped catheter is inserted into the sheath and used to occlude the arteriotomy *(inset)*. Sheath is retracted to just outside the vessel, and a procoagulant solution is delivered through the side port of the sheath.

Other Devices

1. Duett Pro (Vascular Solutions, Minneapolis, MN)[41]: Similar to Mynx (Figure 14-12)
2. EVS Stapling System (Medtronic, Minneapolis, MN)[42]: Similar to StarClose (Figure 14-13)
3. Femoral Introducer Sheath and Hemostasis (FISH) (Morris Innovative, Bloomington, IN): This is a novel device that uses a porcine small intestinal submucosa (SIS) plug partially deployed at the beginning of the procedure with use of an integrated sheath introducer

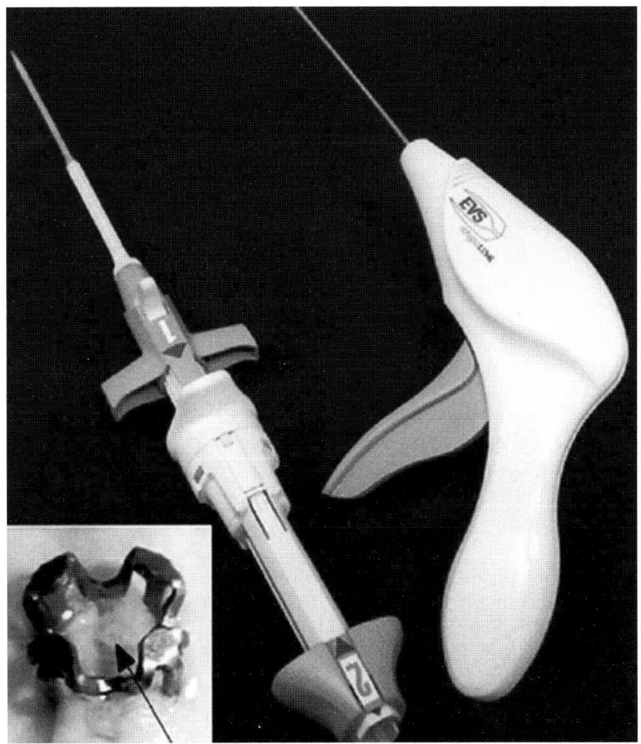

FIGURE 14-13 EVS Stapling System (Medtronic, Minneapolis, MN).

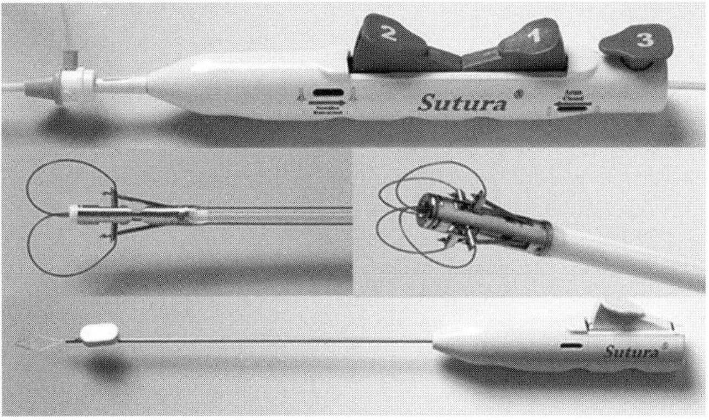

FIGURE 14-14 SuperStitch (Sutura, Fountain Valley, CA). *Top,* Deployment handle inserted through an existing sheath. *Middle,* Single suture for 6F to 8F *(left)* and double suture for 12F to 16F *(right)* closures. *Bottom,* Automated suture-securing device.

system and actively secured with a suture to close the arteriotomy at the conclusion of the procedure (http://www.morrisinnovative.com/fishvideo.html). In its pivotal multicenter clinical trial, mean time to hemostasis (8.9 minutes) and ambulation (2.4 hours) was approximately half that of manual compression cohort.[43]

4. SuperStitch (Sutura, Fountain Valley, CA): Similar to Perclose. This is a suture-mediated closure system available in 6F and 8F sizes.[44] Currently, however, it does not have an on-label indication for percutaneous closure of arteriotomies. A 12F version and the latest version, SuperStitch II, are investigational devices that are seeking Food and Drug Administration indications for use in endovascular aortic repairs (Figure 14-14).

CONCLUSION

There is a large variety of arterial closure devices currently available for management of percutaneous management of puncture sites. Despite the obvious differences in their mechanisms of action, the body of evidence suggests superiority of these devices over conventional manual compression in terms of achieving rapid hemostasis and shorter time to ambulation. Regardless of the apparent ease or simplicity of any one device over another, the success of each device is critically dependent on meticulous technique and patient selection, which are generalizable of any invasive procedure. With further technologic improvements and our own willingness to venture outside of our "comfort zones," adoption of closure devices will likely increase in the near future and even become the new standard of care.

References

1. Phillips WJ, Lee PV: Vascular closure devices: begin with the end in mind, *J Am Coll Cardiol* 51:1416–1417, 2008.
2. Guimaraes M, Uflacker R, Schonholz C, et al: Use of percutaneous closure devices in the removal of central venous catheters from inadvertent arterial catheterizations, *J Cardiovasc Surg (Torino)* 49:345–350, 2008.
3. Shetty SV, Kwolek CJ, Garasic JM: Percutaneous closure after inadvertent subclavian artery cannulation, *Catheter Cardiovasc Interv* 69:1050–1052, 2007.
4. Ozawa A, Chaturvedi R, Lee KJ, et al: Femoral vein hemostasis in children using a suture-mediated closure device, *J Interv Cardiol* 20:164–167, 2007.
5. Leijdekkers VJ, Go HL, Legemate DA, et al: The use of a percutaneous closure device for closure of an accidental puncture of the aortic arch; a simple solution for a difficult problem *Eur J Vasc Endovasc Surg* 32:94–96, 2006.
6. Pullen AJ, Carrell TW, Wilkins CJ, et al: Percutaneous closure devices in synthetic graft punctures: a case for concern? *Eur J Vasc Endovasc Surg* 24:545–546, 2002.
7. Behan MW, Large JK, Patel NR, et al: A randomised controlled trial comparing the routine use of an Angio-Seal STS device strategy with conventional femoral haemostasis methods in a district general hospital, *Int J Clin Pract* 61:367–372, 2007.
8. Arora N, Matheny ME, Sepke C, et al: A propensity analysis of the risk of vascular complications after cardiac catheterization procedures with the use of vascular closure devices, *Am Heart J* 153:606–611, 2007.
9. Martin JL, Pratsos A, Magargee E, et al: A randomized trial comparing compression, Perclose Proglide and Angio-Seal VIP for arterial closure following percutaneous coronary intervention: the CAP trial, *Catheter Cardiovasc Interv* 71:1–5, 2008.

10. Resnic FS, Arora N, Matheny M, et al: A cost-minimization analysis of the angio-seal vascular closure device following percutaneous coronary intervention, *Am J Cardiol* 99(6):766–770, 2007.
11. Bent CL, Kyriakides C, Matson M: Femoral artery stenosis following percutaneous closure using a Starclose closure device, *Cardiovasc Intervent Radiol* 31(4):814–816, 2008.
12. Osborn LA, Sunderman H, Langsfeld M: Common femoral artery stenosis after deployment of vascular clip closure device, *Catheter Cardiovasc Interv* 71:736–737, 2008.
13. Van Den Broek T, Liqui Lung PF, Suttorp MJ, et al: Vascular occlusion as a late complication of the Angio-Seal closure device. A review of literature, *Minerva Cardioangiol* 55:815–819, 2007.
14. Tam J, Given M, Lutjen P, et al: Iatrogenic stenosis following suture-mediated closure device, *Australas Radiol* 51(Suppl:B): 319–323, 2007.
15. Boston US, Panneton JM, Hofer JM, et al: Infectious and ischemic complications from percutaneous closure devices used after vascular access, *Ann Vasc Surg* 17:66–71, 2003.
16. Doyle BJ, Konz BA, Lennon RJ, et al: Ambulation 1 hour after diagnostic cardiac catheterization: a prospective study of 1009 procedures, *Mayo Clin Proc* 81:1537–1540, 2006.
17. Nasu K, Tsuchikane E, Sumitsuji S: PARADISE Investigators: Clinical effectiveness of the Prostar XL suture-mediated percutaneous vascular closure device following PCI: results of the Perclose AcceleRated Ambulation and DISchargE (PARADISE) Trial, *J Invasive Cardiol* 15:251–256, 2003.
18. Smith TP, Cruz CP, Moursi MM, et al: Infectious complications resulting from use of hemostatic puncture closure devices, *Am J Surg* 182:658–662, 2001.
19. Johanning JM, Franklin DP, Elmore JR, et al: Femoral artery infections associated with percutaneous arterial closure devices, *J Vasc Surg* 34:983–985, 2001.
20. Sohail MR, Khan AH, Holmes DR Jr, et al: Infectious complications of percutaneous vascular closure devices, *Mayo Clin Proc* 80:1011–1015, 2005.
21. Derham C, Davies JF, Shahbazi R, et al: Iatrogenic limb ischemia caused by angiography closure devices, *Vasc Endovascular Surg* 40:492–494, 2007.
22. Jang JJ, Kim M, Gray B, et al: Claudication secondary to Perclose use after percutaneous procedures, *Catheter Cardiovasc Interv* 67:687–695, 2006.
23. Siani A, Schioppa A, Flaishman I, et al: Management of acute lower limb ischemia following percutaneous arterial closure device application: our experience, *G Chir* 27:119–122, 2006.
24. Lee WA, Brown MP, Nelson PR, et al: Total percutaneous access for endovascular aortic aneurysm repair ("Preclose" technique), *J Vasc Surg* 45:1095–1101, 2007.
25. Howell M, Villareal R, Krajcer Z: Percutaneous access and closure of femoral artery access sites associated with endoluminal repair of abdominal aortic aneurysms, *J Endovasc Ther* 8:68–74, 2001.
26. Hermiller JB, Simonton C, Hinohara T, et al: The StarClose Vascular Closure System: interventional results from the CLIP study, *Catheter Cardiovasc Interv* 68:677–683, 2006.
27. Rashid MN, Ahmed B, Straight F, et al: Extravascular closure for patients with high-risk femoral anatomy, *J Invasive Cardiol* 20:328–332, 2008.
28. Williams RE, Angel CY, Bourkaib R, et al: Multicenter safety and efficacy analysis of assisted closure after antegrade arterial punctures using the StarClose device, *J Endovasc Ther* 14:498–505, 2007.
29. Ratnam LA, Raja J, Munneke GJ, et al: Prospective nonrandomized trial of manual compression and Angio-Seal and Starclose arterial closure devices in common femoral punctures, *Cardiovasc Intervent Radiol* 30:182–188, 2007.
30. Fowler SJ, Nguyen A, Kern M: Trapping of vascular clip closure device in previously accessed femoral puncture site, *Catheter Cardiovasc Interv* 70:62–64, 2007.
31. Kapoor B, Panu A, Berscheid B: Angio-seal in antegrade endovascular interventions: technical success and complications in a 55-patient series, *J Endovasc Ther* 14:382–386, 2007.
32. Lupattelli T, Clerissi J, Clerici G, et al: The efficacy and safety of closure of brachial access using the AngioSeal closure device: experience with 161 interventions in diabetic patients with critical limb ischemia, *J Vasc Surg* 47:782–788, 2008.
33. Belenky A, Aranovich D, Greif F, et al: Use of a collagen-based device for closure of low brachial artery punctures, *Cardiovasc Intervent Radiol* 30:273–275, 2007.
34. Applegate RJ, Rankin KM, Little WC, et al: Restick following initial Angioseal use, *Catheter Cardiovasc Interv* 58:181–184, 2003.
35. Rastan A, Sixt S, Schwarzwälder U, et al: VIPER-2: a prospective, randomized single-center comparison of 2 different closure devices with a hemostatic wound dressing for closure of femoral artery access sites, *J Endovasc Ther* 15:83–90, 2008.
36. Geyik S, Yavuz K, Akgoz A, et al: The safety and efficacy of the Angio-Seal closure device in diagnostic and interventional neuroangiography setting: a single-center experience with 1,443 closures, *Neuroradiology* 49:739–746, 2007.
37. Andreotti F, Lavorgna A, Coluzzi G, et al: Lost and found: an unusual late complication of the Angio-Seal closure device, *Int J Cardiol* 117:e1–e3, 2007.
38. Dregelid E, Jensen G, Daryapeyma A: Complications associated with the Angio-Seal arterial puncture closing device: intra-arterial deployment and occlusion by dissected plaque, *J Vasc Surg* 44:1357–1359, 2006.
39. Doyle BJ, Godfrey MJ, Lennon RJ, et al: Initial experience with the Cardiva Boomerang vascular closure device in diagnostic catheterization, *Catheter Cardiovasc Interv* 69:203–208, 2007.
40. Scheinert D, Sievert H, Turco MA, et al: The safety and efficacy of an extravascular, water-soluble sealant for vascular closure: initial clinical results for Mynx, *Catheter Cardiovasc Interv* 70:627–633, 2007.
41. Dickey KW: Arterial hemostasis using the Duett sealing device, *Tech Vasc Interv Radiol* 6:85–91, 2003.
42. Caputo RP, Ebner A, Grant W, et al: Percutaneous femoral arteriotomy repair—initial experience with a novel staple closure device, *J Invasive Cardiol* 14:652–656, 2002.
43. Bavry AA, Raymond RE, Bhatt DL, et al: Efficacy of a novel procedure sheath and closure device during diagnostic catheterization: the multicenter randomized clinical trial of the FISH device, *J Invasive Cardiol* 20:152–156, 2008.
44. Eggebrecht H, Naber C, Woertgen U, et al: Percutaneous suture-mediated closure of femoral access sites deployed through the procedure sheath: initial clinical experience with a novel vascular closure device, *Catheter Cardiovasc Interv* 58:313–321, 2003.

SECTION II

IMAGING

CHAPTER

15

Duplex Ultrasonography

J. Dennis Baker

Diagnostic ultrasonography has always had great appeal because it is noninvasive with wide patient acceptance and performing repeat examinations is easy. The duplex scanner was first developed at the University of Washington in the 1970s. The device combined two different diagnostic modalities: a pulsed Doppler detection system and a grayscale ultrasound imaging system. The earliest scanners had limited grayscale resolution, and the image was used primarily to position the Doppler sample volume within the vessel. The severity of stenosis was based on focal changes in the velocity waveform tracings recorded. Important shortcomings of the early devices included limited range of tissue penetration and poor detection of low flow velocities. In spite of the problems with the equipment, duplex scanning rapidly became accepted as the noninvasive test of choice for evaluation of carotid disease. The success of this application led to its subsequent use for detection of lower-extremity venous thrombosis.

The initial interest in the clinical application of duplex scanning to the evaluation of the cervical portion of the carotid artery led to important refinements in the equipment. The second- and third-generation scanners had greatly improved image quality. The better resolution permitted definition of the actual structure of plaques and other disorders. The need for deeper penetration led to production of lower-frequency probes. Problems with Doppler signal processing and sonogram display likewise were addressed, especially the techniques for wraparound display to deal with aliasing. Ways were also developed to increase the sensitivity of detection of very low flow velocities, thus improving differentiation between sluggish flow beyond a very tight area of stenosis and occlusion. These developments enhanced the quality of duplex sonography for carotid and venous work; however, examination of the long segments of peripheral arteries was still tedious. In spite of this difficulty, a few laboratories used ultrasound scanning for the workup of patients with arterial occlusive disease and showed good correlations with angiography.[1-3]

The most important step came with the development of color-flow mapping. This technology made the examination of both the pelvic and the leg vessels much easier. In 1989, Cossman et al.[4] studied lower-extremity arteries to select patients for angioplasty. They reported a close correlation between ultrasound findings and contrast angiographic findings and found high positive and negative predictive values for the detection of both severe stenosis and occlusion. In addition, the ultrasound studies accurately demonstrated the length of areas of arterial occlusion. Before long, many surgeons were investigating the use of duplex scanning as the definitive diagnostic test in determining the treatment plan for peripheral arterial disease, in the same way it had been used for carotid bifurcation lesions.

EXAMINATIONS

Full evaluation of the lower-extremity arteries is best carried out with a scanner having color-flow capability. For most adults, at least two scan heads are necessary: one with a 3- to 3.5-MHz range to provide adequate depth for the iliac branches deep in the pelvis and another with a 5- to 7-MHz range to provide better-resolution imaging for the more superficial arteries in the leg. Examination of the aorta and the iliac branches is best performed after the patient has had an overnight fast to reduce the incidence of difficulties produced by bowel gas. Ramaswami et al.[5] reported that the aortoiliac segment could not be fully studied in 20% of patients, most commonly because of bowel gas or obesity. Routine use of a mechanical bowel preparation routine has been advocated, but this method is rarely used.[6] For patients with normal femoral pulses and normal common femoral artery Doppler waveforms, it may be necessary to examine only below the inguinal ligament, in which case fasting is not required.

A full examination requires careful interrogation of the vessels from the distal aorta to at least the level of the popliteal arteries. Some laboratories include examination of the infrapopliteal branches down to the ankle, but the success rate for obtaining satisfactory assessment of these arteries is variable. The color-flow image is used to locate the diseased areas, but most investigators do not rely on the image to define the severity of stenosis. Doppler velocity waveforms are recorded in the normal regions of the vessels and in the regions of greatest stenosis. The peak systolic velocity ratio (PSVR) is the parameter most commonly used to define severity of stenosis. This value is obtained by dividing the peak systolic velocity in the stenosis by that in the normal portion of the artery. Most vascular laboratories interpret a ratio of greater than 2.0 as indicating stenosis that reduces diameter by more than 50%.[2] Leng and coworkers found the velocity ratio to be a better primary diagnostic criterion than the absolute peak systolic velocity in stenosis of femoropopliteal lesions.[7] The group also found good reproducibility on repeat studies. Some investigators have further refined the criteria to distinguish whether the stenosis is more or less than 75%. Cossman et al.[4] have stated that stenosis of more than 75% is present when the PSVR is more than 4.0 or when the peak velocity in the stenosis is more than 400 cm/s. Gonsalves and Bandyk use the criteria of a PSVR of more than 4.0, a peak systolic velocity of more than 300 cm/s, or an end-diastolic velocity of more than 100 cm/s.[8] Occlusion is shown by lack of color mapping within the lumen and failure to detect a signal with the pulsed Doppler detector. Whenever this occurs, the examiner must take care to change the scanner controls so as to maximize the ability to detect low flow velocities. Failure to optimize the settings is a common reason for an error in the diagnosis of occlusion. When an occlusion is found, one must take care to examine the proximal and the distal end of the involved segment to obtain an accurate measurement of the total length.

An important part of the lower extremity examination is the determination of the specific location of the significant lesion. Within the pelvis, it is possible to estimate the distance from the aortic or the iliac bifurcation. Below the inguinal ligament, there are fewer useful landmarks. One approach is to mark the location of stenoses or the top and the bottom of an occlusion on the skin. Measurement from these reference points to a fixed structure such as the knee joint provides a reproducible mapping.

A variety of factors limit the quality that can be obtained with a study. The massively obese patient presents a real challenge. In many cases, it is not possible to reach the aortoiliac segment, and even reaching the common femoral and the proximal superficial femoral arteries may be difficult. The presence of significant amounts of edema, such as may occur with trauma or immediately after surgery, interferes with obtaining clear images of the vessels. In many of these cases, it is possible to record a suitable Doppler tracing so that a partial examination can be obtained. Freshly placed polytetrafluoroethylene grafts initially have a high content of air, which blocks insonation. As the air is replaced by fluid, the graft becomes transparent to ultrasound, permitting adequate studies to be done. In some patients, this process may take up to 24 hours.

APPLICATIONS

Initial Assessment and Preoperative Evaluation

Ultrasound imaging has long been used to screen for abdominal aortic aneurysm and to define its size when one is found. With the improvements in visualization of the abdominal vessels made possible by lower-frequency transducers, vascular laboratories have been increasingly using duplex scanning for the evaluation of aneurysms. Although bowel gas can interfere with the complete evaluation of visceral vessels, a satisfactory screening examination for an infrarenal aneurysm can often be completed via a flank approach. An advantage of the duplex scan over conventional ultrasonography is the ability to detect aortoiliac occlusion, which often coexists with aneurysmal degeneration. A limitation of all ultrasound imaging studies is the variability in the measurement of vessel size, especially when compared with computed tomograms or magnetic resonance imaging scans. The duplex scan is also useful in the documentation of true and false aneurysms below the inguinal ligament.

Since 1990, arterial duplex scanning has been increasingly used specifically for the evaluation of patients for transluminal angioplasty.[4,9-11] This test was found to have high accuracy in defining the severity of the stenoses, as well as the length of occluded segments. This information permits planning for the specific procedure, including the optimal angiographic approach. The initial intervention planned can be carried out in 84% to 94% of patients.[9-11] Obtaining the noninvasive study helps eliminate the need to perform an initial diagnostic angiogram and then have the patient return later for the definitive treatment. In addition, one can often reduce the extent of the contrast study needed at the time of the angioplasty.

The success of using duplex scanning as the primary diagnostic test in decision making regarding carotid endarterectomy led to evaluation of the feasibility of a similar approach in peripheral arterial operations. In 1990, Kohler et al.[12] carried out a study in which six surgeons developed treatment plans for 29 patients. First, the cases were evaluated using only data from duplex scanning; later, only angiographic data were used. The clinical decisions made in the two settings were found to be very similar. Subsequent papers reported the results of surgery performed without preoperative angiography. Bodily et al.[13] reported successful management of 11 patients who underwent aortoiliac reconstruction based on findings of ultrasound scans. Pemberton and associates reported a 2-year experience that included 85 limbs in 75 patients.[14] It must be noted that, in this study, all patients requiring bypass to the popliteal or the infrapopliteal level underwent routine on-table angiography. There were no complications attributed to the lack of preoperative arteriography, and the authors concluded that the contrast study can be avoided in the majority of patients. Wain and the group from Montefiore Hospital carried out a further study of the feasibility of leg bypass based only on ultrasound scan findings.[15] Duplex mapping predicted the correct distal anastomotic site in 90% of bypasses to the popliteal artery but in only 24% of those to distal sites. At present, the distal bypass is probably the most problematic aspect of lower-extremity reconstruction without preoperative arteriography. An appropriate compromise is to employ on-table selective injection to confirm the status of the proposed distal anastomosis, as reported by Pemberton et al.[14] and later by Ahn et al.[16]

A special case in the preoperative choice of intervention is the failing bypass graft that requires revision to prolong patency. Treiman et al.[17] reviewed the results in 31 grafts that were revised without preoperative angiography and concluded that this was a safe practice.[17] A subsequent study from Oregon challenged this premise, reporting that arteriography contributed to the choice of procedure in 43% of the 205 operations included.[18] In about half the cases for which angiography added to the determination of the specific operation required, the scan showed only a low flow state, and the additional study was needed to locate the lesion to be treated. In the rest of the cases, the angiographic findings helped identify additional stenoses, which were corrected. At present, one can only conclude that critical judgment is required in selecting the patients for whom preoperative angiography can be skipped.

Intraoperative Assessment

For many years, vascular surgeons have used intraoperative completion angiography to evaluate the appearance of a reconstruction. This practice has been most common after carotid endarterectomies and in situ vein bypasses. Since the early 1990s, many surgeons have been changing to duplex scanning for the completion studies. The ultrasound technique has the advantage of providing physiologic data, as well as an image of the involved segments. Experience has shown that in some cases, the additional information helps identify problem areas that might be missed by an arteriogram, especially if only a single exposure is obtained. In 1993, Mewissen et al.[19] reported on the use of duplex scanning to evaluate the results of balloon angioplasty of the superficial femoral and the popliteal arteries. The initial success of the procedure was judged by the findings on the completion angiogram. Duplex scans of the dilated segments showed that 28% had stenosis of more than 50%. Follow-up examinations showed that the lesions that initially had stenosis of more than 50% had only a 15% patency rate at 1 year, compared with an 84% rate for the lesions with stenosis of less than 50%. The authors made a strong plea for the use of completion duplex scanning to determine the results of angioplasty, thus allowing for immediate use of additional treatment to improve the result of the intervention. A small study published the following year by Cluley et al.[20] reported the results of completion duplex scanning and found that 5 of 21 lesions had residual stenosis of more than 50%.[20] Adjunctive procedures were performed at the same sitting for all these patients to eliminate the significant residual stenosis. Gonsalves and Bandyk[8] found that completion scan findings led to additional procedures in 29% of patients undergoing balloon dilatation. They recommend not ending a dilatation procedure so long as the PSVR is more than 2.0 or the peak systolic velocity is more than 180 cm/s. Likewise, Katzenschlager et al.[21] showed a similar advantage to the use of duplex scanning at the time of the intervention. Although ultrasonic evaluation of the results of endovascular procedures has not been widely used, it provides a simple tool, especially in the treatment of lesions below the inguinal ligament.

Follow-Up Studies

From the early days of bypass grafting, surgeons have recognized that pathologic changes develop in a significant number of patients and threaten the longevity of the results. In the 1970s, authors started advocating the use of noninvasive tests to identify grafts at risk.[22] For the first 15 years, surveillance was carried out in most cases by measuring ankle pressures. Improvement in the accuracy of detection of advanced lesions was achieved by means of ultrasound scanning of the length of the entire graft.[23] A number of studies have documented the benefit of identifying a deteriorating graft and repairing it before thrombosis occurs, because the long-term results are superior to those for grafts that are not repaired until thrombosis has occurred. Although there has not been much experience with follow-up testing after endovascular procedures, it is likely that the experience with bypass grafts is relevant to this group of patients. If one accepts the principle that it is preferable to repair a deteriorating lesion before thrombosis develops, then a good case can be made for surveillance of patients who have had dilatation or stent placement below the inguinal ligament. The experience with bypass grafts shows that patients in whom abnormalities are detected on the first postoperative scan have a much higher incidence of the development of occlusion than those in whom findings are initially normal.[24] This principle is likely to apply as well for the patient undergoing angioplasty who has abnormal completion scan findings or a suboptimal appearance on arteriography.

Another application of follow-up ultrasound examinations is the assessment of endovascular grafts used to treat aortic aneurysms. An area of great concern is the endoleak, the persistence of blood flow in the aneurysmal sac outside the graft. The accepted technique for documentation of endoleaks is the contrast-enhanced computed tomographic scan. The finding of any contrast material in the sac outside the graft is defined as abnormal. A few centers have carried out studies focused on evaluating the potential of duplex scanning for surveillance of endovascular aneurysm repairs.[25,26] The ultrasound examination of endografts for postprocedure abnormalities is a difficult procedure. The Endovascular Aneurysm Clinical Trial has reviewed a large number of tests and has found that only a fraction meet all the criteria established for a complete study.[26] When satisfactory scans were obtained, the positive and the negative predictive values were 98% and 82%, respectively, compared with computed tomographic scans. Heilberger et al.[25] reported that results of scanning may be improved with the use of ultrasound contrast material. In addition to detection of endoleaks, the duplex scan can detect other complications, such as endograft kinking, that might limit flow and possibly produce claudication or result in early occlusion. When identified, such problem areas can often be repaired by means of further stenting. The early experience suggests that, with more experience in examination techniques, the duplex scanner may become the tool of choice for routine surveillance of endovascular aneurysm grafts.

NEW DIRECTIONS

Enlarged-Field Images

An important limitation of current duplex scanning techniques is the small size of the field covered by any one image. Unlike with angiography, it is not possible to have a long segment of an artery included on a single view so that the position of a specific lesion can be reproducibly demonstrated relative to fixed landmarks. Especially in the leg, the only way to define the anatomic position of an involved segment is to make external measurements to a fixed point on the extremity. One solution to this problem is real-time extended field-of-view sonography.[27] The system provides for the detection and the correlation of internal landmarks that are used to link adjacent images into a composite. A single image can be constructed that covers up to a 60-cm length of a vessel. Another approach to the wide-field image uses an external three-dimensional referencing system to link a number of adjacent images to form a single long view of a leg artery or a bypass graft.[28] This particular technique was developed to provide reproducible localization of graft lesions from one examination to the next.

Objective Plaque Characterization

For many years, there have been attempts to characterize the nature of a plaque on the basis of its appearance on an ultrasound scan. Experience has shown that lesions with either heavy calcification or dense fibrosis usually have a poor response to balloon dilatation. Ramaswami et al.[29] used ultrasound image densitometry to provide an objective definition of the characteristics of the lower limb plaque. Plaques with low density both showed a greater improvement at the time of balloon dilatation and had lower restenosis rates than images with a higher echogenicity. More studies need to be carried out to corroborate these interesting results; it certainly would be an advantage to be able to predict both initial and long-term results of balloon dilatation before the intervention.

References

1. Jager K, Ricketts H, Strandness D: Duplex scanning for the evaluation of lower extremity arterial disease. In: Bernstein E, editor: *Noninvasive diagnostic techniques in vascular disease*, St. Louis, 1985, CV Mosby, pp 619–631.
2. Kohler T, Nance DR, Cramer MM, et al: Duplex scanning for diagnosis of aortoiliac and femoropopliteal disease: a prospective study, *Circulation* 76:1074–1080, 1987.
3. Legemate D, Teeuwen C, Hoeneveld H, et al: The potential of duplex scanning to replace aorto-iliac and femoropopliteal angiography, *Eur J Vasc Surg* 3:49–54, 1989.
4. Cossman D, Ellison JE, Wagner WH, et al: Comparison of arteriography to arterial mapping with color-flow duplex imaging in the lower extremities, *J Vasc Surg* 10:522–529, 1989.
5. Ramaswami G, Al-Kutoubi A, Nicholaides AN, et al: The role of duplex scanning in the diagnosis of lower limb arterial disease, *Ann Vasc Surg* 13:494–500, 1999.
6. Whiteley M, Fox A, Harris R, Horrocks M: Iso-osmotic bowel preparation improves the accuracy of iliac artery color flow duplex examination, *J R Soc Med* 7:11–17, 1995.

7. Leng G, Whyman MR, Donnan PT, et al: Accuracy and reproducibility of duplex ultrasonography in grading femoropopliteal stenoses, *J Vasc Surg* 17:510–517, 1993.
8. Gonsalves A, Bandyk D: Duplex scanning for lower extremity arterial disease. In: AbuRahma A, Bergan J, editors: *Noninvasive Vascular Diagnosis*, New York, 2000, Springer, pp 241–252.
9. Edwards J, Coldwell DM, Goldman MZ, et al: The role of duplex scanning in the selection of patients for transluminal angioplasty, *J Vasc Surg* 13:69–74, 1991.
10. van der Heijden F, Legemate DA, van Leeuwen MS, et al: Value of duplex scanning in the selection of patients for percutaneous transluminal angioplasty, *Eur J Vasc Surg* 7:71–76, 1993.
11. de Smet A, Visser K, Kitslaar P: Duplex scanning for grading aortoiliac obstructive disease and guiding treatment, *Eur J Vasc Surg* 8:711–715, 1994.
12. Kohler T, Andros G, Porter JM, et al: Can duplex scanning replace arteriography for lower extremity arterial disease? *Ann Vasc Surg* 4:280–287, 1990.
13. Bodily K, Buttorff J, Nordesgaard A, et al: Aorto-iliac reconstruction without arteriography, *Am J Surg* 171:505–507, 1996.
14. Pemberton M, Nydahl S, Hartshorne T, et al: Can lower limb vascular reconstruction be based on colour duplex imaging alone?, *Eur J Vasc Endovasc Surg* 12:452–454, 1996.
15. Wain R, Berdejo GL, Delvalle WN, et al: Can duplex scan arterial mapping replace contrast arteriography as the test of choice before infrainguinal revascularization?, *J Vasc Surg* 29:100–109, 1999.
16. Sarkar R, Ro KM, Obrand DI, Ahn SS: Lower extremity vascular reconstruction and endovascular surgery without preoperative angiography, *Am J Surg* 176:203–207, 1998.
17. Treiman G, Lawrence P, Galt S, Kraiss L: Revision of reversed infrainguinal bypass grafts without preoperative arteriography, *J Vasc Surg* 26:1020–1028, 1997.
18. Landry G, Moneta G, Taylor L Jr, et al: Duplex scanning alone is not sufficient imaging before secondary procedures after lower extremity reversed vein bypass graft, *J Vasc Surg* 29:270–281, 1999.
19. Mewissen M, Kinney EV, Bandyk DF, et al: The role of duplex scanning versus angiography in predicting outcome after balloon angioplasty in the femoropopliteal artery, *J Vasc Surg* 15:860–866, 1992.
20. Cluley S, Brener BJ, Hollier L, et al: Transcutaneous ultrasonography can be used to guide and monitor balloon angioplasty, *J Vasc Surg* 17:23–31, 1993.
21. Katzenschlager R, Ahmadi A, Minar E, et al: Femoropopliteal artery: initial and 6-month results of color duplex US-guided percutaneous transluminal angioplasty, *Radiology* 199:331–334, 1996.
22. Mozersky D, Strandness D, Sumner D: Disease progression after femoropopliteal surgical procedures, *Surg Gynecol Obstet* 135:700–704, 1972.
23. Bandyk D, Johnson B: Duplex surveillance of infrainguinal bypass grafts. In: AbuRahma A, Bergan J, editors: *Noninvasive Vascular Diagnosis*, New York, 2000, Springer, pp 253–267.
24. Mills JL, Bandyk DF, Gahtan V, Esses GE: The origin of infrainguinal vein graft stenosis: a prospective study based upon duplex surveillance, *J Vasc Surg* 21:16–25, 1995.
25. Heilberger P, Schunn C, Ritter W, et al: Postoperative color flow duplex scanning in aortic endografting, *J Endovasc Surg* 4:262–271, 1997.
26. Sato D, Goff CD, Gregory RT, et al: Endoleak after aortic stent graft repair: diagnosis by color duplex ultrasound scan versus computed tomography scan, *J Vasc Surg* 28:657–663, 1998.
27. Sauerbrei E: Extended field-of-view sonography: utility in clinical practice, *J Ultrasound Med* 18:335–341, 1999.
28. Jong J, Beach K, Primozich J, et al: Vein graft surveillance with scanhead tracking duplex ultrasound imaging: a preliminary report, *Ultrasound Med Biol* 24:1313–1324, 1998.
29. Ramaswami G, Tegos T, Nicolaides AN, et al: Ultrasonographic plaque character and the outcome after lower limb angioplasty, *J Vasc Surg* 29:110–121, 1999.

CHAPTER

16

Vascular Laboratory Surveillance After Arterial Intervention

Dennis F. Bandyk

A surveillance program based on duplex ultrasound testing after peripheral arterial intervention can increase long-term patency by identifying and repairing clinically significant lesions. Its successful application requires that a number of conditions be present regarding pathobiology of arterial repair failure and its consequences, arterial testing expertise, and the durability of secondary procedures used to repair duplex-detected lesions. The methodology of surveillance should be tailored to the type of arterial intervention. Clinical reports on the efficacy of duplex ultrasound surveillance have supported its routine use, but controversy of cost-effectiveness remains. Duplex ultrasound surveillance will decrease procedural primary patency resulting from the detection of asymptomatic lesions, but successful lesion repair produces primary-assisted and secondary patency rates significantly higher than if no surveillance was performed. An outcome analysis of the primary, primary-assisted, secondary patency rates after arterial procedure will indicate the benefit (or lack of benefit) of a surveillance program, as well as the appropriateness of the threshold criteria used for secondary interventions.

The rationale for the application of vascular laboratory surveillance after peripheral arterial intervention is straightforward—to confirm technical success of revascularization and to identify and repair developing lesions before failure occurs. Failure of arterial reconstructive procedures whether performed by open repair, arterial bypass, or endovascular intervention (balloon, stent, stent-graft, atherectomy) remains an important clinical problem. For example, the treatment of critical limb ischemia (CLI) requires that a level of arterial perfusion be achieved and maintained to heal lesions and amputation sites or relieve rest pain. The likelihood of failure varies with procedure type, patient characteristics, and disease severity, and when arterial repair thrombosis occurs patient morbidity and health care costs increase. The most common mechanisms of arterial repair failure include technical error, stenosis caused by myointimal hyperplasia, and atherosclerotic disease progression. These vascular conditions are readily identified by duplex ultrasound imaging, and their severity can be classified as mild, moderate, or severe, that is, a critical lesion that should be considered for repair even in the asymptomatic patient. The application of duplex surveillance beginning in the immediate postprocedural period and then repeated at regular intervals thereafter can improve patient outcomes and extend the functional patency of arterial intervention.[1-3]

Several essential elements must exist for a surveillance program to be worthwhile. Vascular testing should be noninvasive and inexpensive and have diagnostic accuracy with high sensitivity to ensure that clinically significant lesions are not missed. It is also necessary that the mechanism(s) of arterial repair failure has a pathology and natural history appropriate for detection by a surveillance protocol. Lesion severity, that is, degree of stenosis, should correlate with risk of failure, and testing should be capable of detecting stenosis progression from mild to severe categories. The incidence of lesion development should be sufficiently common (incidence: 5%-10% or greater) to be cost-effective. Last but vitally important, there must be safe and effective procedures to repair identified lesions. Many if not all "open" and endovascular interventions performed for peripheral atherosclerotic disease in the carotid or lower-limb arterial circulations satisfy the conditions for surveillance to be of clinical benefit. Certainly, if the primary failure mode of arterial repair is the result of myointimal hyperplasia, surveillance and timely repair of lesions that progress to a severe stenosis should enhance long-term patency. Another

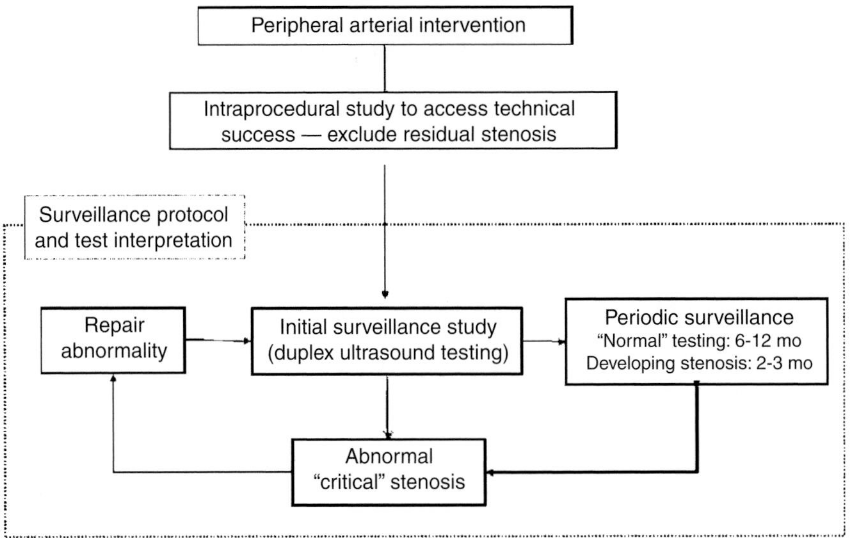

FIGURE 16-1 Schematic of a duplex ultrasound surveillance protocol after peripheral arterial intervention. Components included a procedural study to exclude technical error, initial surveillance using duplex surveillance to identify residual repair abnormality, and then periodic surveillance testing to detect and repair acquired stenotic lesions that meet criteria for severe "critical" stenosis.

important measure of a surveillance program is the incidence of arterial repair failure when testing results are "normal," that is, no anatomic or hemodynamic abnormality is identified. When duplex testing identifies no repair-site stenosis or other anatomic abnormality (aneurysm, mural thrombus) failure should be uncommon, and if thrombosis does occur the cause should be from a condition that testing would not have detected such as cardiac embolus or an acquired hypercoagulable state. When surveillance is properly performed and interpreted, the incidence of unexpected repair failure should be in the range of low (1%-5%/yr)—depending on the arterial repair type.[3-8]

The algorithm for arterial repair surveillance should begin with an intraprocedural study to assess for technical success followed by enrollment in a surveillance protocol with an initial testing several weeks after the procedure (Figure 16-1). The application of duplex testing at operation or after endovascular therapy is an accurate and reliable method to confirm "normal" repair site hemodynamics, exclude residual stenosis, and assess distal arterial perfusion. Normal duplex testing is associated with a low (1%-2%) incidence of angioplasty site or bypass graft thrombosis, as is the development of a critical stenosis in the early postprocedural period. The goal of the initial surveillance study is to complement clinical assessment to determine whether the arterial intervention has been successful and in patients with CLI an appropriate level of arterial perfusion has been achieved. Thus surveillance testing should include both duplex scanning of the arterial repair and indirect physiologic testing (ankle-brachial systolic pressure index [ABI] measurement, pulse volume recordings, digit/toe systolic pressure measurements). The initial examination serves as a baseline for subsequent testing to detect stenosis or other arterial lesion development. The need for routine duplex testing after lower bypass grafting is controversial but a necessary part of surveillance after carotid, renal, and visceral artery interventions. After lower-limb arterial revascularization, duplex testing is more sensitive than clinical assessment, that is, patient recognition of the symptoms associated with procedure failure, physical examination combined with ABI measurement, for detection of developing myointimal hyperplasia or aneurysm degeneration. Myointimal stenosis capable of producing arterial repair failure can develop without symptoms until a high-grade stenosis forms or thrombosis occurs.

It is essential to use objective interpretation criteria to grade lesion severity in a surveillance program. This allows for the application of "threshold" criteria for reintervention or a decision that additional arterial imaging is necessary. Test interpretation with use of three disease categories is sufficient to characterize an arterial repair as "normal" or "abnormal" and further grade a duplex-detected abnormality as one that be followed for progression, that is, intermediate lesion, or should be considered for repair (see Figure 16-1, Table 16-1). The use of combined peak systolic velocity (PSV) and velocity ratio (Vr) thresholds to define the severe (>70%-75% diameter reduction [DR]) stenosis category is recommended. A duplex-detected stenosis with a PSV greater than 300 cm/s and associated turbulent velocity spectra at the lesion is associated with a resting systolic pressure gradient of more than 20 mm Hg and thus meets criteria for hemodynamically significant stenosis.[1,2] Whether duplex testing is used for "screening" or "intervention" decisions depends on

TABLE 16-1 Classification of Stenosis Severity After Arterial Intervention

	Duplex ultrasound surveillance categories		
		Abnormal	
	Normal <50% DR	**Intermediate stenosis 50%-75% DR**	**Severe stenosis >75% DR***
Carotid repair			
EA	PSV <150 cm/s	PSV >150 cm/s	PSV >300 cm/s
		PSV_{ICA}/PSV_{CCA} >2	PSV_{ICA}/PSV_{CCA} >4
			End-diastolic >125 cm/s
Stent	PSV <150 cm/s	PSV >150 cm/s	PSV >300 cm/s
		PSV_{ICA}/PSV_{CCA} >2	PSV_{ICA}/PSV_{CCA} >4
			End-diastolic >125 cm/s
Bypass graft	PSV <180 cm/s	PSV 180-300 cm/s	PSV >300 cm/s
	Vr <2	Vr ≤3.5	Vr >3.5
Peripheral angioplasty	PSV <180 cm/s	PSV 180-300 cm/s	PSV >300 cm/s
		Vr ≤3.5	Vr>3.5
	<60% DR	>60% DR*	
Renal stent	PSV <200 cm/s	PSV >200 cm/s	
	RAR ≤3.5	RAR >3.5	
	<70% DR	>70% DR*	
SMA stent	PSV <300 cm/s	PSV >300 cm/s	

* Threshold for reintervention or additional arterial imaging to confirm stenosis severity.
CCA, Common carotid artery; *DR,* diameter reduction; *EA,* carotid endarterectomy; *ICA,* internal carotid artery; *PSV,* peak systolic velocity; *RAR,* renal-aortic ratio; *Vr,* PSV ratio across stenosis; *SMA,* superior mesenteric artery.

the surveillance application. After visceral (mesenteric, renal) artery angioplasty, the application of duplex testing is primarily as a screening method to identify stent/angioplasty stenosis. Abnormal results from a study should prompt additional confirmatory angiographic imaging and/or pressure gradient measurement to assess lesion severity and clinical significance. After peripheral interventions, duplex testing may be used for management decisions including reintervention. The finding of a greater than 75% duplex-detected stenosis is sufficient anatomic/hemodynamic information, if used in conjunction with limb blood pressure measurements or treadmill exercise testing, to recommend and proceed with a secondary intervention (endovascular or open surgical repair). Typically, the stenotic lesions detected during surveillance are focal in nature and thus amenable to endovascular therapy. At the time of angioplasty, lesion severity will be confirmed and other anatomic features that correlate with technical success and durability can be assessed.

The goal of arterial surveillance is to prolong patency and avoid thrombotic events, as well as other procedure-specific adverse events such as stroke after carotid endarterectomy or stent-angioplasty, amputation after peripheral arterial intervention, and organ ischemia after visceral bypass or angioplasty. Assessment of patency, including intervention-free patency, is relatively straightforward to calculate by using life-table (Kaplan-Meier) methods that take into account duration of follow-up and patient death. Duplex ultrasound is the preferred method to assess arterial repair patency because it is inexpensive, highly accurate, and applicable to the spectrum of carotid, visceral, and peripheral arterial interventions. The primary (freedom from intervention or thrombosis) and secondary (freedom from thrombosis despite intervention, including thrombectomy or thrombolysis) patency rates of a hypothetical procedure X estimated by life-table analysis shown in Figure 16-2 depicts decrease in arterial repair patency with time. Any treatment that can increase secondary patency will improve clinical outcome and should be used. If surveillance is successful, secondary patency rates should be higher than with no surveillance or an ineffective surveillance protocol that does not identify and correct the lesions responsible for failure. Thus assessment of secondary patency rate is an appropriate measure of surveillance efficacy and procedure durability. The improved

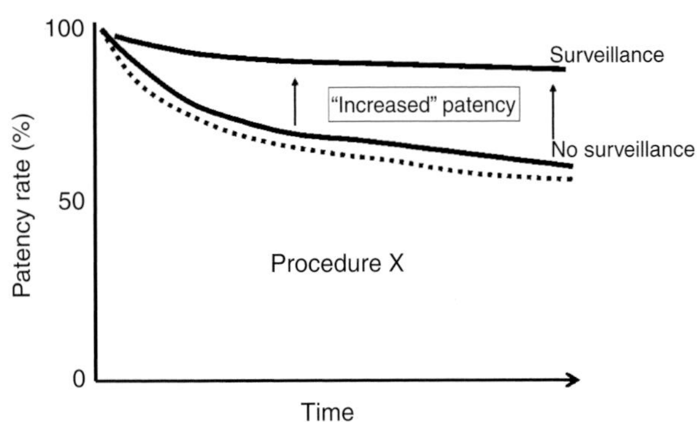

FIGURE 16-2 Primary and secondary patency rates of a hypothetical procedure X, which depicts a greater than 20% increase in secondary patency with the application of a surveillance protocol.

patency with surveillance is due to correction of "identified" lesions that if left unrepaired would lead to thrombosis or failure. The term "assisted-patency" was developed to deal with the "failing" arterial repair/bypass and provide a measure of patency after revision of a patent but "abnormal" arterial intervention. This concept is useful because, in clinical vascular surgery, once thrombosis of an arterial repair or bypass occurs, secondary interventions to restore patency have been shown to not be durable. Thus an important principle of vascular procedure surveillance is to "correct lesions electively to prevent thrombosis from occurring, rather than waiting until thrombosis occurs and then attempting to restore patency and salvage the repair." Peripheral arterial interventions with assisted-primary, that is, intervention-free patency, and secondary patency rates that exceed 80% at 5 years are generally considered to be clinically successful and durable.

The primary, assisted-primary, and secondary patency rates of three "hypothetical" arterial procedures (A, B, and C) that used duplex surveillance to improve outcomes are shown in Figure 16-3. Each procedure has a similar primary patency rate—indicating interventions and/or thrombosis were occurring with loss of "intervention-free patency." By inspecting differences in the assisted-primary and secondary patency curves of each procedure, the benefit or absence of benefit from duplex surveillance can be assessed. After procedure A, surveillance produced a significant increase in both assisted-primary and secondary patency rates—indicating that surveillance and intervention for duplex-detected lesions were successful and prevented thrombosis. By contrast, duplex surveillance after procedure B produced only a minimal increase in assisted-primary and secondary patency rates; thus the efficacy and cost-effectiveness of surveillance was not justified. Surveillance was also not useful after procedure C because only secondary patency was increased. The difference between the assisted-primary and secondary

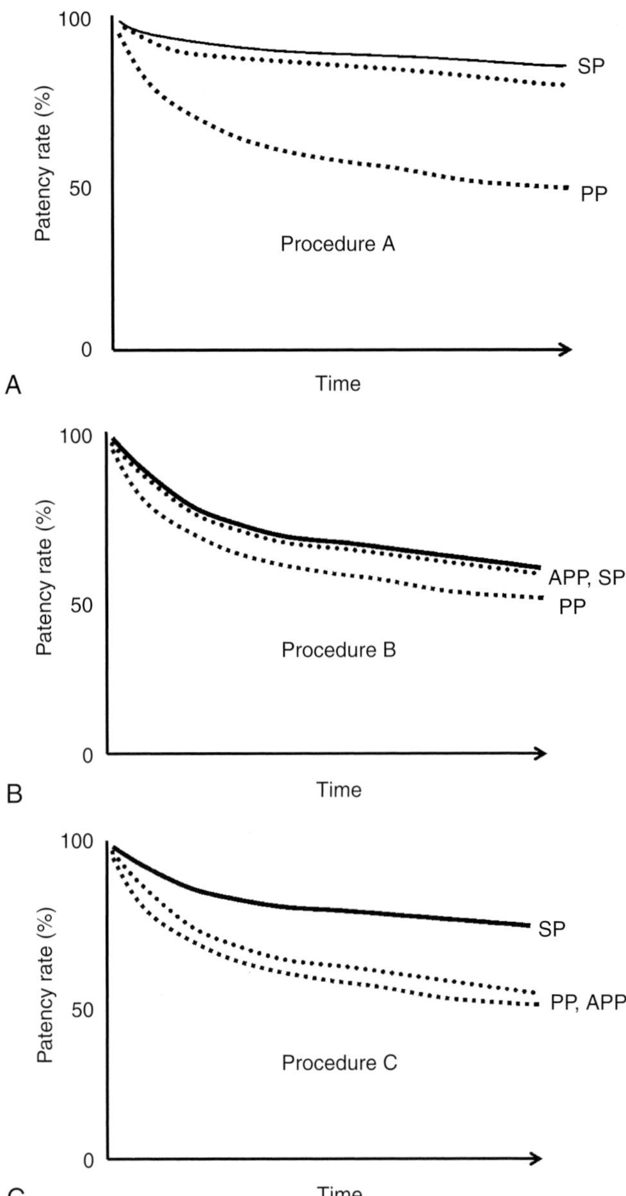

FIGURE 16-3 Primary (*square-box line*, PP), assisted-primary (*dotted line*, APP), and secondary (*solid line*, SP) patency rates of three hypothetical procedures (**A, B,** and **C**) managed in a duplex ultrasound surveillance program. Duplex surveillance and intervention for "severe" stenosis improved assisted-primary and secondary patency rates to >80% only for procedure A. Duplex surveillance was of no benefit in improving patency after procedure B (no significant increase in secondary patency) or procedure C (no significant increase in primary-assisted patency).

patency rate curves indicates the procedure C surveillance protocol did not adequately detect lesions that produced thrombosis, but secondary procedures to restore patency were successful. All the hypothetical procedures depicted demonstrated a progressive decrease in secondary patency rate, that is, failure despite medical treatment, surveillance, and intervention for stenosis or thrombosis, which is known to occur clinically. Interpretation of a secondary patency curve that is minimally increased from the assisted-primary patency curve is that additional interventions for thrombosis to "salvage" the arterial procedure are of marginal benefit. Thus efforts to enhance procedure patency should be directed at measures to avoid thrombosis occurring, that is, repair "threatening" lesions while the repair, angioplasty, or bypass is patent.

The loss of primary patency with time during duplex surveillance deserves additional comment because it is related to several factors: criteria for intervention, thrombosis rate despite surveillance, and compliance by both the patient and physician in adhering to the surveillance protocol including agreeing to a recommendation for intervention. If the threshold for intervention is too high or identified lesions are not repaired, the primary patency rate will be higher and the potential benefit of surveillance less evident. Thus a significant increase in assisted-primary patency compared with primary patency should be present and is supporting evidence that there may be a benefit in repairing lesions before thrombosis occurs. This is especially true when the secondary patency rate curve is similar to the assisted-primary patency curve—indicating that once thrombosis occurs all other secondary interventions were not successful. Duplex surveillance should result in an increase in the number of secondary interventions performed compared with clinical patient follow-up alone; more abnormal but patent arterial repairs will be identified. If the primary and assisted-primary patency curves of a procedure are not significantly different (with use of log-rank analysis), it can be concluded that surveillance did not identify any "clinically" significant lesions. If secondary patency rates are also similar to the primary and assisted-primary patency curves, the clinical benefit of surveillance is lost.

Level 1, evidence-based data proving efficacy of duplex surveillance is limited, and all the clinical trials are subject to criticism in that there was no true control group, that is, no surveillance performed. Because vascular specialists are in agreement with the concept of patient and procedure surveillance, randomized clinical trials have compared outcomes with clinical assessment versus duplex ultrasound surveillance. Criteria for intervention thus differ, but benefits of surveillance can be assessed by inspection of the assisted-primary and secondary patency rates. Shown in Table 16-2 are published life-table patency rates of lower-limb bypass and endovascular procedures in patients enrolled in either a randomized clinical trial or prospective observational study that used duplex ultrasound surveillance. Clinical benefit of surveillance was reported by the authors when assisted-primary patency was significantly ($p < .05$) higher than primary patency, and secondary patency rates both exceeded primary patency by >20% and achieved levels to 80% or greater. These study data indicate that the efficacy of duplex surveillance is dependent on a number of factors—indication for procedure (critical vs. noncritical limb ischemia), criteria for intervention, adherence to protocol, and study design. For a surveillance program to increase long-term patency, vascular testing must be accurate, must be interpreted correctly, and must result in timely, successful repair of duplex-detected lesions that meet "critical" threshold criteria. If secondary interventions do not restore anatomy and hemodynamics to normal, the benefit of surveillance may be lost. When a clinical report extolled the benefit of surveillance, the authors made two observations: unrepaired lesions resulted in thrombosis, and "normal" testing was associated with primary-assisted patency rates in excess of 80% at 3 to 5 years.[2,4,7-10,13]

SURVEILLANCE AFTER LOWER-LIMB ENDOVASCULAR INTERVENTION

The application of duplex surveillance has the potential to improve peripheral endovascular therapy durability by detection of significant residual and recurrent lesions. Late failure of peripheral angioplasty can result from restenosis caused by myointimal hyperplasia within the treated segment or progression of atherosclerosis remote from the percutaneous transluminal angioplasty (PTA) site. On occasion, both disease processes can occur and produce recurrent limb ischemia. The "failing" angioplasty site can be treated by either redilation, stenting, or atherectomy, typically with a prognosis identical to that of a primary procedure. Although an ABI increase is an important criterion of a technically successful procedure, abnormal hemodynamics (increase in peak systolic velocity, turbulent flow) within the angioplasty site affects long-term durability. Measurement of systolic pressure gradient is useful in assessing iliac angioplasty technical success but is not as reliable in identifying residual stenosis after infrainguinal angioplasty. Duplex ultrasound, an accurate method for the detection and classification of peripheral artery stenosis severity, is underused for endovascular therapy assessment and surveillance. The early failure rate of PTA varies widely (9%-47%) because of differences in procedure type, reporting criteria, and testing method. A residual greater than greater than 50% DR stenosis based on duplex criteria (PSV >180 cm/s; Vr >2) has been shown to predict early failure: 15% versus 84% at 1 year.[14] The goal of endovascular surgery should be to "normalize" hemodynamics in the treated artery segment.

Timing of initial assessment after peripheral angioplasty depends on the indication for the PTA procedure. For claudicants and palpable pulses after the

TABLE 16-2 Reported Infrainguinal Arterial Repair Patency Rates Associated With Duplex Ultrasound Surveillance

	Arterial repair patency (%)			
Clinical report/study design	**Primary**	**Assisted-primary**	**Secondary**	**Surveillance benefit**
Lundell et al., 1995[4]				
Prospective, randomized				
Vein bypass	55	78	82	Yes, at 3 yr
Prosthetic	50	55	67	No, at 1 yr
Ihlberg et al., 1998[5]				
Prospective, randomized				
Vein bypass	—	65	71	No, at 1 yr
Davies et al., 2005[9]				
Prospective, randomized				
Vein bypass	67	76	79	No, at 18 mo
Armstrong et al., 2004[10]				
Prospective, observational				
Arm vein	43	91	94	Yes, at 3 yr
Schanzer et al., 2007[11]				
Prospective, observational				
Vein bypass	60	78	81	Yes, at 1 yr
Chauvapun et al., 2008[13]				
Vein bypass	61	84	86	Yes, at 3 yr
Nguyen et al., 2004[6]				
Prospective, observational				
Revised vein bypass	49	76	80	Yes, at 5 yr
Stone et al., 2006[8]				
Prospective, observational				
Popliteal aneurysm repair	68	88	95	Yes, at 3 yr
Keeling et al., 2007[12]				
Retrospective, observational				
Femoropopliteal atherectomy	62	64	76	No, at 1 yr

angioplasty, lower-limb duplex scanning (CPT code 93926) and measurement of ABI within 2 weeks of procedure is sufficient. For CLI, testing before discharge is recommended to verify less than 50% DR residual PTA site stenosis (PSV <180 cm/s), an increase in ABI greater than 0.2 compared with pre-PTA level, and a toe pressure greater than 20 to 30 mm Hg. Subsequent surveillance of "normal" PTA sites, that is, less than 50% stenosis, is recommended at 3 months and then every 6 months thereafter.

An audit of our vascular group's experience demonstrated an abnormal initial duplex surveillance study; that is, an intermediate 50% to 75% DR stenosis (PSV >180 cm/s, Vr >2), was present in 5% to 20% of endovascular arterial interventions (Table 16-3).[12,14,15] A smaller percentage of patients were identified to have a residual high-grade stenosis, that is, PSV above 300 cm/s, Vr above 3.5. When the post-PTA duplex scan identifies a residual stenosis but ABI has increased appropriately, a repeated scan should be performed in 1 to 2 weeks to assess for improvement or deterioration in functional patency. A persistent or progressive PTA site stenosis with velocity spectra of PSV greater than 300 cm/s, Vr greater than 3.5, should be considered for repeated

TABLE 16-3 Incidence of Intermediate and Severe Duplex-Detected Stenosis on Initial Surveillance Testing After Endovascular Intervention in the Femoropopliteal Arterial Segment

Type of endovascular intervention	Intermediate stenosis (PSV >180 cm/s, <300 cm/s)	Severe stenosis (PSV >300 cm/s, Vr >3.5)
Atherectomy (%)	20	5
Balloon angioplasty (%)	10	2
Stent angioplasty (%)	5	2
Stent-graft (%)	<5	0

endovascular therapy depending on the anatomic characteristics/site of the lesion/arterial segment.

Endovascular therapy for advanced, long-segment atherosclerotic disease in the lower limb is more likely to have residual anatomic defects. Clinical success in treating occlusive disease involving the superficial femoral, popliteal, or tibial arteries depends primarily on disease severity as defined by the Transatlantic Inter-societal Consensus (TASC) classification.[16] Treatment of focal occlusive disease (TASC A and B) is associated with higher stenosis-free patency than treatment of diffuse stenotic disease or long segment occlusion (TASC C and D).

Keeling et al.[12] reported 12-month duplex stenosis-free patency of 41% after atherectomy of TASC C and D lesions compared with 76% for TASC A and B lesions. Residual stenosis after PTA of a vein bypass stenosis was demonstrated after 20% of procedures and correlated with a reduced (47%) 2-year stenosis-free patency compared with a 80% patency rate when the angioplasty site had normal hemodynamics (PSV <180 cm/s, Vr <2.5).[15] Although cost-benefit aspects of duplex surveillance after PTA have not been studied, it has been shown that PTA is less expensive than surgical bypass. The ratio of hospital costs of PTA to bypass surgery was 53% for patients treated for claudication but rose to 75% for those with critical ischemia. Because angioplasty failure is expensive, efforts to improve the technical success or durability of these procedures are worthwhile. Although duplex surveillance can identify PTA site stenosis, clinical symptoms and hemodynamic criteria should also be used in the decision for reintervention. Most claudicants with PTA site stenosis will indicate recurrence of exertional leg pain, and, because PTA has a failure mode similar to that of infrainguinal vein bypass, the cost-effectiveness and efficacy of surveillance should be comparable.

After iliac angioplasty, surveillance should include both indirect (clinical status, ABI, femoral artery waveform analysis) and direct (duplex scanning) evaluation of the treated iliac system. If the Doppler velocity waveform of the common femoral artery distal to the treated iliac segment is normal, that is, triphasic or multiphasic, or, in the case of an occluded superficial femoral artery, the waveform is monophasic but the acceleration time is normal (<200 ms), duplex imaging of the iliac angioplasty is not necessary because a hemodynamically significant lesion is unlikely. When the femoral pulse is abnormal or a damped, monophasic femoral artery waveform is identified, direct aortoiliac duplex imaging should be performed. Detection of an iliac lesion by duplex scanning with a PSV greater than 300 cm/s and a Vr greater than 2.0 indicates a hemodynamically failing iliac angioplasty, and the patient should be recommended for arteriography and possible secondary endovascular intervention. Reports of duplex surveillance after iliac angioplasty have demonstrated a 20% incidence of PTA stenosis within 2 years. In a prospective study, duplex surveillance resulted in reintervention in 10% of iliac PTAs and was associated with a secondary patency of 95% at 2 years—4% of the treated iliac segments thrombosed.[2]

Serial clinical evaluation, measurement of limb pressures, and duplex testing at 6-month intervals can reliably identify failing PTAs. Progression to occlusion is uncommon, and essentially all recurrent lesions are amenable to endovascular therapy. If limb pressures and ankle-level Doppler waveforms are normal or unchanged, routine duplex scanning can be avoided, which reduces overall costs. Clinical usefulness of a surveillance algorithm is predicated not only on the ability to detect PTA sites at risk for failure but also the success of reintervention and overall secondary patency. Thrombosis of an iliac PTA in a patient with multilevel disease is more likely to result in CLI than in a patient initially presenting with claudication. Similarly, failure of the treated iliac system also may threaten patency of a downstream lower-limb bypass graft and substantially increase the risk of limb loss. Angioplasty failure is more common in patients with multilevel atherosclerosis, and thus this cohort should be considered "high risk" and be offered duplex ultrasound surveillance. Endovascular treatment of recurrent or de novo iliac stenosis is preferred over attempted secondary recanalization of occluded iliac systems. The utility of surveillance in claudicants is less clear because patency rates after PTA are better in this group, and the ischemic sequelae of treatment site failure may be less significant clinically.

The application of duplex ultrasound surveillance after peripheral arterial intervention remains a decision of the interventionist. The patient cannot request surveillance or perform it adequately himself or herself. Arterial testing and its interpretation within a surveillance protocol can be challenging. Many vascular surgeons are not convinced routine duplex surveillance will benefit their patients or do not have available to them the logistics necessary to conduct a quality surveillance program. Surveillance is during the first 12 months after arterial intervention with subsequent follow-up individualized to the specific patient depending on type of intervention, TASC category, and previous duplex scan findings. The inclusion of duplex surveillance as "part of patient service" has the potential to improve outcome after a variety of open and endovascular arterial procedures.

References

1. Bandyk DF: Surveillance of lower extremity reconstructions: Is it worthwhile and which method should we use? *Perspectives Vasc Surg* 8:20–30, 1995.
2. Back MR, Novotney M, Roth SM, et al: Utility of duplex surveillance following iliac artery angioplasty and primary stenting, *J Endovasc Ther* 8:629–637, 2001.
3. Bandyk DF. Ultrasound assessment following peripheral arterial interventions. In Zwiebel W and Perriloto J editors, *Introduction to vascular ultrasonography,* Philadelphia, 2005, Saunders.
4. Lundell A, Linblad B, Bergvist D, et al: Femoropopliteal-cural graft patency is improved by an intensive surveillance program: a prospective randomized study, *J Vasc Surg* 21:26–33, 1995.
5. Ihlberg L, Luther M, Tierla E, et al: The utility of duplex scanning in infrainguinal vein graft surveillance: results from a randomized controlled study, *Eur J Vasc Endovasc Surg* 16:19–27, 1998.
6. Nguyen LL, Conte MS, Menard MT, et al: Infrainguinal vein bypass graft revision: factors affecting long-term outcome, *J Vasc Surg* 40:916–923, 2004.
7. Tinder C, Chauvapun JP, Bandyk DF, et al: Enhanced efficacy of duplex ultrasound surveillance after infrainguinal vein bypass by identification of characteristics predictive of graft stenosis development, *J Vasc Surg* 48:613–618, 2008.
8. Stone PA, Armstrong PA, Bandyk DF, et al: The value of duplex surveillance after open and endovascular popliteal aneurysm repair, *J Vasc Surg* 41:936–941, 2005.
9. Davies AH, Hawdon AJ, Sydes MR, et al: Is duplex surveillance of value after leg vein bypass grafting? Principle results of the vein graft surveillance randomized trial (VGST), *Circulation* 112:1985–1991, 2005.
10. Armstrong PA, Bandyk DF, Wilson JS, et al: Optimizing infrainguinal arm vein bypass patency with duplex ultrasound surveillance and endovascular therapy, *J Vasc Surg* 40:724–731, 2004.
11. Schanzer A, Hevelone N, Owens CD, et al: Technical factors affecting autogenous vein graft failure: Observations from a large multi-center trial, *J Vasc Surg* 42:104–111, 2007.
12. Keeling WB, Shames ML, Stone PA, et al: Plaque excision with the Silverhawk catheter: Early results in patients with claudication or critical limb ischemia, *J Vasc Surg* 45:25–31, 2007.
13. Mofidi R, Kelman J, Berry O, et al: Significance of the early postoperative duplex result in infrainguinal vein bypass surveillance, *Eur J Vasc Endovasc Surg* 34:327–332, 2007.
14. Mewissen MW, Kinney EV, Bandyk DF, et al: The role of duplex scanning versus angiography in predicting outcome after balloon angioplasty in the femoropopliteal artery, *J Vasc Surg* 15:860–865, 1992.
15. Gonsalves C, Bandyk DF, Avino AJ, et al: Duplex features of vein graft stenosis and the success of percutaneous transluminal angioplasty, *J Endovsc Surg* 6:66–72, 1999.
16. DeRubertis BG, Pierce M, Chaer RA, et al: Lesion severity and treatment complexity are associated with outcome after percutaneous infrainguinal intervention, *J Vasc Surg* 46: 709–716, 2007.

CHAPTER

17

Computed Tomographic Scanning

Mark F. Fillinger

Computed tomographic (CT) scanning has an extremely important role in endovascular surgery, especially with regard to the treatment of aortic aneurysms. In the early development of handmade stent grafts and in the initial clinical trials of commercial endografts, the preoperative workup before aneurysm repair generally required both CT and conventional angiography with a graduated-marker catheter. The reason for this strategy was simple: Each imaging modality provided unique and complementary information critical to the process of patient selection and endograft sizing. Unlike preoperative imaging for open repair, which requires primarily *qualitative* morphologic assessments, preoperative imaging for endovascular repair of abdominal aortic aneurysms (AAAs) also requires a large number of *quantitative* assessments (Figure 17-1). Conventional CT provides relatively accurate diameter measurements, delineates intraluminal thrombus and the extent of the aneurysm, and can display important features such as inflammatory rims, tumors, and other structures that are not imaged well with angiography. In the past, because conventional CT was not accurate in measuring length or evaluating occlusive disease, a complete evaluation required angiography. Angiography provides excellent images of the aortic lumen and the branch vessels, but it cannot provide information about the location or the thickness of intraluminal thrombus. This inability to display thrombus makes it impossible to distinguish between normal-diameter aorta and thrombus-filled aneurysm, so angiography requires the complementary information provided by CT. This imaging strategy provides an adequate evaluation in most cases, but the pitfalls of each modality also create some obstacles to obtaining the detailed measurements required for proper patient selection and stent graft sizing.[1-5] Issues that are minor for open AAA repair can be critical for endovascular AAA repair. For example, a diameter difference of only 2 mm can change the selected graft size, can prevent (or cause) an endoleak, can affect the durability of the attachment site, or can result in rejection or selection of the patient for endovascular repair.

Spiral CT dramatically changed the traditional CT evaluation, however. Spiral or helical CT acquires large quantities of data in far less time than conventional CT because data are acquired continuously while the patient moves through the scanner. Spiral CT has three major advantages: (1) the data can be acquired during a single breath-hold and a single contrast agent bolus; (2) the collimation (beam thickness) can be decreased; and (3) multiplanar reformatting into sagittal, coronal, or arbitrary planes is possible. All these features are key to the evaluation of visceral, renal, and iliac artery occlusive disease. The combination of spiral CT and multiplanar reformatting is often referred to as CT angiography (CTA). This technique can be quite accurate in evaluating the extent of aortic aneurysms, the presence of visceral aneurysms, or the presence of occlusive disease in vessels such as renal or iliac arteries.[6-10] CTA is still a two-dimensional (2-D) representation of a three-dimensional (3-D) structure, but 3-D reconstructions have been created from spiral CT data with use of a variety of techniques.[4,6,7] Clinical experience indicates that 3-D reconstructions with specialized software can increase accuracy, provide additional insight into aneurysm anatomy, and produce a more rapid understanding of complex anatomy.[4,5,11,12] For these reasons, spiral CT with 3-D reconstruction has become the sole preoperative imaging modality for the evaluation of AAA morphology and thoracic aortic pathology in most centers. Regardless of how CT technology is used in an individual center, however, it is a standard component of the workup before endovascular aneurysm repair.

TECHNICAL CONSIDERATIONS

Although this chapter is directed at clinical applications, the technical aspects of spiral CT are the key to its clinical usefulness and deserve a brief overview. Spiral CT data acquisition occurs by rotation of the x-ray source while the gantry (table) moves in a continuous linear fashion. Advances in x-ray tube technology allow continuous x-ray beam transmission in a 360-degree arc for intervals of 30 seconds or more. Combined with linear table movement, the continuous scanning path traces the classic spiral from which the technique derives its name. More important, this technique allows data from a large volume to be acquired rapidly—during a single breath-hold and a single contrast agent bolus—so that motion artifacts and contrast agent load are greatly reduced.

A typical spiral CT scan might use intravenous contrast material injected at 2 to 5 mL/s, a "slice" thickness (x-ray beam thickness or collimation) of 1 to 2 mm, a pitch of 1 to 2 (ratio of table speed in millimeters per second to collimation in millimeters), 20 to 50 seconds of continuous scan time, and an x-ray source that rotates 360 degrees in 1 second. State-of-the-art scanners use multiple rows of detectors to enable thinner collimation and faster scan times. These are referred to as multidetector or multirow scanners. The contrast agent level is monitored manually or automatically so that the scan sequence begins at the appropriate time and location. A scan of this type, covering a volume from the celiac artery to the femoral arteries with good contrast agent levels, can be performed with a contrast agent dose of 90 to 150 mL. These settings produce a spiral CT that acquires raw data over a linear distance of 9 to 50 cm during a single breath-hold. The distance covered by the scan varies greatly and is determined primarily by time (heat) limitations of the x-ray emitter and the degree of "overlap" of the CT slices (which in turn affects the signal-to-noise ratio). Multirow scanners allow scans from clavicles to groins in 20 seconds with 90 to 150 mL of contrast agent.

There are tradeoffs involved in any scan protocol. Techniques directed at covering a large distance (large or "thick" collimation and higher pitch) generally limit the ability to detect accurately small branch vessels and subtle occlusive disease. Notably, the reconstruction interval or the reformat interval (the interval at which axial images are output for display on a workstation or for hard-copy printout) is *not* the same as the x-ray beam thickness (collimation). The data are stored on a computer so that images can be reformatted at arbitrarily small intervals. If collimation is thick, however, "thin" reformat intervals will be of no value. A more thorough review of this topic is beyond the scope of this chapter, but detailed discussions are readily available to interested readers.[13,14]

Image Processing

Sophisticated spiral CT hardware and good CT protocols are important for good results, but the image quality is equally dependent on software. During data acquisition, sophisticated computer algorithms allow the raw data to be stored with an x, y, and z dimension, which permits reformatting of the data into extremely thin axial, coronal, and sagittal sections or "reformats."

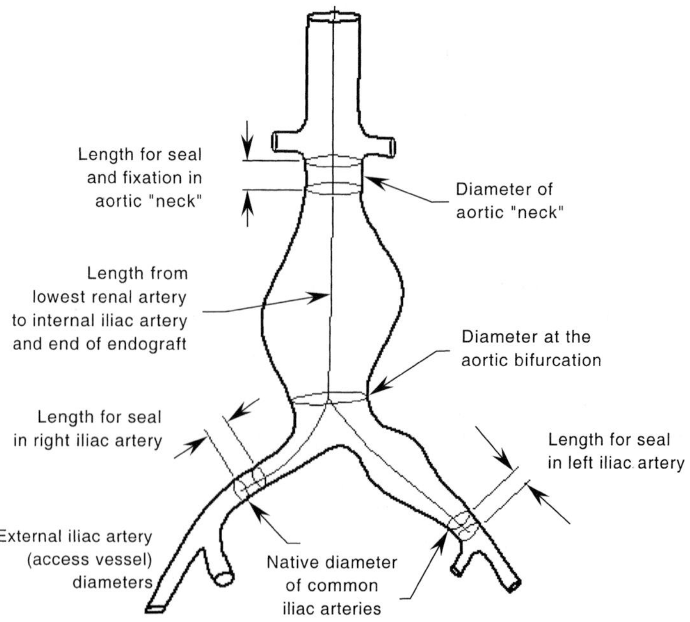

FIGURE 17-1 Measurement considerations for endoluminal repair of an aortic aneurysm using a bifurcated stent graft or an endograft. A large number of measurements are necessary, including the length and the diameter of the proximal aortic neck, the length and the diameter of the distal cuffs, and the length of the two graft limbs.

This technique is commonly referred to as multiplanar reconstructions or multiplanar reformats (MPRs). CTA is the process of acquiring a large number of axial CT images during the "arterial phase" of a single contrast agent bolus, in combination with MPRs to evaluate better the morphology in multiple planes. Although emphasis has recently been placed on 3-D reconstruction, CTA and MPRs, including curvilinear reformats, have greatly increased the accuracy of spiral CT with regard to evaluating occlusive disease and delineating the precise extent of aneurysms.[6-10] A comparison of MPRs, 3-D reconstruction, and conventional angiography is shown in Figure 17-2.

To make the best use of CTA and MPR techniques, a CT workstation is used to scroll through multiple axial, coronal, or sagittal cross sections in a cine mode. This can be very helpful in clarifying the patient's anatomy, following a structure from one slice to the next in rapid succession. A spiral CT data set with thin axial reformats over a large volume generates hundreds of slices, and most spiral CT workstations allow scrolling through every slice in the entire data set. Special workstation capabilities (such as generating 3-D reconstructions) may be available only on the day of the study. Arrangements can usually be made with the radiology department so that the operating surgeon can take advantage of these capabilities post hoc, however.

Other types of reformatting have been used to define better a patient's anatomy. Maximum-intensity projections (MIPs) are constructed by choosing a viewpoint and displaying a 2-D projection of the maximal pixel intensity along the "line of sight," resulting in a view very similar to an angiogram. Three-dimensional reconstructions using a single-object, surface-shaded display (SSD) are also possible with most current spiral CT workstations. Generally, CT workstations use automated computer algorithms that rely on the dramatic difference in density between the contrast agent–filled vessel lumen and the surrounding structures, such as thrombus. Thus a 3-D image of the contrast-enhanced lumen is generated relatively quickly and easily. These automated algorithms cannot generate 3-D images that include thrombus or noncalcified plaque, however, because the computer cannot distinguish these anatomic features of the AAA from adjacent psoas muscle or vena cava. Calcified plaque is often erroneously included in automated 3-D reconstructions of the blood flow because the algorithms have difficulty distinguishing calcified plaque from contrast-enhanced blood. Thus the automated 3-D images generated by most spiral CT scanners are useful for evaluating tortuous

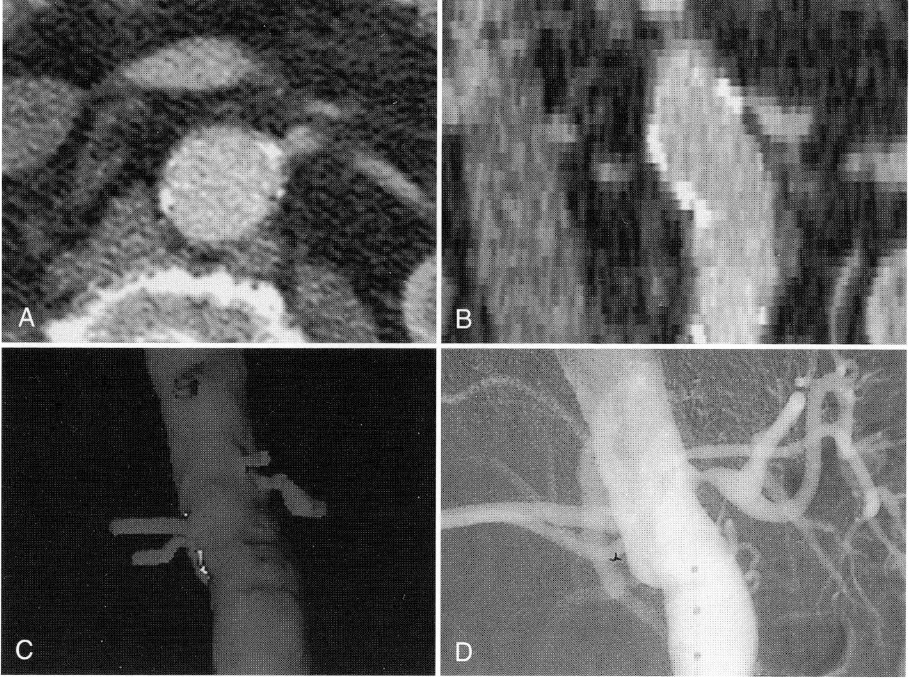

FIGURE 17-2 **A,** Left renal artery stenosis demonstrated by an axial reformat from spiral CT. **B,** Coronal reformat from the same CT. **C,** Multiobject 3-D reconstruction from the same spiral CT data, with plaque made invisible to reveal the stenosis. **D,** Conventional digital subtraction angiography. Even though the 3-D reconstruction can rapidly convey a sense of occlusive disease, it is still important to evaluate the original CT data (in this case, by viewing serial axial and coronal slices). The renal artery origin is seen well in these reformats, but appropriate evaluation requires scrolling through other coronal and axial slices to provide an accurate representation of potential occlusive disease in this vessel. Scrolling through axial and coronal reformats in cine mode would reveal the accessory renal arteries, which are immediately apparent in the 3-D reconstruction.

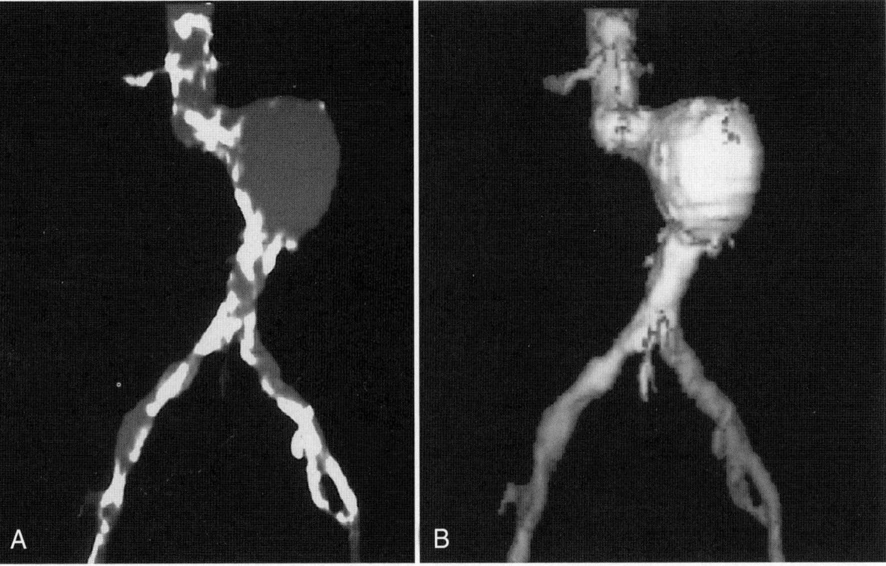

FIGURE 17-3 Different types of reconstruction made possible by spiral CT. **A,** Maximum intensity projection. This technique has the advantage of displaying calcified plaque quite well, but this type of display makes it difficult to determine whether the calcification is causing significant stenosis. **B,** A typical single-object 3-D reconstruction. In this type of reconstruction, contrast-enhanced blood flow and calcified plaque are shown as a single object in the display. This can obscure significant occlusive disease, which can be problematic for device access and fixation.

vessels and aneurysms with little thrombus, but they should not be used to determine the precise extent of the aneurysm or occlusive disease. A comparison of an MIP image and a single-object SSD is displayed in Figure 17-3. Because the spiral CT data are stored digitally in a computer hard drive, viewing the data from many different perspectives is possible without exposing the patient to additional radiation or contrast agent. In some cases, only selected views are typically provided to surgeons. Collaboration with the radiologist directing the CT study or access to the CT workstation allows viewing of the images from any perspective, which can be crucial in cases of ambiguous anatomy.

Advances in Imaging

Because of the limitations of MIPs and single-object SSD, more sophisticated 3-D reconstruction techniques have been developed. Several centers (including Dartmouth-Hitchcock Medical Center) have participated in the development of 3-D imaging systems capable of displaying thrombus and calcified plaque as separate objects. Currently, this involves a semiautomated process in which a trained technician assists the computer in edge detection of structures that are indistinct or ambiguous. This "segmentation" process is still based on the CT density of contrast-enhanced blood flow, thrombus, and calcified plaque, but it avoids some of the artifacts that occur in a computer-generated process devoid of human intervention. The process is more time and labor intensive, but it provides data and images that cannot be obtained by simpler methods. My group and others have found this method of display to be extremely useful in portraying the extent of aneurysmal and occlusive disease.[4,6,11] Multiobject 3-D reconstructions are shown in Figure 17-4 demonstrating some of the advantages of this technology. Although all methods have some limitations, spiral or helical CTA with 3-D reconstruction offers several important benefits before endovascular surgery.[4,5,11,15] Most systems of this type have all the capabilities of advanced spiral CTA and MPR, but the first thing most users notice is how the 3-D reconstruction speeds assimilation of the CT data. With high-quality 3-D reconstructions, a surprising amount of anatomic detail can be demonstrated rapidly.

Although 3-D reconstructions are extremely valuable, they do not diminish the importance of the raw CT images. To have clinical usefulness, 3-D reconstructions must be validated against phantoms of known size and shape. In addition, a 3-D reconstruction system should have a method for displaying the original CT data and the reconstruction simultaneously so that the accuracy of the 3-D reconstruction can be confirmed in every case. This is especially useful when the 3-D reconstruction appears to show an abnormality or in cases of CT artifact. In the system currently used in my institution, the entire spiral CT data set, MPRs, and an interactive 3-D model of the data can be viewed individually and interactively on a personal computer. This format allows scrolling through the full set of CT images, as described

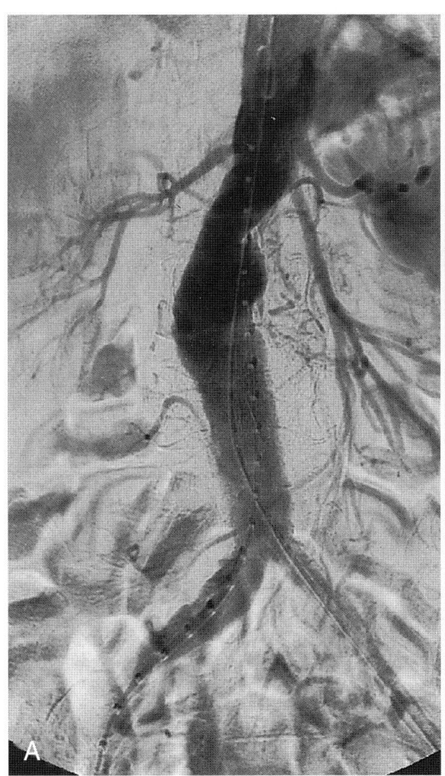

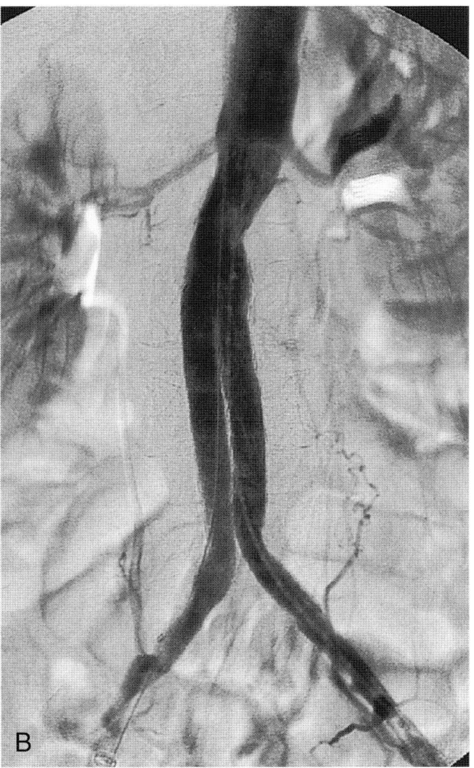

FIGURE 17-4 Angiogram for a patient before **(A)** and after **(B)** endograft deployment. Note confirmation of the lumen morphology and appropriate endograft sizing as determined by the preoperative plan. Despite slight differences in magnification and rotation, the preoperative 3-D reconstruction is obviously an excellent display of the actual anatomy and an excellent prediction of the actual path of the endograft. Note the path of the graduated marker catheter in the predeployment angiogram **(A).** Because the marker catheter has a much smaller diameter than the endograft, the catheter takes a shorter path. In this case, the length measured by the marker catheter was 1 cm shorter than the actual graft path. The 3-D reconstruction measured this length accurately, and the extension planned before surgery was indeed required.

earlier. Unlimited access to the full range of images is extremely useful for initial preoperative planning and for detailed review before the procedure. A computer is kept in the operating room to allow access to the entire imaging data set and the preoperative plan during the procedure.

CLINICAL CONSIDERATIONS

Preoperative Imaging for Endovascular Abdominal Aortic Aneurysm Repair

As stent graft technology has evolved, it has become clear that it places unique demands on preoperative imaging modalities, especially when applied to the repair of AAAs.[1-5,11] Unlike graft selection for conventional AAA repair, stent graft or endograft dimensions must be chosen before the procedure, without direct visualization of the vessel. For a typical bifurcated graft, a large number of precise measurements are necessary, including the length and the diameter of the proximal neck, the length and the diameter of the distal cuffs (usually both common iliac arteries), and the length from the lowest renal artery to the end of the two graft limbs. (See Figure 17-1.)

The consequences of small errors in graft sizing are also quite different from those that occur in open repair. If the endograft diameter is even 1 mm too small or if the length of the "seal zone" is inadequate, there may be insufficient fixation or sealing between the endograft and the vessel wall. Lack of proper sealing allows blood flow around the endograft and into the aneurysm sac—endoleak, or perigraft flow—which has been associated with aneurysm rupture in some cases. Poor graft sizing can also lead to insecure attachment of the stent graft to the vessel, which can lead to graft migration, endoleak, or rupture. Conversely, choosing an overly large endograft diameter can lead to crimping or folding of the excess material, which may also contribute to endoleak. Long-term implications of severe oversizing are unknown, but it may contribute to aortic enlargement. Endografts that are too short or too long may similarly create attachment problems, endoleaks, graft kinking, or occlusion of important branch vessels. Additional components to correct sizing problems lead to increased cost or time and potential morbidity. Thus appropriate sizing and placement of endoluminal grafts require a preprocedure imaging system that can determine the lengths and the diameters of tortuous vessels with a high degree of accuracy. The imaging protocol must also provide the information traditionally required for conventional repair: the precise proximal and distal extent of the aneurysm; the presence of occlusive or aneurysmal disease in the visceral, the renal, or the iliac arteries; the presence of multiple renal arteries or vascular anomalies, including horseshoe kidney; the degree of calcified or noncalcified plaque; and the presence of aortic or iliac dissections. This combination of imaging requirements necessitates techniques that have not been required for conventional open surgery. Initially, these stringent requirements led to the use of both CT and conventional angiography before endovascular repair. With the currently available technology, however, preoperative imaging requirements can be met with entirely noninvasive technology in almost all cases.

Extent of the Aneurysm

One of the most important morphologic considerations for endovascular repair of an aortic aneurysm is proximal and distal extent of disease. CT is generally recognized as the best imaging modality for ascertaining proximal and distal extent of an aortic aneurysm, and spiral CT offers distinct advantages in this respect because the data may be viewed from different perspectives via MPRs and 3-D reconstructions. Three-dimensional reconstructions can be especially helpful in determining the extent of aneurysmal disease and the locations for optimal cross-clamp placement.[6,7] In some systems, 3-D reconstructions and MPRs can even be combined to improve the context of the CT images.

Another important aspect of preoperative evaluation for AAA repair is the assessment of aneurysms in the iliac arteries. In many cases, conventional CT has been poor in this regard, with reported error rates of 16% for the detection of iliac aneurysms.[16] Groups using spiral CT with MPRs alone, however, have noted more than 90% accuracy for the detection of iliac aneurysms.[9] In more than 50 consecutive AAAs evaluated by means of spiral CT with MPRs and 3-D reconstruction before open repair at my institution, we have not missed a single iliac aneurysm (as confirmed by inspection).

Occlusive Disease of the Aortic Branches

Another key aspect in the evaluation of potential candidates for endovascular AAA repair is the extent of occlusive disease in aortic branch vessels. The importance of iliac occlusive disease is obvious: it may prevent access for the deployment device. Mesenteric vascular disease cannot be overlooked, however, because endovascular AAA repair may be contraindicated in a patient with significant superior mesenteric artery disease and a patent inferior mesenteric artery. Renal artery disease is unlikely to be treated before endovascular AAA repair, but its presence is important in patient evaluation. Patients with suspected iliac, renal, or visceral occlusive disease have historically required angiography before AAA repair because the ability to evaluate occlusive disease has been a traditional shortcoming of conventional CT.[17] With conventional CT, tube overheating problems limited the number of slices that could be obtained and the volume of the body that could be covered by the scan. Therefore fewer axial slices were obtained in the visceral and the renal segments, and very few slices were obtained in the iliac segment. The paucity of slices and the tortuosity of the vessels made evaluation of occlusive disease difficult.

Because of the technical considerations mentioned earlier, however, spiral CT can obtain data rapidly over a large 3-D volume and can still provide large numbers of thin multiplanar sections, especially with newer multirow scanners. This ability is key to the evaluation of occlusive disease. Large numbers of thin axial slices make it more likely that stenosis will be seen clearly on axial slices alone. This technique also improves the quality of MPRs and 3-D reconstructions.[14] Thus, with appropriate scan protocols and adequate timing of the contrast agent load, evaluation of iliac occlusive disease with spiral CT is far superior to conventional CT and rivals angiography.[9] Occlusive disease of the iliac arteries is demonstrated in Figure 17-3, even without the multiple views available with typical software. In comparisons at my institution, angiography evaluated iliac artery occlusive disease accurately (defined as 50% or greater stenosis) in 22 of 28 cases (79%). Spiral CT with axial slices alone was accurate in a similar percentage of cases, but spiral CT with MPRs and 3-D reconstruction was correct in all 28 cases.

The evaluation of occlusive disease in the renal and the mesenteric vessels is more difficult than the evaluation of iliac occlusive disease. The vessels are smaller, the stenotic areas are often quite focal, and the vessels may be oriented at odd angles relative to conventional axial slices. Again, spiral CT is superior to conventional CT because of the availability of extremely thin (1 to 2 mm) axial reformats and MPRs. For the visceral segment of the aorta, we generally use a protocol that includes less than 1 mm collimation and a reconstruction interval (reformat interval) of 1 mm for axial images. It is important to reiterate that collimation and reconstruction interval are not synonymous, but both terms are frequently interchanged with the term "thin slices." If the images are acquired by using thick collimation (the thickness of the x-ray beam), it will not be helpful to reconstruct the images at 1-mm intervals. Thus it may be necessary to discuss the goals of the scan with a radiologist to obtain the optimal CT imaging protocol.

Although the acquisition technique is crucial, post hoc reconstruction techniques are also important. It is best to generate views or reformatted slices perpendicular to the long axis of the vessel. Thus the renal arteries are best evaluated with axial, coronal, and 3-D reconstructions, whereas the celiac and superior mesenteric arteries are best depicted in axial, sagittal, and 3-D reconstructions. These special images can be very helpful in the overall evaluation. CT artifacts are possible, including motion artifacts (patient movement during the scan) and partial volume-averaging artifacts (e.g., signal averaging from dense structures such as calcium causing a small rim of adjacent thrombus to have the appearance of contrast-enhanced blood flow).[14] MPRs are often helpful in this regard, however, and I am much more confident when stenosis appears consistently in multiple views. Figure 17-2 demonstrates the usefulness of spiral CT with 3-D reconstruction in the evaluation of renal artery stenosis. I have found that the accuracy of these techniques is similar to that of angiography for visceral and renal artery stenoses (for detecting a stenosis of 50% or greater). Other investigators have also found a high degree of accuracy for renal artery stenoses using spiral CT and MPRs alone, although sensitivities in the 90% range are not universal.[8-10,18-20] In general, however, the accuracy of spiral CT is uniformly superior to reported values for conventional CT.[17] Depiction of visceral artery stenosis appears to be very accurate in most studies.[9,10] Although 3-D reconstructions are helpful, they should not be used to assess renal or visceral artery stenoses in the absence of the "source" CT images.[20] In my experience, a complete evaluation of visceral or renal artery occlusive disease should include a thorough study of all available axial, coronal, and sagittal sections, including magnified views. Magnified and rotated views with and without plaque are helpful, but only multiobject 3-D reconstructions offer these options (see the discussion of technical considerations). Appropriate scanning protocols and detailed evaluation are needed to obtain high-quality results. With state-of-the-art technology, however, angiography is rarely necessary for preoperative evaluation.

Accessory Renal Arteries and Inferior Mesenteric Artery Patency

Another area that has traditionally been difficult for conventional CT is the evaluation of accessory renal arteries and the inferior mesenteric artery. Because of the advantages described earlier, however, spiral CT is quite good at detecting the presence of these vessels and determining whether they are patent. Three-dimensional reconstruction is also helpful in this regard, but the key to accuracy in imaging these vessels is thin collimation (1 to 2 mm), small axial reconstruction intervals (1 mm), and the willingness to scroll through every single axial slice or reformat looking for small branch vessels. Again, small reconstruction intervals are not useful with thick (5 to 10 mm) collimation because a 1-mm vessel is easily "lost" as a result of partial volume averaging (especially if intraluminal contrast is poor). With a 2-mm reconstruction interval, a typical spiral CT scan for AAA evaluation generates hundreds of axial slices. It is not adequate to review a small subset of selected images; the radiologist or the surgeon must sit at the CT workstation and review magnified views of every axial CT reformat in the area of interest.

In my institution, surgeons use specialized software to review each CT slice on a personal computer employing magnified views. The same software allows the review of MPRs to view the vessels in two or three planes and produces 3-D reconstructions that are capable of displaying the blood flow, the thrombus, and the calcified plaque as separate objects. Automated 3-D reconstruction algorithms are unreliable here because the contrast may be poor in small vessels (another form of partial volume averaging), and calcified plaque is sometimes "modeled" as contrast-enhanced blood flow. At present, there are at least three commercially available software-hardware combinations capable of multiobject 3-D reconstructions. Some of these packages allow the separate objects in the 3-D models to be viewed individually and to be rotated so that the structure can be viewed from any angle. I have found this technique useful in detecting the number, the location, and the patency of accessory renal arteries. In a series of more than 50 open AAA repairs with 3-D imaging, my colleagues and I identified all patent accessory renal arteries when compared with operative findings. (See Figure 17-2.) Other groups have noted accuracies of 96% to 100% in the detection of accessory renal arteries.[8,20,21] We have also found this technique to be more accurate than angiography in the determination of inferior mesenteric artery patency, with only one error in more than 50 cases. An example of inferior mesenteric artery patency is shown in Figure 17-3, with less sophisticated imaging software (though it can be seen on the raw CT images).

Stent Graft Sizing

Diameter Measurements

Although CT has typically been the study of choice for diameter measurements, axial CT slices often do not cut through planes perpendicular to the vessel. The resulting elliptical cross sections can make diameter measurements difficult.[32,33] Although one might presume that the narrowest diameter of the elliptical cross section is the "true" diameter, this is not always the case because an aneurysm does not always have a simple cylindrical or conical shape. Thus axial reformats often lead to a slight overestimation of diameter, whereas slices reconstructed perpendicular to the vessel tend to be more accurate.[5,11,15] Simply using sagittal or coronal reconstruction from spiral CT is not always adequate because these sections may not be perpendicular to the vessel either (which may lead to an overestimation of diameter) or may not cut through the center of the vessel (which may produce an underestimation of diameter). The frequency of significant errors is not entirely clear because some problems may not become evident without long-term follow-up.

If graft diameters are estimated solely on the basis of CT, the key considerations are the following: use of spiral CT; use of good CT protocols, including adequate rate and volume of contrast agent injection (to achieve sufficient contrast agent density in the iliac arteries); small reconstruction (reformat) intervals for axial slices; extensive MPRs (sagittal, coronal, and perpendicular to the vessel, if possible); thorough understanding of the aforementioned pitfalls; and recognition of cases in which 3-D reconstruction or other adjunctive procedures are needed. Adjunctive angiography has been considered important for diameter measurements in some centers, but it has recently become clear that angiography tends to underestimate diameter measurements *systematically* by 6% to 17%, even with orthogonal views using a marker catheter and appropriate calibration.[5,11,15] In addition, plaque and thrombus are not seen on angiograms. Angiography therefore complements CT imaging, but measurements are still difficult and often inaccurate. It is also invasive and expensive, and it adds to the preoperative radiation dose for the patient. Intravascular ultrasound has excellent accuracy in diameter measurement, but it too is invasive.

In my experience, the best method of diameter measurement is spiral CTA with MPRs, 3-D reconstructions, and specialized measurement software. This system allows CT data to be displayed in slices reconstructed perpendicular to the vessel axis, which facilitates accurate measurement of lumen diameter by avoiding problems with elliptical cross sections or noncylindrical vessels. It also provides a 3-D context to help decipher ambiguities. In a comparative study using life-size models with shapes similar to actual AAAs, my colleagues and I compared spiral CT alone, angiography with a 1-cm graduated catheter, intravascular ultrasound, and spiral CTA with interactive multiobject 3-D reconstructions and specialized measurement software.[15] Although all these methods produced reasonable results in experienced hands, CTA with 3-D reconstructions and specialized software was the only imaging method that was accurate for *both* diameter and length measurements, thus allowing it to be used reliably as the sole preoperative imaging modality. My center and others have had similar results in a purely clinical setting.[5,11,12,32] To date, my center has had no diameter measurement errors in more than 800 cases. This imaging strategy is also the least expensive and the least invasive, and it gives the patient the lowest preoperative radiation dose.

Length Measurements

Diameter measurements on CT may require some interpretation, but using conventional or even spiral CT to determine the length of a proposed endograft is difficult at best. Thus the current standard is to perform angiography for length measurements and for the evaluation of occlusive disease before endovascular repair. Angiography for the evaluation of iliac occlusive disease has well-known pitfalls, however, because it provides a 2-D projection of a 3-D structure. Interpretation of the true vessel dimensions can be difficult, even with orthogonal or oblique views. Length measurements also have potential pitfalls. To obtain more accurate measurements, angiograms must be performed with graduated-marker catheters (radiodense marks at 1-cm intervals). Unfortunately, the catheter does not usually follow the proposed graft path because it is not the same diameter as the graft. Generally, the catheter takes a path that is shorter than the endograft, but sometimes the marker catheter deviates into a saccular or a tortuous AAA, following a *longer* path than the proposed endograft. The catheter can make these deviations in planes that are not projected on the 2-D image of the angiogram. Thus an educated estimate must be made regarding how far the catheter deviates from the actual path of the endograft, leading to length errors greater than 1 cm in more than 19% of cases.[3,5,11,32,34] In addition, plaque and thrombus are not seen on angiograms. Angiography therefore complements CT imaging, but measurements are still difficult and often inaccurate. If angiography is to be used as the primary method of choosing endograft length, the keys are use of a marker catheter, two orthogonal views without moving the catheter between "runs" (to make it clear when the catheter is bending in a second plane "away" from the observer), and CT to help determine lengths of aortic and iliac "seal zones" or fixation areas (because angiography cannot demonstrate thrombus or plaque within the vessel lumen).

Spiral CT with 3-D reconstruction and specialized measurement software can eliminate most of the problems associated with conventional preoperative length measurement techniques. In the system used at my institution, a software algorithm is used to display the center line of the contrast-enhanced lumen in the aorta and the iliac arteries, which allows length measurements along the central lumen line, even in tortuous iliac segments. Rather than measuring the length of the line drawn in a 2-D projection, the computer software calculates the length from the actual 3-D path. In some situations, an endovascular graft may not follow the center line of the lumen throughout its entire course. For this reason, some centers (including mine) have developed a system in which measurements can be made along a 3-D path defined by the user.[4,5,22,23] A user-defined graft path measurement is most useful for endovascular AAA repair when the aneurysm is saccular and has little intraluminal thrombus, causing the center line to deviate into the saccular portion of the AAA. In test phantoms and in my clinical experience, the centerline and user-defined graft path measurement techniques have eliminated length measurement problems for AAA.[11,15,32,34] My colleagues and I have used this system as the sole preoperative imaging modality for more than 800 endovascular AAA repairs without a significant length or diameter measurement error. Several systems are now commercially available or in development, and at least two commercially available systems have reported success using this type of specialized software for diameter and length measurements.[4,5,11] The key with this technique is to use validated software, to obtain proper training, and initially to confirm measurements using adjunctive modalities.

It is also important to note that in TEVAR the key measurement is generally the outer curve of the proposed endograft, rather than the center line, as in AAA. The difference is that in AAA there are often multiple curves (right, left, anterior, posterior), which often compress the inner curve in a manner that averages in the center line length. In TEVAR, the thoracic aorta frequently follows a single long, sweeping curve. In this case the inner curve of the device is compressed but the outer curve cannot expand. Therefore the overall device length and end point are determined by forces pushing the device to the outer curve. We use software

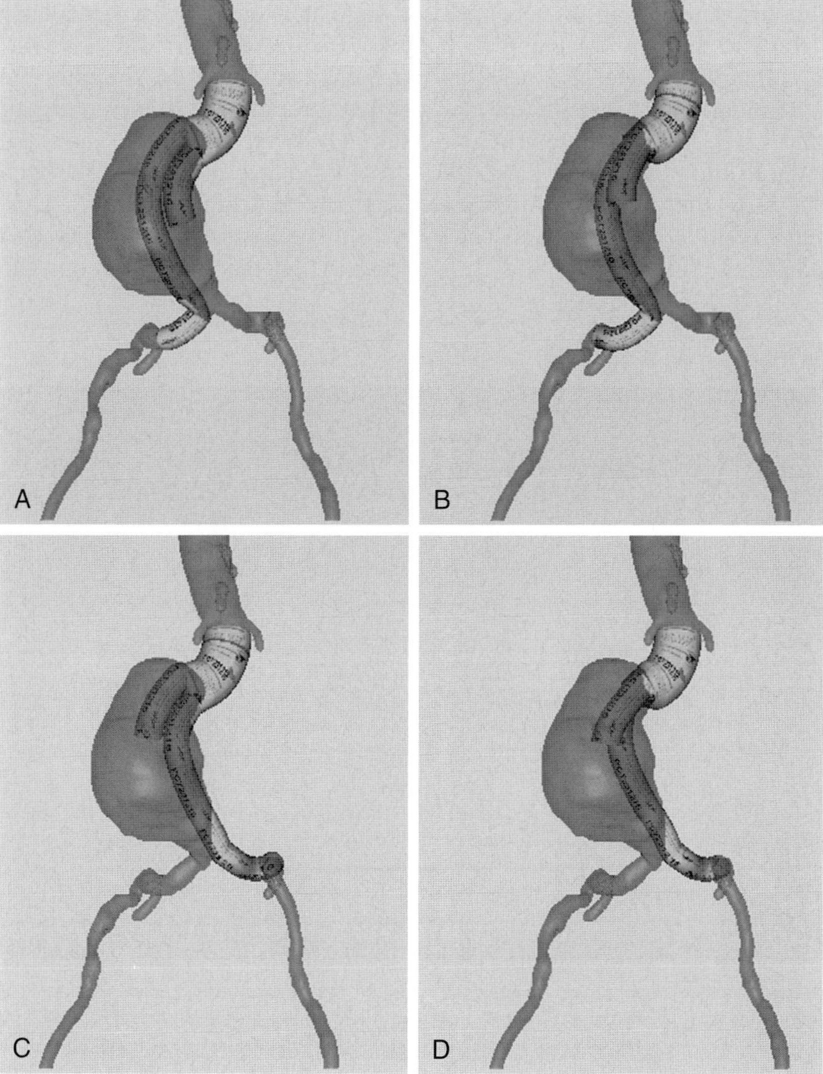

FIGURE 17-5 Simulated "virtual graft" modeled within a patient-specific 3-D model, demonstrating potential pathways when delivered via right (**A** and **B**) or left (**C** and **D**) femoral and with different amount of rotation (e.g., with the docking limb anterior in B and D).

that gives this length in addition to the center line (Figure 17-6).

Special Techniques Potentiated by Three-Dimensional Reconstruction

Another unique innovation made possible by spiral CTA, 3-D reconstructions, and specialized software is a technology termed the "virtual graft," in which the diameter, the length, and the path of a proposed endograft can be simulated in 3-D space.[11,22,32,34] This simulated graft can be displayed within the 3-D model of the AAA or thoracic aortic aneurysm (TAA) and can be used to investigate potential problems with endograft sizing, kinking, compression, and deployment (Figure 17-5). The technique provides a rapid visual assessment of the proposed plan and allows simulation of reversed-limb configurations, anteroposterior limb configurations, alternative access routes, and the effect of different endograft lengths without the need for invasive studies. In my experience, this technique has frequently altered the access route to the contralateral side to minimize potential difficulties with delivery device angulation in the aorta, to aid cannulation of the "docking" limb in a modular graft, to optimize coverage of the common iliac artery, or to eliminate the need for a modular extension (because the distance from the renal artery to the iliac seal zone is different on each side). This method complements the inner/outer curve measurements for TEVAR, in which the outer curve is key.

My colleagues and I have used similar aspects of this system to evaluate the proposed access path for the delivery system and have found it to be extremely helpful (Figure 17-7).[32] Generally, the key parameters for delivery device access are diameter, tortuosity, and occlusive disease (especially calcified plaques). With good imaging, patient selection for delivery device access can "push the margins" slightly on one of these parameters without too much difficulty. Pushing the margins on more than one of these parameters (e.g., focal calcified stenosis but no tortuosity) likely means difficult device access but a high likelihood of success. Pushing the margins on all three of these parameters, however, is likely to result in failure. Other institutions have demonstrated that CTA alone can be quite accurate for the evaluation of iliac artery occlusive disease, but 3-D reconstruction provides rapid visual feedback and visual cues to potential access problems.[9,24] We have found that a stenotic calcified plaque in a tortuous or angulated segment is particularly problematic. As part of evaluating delivery device access, we also use this technology routinely to simulate the C-arm gantry angle that provides optimal endograft deployment in relation to the renal arteries and the internal iliac arteries or in the case of TEVAR, the arch vessels. Angle measurements performed on the CT reformats can also be used for this purpose (Figure 17-8). This avoids the trial-and-error method of finding the

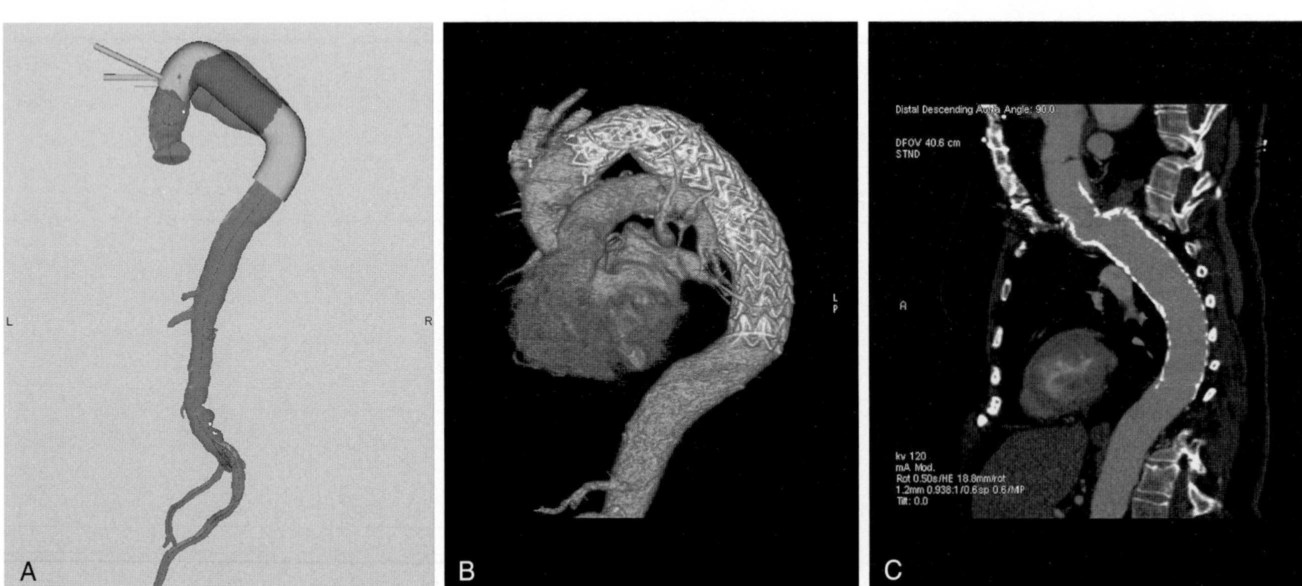

FIGURE 17-6 Virtual graft simulation for thoracic endovascular aortic repair (TEVAR) in a patient with a prior arch reconstruction with "elephant trunk" technique. **A,** The simulation is helpful in determining the correct gantry angles and the distance the stent-graft must travel on the *outer curve*, which will limit the distance covered and is a better approximation of distal landing zone and distance covered than center line. **B** and **C** show postoperative evaluations using volume-rendered 3-D reconstruction **(B)** and curvilinear reformat **(C)** to evaluate structure, deformation, migration, and wall apposition.

appropriate viewing angle for endograft delivery, diminishing the total contrast agent dose, the radiation dose, and the probability of deploying the endograft in a misleading view.

Postoperative Imaging

CT also has a prominent role in postoperative maging after endovascular aneurysm repair. Unfortunately, because there is no single imaging modality that is optimal for postoperative surveillance, a combination of modalities is needed for appropriate evaluation.[23] Current clinical trials use a clinic visit with history and physical examination, ankle–brachial indices, abdominal x-rays (three or four views), and contrast-enhanced CT with or without 3-D reconstruction. Abdominal x-rays are used primarily to evaluate the stent framework for deformation and fractures. CT is used primarily to evaluate stent graft migration, fixation or apposition to the vessel wall, endoleak, branch vessels (renal, mesenteric, and internal iliac arteries), and aneurysm size (diameter and possibly volume). CT can also evaluate stent graft deformation and potential iliac occlusive disease in a manner that may supplement information obtained from ankle/brachial indices and abdominal x-rays. Duplex scans using color Doppler ultrasound or power Doppler can be used to detect aneurysm size and potential endoleak, but accuracy tends to be on the order of 85%.[23,25] Contrast-enhancement agents for intravenous ultrasound may increase accuracy, but duplex scanning is highly operator dependent, subject to difficulties involving bowel gas or obesity, and less accurate in determining migration and stent-vessel apposition. In addition, ultrasonography is generally less accurate than CT for diameter measurements.[23,26]

Contrast-enhanced CT should include the arterial phase at a minimum, with the addition of a noncontrast phase if extensive calcifications are present. Calcifications tend to "average" with low-density thrombus to produce an intermediate density that can be confused with contrast enhancement.[23] A noncontrast CT can be performed with thicker collimation to minimize radiation dose. If the aneurysm enlarges at any point or shows no signs of shrinkage within 1 year, evaluation should be directed at finding a potential endoleak or an attachment site problem. If there is no evidence of endoleak on arterial-phase CT, a venous-phase CT should be performed. The venous-phase spiral CT can

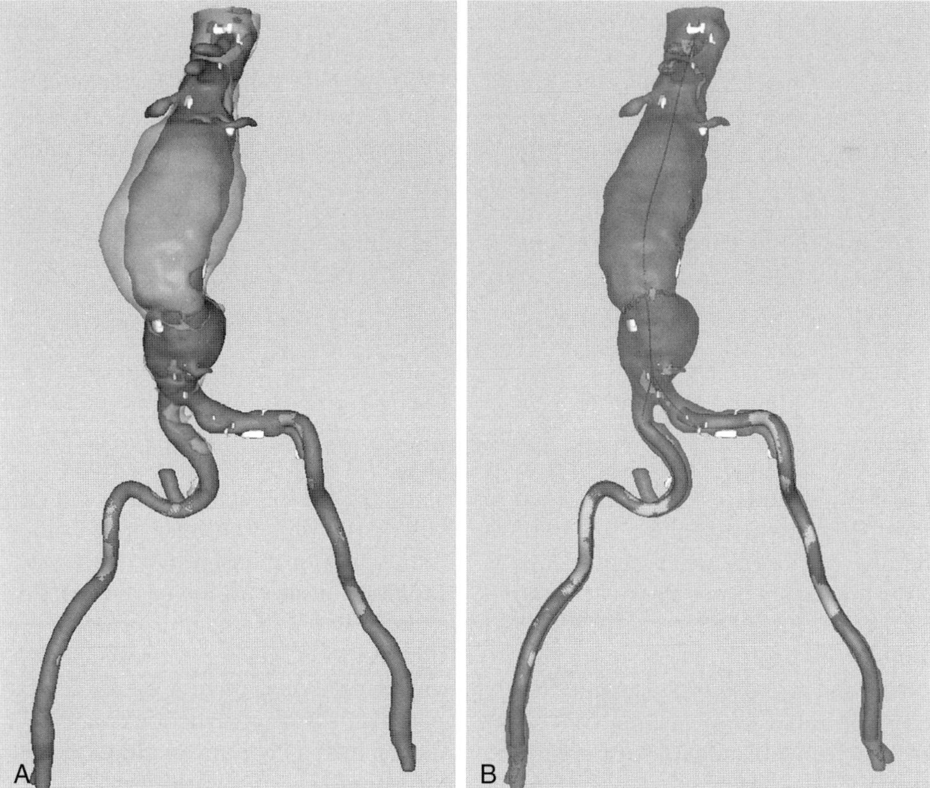

FIGURE 17-7 Simulation of the delivery system diameter within the patient's 3-D reconstruction. This is helpful in evaluating where the diameter of the delivery system may interact in adverse ways with calcific plaque, the native vessel lumen diameter, or tortuosity (see text).

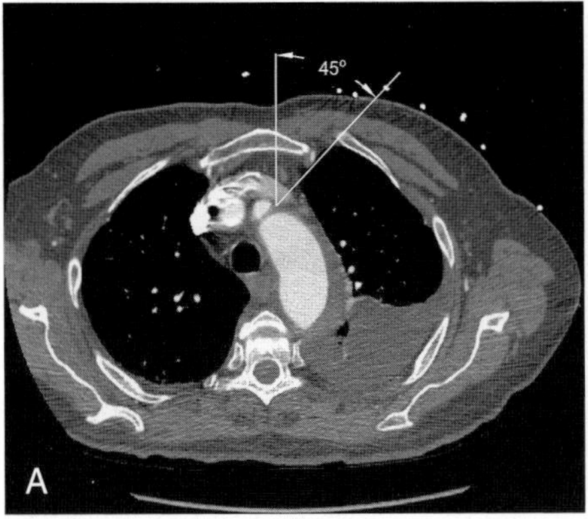

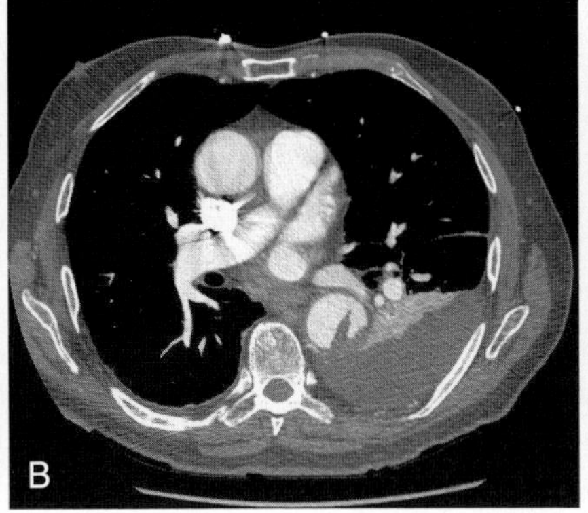

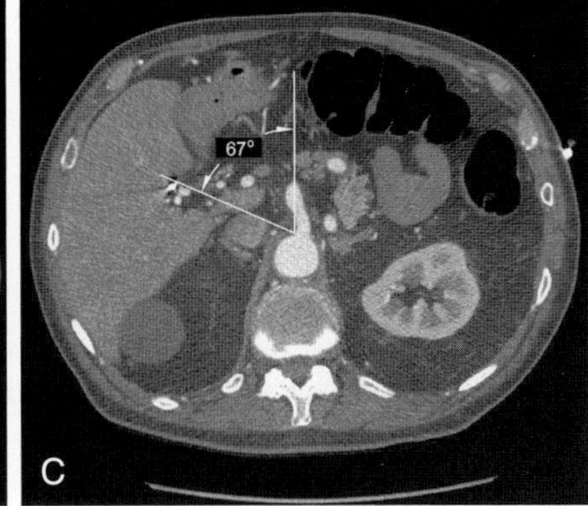

FIGURE 17-8 Thoracic aortic dissection case demonstrating that axial reformats can be used to determine the optimal C-arm gantry for imaging branch vessels such as the left common carotid **(A)** or the celiac **(C)**. **B** shows the primary entry tear in this case, which is more distal to the left subclavian than typical. The dissection and hematoma required implantation of the device just distal to the left common carotid, however, so the gantry angle was planned relative to the carotid artery rather than the subclavian for this case. For EVAR, sagittal reformats can be used in a similar way, in order to make the crucial gantry angle adjustment for the infrarenal neck (avoiding placement of the device too for infrarenal).[32]

be performed with a 2- to 5-minute delay after the arterial phase, again using thicker collimation. The venous-phase technique can detect smaller, late-filling endoleaks that are not easily detected by other means.[23,27] If no endoleak is detected with use of the delayed venous-phase technique, consideration should be given to transmission of pressure without actual flow of contrast material. It has been demonstrated that pressure transmission can occur through thrombus when the stent graft is seated in thrombus rather than seated against the vessel adventitia or when a small hole is sealed with thrombus.[27,28] Three-dimensional reconstruction of CT or magnetic resonance angiography (MRA) data (including special reformats and magnified views) can be quite useful for detecting the source of an endoleak, evaluating appropriate fixation, and detecting shape and volume changes. At present, it appears that aneurysm enlargement is more accurately detected by volume changes than by diameter changes.[23,29]

Currently, most recommend CTA with or without 3-D reconstruction at 1 month and then either 6 or 12 months, depending on results. Once there is an endoleak and/or the aneurysm is clearly shrinking as evidenced by CT or MRI, follow-up can be changed to annual duplex scan. More frequent follow-up or intervention is generally required when endoleak is detected or when the aneurysm is not clearly shrinking. In particular, spiral CT with 3-D reconstruction and volume measurement is useful when there is no evidence of endoleak and the aneurysm is not clearly shrinking. Because a number of problems can occur more than 1 year after endovascular AAA repair, the physician should emphasize the importance of long-term follow-up even if the endograft is functioning perfectly after 1 year.[30]

IMAGING PROTOCOLS

Imaging expertise can vary greatly from one institution to another, and imaging protocols generally reflect that fact. Clinical investigations of spiral CT with 3-D reconstruction continue for endovascular repair of aortic aneurysms. In my institution, this technology has almost entirely eliminated the need for angiography before open and endovascular repair of thoracic or abdominal aortic aneurysms. (Preoperative angiography is used for fewer than 5% of endovascular cases.) CTA with 3-D reconstructions and specialized software has been extremely accurate for endograft sizing and has reliably demonstrated important anatomic features such as accessory renal arteries, inferior mesenteric artery patency, patency of lumbar arteries, common iliac artery dissections, and complex anatomic relationships that were either unclear or not demonstrated at all on conventional CT or angiographic imaging. This technique is not perfect, however, and it requires special software, a dedicated radiologist-technologist-surgeon team, and possibly a commercial service to produce quality results. At this point, spiral CT with 3-D reconstruction and specialized software has emerged as the standard for the evaluation of patients before endovascular AAA repair because of its unique imaging capabilities, superior measurement accuracy, lower cost, lower radiation dose, and lower patient morbidity.

Postoperative imaging protocols require a combination of modalities for appropriate evaluation, and these protocols should include spiral CT. In the postoperative period, 3-D reconstructions and specialized measurements such as volume evaluation will probably become commonplace only for selected patients with endoleak, stent graft deformation, or failure of the aneurysm to decrease in size.

MAGNETIC RESONANCE ANGIOGRAPHY

MRA is not commonly used for the evaluation of patients before endovascular AAA repair, in part because it does not provide sufficient contrast between aortic lumen, thrombus, and calcified plaque. In particular, because calcium is poorly imaged with MRA, noncontrast CT is required as an adjunctive study to avoid missing large calcified plaques at attachment sites.[14] More recently, the use of intravenous gadolinium infusion has provided better contrast for the lumen, making MRA images easier to interpret by decreasing flow artifact. Reconstructions from multiple views give relative 3-D spatial information and help resolve some image artifacts. Because rotated images still fall far short of the detailed measurement capabilities needed for endovascular AAA repair, however, specialized software for true 3-D reconstructions is still necessary if adjunctive studies are to be avoided. Fortunately, many of the specialized systems developed for the 3-D reconstruction of spiral CT data can also be used with MRA data.

Other factors still limit MRA in this particular application, however. One of the limiting factors is the volume that needs to be imaged. Ideally, the evaluation should extend from the celiac artery to the common femoral arteries. The time needed to cover this volume and patient claustrophobia can be limiting factors for this study. More important, MRA still provides a less detailed display of intraluminal thrombus, although this is improving. Because the extent and the thickness of calcified and noncalcified plaque are very important for evaluating potential seal zones and the access path of the delivery device, poor or unreliable contrast for plaque is a major problem. Last, MRA generally uses a 256 × 256 data matrix that provides roughly half the resolution of CT with a similar field of view. This problem is also being resolved with the latest hardware and software.

Despite all these limitations, however, MRA can be used successfully in this setting.[31] The keys to this modality are gadolinium enhancement, provided renal function is normal, reconstruction of multiple views, use of 3-D reconstructions and specialized software when available, good protocols to provide thin slices and adequate resolution, and liberal use of adjunctive studies. Because of its cost and limitations, MRA is less useful than CT, and gadolinium cannot be used for patients with severe renal insufficiency as a result of nephrogenic sclerosing fibrosis. With current technology, adjunctive studies such as CT without contrast (to view calcified plaque), carbon dioxide angiography or intravascular ultrasound (to confirm measurements), and duplex scanning (to evaluate occlusive disease in selected cases) are likely to be necessary. Such studies can be helpful in determining whether apparent defects are disease or artifact.

SUMMARY

Preoperative imaging for endovascular AAA repair is much more demanding than that required for open repair. As with any surgical procedure, patient selection and preoperative planning are at least as important as technical skill and at least as difficult to learn. Spiral CT is a necessary component of the preoperative evaluation of aortic aneurysm morphology, and techniques such as MPR and 3-D reconstruction are helpful in many cases and crucial in others. There are a number of anatomic features that range from critically important to extremely helpful when planning aortic aneurysm repair, and precise anatomic information can alter the operative plan or the risk-benefit ratio of the procedure. In the past, preoperative evaluation for endovascular aortic aneurysm repair required a combination of CT and conventional angiography with a graduated-marker catheter. Currently, however, the preoperative workup can be completed noninvasively by using state-of-the-art spiral CT with MPRs, interactive 3-D reconstruction, and specialized software. Access to a CT workstation or specialized software is helpful for most anatomic features and is crucial for evaluating visceral occlusive disease, accessory renal arteries, and inferior mesenteric arteries. With appropriate protocols and software, spiral CT with MPRs and multiobject 3-D reconstruction is more accurate than conventional CT or angiography for endograft sizing and is the gold standard. Preoperative angiography will be reserved for highly selected patients and oriented toward a therapeutic rather than a diagnostic role.

ACKNOWLEDGMENTS

I would like to thank M25, West Lebanon, NH—including D. T. Chen, PhD), which has been the focal point for development of the vascular 3-D reconstruction capabilities used at my institution. M25 has provided grant and research support for these development efforts. I have no other potential conflicts of interest. An expression of thanks also goes to Robert F. Jeffery, MD, and Richard Morse, MD (Department of Radiology), who diligently worked on optimizing spiral CT protocols for our institution and provided technical assistance in downloading spiral CT data for 3-D reconstructions in the early days of development.

References

1. Parodi J: Endovascular repair of abdominal aortic aneurysms and other arterial lesions, *J Vasc Surg* 21:549–557, 1995.

2. Chuter TA, Green RM, Ouriel K, DeWeese JA: Infrarenal aortic aneurysm structure: implications for transfemoral repair, *J Vasc Surg* 20:44–50, 1994.
3. Beebe HG, Jackson T, Pigott JP: Aortic aneurysm morphology for planning endovascular aortic grafts: limitations of conventional imaging methods, *J Endovasc Surg* 2:139–148, 1995.
4. Fillinger MF: Utility of spiral CT in the preoperative evaluation of patients with abdominal aortic aneurysms. In: Whittemore AD, editor: *Advances in Vascular Surgery,* St. Louis, 1997, Mosby, pp 115–131.
5. Broeders I, Blankensteijn J, Olree M, et al: Preoperative sizing of grafts for transfemoral endovascular aneurysm management: a prospective comparative study of spiral CT angiography, arteriography, and conventional CT imaging, *J Endovasc Surg* 4:252–261, 1997.
6. Balm R, Eikelboom BC, van Leeuwen MS, Noordzij J: Spiral CT-angiography of the aorta, *Eur J Vasc Surg* 8:544–551, 1994.
7. Rubin GD, Walker PJ, Dake MD, et al: Three-dimensional spiral computed tomographic angiography: an alternative imaging modality for the abdominal aorta and its branches, *J Vasc Surg* 18:656–665, 1993.
8. Van Hoe L, Baert AL, Gryspeerdt S, et al: Supra- and juxtarenal aneurysms of the abdominal aorta: preoperative assessment with thin-section spiral CT, *Radiology* 198:443–448, 1996.
9. Raptopoulos V, Rosen MP, Kent KC, et al: Sequential helical CT angiography of aortoiliac disease, *AJR Am J Roentgenol* 166:1347–1354, 1996.
10. Cikrit DF, Harris VJ, Hemmer CG, et al: Comparison of spiral CT scan and arteriography for evaluation of renal and visceral arteries, *Ann Vasc Surg* 10:109–116, 1996.
11. Fillinger MF: New imaging techniques in endovascular surgery, *Surg Clin North Am* 79:451–475, 1999.
12. Beebe HG, Kritpracha B, Serres S, et al: Endograft planning without preoperative arteriography: a clinical feasibility study, *J Endovasc Ther* 7:8–15, 2000.
13. Zeman RK, Brink JA, Costello P, et al: *Helical/Spiral CT: A Practical Approach,* New York, 1995, McGraw-Hill.
14. Fillinger MF: Computed tomography, CT angiography and three-dimensional reconstruction for the evaluation of vascular disease. In: Rutherford RB, editor: *Rutherford's Textbook of Vascular Surgery,* Philadelphia, 1999, W.B. Saunders, pp 230–268.
15. Farber A, Fillinger MF, Connors J, et al: *Comparison of angiography, intravascular ultrasound and three dimensional CT for morphologic evaluation in a three dimensional aneurysm model,* 1998, Paper presented at the International Society for Endovascular Interventions, Scottsdale, AZ, February 17.
16. Todd GJ, Nowygrod R, Benvenisty A, et al: The accuracy of CT scanning in the diagnosis of abdominal and thoracoabdominal aortic aneurysms, *J Vasc Surg* 13:302–310, 1991.
17. Salaman RA, Shandall A, Morgan RH, et al: Intravenous digital subtraction angiography versus computed tomography in the assessment of abdominal aortic aneurysm, *Br J Surg* 81:661–663, 1994.
18. Galanski M, Prokop M, Chavan A, et al: Renal arterial stenoses: spiral CT angiography, *Radiology* 189:185–192, 1993.
19. Kaatee R, Beek FJ, Verschuyl EJ, et al: Atherosclerotic renal artery stenosis: ostial or truncal? *Radiology* 199:637–640, 1996.
20. Rubin GD, Dake MD, Napel S, et al: Spiral CT of renal artery stenosis: comparison of three-dimensional rendering techniques, *Radiology* 190:181–189, 1994.
21. Costello P, Gaa J: Spiral CT angiography of abdominal aortic aneurysms, *Radiographics* 15:397–406, 1995.
22. Fillinger MF, Robbie PJ, McKenna MA, et al: The "virtual" graft: preoperative simulation of endovascular grafts using spiral CT with interactive three-dimensional reconstructions, *J Endovasc Surg* 4(suppl I):10, 1997.
23. Fillinger MF: Postoperative imaging after endovascular AAA repair, *Semin Vasc Surg* 12:327–338, 1999.
24. Rieker O, Düber C, Neufang A, et al: CT angiography versus intraarterial digital subtraction angiography for assessment of aortoiliac occlusive disease, *AJR Am J Roentgenol* 169:1133–1138, 1997.
25. Sato DT, Goff CD, Gregory RT, et al: Endoleak after aortic stent graft repair: diagnosis by color duplex ultrasound scan versus computed tomography scan, *J Vasc Surg* 28:657–663, 1998.
26. Thomas PR, Shaw JC, Ashton HA, et al: Accuracy of ultrasound in a screening programme for abdominal aortic aneurysms, *J Med Screen* 1:3–6, 1994.
27. Schurink GW, Aarts NJ, Wilde J, et al: Endoleakage after stent-graft treatment of abdominal aneurysm: implications on pressure and imaging—an in vitro study, *J Vasc Surg* 28:234–241, 1998.
28. Marty B, Sanchez LA, Ohki T, et al: Endoleak after endovascular graft repair of experimental aortic aneurysms: does coil embolization with angiographic "seal" lower intraaneurysmal pressure? *J Vasc Surg* 27:454–462, 1998.
29. Balm R, Kaatee R, Blankensteijn JD, et al: CT-angiography of abdominal aortic aneurysms after transfemoral endovascular aneurysm management, *Eur J Vasc Endovasc Surg* 12:182–188, 1996.
30. Umscheid T, Stelter WJ: Time-related alterations in shape, position, and structure of self-expanding, modular aortic stent-grafts: a 4-year single-center follow-up, *J Endovasc Surg* 6:17–32, 1999.
31. Fox AD, Whiteley MS, Murphy P, et al: Comparison of magnetic resonance imaging measurements of abdominal aortic aneurysms with measurements obtained by other imaging techniques and intraoperative measurements: possible implications for endovascular grafting, *J Vasc Surg* 24:632–638, 1996.
32. Wyers MC, Fillinger MF, Schermerhorn ML, et al: Endovascular repair of abdominal aortic aneurysm without preoperative arteriography, *J Vasc Surg* 38:730–738, 2003.
33. Fillinger MF, Racusin J, Baker RK, et al: Anatomic characteristics of ruptured abdominal aortic aneurysm on conventional CT scans: implications for rupture risk, *J Vasc Surg* 39:1243–1252, 2004.
34. Whittaker DR, Dwyer J, Fillinger MF: Prediction of altered graft path during endovascular abdominal aortic aneurysm repair, *J Vasc Surg* 41:575–583.

CHAPTER

18

Computed Tomographic Angiography in Peripheral Arterial Occlusive Disease

Nicolas A. Nelken

Ever since Moniz introduced the angiogram in 1927, a two-dimensional visual metaphor for the vascular system has been the foundation of vascular imaging. Thus far, angiography has been considered the "gold standard" of vascular imaging in spite of the fact that physiologic function depends on three-dimensional parameters (Poiseuille's law), only loosely associated with the two-dimensional representations. Vascular surgeons speak routinely of "diameter stenosis," an essentially one-dimensional concept, the physiologic consequence of which is dependent entirely on the assumption that stenoses are symmetric. We know of course that they are not. Diameter stenosis persists as a basic concept because many seminal and hard-to-duplicate randomized controlled trials have been performed with use of a diameter-stenosis standard that forms the foundation of much clinical decision-making (e.g., Asymptomatic Carotid Atherosclerosis Study, North American Symptomatic Carotid Endarterectomy, [NASCET]). Despite its problems, the explanation is that until now the resolution of angiography far exceeded that of any other modality. By comparison, duplex ultrasound depends primarily on functional physiologic parameters to complement the visual parameters seen well on angiograms. Although ultrasound physiologic data have been shown to be very accurate, vascular laboratory imaging itself is far inferior to angiographic imaging.

True three-dimensional data acquisition began with computed tomography (CT), which revolutionized medicine in the 1970s, culminating in the Nobel prize in medicine for Sir Godfrey Hounsfield (for whom the basic unit of radiopacity is named) and Dr. Allan Cormack in 1979. With subsequent generations of CT scanners, consistently more detailed data sets have become available. The improvements in cross-sectional imaging have developed hand-in-hand with vast improvements in computational power. Only recently has image quality advanced to the degree in which the information available through these methods rivals and complements that available with digital subtraction angiography (DSA).

CT angiography (CTA) used to be thought of as a sequence of contiguous axial images that were really *mentally* reconstructed into an understanding of vascular anatomy by the user. Today, however, high-speed workstations allow two-dimensional and three-dimensional reconstructions of isotropic (definition: having the same qualities in all directions) data sets. These sets are then postprocessed in almost any projection, with numerous different rendering protocols, each of which offers different diagnostic advantages. The data can be thought of as a three-dimensional cubic matrix to be explored by the clinician.[1]

Far more than just creating beautiful reconstructions, understanding the basis and importance of these projections and renderings has finally allowed quantum improvements in diagnostic power especially within the last few years.[2]

As an additional consequence of technologic power, some authors claim that CTA is now a relatively operator-independent study.[3,4] In fact, this is one of its purported advantages over DSA or duplex and sounds attractive to nonvascular specialists ordering tests. In-house CT technicians are easily trained to perform good-quality scans. As long as certain reliable protocols are followed, the data sets obtained will contain the information one is looking for. However, proper *display* of this vast amount of information in a format that is intuitive and understandable to the referring clinician is truly an art form and is far from operator independent. Improper projection can display information that is frankly misleading (as will be demonstrated in this chapter), and without specialized understanding of vascular disease a lot of information can be missed. Learning the basis of different projections and attendant artifacts is fundamental in understanding their meaning and assessing their accuracy. Nonetheless, universal perception that CTA is operator independent will certainly encourage its usage. Because of the expertise necessary to accurately analyze a complex study, some vascular surgeons have even made the converse argument that reading CTA studies should fall under the aegis of the vascular laboratory.[5] The financial implications of this aside, it is clear that the information obtained from these studies requires detailed understanding of vascular disease and a substantial time commitment; these are certainly not "operator-independent" studies.

This chapter is about the technologic foundations of CTA, understanding the basis of numerous projections and rendering protocols, and its current clinical uses.

HISTORY

The history of contemporary CTA really began with helical CT, which was a fundamental departure from the straightforward axial data sets of older CTs. Mathematically based three-dimensional reconstructions instead of simple axial slices allowed greatly increased plasticity of reconstruction. In helical CT, the patient moves continuously through the rotating gantry creating a "spiral" data set. Because "volumetric" data sets were created, this allowed overlapping reconstructions that improved resolution. There was no longer the limitation of a simple one-to-one relationship between detector size and slice thickness during reconstruction. Unfortunately, a single detector subtends such a small distance that in spite of increases in gantry rotation speed, contrast boluses small enough to be nontoxic outrun the gantry within about 30 to 40 cm, not to mention limitations in breath holding. This means that to obtain an angiogram from the distal thoracic aorta to the pedal arteries a single-detector CT scanner would require multiple boluses and acquisitions. The contrast dose notwithstanding, each subsequent acquisition would suffer from the previously injected and distributed contrast, which would opacify not only arteries but also veins and the tissues themselves. As gantry speeds reached their limitations, single-detector acquisitions were still far from adequate.

Technically, there is another problem with single-detector acquisition. Although the x-ray tube generates x-rays in all directions from its point source, only a small fraction of these emitted x-rays pass between the collimators. Estimates in the late 1990s demonstrated that approximately 5.5% of the total energy emitted by the tube passed through the collimators for a section thickness of 10 mm, and even less for thinner sections (the rest is wasted as heat). Therefore there were also physical limitations resulting from heat generation for long exposures. This created a trade-off of longitudinal resolution (z-axis) and scanning time. The solution was to create adjacent detector arrays that allowed the collimators to be opened wider with use of a larger proportion of the output of the tube. Therefore each rotation captures more simultaneous slices without any change in the generation of heat[6] (Figure 18-1). Generally, as the number of detectors increases, the thickness of each detector gets smaller, but there is not a linear relationship between the number of detectors in their size (range: 5 to 0.625 mm). There is, however, a considerably longer distance examined in a single rotation with larger numbers of detectors. Therefore longitudinal acquisition is far faster, and the bolus of contrast can be followed all the way from the thoracic aorta to the toes within the technical limitations of the tube. The current generation of 64-slice scanners is so fast that artificial means to slow down data acquisition are necessary not to outrun the bolus itself. Some scanners are even able to do duplicate acquisitions on a single contrast bolus, thereby giving some small measure of temporal information as well. Over the last 10 years there has been introduction of 2-, 4-, 8-, 16-, and 64-slice scanners (256-slice experimental scanners), each generation adding to the functionality of the one before. As is typical in periods of rapid technologic change, the literature evaluating these changes lags behind what is available in the marketplace. The most complete meta-analysis of comparisons between CTA and DSA was published in 2007 and does not even contain data from 64-detector scanners.[1]

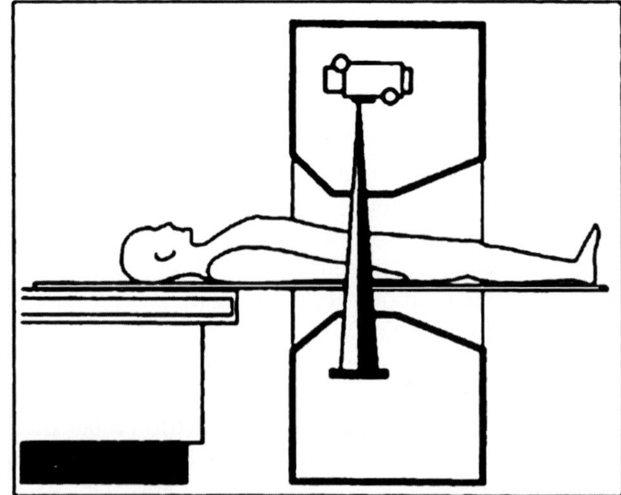

FIGURE 18-1 Cartoon demonstrating the effect of increasing the number of detectors on data acquisition in CT. *(From Weg N, Scheer MR, Gabor MP: Liver lesions: improved detection with dual-detector-array CT and routine 2.5-mm thin collimation,* Radiology *209:417-426, 1998.)*

TECHNICAL NOTES

Geoffrey Rubin of Stanford, one of the pioneers of multidetector CTA, declared back in 2003 that multidetector-row CT was "faster, longer, better" in comparison with single-slice CT.[7] Regarding "faster" and "longer," even in 2003 with four-detector—row scanners and 2.5-mm collimations, a distance of 1300 mm from the thoracic aorta to the feet could be covered in less than 70 seconds. As far as "better" is concerned, to quote Rubin, "We have not found one situation in which single-detector scanning would be better."

Isotropic data sets are basically three-dimensional cubic arrays. With thicker-sliced older CTs, the z-axis (length) data were substantially less detailed than the x-or y-axis data points. In other words, the length of the data elements in the z-axis was considerably longer than in the x or y axes. Multiplanar reformatting of older single-slice CT images therefore demonstrated considerable loss of detail and severe pixilation ("jaggies") compared with axial slices. The thinner slices associated with today's multidetector arrays allow true isotropic multiplanar reconstructions without loss of detail. With the processing speed of modern workstations, manipulation of these planes can occur in real time without angle restriction (Figure 18-2).

Each three-dimensional rendered data volume is called a voxel (a three-dimensional "pixel"). Contemporary machine acquisition protocols manipulate gantry rotation speed, pitch (P = Table feed/Collimation), and contrast bolus timing to create their data sets. As can be seen by looking at Figure 18-1, there is some parallax associated with covering the multidetector row from a single x-ray point source. This fact, and the overlap created by variation in pitch, are accounted for in the detailed reconstruction mathematics within the workstations. These complex mathematical reconstructions allow the creation of different-sized voxels even within the same data set. Typical modern studies can produce up to 5000 slices. The data sets associated with these huge studies are so large that not all departments are able to archive them all, and simplified data sets are sometimes kept long term. This requires that detailed reconstructions be performed by the radiologist acutely after the study is done and before archiving the smaller data sets.

CAPABILITIES OF MULTIDETECTOR SCANNERS

The last few years have seen very rapid development of generations of CT scanners. Each has its limits as described here.

Four detector: The thinnest effective section thickness is approximately 4 × 2 .5 mm (collimation). Image reconstruction however may allow slices as small as 1 to 2 mm to be examined as a result of overlap. Four-detector scanners generally do not support resolution good enough for very small arterial branches or tibial or pedal arteries unless the vessels are normal or unusually large and uncalcified. They are also too slow to follow a contrast bolus from the thoracic aorta to the feet in a single acquisition unless fairly thick 2.5-mm slices are obtained.

Eight detector (8 × 1.25-mm collimation): Longitudinal scan time is similar to that of a four-channel scanner, though resolution is better. High resolution as opposed to standard resolution imaging can be performed in limited ranges (1.25-mm thickness collimation, reconstructed at 0.8 mm). With increased gantry rotation speeds, however, this is about the smallest number of channels able to cover the entire vascular system in a single acquisition at the standard resolution of 2.5 mm.

Sixteen detector (16 × 1.25- to 16 × 1.5-mm collimation): Provides the same resolution as an eight-detector scanner but is substantially faster. Collimation is pretty much the same per detector as an eight-channel machine, but twice the distance is covered per revolution. Because 16-detector scanners are fast enough to the outrun the contrast bolus it is no longer necessary to choose maximum pitch or gantry rotation speed. At 16 channels limitations are determined by patient anatomy rather than machine capabilities. This is the least number of channels that allows a true isotropic data set. Configuration (16 × 1.25 mm) will easily allow full coverage from the thoracic aorta to the feet. Narrower slice acquisition time is again slower. At this level of detail, it may be expedient to reconstruct a lower resolution than the data set might allow depending on the power of the workstation or PACS unit (1.25 mm), permitting faster reconstruction and smaller files. The radiologist can always come back later if clinically necessary and reconstruct a high-resolution data set. Higher resolution data sets can paradoxically increase noise in the abdomen because of motion artifacts.

Sixty-four detector (64 × 0.6 mm or 64 × 0.625 mm): Pitch and gantry rotation speed control is necessary because of the potential for outrunning the contrast bolus. The maximum resolution is an amazing 0.6 mm spaced every 0.4 mm. These resolutions are best for patients with very advanced peripheral arterial occlusive disease, especially in the tibial and pedal arteries. Storage can be a problem because of the immense size of these files. Some institutions save less detailed 1.5- to 2-mm—thick images to PACS and only use the submillimeter sections for data viewing and selected permanent

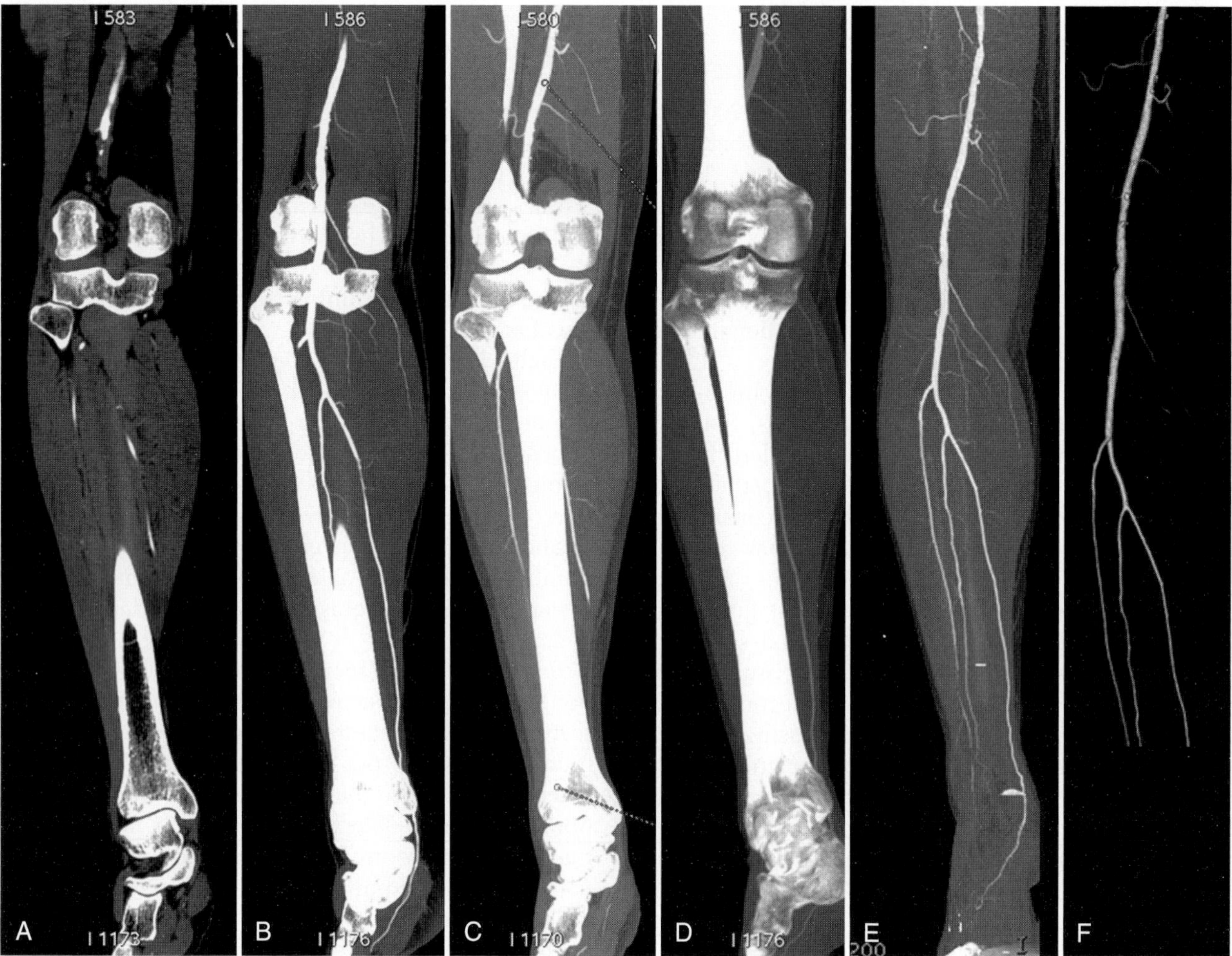

FIGURE 18-2 **A,** MPR represents a single plane of voxels, one voxel thick. It represents a true planar cross section. Vessels are seen only as they intersect with this plane. Isotropic data sets allow rendering of any chosen viewing angle. **B,** MIP, in this case a thin section of 1 cm. The highest intensity voxel represented by a "ray" pointed at the viewer within this thin "slice" is shown. Obviously bone density overshadows all other densities. Where the vessels can be seen without bone corresponds to areas in which there is no bone within the slice. **C,** MIP, 2 cm slice; bone is represented progressively more and the vessels hidden. **D,** MIP, full-thickness slice. This includes the entire volume of the lower extremity, but bone hides almost all vascular detail. **E,** MIP, full-thickness slice, with automatic removal of bone densities. The program removes calcium by complex algorithms related to Hounsfield units. Newer workstations also compute complex anatomic relationships related to contiguous structures to perform more complete bone removal. This projection is metaphorically the most like contrast DSA and is probably the most helpful for quick communication between clinicians. Advanced analysis, however, may be considerably more accurate with use of other projections. **F,** VR: three-dimensional reconstruction of vascular elements with bone subtracted.

reformatted images. Gantry rotation can be as fast as three rotations per second in the newer machines.

Compared with single-detector CT scans, multidetector scans often deliver more radiation. Nonetheless, the total radiation dose is only about 20% of the total dose of DSA.

ACQUISITION PROTOCOLS

A typical complete protocol includes five basic steps[3]:

1. *Topogram:* This is a quick initial scan projected in two dimensions and looks like a plain radiograph to determine the anatomic start and stop locations of subsequent runs. Programming of the subsequent acquisitions is done pictorially on these topograms.
2. *Nonenhanced acquisition:* This portion is especially useful in patients with a lot of calcification. Sometimes it is very important to compare the nonenhanced acquisition with the enhanced acquisition in specific areas under question, especially in situations with poor distribution of contrast resulting from proximal stenosis or occlusion.
3. *Test, or triggering, bolus:* A small bolus of contrast is given to establish "the contrast medium transit time" (the time between intravenous injection and arrival of

contrast in the aorta), usually between 12 and 40 seconds depending on the cardiovascular status of the patient. Some protocols allow manual timing of scan initiation, and others look for changes in attenuation in a defined region to automatically begin the scan. This initiating region is usually within the distal thoracic aorta for peripheral vascular studies. Further refinement of scan parameters can be achieved with a second timing bolus detected at the popliteal arteries to calculate transit times in the diseased segments. Peripheral atherosclerotic disease can make timing tricky because of overall delays in contrast circulation, as well as asymmetric filling resulting from specific occlusive patterns. The more complex the patient, the more useful a second timing bolus in the popliteal arteries will be. The aortopopliteal bolus transit time is quite variable (between 4 and 24 seconds). This corresponds with table speeds ranging from 29 mm/s to 177 mm/s. Given the spectacular processing power of today's workstations, timing is able to be adjusted for almost all circulatory problems. To minimize toxicity, the contrast bolus injection is scheduled to end 10 seconds before the end of the scan. Contrast injections between 80 and 140 mL are generally given at 3 to 5 mL/s. Biphasic injections even out the attenuation values in the aorta. To conserve contrast, a late saline chasing bolus improves contrast delivery at the tail end of the contrast bolus. Scanning too early leaves unopacified areas and too late results in opacification of the venous system and surrounding tissues. Needless to say, many different scan protocols are listed in the literature.

4. *Contrast acquisition:* This is the actual study individualized on the basis of the findings of the first three steps.
5. *Optional late-phase acquisition:* This either can be preprogrammed or can be conditional depending on whether there is adequate contrast filling at the end of the first acquisition. If conditional, the technician has to be very quick in identifying the need for a late-phase acquisition so that the machine can respond in time. Late-phase rescanning is useful in patients with very asymmetric disease resulting in large transit time differences between the lower extremities.

VIEWING

Current workstations offer a large menu of reconstruction options. Although somewhat bewildering at first, each projection has significant advantages and disadvantages that need to be understood properly. Although vascular imaging is primarily related to assessment of stenosis and occlusion, anatomic relationships can be viewed by CTA that are completely absent in DSA. Many proprietary workstations now exist for reformatting CT data, which are usually collected in a single universal data format called DICOM. Unfortunately, although DICOM is a standard, subtle differences in data management between companies exist that sometimes make translation difficult between different systems. The newest generations of scanners have proprietary workstations and software optimized for their own machines.

Two-Dimensional Reconstructions

Axial Sections

The number of slices produced by even a moderate contemporary study is much too large to be able to be represented on film. Workstation viewing or viewing over a PACS system is now the norm with use of a "page" system where each subsequent slice is viewed sequentially as if turning pages of a book. With very rapid image reconstruction, the slices can be examined back and forth. The skilled user can then reconstruct the anatomic relationships mentally. Rapid flipping between images allows conceptualization of longitudinal (z axis) findings, and each individual slice is examined for detail. Axial reconstruction may or may not be orthogonal or parallel to the vessels in question. Therefore assessments of degree of stenosis may be affected by obliquity. Axial sections are standard and are generally the first reconstructions brought up in any study. Because of the overlapping of acquisition slices, which depends on pitch and detector size, the size and thickness of the reconstructed axial images are not necessarily the same as those of the raw acquired images and can be manipulated on the basis of postprocessing parameters. (*Example*: M2S images are reconstructed in 1-mm increments even though 2.5-mm sections are usually sent.)

Multiplanar Reformatting

With a true isotropic system, a three-dimensional matrix of voxels can be created. Multiplanar reformatting (MPR) refers to the ability to manipulate the plane of view transecting this matrix. Workstations allow examination in any plane in real time (see Figure 18-2). Review planes are easily manually manipulated to examine structures at different angles, and this can be done "on the fly." Most MPR images are metaphorically considered thin sections that only represent the most superficial voxels. In other words each voxel can be considered opaque (one can only see the most superficial voxel in the plane). With respect to blood vessels, true longitudinal and true transverse sections are the most useful. Orthogonal, 90-degree transverse sections with respect to the center line are best for examining

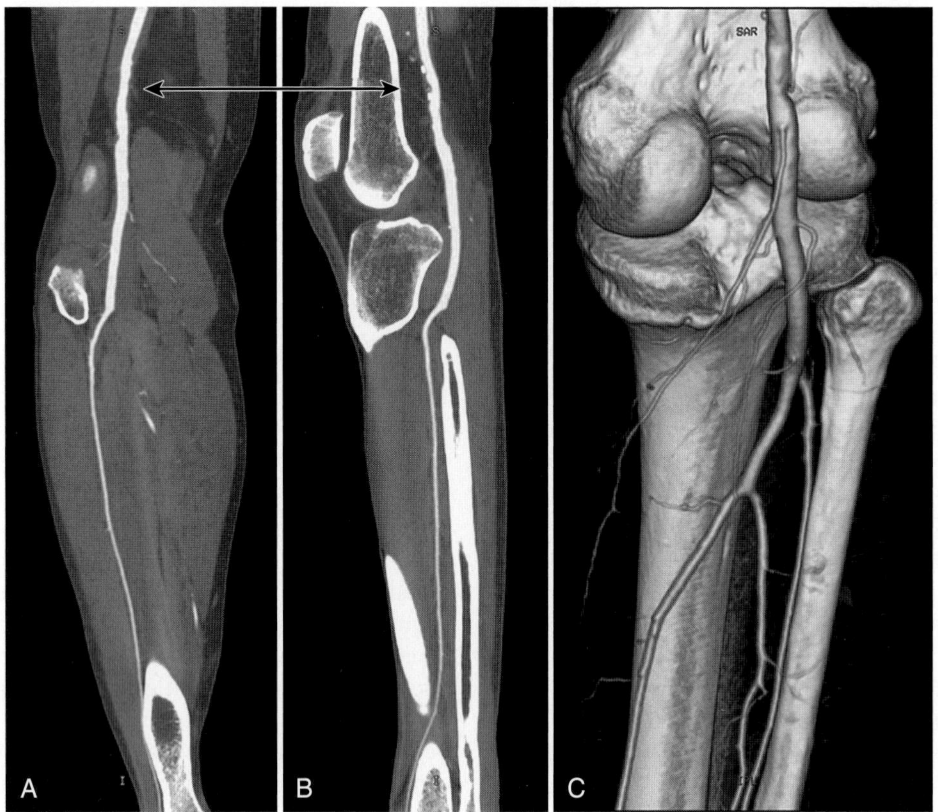

FIGURE 18-3 **A,** CPR. MPR is "warped" according to the centerline of the popliteal and anterior tibial arteries. This allows longitudinal views of arteries as they penetrate bony landmarks and allows views of vessels that might be obscured in MIPs. **B,** The same CPR as in **A** but from a different angle. Angles of view are important. Note the irregular thrombus visible in the above-the-knee popliteal artery in **B** that is not visible in **A** *(double-headed arrow).* **C,** Complex angled view of a VR of the same data set as **A** and **B** to demonstrate the anterior tibial artery penetrating the interosseus septum.

slice-by-slice stenosis measurements. Data show that true orthogonal transverse measurements of stenosis are the most accurate, but the angle of the each slice may be different from its nearest neighbor in a tortuous artery.[8] This may be very hard to do manually. True longitudinal segments are only useful insofar as a vessel is straight enough to be represented on a single plane, but very few actual blood vessels meet these criteria. In addition, because stenoses are rarely truly symmetric, even if a true longitudinal segment could be found, a different stenosis measurement would result depending on the rotation of the plane around the vessel centerline. This is akin to multiple gantry acquisitions in DSA, but in CTA it is possible to rapidly examine the full 360-degree rotation.

Curved Planar Reformatting

With these limitations in mind, it is possible to "bend" the planes represented in MPR (Figure 18-3). In vascular studies, these planar deformations are best related to the curvature of the vessel itself. The best way to anticipate the proper angle is to base these reformations on the centerline of the vessel. Numerous algorithms exist to calculate the centerline with various degrees of accuracy. Centerline calculations are subject to a whole host of artifacts. Ulcers, branching, and calcification can all affect centerline measurements. However, transverse curved planar reformatting (CPR) (90 degrees off the centerline) allows very accurate slice-by-slice evaluation of stenosis. Curved planar transverse reformations have been demonstrated to improve sensitivity and specificity over axial images compared with DSA. Ota et al.[9] noted an increased sensitivity from 89% to 97% and specificity from 96% to 100% in CPRs using a four-detector scanner. Transverse viewing also allows a detailed examination of the qualities of the plaque in very high-resolution images. Careful manipulation of the viewing window (essentially brightness and contrast but based on Hounsfield units) allows the best evaluation of plaque and lumen. With very calcified vessels this has to be done carefully. "Blooming" of high-density signals (calcification or stents) may artifactually display more stenosis than is actually present.[8]

Longitudinal CPR images can be produced parallel to centerlines (Figure 18-4, *C, D,* and *E*). In other words the plane of the image bends and follows the artery at each

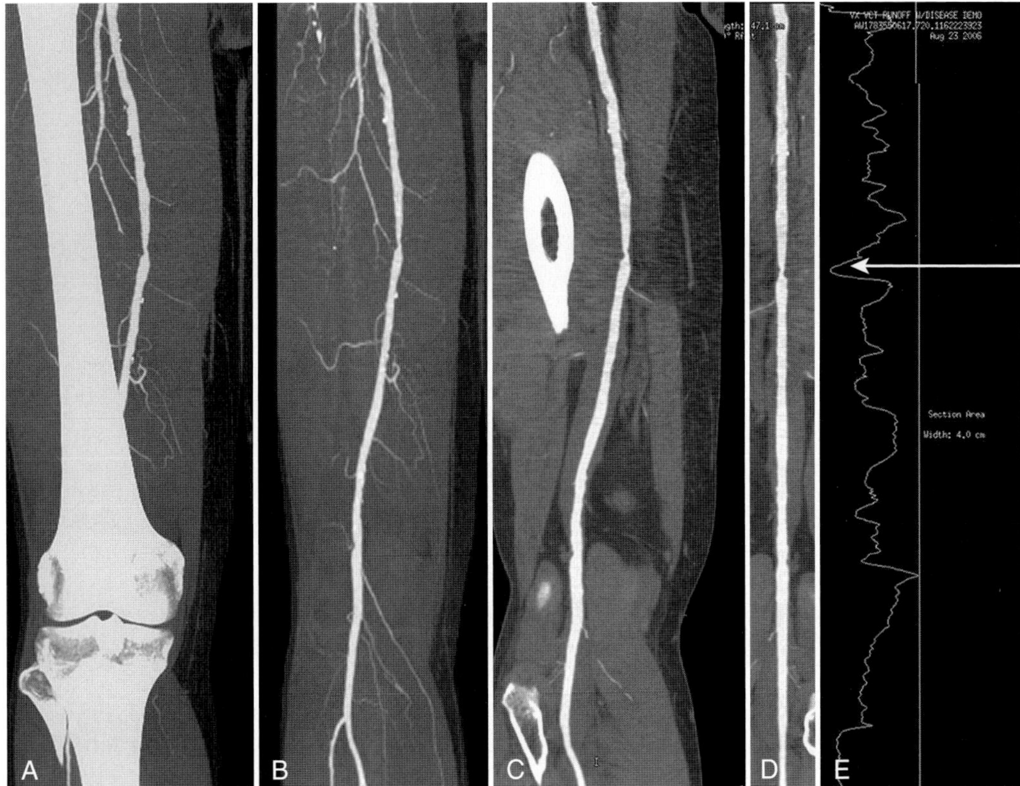

FIGURE 18-4 **A,** MIP without bone subtraction. **B,** MIP with bone subtraction. **C,** CPR image. Plane is "warped" in the plane of view. Note that below the knee the centerline follows the tibioperoneal trunk and not the anterior tibial artery. **D,** CPR image. Plane is "warped" symmetrically around the centerline of the vessel creating a straight-line representation of the vessel. Even this image can be viewed in 360 degrees of rotation. This rotation is sometimes necessary to view asymmetric stenoses. **E,** Longitudinal running calculation of the cross-sectional area of the vessel along the centerline shown in **D.** *Arrow* points to the level of the stenosis at Hunter's canal demonstrated in **A** through **E.**

point along the centerline. This projection is useful for finding the most stenotic segment of artery at a glance but may still need to be rotated about the centerline axis to find a projection that demonstrates the asymmetric stenosis most clearly (see Figure 18-3, *A,* and *B*). Longitudinal CPR projections are also very useful in eliminating the bone artifacts. A good example of this is evaluation of the anterior tibial artery from its origin through the interosseous membrane between the tibia and fibula (see Figure 18-5).

Maximum Intensity Projection

Maximum intensity projections (MIPs) are metaphorically very similar to DSAs. Instead of merely a plane, they can be thought of as a thick slice of partially transparent voxels through which imaginary rays are pointed at the viewer. In fact MIPs are somewhere between surface and volume rendering in concept. These rays are affected by the attenuation of each voxel along their path[1] (see Figure 18-2). MIPs represent the highest attenuation voxel along the path of each ray. As in DSA, the highest density structure within the path of the x-ray affects the image the most. The advantage of MIPs is that the projection is very much what most clinicians are used to seeing. They are flat projections that look like unsubtracted angiographic projections.[10] In heavily calcified or stented vessels, however, the lumen is impossible to see because the attenuation of the calcium is what is preferentially represented in the view (see Figure 18-5). Unlike angiograms, in which the ultimate attenuation is based on a sum of attenuation through the volume, because MIPs merely project the maximum attenuation along the path they really do not represent exactly the same thing. Bone also needs to be removed either manually or algorithmically from the chosen slice or it too will be represented in the projection obliterating the image of the lumen (see Figures 18-2 and 18-4, *A* and *B*). This may require substantial and time-consuming "slab editing" at the workstation to remove nearby high-attenuation tissues.

Because each pixel in the image represents the highest attenuation voxel in the slice, these images appear very flat. Three-dimensional structures are not well represented with MIPs although they can be rotated in real time on current workstations creating an illusion of depth. If there is opacification of venous and arterial structures together, they can appear to be in the same plane. Conversely, collateral networks and vessels are

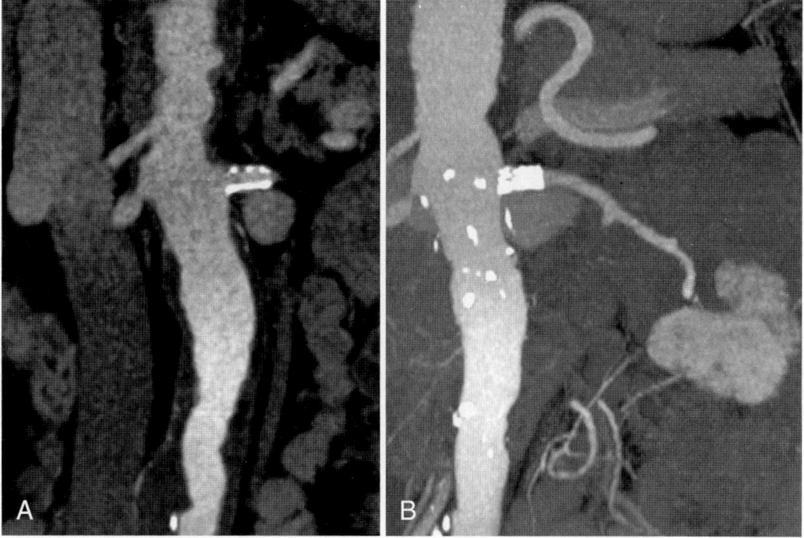

FIGURE 18-5 **A,** MPR image of a renal stent. The renal artery is only seen over a short distance because it leaves the plane of the image. However, the lumen can be seen within the stent. **B,** MIP image of a renal stent. Although the entire course of the renal artery is visible, the thickness of the slice obliterates one's ability to detect luminal diameter within the stent because density of the stent itself is projected over that of the lumen.

prominently displayed with MIPs. MIPs are very easy to produce in real time but need to be evaluated carefully.

Three-Dimensional Reconstructions

Much of the "wow factor" associated with CTA is related to spectacular images that appear to represent detailed anatomic dissections in three dimensions.[3,11] Careful evaluation of the construction of these images, however, reveals that all represented parameters are conscious choices.[1] Careless choices in reconstruction can provide very misleading images. Each rendering undergoes three basic steps:

1. *Volume formation:* Creating the three-dimensional volume, stacking of data slices, sizing the voxels, removing artifacts such as, for example, the CT table
2. *Classification:* Assignation of color and other visual properties to each voxel. This usually involves separating different tissue types on the basis of Hounsfield units (Figures 18-6 and 18-7).
3. *Image projection:* Two-dimensional display of three-dimensional data in a manner selected by the user.

In addition, three-dimensional rendering is basically performed in two separate ways, called surface rendering and volume rendering.

Surface Rendering (Binary)

This is essentially a threshold phenomenon.[8] Each voxel is assigned a Hounsfield value in three-dimensional space. Those voxels that exceed this assigned value (or threshold) are represented as opaque and those that do not are clear. The opaque voxels then define a shape that is shaded by applying virtual light and shading to the shape to make it easier and more intuitive to view. A surface is defined as the boundary between voxels of one tissue type (or density) and those of another. Surface rendering provides images that are basically monochromatic and reveal nothing about what is behind the opaque structures. By definition, threshold rendering is incompatible with volume averaging. And yet the interfaces between tissues of different attenuation that define these surfaces are precisely in the locations where volume averaging of voxels is likely to occur. This is the basis of much of the artifact obtained by surface rendering, which can include irregular shapes, "holes," and "floating fragments." Its detail is limited to an expression of the average attenuation within the volume of each voxel. Because opaque voxels hide information behind them, surface rendering is truly two-dimensional in spite of the way it looks, and it requires far less computational power than volume rendering (described next). Surface rendering used to be more popular when computational power was less than it is today.

Volume Rendering (Semitransparent)

Although superficially similar to surface rendering, volume rendering (VR) continuously represents the attributes of the entire data set in three dimensions.[8] As a result, computational demands are extremely high. Each voxel not only represents an average of its attenuation but is affected by its relation to its nearest neighbors. As a result, and because of overlapping acquisition slices, a more sophisticated representation can be made of structures in three dimensions. Overall rendering is not a strict threshold phenomenon anymore; there is actually more information in the data set than just an average value for each voxel. For example, if the voxel lies in the transition zone between one tissue, the density of which would be

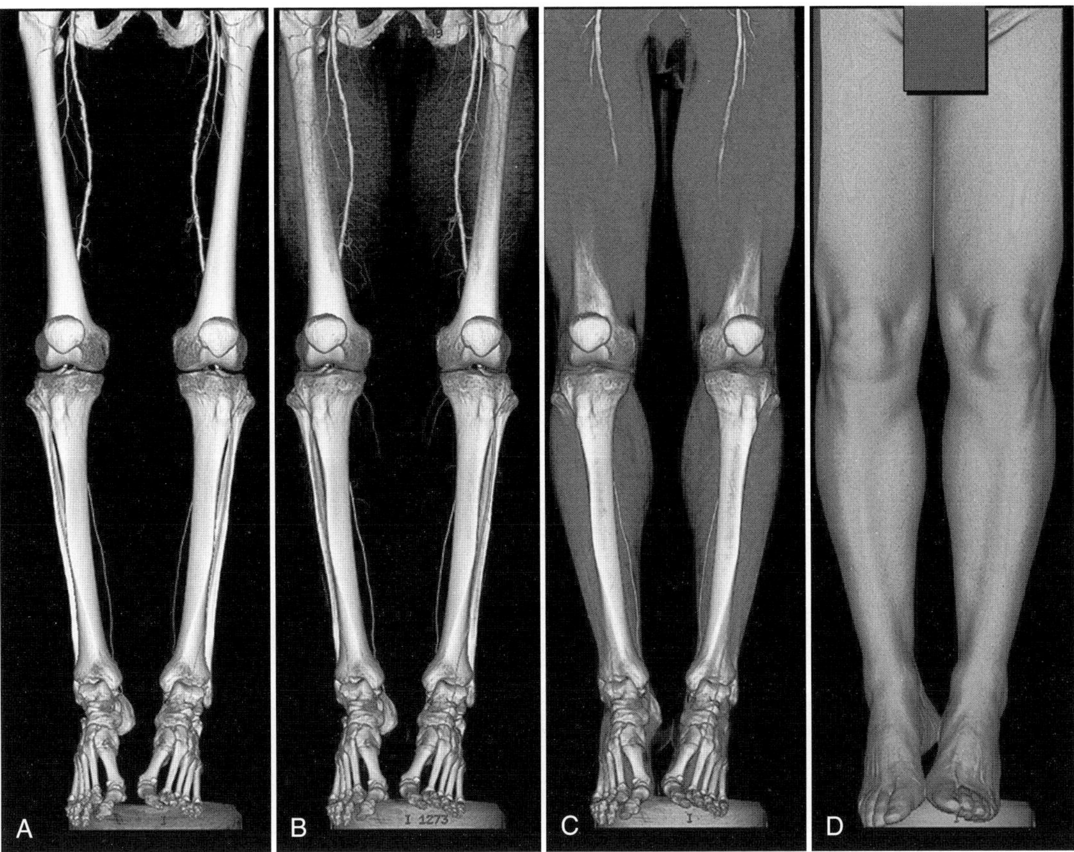

FIGURE 18-6 VR: progressive opacity of elements of decreasing density (Hounsfield units). Note that in these truly volume-rendered images, structures of higher density remain the same color and opacity throughout all the images but that progressive opacity of less-dense images is overlaid. Colors are assigned to different densities to make anatomic sense to the viewer (note bone, muscle, and skin). They can be arbitrarily assigned.

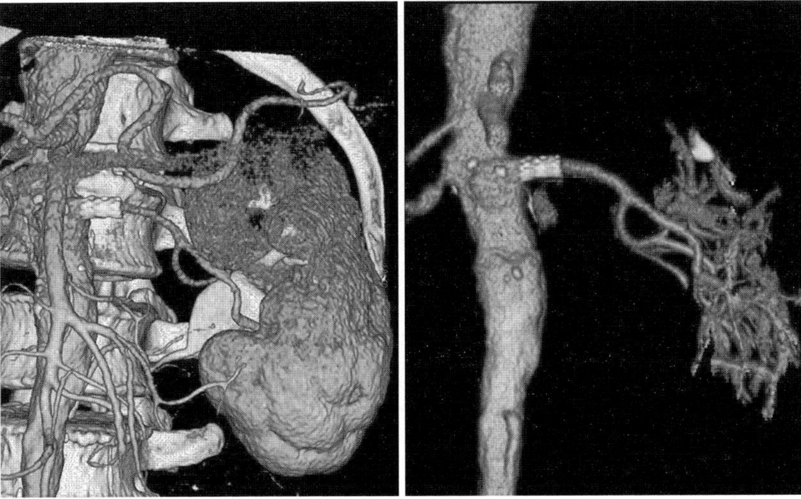

FIGURE 18-7 Two different VRs of the renal artery from the same data set. Newer algorithms allow structures to be "grown" from chosen data points to isolate different types of structures such as vessels, bones, and organs.

represented as white, and another, the density of which would be represented as red, the voxel in question would be represented in a specific pink hue that reflected the percentage contribution of each tissue type within that particular volume. In addition to color and shading, degrees of opacity can be determined to bring out or hide voxels with certain characteristics. Partial opacity allows true demonstration of the entire volume. The virtual light and shading are no longer just surface phenomena but also virtually penetrate three-dimensional structures depending on opacity.

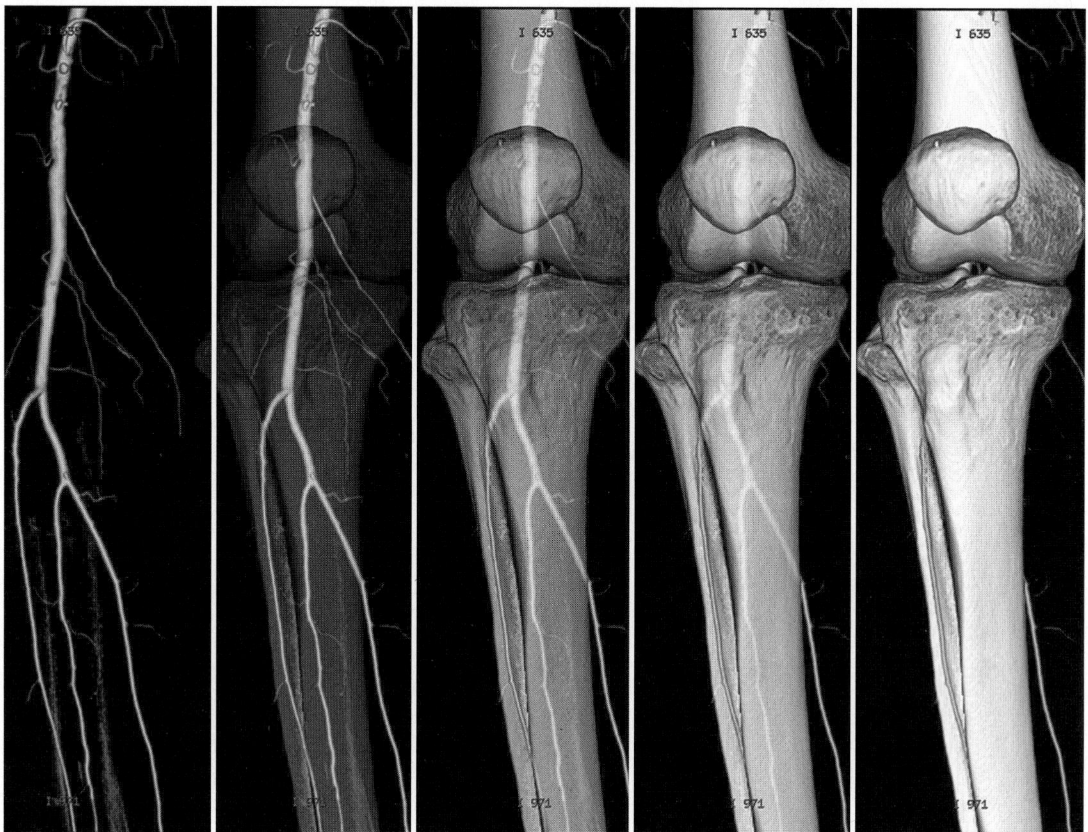

FIGURE 18-8 Progressive opacity of elements of bone density, keeping elements of vascular density the same. Note position of the anterior tibial and posterior tibial arteries with respect to the bony elements.

This degree of programmability is also useful for the removal of the bony structures (Figure 18-8). The attenuation of bone and calcifications is distinct from that of all other tissues. By describing the range of attenuation represented by bone, the bones can actually be removed from the reconstruction. Unfortunately, this also sometimes removes calcifications from reconstructions of the blood vessels. The bones can also be subtracted in the same way that DSA images are subtracted by comparing the precontrast and postcontrast images. Sophisticated programming also uses contiguity of structures to determine what is bone and what is calcification even though there is an overlap in density.

Additionally, there are numerous tools that allow clipping of images and examination of user-defined slices to eliminate irrelevant aspects of the scan.

Three-dimensional imaging is much more useful for planning approaches and understanding anatomic relationships than it is for calculating stenoses, where it can be frankly misleading. Rendered images are dependent on color and opacity determinations. These two qualities describe what is known as a "trapezoid" (defined as a continuum of these two orthogonal parameters), and it has been shown that this determination of the trapezoid strongly affects vascular lumen measurements because opacity can cause portions of rendered arteries to disappear (Figure 18-9).

Approach to Evaluating Computed Tomography Angiogram

"Volume visualization" is a term applied to the way that studies are clinically approached today. The entire case is approached as a "volume of information" to be reviewed as appropriate instead of going through individual two-dimensional images with selected multiplanar reconstructions.[8] It should be obvious from the preceding description that representation of the anatomy is heavily affected by choices. It should also be obvious that these reconstructions take time. Therefore at least one person in the radiology department needs to be heavily focused on CTA to properly use the immense capabilities of the current generation of scanners. In some high-volume centers this person can be a technician but obviously needs to be sophisticated and well supervised. Because this is a chapter for clinicians involved primarily in vascular intervention, and not primarily radiologists, it is unlikely that the reader is going to be making those choices (although I would highly recommend that you learn how). Especially in an environment

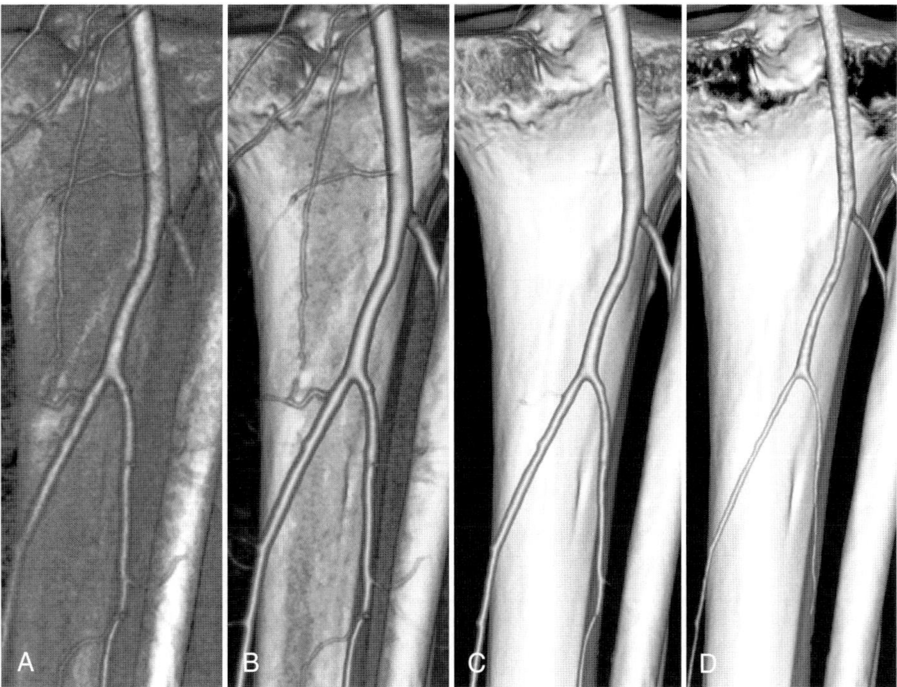

FIGURE 18-9 A-D, Successive changes in rendering parameters has the unintended effect of severely changing the size of the rendered vessel. Although VR is excellent in displaying anatomic relationships, it is not a reliable way to measure vascular diameters.

in which only a partial data set is archived, the relationship needs to be developed between the postprocessing radiologist and the vascular interventionist so that the most accurate and useful data are presented and understood before the detailed data are thrown out. Some form of local standardization is useful.

COMPARISONS BETWEEN MODALITIES

Digital Subtraction Angiography

DSA is the de facto gold standard of vascular imaging. Studies are therefore reported with respect to sensitivity, specificity, and accuracy compared with DSA. Although the detail of a DSA study is extremely high, we know that DSA is not a perfect representation of the anatomy. Therefore in spite of the fact that research comparisons use DSA as a statistical standard, there are clearly situations in which CTA is more accurate than DSA. The superiority of three-dimensional imaging has been shown before in other examples. Pan et al.[12] compared angiographic images with duplex and magnetic resonance angiography (MRA) using latex casts of explanted carotid artery specimens as a true standard. They showed as far back as 1995 that DSA was less accurate than both other modalities. The most obvious explanation relates to the fact that real stenoses tend to be irregular. The stenosis demonstrated on DSA depends on the angle of view. Orthogonal view DSA is often performed during carotid angiography but rarely done in any other situation. We know that iliac and common femoral plaque tends to be located on the posterior wall, and yet the usual anteroposterior (AP) and oblique DSA images frequently miss the contribution of these AP stenoses. These stenoses are revealed subtly by decreased opacity of dye column, something that is very hard to accurately measure. Because of the unlimited incident angles possible with CTA, a more faithful demonstration of stenosis is possible. The clinician just has to know to look for them. Vascular laboratory studies often do find stenoses that are hard to see on DSA, but it is likely that CTA will turn out to be more reliable in the pelvis.

Comparisons with DSA are complicated by the fact that they depend on the generation of CT scanner examined.[13-15] Refer to Tables 18-1 and 18-2 for sensitivity and specificity data in the literature.[13] More recent articles demonstrate sensitivities and specificities in the 90% to 95% range with very small interobserver variability.[14,16] In addition, comparisons usually take a histogram approach, comparing detection of (1) normal, (2) nonhemodynamically significant stenosis (<50%), (3) hemodynamically significant stenosis (50%-99%), and (4) occlusion, rather than finer distinctions.[17] Noncalcified vessels demonstrate considerably better agreement with DSA than heavily calcified vessels.[9]

TABLE 18-2 Pooled Estimates of Sensitivity and Specificity for Subdivisions of Arterial Tract of Lower Extremities*

Study and Year	Tract	Sensitivity (%)	Specificity (%)
Mesurolle et al, 2004 (19)	Aortoiliac	100 (18/18)	97 (29/30)
Portugaller et al, 2004 (21)	Aortoiliac	92 (24/26)	95 (212/224)
Willmann et al, 2005 (25)	Aortoiliac	95 (74/78)	98 (267/273)
Pooled results*		96 (92,100)	97 (94,99)
Mesurolle et al, 2004 (19)	Femoropopliteal	97 (31/32)	93 (55/59)
Portugaller et al, 2004 (21)	Femoropopliteal	98 (62/63)	70 (26/37)
Willmann et al, 2005 (25)	Femoral	98 (99/101)	94 (199/211)
Pooled results†		98 (96,100)	89 (80,98)
Mesurolle et al, 2004 (19)	Infrapopliteal	43 (3/7)	86 (19/22)
Portugaller et al, 2004 (21)	Infrapopliteal	90 (154/172)	74 (161/218)
Willmann et al, 2005 (25)	Popliteocrural	96 (177/184)	95 (494/518)
Pooled results†		90 (81,99)	85 (69,100)

From Heijenbrok-Kal MH, Kock MC, Hunink MG: Lower extremity arterial disease: multidetector CT angiography meta-analysis, Radiology *245:433-439, 2007.*
Note.—Except where indicated, numbers in parentheses are numbers of segments. Differences between the tract subdivisions were not statistically significant. Excellent sensitivity and specificity by region except in the infrapopliteal segments. The study by Mesurolle et al.[15] with 43% sensitivity and 86% specificity in the infrapopliteal region was done with a two-detector scanner and demonstrated considerably poorer results than Portugaller (four detector) and Willmann et al.[16] (16 detector) *(red box).* These differences were not apparent in the aortoiliac or femoropopliteal region.
* *Reference numbers are from the source of the table and are not included in this chapter.*
† *Numbers in parentheses are 95% CIs.*

Radiation

Numerous studies have shown that total radiation with CTA is considerably less than with DSA: radiation dose 1.6 to 3.9 mSv for CTA versus 6.4 to 16.0 mSv for DSA. On average there is four to five times less radiation than with DSA.[16]

Intervention

DSA allows simultaneous intervention, not usually possible with CTA. Depending on work flows, CTA may be completely unnecessary. In our practice, we performed diagnostic angiography at the same time as our interventions. We usually have duplex data and clinical history, which are enough to make a decision whether intervention should be attempted or not. The DSA is performed as part of the intervention. Very rarely do we perform DSA for diagnostic purposes only.[18] In the words of George Andros, "Angiography is a strategic, not a diagnostic study" (personal communication, 1995).

Contrast Use

Studies of CTA report between 80 and 180 mL of full-strength iodinated contrast. Routine DSA studies report contrast use within the same order of magnitude. This underscores a major difference in the way DSA is performed in the literature versus the way that it is performed in our practice. Most articles in the literature are interested in comparing the diagnostic accuracy of both studies compared side by side. In fact, by the time a "strategic" angiogram is obtained for the purpose of intervention, a full aortogram with runoff defining the entire vascular system is usually not even necessary because history and duplex have answered many of the questions already. We often performed targeted aortograms with runoffs using very dilute contrast (Visipaque diluted 1:5) with totals of only 15 to 20 mL of contrast (a philosophy that would rancor some radiologists). There is no question that the dilute contrast use would not stand up to a side-by-side comparison when looking at complete studies. These comparisons, however, are slightly artificial. A strategic angiogram with complex interventions, especially supplemented with carbon dioxide, can be done with less than 30 mL of contrast. The parameters of CTA, however, are pretty well defined in terms of contrast use. Use of lesser degrees of contrast produces attenuations of the lumen that are not separable from other tissues. Theoretically, subtraction techniques are possible, and perhaps more dilute boluses may be useful in the future using differences between the unenhanced and contrast-enhanced scans. Because of considerable time delays between the two separate scans, subtraction might be technically difficult, unlike DSA, in which the mask is subtracted from the same run.

Availability

Once the initial protocols have been verified in an institution, CT angiograms are much faster and more available than DSA. DSA requires a specialized team.

For this reason, they have become very popular in trauma surgery.[19]

Temporal Resolution

CTA provides very little temporal data. DSA and duplex are far better. The direction and timing of blood flow is very well demonstrated by DSA. For example, rapid filling of a profunda femoris with comparatively slower filling of the superficial femoral artery is circumstantial evidence of hemodynamically significant obstruction distal to the field of view, even if you cannot actually see where it is. CTA, however, takes views of arteries in which filling of contrast is already completed.

Occlusions

Conversely, the filling of open vessels immediately distal to an occlusion is better with CT angiograms than with DSA.[11] Demonstration and characterization of reentry sites distal to a chronic total occlusion may be better understood with CTA for this reason.

Cost

Although CT angiograms are far from cheap, they are far less expensive than DSA because of DSA's invasive nature, use of special procedure room, and recovery. CT angiograms are very fast and, once the patient is in the suite, can be completed in about 15 minutes without the need for recovery.

Viewing Angle

CT angiograms offer essentially unlimited viewing angles. Not only this, but changes in angles can be performed as a postprocessing function after the patient has gone home. DSA is dependent on understanding the anatomy at the time of the study. Although rotational angiography now exists with sophisticated three-dimensional reconstruction, its use is limited by large contrast requirements for each 16-inch stage.

Extravascular Structures

DSA provides essentially no direct information about extravascular structures. CT angiograms are very useful in imaging conditions such as popliteal entrapment or tumor compression.

Complication Rates

DSA complication rates are 1% to 2% (more depending on the complexity of the study) whereas CTA complication rates are very low. Really the only potential serious complication relates to contrast nephropathy or contrast allergy. Because contrast use in DSA and CTA are the same in the literature, this will be the same between modalities. Because we use far less contrast in our studies, we hope that our contrast nephropathy rates will be less than those in the literature. CTA is not a good study to perform in a patient with borderline renal function.

Magnetic Resonance Angiography

Artifacts from metallic stents and joint prostheses limit the usefulness of MRA. Patients with pacemakers are also not candidates for MRA. Contemporary CT angiogram voxels are smaller and more detailed than in MRA.[20] In addition, surrounding bony structures are not well seen on MRA. This can be a real drawback in cerebrovascular studies in helping decide between carotid endarterectomy versus stenting if that decision depends on the location of the stenosis. Similarly, calcifications and mural thickness are also not well seen on MRA. This may make the flow lumen easier to pick out from the surrounding vessel wall, but awareness of calcification is very important to procedural planning. Conversely, diffuse calcification may result in overestimation of the degree of stenosis with CTA especially if there is too much reliance on MIP images.[9] MRA also suffers from flow artifacts and venous overlay depending on the protocol used.

MRA also takes considerably longer to perform than multislice CTA; patient compliance is more of a problem with respect to motion artifacts and claustrophobia. With the recent advent of concern over contrast-induced nephrogenic fibrosing dermopathy associated with gadolinium, much of the advantage of MRA in patients with renal insufficiency has been lost.[21] CTA obviously delivers radiation, though the total amount delivered is better than DSA (see previous discussion).

DUPLEX

Duplex is very operator dependent. Most vascular specialists understand clearly which studies are done better than others within their own vascular laboratories and which technicians excel at which protocols. But duplex is also much less expensive than any of the other modalities. It delivers no harmful contrast or radiation doses as compared with all other modalities. Duplex is the least "anatomic" and the most "physiologic" of the vascular diagnostic studies. It is likely that CTA will decrease some use of the vascular laboratory as it becomes more popular, but those questions that duplex answers best are not well demonstrated by CTA. Turbulence, stenotic jets, and dynamics of flow in different parts of the cardiac cycle are all things that CTA is unable to assess. Duplex accuracy is considerably decreased in overweight patients, especially in the abdomen or pelvis. CTA is also easier to perform in patients in the immediate postoperative period because of the presence of bandages and local pain or tenderness. Shadowing from calcifications makes accurate

TABLE 18-1 Selected Characteristics of Included Studies*

Study and Year	No. of Sections	Section Thickness (mm)	Arterial Tract	No. of Patients†	Mean Patient Age (y)	Proportion of Men (%)	Sensitivity (%)‡	Specificity (%)‡
Puls et al, 2001 (16)	4	2.5	Aorta to ankles	31 (186)	53	55	89 (56/63)	86 (106/123)
Ofer et al, 2003 (5)	4	3.2	Superior mesenteric artery to pedal arteries	18 (410)	64	83	91 (110/121)	92 (267/289)
Heuschmid et al, 2003 (17)	4	3	Aorta to ankles	23 (568)	66	65	91 (136/149)	90 (379/419)
Martin et al, 2003 (6)	4	5	Celiac artery to toes	41 (1312)	67	68	90 (327/365)	94 (886/947)
Catalano et al, 2004 (18)	4	3	Diaphragm to feet	50 (1137)	67	78	99 (251/254)	97 (860/883)
Mesurolle et al, 2004 (19)	2	5	Celiac artery to 10 cm below trifurcation	16 (168)	64	88	91 (52/57)	93 (103/111)
Ota et al, 2004 (20)	4	2	L2 vertebra to calf	24 (470)	69	96	99 (121/122)	99 (345/348)
Portugaller et al, 2004 (21)	4	NR	Aorta to ankles	50 (740)	68	84	92 (240/261)	83 (399/479)
Bul et al, 2005 (22)	4	2	Celiac artery to toes	25 (718)	63	96	90 (159/177)	86 (466/541)
Edwards et al, 2005 (23)	4	3.2	Aorta to ankles	44 (1042)	68	68	79 (213/270)	93 (721/772)
Fraioll et al, 2005 (24)	4	3	Xiphoid process to feet	25 (475)	59	72	93 (55/59)	94 (393/416)
	4	3	Xiphoid process to feet	25 (475)	64	88	94 (47/50)	95 (405/425)
	4	3	Xiphoid process to feet	25 (475)	71	68	91 (60/66)	96 (392/409)
Willmann et al, 2005 (25)	16	0.75	Aorta to anides	39 (1365)	65	69	96 (350/363)	96 (960/1002)

From Heijenbrok-Kal MH, Kock MC, Hunink MG: Lower extremity arterial disease: multidetector CT angiography meta-analysis, Radiology *245:433-439, 2007.*

NOTE: The pooled sensitivity and specificity for all studies were 92% (95% confidence interval [CI]: 89%, 95%) and 93% (95% CI: 91%, 95%), respectively. NR = not reported. Although this table was published as recently as 2007 no 64-slice scanners were evaluated. Also notice that section thickness was large by today's standards.

* Reference numbers are from the source of the table and are not included in this chapter.

† Numbers in parentheses are the number of segments.

‡ Sensitivity and specificity were determined for the detection of a stenosis of 50% or greater. Numbers in parentheses are numbers of segments.

assessment of portions of the arterial lumen difficult with duplex, although calcium artifacts also obscure CT angiograms. Proper tracking of a contrast bolus, however, allows distinction between contrast enhancement and calcification based on Hounsfield units.

OTHER ISSUES

CTA may be an excellent modality for assessment of diseased bypass grafts, especially those within the abdomen and pelvis.[22] Indications for CTA of bypass grafts include

1. Is the graft in the correct location?
2. What extravascular structures may be compressing the graft?
3. Evaluation of anastomotic stenosis, made more accurate by multiplanar reformatting and true axial reconstructions
4. Is the graft at risk for rupture, and into what planes?
5. Is the graft infected? Axial images are superb at detecting air or pus.
6. Anatomic location of pseudoaneurysms to help plan repair

The advent of routine use of CTA means that the overall use of DSA will decrease. This will have training implications related to the fact that DSA will be reserved for more complex interventions, and the simple routine angiograms will slowly disappear. Therefore simulators will become an ever more important tool in the training of residents and fellows. Beginning one's career with complex cases runs the risk of increasing complication rates. It may also affect societal recommendations regarding interventional training. Already, the large number of diagnostic carotid arteriograms demanded by some societies runs counter to standard management of carotid disease with duplex and MRA.

CONCLUSION

CTA demonstrates excellent correlation with DSA in studies of older generations of scanners. These correlations will only strengthen as the technology improves. Although spectacular images are currently easily obtained with current-generation multislice CT scanners, understanding the strengths and weaknesses of a whole host of different projections and renderings is fundamental to critical and meaningful use of the technology. The richness of data available requires that the person reading the study be very well versed in vascular dynamics and that the clinician fully understand not only what the technology can tell about a vascular bed but also how it can lead one astray.

At stake in these studies may be the whole notion of a two-dimensional gold standard in a three-dimensional system. As real fluid systems are constrained by three-dimensional structures, imaging and then perhaps modeling may substantially change with the availability of high-resolution isotropic data sets. For numerous reasons, the data available with CTA may actually be better than angiography, but treatment decisions are currently based on a vast experience with DSA and will take some time to change just as the changes brought on by physiologic measurements in the vascular laboratory have changed practice in the last 30 years.

References

1. Fishman EK, Ney DR, Heath DG, et al: Volume rendering versus maximum intensity projection in CT angiography: what works best, when, and why, *Radiographics* 26:905–922, 2006.
2. Hiatt MD, Fleischmann D, Hellinger JC, Rubin GD: Angiographic imaging of the lower extremities with multidetector CT, *Radiol Clin North Am* 43:1119–1127, ix, 2005.
3. Fleischmann D, Hallett RL, Rubin GD: CT angiography of peripheral arterial disease, *J Vasc Interv Radiol* 17:3–26, 2006.
4. Duddalwar VA: Multislice CT angiography: a practical guide to CT angiography in vascular imaging and intervention, *Br J Radiol* 77(Spec No 1):S27–S38, 2004.
5. Dawson DL: Should we incorporate CT and MR angiography into our vascular laboratories? In *Western Vascular Society annual meeting*, Napa, CA, September 13–16, 2008, Silverado Resort.
6. Weg N, Scheer MR, Gabor MP: Liver lesions: improved detection with dual-detector-array CT and routine 2.5-mm thin collimation, *Radiology* 209:417–426, 1998.
7. Rubin GD: MDCT imaging of the aorta and peripheral vessels, *Eur J Radiol* 45(suppl 1):S42–49, 2003.
8. Lell MM, Anders K, Uder M, et al: New techniques in CT angiography, *Radiographics* 26(suppl. 1):S45–62, 2006.
9. Ota H, Takase K, Igarashi K, et al: MDCT compared with digital subtraction angiography for assessment of lower extremity arterial occlusive disease: importance of reviewing cross-sectional images, *AJR Am J Roentgenol* 182:201–209, 2004.
10. Kang PS, Spain JW: Multidetector CT angiography of the abdomen, *Radiol Clin North Am* 43:963–976, vii, 2005.
11. Chin AS, Rubin GD: CT angiography of peripheral arterial occlusive disease, *Tech Vasc Interv Radiol* 9:143–149, 2006.
12. Pan XM, Saloner D, Reilly LM, et al: Assessment of carotid artery stenosis by ultrasonography, conventional angiography, and magnetic resonance angiography: correlation with ex vivo measurement of plaque stenosis, *J Vasc Surg* 21:82–88, discussion 88–89, 1995.
13. Heijenbrok-Kal MH, Kock MC, Hunink MG: Lower extremity arterial disease: multidetector CT angiography meta-analysis, *Radiology* 245:433–439, 2007.
14. Sun Z: Diagnostic accuracy of multislice CT angiography in peripheral arterial disease, *J Vasc Interv Radiol* 17:1915–1921, 2006.
15. Mesurolle B, Qanadli SD, El Hajjam M, et al: Occlusive arterial disease of abdominal aorta and lower extremities: comparison of helical CT angiography with transcatheter angiography, *Clin Imaging* 28:252–260, 2004.
16. Willmann JK, Baumert B, Schertler T, et al: Aortoiliac and lower extremity arteries assessed with 16-detector row CT angiography: prospective comparison with digital subtraction angiography, *Radiology* 236:1083–1093, 2005.

17. Catalano C, Fraioli F, Laghi A, et al: Infrarenal aortic and lower-extremity arterial disease: diagnostic performance of multi-detector row CT angiography, *Radiology* 231:555–563, 2004.
18. Lookstein RA: Impact of CT angiography on endovascular therapy, *Mt Sinai J Med* 70:367–374, 2003.
19. Fleiter TR, Mervis S: The role of 3D-CTA in the assessment of peripheral vascular lesions in trauma patients, *Eur J Radiol* 64:92–102, 2007.
20. Prokop M: Multislice CT angiography, *Eur J Radiol* 36:86–96, 2000.
21. Canavese C, Mereu MC, Aime S, et al: Gadolinium-associated nephrogenic systemic fibrosis: the need for nephrologists' awareness, *J Nephrol* 21:324–336, 2008.
22. Toomay SM, Dolmatch BL: CT angiography of lower extremity vascular bypass grafts, *Tech Vasc Interv Radiol* 9:172–179, 2006.

CHAPTER

19

Magnetic Resonance Imaging and Angiography

Grace J. Wang, Harold Litt, Jeffrey P. Carpenter

As endovascular approaches to treating arterial lesions increase, the reliance on noninvasive preoperative imaging to guide therapy has also increased. Information garnered from preoperative evaluation helps to determine access strategy and avoidance of excessive fluoroscopy and contrast usage. Magnetic resonance angiography (MRA) has become an accepted mode for evaluation of renovascular and peripheral vascular disease because it has been demonstrated to be accurate, cost-effective, and simple to perform. As the technique of MRA has evolved, it is being used more and more for other pathologies as well, including carotid stenosis, thoracic and abdominal aneurysms, and aortic dissection. MRA and magnetic resonance venography (MRV) have also demonstrated usefulness in the evaluation of central venous thrombosis, deep venous thrombosis (DVT), mesenteric arterial and venous disease, thoracic outlet syndrome, potential renal donors, and postoperative transplant grafts. Even rarer diseases, such as large-vessel vasculitis, connective tissue disorders, and pulmonary arteriovenous malformations, can be accurately diagnosed and assessed by MRA. Additionally, MRA is noninvasive, uses a contrast medium that is nonnephrotoxic, and induces little allergic reaction. Although the discovery of the devastating disease process nephrogenic systemic fibrosis (NSF) linked to gadolinium exposure in patients with renal insufficiency has curbed enthusiasm for its use in the avoidance of nephrotoxicity, MRA will continue to be an important diagnostic modality for evaluating vascular disease, as well as an important adjunct for preprocedural planning.

MAGNETIC RESONANCE IMAGING TECHNIQUE

Magnetic resonance (MR) images are created by using an external magnetic field, magnetic field gradients, and an applied oscillating magnetic field known as the radiofrequency field (RF). Combining these three types of applied magnetic fields allows the production of signals from inside patients that can then be used to create MR images.

The contrast in MR images depends on the characteristics of the object being imaged, as well as the specifics of the sequence itself. Images are typically referred to as either T1 or T2 weighted. T2-weighted images display simple fluids such as urine, bile, or cerebrospinal fluid as bright and other tissues with lower signal. T2-weighted imaging is one of the basic sequences for tumor imaging but is not used for angiographic imaging. MRA and MRV examinations are performed with T1-weighted image sequences. Things that are bright on T1-weighted images are bright on MRA images as well, including fat, methemoglobin, flow effects, and MR imaging (MRI) contrast33.

MAGNETIC RESONANCE ANGIOGRAPHY AND MAGNETIC RESONANCE VENOGRAPHY

Noncontrast Magnetic Resonance Angiography

Contrast-enhanced methods have been favored because of their ability to achieve higher spatial resolution. However, the recent description of NSF in patients with poor renal function who have received gadolinium diethylenetriaminepentaacetic acid (DTPA) has led to a renewed interest in noncontrast techniques, such as time-of-flight (TOF) imaging.[1-5]

TOF angiography uses a rapid T1-weighted pulse sequence in sequentially acquired two-dimensional (2-D) slices or a three-dimensional (3-D) imaging slab. When data are gathered rapidly, the protons within the slice lose much of their magnetization. The rapid imaging does not degrade any protons outside of the slice, however. When the fully magnetized protons in a vessel flow into the slice of interest they produce more signal than the surrounding tissue. This results in an image where the blood flowing into the slice is bright and the surrounding tissue is relatively dark.

Recent developments in noncontrast MRA include steady state free procession (SSFP), arterial spin labeling (ASL), and half-Fourier fast spin-echo imaging (HASTE) with flow spoiled gradients. These techniques use combinations of different methods that accentuate the signal of flowing blood and attenuate the signal from nonmoving structures and tissue with signal characteristics different than blood. By applying additional pulses to null the signal from other tissue with bright signal, such as fat and simple fluid, images of the vessels can be obtained with high contrast. These techniques have the potential to replace contrast-enhanced MRA.

Contrast-Enhanced Magnetic Resonance Angiography

Currently, Food and Drug Administration (FDA)–approved MR contrast agents include variants of Gd-DTPA and Gd-BOPTA, in which the rare earth element gadolinium is chelated to another substance to avoid release of toxic free gadolinium into the body. These agents shorten the T1 signal of the protons in the local vicinity thereby making them more conspicuous on T1-weighted imaging sequences. Gadolinium-based contrast has decreased nephrotoxicity and a lower incidence of contrast reactions compared with standard agents used for arteriography.[6-10]

Step-Table Magnetic Resonance Angiography

When one is imaging the aorta or the lower extremity runoff, acquisition of data from the entire area of interest can be impractical and lead to decreased image quality. Step-table acquisition, in which portions of the anatomy of interest are imaged sequentially, can circumvent these issues. For example, a peripheral runoff study may include four step-table stations: abdomen/pelvis, thighs, calves, and feet.

Step-table MRA requires additional hardware, including a set of MRI coils for optimal imaging of each anatomic segment and (usually) optional software to control the automated table motion. A disadvantage of the step-table technique may be a longer total acquisition time, leading to venous contamination in the later stations.

Three-Dimensional Image Reconstruction

Contrast-enhanced MRA is performed as a 3-D imaging sequence. Three-dimensional imaging sequences are typically faster and have higher resolution than noncontrast angiograms. The higher resolution of 3-D methods allows for the use of multiplanar reformatting (MPR). MPR is a manipulation of the data to create images from multiple views that optimize the visualization of anatomy or pathology. Images can be processed with many types of algorithms to display the 3-D data to best advantage. Maximum intensity projection[11] (MIP) is the most commonly used algorithm for reconstructing 3-D MRA images. Volume rendering (VR) is another display method that has been developed and has been demonstrated to be equivalent or superior to MIP for both MRA and computed tomographic angiography of several vascular territories.[12-14]

CLINICAL APPLICATIONS OF MAGNETIC RESONANCE ANGIOGRAPHY

Renovascular Disease

Three-dimensional gadolinium-enhanced MRA has become a clinical standard for the evaluation of renovascular disease.[15] Additionally, MRI techniques offer the added benefit of soft tissue imaging so that concurrent assessment of renal size and coexisting parenchymal disease can be performed. It is most commonly used for the assessment of atherosclerotic renal artery stenosis. However, as MRA has matured, it has proved to be useful in evaluating more subtle renal vascular conditions such as fibromuscular dysplasia, renal artery aneurysms, and accessory renal arteries.[1] The detection of accessory arteries is particularly important for the assessment of potential living renal donors.[16-18]

Approximately 25% of the middle-aged white and African-American population in the United States have high blood pressure.[19] Renal artery stenosis is the most common cause of secondary hypertension, and approximately 1% of those people with hypertension will have renal artery stenosis.[20] Because renal artery stenosis is potentially curable,[21-23] it is critical that appropriate screening tests exist for those at risk. Three-dimensional contrast-enhanced MRA has a sensitivity of 94% and a specificity of 93%.[1] In addition, it has been shown that when MRA is used to plan a renal artery intervention both the number of pretreatment angiograms and the total amount of contrast were reduced.[24]

As shown in Figure 19-1, the majority of renal artery stenoses are in the ostial segments of the renal arteries.[25] As methods for 3-D contrast-enhanced MRA have improved, diseases that are not typically near the renal artery origin have been more commonly diagnosed by MRA. These include fibromuscular dysplasia[26,27] shown in Figure 19-2.

Accessory renal arteries occur in nearly 45% of cases,[28] and their diagnoses can be important in screening candidates for renal donation.[16-18] MRI and MRA have been shown to be a very cost-effective method of evaluating potential renal donors.[29]

Peripheral Vascular Disease

MRA has become a standard method of evaluation for peripheral vascular disease.[30] The prevalence is approximately 3% in those greater than 55 years of age but increases to 11% for those over 65 years and up to as high as 20% for those over 70 years of age.[31] MRA has been demonstrated to be effective in the preoperative evaluation of patients[32,33] with peripheral vascular disease including imaging the inflow vessels[33] and evaluating any stenoses[34] as shown in Figure 19-3. The sensitivity of detecting hemodynamically significant stenoses is 99.5% and the specificity is 98.8% when compared with digital subtraction angiography (DSA).[34] In addition, MRA has been shown to be effective in imaging suitable target vessels including vessels not seen by conventional catheter angiography.[34,35] MRA is also a cost-effective method to evaluate a patient with peripheral vascular disease.[36]

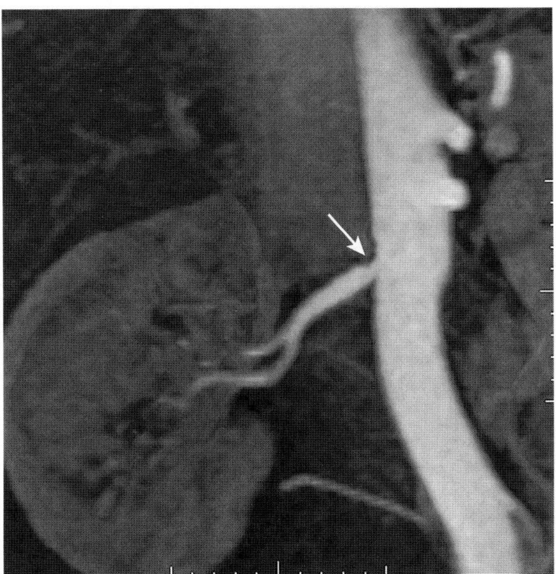

FIGURE 19-1 Coronal 3-D MRA showing an ostial renal artery plaque *(white arrow).*

As MR technology develops, MRA evaluation of peripheral vascular disease continues to improve.[36-39] Stepping table examinations have increased the speed and resolution of the examination. This has allowed for improved visualization of smaller distal vessels, as well as dedicated arterial phase imaging of the feet. As mentioned previously, MRA has been shown to be superior to DSA in the evaluation of distal vessels in some cases.[34,35] A study in 37 patients indicated that MRA depicts significantly more vascular segments in the foot than DSA (p ~0.0001).[39]

In addition to the value of MRA for diagnosis and pretreatment planning, MRA may be used in the evaluation of patients after therapy.[40-42] The normal appearance of a femoral-to-popliteal bypass graft is shown in Figure 19-4. MRA can be used to assess graft patency and stenosis. Figure 19-5 demonstrates narrowing at the distal end of a femoral-to-popliteal bypass graft. MRA is also a powerful technique to demonstrate complications of graft placement such as pseudoaneurysm formation. Even very small grafts with very distal touchdown points can be evaluated with MRA, as shown in Figure 19-6.

Carotid Vascular Disease

MRA is becoming an increasingly used method of evaluating carotid artery atherosclerosis. For a stenosis

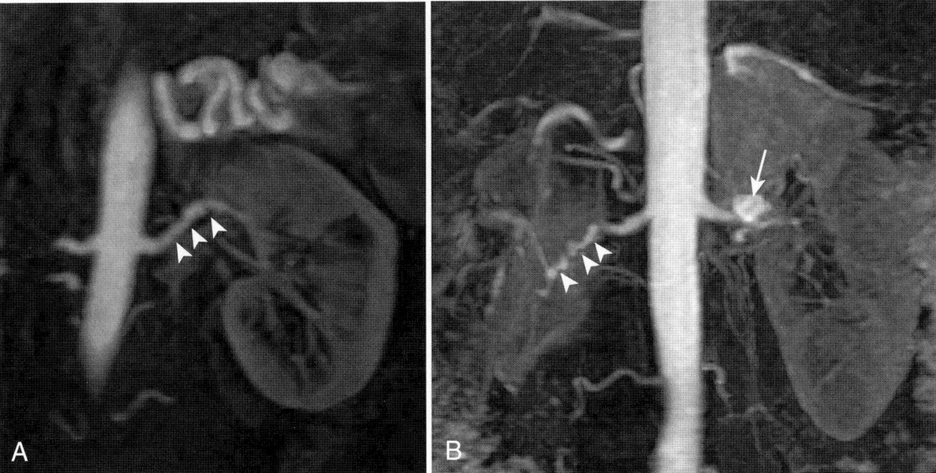

FIGURE 19-2 **A,** Coronal 3-D MRA showing subtle fibromuscular dysplasia *(white arrowheads).* Note that the disease is isolated to the distal portion of the main renal artery. **B,** Coronal 3-D MRA showing right-sided fibromuscular dysplasia *(white arrowheads)* and a left-sided renal artery aneurysm *(white arrow).* Renal artery aneurysms may occur in patients with fibromuscular dysplasia.

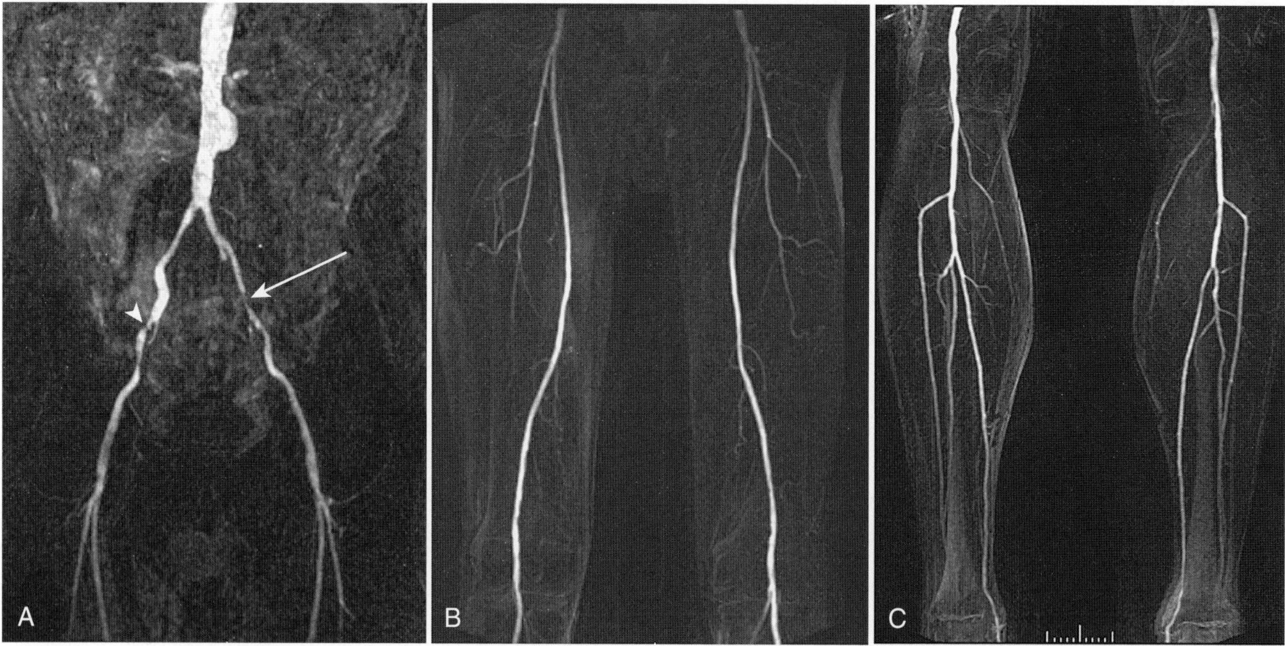

FIGURE 19-3 Coronal 3-D MRA step-table examination showing bilateral iliac disease **(A)** within the right external (*white arrowhead*) and left external *(white arrow)* iliac arteries. Note the excellent detail in the thigh **(B)** and calf **(C)** stations of the examination.

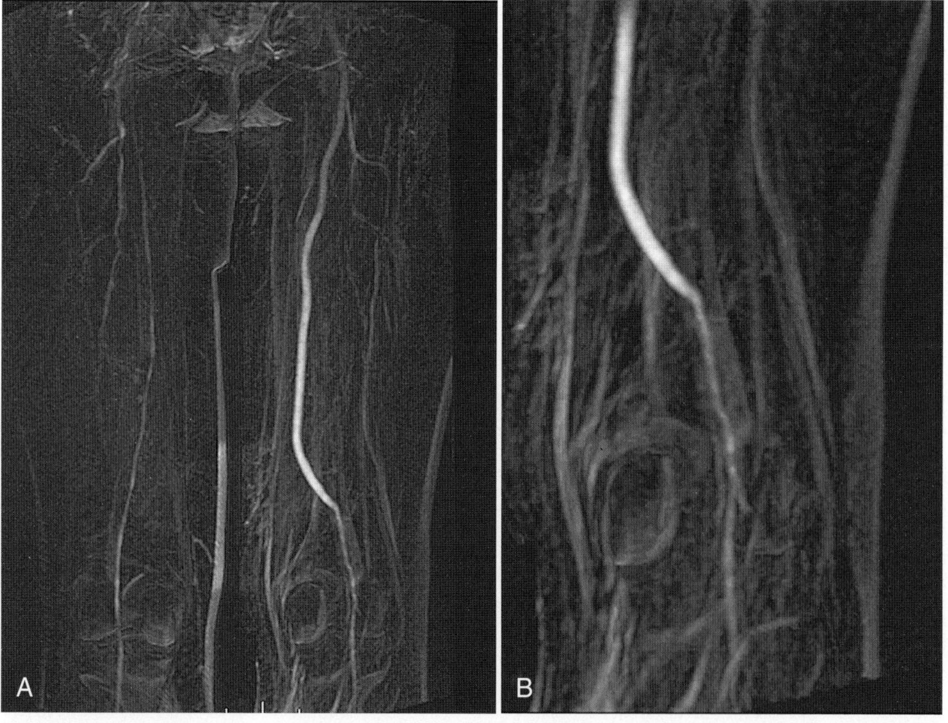

FIGURE 19-4 **A,** Coronal 3-D MRA thigh station of a femoral-to-popliteal bypass graft. Note the contralateral disease of the superficial femoral artery. **B,** An oblique reformatted image shows the normal touchdown of the graft.

with 70% to 99% narrowing, MRA has a reported sensitivity of 95% and a specificity of 90%.[43] For all stenoses MRA has a reported sensitivity of 98% and a specificity of 86%.[44] Several authors conclude that the performance of MRA warrants its use as a tool to plan operative or interventional revascularization.[45,46] A 3-D MRA of the carotid and vertebral arteries is shown in Figure 19-7.

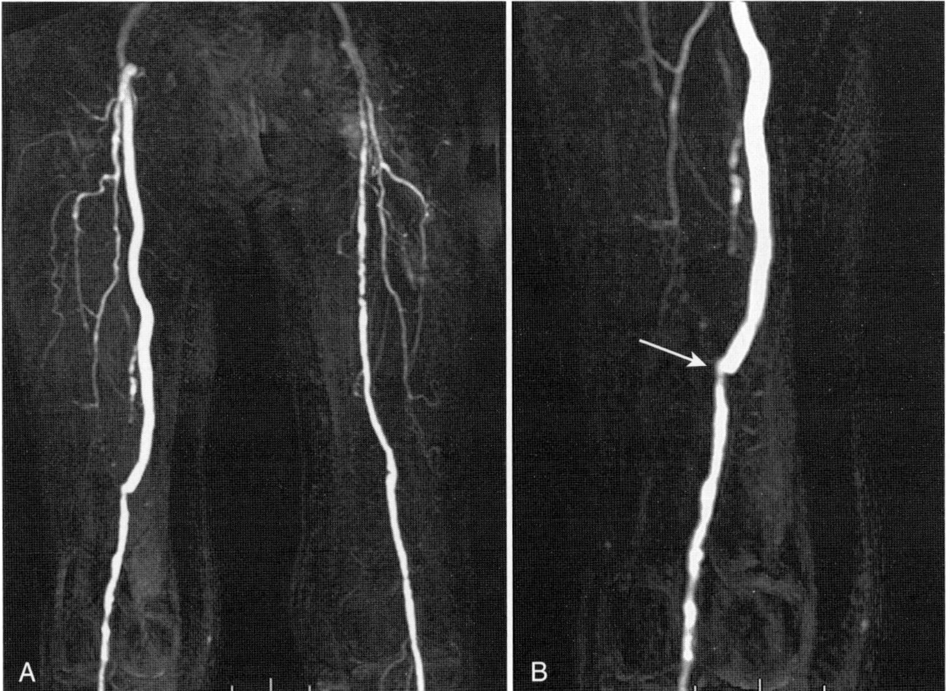

FIGURE 19-5 **A,** Coronal 3-D MRA thigh station of a femoral-to-popliteal bypass graft. Note the contralateral disease of the superficial femoral artery. **B,** An oblique reformatted image shows the narrowing at the touchdown of the graft *(white arrow).*

Aortic Vascular Disease

Contrast-enhanced 3-D MRA has been used to assess the aorta in patients with many different aortic pathologies.[47-50] The evaluation of the aortic arch by contrast-enhanced MRA may be superior to that of any other technique.[51] See Figure 19-8. Other diseases that are routinely evaluated by MRA at some centers include aortic dissection[47,52-54] as shown in Figure 19-9 and aneurysms.[47] MRA has also been used for the evaluation of patients with connective tissue disorders,[55] preoperative assessment for aortic stent graft placement,[56,57] and detection of endoleak in patients after aortic stent graft placement.[58,59]

Dynamic MRA is a technique that has recently been introduced as a more appropriate modality for the assessment of aortic remodeling after stent-graft repair.[60] By timing image acquisition with the cardiac cycle, differences in pulsatile aortic distension along different axes can be determined. These data will be important in assessing the durability of endovascular stent graft repair of aneurysms, as well as providing information for future endograft design.

Mesenteric Vascular Disease

The most common use of MRA to evaluate mesenteric vascular disease is in the evaluation of patients with suspected intestinal angina or chronic mesenteric ischemia.[61] MRA is 95% and 97% accurate for characterizing proximal disease of the superior mesenteric artery[62] in cases of chronic mesenteric ischemia.

MRA is also useful to evaluate more complex diseases of the mesenteric vasculature. The median arcuate ligament originates anteriorly from the aorta at the T12 level. During end expiration, the ligament can compress the proximal portion of the celiac axis, which can lead to a false impression of proximal celiac stenosis. MRA can be useful to demonstrate the effect of the arcuate ligament during a single examination.[88]

MRV is also useful in detecting mesenteric venous thrombosis and has been suggested as a superior method to mesenteric catheter angiography.[63] Figure 19-10 shows the portal vein, splenic vein, superior mesenteric vein, and inferior mesenteric venous branches occluded with thrombus.

Venous Vascular Disease

MRV is a powerful technique to evaluate both central[64,65] and deep[66-68] venous structures. Central venous structures, in particular the superior vena cava, can be evaluated with 3-D methods with 100% sensitivity for the detection of thrombus compared with DSA.[65] MRV was also able to demonstrate DVT in 20% of patients with a pelvic DVT and negative results on ultrasound examination.[67]

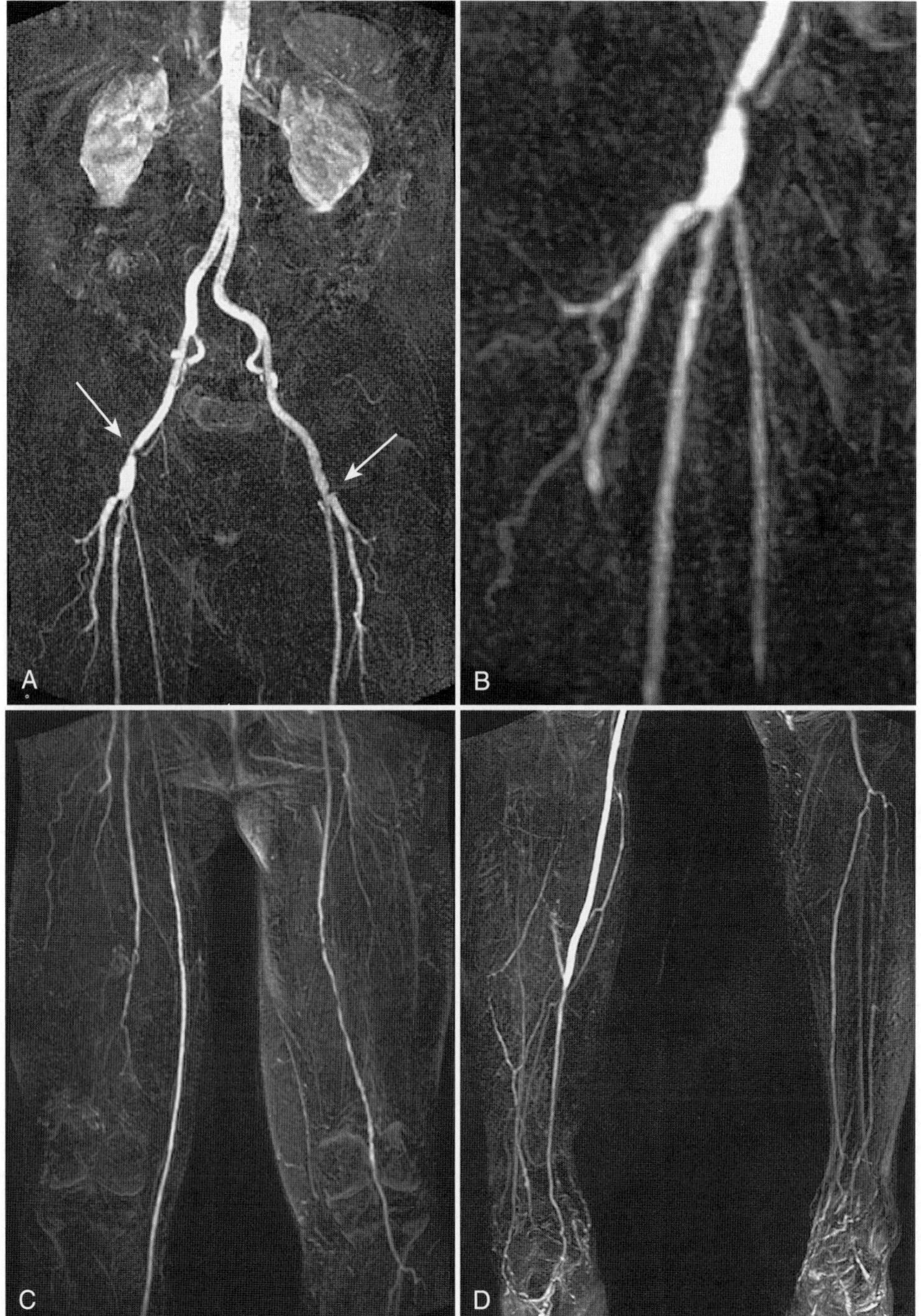

FIGURE 19-6 **A,** Coronal 3-D MRA showing bilateral common femoral disease *(white arrows)*. The origin of a right saphenous vein graft is seen. **B,** An oblique reformatted image shows the origin of the graft and disease in the distal common femoral. **C,** Coronal 3-D MRA thigh station showing the course of the vein graft. **D,** Coronal 3-D MRA calf station showing the touchdown of the graft on the posterior tibialis artery.

See Figure 19-11 for a depiction of inferior vena cava (IVC) thrombus.

Other Applications

MRA can be used to assess a variety of vascular pathologies. It can be performed to evaluate patients with suspected thoracic outlet syndrome if the appropriate image sequences can be combined with maneuvers to elicit the symptoms.[69] MRA is also useful for the assessment of potential renal donors.[16-18] After surgery, it can be useful in the assessment of suspected failure of the arterial or venous anastomoses of the transplant graft.[5,70] Less-common diseases such as large vessel vasculitis, as well as the response to therapy, can also be assessed via MRA.[71] Pulmonary arteriovenous malformations

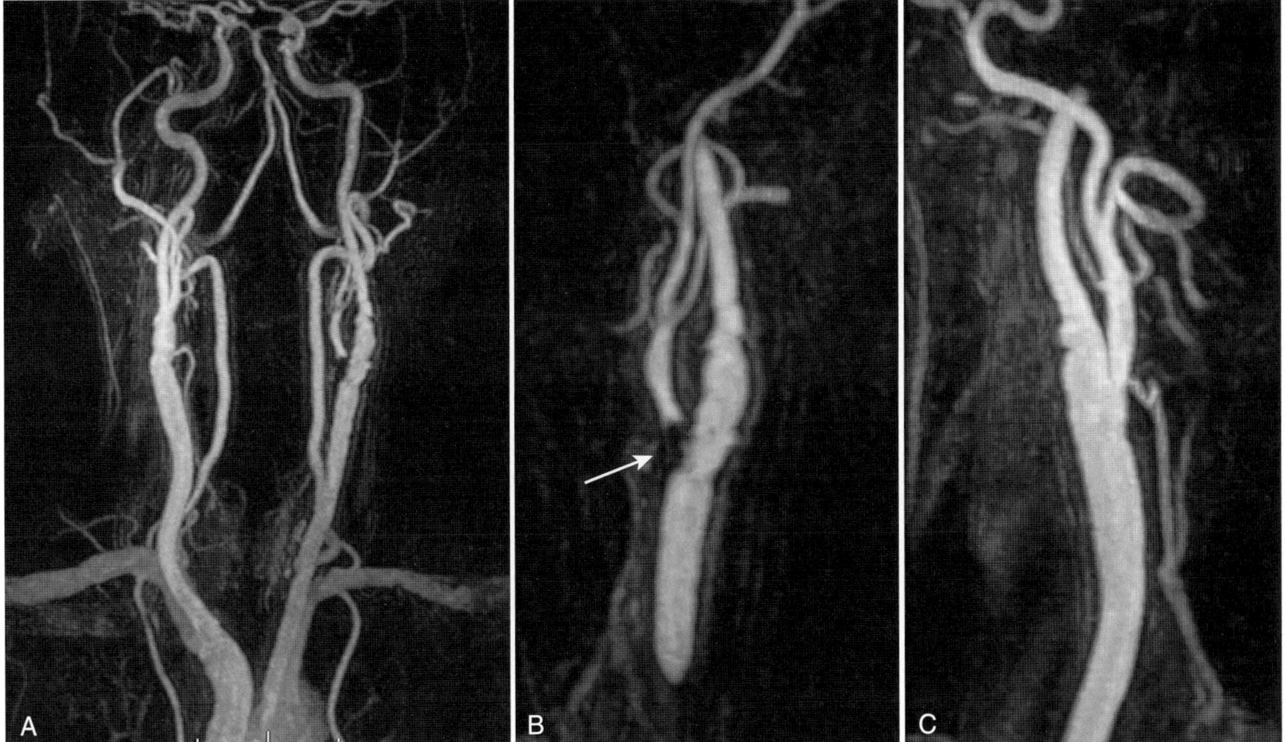

FIGURE 19-7 **A,** Coronal 3-D MRA of the carotid and vertebral arteries. **B,** Oblique sagittal reformatted MRA showing the high-grade narrowing (*arrow*) at the origin of the left external carotid artery and mild disease of the left internal carotid artery. **C,** Oblique sagittal reformatted MRA showing the right carotid bifurcation with only mild disease in the proximal right internal carotid.

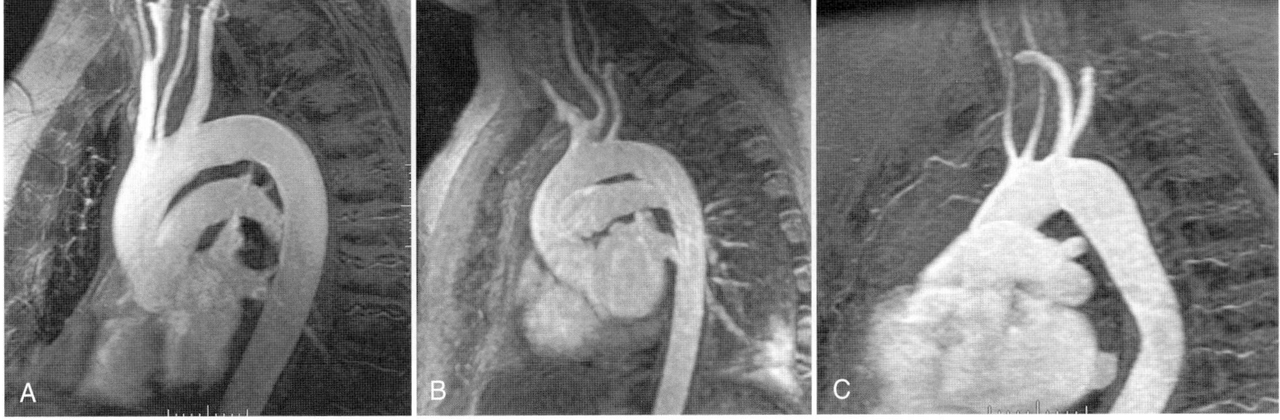

FIGURE 19-8 **A,** Sagittal oblique reformatted MRA of a normal aortic arch. **B,** Sagittal oblique reformatted MRA of a bovine arch. **C,** Sagittal oblique reformatted image of a very rare arch anomaly, bicarotid truncus. All four vessels arise separately from the arch. The carotids arise anteriorly and the subclavians posteriorly.

and their feeding arteries and veins can also be characterized.[72,73]

LIMITATIONS OF MAGNETIC RESONANCE

There are several common artifacts and/or pitfalls associated with MRA. Knowledge of these limitations is important in interpreting MRA results.

Fat Saturation in Chest Magnetic Resonance Angiography

Suppressing the signal from fat may be advantageous, because fat will have high signal on the T1-weighted images used for MRA. Within the chest, there are intravascular water protons in blood vessels that are adjacent to the lung. When the resonance frequency of the water protons shifts to the same range where fat protons resonate, fat suppression will result in

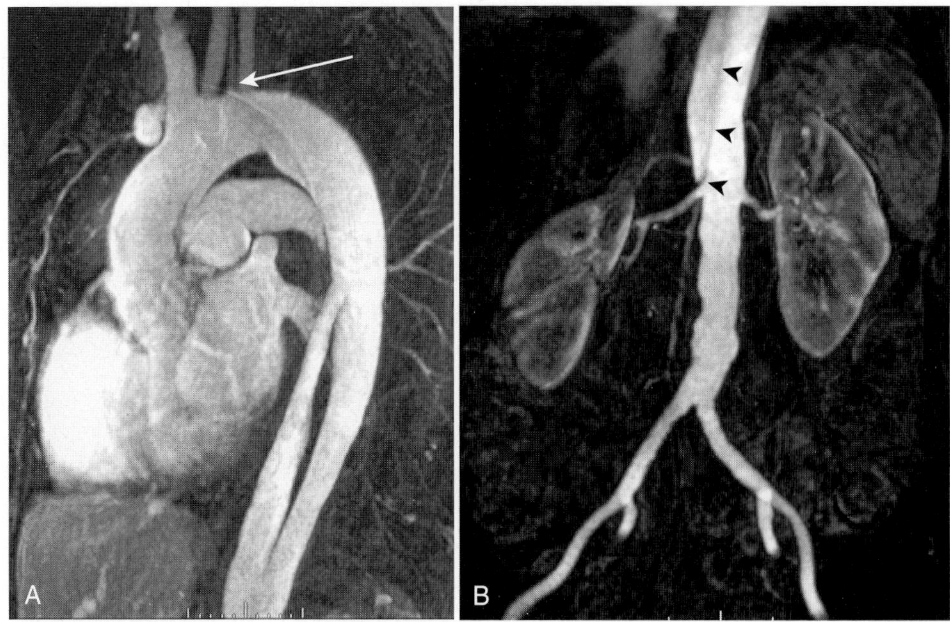

FIGURE 19-9 **A,** Sagittal oblique reformatted MRA showing a type B dissection. The origin of the flap and filling of the proximal false lumen are seen. A separate origin of the left vertebral artery is seen from the aortic arch *(white arrow).* **B,** Coronal 3-D MRA obtained during the same examination as the chest station with use of step-table technique. The dissection flap *(black arrowheads)* terminates just above the origin of the right renal artery.

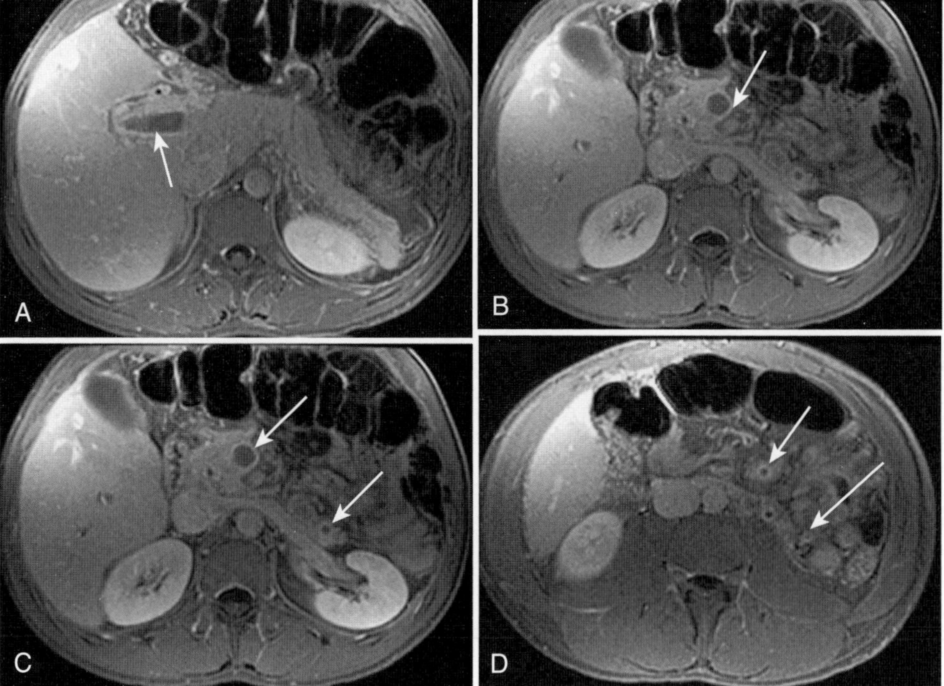

FIGURE 19-10 **A,** 2-D T1-weighted postcontrast MRI showing portal venous thrombus *(white arrow).* **B,** 2-D T1-weighted postcontrast MRI showing splenic venous thrombosis *(white arrow).* **C,** 2-D T1-weighted postcontrast MRI showing superior mesenteric vein (SMV) and inferior mesenteric vein (IMV) thrombus *(white arrows).* **D,** 2-D T1-weighted postcontrast MRI showing small distal branches of the SMV and IMV filled with thrombus *(white arrows).*

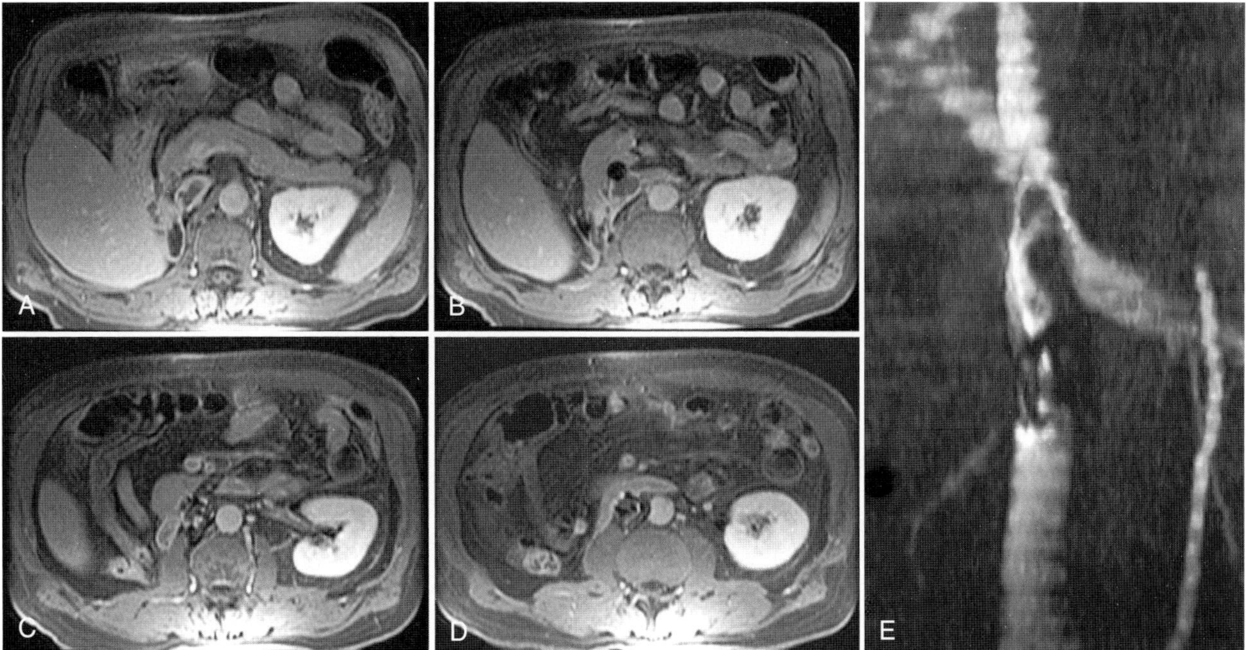

FIGURE 19-11 **A-D,** 2-D T1-weighted postcontrast MRI showing IVC thrombus in and superior to an IVC filter. **E,** Coronal MIP of the corresponding stack of 2-D TOF images again showing the IVC filter below the left renal vein and the thrombus as a filling defect in the flow extending superiorly.

suppression of the water signal instead.[74] Thus a vessel that is patent may appear occluded or a vessel that is occluded may not be accurately assessed.

Susceptibility Artifact From Concentrated Gadolinium

At high concentrations, MR contrast behaves like a metallic object and produces an artifact on surrounding tissues. These concentrations occur during the injection of pure contrast and are seen at the origin of the great vessels[75] or in the subclavian artery during initial passage of injected contrast through the adjacent vein.[76] If artifact is suspected to be the cause of an apparent stenosis, repeating the sequence immediately should demonstrate resolution, as contrast in the adjacent vein becomes more dilute.

High Intravascular Signal From Thrombus Containing Methemoglobin

The appearance of thrombus varies depending on both the redox state of the hemoglobin molecule and the integrity of the red blood cell wall. At a certain state in its evolution, clotted blood will pass through a state of either intracellular or extracellular methemoglobin. This state typically occurs in the subacute phase (1-14 days) of a blood clot.[77] When the clot contains large amounts of methemoglobin, the signal may be high on T1-weighted images, which can mimic intravascular contrast. Precontrast T1-weighted imaging in these cases can be used to identify thrombus.

CONTRAINDICATIONS TO MAGNETIC RESONANCE IMAGING

Nephrogenic Systemic Fibrosis

Gadolinium-containing contrast agents have long been regarded as safer for patients with impaired renal function, because they were associated with a lower incidence of contrast-induced nephropathy (CIN) than iodinated contrast at the doses used for clinical imaging.[78,79] Later studies showed that very high doses of gadolinium might be associated with CIN.[80-82]

NSF, previously known as nephrogenic fibrosing dermopathy (NFD), is a disease with primarily dermatologic manifestations, although findings in other organs have now been reported.[83-85] NSF is characterized by thickening of the skin and hyperpigmentation of the extremities and trunk. Patients with more severe involvement may have systemic manifestations including organ fibrosis affecting the heart, kidney, and liver, in some cases leading to death. All reported cases have occurred in patients with renal insufficiency, primarily in those with chronic renal failure, although cases have been described in acute renal failure, particularly in association with hepatorenal syndrome or liver transplantation.[86] There is no specific treatment for NSF other than improving kidney function through kidney transplantation, although steroids and other anti-inflammatory treatments have been used, along with hemodialysis and photopheresis.[87-90]

Although the first cases of NSF were described in 2000,[91] a possible association between NSF and exposure of patients with renal insufficiency to gadolinium-containing contrast agents was not proposed until 2006, when five cases were reported in a cohort of dialysis patients who had undergone MRA.[92] Since that time, several hundred cases have been reported, in patients both receiving and not receiving dialysis.[93] Predisposing factors include metabolic acidosis, receiving a larger dose of gadolinium contrast agent, repeated contrast-enhanced studies, proinflammatory conditions, and recent vascular procedures, including surgery. All but five documented cases of NSF have been in patients exposed to gadolinium contrast agents, and thus far there have been no documented cases of NSF in patients with normal renal function. In those with normal renal function, gadolinium agents are cleared rapidly by the kidneys, but residence time may be increased 100-fold in those with markedly impaired renal function. It is currently unknown whether repeated exposure to gadolinium agents could induce NSF even in those with normal renal function,[93-95] but the histologic finding of gadolinium deposition in affected tissues supports the mechanism, as does the association with proinflammatory states.[96] An estimate of the glomerular filtration rate to guide the clinician's decision to use contrast-enhanced MRA can be obtained from the Modified Diet in Renal Disease Study Group equation.[97]

Pacemakers and Implanted Devices

The degree of safety is ensured by maintaining the appropriate environment around the magnet and through careful screening of the patients. There are a number of implanted metallic devices that are not safe in or near an MRI magnet. These include implanted pumps or neurostimulators, cochlear implants, and some intracranial aneurysm clips. One should review reference books,[98] published articles,[99] and websites[100] before considering MRI for a patient with an implanted device.

Implanted pacemakers and defibrillators had long been considered absolute contraindications to MRI[101]; however, several recent studies have demonstrated that some patients with pacemakers and defibrillators can be imaged safely under carefully controlled conditions. The risks in imaging patients with pacemakers or defibrillators include patient- and device-related complications, although the factor of greatest concern is whether the patient's underlying cardiac rhythm would be able to tolerate the pacemaker ceasing to function while in the magnet, where immediate treatment may be more difficult. In general, factors that entail greater risk include a pacemaker-dependent patient, pacemaker generator implanted before 2000 (some older models appear more susceptible to an electrical reset to default parameters while in the magnet), presence of an implantable cardioverter defibrillator (ICD), and inclusion of the pacemaker/ICD generator and/or leads in the RF field.

Vascular Stents, Filters, and Coils

The majority of implantable vascular stents, filters, and coils have been shown to be "MR safe" or, with use of terminology developed by the American Society for Testing and Materials International, "MRI conditional,"[100] that is, they are not subject to significant forces when placed inside the magnet and have been demonstrated to pose no known hazards. One exception is the Zenith AAA stent graft system (Cook Medical, Bloomington, IN), which is made of stainless steel, has been shown to be subject to significant forces in in vitro testing, and is therefore characterized as MR unsafe.[100] This stent has not been systematically studied in vivo; however, retrospective results from a small cohort of 11 patients with Zenith stent grafts who underwent a total of 20 MR examinations (including 10 of the abdomen, pelvis, or spine) reported no ill effects.[102]

IVC filters and vascular embolization coils are composed of either nonferromagnetic alloys such as nitinol or weakly ferromagnetic stainless steel. Neither of these materials is subject to significant force when exposed to MRI, and all IVC filters tested are classified as MRI safe or conditional. As with stents, device manufacturers recommend waiting up to 8 weeks after device placement before performing MRI, because this is thought to be the amount of time needed for stable incorporation into the vessel wall; however, there are no specific data to justify this policy. Stents, filters, and coils composed of nonferromagnetic materials may be safely imaged immediately after placement. For weakly ferromagnetic devices, the decision to perform MRI within 6 to 8 weeks after placement should be accompanied by consideration of the potential risks versus the benefits of the information that the study will provide.[103]

NEW ADVANCES IN MAGNETIC RESONANCE TECHNOLOGY

Three-Tesla Magnetic Resonance Angiography

MR systems with magnets up to 3 tesla (3 T) are now FDA approved. Use of a 3-T magnet can result in increased spatial resolution or decreased time in image acquisition. Preliminary studies have shown improved image quality and accuracy of 3-T MRA compared with 1.5 T for imaging of the renal, carotid, and supra-aortic arteries.

Plaque Imaging

MRA enables one to visualize arterial stenoses caused by atherosclerotic disease. MRI provides information regarding the soft tissue characteristics of the atherosclerotic plaque. There are several methods available for plaque imaging, including noncontrast techniques, the use of gadolinium DTPA and other typical contrast agents, and imaging with contrast agents that concentrate specifically in atherosclerotic plaque.[104-108]

Carotid plaque has been the subject of many imaging investigations. Multispectral imaging, which combines information from sequences with T1, T2, and proton density weighting, has allowed discrimination of the various components of carotid atherosclerotic plaques, including the lipid core and fibrous cap, and distinction between necrotic, calcified, and hemorrhagic plaques.[104]

Contrast-enhanced imaging has also been used to quantify the degree of neovascularity of an atherosclerotic plaque, which may be related to vulnerability or likelihood of rupture. Currently under development are MR molecular imaging agents that specifically bind to components of atherosclerotic plaque or vessel walls, such as integrins.[109]

SUMMARY

MRA is an accepted mode of evaluation of a diverse set of vascular and cardiovascular diseases. Paralleling the growing need for accurate preoperative assessment, MRA technique has evolved, offering better special resolution and faster data acquisition. In the era of aortic stent grafts, coronary stents, and defibrillators, physicians should review potential adverse events before ordering MRI/MRA. Contrast-based MRA should likewise be ordered with caution in patients with renal insufficiency.

References

1. Tan KT, van Beek EJ, Brown PW, et al: Magnetic resonance angiography for the diagnosis of renal artery stenosis: a meta-analysis, *Clin Radiol* 57:617–624, 2002.
2. Meaney JF: Magnetic resonance angiography of the peripheral arteries: current status, *Eur Radiol* 13:836–852, 2003.
3. Hood MN, Ho VB, Foo TK, et al: High-resolution gadolinium-enhanced 3D MRA of the infrapopliteal arteries: lessons for improving bolus-chase peripheral MRA, *Magn Reson Imaging* 20:543–549, 2002.
4. Sharafuddin MJ, Stolpen AH, Sun S, et al: High-resolution multiphase contrast-enhanced three-dimensional MR angiography compared with two-dimensional time-of-flight MR angiography for the identification of pedal vessels, *J Vasc Interv Radiol* 13:695–702, 2002.
5. Johnson DB, Lerner CA, Prince MR, et al: Gadolinium-enhanced magnetic resonance angiography of renal transplants, *Magn Reson Imaging* 15:13–20, 1997.
6. Spinosa DJ, Angle JF, Hartwell GD, et al: Gadolinium-based contrast agents in angiography and interventional radiology, *Radiol Clin North Am* 40:693–710, 2002.
7. Srodon P, Matson M, Ham R: Contrast nephropathy in lower limb angiography, *Ann R Coll Surg Engl* 85:187–191, 2003.
8. Rieger J, Sitter T, Toepfer M, et al: Gadolinium as an alternative contrast agent for diagnostic and interventional angiographic procedures in patients with impaired renal function, *Nephrol Dial Transplant* 17:824–828, 2002.
9. Freed KS, Leder RA, Alexander C, et al: Breakthrough adverse reactions to low-osmolar contrast media after steroid premedication, *AJR Am J Roentgenol* 176:1389–1392, 2001.
10. Lieberman PL, Seigle RL: Reactions to radiocontrast material: anaphylactoid events in radiology, *Clin Rev Allergy Immunol* 17:469–496, 1999.
11. Sun Y, Parker DL: Performance analysis of maximum intensity projection algorithm for display of MRA images, *IEEE Trans Med Imaging* 18:1154–1169, 1999.
12. Persson A, Brismar TB, Lundström C, Dahlström N, Othberg F, Smedby O: Standardized volume rendering for magnetic resonance angiography measurements in the abdominal aorta, *Acta Radiol* 47(2):172–178, 2006 Mar.
13. Smedby O, Oberg R, Asberg B, et al: Standardized volume-rendering of contrast-enhanced renal magnetic resonance angiography, *Acta Radiol* 46(5):497–504, 2005 Aug.
14. Vogt FM, Ajaj W, Hunold P, Herborn CU, Quick HH, Debatin JF, Ruehm SG: Venous compression at high-spatial-resolution three-dimensional MR angiography of peripheral arteries, *Radiology* 233(3):913–920, 2004 Dec.
15. Marcos HB, Choyke PL: Magnetic resonance angiography of the kidney, *Semin Nephrol* 20(5):450–455, 2000.
16. Hussain SM, Kock MC, Jzermans JN, et al: MR imaging: a "one-stop shop" modality for preoperative evaluation of potential living kidney donors, *Radiographics* 23:505–520, 2003.
17. Israel GM, Lee VS, Edye M, et al: Comprehensive MR imaging in the preoperative evaluation of living donor candidates for laparoscopic nephrectomy: initial experience, *Radiology* 225: 427–432, 2002.
18. Monroy-Cuadros M, McLaughlin K, Salazar A, et al: Assessment of live kidney donors by magnetic resonance angiography: reliability and impact on outcomes, *Clin Transplant* 22(1):29–34, 2008 Jan-Feb.
19. He J, Klag MJ, Appel LJ, et al: Seven-year incidence of hypertension in a cohort of middle-aged African Americans and whites, *Hypertension* 31:1130–1135, 1998.
20. Derkx FHM, Schalekamp MADH: Renal artery stenosis and hypertension, *Lancet* 344:237–239, 1994.
21. Baumgartner I, von Aesch K, Do DD, et al: Stent placement in ostial and nonostial atherosclerotic renal arterial stenoses: a prospective follow-up study, *Radiology* 216:498–505, 2000.
22. Bush RL, Najibi S, MacDonald MJ, et al: Endovascular revascularization of renal artery stenosis: technical and clinical results, *J Vasc Surg* 33:1041–1049, 2001.
23. Henry M, Amor M, Henry I, et al: Stents in the treatment of renal artery stenosis: long-term follow-up, *J Endovasc Surg* 6:42–51, 1999.

24. Sharafuddin MJ, Stolpen AH, Dixon BS, et al: Value of MR angiography before percutaneous transluminal renal artery angioplasty and stent placement, *J Vasc Interv Radiol* 13:901–908, 2002.
25. Kaatee R, Beek FJ, Verschuyl EJ, et al: Atherosclerotic renal artery stenosis: ostial or truncal? *Radiology* 199:637–640, 1996.
26. Birrer M, Do DD, Mahler F, et al: Treatment of renal artery fibromuscular dysplasia with balloon angioplasty: a prospective follow-up study, *Eur J Vasc Endovasc Surg* 23:146–152, 2002.
27. Gilfeather M, Holland GA, Siegelman ES, et al: Gadolinium-enhanced ultrafast three-dimensional spoiled gradient-echo MR imaging of the abdominal aorta and visceral and iliac vessels, *Radiographics* 17:423–432, 1997.
28. Debatin JF, Sostman HD, Knelson M, et al: Renal magnetic resonance angiography in the preoperative detection of supernumerary renal arteries in potential kidney donors, *Invest Radiol* 28:882–889, 1993.
29. Nelson HA, Gilfeather M, Holman JM, et al: Gadolinium-enhanced breathhold three-dimensional time-of-flight renal MR angiography in the evaluation of potential renal donors, *J Vasc Interv Radiol* 10:175–181, 1999.
30. Velazquez OC, Baum RA, Carpenter JP: Magnetic resonance angiography of lower-extremity arterial disease, *Surg Clin North Am* 78:519–537, 1998.
31. Dillavou E, Kahn MB: Peripheral vascular disease: Diagnosing and treating the 3 most common peripheral vasculopathies, *Geriatrics* 58:37–42, 2003.
32. Carpenter JP, Baum RA, Holland GA, et al: Peripheral vascular surgery with magnetic resonance angiography as the sole preoperative imaging modality, *J Vasc Surg* 20:861–871, 1994.
33. Carpenter JP, Owen RS, Holland GA, et al: Magnetic resonance angiography of the aorta, iliac and femoral arteries, *Surgery* 116:17–23, 1994.
34. Steffens JC, Schafer FK, Oberscheid B, et al: Bolus-chasing contrast-enhanced 3D MRA of the lower extremity: Comparison with intraarterial DSA, *Acta Radiol* 44:185–192, 2003.
35. Owen RS, Carpenter JP, Baum RA, et al: Magnetic resonance imaging of angiographically occult runoff vessels in peripheral arterial occlusive disease, *N Engl J Med* 326:1577–1581, 1992.
36. Visser K, Kuntz KM, Donaldson MC, et al: Pretreatment imaging workup for patients with intermittent claudication: a cost-effectiveness analysis, *J Vasc Interv Radiol* 14:53–62, 2003.
37. Konkus CJ, Czum JM, Jacobacci JT: Contrast-enhanced MR angiography of the aorta and lower extremities with routine inclusion of the feet, *AJR Am J Roentgenol* 179:115–117, 2002.
38. Hood MN, Ho VB, Foo TK, et al: High-resolution gadolinium-enhanced 3D MRA of the infrapopliteal arteries: lessons for improving bolus-chase peripheral MRA, *Magn Reson Imaging* 20:543–549, 2002.
39. Hofmann WJ, Forstner R, Kofler B, et al: Pedal artery imaging: a comparison of selective digital subtraction angiography, contrast enhanced magnetic resonance angiography and duplex ultrasound, *Eur J Vasc Endovasc Surg* 24:287–292, 2002.
40. Heverhagen JT, Wagner HJ, Bandorski D, et al: Magnetic resonance phase contrast velocity measurement for non-invasive follow up after percutaneous transluminal angioplasty, *Vasa* 31:235–240, 2002.
41. Heverhagen JT, Kalinowski M, Schwarz U, et al: Quantitative human in vivo evaluation of high resolution MRI for vessel wall morphometry after percutaneous transluminal angioplasty, *Magn Reson Imaging* 18:985–989, 2000.
42. Coulden RA, Moss H, Graves MJ, et al: High resolution magnetic resonance imaging of atherosclerosis and the response to balloon angioplasty, *Heart* 83:188–191, 2000.
43. Nederkoorn PJ, van der Graaf Y, Hunink MG: Duplex ultrasound and magnetic resonance angiography compared with digital subtraction angiography in carotid artery stenosis: A systematic review, *Stroke* 34:1324–1332, 2003.
44. Lenhart M, Framme N, Volk M, et al: Time-resolved contrast-enhanced magnetic resonance angiography of the carotid arteries: diagnostic accuracy and inter-observer variability compared with selective catheter angiography, *Invest Radiol* 37:535–541, 2002.
45. Westwood ME, Kelly S, Berry E, et al: Use of magnetic resonance angiography to select candidates with recently symptomatic carotid stenosis for surgery: Systematic review, *BMJ* 324 (7331):198–222, 2002.
46. Cosottini M, Pingitore A, Puglioli M, et al: Contrast-enhanced three-dimensional magnetic resonance angiography of atherosclerotic internal carotid stenosis as the noninvasive imaging modality in revascularization decision making, *stroke* 34(3): 660–664, 2003.
47. Roberts DA: Magnetic resonance imaging of thoracic aortic aneurysm and dissection, *Semin Roentgenol* 36:295–308, 2001.
48. Carr JC, Finn JP: MR imaging of the thoracic aorta, *Magn Reson Imaging Clin North Am* 11:135–148, 2003.
49. Ho VB, Corse WR: MR angiography of the abdominal aorta and peripheral vessels, *Radiol Clin North Am* 41:115–144, 2003.
50. Vogt FM, Goyen M, Debatin JF: MR angiography of the chest, *Radiol Clin North Am* 41:29–41, 2003.
51. Carpenter JP, Holland GA, Golden MA, et al: Magnetic resonance angiography of the aortic arch, *J Vasc Surg* 25:145–151, 1997.
52. Fernandez GC, Tardaguila FM, Duran D, et al: Dynamic 3-dimensional contrast-enhanced magnetic resonance angiography in acute aortic dissection, *Curr Probl Diagn Radiol* 31:134–145, 2002.
53. Leiner T, Elenbaas TW, Kaandorp DW, et al: Magnetic resonance angiography of an aortic dissection, *Circulation* 103:E76–E78, 2001.
54. Hartnell GG: Imaging of aortic aneurysms and dissection: CT and MRI, *J Thorac Imaging* 16:35–46, 2001.
55. Kawamoto S, Bluemke DA, Traill TA, Zerhouni EA: Thoracoabdominal aorta in Marfan syndrome: MR imaging findings of progression of vasculopathy after surgical repair, *Radiology* 203:727–732, 1997.
56. Engellau L, Albrechtsson U, Dahlstrom N, et al: Measurements before endovascular repair of abdominal aortic aneurysms: MR imaging with MRA vs. angiography and CT, *Acta Radiol* 44:177–184, 2003.
57. Neschis DG, Velazquez OC, Baum RA, et al: The role of magnetic resonance angiography for endoprosthetic design, *J Vasc Surg* 33:488–494, 2001.
58. Cejna M, Loewe C, Schoder M, et al: MR angiography vs CT angiography in the follow-up of nitinol stent grafts in endoluminally treated aortic aneurysms, *Eur Radiol* 12:2443–2450, 2002.
59. Insko EK, Kulzer LM, Fairman RM, et al: MR imaging for the detection of endoleaks in recipients of abdominal aortic stent-grafts with low magnetic susceptibility, *Acad Radiol* 10:509–513, 2003.
60. van Herwaarden JA, Bartels LW, Muhs BE, et al: Dynamic magnetic resonance angiography of the aneurysm neck: conformational changes during the cardiac cycle with possible consequences for endograft sizing and future design, *J Vasc Surg* 44(1):22–28, 2006.
61. Cognet F, Salem DB, Dranssart M, et al: Chronic mesenteric ischemia: imaging and percutaneous treatment, *Radiographics* 22:863–880, 2002.

62. Carlos RC, Stanley JC, Stafford-Johnson D, et al: Interobserver variability in the evaluation of chronic mesenteric ischemia with gadolinium-enhanced MR angiography, *Acad Radiol* 8:879–887, 2001.
63. Bradbury MS, Kavanagh PV, Bechtold RE, et al: Mesenteric venous thrombosis: diagnosis and noninvasive imaging, *Radiographics* 22:527–541, 2002.
64. Kroencke TJ, Taupitz M, Arnold R, et al: Three-dimensional gadolinium-enhanced magnetic resonance venography in suspected thrombo-occlusive disease of the central chest veins, *Chest* 120:1570–1576, 2001.
65. Thornton MJ, Ryan R, Varghese JC, et al: A three-dimensional gadolinium-enhanced MR venography technique for imaging central veins, *AJR Am J Roentgenol* 173:999–1003, 1999.
66. Stern JB, Abehsera M, Grenet D, et al: Detection of pelvic vein thrombosis by magnetic resonance angiography in patients with acute pulmonary embolism and normal lower limb compression ultrasonography, *Chest* 122:115–121, 2002.
67. Spritzer CE, Arata MA, Freed KS: Isolated pelvic deep venous thrombosis: relative frequency as detected with MR imaging, *Radiology* 219:521–525, 2001.
68. Evans AJ, Sostman HD, Witty LA, et al: Detection of deep venous thrombosis: prospective comparison of MR imaging and sonography, *J Magn Reson Imaging* 6:44–51, 1996.
69. Demondion X, Bacqueville E, Paul C, et al: Thoracic outlet: assessment with MR imaging in asymptomatic and symptomatic populations, *Radiology* 227:461–468, 2003.
70. Fang YC, Siegelman ES: Complications of renal transplantation: MR findings, *J Comput Assist Tomogr* 25:836–842, 2001.
71. Atalay MK, Bluemke DA: Magnetic resonance imaging of large vessel vasculitis, *Curr Opin Rheumatol* 13:41–47, 2001.
72. Goyen M, Ruehm SG, Jagenburg A, et al: Pulmonary arteriovenous malformation: characterization with time-resolved ultrafast 3D MR angiography, *J Magn Reson Imaging* 13:458–460, 2001.
73. Maki DD, Siegelman ES, Roberts DA, et al: Pulmonary arteriovenous malformations: three-dimensional gadolinium-enhanced MR angiography—initial experience, *Radiology* 219:243–246, 2001.
74. Siegelman ES, Charafeddine R, Stolpen AH, et al: Suppression of intravascular signal on fat-saturated contrast-enhanced thoracic MR arteriograms, *Radiology* 217:115–118, 2000.
75. Tirkes AT, Rosen MA, Siegelman ES: Gadolinium susceptibility artifact causing false positive stenosis isolated to the proximal common carotid artery in 3D dynamic contrast medium enhanced MR angiography of the thorax: A brief review of causes and prevention, *Int J Cardiovasc Imaging* 19:151–155, 2003.
76. Neimatallah MA, Chenevert TL, Carlos RC, et al: Subclavian MR arteriography: Reduction of susceptibility artifact with short echo time and dilute gadopentetate dimeglumine, *Radiology* 217:581–586, 2000.
77. Insko EK, Siegelman ES, Stolpen AH: Subacute clot mimicking flow in a thrombosed arterial bypass graft on two-dimensional time-of-flight and three-dimensional contrast-enhanced MRA, *J Magn Reson Imaging* 11:192–194, 2000.
78. Tombach B, Bremer C, Reimer P, et al: Renal tolerance of a neutral gadolinium chelate (gadobutrol) in patients with chronic renal failure: results of a randomized study, *Radiology* 218:651–657, 2001.
79. Kaufman JA, Geller SC, Waltman AC: Renal insufficiency: gadopentetate dimeglumine as a radiographic contrast agent during peripheral vascular interventional procedures, *Radiology* 198:579–581, 1996.
80. Prince MR, Arnoldus C, Frisoli JK: Nephrotoxicity of high-dose gadolinium compared with iodinated contrast, *J Magn Reson Imaging* 6:162–166, 1996.
81. Sam AD 2nd, Morasch MD, Collins J, et al: Safety of gadolinium contrast angiography in patients with chronic renal insufficiency, *J Vasc Surg* 38:313–318, 2003.
82. Erley CM, Bader BD, Berger ED, et al: Gadolinium-based contrast media compared with iodinated media for digital subtraction angiography in azotaemic patients, *Nephrol Dial Transplant* 19(10):2526–2531, 2004.
83. Saab G, Abu-Alfa A: Nephrogenic systemic fibrosis: Implications for nephrologists, *Eur J Radiol* 66(2):208–212, 2008.
84. Broome DR: Nephrogenic systemic fibrosis associated with gadolinium based contrast agents: A summary of the medical literature reporting, *Eur J Radiol* 66(2):230–234, 2008.
85. Prchal D, Holmes DT, Levin A: Nephrogenic Systemic Fibrosis: The story unfolds, *Kidney Int* 73(12):1335–1337, 2008.
86. Broome DR, Girguis MS, Baron PW, et al: Gadodiamide-associated nephrogenic systemic fibrosis: why radiologists should be concerned, *AJR Am J Roentgenol* 188(2):586–592, 2007.
87. Mathur K, Morris S, Deighan C, et al: Extracorporeal photopheresis improves nephrogenic fibrosing dermopathy/nephrogenic systemic fibrosis: Three case reports and review of literature, *J Clin Apheresis* 23(4):144–150, 2008.
88. Okada S, Katagiri K, Kumazaki T, et al: Safety of gadolinium contrast agent in hemodialysis patients, *Acta Radiol* 42:339–341, 2001.
89. Yerram P, Saab G, Karuparthi PR, et al: Nephrogenic systemic fibrosis: a mysterious disease in patients with renal failure: role of gadolinium-based contrast media in causation and the beneficial effect of intravenous sodium thiosulfate, *Clin J Am Soc Nephrol* 2:258–263, 2007.
90. Knopp EA, Cowper SE: Nephrogenic systemic fibrosis: early recognition and treatment, *Semin Dial* 21(2):123–128, 2008.
91. Cowper SE, Robin HS, Steinberg SM, et al: Scleromyxoedema-like cutaneous diseases in renal-dialysis patients, *Lancet* 356:1000–1001, 2000.
92. Grobner T: Gadolinium: a specific trigger for the development of nephrogenic fibrosing dermopathy and nephrogenic systemic fibrosis? *Nephrol Dial Transplant* 21(4):1104–1108, 2006.
93. Peak AS, Sheller A: Risk factors for developing gadolinium-induced nephrogenic systemic fibrosis, *Ann Pharmacother* 41(9):1481–1485, 2007.
94. Sadowski EA, Bennett LK, Chan MR, et al: Nephrogenic systemic fibrosis: risk factors and incidence estimation, *Radiology* 243(1):148–157, 2007.
95. US FDA Center for Drug Evaluation and Research. Information on Gadolinium-Containing Contrast Agents [US FDA website]. Available at http://www.fda.gov/cder/drug/infopage/gcca/default.htm, accessed November 4, 2007, 2007.
96. Thakral C, Alhariri J, Abraham JL: Long-term retention of gadolinium in tissues from nephrogenic systemic fibrosis patient after multiple gadolinium-enhanced MRI scans: case report and implications, *Contrast Media Mol Imaging* 2:199–205, 2007.
97. Levey AS, Bosch JP, Lewis JB, et al: A more accurate method to estimate glomerular filtration rate from serum creatinine: a new prediction equation. Modification of Diet in Renal Disease Study Group, *Ann Intern Med* 130(6):461–470, 1999.
98. Shellock FG, Kanal E: *Magnetic Resonance: Bioeffects, safety, and patient management,* ed 2, Philadelphia, 1996, Lippincott Williams & Wilkins.
99. Shellock FG: Magnetic resonance safety update 2002: Implants and devices, *J Magn Reson Imaging* 16:485–496, 2002.
100. American Society for Testing and Materials (ASTM) International: *ASTM F2503–05: Standard practice for marking medical devices and other items for safety in the magnetic resonance environment*, West Conshohocken, Pa, http://www.astm.org; 2005, 2005, ASTM International.

101. Levine GN, Gomes AS, Arai AE, et al: Safety of magnetic resonance imaging in patients with cardiovascular devices: an American Heart Association scientific statement from the Committee on Diagnostic and Interventional Cardiac Catheterization, Council on Clinical Cardiology, and the Council on Cardiovascular Radiology and Intervention: endorsed by the American College of Cardiology Foundation, the North American Society for Cardiac Imaging, and the Society for Cardiovascular Magnetic Resonance, *Circulation* 116:2878–2891, 2007.
102. Hiramoto JS, Reilly LM, Schneider DB, et al: The effect of magnetic resonance imaging on stainless-steel Z-stent–based abdominal aortic prosthesis, *J Vasc Surg* 45(3):472–474, 2007.
103. Gerber TC, Fasseas P, Lennon RJ, et al: Clinical safety of magnetic resonance imaging early after coronary artery stent placement, *J Am Coll Cardiol* 42(7):1295–1298, 2003.
104. Yuan C, Mitsumori LM, Ferguson MS, et al: In vivo accuracy of multispectral magnetic resonance imaging for identifying lipid-rich necrotic cores and intraplaque hemorrhage in advanced human carotid plaques, *Circulation* 104:2051–2056, 2001.
105. Cai JM, Hatsukami TS, Ferguson MS, et al: Classification of human carotid atherosclerotic lesions with in vivo multi-contrast magnetic resonance imaging, *Circulation* 106: 1368–1373, 2002.
106. Wasserman BA, Smith WI, Trout HH III, et al: Carotid artery atherosclerosis: in vivo morphologic characterization with gadolinium-enhanced double-oblique MR imaging initial results, *Radiology* 223:566–573, 2002.
107. Yuan C, Kerwin WS, Ferguson MS, et al: Contrast-enhanced high resolution MRI for atherosclerotic carotid artery tissue characterization, *J Magn Reson Imaging* 15:62–67, 2002.
108. Kooi ME, Cappendijk VC, Cleutjens KB, et al: Accumulation of ultrasmall superparamagnetic particles of iron oxide in human atherosclerotic plaques can be detected by in vivo magnetic resonance imaging, *Circulation* 107:2453–2458, 2003.
109. Langer HF, Haubner R, Pichler BJ, et al: Radionuclide imaging: a molecular key to the atherosclerotic plaque, *J Am Coll Cardiol* 52(1):1–12, 2008.

CHAPTER

20

Angiography

Robert J. Feezor, James Caridi, Irvin Hawkins, Jr., [†]James M. Seeger

Contrast angiography has been an integral part of the evaluation of patients requiring vascular reconstruction for years. It provides detailed anatomic information about the location and the extent of the lesion or lesions causing the hemodynamic abnormality responsible for the patient's symptoms. Such information is essential to the proper planning of open surgical arterial reconstructive procedures. Additionally, with the emergence of endovascular therapy, the role of angiography has become even more vital: it is not only an aid in diagnosis and planning, but a means to direct therapy. In general, angiography defines the anatomy of the target lesion to be treated—whether that treatment is with balloon angioplasty, endoluminal stenting, or some other endovascular therapy such as cryoablation, laser, or an atherectomy device or open surgical bypass.

To adequately interpret the images generated from angiography, clinicians must possess more than a cursory knowledge of the mechanics of how each image is derived, including the shortcomings and pitfalls of each angiography technique. The primary limitation, of course, is that, despite any high-quality image generated, that image still is an indirect evaluation of a pathologic lesion within a vessel wall using a two-dimensional "lumenogram." Losing sight of this fact may cause the misinterpretation of images, a flaw that can have serious consequences.

Clearly, the use of contrast angiography in patients with peripheral vascular disease, cerebrovascular disease, or aneurysmal disease has significant risks, and these, in general, fall into three specific categories: the radiation exposure required for image acquisition; the local vessel trauma necessary to introduce diagnostic or therapeutic devices; and the adverse sequelae of the contrast medium, whether that is an allergic reaction or the exaggeration of a known contrast agent toxicity (e.g., nephrotoxicity from iodinated contrast agents). The risk of each of these can be minimized but not eliminated entirely. Additionally, an alteration in technique may provide equal quality imaging with a smaller risk. For example, use of digital subtraction angiography (DSA) has several advantages over standard cut-film angiography: increased contrast agent resolution, requiring decreased volumes of angiographic contrast material; real-time display of images; and digital manipulation of images to improve contrast agent density and to integrate multiple frames to produce a composite diagnostic image. To minimize local trauma, interventionalists habitually use the smallest-diameter devices that will serve the purposes needed; additionally, industry seeks to devise therapeutic devices that can be implanted or used in smaller-diameter delivery devices. To limit the toxicity of the contrast medium, some investigators have attempted, with modest successes, to use nonionic liquids and carbon dioxide (CO_2) gas as contrast agents. Although the images obtained can be relatively high quality, use of these contrast agents is not widespread as of yet.

This chapter addresses basic principles of angiography and briefly discusses noninvasive and invasive techniques of imaging. Additionally, we discuss the indications and a great deal of the complications of contrast angiography. Last, we review some larger-scale issues of radiation safety and the various types of equipment used in contrast angiography.

ALTERNATIVES TO STANDARD CONTRAST ARTERIOGRAPHY

Standard contrast arteriography is invasive, uncomfortable, and expensive. In addition, as previously noted, the two-dimensional lumenogram of the vascular tree provided by contrast angiography is a less-than-ideal method by which to evaluate vascular anatomy and pathology. Because of these factors and the risks associated with standard contrast angiography, newer

[†]Deceased.

vascular imaging techniques, including arterial duplex ultrasonography, computed tomography (CT) angiography (CTA), and magnetic resonance (MR) arteriography (MRA), are being investigated. These techniques will be briefly discussed to provide a perspective for standard contrast angiography, the focus of this chapter.

Arterial Duplex Ultrasonography

Ultrasonography has emerged as a viable alternative to invasive arterial imaging in certain circumstances. The risk and cost to the patient are significantly less; however, ultrasonography is even more operator dependent than standard angiography. Arterial duplex ultrasound imaging is used for carotid bifurcation lesion imaging and carotid endarterectomy planning in up to 80% of patients in many centers. Several reports have shown that arterial duplex ultrasound imaging also provides adequate information for surgical arterial reconstruction planning in up to 90% of patients with symptoms of lower-extremity arterial occlusive disease.[1] Additionally, it is now possible to use duplex ultrasound imaging as the sole imaging technique during the conduct of peripheral endovascular interventions. Ascher et al.[2] used duplex to guide angioplasty and stent placement for 253 lesions in 196 patients with femoral-popliteal occlusive disease and reported a technical success rate of 93%, with all of the failures associated with lesions designated as Trans-Atlantic Inter-Society Consenus (TASC) C or TASC D. Duplex arterial ultrasound has also been used in some centers as a completion imaging tool after distal bypass procedures, with objective predictive capabilities based on the velocities detected.[3] Although again operator dependent, intraoperative duplex ultrasound has been reported to be quick and easily performed; Hansen et al.[4] noted that the mean duration of intraoperative completion duplex after renal artery bypass or endarterectomy was 4.5 minutes. Last, in certain circumstances, duplex ultrasound has begun to replace conventional contrast imaging for surveillance after endoluminal abdominal aortic aneurysm (AAA) therapy. Sandford et al.[5] used duplex ultrasonography in direct comparison with contrast CT scanning and found the specificity of duplex to be 91%; moreover, none of the endoleaks seen by CT but not by duplex were type I, and none required intervention.

Computed Tomography Angiography

In its early years, CT scanning technology with four-section CT scanners prohibited their use for vascular imaging. However, with the advent of 16-, 64-, and now 128-section CT scanners, their use for arterial imaging has become commonplace and, in the realm of aneurysmal disease, requisite. Willman et al.[6] compared 16-section CT images with conventional DSA in 39 patients with peripheral vascular occlusive disease and showed that the sensitivity and specificity of the CT images was 96% and 97%, respectively, for lesions thought to be hemodynamically significant. Notably, they also found the amount of radiation required to be much less for the CT examination (1.6-3.9 mSv vs. 6.4-16.0 mSv). Post-processing of the images generated can also be performed, allowing three-dimensional modeling of the images (Figure 20-1). The potential disadvantages for CTA, in general, include not only the need for ionizing radiation but also the potential for nonvisualization of the distal vasculature because of intense calcification of the vessel walls, metal artifact, or mistiming of the contrast bolus.[7] In our clinical practice, this final point has been the largest reason limiting the utility of CTA for imaging the infrageniculate vessels, which commonly is required in patients with proximal obstructive lesions as well. This is compounded by the fact that patients often have concomitant cardiac dysfunction that limits the delivery of the contrast bolus to the distal circulation. In essence, then this creates a situation where the contrast bolus is timed correctly for the aortoiliac system, but, as it is followed distally, the CT head "outruns" the bolus of contrast and the vessels are not opacified. Although these technique limitations potentially can be overcome, the main limitation of CTA, clearly, is the inability to use this imaging technique for guidance during endovascular therapeutic maneuvers.

Magnetic Resonance Angiography

Although perhaps not as prevalent as CT imaging, the use of MR to image the vasculature has been advocated recently. In 2001, Koelemay et al.[8] published a meta-analysis of the use of MRA in evaluation of lower-extremity peripheral vascular occlusive disease of 1090 patients. For the detection of 50% or greater stenosis up to occlusion, MRA had a 90% sensitivity, which was increased to 94% with the use of gadolinium. In all the individual studies reviewed, the comparison was made with either conventional angiography or DSA. With use of a "hybrid" approach of a noncontrasted and then contrasted MR, more distal vasculature may be better visualized.[9] However, the problems associated with use of gadolinium as a contrast agent have received much attention of late and will be addressed later.

CONTRAST ANGIOGRAPHY IN PERIPHERAL VASCULAR DISEASE

Contrast angiography remains the mainstay for imaging of the peripheral vascular tree in patients with peripheral vascular disease and, in fact, has become even more important with the advance of

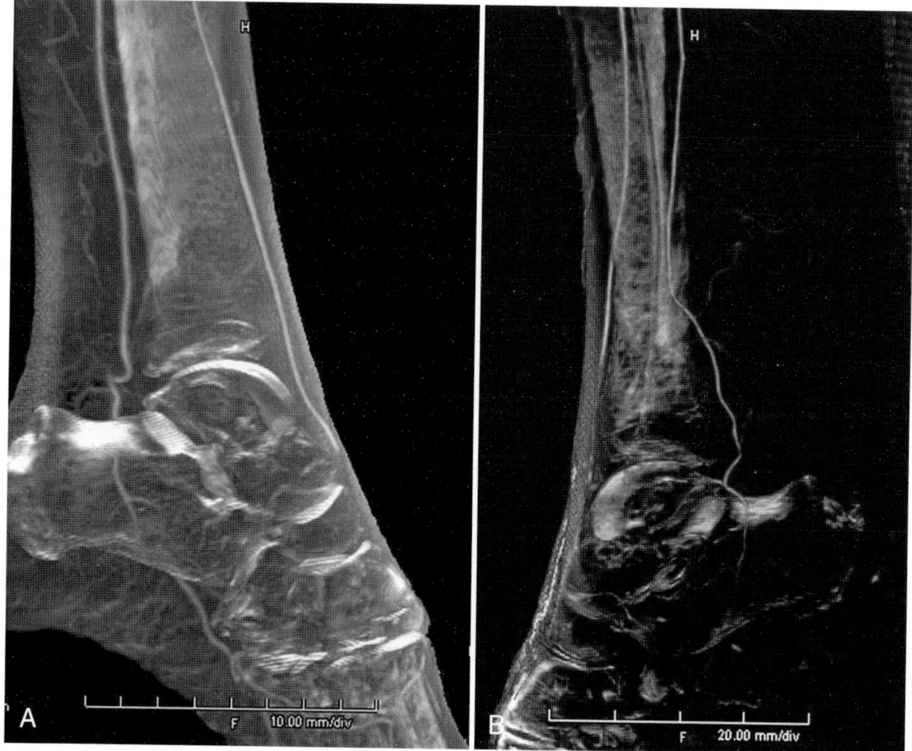

FIGURE 20-1 **A,** Multi-planar reformation of CT angiogram showing the pedal vessels, including the dominant posterior tibial artery, which continues on the sole of the foot. **B,** Three-dimensional reconstruction of the same data set can provide radiographic clues of the nature of the vessels.

endovascular technology. Although symptomatic peripheral vascular disease is a manifestation of hemodynamic rather than anatomic abnormalities, identification of the anatomic lesions responsible for these hemodynamic changes is a vital part of surgical and endovascular reconstructive procedures. Pretreatment visualization of the peripheral vascular tree using contrast arteriography allows selection of the modalities most likely to produce successful correction of the hemodynamic abnormality responsible for the patient's symptoms and appropriate planning of the therapeutic procedure. Repeated studies have shown that more focal lesions, particularly more proximal (i.e., in the aortoiliac segment versus the infrageniculate segment), are more amenable to durable endovascular solutions. Intraprocedure angiography (intraoperative arteriography, fluoroscopy with contrast agent injection during endovascular procedures) also provides information necessary for the guidance of both operative and endovascular revascularization procedures, and completion angiography documents the anatomic technical excellence of any vascular reconstruction.

Basic Principles of Invasive Imaging Using Contrast Angiography

Visualization of vascular anatomy with contrast angiography is based on the principle of passing x-ray beams through the patient and having these beams strike a receiver after the administration of an intravascular contrast agent to the area of interest. Not surprisingly, therefore, the image generation is dependent on successful delivery of the contrast agent to the area being studied and a difference between the radiopacity of the intraluminal contrast agent and the surrounding structures. Liquid contrast agents (both ionic and nonionic) are radiopaque and mix with blood to decrease the transmission of the x-rays through the blood. Conversely, CO_2 gas is radiolucent and displaces blood from the arterial lumen, so that x-ray transmission is increased. The simplest form of an x-ray receiver is a plain film, which is what is used in the classic "cut-film" angiography. Alternatively, the receiver can be coupled with an image intensifier, which is typically used in an interventional or angiographic suite for fluoroscopy and DSA (to be discussed later).

Vessel Access for Contrast Delivery

Regardless of the type of contrast chosen, the particular vascular bed being imaged, or the goals of the imaging (diagnostic or therapeutic), a common early denominator in the procedure is successful vascular access. Despite the ever-increasing complexity of percutaneous interventions, access-related complications historically are the most prevalent among all complications of endovascular procedures. In aggregate, the average incidence of complications with endovascular AAA repair is 15%, and the vast majority of these are local, not systemic, suggesting groin access site complications.[10]

Percutaneous vascular access using the standard Seldinger technique is employed for all forms of arteriography. It has been our practice to start with a small, 21-gauge needle and a 3F or 4F catheter and to confirm intraluminal guidewire/catheter placement with hand-injected contrast and digital fluoroscopy. For most arterial work, the preferred access site is the common femoral artery (CFA), which is typically 4 to 8 cm in length.[11] If the arteriogram is performed for lower-extremity arterial occlusive disease, the CFA in the less symptomatic extremity is usually selected to allow for antegrade angiography and intervention across the aortic bifurcation of the symptomatic extremity. An alternative is an antegrade approach, puncturing ipsilateral to the more symptomatic extremity, but this requires careful positioning of the needle to reach the CFA proper. Additionally, obesity is a relative contraindication to an antegrade approach. As compared with upper-extremity access, transfemoral access is associated with low morbidity. AbuRahma et al.[12] cited a major complication rate of 1.3% among 588 patients undergoing angiography, of whom 93% had a transfemoral approach.

Some interventions are better suited for brachial access because of either anatomic angles (i.e., the downward trajectory of the superior mesenteric artery off the aorta) or the intrinsic pathologic process being studied (i.e., angiography in the setting of infrarenal aortic occlusion). Brachial artery cannulation is only modestly more challenging from a technical standpoint but appears to be associated with a significantly higher incidence of complications. Basche et al.[13] reviewed their series of 156 catheter interventions using transbrachial access and found 3 (1.9%) complications, 2 of which were local hematomas managed conservatively. In contrast, Hammacher et al.[14] systematically studied perfusion distal to brachial artery catheterization sites in 502 patients and found that 5.8% of patients had post-procedural complaints potentially contributed to by malperfusion. Additionally, 19% had wrist-brachial indexes of less than 0.85, suggesting some degree of brachial artery stenosis or occlusion. Axillary artery cannulation, which was previously very popular, likely because of the larger size of the vessel and thus the potential for use of relatively larger diagnostic and interventional devices, has largely been abandoned as a result of the risk of access-related complications. Indeed, Chitwood et al.[15] retrospectively reviewed 842 cases of transaxillary arteriography, identifying 19 (2.3%) complications including 14 nerve injuries, 4 hematomas or pseudoaneurysms, and 1 axillary artery thrombosis. Similarly, a translumbar approach may also be employed with use of a fine needle for initial vessel access, followed by introduction of a 4F catheter, although this technique is now seldom used for diagnostic angiography, again because of the significant potential for complications and the limited flexibility this access site offers. Translumbar direct aortic access is now essentially only used for endovascular procedures, with its sole remaining practical use being therapeutic maneuvers to treat a lumbar-based type II endoleak after endovascular exclusion of an AAA.

After the introduction of a small-diameter sheath (usually no larger than 5F for diagnostic angiography), the selection of a catheter for contrast delivery is based on the vessel access site and the location of the diseased vessel to be studied. For diagnostic angiography of the abdominal aorta and the bilateral lower extremities, a small (4F) catheter is adequate. Pigtail catheters and variations of the shepherd-hook catheter are used for aortography. The Omni Flush (AngioDynamics, Queensburg, NY), a type of shepherd-hook catheter with multiple side-holes, also permits catheterization of the contralateral iliac artery and easily "feeds" distally to the CFA. Other shaped catheters may be used for "superselective" vessel catheterization, including visceral artery catheterization.

Historically, vascular surgeons and interventionalists used intravenous injection of contrast to image a particular area of vasculature in patients for whom arterial access was either too difficult or risky. This relied on a reasonable cardiac output to deliver the contrast to the area being studied. The newer DSA equipment can provide excellent images of even the pedal arteries after intravenous injections of 30 to 40 mL of iodinated contrast agent in some patients. A reported advantage of intravenous contrast injection is the fact that all collaterals tend to fill, which can provide additional detail of complex postsurgical anatomy. If renal function is normal, as many as five or six injections can be used to obtain images of the entire abdomen and the lower-extremity vasculature. However, in the era of high-quality CT scanning, this same diagnostic purpose can be accomplished with use of a single bolus of contrast. Additionally, like CTA, angiography using intravenous injection is limited by timing and adequate contrast delivery particularly in lower extremities with significant occlusive disease.

Contrast Media

Presently available iodinated liquid contrast agents include high-osmolar ionic agents, low-osmolar nonionic agents, and low-osmolar ionic hybrid agents. Additionally, CO_2 gas can be used as an angiographic contrast agent (discussed later in this chapter). The factors that influence the choice of contrast agents are, to a large extent, related to patient comfort and to the patient's underlying medical conditions. Compared with nonionic contrast agents, iodinated ionic contrast agents produce more allergic reactions and side effects, the most frequent being nausea, vomiting, urticaria, pruritus, and edema. Indeed, ionic agents have been reported to produce hypersensitivity reactions in up to 25% of patients with a history of contrast-agent allergy.[16] Acute renal dysfunction after arteriography using iodinated ionic contrast agents has also been reported to occur in 11% of patients with peripheral vascular disease and in 62% of patients with preexisting elevation of the serum creatinine level above 2.0 mg/dL.[17] Additional risk factors associated with contrast-induced nephrotoxicity include diabetes mellitus, the volume of contrast material used, and the degree of serum creatinine elevation.[18] Although animal studies have shown nonionic contrast agents to be less nephrotoxic, a randomized comparison of ionic and nonionic iodinated contrast agents used during cardiac catheterization failed to demonstrate such a benefit in humans.[19] The cost of the various contrast agents is also a concern, with nonionic contrast agents costing 20 times more than ionic contrast agents. We now almost exclusively use iodixanol (Visipaque, GE Healthcare, Princeton, NJ), which produces minimal patient discomfort. This is important for DSA imaging because it minimizes patient movement resulting from discomfort, which degrades the DSA image.

The technique of image acquisition is also directly related to the volume of contrast required. It is now routine to conduct endovascular surgical procedures with use of DSA, which reduces the amount of contrast agent needed for any single angiogram. Even still, the repeated contrast agent injections needed to visualize the vessels during an endovascular procedure can lead to a significant volume of contrast material being administered. The volume of contrast agent required for adequate visualization of some smaller arteries (e.g., infrapopliteal or pedal arteries) can also be large because of variability in flow in and around stenotic vessels. This volume can be minimized, by positioning the injection catheter as close to the identified lesion as possible (e.g., placing the catheter in the distal external iliac artery for superficial femoral artery [SFA] lesions instead of the distal aorta). DSA also has the capacity to minimize the "guesswork" of matching contrast delivery to the area of interest with image acquisition sequence, and, furthermore, digital subtraction allows the user to remove overlying interfering bone and soft tissue, which may decrease the total number of angiogram runs necessary to adequately visualize the vessels being examined.

Contrast Injection Systems

Contrast agents can be delivered either by hand injection or by a mechanical injector. Deciding which to use depends on the reason for the angiogram and the area of the vascular tree being studied. Diagnostic angiography is usually done with a mechanical injector so that significant contrast can be delivered to provide detailed images of a large area of the vascular tree. Additionally, aortic angiography, particularly in the thoracic aorta, requires a machine injector to infuse sufficient volume of contrast to opacify a large-diameter blood vessel, despite a large volume of blood flowing through the vessel. Selective angiography of smaller secondary aortic and visceral branches and smaller distal arteries can often be done adequately by using hand injection. Hand injection of contrast agent is also most commonly used for angiographic guidance and preliminary assessment of technical success during endovascular procedures, for reasons of convenience, as well as flexibility. However, final documentation of a completed endovascular procedure, particularly stent graft repair of aortic pathologies, is usually done with a mechanical injector to provide the most detailed angiogram possible.

Image Quality

The most significant factors influencing the quality (and therefore the accuracy) of images of the peripheral vascular system obtained with use of contrast angiography are spatial resolution, contrast resolution, distortion, and parallax. In general, these principles are more vital when interventions are planned and when the target vessels (and lesions) are small. *Spatial resolution* refers to the sharpness of detail and the ability to resolve small vessels, instruments, or adjacent structures. Diminished spatial resolution can be caused by motion artifact or "noise" in the DSA circuitry. Motion artifact can be minimized by use of sedation or use of contrast agents associated with limited patient discomfort (see previous discussion). *Contrast resolution* refers to the ability to resolve structures based on differences in their density or radiopacity; in other words, it is the ability to distinguish the vessel of interest with the background structures. *Distortion* results from less precise focusing of the electron beam in an image intensifier at its periphery than at the center. Associated with this is a decrease in image brightness toward the image periphery, which is referred to as *vignetting*. Both of these problems are minimized in today's high-resolution angiography systems but may be present in some older imaging systems. Last, *parallax* is the differences in lesion geometry caused by changes in the relation of the patient and the image intensifier. To minimize parallax, the lesion of interest should be kept in the center of the field of view.

Image Documentation Techniques

Cut-Film Angiography

Documentation of contrast angiogram images can be done with use of either x-ray film or computerized digital processing (DSA). In the case of conventional cut-film angiography, variable tissue density, enhanced by arterial contrast agents, alters the amount of radiation striking a phosphorescent screen, which emits photons (light) in proportion to the amount of x-rays received. These photons then expose photographic film coated with a light-sensitive emulsion that, after development, produces a plain radiograph. Grids consisting of alternating layers of lead and radiolucent materials are often interposed between the x-ray beam and the screen-film combination to absorb scattered radiation that might degrade the clarity of the image.[20]

Because blood flow, and thus contrast agent movement, is a dynamic process, the film must be changed after each image is acquired. This can be achieved by one of several film changers that are capable of filming at three to six films (frames) per second. The timing and the rapidity of contrast agent injection and the film framing speed necessary to image the vascular tree accurately vary from one organ to another, depending on the volume of the organ's vascular bed and the flow of blood through that bed. The larger the bed or the slower the blood flow through the bed, the slower the contrast agent injection and the film framing rates should be. Alternatively, changes in the contrast agent column image can be recorded by using a cine filming technique such as that commonly employed in cardiac angiography suites, if the area of interest is less than a foot in diameter. Cut-film angiograms provide large, high-resolution, detailed images of the peripheral vascular tree. These images are particularly useful in planning surgical procedures because vessel image size and relationship to bony landmarks closely approximate surgical findings (i.e., minimal parallax). However, because cut-film techniques require development of the film before the angiographic images can be reviewed, they are of limited value during endovascular procedures. Furthermore, when cut films are used, subtraction must be done manually and road-mapping is not possible, making this documentation technique impractical for guidance during endovascular procedures.

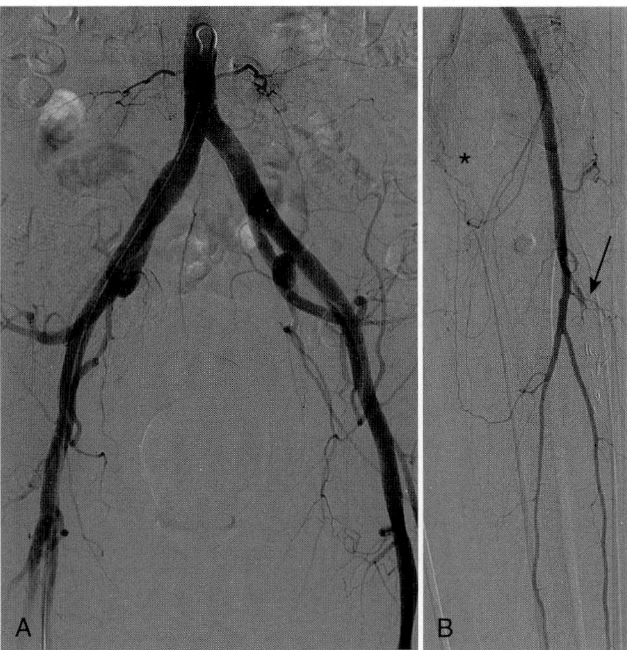

FIGURE 20-2 DSA of **(A)** distal abdominal aorta and iliac arteries and **(B)** the popliteal and tibial arteries. **A,** The pelvic vessels imaged in this manner show no lesions that have the appearance of hemodynamic significance. **B,** Although the popliteal and two tibial vessels show no apparent disease, the anterior tibial artery *(arrow)* is occluded. Although faint, it is still possible to delineate the knee joint *(*)*.

Digital Subtraction Angiography

DSA involves transmission of a video image of the output screen of the image intensifier to a computer, where that image is digitized, subtracted from static tissues, and recorded or printed (Figure 20-2, *A*). The image intensifier tube used in fluoroscopy is essentially a large vacuum tube that receives, concentrates, and brightens the x-ray image. It then produces an electronic image that can be transmitted to a monitor or a computer. The image intensifier contains an input screen with a layer of cesium chloride overlying a photocathode layer. Received x-rays cause the cesium chloride to emit light that strikes the photo-cathode, which then emits electrons. This electron beam is then focused and accelerated toward an output screen coated with zinc cadmium sulfide. When struck by electrons, this screen emits light, which traverses a lead glass window to remove the radiation, after which it is converted into an electronic image by a video camera and is displayed on a television monitor.[20] The output screen image can also be transmitted to a computer and can be electronically digitized for subsequent manipulation to produce near real-time subtracted images. This processed image is then sent to the recording device, usually digitally. After the initial recording, it is often possible to alter the image contrast and background to enhance visualization (postprocessing of the images). The vast majority of angiographic suites are now equipped with digital imaging systems consisting of an image intensifier, a high signal-to-noise–ratio camera, a computer, and a high-resolution television monitor.

DSA often allows better demonstration of small, infrapopliteal, and pedal vessels (Figure 20-2, *B*) and can be done with smaller volumes of contrast medium than cut-film angiography. The rapidity of image retrieval and hence analysis improve the flow of the procedure. Care must be taken, however, in interpreting DSA images and using them for reconstruction planning because the lack of landmarks in many subtracted images can lead to errors in determining the location of lesions (Figure 20-2, *B*). Additionally, the small actual size of the displayed vessels may mislead physicians in the judgment of the appropriateness of vessels as reconstructive targets.

DSA also lends itself to road-mapping, in which a digitally subtracted initial image outlining the vessel being treated is displayed as a background image over which a real-time fluoroscopic image is projected. This type of processing significantly aids in the guidance of endovascular procedures by allowing placement of devices such as balloons and stents within lesions previously identified by angiography. When using this technique, the relationship between the image intensifier and the patient must remain stable; if the patient, the table, or the x-ray tube moves, the real-time fluoroscopic image will no longer be precisely spatially related to the road-mapped image. This could lead to arterial damage or maldeployment of the balloon or stent, with potentially catastrophic results.

Film Interpretation and Hemodynamic Assessment

Images of the peripheral vascular tree produced by contrast angiography are two-dimensional "lumenograms" and thus subject to significant limitations when used for the evaluation of patients with peripheral vascular disease. Despite this, contrast angiography provides an "accurate" representation of the vascular tree when compared with findings during surgical arterial reconstruction, so long as certain caveats are kept in mind. In general, areas of vessel stenosis, occlusion, or dilatation are easily identified from high-resolution cut-film or DSA images. However, stenosis caused by atherosclerotic plaque is usually not concentric, so that a vessel significantly narrowed by posterior plaque may appear relatively normal on a standard anterior-posterior view. Because of this, in general, contrast arteriography underrepresents the degree of occlusive disease present in the vascular beds above the inguinal ligament. Overlying, less diseased arteries, collaterals, or bone can also obscure a site of significant stenosis or a short-segment occlusion of certain vessels, such as the deep femoral artery, particularly when cut-film images are obtained. Three-dimensional knowledge of anatomic relationships minimizes this source of error. For instance, the common femoral bifurcation is best imaged at a projection of 30 degrees off the straight anterior-posterior axis (Figure 20-3, *A*), thereby rotating the proximal SFA off the proximal profunda femoris artery. Similarly, the iliac bifurcation is traditionally best viewed 30 degrees contralateral to the side being imaged (see Figure 20-3, *B*). These maneuvers are even more vital in endovascular therapies, whether trying to seat a stent in the ideal location for occlusive disease or determining the length of an iliac limb of an endovascular abdominal aneurysm exclusion device so as not occlude the hypogastric origin (see Figure 20-3, *B*). Even without rotational changes in images, there can be very subtle clues to the presence and geometry of an atherosclerotic lesion, even if that lesion is due posterior in the line of "sight." For instance, a relative decrease in the opacity of the contrast agent column in a segment of a vessel compared with adjacent segments is suggestive of a posterior plaque or possibly dissection, and the operator may then choose to oblique the image intensifier to demonstrate these areas of stenosis, dissection, or other flow-limiting pathology (Figure 20-4).

Accurate demonstration of occlusion or long-segment stenosis of infrainguinal arteries can be difficult, especially in patients with severe arterial occlusive disease above the inguinal ligament that limits contrast agent delivery to the extremity. Therefore, in contrast to the

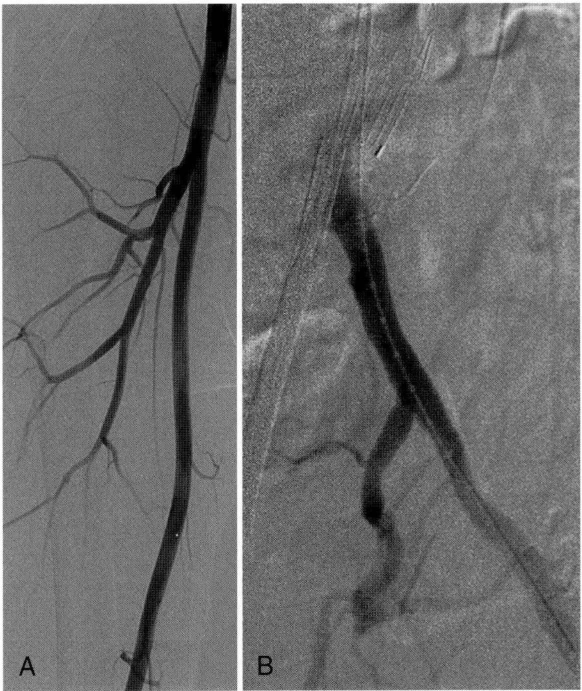

FIGURE 20-3 Rotation of the image-intensifier off the straight anterior-posterior line, in essence, "splays" out the bifurcation of vessels such as the **(A)** common femoral artery and **(B)** common iliac artery. Our standard projection is 30 degrees, which in this case allows visualization of the proximal aspects of each of these vessels.

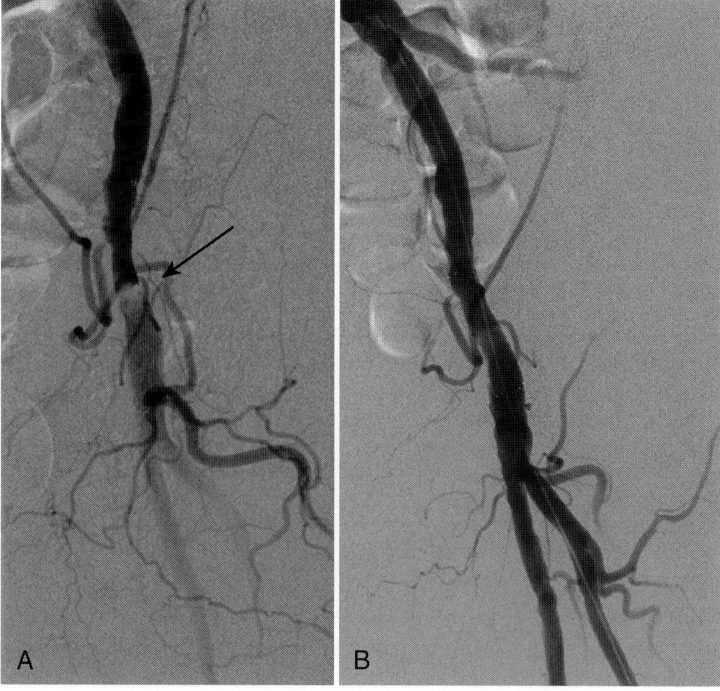

FIGURE 20-4 **A,** In a straight anterior-posterior projection, a flow-limiting dissection can be seen as a diminution of opacification of the vessel (arrow). **B,** After endovascular therapy, the contrast column is more uniform, suggesting resolution of the hemodynamic insult.

aortoiliac segment, angiographic images of the infrainguinal segment often overrepresent the degree of occlusive disease present, primarily by failing to identify patent infrainguinal or infrapopliteal arteries because of poor contrast delivery to patent vessels. This problem can be suggested by a gradually diminishing contrast agent column in the proximal portion of a vessel, by a lack of visualization of collateral vessels in the same area, or by a lack of correlation between the angiographic images and the patient's symptoms or vascular laboratory studies (e.g., an ankle–brachial index of 0.4 in an extremity with no patent vessels visualized or a good Doppler signal in a posterior tibial artery that is not visualized). Almost counterintuitively, more proximal injection of contrast may be necessary to demonstrate distal vasculature in these settings. The best example of this is in patients with complete aortic occlusion, wherein the common femoral arteries are visualized only by injection of contrast in the aortic arch to allow contrast to traverse the mammary and epigastric arteries to reach the lower extremities. Conversely, intraoperative arteriography with direct contrast agent injection into the popliteal or the infrapopliteal arteries may be necessary to identify patent infrapopliteal arteries not seen on preoperative studies. Indeed, we have found that intraoperative prebypass arteriography changes the operative plan developed from the preoperative contrast arteriogram in up to 20% of patients undergoing popliteal and infrapopliteal bypass procedures, largely by demonstration of a more suitable target vessel for a bypass.[21]

Finally, because arterial occlusive disease is commonly diffuse and images of the vascular tree may not demonstrate an obvious area of severe stenosis or occlusion to explain the patient's symptoms and abnormal results of hemodynamics testing, the determination of the hemodynamic significance of a particular area of disease can be difficult with use of anatomic information alone. Assessment of pressure measurements above and below the identified areas of occlusive disease both before and after runoff vasodilatation (with use of intra-arterial papaverine or nitroglycerin) is therefore an excellent adjunct to anatomic imaging that can be done simply by attaching a pressure transducer to the angiographic catheter. However, when measuring pressure within a lumen, it is important to give consideration to the diameter of the catheter, which may be traversing a stenosis and thereby occluding it further and producing an artificial "pressure gradient."

Complications

Complications associated with contrast angiography can be divided into those related to vessel access and injection catheter placement (e.g., vessel injury, hematoma, pseudoaneurysm, embolization, and injury to adjacent structures) and those related to contrast agent injection (e.g., allergic reactions and nephrotoxicity for iodinated contrast agents, as previously discussed). Endovascular procedures such as balloon angioplasty, stent placement, and stent graft repair can also be associated with injury of the treated artery (e.g., dissection or rupture) or device misplacement, but this last subset of complications is not directly related to angiography and is not discussed here. The risk for complications associated with angiography can also be stratified on the basis of the underlying condition for which the angiogram is done. The highest rates of complications occur in patients with aortic dissection, mesenteric ischemia, gastrointestinal bleeding, or symptomatic carotid disease, and the lowest rates occur in patients with trauma or aneurysmal disease.[22] Furthermore, there is a significant difference in the incidence of complications among the three most common angiographic access sites: femoral artery, 1.73%; infrarenal aorta (translumbar approach), 2.89%; and axillary artery, 3.29%.[23] We think that the complication rate associated with vessel access can be considerably reduced by using micropuncture access (21-gauge needles), small platinum-tipped 0.018-inch guidewires, and 3F to 4F catheters, although admittedly the data supporting this are limited.

Access Site Complications

Bleeding and a hematoma occurring at the arterial puncture site are the most common complication associated with contrast angiography, and the risk of development of this complication is directly related to the size of the arterial puncture. This is evidenced by the incidence of hematoma formation with small catheters used for diagnostic angiography being much lower than the incidence of this problem occurring when larger introducer sheaths are used for intervention. Although the size of endovascular devices has decreased, a 6F or larger sheath is still required for most endovascular therapeutic procedures, compared with a 3F to 4F sheath required for diagnostic angiography. The risk of access site bleeding complications can be minimized by using as small a catheter as possible for diagnostic angiography and as small a sheath as possible for endovascular procedures and by adequately compressing the access site after the contrast agent delivery catheter or sheath has been removed. Use of percutaneous arterial sealing devices also appears to decrease the risk of access site bleeding when larger access catheters and sheaths are used. We presently use the Angio-Seal device (St. Jude Medical, Minneapolis, MN) for diagnostic and interventional angiography procedures when sheaths smaller than 8F are used and the Perclose A-T device (Abbott Vascular, Abbott Park, IL) in procedures requiring larger sheaths. Other closure devices for the arterial puncture site are also available. In general, all of these devices are highly successful and have a short learning curve. The Angio-Seal device uses a collagen plug attached to a bioabsorbable foot-plate to seal the arteriotomy. Eggebrecht et al.[24] prospectively assessed the use of the Angio-Seal device in 180 consecutive patients; more than 95% had successful deployment of the device, more than 90% had immediate hemostasis, and the rate of major access site complications was approximately 2%. The Perclose A-T device delivers polyester suture to the arteriotomy by introducing two small needles into the wall of the vessel from the lumen, and, with use of a pretied knot, cinching the suture down to appose the vessel walls. This device can be placed either before or after an intervention. In a randomized study of use of this suture-mediated closure device versus manual compression, patients with the Perclose device had shorter time to hemostasis, ambulation, and discharge.[25] Additionally, there were six access site complications in the Perclose group, only two of which were classified as major (3.8%), and, notably, there was no difference in the rates of complication between manual compression and the device. Koreny et al.[26] reviewed randomized trials that used six commercially available vascular access closure devices and, in nearly 4000 patients, found no difference between patients who had closure devices and those who received manual compression in the incidence of groin hematomas, iatrogenic arteriovenous fistulae, bleeding, or pseudoaneurysm. However, the time to hemostasis was, on average, 17 minutes shorter for the patients having closure devices.

Most groin hematomas that form—irrespective of the presence of a closure device—are small and resolve spontaneously; only those hematomas that continue to expand or are large enough to threaten the viability of the overlying skin require surgical evacuation. On the other hand, retroperitoneal hematomas or retroperitoneal hemorrhage caused by bleeding from an external iliac artery access site often requires surgical evacuation and arterial repair because arterial compression after catheter removal is difficult in this location. Because of the difficulty in gaining surgical control of a bleeding external iliac artery, injuries in this location are often managed by using a contralateral groin puncture and either endoluminal therapy with a covered stent or an intravascular balloon for inflow control. Fortunately, this most serious access-related complication can be minimized by visualizing bony landmarks before attempting vascular access. As stated previously, the CFA is the target vessel for most access, and its anatomic location allows for ease of monitoring for access site hematomas (in the non–morbidly obese patient). Additionally, the juxtaposition of the vessel to underlying bone allows for compressibility should any minor bleeding occur.

As access site hematomas resolve, a pseudoaneurysm caused by failure of the arterial puncture site to seal occasionally becomes evident (Figure 20-5). Most such pseudoaneurysms resolve spontaneously if the patient is not anticoagulated on a long-term basis. Because

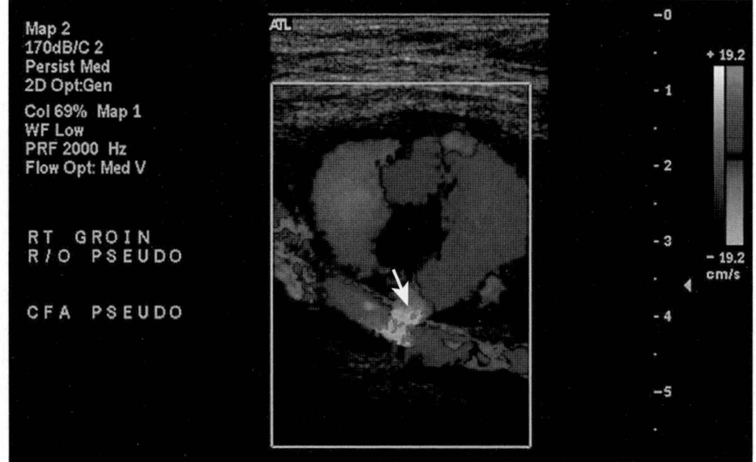

FIGURE 20-5 Pseudoaneurysm arising off the CFA after arterial puncture as demonstrated by duplex sonography. The *arrow* depicts the neck of the pseudoaneurysm.

ultrasound-directed compression or even ultrasound-guided thrombin injection occludes the majority of pseudoaneurysms that do not spontaneously resolve, surgical repair is rarely required.[27] Thus, in those patients without hemodynamic instability, skin compromise, or distal perfusion compromise, we advocate a conservative approach to access site bleeding complications, particularly to femoral pseudoaneurysms, unless they are progressive or there is a concern for infection.

Trauma to the arterial wall from initial arterial puncture or subsequent intimal dissection from guidewire or catheter passage also occasionally complicate angiography. Intimal dissection usually occurs during initial guidewire or catheter passage, which should be done under fluoroscopic control. Recognition of a subintimal position of the guidewire or the catheter and redirection into the lumen can limit the consequences of this complication. If the access is approached via a retrograde manner, the iatrogenic dissection is also against the direction of blood flow and hence has a smaller likelihood of hemodynamic significance. When small, these dissections heal spontaneously in the majority of cases. Occasionally, however, thrombosis of the artery can occur from either trauma at the puncture site or subintimal catheter or guidewire passage, especially in the presence of significant underlying occlusive disease. Arterial thrombosis caused by intimal dissection can be treated by means of thrombolysis and endoluminal stent placement. In contrast, arterial thrombosis caused by injury at the puncture site usually requires surgical thrombectomy and repair.

Distal Embolization

Embolic events can occur with any endovascular manipulation, including diagnostic angiography. Arterial mural thrombus or plaque as well as thrombus formed adjacent to a catheter or a guidewire can be dislodged during arterial access, guidewire or catheter manipulation, and catheter removal. Treatment of this complication can range from immediate operative or endovascular intervention to catheter-directed thrombolysis alone to expectant medical management, depending on the area of involvement and the severity of ischemia resulting from the embolic event. In the majority of cases, the embolic material consists of plaque debris or small pieces of thrombus, which embolize to the digital arteries of the foot. This is managed medically with aspirin and analgesics. Eventual resolution or progression to only small areas of dry gangrene can be expected in most patients, although the course can be protracted (months) and the discomfort caused to the patient may be significant. Larger emboli that cause limb- or organ-threatening ischemia must be treated aggressively with either thrombolysis or surgical or endovascular thrombectomy, depending on the degree of ischemia present and the patient's comorbidities.

Contrast Reactions

Although this topic has been briefly mentioned previously, it bears revisiting. The overall estimated rate of reactions from the administration of intravenous contrast may be as high as 60%.[17] Serious reactions from contrast can be either side effects (nephrotoxicity) or allergic reactions (urticaria, anaphylaxis). Recently, much has been written regarding the best prophylactic strategy for reducing the nephrotoxicity of contrast usage, including hydration, *N*-acetylcysteine, theophylline, and alkalinization. A recent meta-analysis of 41 randomized, controlled trials looking at these and other potentially preventative medications found that *N*-acetylcysteine and theophylline reduced the risk for contrast-induced nephropathy, with relative risks of 0.62 and 0.49, respectively.[28] It is our practice to prescribe oral *N*-acetylcysteine 600 mg twice daily the day before and the day of a procedure in patients with abnormal estimated glomerular filtration rates but not yet receiving dialysis. Additionally, we administer alkalinized intravenous fluid before, during, and after the procedures. To combat the unfortunate circumstance of having an allergic reaction to contrast, we query all patients about a history of such an allergy and then clarify the specific allergic reaction. For mild or moderate reactions, we will then premedicate patients with corticosteroids and antihistamines before the procedure. However, for severe reactions (anaphylaxis), we seek alternative imaging techniques but, if forced, administer steroids in large doses at the beginning of the procedure.

Carbon Dioxide Angiography

Hawkins[29] described the initial use of intraarterial CO_2 gas as a contrast agent for diagnostic peripheral angiography in 20 patients in 1982. Subsequently, the development of more sophisticated instruments and supporting software, including DSA systems, stacking software, tilting examination tables, and reliable CO_2 delivery systems has made CO_2 angiography a viable alternative to iodinated contrast agent studies in certain instances. Furthermore, CO_2 gas used as an arterial contrast agent has been demonstrated to have no allergenic potential, to produce no renal toxicity (with appropriate use), and to be extremely inexpensive.

Basic Principles

An arterial image is produced when CO_2 gas displaces flowing blood within a vessel, allowing the detection of small differences in radiographic density between the gas and the surrounding soft tissue. Therefore diagnostic accuracy of this technique is dependent on the degree of blood displacement by the CO_2 gas within the vessels of interest. CO_2 gas is extremely buoyant, and this buoyancy produces preferential filling of nondependent portions of vessels unless adequate columns of CO_2 gas are used to displace flowing blood completely. Thus incomplete blood displacement may occur in aneurysmal or large-diameter vessels such as the aorta, and the more posteriorly located left renal and lumbar branches may not be visualized with the patient in the usual supine position. In contrast, the left renal artery should always fill if the patient is placed in the right lateral decubitus position and is imaged with cross-table lateral DSA. Also, selective renal artery injections (10 to 20 mL) with the patient supine will fill the renal artery and will reflux into the aorta to allow assessment of ostial lesions. Anterior arteries such as the celiac axis and the superior and inferior mesenteric arteries are easily imaged with the patient in the supine position, again using cross-table imaging.

The buoyancy of CO_2 gas also alters the way in which the "contrast agent" exits the catheter: whereas iodinated contrast agents progress from the catheter tip following the flow of blood, CO_2 will diffuse proximally and distally from the catheter tip. From a practical standpoint, when using CO_2 angiography, the catheter tip therefore should be placed in the center of the imaging beam to maximize visualization. Carbon dioxide gas is also 400 times less viscous than iodinated contrast material, and this low viscosity facilitates filling and increases the likelihood of imaging distal vessels in patients with severe arterial occlusive disease. Additionally, the low viscosity of CO_2 gas allows its delivery through small-diameter catheters (2F to 3F) and through the narrow space between guidewires and catheters and various endovascular devices. The use of a Tuohy-Borst fitting permits rapid injection of CO_2 gas between the guidewire and the catheter, thereby simplifying real-time imaging of catheter or device position.

Carbon Dioxide Delivery

The compressibility of CO_2 gas makes it difficult for the operator to know the exact volume of gas being injected. Because the volume of a perfect gas varies inversely with pressure (Boyle's law), small volumes of gas delivered from pressurized CO_2 gas cylinders assume large volumes when exposed to pressures within the arterial tree. Therefore syringes loaded under pressure from a CO_2 cylinder contain an indeterminate volume of CO_2 gas, which can potentially result in an excessive dose of CO_2 being delivered to the patient. Furthermore, hand delivery of CO_2 gas can be explosive if blood (or any liquid) is present in the delivery catheter immediately before injection, resulting in compression of the CO_2 gas during delivery. In vitro testing of hand and mechanically driven syringes connected to fluid-filled angiographic catheters of various diameters has demonstrated that 95% of the volume of the CO_2 gas within a 100-mL syringe is delivered in the last 0.5 second of a 4-second controlled injection. This results in extremely high flow rates of CO_2 that can cause intimal injury at injection sites. These problems have been circumvented with the development of a dedicated mechanical CO_2 injector and a closed plastic bag hand delivery system that can deliver noncompressed controlled volumes of CO_2 gas.

Imaging Technique

The low density of CO_2 requires subtraction and electronic enhancement, available in DSA equipment, to produce adequate CO_2 arteriography. We currently use a 1024 × 1024–pixel DSA system acquiring three to four frames per second with a 60-ms pulse width. Images are postprocessed if needed by compiling multiple digital images into a single composite image with use of a stacking software program and a function that is specific for CO_2 (Toshiba America Medical Systems, Tustin, CA). The stacking software is used to overcome fragmentation of the CO_2 gas column by flowing blood, particularly in the distal extremity vessels, and, with use of this technique, adequate visualization of the ankle and the foot arteries can be provided after injection of as little as 10 mL of CO_2 gas. As with conventional angiography, bowel gas motion and patient movement can degrade the resolution of stacked images.

Lower-extremity arteriography is performed with the patient initially supine on a tilting angiographic table. Twenty to 40 mL of CO_2 at 40 mL/s is used for initial runoff imaging, with multiple injections performed to film the pelvis, the thigh, the knee, the lower legs, and the feet. For adequate filling of tibial and distal arteries, elevation of the feet by 10 to 20 degrees may be necessary. If filling of the pedal vessels is poor but gas bubbles can be seen, the cause is frequently inadequate delivery of the CO_2 gas for imaging of the vessel of interest, and an attempt should be made to alter CO_2 delivery rather than increasing the injectate volume. If the distal vessels in the extremity contralateral to the access site are poorly imaged, the injection catheter is advanced over the iliac bifurcation into the contralateral CFA or the SFA. If the distal vessels in the extremity ipsilateral to the access site are poorly visualized, the catheter is retracted close to the puncture site. Twenty milliliters of CO_2 gas is then injected at 10 mL/s, giving 100 to 150 mcg of nitroglycerin intraarterially just before the injection; if filling is still poor, a larger volume of CO_2 gas (40 to 60 mL) can be used. Larger volumes plus intraarterial nitroglycerin decrease "breakup" of CO_2 gas into bubbles and frequently provide good distal vessel images without stacking software. Thirty-five to 50 mL of CO_2 gas is delivered in approximately 0.5 second for aortography, while selective injections of 5 to 10 mL over 0.5 to 1.0 second or 5 to 20 mL of CO_2 over 0.5 to 2.0 seconds delivered with a shepherd-hook catheter in the renal or mesenteric artery ostia are used for visceral artery imaging.

Accuracy

More than 1500 patients have undergone angiography with use of CO_2 gas and DSA techniques at the University of Florida since 1981. Early experience with CO_2 arteriography was hampered by poor-quality images and required large volumes of CO_2 gas to produce only fair images of the aorta and poor visualization of the more distal vessels.[29] Subsequent improvements in delivery and imaging equipment and in technique have allowed good-quality diagnostic images of the lower-extremity arterial tree to be obtained in most patients while using smaller volumes of CO_2 gas. In a 1993 review of 115 high-risk patients undergoing CO_2 arteriograms, we found that 91% of the CO_2 studies were of good or excellent quality and that there was agreement between findings of CO_2 and contrast arteriograms in 95% of cases.[30] CO_2 image quality was best in the aorta and in the iliac, the renal, and the mesenteric arteries in that study and was judged to be of good or excellent quality in 90% of femoral arteries as well. Use of stacking programs provided adequate imaging of infrapopliteal arteries in 70% of CO_2 arteriograms, and accurate therapeutic plans could be developed on the basis of CO_2 studies alone in 92% of cases. More recently, further enhancements in imaging technique and routine use of intra-arterial nitroglycerin have improved imaging of infrapopliteal and pedal arteries. No allergic reactions were reported, and only a single patient who received CO_2 and supplemental contrast agent had an increase in serum creatinine level after angiography. Because 79% of patients included in our study had a history of contrast agent allergy or preexisting renal insufficiency, use of CO_2 markedly decreased the risks associated with arteriography in those patients.

Some groups have also attempted CO_2-guided endovascular repair of AAAs. Chao et al.[31] analyzed 16 patients whose endovascular AAA repair was performed primarily with CO_2 but supplemented with intravenous contrast. All procedures were successful, but only 3 were able to be done purely with CO_2. However, compared with a contemporaneous cohort of standard endovascular AAA repairs, the mean volume of contrast used was much smaller (27 mL vs. 148 mL, $p < 0.0005$).

Safety

Because intravenous injections of CO_2 were used routinely for the detection of pericardial effusion in the 1950s without significant problems, peripheral arterial injections of CO_2 should be associated with minimal risk of gas embolism. CO_2 bubbles have to pass through at least one capillary bed likely becoming trapped before reaching the right side of the heart, the pulmonary microvasculature, or the coronary and cerebral circulation. Furthermore, because the solubility of CO_2 in blood is 20 times that of oxygen, the dissolution of CO_2 bubbles in blood occurs more rapidly than that of air bubbles. Peripheral intraarterial injection of CO_2 gas could also theoretically lead to ischemic injury to peripheral organs by trapping gas bubbles within the vasculature of an organ, leading to vessel occlusion. Although small CO_2 bubbles are likely to pass through nutrient arteries, the buoyancy of larger bubbles could lead to gas trapping within larger arteries particularly in nondependent portions of organs or in any nonhorizontal artery in which the buoyant force of bubbles equals the momentum force of antegrade blood flow. In addition, larger bubbles may dissolve more slowly than small bubbles because of a lower surface area–to–volume ratio and thereby a proportionally smaller surface area over which gas transport to blood can occur.

Because of these theoretical concerns, we evaluated the potential for ischemic injury in several organ systems caused by nutrient artery occlusion by CO_2 bubbles after intraarterial injection. Injections of 7 mL/kg (about 10 times the normal human dose) of CO_2 gas directly into canine renal arteries resulted in no decrease in renal blood flow or renal function as measured by Tc 99m dimercaptosuccinic acid and sodium iodohippurate I 131 scans done within 24 hours after CO_2 injections.[32] Furthermore, no microscopic changes in the endothelium of major renal arteries or in the glomeruli were seen by means of scanning or transmission electron microscopy when CO_2 injections were done with the animal supine. Only when the kidney was vertically positioned above the injection site and multiple injections in the same kidney were done were changes compatible with minimal acute tubular necrosis seen via transmission electron microscopy. This minimal injury appears to be due to prolonged CO_2 trapping within the kidney, based on a preliminary ultrasound study demonstrating clearance of injected CO_2 from the renal cortex of kidneys positioned vertically within approximately 2 minutes, compared with 30 seconds when the kidney is in a horizontal position. Thus renal injection of CO_2 is well tolerated despite apparent transport of CO_2 gas through the renal microvasculature.

In contrast, the effects of CO_2 gas in the cerebral circulation are unresolved. Direct injection of CO_2 into the carotid arteries of rats in a study from the University of Florida resulted in significant neurologic deficit, and histologic examination of brain tissue revealed multifocal ischemic infarction and disruption of the blood-brain barrier.[33] In contrast, Shifrin et al.[34] reported no immediate electroencephalographic changes or any neurologic deficits occurring after aortic arch and carotid injections of 3 to 5 mL/kg CO_2 in dogs. Dimakakos et al.[35] injected 3 mL/kg of CO_2 intraarterially in each of 25 rabbits. MR imaging was done before and after the injections, and all animals were killed and a pathologic examination was done on their brains. There were no neurologic sequelae clinically, no pathologic findings on MR imaging, and no abnormal findings on the autopsy specimens. Kozlov et al.[36] catheterized bilateral carotid arteries in 14 pigs, with one side being the control for the other in each animal. A single injection of CO_2 did not produce any neurologic symptoms, but multiple successive boluses of CO_2 resulted in adverse events in every animal tested. These events included seizure activity, cardiopulmonary arrest, hemorrhagic cerebral infarcts, and breakdown of the blood-brain barrier as detected on histologic staining. Further animal studies are needed to determine fully the neurotoxic risk of cerebrovascular CO_2 exposure, but, at present, we avoid injection of CO_2 gas into regions where it can reach the cerebral circulation.

Complications

Adverse events associated with diagnostic and therapeutic vascular imaging in humans using CO_2 gas have been rare in our experience. Trapping of CO_2 gas and subsequent vapor lock phenomena have resulted in complications in only three patients undergoing peripheral angiography of the aorta and the lower-extremity arteries with use of CO_2 gas contrast material. One patient in our series with a large infrarenal aortic aneurysm received 2000 mL of CO_2 over 30 minutes for imaging of the runoff vasculature and had transient diarrhea likely caused by CO_2 trapping anteriorly in the aneurysm and vapor lock within a patent inferior mesenteric artery.[37] Immediate sigmoidoscopy suggested ischemic changes, but a mucosal biopsy performed at the time showed normal findings, and no gross colonic abnormalities were noted 3 weeks later during surgical aneurysm repair. Two other cases of mesenteric ischemia after CO_2 aortography have been reported from other institutions—one case of transient colon ischemia (similar to our case) and one case resulting in livedo reticularis of the lower torso, rhabdomyolysis, massive intestinal infarction, and death.[38,39] Because CO_2 gas combines with water to produce carbonic acid, intravascular injection of acidic saline solution or possibly contamination with air may have contributed to clinical ischemia in the last patient described. Regardless, currently, in patients undergoing evaluation for intestinal ischemia, we inject only 10 mL of CO_2 into the mesenteric vessels and wait 5 minutes or more between injections. In addition, during runoff examinations with distal aortic injections, if the inferior mesenteric artery is well filled, the injection catheter is advanced over the bifurcation and is later retracted to the puncture site for subsequent lower-extremity studies, with each leg examined separately to avoid repeated left part of the colon exposure to CO_2.

Two patients also had transient manifestations of vapor lock in the right ventricular outflow tract during transjugular intrahepatic portasystemic shunt (TIPS) procedures in our series.[37] Stopcock malpositioning caused large-volume (1200 to 3000 mL) delivery of CO_2 in one case and inadvertent injection of room air in another. Hemodynamic compromise, electrocardiographic changes, and symptoms resolved within 1 minute after left lateral decubitus positioning in each case. Finally, transient unconsciousness (20 seconds) occurred in one of our patients undergoing CO_2 arteriography for evaluation of an axillofemoral bypass when he accidentally raised his head above the level of the CO_2 injection. A similar transient neurologic event was reported from another institution during CO_2 angiographic evaluation of an arm dialysis shunt, when CO_2 refluxed into the cerebral circulation.[40] Last, pain associated with CO_2 injections may be significant. Kessel et al.[41] reported on 50 consecutive patients who underwent CO_2 angiography and noted that two had significant pain during injection, and, in one of these cases, the pain was so severe that the procedure had to be aborted.

Contraindications

Although we have not seen untoward effects in patients with chronic obstructive pulmonary disease (COPD), severe COPD with evidence of CO_2 retention on blood gas analysis is a relative contraindication to CO_2 angiography. However, both Bettman and Weaver and their colleagues[42,43] demonstrated no increase in the partial pressure of CO_2 in arterial blood gas samples after CO_2 arteriography, and five patients in the series of Weaver et al. had significant COPD. Regardless, when patients with COPD undergo CO_2 arteriography, we increase the time between CO_2 injections to greater than 2 minutes and decrease the total volume of CO_2 injected. We also do not use CO_2 angiography to evaluate cerebral or upper-extremity vasculature because of the previously described potential risk for neurotoxicity. Furthermore, because of the potential for retrograde embolization of CO_2 gas bubbles into cerebral arteries with the injection of CO_2 into the upper-extremity vasculature or into bypasses connected to these vessels, CO_2 arteriography has been limited to evaluation of arteries below the level of the diaphragm at our institution.

Gadolinium as a Contrast Agent

Gadolinium is classified as a rare earth element, one of the lanthanide series. It has seven unpaired electrons, which makes it a powerful contrast agent in MR imaging. However, it inhibits calcium channels and hence is associated with significant cardiovascular and neurologic toxicity. Additionally, for patients with renal dysfunction, the association of gadolinium administration and the development of nephrogenic systemic fibrosis (NSF) has been widely publicized of late. As such, any procedure performed with gadolinium should be approached with caution.

Gadolinium has been used as an intraarterial contrast agent in patients with a significant contraindication to iodinated compounds, which most often in our practice is due to the documentation of a significant allergy to iodinated contrast. Wagner et al.[44] compared the feasibility of gadolinium as a contrast agent in patients with direct contraindications to other contrast agents and were able to successfully perform diagnostic angiography in 15 cases and therapeutic interventions in another 15 cases. However, they found that the images obtained were inferior to images using standard contrast agents. It also remains unclear whether gadolinium is more toxic than standard iodinated contrast. Nyman et al.[45] reviewed equal-attenuating doses of gadolinium-based and iodinated contrast agents and found that, at least in mice, the general toxicity of gadolinium was six to 25 times greater than that of iodinated contrast. However, Kane et al.[46] examined the nephrotoxic effects of these agents in patients with renal dysfunction who were undergoing percutaneous renal angioplasty and reported the incidence of postprocedure serum creatinine elevation to be less in patients administered gadolinium (5.3%) compared with patients administered iodinated contrast (20.6%).

Nephrogenic Systemic Fibrosis

Formerly called nephrogenic systemic dermopathy because of the predominance of skin manifestations noted in the original cases, NSF was first observed in 1997 and reported in 2000.[47] The purported mechanism of NSF is the deposition of free gadolinium in body tissues resulting from prolonged gadolinium clearance in patients with renal dysfunction. Once deposited, gadolinium remains trapped in the tissue on account of its poor water solubility. Although only some of the commercially available gadolinium chelates have been associated with NSF, the Food and Drug Administration (FDA) has warned that all gadolinium compounds should be used in patients with severe renal dysfunction only if absolutely necessary.[48] The clinical manifestations of NSF include a symmetric thickening of the skin, with lower extremities affected in 97% of cases, followed by upper extremities in 77%, and the torso in 30%.[49] This fibrotic reaction can progress to involve deeper tissues, resulting in joint contractures and immobility,[50,51] and has been reported to be the cause of respiratory distress resulting from involvement of the diaphragm.[52] NSF is also associated with a significant hypercoagulable state with manifestations of deep venous thromboses, pulmonary emboli, thrombosis of arteriovenous fistulae, or atrial thrombi.

The treatment of NSF is largely unsuccessful, although improvement of renal function (e.g., with renal transplantation) appears to have some benefit in afflicted patients. Efforts such as radiation with ultraviolet light, treatment with sodium thiosulfate, extracorporeal photopheresis, and intravenous immunoglobulin have been tried with sporadic success. Even the recommendation by the FDA to initiate hemodialysis after gadolinium administration is weak, and, although other organizations such as the American College of Radiology have advocated this "treatment," there are no data to support this recommendation.[48] However, all agencies do advocate using the minimum dosage required and to avoid repeated gadolinium administration within a week's time.

RADIATION SAFETY

Contrast angiography involves the use of ionizing radiation, regardless of the technique used to record the image. Fortunately, DSA uses relatively low-dose techniques, and modern equipment is efficient at achieving high-quality images with low dosages of radiation. Endovascular therapies, however, involve a higher total dose of radiation because of the length of the procedures, and the cumulative dose administered during a long diagnostic procedure is also not negligible. Adequate lead shielding is essential for health care workers and patients, and the dose of radiation during a procedure should be minimized by using digital procedures such as road-mapping, last-image hold, and pulsed fluoroscopy. Proper calibration and monitoring of equipment to avoid excessive radiation exposure and compulsive radiation monitoring of all personnel involved in arteriography and endovascular procedures are also essential. Finally, it is important to remember that no safe lower level of radiation exposure has been demonstrated, and repeated exposure to even small doses of ionizing radiation over a prolonged period can result in cumulative doses that are significant.

FIXED VERSUS PORTABLE EQUIPMENT

Traditional operating rooms typically have imaging systems that consist of a portable C-arm system with a high-output, high-heat-capacity x-ray tube; a 12-inch image intensifier; and a sophisticated digital processing system that provides last-image hold, DSA, and road-mapping. In addition, a cantilevered or dual-end-supported radiolucent operating table with a floating top for position changes and an appropriate array of guidewires and catheters should be available. With such equipment, angiography and current endovascular procedures can be performed successfully in a standard operating room.

Traditional radiology suites that contain fixed, higher-resolution imaging systems are poorly designed for open surgical or open endovascular procedures because of limited space, poor lighting, limited access to core surgical facilities, lack of a controlled sterile environment, inadequate sterilization facilities, and quite often staff who are not familiar with the degree of sterility required for open surgical procedures. Conversely, as noted, most operating rooms lack sophisticated x-ray equipment capable of providing high-quality fluoroscopic and digital images; a flexible easy-to-use radiolucent surgical table; and a readily available, full variety of guidewires and catheters.

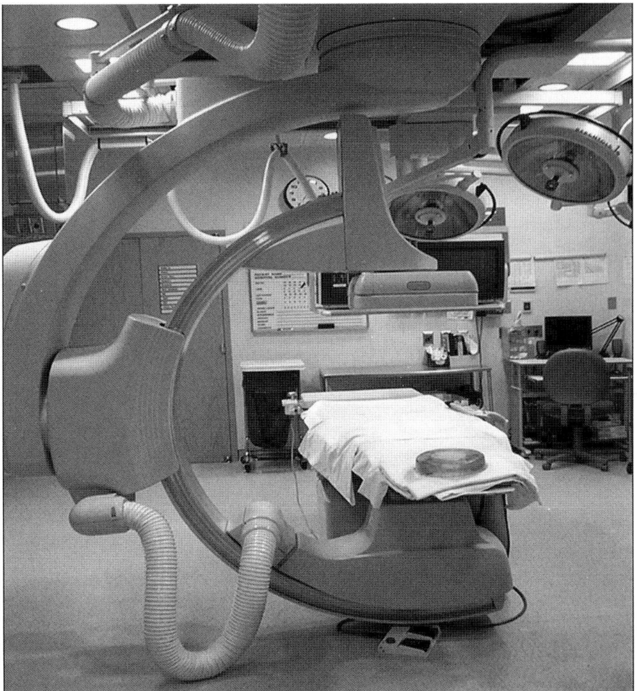

FIGURE 20-6 An example of a converted traditional operating room that has been equipped with a mounted C-arm, sophisticated imaging software, and a movable table. The room also houses a standard anesthesia machine and is large enough to perform full cardiopulmonary bypass if needed.

The best solution for these conflicting problems is a melding of these complementary technologies in an endovascular suite specifically designed for such procedures (Figure 20-6). Operating room–compatible fixed angiography systems are available from several companies, although the initial cost is somewhat prohibitive for widespread adoption without the overt commitment to design or maintain an aggressive endovascular program. The modern surgical and angiography suite is well suited to perform diagnostic angiography, as well as therapeutic endovascular procedures, from tibial angioplasty to thrombolysis to thoracic stenting. The fixed equipment in the suite includes a high-power, high-heat-capacity, rapid-cooling x-ray tube; a large image intensifier capable of complex angulation in multiple planes, and variation of the source-to-intensifier distance; a cantilevered radiolucent table that is easily moved; convenient high-resolution video monitors; and immediately available film and electronic image processing equipment. This equipment also has good image quality and good spatial and contrast resolution, allowing lower radiation and contrast doses, and is less technician dependent.

References

1. Ligush J Jr, Reavis SW, Preisser JS, et al: Duplex ultrasound scanning defines operative strategies for patients with limb-threatening ischemia, *J Vasc Surg* 28:482–490, discussion 490–481, 1998.
2. Ascher E, Marks NA, Hingorani AP, et al: Duplex-guided endovascular treatment for occlusive and stenotic lesions of the femoral-popliteal arterial segment: a comparative study in the first 253 cases, *J Vasc Surg* 44:1230–1237, discussion 1237–1238, 2006.
3. Rzucidlo EM, Walsh DB, Powell RJ, et al: Prediction of early graft failure with intraoperative completion duplex ultrasound scan, *J Vasc Surg* 36:975–981, 2002.
4. Hansen KJ, O'Neil EA, Reavis SW, et al: Intraoperative duplex sonography during renal artery reconstruction, *J Vasc Surg* 14:364–374, 1991.
5. Sandford RM, Bown MJ, Fishwick G, et al: Duplex ultrasound scanning is reliable in the detection of endoleak following endovascular aneurysm repair, *Eur J Vasc Endovasc Surg* 32:537–541, 2006.
6. Willmann JK, Baumert B, Schertler T, et al: Aortoiliac and lower extremity arteries assessed with 16-detector row CT angiography: prospective comparison with digital subtraction angiography, *Radiology* 236:1083–1093, 2005.
7. Lopera JE, Trimmer CK, Josephs SG, et al: Multidetector CT angiography of infrainguinal arterial bypass, *Radiographics* 28:529–548, 2008, discussion 549.
8. Koelemay MJ, Lijmer JG, Stoker J, et al: Magnetic resonance angiography for the evaluation of lower extremity arterial disease: a meta-analysis, *JAMA* 285:1338–1345, 2001.
9. Ersoy H, Rybicki FJ: MR angiography of the lower extremities, *AJR Am J Roentgenol* 190:1675–1684, 2008.
10. Rutherford RB, Krupski WC: Current status of open versus endovascular stent-graft repair of abdominal aortic aneurysm, *J Vasc Surg* 39:1129–1139, 2004.
11. Schneider P: *Endovascular skills: guidewire and catheter skills for endovascular surgery*, ed 2, New York, 2003, Marcel Dekker, Inc.
12. AbuRahma AF, Elmore M, Deel J, et al: Complications of diagnostic arteriography performed by a vascular surgeon in a recent series of 558 patients, *Vascular* 15:92–97, 2007.
13. Basche S, Eger C, Aschenbach R: The brachial artery as approach for catheter interventions: indications, results, complications, *Vasa* 33:235–238, 2004.
14. Hammacher ER, Eikelboom BC, van Lier HJ, et al: Brachial artery lesions after cardiac catheterisation, *Eur J Vasc Surg* 2:145–149, 1988.
15. Chitwood RW, Shepard AD, Shetty PC, et al: Surgical complications of transaxillary arteriography: a case-control study, *J Vasc Surg* 23:844–849, discussion 849–850, 1996.
16. Katayama H, Yamaguchi K, Kozuka T, et al: Adverse reactions to ionic and nonionic contrast media: a report from the Japanese Committee on the Safety of Contrast Media, *Radiology* 175:621–628, 1990.
17. Martin-Paredero V, Dixon SM, Baker JD, et al: Risk of renal failure after major angiography, *Arch Surg* 118:1417–1420, 1983.
18. Gomes AS, Baker JD, Martin-Paredero V, et al: Acute renal dysfunction after major arteriography, *AJR Am J Roentgenol* 145:1249–1253, 1985.
19. Schwab SJ, Hlatky MA, Pieper KS, et al: Contrast nephrotoxicity: a randomized controlled trial of a nonionic and an ionic radiographic contrast agent, *N Engl J Med* 320:149–153, 1989.
20. Deutsch L–S: Angiography and fluoroscopy during endovascular surgery. In Ahn S, Moore W, editors: *Endovascular surgery*, Philadelphia, 1992, W.B. Saunders230–268.
21. Huber TS, Back MR, Flynn TC, et al: Intraoperative prebypass arteriography for infrageniculate revascularization, *Am J Surg* 174:205–209, 1997.
22. Caro JJ, Trindade E, McGregor M: The risks of death and of severe nonfatal reactions with high- vs low-osmolality contrast media: a meta-analysis, *AJR Am J Roentgenol* 156:825–832, 1991.
23. Hessel SJ, Adams DF, Abrams HL: Complications of angiography, *Radiology* 138:273–281, 1981.
24. Eggebrecht H, Haude M, von Birgelen C, et al: Early clinical experience with the 6 French Angio-Seal device: immediate closure of femoral puncture sites after diagnostic and interventional coronary procedures, *Catheter Cardiovasc Interv* 53:437–442, 2001.
25. Starnes BW, O'Donnell SD, Gillespie DL, et al: Percutaneous arterial closure in peripheral vascular disease: a prospective randomized evaluation of the Perclose device, *J Vasc Surg* 38:263–271, 2003.
26. Koreny M, Riedmuller E, Nikfardjam M, et al: Arterial puncture closing devices compared with standard manual compression after cardiac catheterization: systematic review and meta-analysis, *JAMA* 291:350–357, 2004.
27. Kang SS, Labropoulos N, Mansour MA, et al: Percutaneous ultrasound guided thrombin injection: a new method for treating postcatheterization femoral pseudoaneurysms, *J Vasc Surg* 27:1032–1038, 1998.
28. Kelly AM, Dwamena B, Cronin P, et al: Meta-analysis: effectiveness of drugs for preventing contrast-induced nephropathy, *Ann Intern Med* 148:284–294, 2008.
29. Hawkins IF: Carbon dioxide digital subtraction arteriography, *AJR Am J Roentgenol* 139:19–24, 1982.
30. Seeger JM, Self S, Harward TR, et al: Carbon dioxide gas as an arterial contrast agent, *Ann Surg* 217:688–697, discussion 697–688, 1993.
31. Chao A, Major K, Kumar SR, et al: Carbon dioxide digital subtraction angiography—assisted endovascular aortic aneurysm repair in the azotemic patient, *J Vasc Surg* 45:451–458, discussion 458–460, 2007.
32. Hawkins IF Jr, Mladinich CR, Storm B, et al: Short-term effects of selective renal arterial carbon dioxide administration on the dog kidney, *J Vasc Interv Radiol* 5:149–154, 1994.
33. Coffey R, Quisling RG, Mickle JP, et al: The cerebrovascular effects of intraarterial CO_2 in quantities required for diagnostic imaging, *Radiology* 151:405–410, 1984.
34. Shifrin EG, Plich MB, Verstandig AG, et al: Cerebral angiography with gaseous carbon dioxide CO_2, *J Cardiovasc Surg (Torino)* 31:603–606, 1990.
35. Dimakakos PB, Stefanopoulos T, Doufas AG, et al: The cerebral effects of carbon dioxide during digital subtraction angiography in the aortic arch and its branches in rabbits, *AJNR Am J Neuroradiol* 19:261–266, 1998.
36. Kozlov DB, Lang EV, Barnhart W, et al: Adverse cerebrovascular effects of intraarterial CO_2 injections: development of an in vitro/in vivo model for assessment of gas-based toxicity, *J Vasc Interv Radiol* 16:713–726, 2005.
37. Caridi JG, Hawkins IF Jr: CO_2 digital subtraction angiography: potential complications and their prevention, *J Vasc Interv Radiol* 8:383–391, 1997.
38. Rundback JH, Shah PM, Wong J, et al: Livedo reticularis, rhabdomyolysis, massive intestinal infarction, and death after carbon dioxide arteriography, *J Vasc Surg* 26:337–340, 1997.
39. Spinosa DJ, Matsumoto AH, Angle JF, et al: Transient mesenteric ischemia: a complication of carbon dioxide angiography, *J Vasc Interv Radiol* 9:561–564, 1998.

40. Ehrman KO, Taber TE, Gaylord GM, et al: Comparison of diagnostic accuracy with carbon dioxide versus iodinated contrast material in the imaging of hemodialysis access fistulas, *J Vasc Interv Radiol* 5:771–775, 1994.
41. Kessel DO, Robertson I, Patel JT, et al: Carbon-dioxide–guided vascular interventions: technique and pitfalls, *Cardiovasc Intervent Radiol* 25:476–483, 2002.
42. Bettmann MA, D'Agostino R, Juravsky LI, et al: Carbon dioxide as an angiographic contrast agent: a prospective randomized trial, *Invest Radiol* 29(Suppl 2):S45–46, 1994.
43. Weaver FA, Pentecost MJ, Yellin AE, et al: Clinical applications of carbon dioxide/digital subtraction arteriography, *J Vasc Surg* 13:266–272, discussion 272–263, 1991.
44. Wagner HJ, Kalinowski M, Klose KJ, et al: The use of gadolinium chelates for X-ray digital subtraction angiography, *Invest Radiol* 36:257–265, 2001.
45. Nyman U, Elmstahl B, Leander P, et al: Are gadolinium-based contrast media really safer than iodinated media for digital subtraction angiography in patients with azotemia? *Radiology* 223:311–318, 2002, discussion 328–319, .
46. Kane GC, Stanson AW, Kalnicka D, et al: Comparison between gadolinium and iodine contrast for percutaneous intervention in atherosclerotic renal artery stenosis: clinical outcomes, *Nephrol Dial Transplant* 23:1233–1240, 2008.
47. Cowper SE, Robin HS, Steinberg SM, et al: Scleromyxoedema-like cutaneous diseases in renal-dialysis patients, *Lancet* 356:1000–1001, 2000.
48. Penfield JG, Reilly RF Jr: What nephrologists need to know about gadolinium, *Nat Clin Pract Nephrol* 3:654–668, 2007.
49. Mendoza FA, Artlett CM, Sandorfi N, et al: Description of 12 cases of nephrogenic fibrosing dermopathy and review of the literature, *Semin Arthritis Rheum* 35:238–249, 2006.
50. Gilliet M, Cozzio A, Burg G, et al: Successful treatment of three cases of nephrogenic fibrosing dermopathy with extracorporeal photopheresis, *Br J Dermatol* 152:531–536, 2005.
51. Levine JM, Taylor RA, Elman LB, et al: Involvement of skeletal muscle in dialysis-associated systemic fibrosis (nephrogenic fibrosing dermopathy), *Muscle Nerve* 30:569–577, 2004.
52. Kucher C, Steere J, Elenitsas R, et al: Nephrogenic fibrosing dermopathy/nephrogenic systemic fibrosis with diaphragmatic involvement in a patient with respiratory failure, *J Am Acad Dermatol* 54:S31–S34, 2006.

CHAPTER

21

Intravascular Ultrasound

Arash Keyhani, George Kopchock, Rodney A. White

Intravascular ultrasound (IVUS) has developed rapidly from being predominantly a research tool to being a highly useful clinical tool in interventional centers that focus on the evaluation and the application of endovascular technologies. Advances in instrumentation and technology along with positive clinical data have contributed to the wider use of IVUS. For many interventional specialists, IVUS is an invaluable part of their endovascular armamentarium. This chapter reviews the principles of IVUS imaging and emphasizes the clinical application in endovascular interventions.

IVUS IMAGING SYSTEMS

In the 1990s, several advances in imaging quality and catheter design were made. Image resolution is a function of transducer frequency; the higher the transducer frequency, the finer the resolution. For example, transthoracic echocardiography routinely uses a frequency of 2.5 MHz with a resolution of 2 to 4 mm, whereas transesophageal echocardiography uses a frequency of 5 MHz with a resolution of 1 to 2 mm. The 10- to 30-MHz IVUS transducers currently used to image vessels have a resolution of approximately 0.1 to 0.15 mm (120 to 150 μm). Additionally, the depth of penetration is inversely proportional to the frequency. For thoracic and abdominal aortic imaging, 8- to 12-MHz catheters are typically used whereas the 20- and 30-MHz catheters are used for smaller-diameter vessels such as the iliac and coronary arteries. To obtain a 360-degree cross-sectional image, the ultrasound beam must be scanned through a full circle, and the beam direction and deflection on the display must be synchronized. This can be achieved by mechanically rotating the imaging elements or by using electronically switched arrays.

Electronically Switched Transducers

By using electronically switched arrays, or phased arrays, an intravascular catheter with a number of stationary elements was constructed in the early 1970s.[1] This type of IVUS catheter consists of elements arranged in a circular array mounted on the tip of a catheter. These elements produce real-time intraluminal images in a plane perpendicular to the long axis of the catheter and provide a full 360-degree image of the blood vessel. Current catheter design incorporates a miniature integrated circuit into the tip, which provides sequenced transmission and reception without requiring numerous electrical circuits traveling the full length of the catheter. In addition to reducing the amount of electronic noise, this modification simplifies the manufacturing complexity and improves the flexibility of the catheter.

Current phased-array IVUS catheters use frequencies in the range of 10 to 40 MHz. The most common catheter currently used for large-diameter aortic procedures is an 8.2F, 10-MHz catheter that tracks over a 0.035-inch wire (Figure 21-1). A problem with these imaging catheters (common with all high-frequency ultrasound devices to some extent) is the inability to image structures in the immediate vicinity of the transducer. Because the imaging crystals in a phased-array configuration are in almost direct contact with the structure being imaged, a bright circumferential artifact known as "ring down" surrounds the catheter. Although this effect is seen in transcutaneous ultrasound imaging, it is not a significant problem because the structures of interest are generally at some distance from the transducer. Because IVUS devices use higher frequencies than transcutaneous arrays, the ring-down artifact can be a substantial problem since the imaging component is much closer to the target structure. If the catheter remains in a central position within the blood vessel during imaging, only blood echoes immediately surrounding the imaging assembly will be lost. The ring-down artifact can be electronically

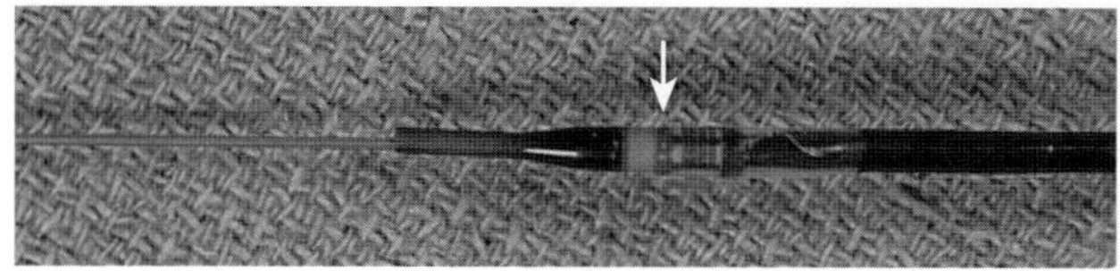

FIGURE 21-1 The Volcano Vision PV 8.2F, 10-MHz phased-array IVUS catheter introduced over a 0.035-inch guidewire. The 64 linear crystals *(arrow)* are positioned at the tip of the catheter. *(Courtesy Volcano Therapeutics, Rancho Cordova, CA.)*

removed, but structures within the region that is masked will not be seen. In large and medium-sized vessels (aortoiliac), this is not usually a problem because the clinicians can usually reposition the guidewire to remove the catheter off the vessel wall.

Mechanical Transducers

The first prototypes of mechanical intraluminal ultrasound imaging devices were used in gastrointestinal and transesophageal imaging.[2,3] Refinements in transducer manufacturing and computerized image processing have led to the development of the current low-profile, high-quality intravascular configurations.

Mechanical transducers use a transducer located at the tip of the catheter, which uses a flexible high-torque cable that extends the length of the device. The transducer is angled slightly forward and perpendicular to produce a cone-shaped ultrasound beam, resulting in an image of the vessel that is slightly forward or in front of the transducer assembly. In rotating transducer devices, ultrasound frequencies between 10 and 30 MHz are generally used, although some experimental devices using frequencies up to 45 MHz produce excellent images of human arteries.

One advantage of this configuration is that the distance between the transducer and the vessel lumen partially eliminates the ring-down artifact and the poor near-field resolution. The scan converter in the image processing unit compensates for this nonimaging portion of the beam and generates images beginning precisely at the surface of the catheter. In the rotating transducer and multiple array devices, a part of the ring-down region in the near-field zone of the beam occurs outside the catheter, so that it is not possible to image clearly in this area. Mechanical imaging catheters suffer from less image loss as described above.[4]

Other potential disadvantages of mechanical systems include the need for imaging chamber flushing and mechanical artifacts caused by the parallel guidewire, which is necessary for combined use with guidewires or as part of a combined therapeutic catheter system. Current disposable mechanical catheters require a saline- or water-filled imaging chamber. This chamber must be rendered and maintained bubble free to allow adequate imaging. Should a bubble appear, the image will be distorted or destroyed, and it may be necessary to flush the catheter to clear the bubble from the chamber.

Phased-array catheters can be constructed with a central lumen suitable for a guidewire, whereas mechanical devices require a coaxial monorail configuration because the imaging assembly cannot accommodate a central lumen. The difference in possible locations of the guidewire is not particularly important when imaging larger vessels or arteries before intervention. In small vessels such as the coronary arteries or after intervention (which may result in irregularities in the vessel wall), a centrally placed guidewire may be advantageous in passing the imaging catheter through the arterial segment.

CATHETER TECHNIQUES

Optimizing Image Quality and Accuracy

Although there are differences between mechanical and phased-array catheters, the techniques for obtaining optimal IVUS images are applicable to both.

Guidewire Use

Several of the IVUS catheters can be passed over a guidewire (0.014- to 0.038-inch in diameter), which allows more controlled maneuvering of the device within the lumen of the vessel from a remote introduction site, particularly in tortuous or tightly stenotic vessels. The mechanical rotating catheters use a variety of monorail and coaxial guidewire channels for over-the-wire applications, which can limit the tractability in tortuous arteries. Phased-array devices use a central guidewire channel, which offers an advantage in passing catheters through tortuous or narrowed vessels. When IVUS is used to image vessels before and after interventions such as balloon angioplasty or stent deployment, use of a guidewire is essential to allow manipulation of the catheters and repeated crossing of the lesion without further disruption of the angioplasty or stent site.

Rotational Orientation

It may be important to orient the IVUS catheter within the vessel so that anteroposterior accuracy can be achieved. The most successful method of maintaining orientation is the establishment of correct alignment in reference to the constant anatomic landmarks when used in phased-array transducers. When the aortoiliac segments are being imaged via a femoral puncture site, the common iliac arteries can be positioned side by side on the screen. Occasionally, this anatomic arrangement is not true, especially with tortuous dilated vessels, and the alignment must be checked against other parameters. The posteromedial position of the internal iliac artery

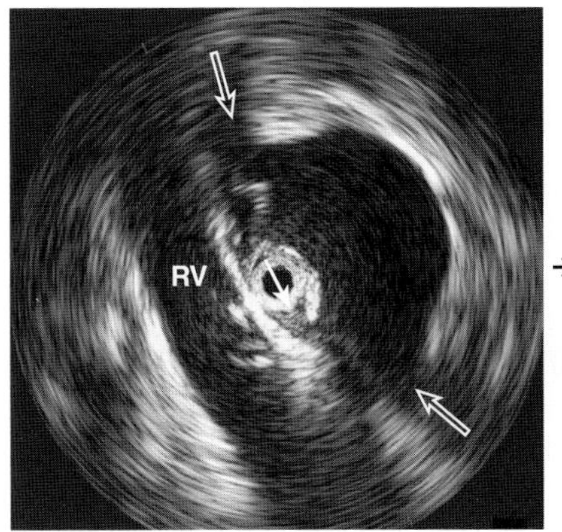

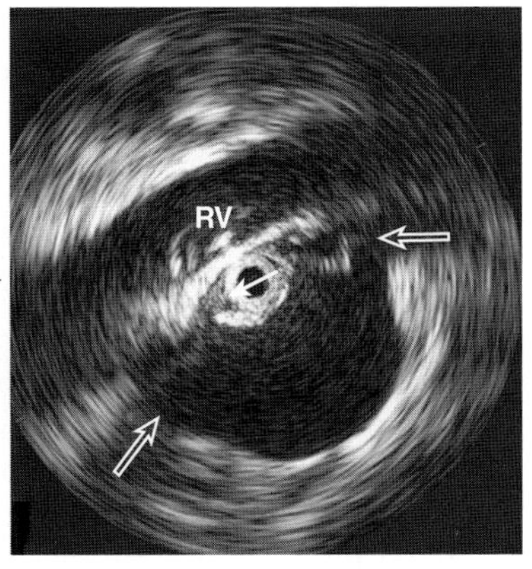

FIGURE 21-2 The IVUS imaging of the abdominal aorta at the level of the renal arteries *(white arrows)* reveals that the image is rotated posterior in reference to the anterior-positioned renal vein *(RV)*. The image can be rotated to place the renal vein in an anterior location, providing correct anterior-posterior alignment during the aortic interrogation.

orifices and the known position of the catheter at the site of insertion are used to determine rotational alignment of the device. The anterior location of visceral vessels (i.e., celiac, superior mesenteric, and renal arteries and renal vein) is also useful when imaging is done in the abdominal aorta (Figure 21-2). Because the catheters are rotationally rigid, there is very little loss of orientation during torquing and manipulation.

Centering and Flexion

Image quality is best when the catheter is parallel to the vessel wall (i.e., the ultrasound beam is directed at an angle 90 degrees to the luminal surface), whereas minor angulations may affect the luminal shape and the dimensional accuracy. Eccentric positioning causes the vessel wall nearer the imaging chamber to appear more hyperechoic than the distant wall, resulting in an artifactual difference in wall thicknesses.

Catheter centering is especially difficult in tortuous vessels, and rotational alignment may also be partly lost as the catheter meanders through the vessel. The best-quality images are obtained as the catheter is withdrawn through the lumen rather than during advancement. The slight tension produced during withdrawal straightens the catheter, and the tip tends to find the center of the vessel if there is no gross tortuosity. As vessel tortuosity or angulation increases, the catheter tends to assume a direct course through the lumen, resulting in more eccentric imaging. Eccentric positioning may affect the true luminal shape and dimensional accuracy. Therefore the minimal diameter (i.e., minor axis) should be used to measure vessel diameter. This has been previously described to represent an accurate measurement in angled images or tortuous anatomy.[5]

Longitudinal Gray-Scale Image Reconstruction

The longitudinal gray scale is reconstructed by mechanically withdrawing the catheter through the desired vessel at a controlled rate. A computer processor takes the cross-sectional images and stacks them into longitudinal image. The plane of section can be varied at every degree of axial rotation (e.g., anteroposterior, lateral, or oblique) or coronal alignment. The luminal profile can be examined, providing data similar to that found via angiography but with an almost limitless number of available projections. A more important feature of two-dimensional (2-D) longitudinal reconstruction, versus angiography, is its display of the transmural blood vessel morphology. An image of the entire vessel is produced rather than only the luminal profile that contrast angiography provides.

The 2-D gray-scale image is especially useful because it displays the luminal and the transmural morphology in true multiple gray scale. The differentiation of plaque, normal tissue, thrombus, dissections, and flaps is often much better appreciated in the 2-D longitudinal image.

IMAGE INTERPRETATION

The images produced by IVUS catheters not only outline the luminal and the adventitial surfaces of normal arterial segments but also have the potential to discriminate between normal and diseased vessel wall.

Tissue Characterization

In muscular arteries, distinct sonographic layers are visible, with the media appearing as an echolucent layer sandwiched between the more echodense intima and adventitia (Figure 21-3).[6] The internal and the external elastic laminae and adventitia are considered to be the backscatter substrates for the inner and the outer echodense zones.[6,7] Precise measurement of the adventitia may be difficult unless the vessel is surrounded by tissues of differing echogenicity (e.g., echolucent fat). Smooth muscle in the media is echolucent, whereas collagen in the adventitia and elastin in the intima are echodense. Small intimal lesions are also quite well defined in muscular arteries because of the fibrous tissue content, whereas large or complex plaques may compress or shadow the medial detail. The three-layer vessel image seen in muscular arteries may be lost in smaller distal arteries and larger elastic arteries because the increased elastin content makes the media echodense. In medium-sized vessels such as the femoral artery, the media is visible but is thinner than in more central vessels.

Gussenhoven et al.[7] described four basic plaque components, which can be distinguished by using 40-MHz IVUS in vitro: (1) echolucent (representing a lipid deposit or a lipid "lake"), (2) soft echoes (representing fibromuscular tissue and intimal proliferation, including varying amounts of diffusely dispersed lipid), (3) bright echoes (representing collagen-rich fibrous tissue), and (4) bright echoes with acoustic shadowing (representing calcified tissue). In addition to characterization of atherosclerotic plaque, IVUS can frequently distinguish thrombus from normal vessel wall or minimal occlusive disease. Fresh thrombus usually appears as a highly echogenic homogeneous mass with varying shadowing (image attenuation) beyond its location. Older thrombus can be difficult to differentiate from a fibrous atheromatous lesion but is usually less echogenic and very homogeneous.

For soft tissue, the absorption coefficient for ultrasound energy is proportional to the frequency, whereas for hard tissue it is proportional to the square of the frequency.[8] IVUS devices therefore are sensitive in differentiating between calcified and noncalcified vascular lesions. Because the ultrasound energy is strongly reflected by calcific plaque, the latter appears as a bright image with dense acoustic shadowing behind it. For this reason, the exact location of the media and the adventitia

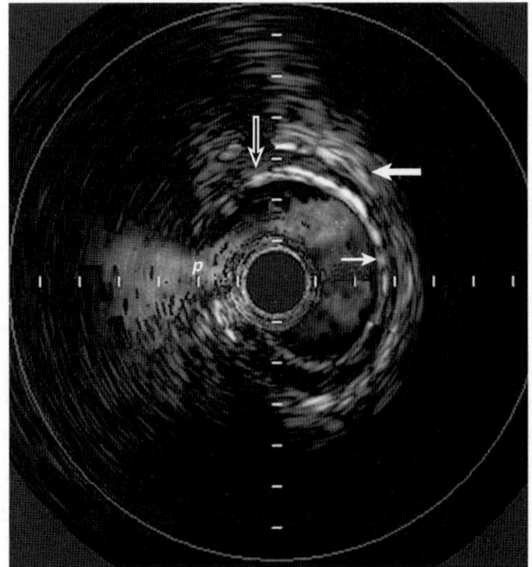

FIGURE 21-3 IVUS imaging of a femoral artery after endovascular access. The three distinct layers of the artery—intima *(small white arrow)*, muscular layer *(open arrow)*, and the adventitia *(solid arrow)*—are well delineated. The image also defines an area of a pseudoaneurysm *(p)* after the femoral artery was percutaneously accessed.

cannot be seen in segments of vessels containing heavily calcific disease, and dimensions must be estimated by interpolation of adjacent size data.

Dimensional Morphology and Lesion Distribution

Several authors have observed that intraluminal ultrasound determines the dimensions of the luminal diameter and the wall thickness of normal or minimally diseased arteries both in vitro and in vivo, and they have found the method to be accurate within 0.05 mm.[6-17] Determination of the outside diameter of the vessels may be less accurate, with a margin of error in some cases of up to 0.5 mm. Additional studies have compared IVUS with uniplanar angiography to determine the luminal dimensions of normal and moderately atherosclerotic human arteries.[11,18,19] Uniplanar angiography can be quite accurate in defining luminal cross-sectional area if the vessel is circular, as it is in most normal and mildly diseased arteries. Clinically significant atherosclerotic occlusive disease is usually eccentrically positioned in the arterial lumen, and the lumen may be either circular or elliptical, although most are circular.[20-22] If the lumen is elliptical, biplanar angiography is needed to define luminal cross-sectional areas more accurately and to calculate percent area stenosis.[23]

Investigations have also shown that luminal cross-sectional areas calculated via IVUS correlate very well with those obtained via angiography in normal or minimally diseased peripheral and coronary arteries.[18] In most studies in which imaged lumina have been only mildly elliptical, cross-sectional areas evaluated with angiography and those measured via IVUS correlate significantly, whereas in some severely diseased arteries with elliptical lesions the luminal cross-sectional area calculated by means of angiography is less accurate. In elliptical lumina, the cross-sectional area calculated by means of angiography is usually greater than that measured by means of IVUS.

In addition to its limitations in defining luminal dimensions of elliptical vessels, angiography gives no information about vessel wall morphology aside from calcification or aneurysms visualized on the plain x-ray films.

APPLICATION IN ENDOVASCULAR INTERVENTIONS

Diagnostic Application

IVUS is most often used in conjunction with other procedures such as angiography and angioplasty. In cases where contrast angiography is contraindicated or the computed tomographic (CT) scan is inconclusive, IVUS can be used as the sole diagnostic tool. This is especially true in cases such as thoracic aneurysms and dissections where intravascular imaging provides more information about pathology of the aneurysm and points of entry and reentry in dissection flaps (Figure 21-4). The IVUS pull-through identifies the proximal landing zone, the diameter of the landing zone, and the overall length between the proximal and distal landing zones. On the basis of this information, the endoluminal graft can be positioned at the marked location and deployed without the need of large amounts of contrast.

Peripheral Vascular Interventions

Stenoses and Cross-Sectional Area

By providing transmural imaging of the arterial wall, IVUS offers a new perspective on the development, the distribution, and the cross-sectional analysis of plaque morphology and volume quantitation. In the same vessel, luminal volume may be identical along the vessel, but some segments may have significant plaque volume whereas others have no apparent disease. This phenomenon has been well documented by the inspection of diseased vessels by several investigators; it is a consequence of the overall enlargement of the arterial wall to accommodate atherosclerotic plaque while preserving luminal volume during the early evolution of disease.[20-22,24] Vessel enlargement occurs until about 40% of the lumen is occupied by plaque; at this point, luminal volume is usually compromised by further lesion development.

IVUS offers an additional important perspective of diseased vessels, in contrast to angiography, which outlines only the luminal area. In an artery that has disease at only one site, angiography identifies the degree of luminal narrowing quite accurately by demonstrating the degree of constriction produced by the lesion. In diffusely diseased arteries with an accumulation of plaque in all segments, estimation of the degree of luminal compromise by comparison with adjacent normal-caliber arteries grossly underestimates the total plaque volume (Figure 21-5).

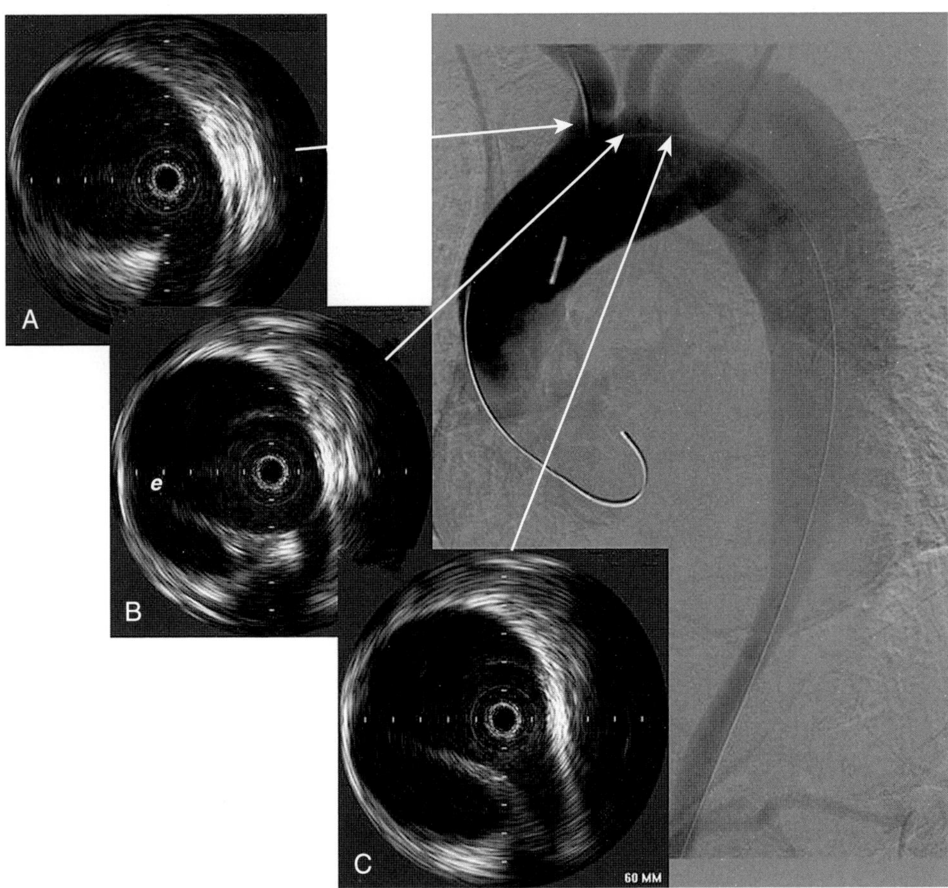

FIGURE 21-4 Evaluation of the proximal fixation point for a thoracic dissection. The cross-sectional IVUS imaging demonstrates the origin of the arch vessels (innominate **[A]**, carotid **[B]**, left subclavian **[C]**) relative to the dissection. The entry tear *(e)* of the dissection starts at the junction between the left carotid and left subclavian artery. The patient required a carotid-carotid bypass before placement of an endoluminal graft distal to the origin of the innominate artery.

Balloon Angioplasty and Stent Deployment

IVUS can provide useful information for both preprocedural and postprocedural assessment of peripheral vascular interventions. It provides information about the cross-sectional diameter and the morphology of the arterial wall. Assessment of wire location whether being intraluminal or subintimal in a dissection plane can be better delineated with IVUS before further intervention.

Since the 1980s, intravascular stenting has been considered a possible method of reducing the complications of angioplasty related to vessel wall recoil, intimal flaps, medial dissection, and spasm. Essential requirements for successful stenting are correct initial positioning and complete deployment at the time of balloon expansion.[25] Incomplete expansion, not detected by angiography but identified by IVUS, has been reported to occur in up to 20% to 40% of cases of stent deployment.[26] By using intraluminal ultrasonography to image the vessel before stent insertion, the exact location, the shape, and the dimensions of the arterial disorders can be identified, including flaps, dissections, and stenoses. Incomplete stent deployment, as evidenced by incomplete apposition of the stent struts to the vessel wall, may be associated with an increased incidence of vessel thrombosis and stent migration. Figure 21-6 shows IVUS imaging from a case of an inadequately deployed superior vena cava stent. The stent appears to be undersized and have poor stent-to-wall apposition increasing concerns for stent migration. The angiographic imaging performed had demonstrated widely patent stent with good apposition.

Vena Caval Filter Placement

Traditionally, venal caval filters (inferior vena cava [IVC]) have been placed in the interventional suite with the aid of venography and x-ray examination. In critically ill patients requiring vena caval filter placement the challenge of medical stabilization and transportation of the patients can sometimes delay the placement of the filter. The placement of filters can be technically performed at the bedside with the use of a portable IVUS system and introducer sheath and wire. This eliminates the need for portable x-ray equipment and venograms. The IVUS can correctly identify the renal veins that are in proximity to the renal artery (Figure 21-7).[27] The renal artery typically appears as an echodense structure usually crossing underneath the vena cava. Once the renal veins have been identified, the distance from the introducer sheath to the area of interest is marked on the IVUS catheter. The filter catheter is then advanced to the same distance, and the filter

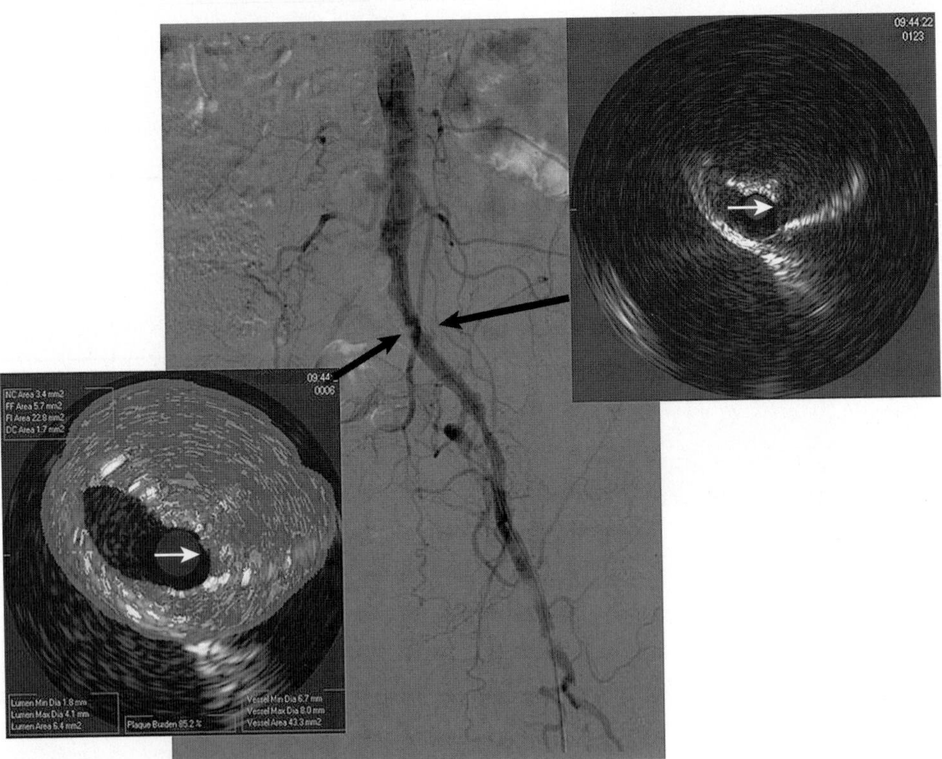

FIGURE 21-5 Angiographic and IVUS imaging of the left aortoiliac segment. The angiogram reveals area of stenosis relative to the diseased proximal and distal iliac artery. The virtual histology *(left image)* delineates the true flow lumen versus the atherosclerotic (colors not shown) segment. The area of stenosis is calculated to be 85% with the arterial diameter of 8 mm. The proper balloon and stent diameter can be chosen from the information obtained in the cross-sectional imaging of the vessel.

is then deployed. The precise locations of the renal veins are better visualized with ultrasound than with venography because the contrast jet is moving away from the renal veins.

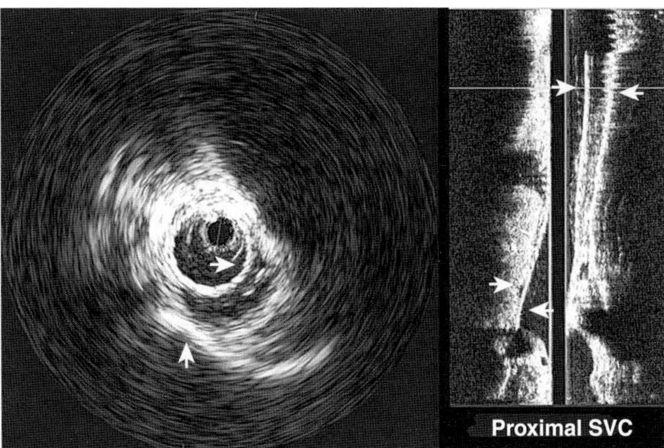

FIGURE 21-6 IVUS interrogation of the superior vena cava (SVC). The cross-sectional view, *left,* reveals the poor apposition of the stent to the caval wall. The 2-D gray-scale longitudinal imaging highlights the poor apposition of the stent against the distal SVC wall *(upper arrows),* whereas there is adequate stent-to-wall apposition more proximally (*lower arrows*). The stent deployed appears to be undersized for the SVC, and concerns for stent migration are imminent.

Abdominal Aortic Aneurysms

IVUS can be an important tool used during endovascular management of abdominal aortic aneurysms. In most situations the preprocedural assessment of the endoluminal graft (ELG) can be determined by the spiral CT scan imaging. The information obtained can be confirmed with the aid of IVUS to determine the proximal and distal landing points, the morphology of the arterial wall, and the length for optimal device selection. In addition, detailed information such as the intraluminal morphology (i.e., degree of thrombus load, calcification) can be better delineated with the IVUS imaging because it provides a true intraluminal imaging of the vessel. In our practice the IVUS catheter position is recorded in relation to the radiopaque ruler placed behind the patient's spine. The fluoroscopic imaging is placed to center the IVUS catheter and eliminate the parallax created. This allows creation of a road map in determining the location of the renal arteries along with the hypogastric arteries before placement of the ELG. Therefore the total fluoroscopic time and radiation along with contrast load is dramatically reduced.

Additionally, the lengths of different key locations can be determined. The IVUS is brought and positioned to the level of the lowest renal artery. The operator then places the finger over the IVUS catheter at its location

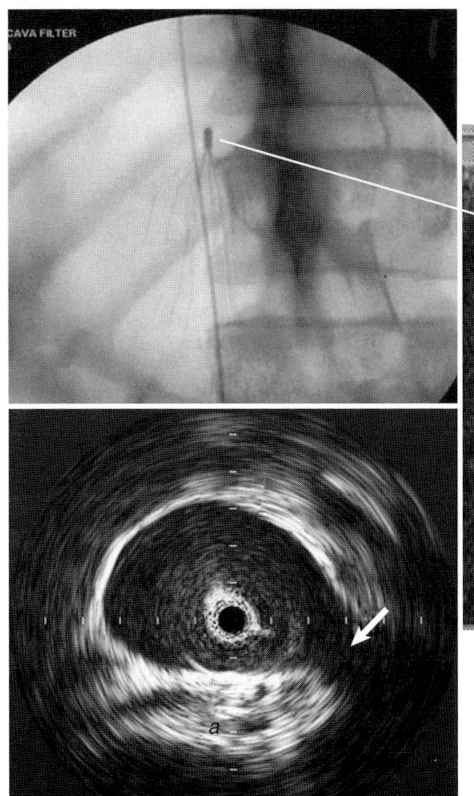

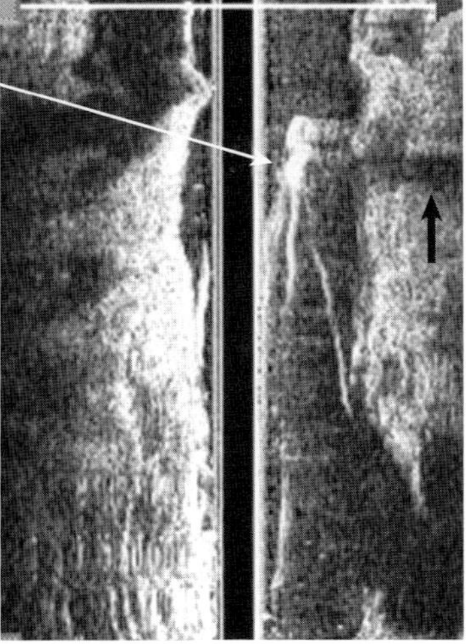

FIGURE 21-7 Imaging obtained after IVUS interrogation of the inferior vena cava. The renal vein *(black arrow)* is visualized entering the vena cava. The renal artery *(a)* can be seen crossing underneath the vena cava. The 2-D grayscale longitudinal imaging shows the inferior vena cava filter deployed at the level of the renal vein.

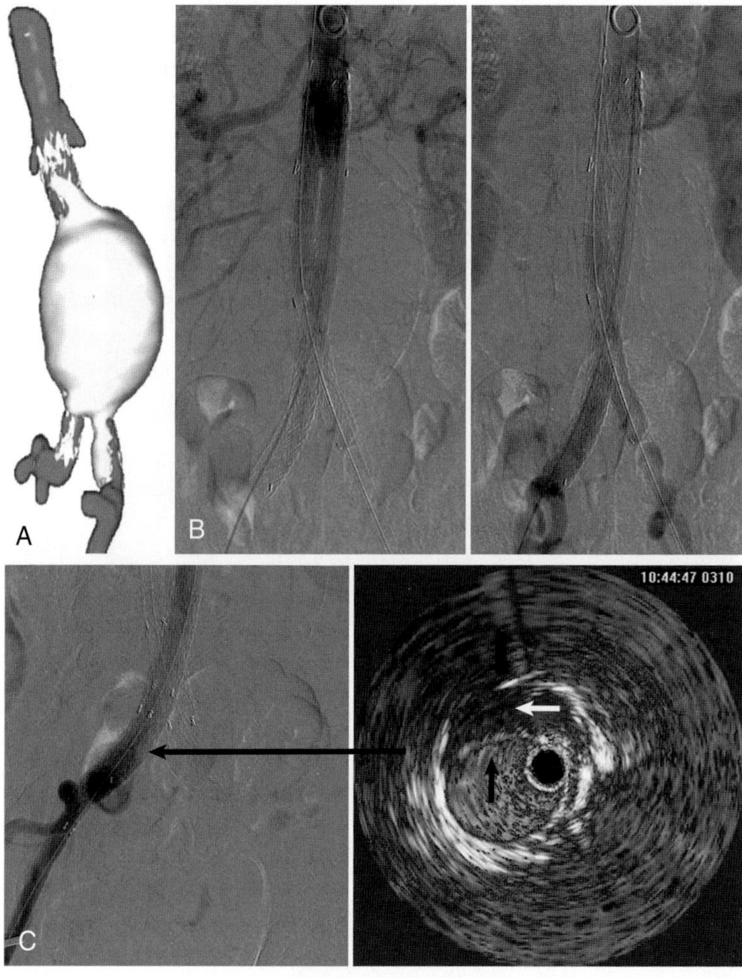

FIGURE 21-8 **A,** Aneurysm of the abdominal aorta found to have aneurysm sac expansion without any evidence for an endoleak on CT scan reconstruction. **B,** Angiography of the aorta reveals no evidence for an endoleak. **C,** IVUS interrogation of the aorta and iliac arteries was performed. The right iliac limb reveals poor stent-to-wall apposition with evidence for an endoleak *(black and white arrows, right lower arrow).* After realignment of the right iliac limb sac regression was seen with follow-up CT scans.

exiting the introducer sheath. The catheter is slowly pulled back until the start of the aneurysm. This allows for the measurement of the proximal fixation length. The catheter is pulled farther back until the level of the aortic bifurcation is determined. This is the second length that is measured. The final pullback is performed to the level of the iliac bifurcation. This allows for the total aortoiliac length measurement and determination of the best ELG length.

After determining the aortic wall morphology, the diameter of each key vessel, and the total length of the artery, the ELG device can be positioned at the level of the renal arteries and a small run angiogram can be performed to confirm the infrarenal fixation point relative to the ELG. Once the ipsilateral limb is deployed, the contralateral gate is typically cannulated with a soft-tip guidewire such as a glide wire. The IVUS catheter can then be advanced over the wire to confirm intraluminal cannulation of the contralateral limb along with position of the ELG relative to the renal arteries and the stent-to-wall apposition. There have been cases in our practice where the wire appeared to be inside the graft but was confirmed to be extraluminal with the IVUS. The stent-to-wall apposition can be well delineated with the IVUS to prevent any potential for type I endoleak that can sometimes be mistaken for a type II endoleak on the final angiographic run (Figure 21-8).

Dissections and Flaps

Since the first reported treatment of thoracic dissection with an ELG in 1999, thoracic dissections are being treated in many large major medical centers. This is one of the most recognized disease entities where IVUS imaging is an invaluable part of the endovascular management. Other accepted diagnostic techniques for evaluating acute aortic dissection (e.g., angiography, computed tomography, magnetic resonance imaging, and transesophageal and transthoracic echocardiography) have limitations related to the technique of image production and resolution. IVUS imaging provides an expedient method of defining the anatomic location and the size of the dissecting transmural vessel by allowing visualization of the vessel lumen and the wall at the time of intervention without requiring additional intravenous contrast agent administration.

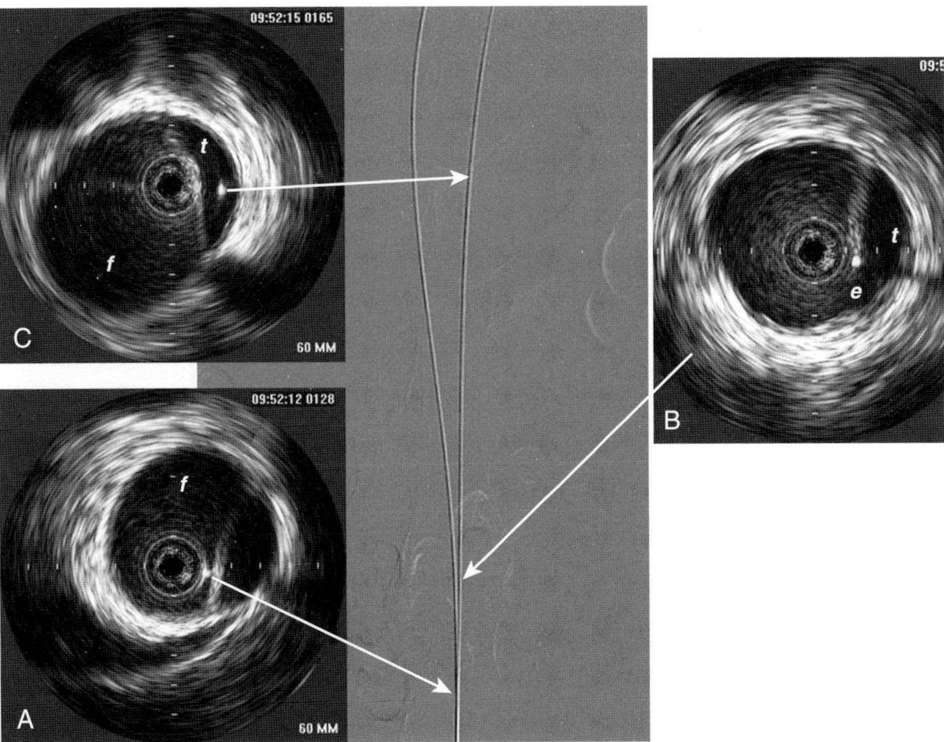

FIGURE 21-9 IVUS imaging of the distal aorta demonstrating access wire into true and false lumens. **A,** The IVUS imaging reveals the IVUS catheter placed into the false lumen *(f)* with the starter wire *(arrow)* remaining in the false lumen *(f)*. **B,** IVUS imaging demonstrating an entry site *(e)* with the starter wire entering into the true lumen *(t)*. **C,** IVUS imaging with the starter wire remaining in the true lumen *(t)* with the IVUS catheter in the false lumen *(f)*.

Several parameters are required for successful identification of the extent and the possible treatment of acute aortic dissection by means of endoluminal stenting.[28] These parameters include (1) the site of the proximal entry point and the distal extent of the dissection, (2) the relationship of the false lumen to major aortic branches, (3) the measurement of aortic dimensions to allow selection of correct stent size, and (4) the confirmation that the stent is being deployed in the true lumen to obliterate the false lumen.[1-3,29] The ability of IVUS to identify luminal and vessel wall abnormalities that are not readily apparent on conventional angiographic studies provides a new dimension to future diagnostic evaluations and therapeutic interventions.

Guidewire access into the true lumen is essential for the successful treatment of acute and chronic thoracic dissections. The unpredictable course of a dissection plane with multiple entry and reentry points can make the passage of a guidewire into the true lumen very difficult to visualize with angiography. IVUS interrogation is an essential tool that aids with the cannulation of the true lumen leading to a successful ELG management of a dissection. In our practice, the passage of the guidewire is confirmed from its introduction site all the way into the ascending aorta. This involves placing the IVUS catheter over the introducer wire while advancing the wire and the IVUS catheter as a unit and visualizing the path of the wire. This technique must be done with the wire a few millimeters past the stiff IVUS probe tip to avoid a tear into the aorta. Successful access of the true lumen may require multiple attempts of manipulation and readvancement through the dissection plane (Figure 21-9).

Additional information provided with the IVUS includes the relationship of the major aortic branches in relationship to the dissected plane. It is crucial to determine the origin of each major aortic vessel in relationship to the true and false lumen before treatment. If the dissection extends into the branched vessels, flow must be maintained after treatment. This information can be determined precisely from the IVUS interrogation along with the change in flow determined after ELG deployment. As Figure 21-10 demonstrates, the patient has limited flow into the superior mesenteric artery and renal arteries from the compromised true lumen after an acute dissection. After the deployment of the ELG to exclude the proximal entry site, the patient had expansion of the true lumen with improved flow into the visceral organs.

Imaging of the Thoracic Arch

Large numbers of thoracic aortic pathologies require placement of the ELG into the thoracic arch for proper treatment. The sharp angulations of the thoracic arch in addition to the short distance between the origin of each great vessel limit the use of contrast angiography as the sole imaging modality for these ELG procedures. Additional variables such as the anomalous origin of the great vessels, the diffuse thoracic aortic pathologies, and the noncircular cross-sectional area of the thoracic arch lend to the usage of IVUS for successful diagnostic and posttherapeutic imaging modality. The utility of IVUS imaging is very crucial for successful treatment of aortic pathologies.

In placement of the ELG into the thoracic arch, three key imaging components are needed. These include (1) the initial mapping of the great vessels in relationship to

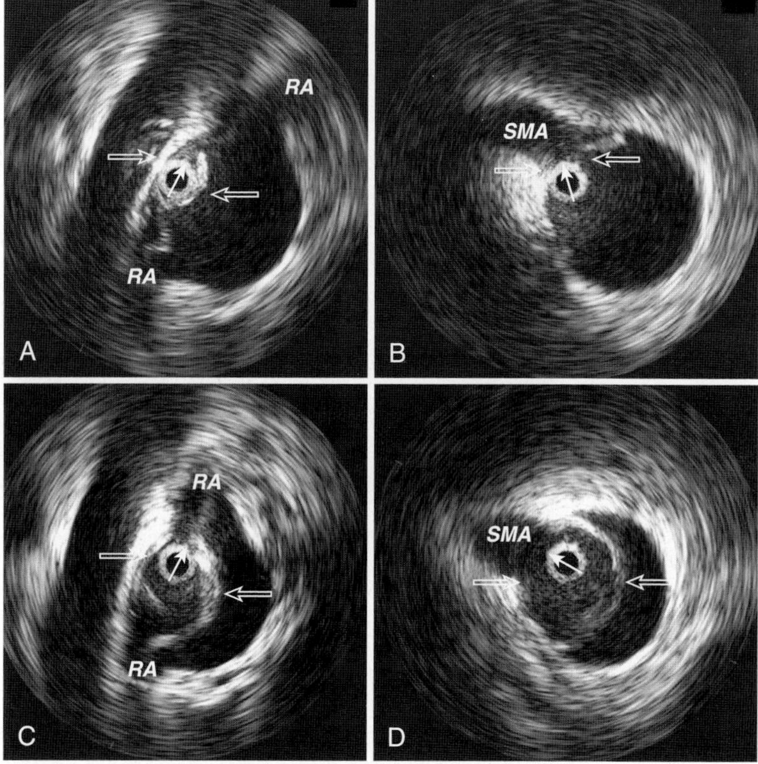

FIGURE 21-10 IVUS imaging for acute type B dissection. **A** and **B,** Imaging at the renal arteries *(RA)* and superior mesenteric artery *(SMA)* shows limited flow through the true lumen *(black arrows).* **C** and **D,** After endoluminal exclusion of the proximal reentry site, there is expansion of the true lumen with improved visceral flow.

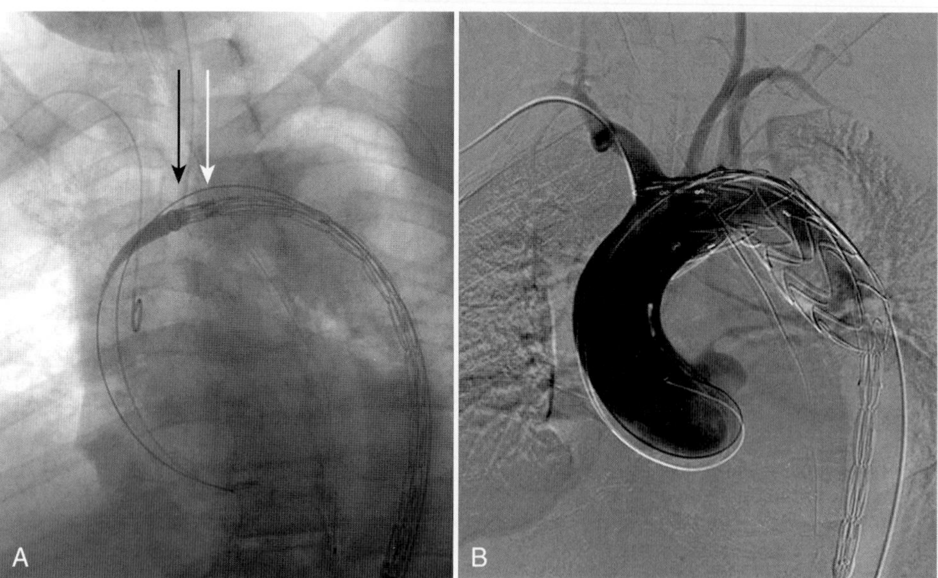

FIGURE 21-11 Thoracic arch imaging. **A,** The innominate *(black arrow)* and the left carotid artery *(white arrow)* have been marked on the fluoroscopic screen after IVUS interrogation. The entire arch imaging was obtained by IVUS without the initial usage of contrast. **B,** The device is partially deployed, and the first angiographic run is performed to confirm location of the arch vessels. This technique limits the contrast load while providing an accurate method for mapping the arch vessels.

the thoracic arch, (2) determination of the correct arch diameter, and (3) morphology and the distance of the landing zone. The cross-sectional view obtained along with the 2-D gray scale formatted in IVUS imaging will provide the above information needed. As Figure 21-11 demonstrates, the IVUS can define the origin of the vessels relative to the thoracic arch and the locations marked on the fluoroscopic screen without usage of contrast angiography. The device can be delivered to the desired location and partially deployed before contrast administration. Before complete deployment, the location can be confirmed with angiography. This technique allows for optimization of the imaging modality and limiting the contrast load and x-ray radiation.

After deployment IVUS interrogation of the aorta will provide information about the stent-wall apposition, location of the stent relative to the great vessels, and concerns for in-stent collapse (Figures 21-12 and 21-13).

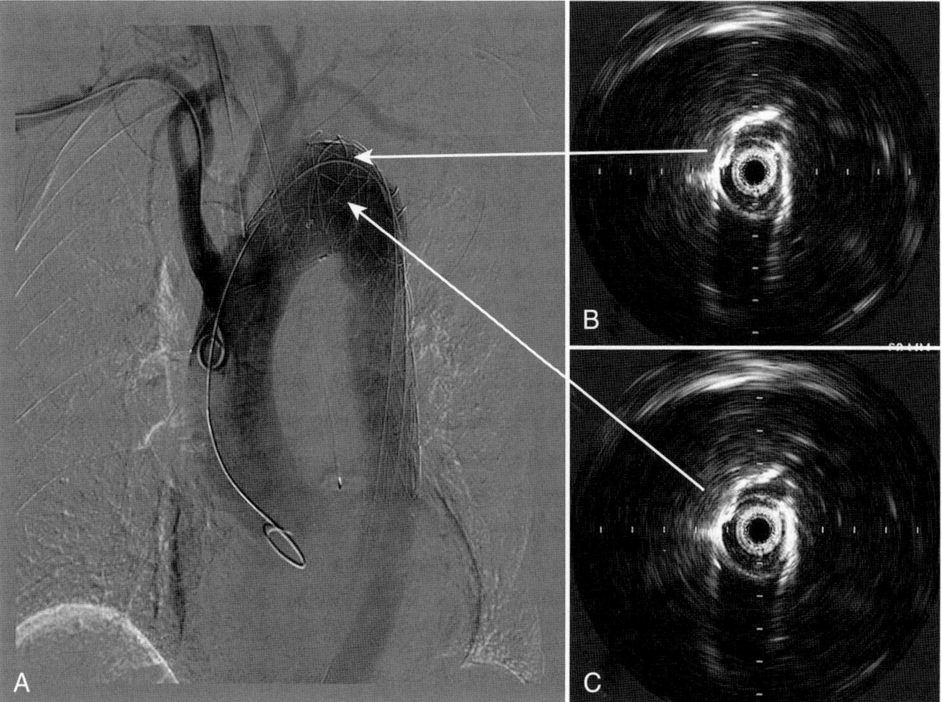

FIGURE 21-12 **A,** Thoracic angiography after deployment of endoluminal graft for exclusion of a proximal descending thoracic aneurysm. The angiographic imaging shows no evidence of an endoleak with an adequate flow into the stent. **B** and **C,** The IVUS interrogation reveals areas of in-stent collapse at the bend of the thoracic arch *(arrows)*. This was successfully treated with balloon angioplasty.

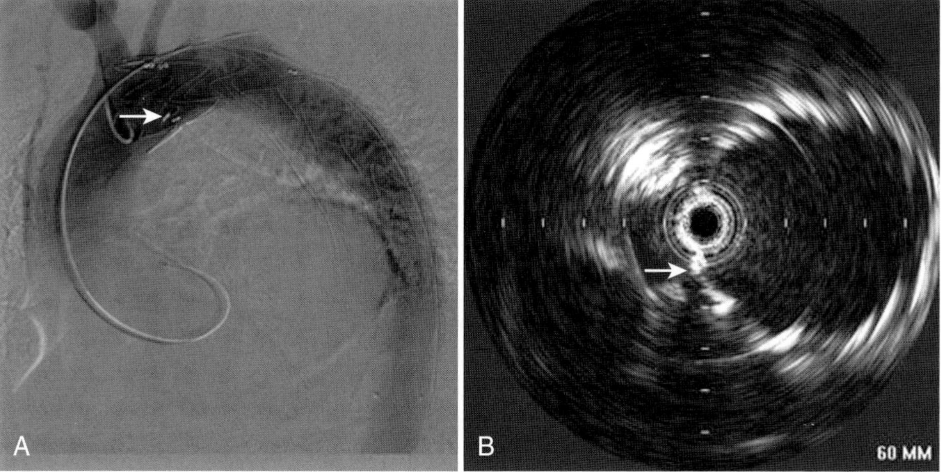

FIGURE 21-13 Selected cross-sectional images of the thoracic arch after ELG deployment. **A,** The angiographic imaging is inconclusive for showing coverage of the left carotid artery origin (*white arrow* delineates beginning of the covered segment of graft). **B,** The IVUS imaging reveals (1) closed graft fabric over the left carotid artery *(white arrow)* and (2) good stent-wall apposition of the ELG.

References

1. Bom N, Lancee CT, Van Egmond FC: An ultrasonic intracardiac scanner, *Ultrasonics* 10:72–76, 1972.
2. Wild JJ, Reid JM: Ultrasonic rectal endoscope for tumor location, *Am Inst Ultrasonics Med* 4:59–66, 1955.
3. Ebina T, Oka S, Tanaka M, et al: The diagnostic application of ultrasound to the disease in mediastinal organs. Ultrasonotomography for the heart and great vessels, *Sci Rep Res Inst Tohoku Univ* 12:199–217, 1965.
4. Yock PG, Linker DT, Angelsen BAJ: Two-dimensional intravascular ultrasound: technical development and initial clinical experience, *J Am Soc Echocardiogr* 2:296–304, 1989.
5. Cavaye DM, White RA, Kopchok GE, et al: Three dimensional intravascular ultrasound imaging of normal and diseased, canine and human arteries, *J Vasc Surg* 16:509–519, 1992.
6. Gussenhoven EJ, Essed CE, Lancee CT: Arterial wall characteristics determined by intravascular ultrasound imaging: an in-vitro study, *J Am Coll Cardiol* 14:947–952, 1989.
7. Gussenhoven WJ, Essed CE, Frietman P, et al: Intravascular echographic assessment of vessel wall characteristics: a correlation with histology, *Int J Cardiovasc Imaging* 4:105–116, 1989.
8. West AI: Endovascular ultrasound. In: Moore WS, Ahn SS, editors: *Endovascular Surgery*, Philadelphia, 1989, W.B. Saunders Co, pp 518–525.
9. Kopchok GE, White RA, Guthrie C, et al: Intraluminal vascular ultrasound: preliminary report of dimensional and morphologic accuracy, *Ann Vasc Surg* 4:291–296, 1990.
10. Kopchok G, White R, White G: Intravascular ultrasound: a new potential modality for angioplasty guidance, *Angiology* 41: 785–792, 1990.
11. Nissen SE, Gurley JC, Grines CL, et al: Comparison of intravascular ultrasound and angiography in quantitation of coronary dimensions and stenoses in man: impact of lumen eccentricity [abstract], *Circulation* 82(suppl III):440, 1990.
12. Tabbara M, Kopchok G, White R: In vitro and in vivo evaluation of intraluminal ultrasound in normal and atherosclerotic arteries, *Am J Surg* 160:556–560, 1990.
13. Meyer CR, Chiang EH, Fechner KP, et al: Feasibility of high resolution intravascular ultrasonic imaging catheters, *Radiology* 168:113–116, 1988.
14. Yock PG, Johnson EL, Linker DT: Intravascular ultrasound development and clinical potential, *Am J Card Imaging* 2:185–193, 1988.
15. Nissen SE, Grines CL, Gurley JC, et al: Application of new phased-array ultrasound imaging catheter in the assessment of vascular dimensions, *Circulation* 81:660–666, 1990.
16. Neville RF, Bartorelli AL, Leon MB, et al: Validation and feasibility of in vivo intravascular ultrasound imaging with a new flexible catheter, *Surg Forum ACS* 75:314–316, 1989.
17. Mallery JA, Tobis JM, Griffith J, et al: Assessment of normal and atherosclerotic arterial wall thickness with intravascular ultrasound imaging catheter, *Am Heart J* 119:1392–1400, 1990.
18. Tabbara MR, White RA, Cavaye DM, Kopchok GE: In-vivo comparison of intravascular ultrasound and angiography, *J Vasc Surg* 14:496–504, 1991.
19. Tobis JM, Mahon D, Lehmann K, et al: The sensitivity of ultrasound imaging compared with angiography for diagnosing coronary atherosclerotic lesions [abstract], *Circulation* 82(suppl III):439, 1990.
20. Zarins C, Zatura MA, Glagov S, et al: Correlation of postmortem angiography with pathologic anatomy: quantitation of atherosclerotic lesions. In: Bond MG, Insull W, Glagov S, editors: *Clinical diagnosis of atherosclerotic disease*, New York, 1983, Springer-Verlag, pp 283–306.
21. Roberts RW: Coronary arteries in coronary heart disease: morphologic observations, *Pathobiol Annu* 5:249–259, 1975.
22. Waller BF: The eccentric coronary atherosclerotic plaque: morphologic observations and clinical relevance, *Clin Cardiol* 12:14–20, 1989.
23. Sumner DS, Russell JB, Miles RD: Pulsed Doppler arteriography and computer assisted imaging of carotid bifurcation. In: Bergan JJ, Yao JST, editors: *Cerebrovascular insufficiency*, New York, 1983, Grune & Stratton, pp 115–135.
24. Glagov S, Weisenberg E, Zarins C, et al: Compensatory enlargement of human atherosclerotic coronary arteries, *N Engl J Med* 316:1371–1375, 1987.
25. White RA, Verbin C, Kopchok G, et al: Role of cinefluoroscopy and intravascular ultrasound in evaluating the deployment of experimental endovascular prostheses, *J Vasc Surg* 21:365–374, 1995.
26. Katzen BT, Benenati JF, Becker GJ, et al: Role of intravascular ultrasound in peripheral atherectomy and stent deployment [abstract], *Circulation* 84(suppl II):2152, 1991.
27. Oppat WF, Chiou AC, Matsumura J: Intravascular ultrasound–guided vena cava filter placement, *J Endovasc Surg* 6:285, 1999.
28. Cavaye DM, White RA, Lerman RD, et al: Usefulness of intravascular ultrasound imaging for detecting experimentally induced aortic dissection in dogs and for determining the effectiveness of endoluminal stenting, *Am J Cardiol* 69:705–707, 1992.
29. Lockwood GR, Ryan LK, Foster FS: High frequency intravascular ultrasound imaging. In: Cavaye DM, White RA, editors: *Arterial imaging: modern and developing technology*, London, 1993, Chapman & Hall, pp 125–128.

CHAPTER

22

Duplex-Guided Infrainguinal Interventions

Enrico Ascher, Anil P. Hingorani, Natalie Marks

Over the last 12 years our group has collected an extensive experience with preoperative duplex arteriography of lower extremities as a sole imaging modality.[1,2] We have learned that duplex scanning offers multiple unique features such as (1) arterial visualization regardless of its patency, (2) imaging of the arterial wall, (3) real-time visualization in presence of limb motion, (4) up to five times magnification, (5) instant precise measurements, and (6) readily available various hemodynamic parameters such as flow direction, velocity, and waveform. This has translated into the use of duplex imaging for guidance of various venous and arterial therapies (interventional vascular ultrasound).

Indeed, preliminary experiments with transcutaneous ultrasound in guidance of infrainguinal arterial procedures described by Ahmadi et al.[3] and Ramaswami et al.[4] persuaded us to further extend this approach and implement duplex guidance for endovascular interventions in our institution. This exciting novel technique turned out to be feasible, effective, and safe. Over the last 5 years we were able to complete duplex-guided lower-extremity angioplasties of femoral-popliteal arterial segment in 360 cases, infrapopliteal arteries in 80 cases, and infrainguinal arterial bypasses in an additional 47 cases.[5-9] In addition, we successfully used duplex-guided interventions to treat 40 nonmaturing or failing upper-extremity arteriovenous fistulas.[10,11] Duplex-assisted balloon angioplasties and stenting of 41 internal carotid arteries represent yet another unique application of this approach.[12,13] Herein we describe our experience with these procedures.

INFRAINGUINAL ARTERIAL ANGIOPLASTIES

Preoperative Evaluation

In our institution arterial balloon angioplasty is offered to patients on the basis of the results of preoperative duplex imaging only. Preoperative duplex arteriography in our ICAVL-accredited vascular laboratory is performed by experienced registered vascular technologists (RVTs) and includes assessment of pattern and extent of occlusive disease in the femoral-popliteal arterial segment, as well as infrapopliteal arteries. Aortoiliac stenoses are ruled out by analysis of the common femoral artery (CFA) spectral waveform. Biphasic or monophasic waveform of the CFA warrants duplex assessment of the aortoiliac segment. Those with triphasic waveform in the CFA do not require further evaluation. Patients with significant ipsilateral suprainguinal stenoses are subjected to adjunctive iliac balloon angioplasty.

TransAtlantic Inter-Society Consensus (TASC) classification can be used for morphologic description of femoral-popliteal lesions. The length of the occluded and stenotic lesions is measured knowing that L7-4 MHz probe foot has a length of 4 cm and adding lengths of insolated images or by marking the beginning and end of the lesion on the skin with use of duplex image and measuring it with a tape. "Flush" arterial occlusions are defined as a totally occluded vessel within the first 5 mm of its origin.

Technique

Duplex guidance should be performed by experienced vascular technologists with an extensive expertise in preoperative duplex arteriography. Guidance of balloon angioplasty procedures requires the technologist to be gowned and gloved and the duplex scanner's keyboard covered by a sterile film. We used an HDI 5000 scanner with SonoCT feature (Philips Medical Systems, Bothell, WA) routinely. A variety of scan heads inserted in a sterile plastic sleeve with coupling gel were used to insonate the arteries according to the anatomic location and depth. Generally, the arteries on the thigh and calf (1-4 cm deep) are being assessed with a linear 7-4 MHz probe. More superficial (<1 cm deep) arterial structures at the ankle and foot can be insonated by a compact linear 15-7 MHz "hockey stick" probe. Addition of a curved 5-2 MHz transducer is necessary for visualization of deeper arterial segments including distal superficial femoral artery (SFA) and above-the-knee popliteal artery (PA).

All duplex-guided procedures in our institution were performed in the operating room with the patient under local anesthetic infiltration of the puncture site and light sedation. One of the distinct differences of the proposed technique is the possibility to perform the majority of the procedures via an ipsilateral puncture. Ipsilateral approach for infrainguinal interventions has several advantages: (1) shorter and therefore more easily manipulated endovascular devices, (2) avoidance of potential difficulties and complications of aortoiliac disease and variable anatomy, and (3) prevention of potential complications of contralateral groin puncture. Duplex guidance helps avoid dissections, posterior wall puncture, bleeding, and other potential problems associated with blind arterial puncture.

Ipsilateral CFA access is possible in the majority of cases. In our experience with 360 femoral-popliteal angioplasties 328 (91%) cases were performed via ipsilateral CFA whereas contralateral cannulation was necessary in the remaining 32 cases (9%). Contralateral CFA access required fluoroscopy (alone in 6 cases and with 10-20 mL of contrast in the remaining 26 cases) for the ipsilateral common iliac artery cannulation. Contraindications to antegrade ultrasound-guided CFA puncture are high bifurcation and/or deep location (≥3 cm from the skin).

After successful ipsilateral CFA cannulation, a guidewire is directed into the proximal SFA, across the diseased segment(s), and parked at the tibioperoneal trunk or one of the tibial arteries under duplex guidance. In cases of contralateral CFA access, fluoroscopy is used to cross the aortic bifurcation. After the guidewire is identified by duplex in the ipsilateral proximal CFA, the procedure should be continued with duplex guidance as described above.

In cases of femoral and/or popliteal occlusions, a directional catheter supporting the guidewire is pointed against the wall 3 to 5 mm proximally to the occlusion to initiate subintimal dissection. Wire loop formation is confirmed by duplex imaging. The advancement of the wire through the occlusion is followed to the patent arterial segment identified by the presence of color signal in the lumen. Reentry attempts should be initiated within the first 1 to 2 cm after flow reconstitution to minimize the length of angioplasty. The arterial segment with the least amount of calcification and thinnest intima-media layer should be preferably chosen for reentry. If the guidewire fails to enter the true lumen after several attempts, the directional catheter should be advanced and pointed toward the lumen for additional wire support. Reentry efforts are usually continued cautiously to prevent extension of the dissection plane to the PA below the knee. We always tried to spare the outflow artery for possible femoral-popliteal bypass in the case of subintimal angioplasty failure. After the guidewire enters the true arterial lumen, its position is confirmed with color flow imaging in both longitudinal and transverse views.

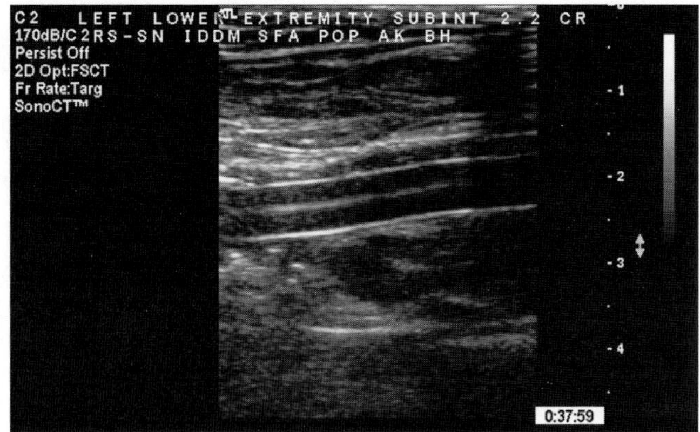

FIGURE 22-1 Gray-scale image of a 6-mm balloon fully inflated in the SFA. Note the hypoechoic plaque shifted by the balloon *(arrow)* in the stretched artery.

The diseased segment(s) is then balloon dilated under duplex guidance (Figure 22-1). Balloon diameter and length can be chosen according to direct arterial measurements obtained by duplex. Duplex image magnification (up to five times) and small error of the measurements (0.1 mm) provide precise measurements of the arterial diameter, as well as lumen and wall thickness, and therefore eliminate oversizing or undersizing of balloons and stents.

A detailed duplex examination of the entire treated segment should be performed after removal of the balloon angioplasty catheters to identify possible areas of residual disease, thrombi, plaque dissection, or recoil. Residual disease and plaque recoils are identified as luminal defects partially obstructing the flow (Figure 22-2). Partial or occlusive arterial thrombi have anechoic intraluminal appearance. Dissections can be diagnosed by identification of bidirectional flow pattern or divided flow with clearly different velocities as shown by color Doppler (Figure 22-3). All suspected abnormalities are carefully evaluated by direct diameter reduction measurement on color and/or power images, as well as spectral analyses including peak systolic velocities (PSV) ratios. Luminal defects of >30% diameter reduction with PSV ratio ≥2 across the stenosis can be treated by placement of self-expanding stents under duplex guidance (Figure 22-4). Significant technical defects were treated with a variety of stents (from one to five per case) in 233 of 342 cases

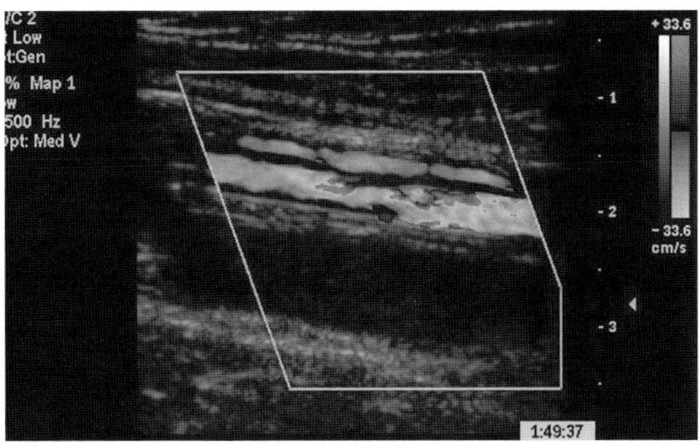

FIGURE 22-2 Color image of plaque recoil after balloon deflation in the SFA creating 60% diameter reduction (measured).

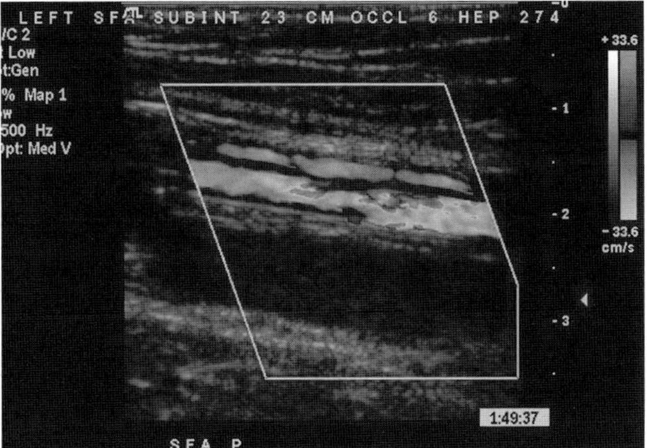

FIGURE 22-3 Color image of plaque dissection after balloon deflation in the SFA.

(68%). Finally, infrapopliteal arteries are insonated to reassure absence of embolization or thrombosis.

Technical Success and Predictors of Technical Failure of Femoral-Popliteal Duplex-Guided Balloon Angioplasty

The overall technical success in our experience was 95% (342/360 cases), and it was 100% for TASC class A and B lesions, 96% (236/245 cases) for TASC class C lesions, and 74% for TASC class D lesions (26/35 cases) ($p < 0.0001$). Of the 17 cases where subintimal SFA/PA duplex-guided balloon angioplasty (DGBA) failed, only 2 (12%) were successfully completed under fluoroscopy guidance. Comparison of multiple risk factors such as age, presence of diabetes (12%), chronic renal insufficiency (CRI) (11%), combination of both diabetes mellitus and CRI (13%), or hemodialysis (38%) in these patients revealed that only hemodialysis was a statistically significant predictive factor of technical failure for duplex-guided subintimal angioplasties ($p < 0.04$).

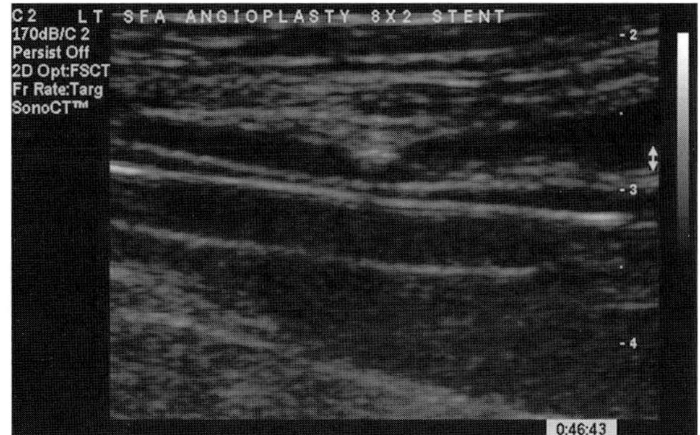

FIGURE 22-4 Gray-scale image of a self-expandable stainless steel stent deployed under ultrasound guidance in the SFA to treat plaque dissection.

Thromboembolic Complications

It was encouraging to see that some of the complications associated with balloon angioplasty, such as embolization or thrombosis, could be accurately identified by duplex examination and successfully corrected under duplex guidance. Completion duplex scans of the treated segment and infrapopliteal arteries identified 10 (2.9%) cases of thromboemboli. The proximal thrombus end was located at the below-the-knee PA in 2 cases, tibioperoneal trunk in 7 cases, and peroneal artery in the remaining case. Six of these cases were treated with duplex-guided suction thrombectomy and intra-arterial pulse-sprayed infusion of thrombolytic agent, and the remaining 4 cases resolved after thrombolysis only.

Follow-up, Patency, and Limb Salvage

Arterial duplex scans are routinely performed before hospital discharge and during follow-up visits in our office at 1 month after procedure, and every 3 to 4 months thereafter. Severe recurrent stenoses are identified by arterial diameter reduction ≥70% measured and local PSV step-up of greater than 3. Absent color or power in the arterial lumen documents total occlusions.

Mean duration of follow-up was 12 ± 8.3 months (range from 1-41 months). Six-month patency rates for TASC class A, B, C, and D lesions were 90%, 74%, 71%, and 64%, respectively. Twelve-month patency rates for TASC class A, B, C, and D lesions were 90%, 59%, 52%, and 46%, respectively. Overall limb salvage rates were 94% and 90% at 6 and 12 months, respectively (two amputations).

Adjunctive Infrapopliteal Balloon Angioplasties

Endovascular interventions for the infrapopliteal vessels are not widely accepted as the standard of care.[14-16] The reluctance to treat tibial vessels originates mostly from the limited patency rates achieved with this technique and uncertain long-term results. We believe that infrapopliteal balloon angioplasties may be beneficial in several settings: (1) runoff improvement during balloon angioplasty of femoral-popliteal arterial segment, (2) in patients with critical ischemia and multiple comorbidities unsuitable for bypass surgery, and (3) in patients with inadequate autogenous vein for bypass operation.

Our overall experience with infrapopliteal angioplasties included 80 arteries in 54 cases (15% of all infrainguinal arterial balloon angioplasty cases). All infrapopliteal angioplasties were attempted after completion of more proximal femoral-popliteal procedures to improve the runoff. Seventy cases (88%) had arterial stenoses (48 tibioperoneal trunks, 10 peroneal arteries, 7 posterior tibial arteries, and 5 anterior tibial arteries). The remaining 10 cases (12%) had arterial occlusions (4 tibioperoneal trunks, 5 peroneal arteries, and 1 anterior tibial artery). Low-profile balloons of appropriate diameter (2 to 4 mm) and length were used for the infrapopliteal angioplasties. The diseased arterial segments are balloon dilated starting from the most distal lesion.

A careful completion infrapopliteal duplex examination should be performed in each case for detection of possible plaque recoils, dissections, or distal thromboemboli. Hemodynamically significant plaque recoils (diameter reduction of greater than 30%, a PSV step-up of greater than 2, or both) can be successfully treated with cutting balloons. Immediate technical success was achieved in 77 of 80 treated infrapopliteal arteries, with an overall success rate of 96%. Failure of the wire to cross 2 stenotic peroneal lesions and 1 occlusion of peroneal artery accounted for the remaining 3 failure cases. Residual defects after angioplasty were documented in 10 (13%) of 77 infrapopliteal arteries. However, none of these cases was hemodynamically significant by duplex criteria. The 6- and 12-month patency rates of balloon-dilated infrapopliteal arteries were 78% and 66%, respectively.

DUPLEX–GUIDED ANGIOPLASTY OF INFRAINGUINAL ARTERIAL BYPASS GRAFTS

The long-term patency of lower-extremity bypasses and limb salvage rates are significantly dependent on diagnosis and timely repair of recurrent stenoses.[17-19] Modern duplex scanners provide reliable diagnostic information by identification of exact location and extent of bypass stenosis sites. Endovascular treatment of failing bypasses has been proved to have results and postprocedure patency rates comparable with those of the surgical approach.[20-26] Although fluoroscopic guidance for these treatments is considered standard, one of the major limitations of balloon angioplasty procedures under fluoroscopic guidance is lack of hemodynamic information.

Duplex guidance offers several indispensable technical advantages. Measurements of graft and arterial depth and diameter and precise localization of the stenotic lesions in reference to the anastomotic sites assist the best access site selection for the procedure. Direct visualization of the access site ensures precise entry of the arterial puncture needle and prevention of dissections, posterior wall bleeding, and other arterial injuries. This technique is especially beneficial in obese patients and previously operated groins when pulse identification becomes more difficult.

Patient Population

Forty-seven DGBA procedures were performed in 36 patients in our institution. Primary interventions were performed in 31 cases, first-redo angioplasties in 11 cases, second-redo angioplasties in 3 cases, third redo in 1 case, and fourth redo in the remaining case. Nineteen patients (53%) had renal insufficiency (serum creatinine level $\geq$1.5 mg/dL). Of the 47 attempted balloon angioplasties included in this study, 36 (77%) were performed in vein grafts and 11 (23%) were in polytetrafluoroethylene (PTFE) grafts. Nineteen autologous grafts were CFA to PA (7) and infrapopliteal (12) bypasses, 11 were SFA to PA (4) and infrapopliteal (7) bypasses, and the remaining 6 were PA to PA (3) and infrapopliteal (3) bypasses. Of the 11 prosthetic grafts 1 was femoral-femoral bypass, 7 were CFA to popliteal (4) and infrapopliteal (3) bypasses, and the remaining 3 were SFA to popliteal bypasses. Bypass operations were performed from 3 to 78 months before the current procedure (mean 28 $\pm$ 21 months).

Preoperative Evaluation

Diagnosis of a failing graft was made on the basis of preoperative duplex scans performed during routine office follow-up visits in our vascular laboratory. Follow-up graft duplex scan protocol included insonation of the entire bypass conduit and infrainguinal inflow and outflow arteries for at least 3-cm length proximal and distal to the anastomotic sites. After color and/or power imaging in the longitudinal plane, the following points were evaluated with spectral analysis: proximal artery; proximal anastomosis; proximal, mid, and distal bypass conduit; distal anastomosis; and distal artery. Any areas of color aliasing created by elevated velocities were also assessed for calculation of PSV step-up ratios to estimate stenosis degree. Biphasic or monophasic waveform detected in the inflow artery warranted insonation of the more proximal ipsilateral arteries extended up to the ipsilateral common iliac artery. Graft duplex scans identified at least one severe stenosis along the bypass conduit or in the native inflow and/or outflow arteries in all cases. Stenosis was characterized as severe when local diameter reduction was measured to be ≥70% on color or power angio image and the corresponding PSV step-up across the lesion was ≥3 (Figure 22-5). Twenty-two balloon angioplasties (47%) were performed on a single stenosis, and the remaining 25 cases (53%) had a mean of 2.9 ± 1 stenoses (range 2-5). The most significant stenotic lesion was found to be at the proximal inflow artery in 8 cases, bypass conduit in 26 cases, and distal outflow artery in the remaining 13 cases. Highest PSVs at the areas of stenosis were recorded and compared before and after procedure. Additionally, we routinely measure preoperative bypass volume flows (VF) × 3 in all cases and report mean value. VF is automatically calculated by the scanner's software using color duplex image and spectral analysis at the non-tapered bypass segment with Doppler angle adjusted at 60 degrees and sample volume equal to or larger than lumen outlined by the calipers.

Technique

All procedures were performed with use of the same technique as described earlier for the arterial infrainguinal duplex-guided balloon angioplasties. Overall, ipsilateral arterial access was possible in 34 cases (72%), and the remaining 13 cases required a contralateral femoral puncture. Femoral artery (15 ipsilateral; 13 contralateral) was used as an access site in 28 cases. The remaining 19 balloon angioplasty procedures were carried out through direct graft puncture (10 venous and 9 PTFE). Duplex scanning was the only imaging tool used to visualize and manipulate all endovascular instrumentation during the 34 procedures (72%) performed via the ipsilateral access. Five of 13 cases (38%) with contralateral CFA punctures in patients with elevated serum creatinine level (≥1.5 mg/dL) did not require contrast use for the cannulation of their ipsilateral iliac artery, which was completed with fluoroscopy guidance only.

In all cases the guidewire supported by a directional catheter of appropriate caliber was advanced from the ipsilateral femoral artery through the bypass conduit to the distal outflow artery under direct duplex visualization.

Duplex measurements of bypass or arterial diameter and lesion extension allowed the precise selection of balloons' caliber and lengths. Cutting balloons (Figure 22-6) used in 25 cases (48%) allowed us to successfully treat recoiling lesions.

Thorough completion duplex examinations followed the removal of balloon angioplasty catheters in all cases. Sagittal and transverse planes of scanning were used for identification of residual stenoses or recoils. A unique feature of a real-time ultrasound image is hemodynamic monitoring of the intervention. Spectral waveform and PSV ratios are essential for assessment of hemodynamic significance of dissections or recoils. Technical success was defined as patency and absence of diameter reduction areas with PSV ratio ≥2 along the bypass, as well as inflow and outflow arteries. Whenever a PSV ratio greater than 2 was registered suggesting residual stenosis or recoil greater than 50%, repeated inflations of larger balloons (if allowed by the adjacent arterial or bypass diameter) or cutting balloons were applied to the corresponding location.

Bypass VF measurements were obtained immediately after completion of the procedure as described earlier for preoperative measurements. VF average value ± SD, as

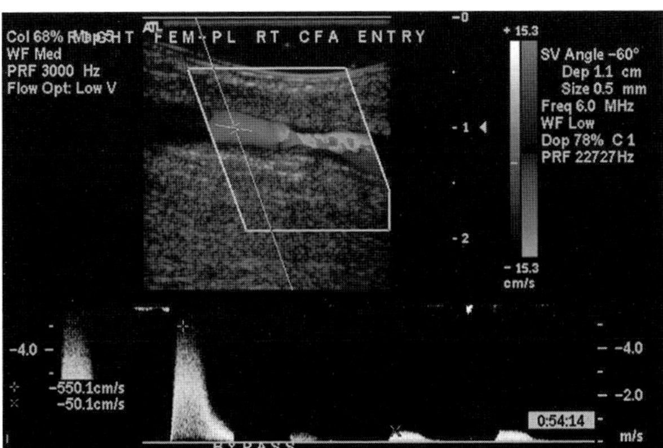

FIGURE 22-5 Doppler spectral analysis obtained at the distal femoral to dorsalis pedis artery vein bypass graft demonstrated critical stenosis by PSV step-up ratio of 11 (550 cm/s over 50 cm/s).

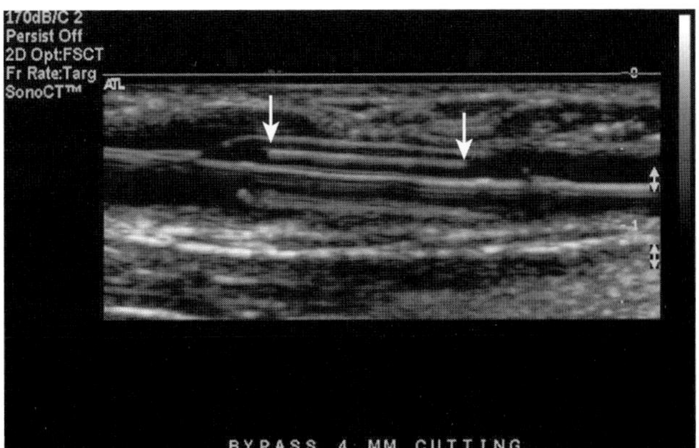

FIGURE 22-6 Fully inflated cutting balloon (4 mm diameter × 15 mm length) placed across the stenosis depicted in Figure 22.5. *White arrows* point to the balloon's blade.

well as ranges, were recorded and compared with the preoperative data. There were no intraoperative contrast arteriograms performed after DGBA procedures in these patients.

Intraoperative Technical Success

Overall technical success in our experience was 98% (46/47 cases). One technical failure was encountered in a case of a popliteal to plantar vein bypass in which the plantar artery anastomosis stenosis could not be crossed with the guidewire because of extreme tortuosity. Two cases of the inflow SFA dissections after balloon angioplasty were successfully treated by placement of self-expanding stents under duplex guidance. We did not use stents along the bypasses conduit in any of these 47 cases.

Early Postoperative Complications

Overall local complication rate was 4% (two cases). In one vein bypass a pseudoaneurysm developed at the site of rupture by cutting balloon, which was repaired by patch angioplasty. One patient receiving warfarin (Coumadin) had a persistent CFA pseudoaneurysm at the puncture site that required open repair after two unsuccessful thrombin injection attempts.

Duplex-Measured Hemodynamic Parameters

PSV obtained at the tightest stenosis level decreased in all 46 successful cases from preoperative 408 ± 148 cm/s (range 191-807 cm/s) to 97 ± 29 cm/s (range 53-152 cm/s) after angioplasty procedures (p <0.0001). On the other hand, bypass VF in all cases increased from preoperative 66 ± 38 mL/min (range 9-144 mL/min) to postoperative 137 ± 72 mL/min (range 52-900 mL/min) (p <0.0001).

Patency and Limb Salvage Rates

Average follow-up was 29 ± 14 months (range 3-46 months). Overall 6- and 12-month primary patency rates were 70% and 50%, respectively. Of the 10 patients whose procedures were performed via direct vein bypass access, 3 (30%) had restenosis at the puncture site.

DUPLEX-GUIDED ANGIOPLASTY OF FAILING OR NONMATURING ARTERIOVENOUS FISTULAS

Arteriovenous (AV) hemodialysis access fistulas are known to be predisposed for development of multiple stenoses and eventual failure during their lifetime.[27-29] Patency and functional ability of autologous AV fistulas have a tremendous influence on quality of life and survival for dialysis-dependent patients with chronic renal failure. Over the last decade, endovascular interventions have become the primary treatment option and almost entirely replaced surgical repair of failing or nonmaturing permanent dialysis accesses.[30-32] Although contrast administration may not be harmful for individuals receiving hemodialysis, patients with borderline renal function and nonmaturing AV accesses present a therapeutic challenge.[33,34] Additionally, an allergy to contrast material makes the endovascular treatment option in some of these patients more challenging.

Despite very high flow creating a substantial current, real-time imaging facilitates accurate position and monitoring of balloon location in relation to stenosis. Real-time Doppler spectral analysis assures confirmation of hemodynamic significance of the stenosis after balloon deflation, presence of recoil, and need for stenting. Residual stenoses caused by elastic recoil were detected in 6 of 11 cases in this series (55%). These recoiling lesions were successfully treated with cutting balloons in 4 cases, larger-diameter conventional balloon in 1 case, and self-expanding stent implanted in the remaining case.

Patients

We performed 40 duplex-guided balloon angioplasties of autologous AV fistulas in 32 patients with CRI. These were 17 men and 15 women with mean age 68.5 ± 10.3 years (range 38-85 years). The 40 fistulas included 27 radial-cephalic, 12 brachial-cephalic, and 1 brachial-basilic. Of these, 17 accesses were failing and 23 were nonmaturing fistulas in patients who were not yet receiving dialysis.

Preoperative Evaluation

Diagnosis of failing or nonmaturing AV access was established on the basis of a combination of physical examination (decreased thrill, present pulse), dialysis success (prolonged dialysis, suboptimal creatinine clearance, prolonged after-dialysis bleeding), and results of duplex scanning. Distinctive flow patterns such as very high velocities (often ≥ 500 cm/s) and major turbulence inherent to AV accesses present a diagnostic challenge for duplex surveillance. Although sonographic criteria indicating AV access abnormalities remain inconsistent, contemporary high-resolution ultrasound scanners and growing technical expertise among vascular technologists established duplex scanning as a very reliable diagnostic tool in detection of failing or nonmaturing AV accesses. Duplex criteria defining compromised AV access included presence of severe stenoses (>70%)

measured on color image and confirmed by PSV ratio of ≥3 in the inflow artery, anastomosis, along the access conduit (Figure 22-7), or in the outflow vein. VF measurements were routinely obtained in a nontapered fistula segment, at least 3 cm away from the anastomosis with use of the same method as described for infrainguinal bypasses. B-mode imaging of the entire fistula added information regarding presence of luminal webs and "frozen" venous valves creating flow obstruction (Figure 22-8). Highest PSVs at the most significant stenosis were recorded and compared with postprocedure values.

The mean number of stenoses was 1.9 ± 1.1 (range 1-5 per AV access).

Technique

Duplex guidance of AV access interventions has multiple and distinctive advantages. Real-time visualization of an AV access stenoses and skin marking make possible identification of the most advantageous access site. This choice is made with consideration of multiple factors such as stenoses locations in relation to anastomosis, fistula diameter, depth and tortuosity, and flow direction. Superficial location and direct visualization with ultrasound makes cannulation targeted and easy.

The first 10 cases were performed in the operating room and the remaining 30 in the outpatient office setting. After the patient was comfortably positioned on the operating table, the ipsilateral upper extremity and neck were prepped and draped in the usual sterile manner. A Philips HDI 5000 scanner with SonoCT feature used for all cases was placed on the side of intervention providing good monitor visibility for both surgeon and vascular technologist; the keyboard was covered with a sterile plastic cover. We found it useful to have two scan heads enclosed in sterile plastic and simultaneously available on the field because of anatomic and hemodynamic features inherent in an AV access. A CL 15-7 MHz transducer was used for insonation of superficial structures (<2 cm deep) and an L7-4 MHz probe was used for deeper (≥2 cm) objects and for measurements of very high velocities present in the AV access.

We were able to complete all procedures via ipsilateral access under local anesthesia. All AV accesses were cannulated under duplex guidance at least 5 cm away from the most proximal stenosis. We attempted to select the access site proximal to the stenosis to use high AV access blood flow as an ally for wire manipulation through tortuosity. Unfortunately, this was possible in only 3 cases (8%). Two more cases required placement of two access sheaths in opposite directions to address venous and arterial stenoses. The remaining 35 cases were accessed via distal fistula puncture, and the stenoses were addressed in a retrograde fashion.

Guidewire and then balloon catheter passage and inflation were performed under duplex guidance. Duplex measurements of arterial/venous lumen diameter adjacent to stenosis helped determine balloon diameters. High-resolution B-mode duplex images of arterial and venous wall allow precise selection of proper diameter and length of balloons and stents. We found proper selection of balloons to be extremely important in prevention of AV access and vein overextension and avoidance of rupture while providing adequate dilation of stenotic areas. We used Ultrathin, Symmetry, or Sterling balloons of various sizes (3-8 mm).

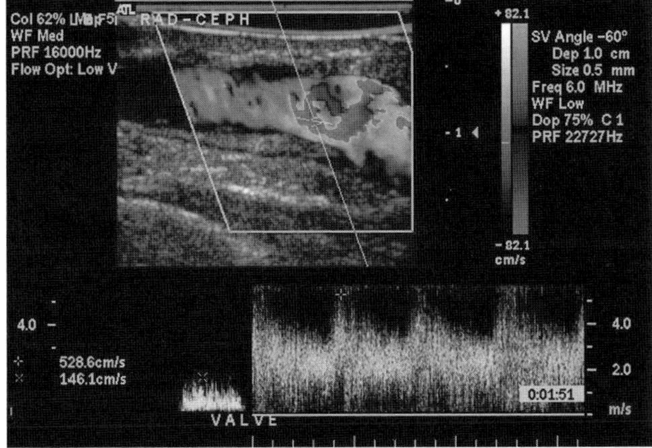

FIGURE 22-7 Intraoperative Doppler spectral analysis (note highest PSV 528.6 cm/s and PSV ratio of 3.6 as compared with the prestenotic PSV 146.1 cm/s) identified severe stenosis in the proximal radial-cephalic fistula at the wrist level. *(From Marks N, Ascher E, Hingorani AP: Duplex-guided repair of failing or nonmaturing arterio-venous access for hemodialysis,* Perspect Vasc Endovasc Ther *19:50-55, 2007.)*

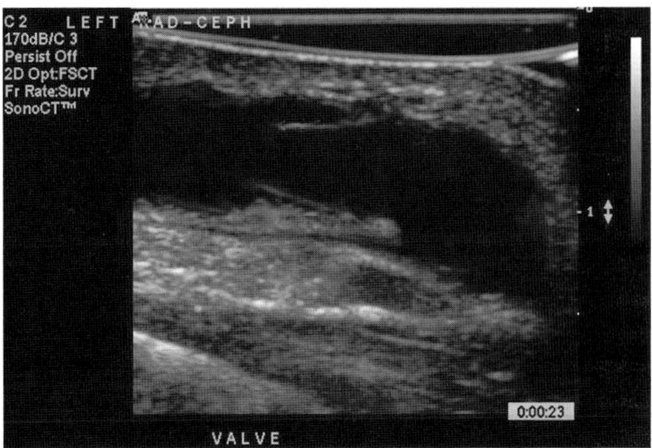

FIGURE 22-8 Intraoperative B-mode image with SonoCT feature depicts both leaflets of the "frozen" valve creating severe stenosis from Figure 22.2. *(From Marks N, Ascher E, Hingorani AP: Duplex-guided repair of failing or nonmaturing arterio-venous access for hemodialysis,* Perspect Vasc Endovasc Ther *19:50-55, 2007.)*

All cases had intraoperative completion duplex scans before access sheath removal. Adequacy of procedures was confirmed by absence of residual stenoses on color and/or power image and measurements of VF and PSV ratios.

Technical Success

All procedures were completed under duplex guidance alone. One patient with small (3-4 mm in diameter), deep (2 cm from the skin level) brachial-basilic AV fistula had a completion contrast arteriogram that confirmed duplex findings. There were no intraoperative or postoperative local complications in these patients. Eight recoiling lesions (20%) were successfully treated with cutting balloons.[35] One additional patient (2.5%) with brachial-cephalic fistula and recoiling lesion at the junction of cephalic and axillary veins required duplex guided placement of a self-expandable stent.

Comparison of Preprocedure and Postprocedure Duplex-Measured Hemodynamic Parameters

Mean preoperative PSV obtained at the most significant stenosis was 563 ± 100 cm/s (range 370-760 cm/s), and it was 200 ± 74 cm/s (range 62-354 cm/s) after procedure ($p < 0.0001$). Mean preoperative VF was 411 ± 279 mL/min (range 50-980 mL/min), and it was 935 ± 360 mL/min (range 370-1520 mL/min) after balloon angioplasty ($p < 0.01$).

Complications and Mortality

One patient had a focal venous rupture with minimal bleeding controlled by manual pressure for 30 minutes. There were no 30-day mortalities; one patient with multiorgan failure died at 4 months after AV access angioplasty.

DUPLEX-ASSISTED INTERNAL CAROTID ARTERY ANGIOPLASTY

Superficial location of the cervical carotid arteries and up to five times magnification provided by contemporary duplex scanners result in exceptional clarity and detail resolution of ultrasound images. Duplex scanning of the carotid arteries has established itself as a reliable preoperative imaging modality for evaluation of degree, location, and extent of carotid stenoses in the neck.[36,37]

Hypothetically, the combination of clear-cut duplex images and real-time spectral analyses can offer data superior to the arteriography during multiple steps of the carotid balloon angioplasty and stenting (CBAS) procedure, including (1) selection of exact balloon and stent diameter and length, (2) exact position of the balloons and stents regardless of the artifacts created by patient's breathing and movements, (3) confirming the apposition of the stent to the arterial wall, and (4) hemodynamic and B-mode verification of the procedure success.

On the other hand, duplex insonation of the aortic arch is restricted by the chest wall anatomy, and fluoroscopic guidance is necessary for manipulation of the wires and catheters in the aorta, as well as cannulation of the aortic branches. One more maneuver requiring fluoroscopy is cerebral protection device placement in the intracranial internal carotid artery (ICA).

Combination of both imaging modalities allowed us to perform a series of 41 duplex-assisted CBAS procedures described in the following section.

Patient Population

Forty patients who were seen with severe (>70%) ICA stenoses underwent 41 carotid angioplasty and stenting procedures in our institution. Twenty-seven lesions (66%) were primary, 11 (27%) were recurrent stenoses after carotid endarterectomy (CEA), and the remaining 3 (7%) were restenoses after prior ICA angioplasties. Fifteen stenoses were symptomatic (37%).

There were 27 men (68%) and 13 women (32%) with a mean age of 73 ± 10 years (range 44-92 years) in this group. Twenty-four patients (59%) had elevated serum creatinine levels (≥1.5 mg/dL), and two additional patients had a history of allergy to contrast material.

Preoperative Imaging

Carotid duplex mapping was the only preprocedure imaging modality. Duplex mapping protocol included (1) ICA stenosis degree measurements in sagittal (Figure 22-9) and transverse planes with use of representative color and/or power images, (2) measurements of disease-free distal common carotid artery (CCA) and ICA lumen, (3) measurements of the plaque extension, (4) identification of severe tortuosity of the cervical ICA (angulation of >90 degrees), and (5) reporting the CCA and ICA calcifications.

Technique

We performed all cases in the operating room with help of an ATL HDI 5000 scanner (Phillips Medical Systems) with SonoCT feature. A linear 7-4 MHz probe was chosen to insonate the CFA, CCA, and its branches. A digital mobile fluoroscopic imaging system with road-map capabilities was used in all cases. The duplex scanner was positioned contralateral to the C-arm at the

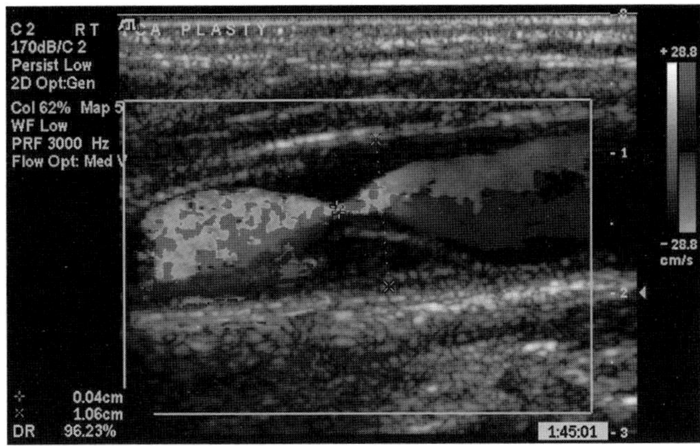

FIGURE 22-9 Color Doppler image of the proximal ICA outlining a critical stenosis (96%) proximally to the previously placed stent. *(From Ascher E, Hingorani AP, Marks N: Duplex-assisted internal carotid artery balloon angioplasty,* Perspect Vasc Endovasc Ther *19:41-47, 2007.)*

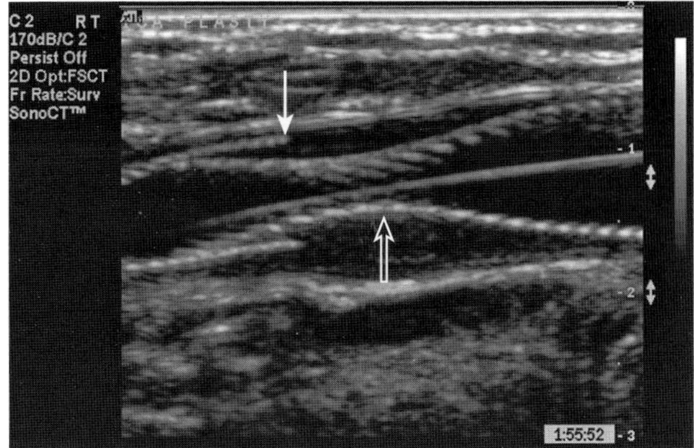

FIGURE 22-10 New stent *(open arrow)* deployed from the old stent *(white arrow)* across the restenosis lesion in the proximal ICA and distal CCA. *(From Ascher E, Hingorani AP, Marks N: Duplex-assisted internal carotid artery balloon angioplasty,* Perspect Vasc Endovasc Ther *19:41-47, 2007.)*

patient's head; the monitor was turned to ensure the best visibility by the interventionist. It is absolutely crucial for the vascular technologist providing duplex imaging during this procedure to have an extensive experience in duplex scanning of the carotid arteries and understanding of various carotid arterial pathologies, as well as their effect on duplex findings. One should not attempt or continue duplex guidance of the CBAS procedure unless the images of the diseased arterial segment and the carotid bifurcation are unquestionably excellent. ICA disease with severe arterial calcification creating shadows covering the lumen for >5 mm should not be treated with duplex-assisted CBAS.

The retrograde cannulation of the CFA was achieved under direct duplex visualization. Manipulation of the guidewire in the iliac arteries and abdominal and thoracic aorta was performed with fluoroscopic assistance. The Bern selective angiographic catheter (Boston Scientific, Miami, FL) or Vitek cerebral catheter (Cook Medical, Bloomington, IN) was used in this series for selective catheterization of the ipsilateral CCA. After the guidewire was visualized in the CCA by duplex, it was directed into the external carotid artery (ECA) with use of the same directional catheter. The next step was a Glidewire wire exchange for a stiff Amplatz (Boston Scientific) wire to allow introduction of a 6F Shuttle SL introducer sheath (Cook Inc.), which was positioned in the CCA about 2 to 3 cm proximal to the carotid bifurcation. All described maneuvers in the neck were completed with duplex visualization alone. The FilterWire embolic protection system (Boston Scientific) was negotiated into the distal cervical ICA beyond the stenosis under ultrasound guidance as well. Further advancement of the filter, its placement, and deployment 4 to 6 cm distal to the ICA stenosis was guided by fluoroscopy.

Next step was duplex-guided dilation of the ICA lesion with a 3- or 4-mm monorail balloon. After this step, a biliary monorail Wallstent (Boston Scientific Corp.) was positioned across the stenosis and deployed under ultrasound visualization (Figure 22-10). A larger balloon (5 or 6 mm in diameter) was inflated once or twice to improve its apposition against the wall and eliminate any residual stenosis. Postprocedure completion duplex scan confirmed (1) wide patency of the native and stented CCA and ICA segments, (2) adequate stent apposition, and (3) absence of dissections, flaps, thrombi, or other potential abnormalities (Figure 22-11). Completion ICA arteriograms with a small amount of contrast material were performed for medicolegal reasons and correlation with duplex results as per surgeon's preference.

Intraoperative Technical Findings

Completion duplex scans confirmed technical success in all cases. Aortic arch arteriograms were necessary to assist with difficult ipsilateral CCA cannulations in 7 cases (17%). Completion ICA arteriograms were obtained in 26 cases (63%) with 10 to 15 mL of contrast (Magnevist, Berlex Laboratories, Wayne, NJ, in 4 cases; Visipaque, Amersham Health, Princeton, NJ, in 22 cases) to validate the duplex findings. Adequate stent apposition and stenosis dilation were achieved in all cases. Biplanar postprocedural cerebral arteriograms performed in 30 patients (73%) for medicolegal reasons did not reveal any defects.

Postprocedure Mortality and Morbidity

There were no early (30 day) postprocedure mortalities. One patient had an ipsilateral stroke (2.4%) with

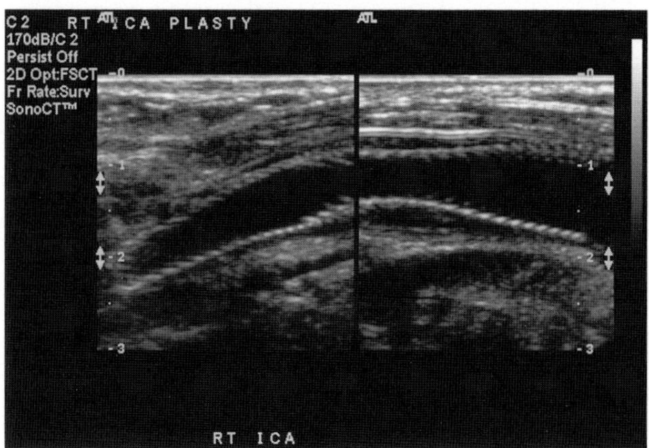

FIGURE 22-11 Gray-scale image of both stents (old in the distal ICA and newly placed in the proximal ICA and distal CCA) demonstrated sufficient stent apposition. *(From Ascher E, Hingorani AP, Marks N: Duplex-assisted internal carotid artery balloon angioplasty,* Perspect Vasc Endovasc Ther *19:41-47, 2007.)*

almost complete clinical recovery in 4 months (mild residual hand weakness). This event occurred during the second balloon inflation in the stent. Nevertheless, intraoperative biplanar cerebral arteriogram did not reveal any abnormalities in this patient.

Follow-Up

All patients were advised to have duplex scans performed in our vascular clinic every 6 months after CBAS procedure. Mean follow-up after duplex-assisted CBAS was 21 $\pm$ 14 months (range 6-46 months). One patient had restenosis at 9 months in the proximal end of the stent and underwent repeated duplex-assisted CBAS.

CONCLUSION

Unquestionably, duplex-guided arterial interventions are particularly beneficial for patients who are allergic to contrast material and for those with CRI. As vascular surgeons become busier with endovascular procedures, they will be more exposed to the deleterious effects of radiation.[38] Unfortunately, these effects are cumulative and permanent and may cause a delayed onset of symptoms. Our experience with the variety of duplex-guided and duplex-assisted vascular interventions makes us believe that the proposed technique is feasible, is safe, and has great potential. We anticipated that some of these procedures will eventually be performed in the vascular laboratory or in an office practice setting.

References

1. Ascher E, Hingorani A, Markevich N, et al: Lower extremity revascularization without preoperative contrast arteriography: experience with duplex ultrasound arterial mapping in 485 cases, *Ann Vasc Surg* 16(1):108–114, 2002. Epub 2002 Jan 17.
2. Ascher E, Hingorani A, Markevich N, et al: Role of duplex arteriography as the sole preoperative imaging modality prior to lower extremity revascularization surgery in diabetic and renal patients, *Ann Vasc Surg* 18(4):433–439, 2004.
3. Ahmadi R, Ugurluoglu A, Schillinger M, et al: Duplex ultrasound-guided femoropopliteal angioplasty: initial and 12-month results from a case controlled study, *J Endovasc Ther* 9(6):873–881, 2002.
4. Ramaswami G, Al-Kutoubi A, Nicolaides AN, et al: Angioplasty of lower limb arterial stenoses under ultrasound guidance: single-center experience, *J Endovasc Surg* 6(1):52–58, 1999.
5. Ascher E, Marks NA, Schutzer RW, et al: Duplex-guided balloon angioplasty and stenting for femoropopliteal arterial occlusive disease: an alternative in patients with renal insufficiency, *J Vasc Surg* 42(6):1108–1113, 2005.
6. Ascher E, Marks NA, Hingorani AP, et al: Duplex-guided endovascular treatment for occlusive and stenotic lesions of the femoral-popliteal arterial segment: a comparative study in the first 253 cases, *J Vasc Surg* 44(6):1230–1237, 2006.
7. Ascher E, Hingorani AP, Marks NA: Duplex-guided angioplasty of lower extremity arteries, *Perspect Vasc Endovasc Ther* 19(1): 23–31, 2007.
8. Ascher E, Marks NA, Hingorani AP, et al: Duplex-guided balloon angioplasty and subintimal dissection of infrapopliteal arteries: early results with a new approach to avoid radiation exposure and contrast material, *J Vasc Surg* 42(6):1114–1121, 2005.
9. Marks NA, Hingorani AP, Ascher E: Duplex-guided balloon angioplasty of failing infrainguinal bypass grafts, *Eur J Vasc Endovasc Surg* 32(2):176–181, 2006.
10. Marks N, Ascher E, Higorani AP: Treatment of failing lower extremity arterial bypasses under ultrasound guidance, *Perspect Vasc Endovasc Ther* 19(1):34–39, 2007.
11. Marks N, Ascher E, Hingorani AP: Duplex-guided repair of failing or nonmaturing arterio-venous access for hemodialysis, *Perspect Vasc Endovasc Ther* 19(1):50–55, 2007.
12. Ascher E, Hingorani AP, Marks N: Duplex-assisted internal carotid artery balloon angioplasty, *Perspect Vasc Endovasc Ther* 19(1):41–47, 2007.
13. Ascher E, Marks NA, Schutzer RW, et al: Duplex-assisted internal carotid artery balloon angioplasty and stent placement: a novel approach to minimize or eliminate the use of contrast material, *J Vasc Surg* 41(3):409–415, 2005.
14. Dorros G, Jaff MR, Dorros AM, et al: Tibio-peroneal trunk (outflow lesion) angioplasty can be used as primary treatment in 235 patients with critical limb ischemia: five-year follow-up, *Circulation* 104:2057–2062, 2001.
15. Kudo T, Chandra FA, Ahn SS: The effectiveness of percutaneous transluminal angioplasty for the treatment of critical limb ischemia: a 10-year experience, *J Vasc Surg* 41(3):423–435. discussion 435, 2005.
16. Clair DG, Dayal R, Faries PL, et al: Tibial angioplasty as an alternative strategy in patients with limb-threatening ischemia, *Ann Vasc Surg* 19(1):63–68, 2005.
17. Nguyen LL, Conte MS, Menard MT, et al: Infrainguinal vein bypass graft revision: factors affecting long-term outcome, *J Vasc Surg* 40(5):916–923, 2004.
18. Bandyk DF, Bergamini TM, Towne JB, et al: Durability of vein graft revision: the outcome of secondary procedures, *J Vasc Surg* 13(2):200–208, 1991.

19. Sullivan TR Jr, Welch HJ, Iafrati MD, et al: Clinical results of common strategies used to revise infrainguinal vein grafts, *J Vasc Surg* 24(6):909–917, 1996.
20. Calligaro KD, Syrek JR, Dougherty MJ, et al: Selective use of duplex ultrasound to replace preoperative arteriography for failing arterial vein grafts, *J Vasc Surg* 27(1):89–94, 1998.
21. Dougherty MJ, Calligaro KD, DeLaurentis DA: The natural history of "failing" arterial bypass grafts in a duplex surveillance protocol, *Ann Vasc Surg* 12(3):255–259, 1998.
22. van der Heijden FH, Legemate DA, van Leeuwen MS, et al: Value of duplex scanning in the selection of patients for percutaneous transluminal angioplasty, *Eur J Vasc Endovasc Surg* 7(1):71–76, 1993.
23. Bandyk DF, Mills JL, Gahtan V, et al: Intraoperative duplex scanning of arterial reconstructions: fate of repaired and unrepaired defects, *J Vasc Surg* 20:426–433, 1994.
24. Rzucidlo EM, Walsh DB, Powell RJ, et al: Prediction of early graft failure with intraoperative completion duplex ultrasound scan, *J Vasc Surg* 36(5):975–981, 2002.
25. Avino AJ, Bandyk DF, Gonsalves AJ, et al: Surgical and endovascular intervention for infrainguinal vein graft stenosis, *J Vasc Surg* 29(1):60–70, 1999.
26. Carlson GA, Hoballah JJ, Sharp WJ, et al: Balloon angioplasty as a treatment of failing infrainguinal autologous vein bypass grafts, *J Vasc Surg* 39(2):421–426, 2004.
27. USRDS: Excerpts from the United States Renal Data System 1998 annual data report. Incidence and prevalence of ESRD, *Am J Kidney Dis* 32(suppl 1):S38–S49, 1998.
28. Beathard GA, Settle SM, Shields MW: Salvage of the nonfunctioning arteriovenous fistula, *Am J Kidney Dis* 33:910–916, 1999.
29. Vorwerk D: Percutaneous interventions to support failing hemodialysis fistulas and grafts, *Kidney Blood Press Res* 20:145–147, 1997.
30. Cavagna E, D'Andrea P, Schiavon F, et al: Failing hemodialysis arteriovenous fistula and percutaneous treatment: imaging with CT, MRI and digital subtraction angiography, *Cardiovasc Intervent Radiol* 23:262–265, 2000.
31. Dougherty MJ, Calligaro KD, Schindler N, et al: Endovascular versus surgical treatment for thrombosed hemodialysis grafts: a prospective, randomized study, *J Vasc Surg* 30(6):1016–1023, 1999.
32. Hingorani A, Ascher E, Kallakuri S, et al: Impact of reintervention for failing upper-extremity arteriovenous autogenous access for hemodialysis, *J Vasc Surg* 34(6):1004–1009, 2001.
33. Parfrey PS, Griffiths SM, Barrett BJ, et al: Contrast material-induced renal failure in patients with diabetes mellitus, renal insufficiency, or both: a prospective controlled study, *N Engl J Med* 320(3):143–149, 1989.
34. Lautin EM, Freeman NJ, Schoenfeld AH, et al: Radiocontrast-associated renal dysfunction: incidence and risk factors, *Am J Roentgenol* 157(1):49–58, 1991.
35. Singer-Jordan J, Papura S: Cutting balloon angioplasty for primary treatment of hemodialysis fistula venous stenoses: preliminary results, *J Vasc Interv Radiol* 16(1):25–29, 2005.
36. Wain RA, Lyon RT, Veith FJ, et al: Accuracy of duplex ultrasound in evaluating carotid artery anatomy before endarterectomy, *J Vasc Surg* 27(2):235–242; discussion 242–244, 1998.
37. Roth SM, Back MR, Bandyk DF, et al: A rational algorithm for duplex scan surveillance after carotid endarterectomy, *J Vasc Surg* 30(3):453–460, 1999.
38. Lipsitz EC, Veith FJ, Ohki T, et al: Does the endovascular repair of aortoiliac aneurysm pose a radiation safety hazard to vascular surgeons? *J Vasc Surg* 32(4):704–710, 2000.

SECTION III

AORTOILIAC ARTERIAL OCCLUSIVE DISEASE

CHAPTER

23

Thrombolysis in Aortoiliac Arterial Occlusive Disease

Edward B. Diethrich, Donald B. Reid

Thrombolysis is a very useful treatment option to have in patients who present with aortoiliac thrombosis because of its ability to treat the major vessels supplying the lower limbs without the disadvantages of open surgery. The minimally invasive approach is at the heart of endovascular surgery, and the techniques that allow the endovascular surgeon to treat the arterial thrombosis from a distant access site also allow other interventions such as angioplasty and stenting or endoluminal grafting. Thrombolysis allows percutaneous treatment of the arteries and the underlying disease that has caused the vessel thrombosis. The disadvantage of thrombolysis is that it takes time to dissolve clot, particularly in the large vessels of the aortoiliac segment, and not all patients with acutely ischemic legs can afford to wait this long. Therefore good clinical judgment is needed to decide to commence thrombolytic therapy instead of open vascular surgery, and frequent reassessments during the course of thrombolysis are required. Knowledge and understanding of the mechanism of fibrinolysis, the differences between the various lytic agents, the necessary perioperative monitoring, and the risk of complications help the endovascular surgeon to apply treatment appropriately. This chapter reviews the indications for and applications of thrombolysis in aortoiliac occlusive disease in detail and includes case illustrations and a review of the literature.

BRIEF HISTORY OF THROMBOLYSIS

In 1933, Tillett and Garner at Johns Hopkins Hospital, Baltimore, noted that culture filtrates of hemolytic streptococci rapidly liquefied the fibrin clot of normal human plasma.[1] Tillett later used streptokinase to dissolve loculated hemothoraces in the 1940s, and, in 1956, Cliffton at Cornell in New York described the first clinical use of intravenous thrombolytic therapy in two separate reports.[2,3] Although his results with streptokinase were variable and bleeding complications were frequent, Cliffton tried to dissolve thrombi in many regions: venous thrombi, pulmonary emboli, retinal occlusions, and even carotid artery thrombi.

In 1963, the first cases of intra-arterial streptokinase were described.[4] The very first case involved a woman who was seen with a grossly ischemic arm. An intra-arterial catheter was introduced into her brachial artery, and, over a weekend, the catheter was slowly advanced and serial angiography performed. When the catheter had reached the wrist and the digital arteries had successfully opened, the lysis was stopped. This new treatment was expensive at the time, and, afterward, the woman's husband hailed her as "the woman with the golden arm."

Up until this time in the early 1960s, the results of treatment for arterial thrombosis and embolism were very poor. Arteries used to be opened surgically above and below the occlusion and saline solution injected to try and wash out the clot. The introduction of streptokinase was, therefore, a promising development and probably the first endovascular procedure performed; however, the introduction by Fogarty of the embolectomy catheter transformed the surgical management of arterial thrombosis, and interest in thrombolysis waned for many years.[5] Thrombolysis took hours or days to complete, and, in a patient with an ischemic limb, vascular surgical treatment was thought to be more effective.[6]

THE MECHANISM OF THROMBOLYSIS

When the coagulation cascade is triggered through either the intrinsic or extrinsic pathway, the result is the conversion of prothrombin to thrombin. Thrombin itself then converts the soluble fibrinogen to insoluble fibrin. Fibrin acts as a molecular glue, binding red and white blood cells and activated platelets to form a thrombus.

During the formation of this thrombus, plasminogen is incorporated into the clot. This is referred to as "bound plasminogen," as opposed to "circulating plasminogen" in plasma. It is this bound plasminogen that, after its activation, breaks up the clot. Plasmin is the active molecule that breaks the fibrin strands to dissolve thrombus. All the thrombolytic agents in clinical use work by activating this precursor to plasmin. They are, therefore, termed "plasminogen activators."[7,8]

One problem of the earlier thrombolytic agents was that they also activated circulating plasminogen. leading to a degradation of plasma fibrinogen and other clotting factors such as factors V and VIII. On the other hand, fibrin-specific agents such as tissue plasminogen activator (t-PA) and tenecteplase (TNK) preferentially activate the fibrin-bound plasminogen. In theory, this should reduce bleeding complications.

THROMBOLYTIC AGENTS

All of the thrombolytic agents are similar in their action. Different agents have been developed over the years, as a faster speed of action and fewer complications are sought.

Streptokinase

Streptokinase was the first agent to be used, initially at a "low dose" (5000 international units per hour) infused over hours or days[4]; however, subsequent studies of catheter-directed lytic therapy showed a higher rate of bleeding complications with streptokinase than with urokinase or t-PA.[9,10] Furthermore, some patients had an immune response to streptokinase, which prevented its use on future occasions. These two difficulties, together with the development of more specific agents, have effectively stopped the use of streptokinase in clinical practice.

Urokinase

Urokinase is an endogenous activator, which is produced by kidney cells and can be recovered from urine.[11] It directly activates plasminogen and is now manufactured with use of recombinant DNA technology.[12] Prourokinase has also been manufactured by recombinant technology, is more fibrin specific, and does not lower levels of circulating plasminogen to the same extent as urokinase.[13] Urokinase was used widely in the United States as the agent of choice for nearly 20 years until its use was suspended by the Food and Drug Administration in late 1998 because of manufacturing concerns.

Tissue Plasminogen Activator and Tenecteplase

t-PA is a naturally occurring agent produced by endothelial cells. It is very fibrin specific and tends not to lower circulating plasminogen. Recombinant t-PA became the agent of choice after the withdrawal of urokinase in the United States.[8,14] TNK—t-PA (tenecteplase) is a genetically engineered variant of t-PA and is faster acting with a longer half-life than recombinant t-PA. This means that TNK can be administered more easily as a single bolus, rather than as an infusion over time. TNK is even more fibrin specific than recombinant t-PA and does not lower fibrinogen or circulating plasminogen to the same extent.[15] At the Arizona Heart Hospital, it has become our agent of choice in the coronary artery because data in the literature indicate it has a better safety profile than t-PA.[16]

In truth, there is very little difference between the commercially available agents. Increasing the dose may increase the speed of lysis but not the percentage of complete lysis over time. Higher doses also seem to increase the bleeding complications without the added benefit to total clot lysis.[8] Although studies of efficacy and safety have been done for coronary artery thrombolysis, they have not been performed in the peripheral arterial regions. Very large studies indeed would be required; as an example, nearly 17,000 patients were needed to show the enhanced safety profile for TNK over t-PA in the coronary arteries.[16] Under such circumstances, the choice of lytic agent for peripheral interventionalists will depend on individual preference, experience, and cost.

INDICATIONS FOR THROMBOLYSIS IN THE AORTOILIAC SEGMENT

Patients with acute thrombosis or embolism of the aortoiliac arteries presenting within 24 to 48 hours are the most suitable cases for thrombolytic therapy, as long as the duration of thrombolysis itself does not risk the viability of the limb. Thrombolysis of the iliac arteries is a relatively straightforward procedure, but the time required to lyse a completely occluded aorta makes this an uncommon treatment. The use of lysis for occluded limbs of aortobifemoral grafts, occluded iliac stents, and endoluminal grafts has increased in recent years.[17] With the expansion of endovascular surgery, many more patients with aortoiliac disease are being treated than in the past. When a patient is seen with thrombosis of an endovascular stent or stent graft, the mind-set now is to treat this by using endovascular techniques. Once the clot has been lysed, any underlying disease can be immediately treated with use of an endovascular approach. Therefore the ability to perform thrombolysis in the aortoiliac segment is of great advantage to the endovascular surgeon.

PATIENT MANAGEMENT

A thorough clinical history and examination should be performed in every patient being considered for thrombolysis treatment of an occlusion of the aortoiliac segment. A history of myocardial infarction or atrial fibrillation, or even an aortic aneurysm, may point directly to the cause. A history of thrombolysis, polycythemia, or recent cessation of anticoagulation may be present. Conversely, a history of a recent stroke or bleeding diathesis is a relative contraindication to thrombolysis. Informed consent is, therefore, of crucial importance because some patients have unexpected bleeding complications.

Clinical examination may also detect aortic aneurysms, arterial bruits, or the presence or absence of disease in the contralateral iliac segment. Such findings may point toward either embolism or thrombosis. So, too, can a neurologic examination help with diagnosis; some patients with acute limb ischemia are seen with a simultaneous stroke.

Before beginning thrombolysis, a coagulation screen with full blood cell count and urea and electrolytes should be performed as a baseline to be referred to during treatment. In patients with a history of contrast allergy, careful judgment is required, and the administration of steroids is necessary. Modern imaging can provide an accurate diagnosis of the site of the thrombosis in the aortoiliac segment. We routinely use multislice (64) detector computed tomographic (CT) angiography in patients seen with aortoiliac occlusion. This means that a planned approach to the route of access for thrombolysis does not hinder treatment, because bleeding during lysis from an arterial puncture after diagnostic angiography may mean that thrombolytic treatment has to be abandoned.

TECHNIQUES FOR ADMINSTERING LYTIC AGENTS

Access

Thrombolytic therapy is ideally performed in an endovascular suite with modern imaging and good patient monitoring. There are three different ways of gaining endovascular access to perform lysis for aortoiliac thrombosis. In general, the closer the puncture site is to the area undergoing thrombolysis, the easier it is to maneuver the guidewire and catheters. A retrograde femoral artery approach is the most commonly used. It is wise at this time to consider the use of ultrasound assistance to gain arterial access. Multiple attempts at a weak or absent femoral pulse are likely to be subsequently regretted. Retrograde femoral access from the contralateral side may occasionally be useful, particularly if endovascular treatment is likely to progress distally into the superficial femoral artery or beyond. For an aortic occlusion, a retrograde brachial artery approach is generally preferred. Once again, ultrasound assistance here is helpful. The abdominal aorta can be demonstrated with aortography from the renal arteries to the bifurcation, and, in this circumstance, manipulation of the catheter from above into the lower aorta, mesenteric, and renal arteries may be required.

No matter where the lesion is in the aortoiliac segment, safe access is maintained with a low-profile sheath. The guidewire and then the thrombolytic catheter are advanced into the thrombus. At this stage, an attempt is made to pass the guidewire completely through the occluded lesion to determine the likelihood of endovascular success. If the guidewire crosses easily, the presence of soft thrombus is probable and lysis is more likely to succeed. Then, the guidewire is withdrawn to allow the thrombolytic agent to be administered. There are a variety of infusion catheters with either a straight tip or side holes. Straight catheters allow delivery to only a small area of the thrombus, whereas catheters with side holes permit more direct access to a long thrombus. We use 5F Unifuse catheters (Angiodynamics, Queensbury, NY) because the side holes are available on different catheters from 10 to 50 cm in length.

Infusion of Thrombolytic Agents

There are a variety of regimens, depending on the thrombolytic agent and the clinical preference of the institution. We use TNK and have found the following protocol useful.[8]

Agent Preparation

1. Reconstitute the 50-mg lyophilized vial of TNK (Genentech Inc., San Francisco, CA) in 10 mL of sterile water (5 mg/mL).
2. Take 1 mL (5 mg) and dilute in 499 mL of normal saline solution, giving a final concentration of 0.01 mg/mL.
3. For acute arterial thrombus, infuse at 25 to 50 mL/hr (0.25-0.5 mg/hr).

Bolus Administration

An initial bolus of 5 mg given throughout the clot can speed up the process. To do this, dilute 1 mL (5 mg) of the reconstituted TNK in 20 mL of normal saline solution and lace the clot, making sure not to displace any thrombus, which may cause an embolus. For infusions that are expected to continue overnight, lacing may not be necessary (no clear data exist to suggest that bolus administration of TNK is more effective than simple infusion at recommended doses).

Heparin Administration

Low-dose heparin (200-400 units/hr) is given through the sheath to prevent pericatheter thrombosis.

PATIENT MONITORING

After the placement of a thrombolytic catheter and the start of the lytic infusion, the patient is transferred to the ward for close observation because most cases of iliac artery thrombosis will take 12 to 24 hours. In practice, most hospitals use an intensive-care bed, where the patient is monitored closely in case of bleeding complications. Pulse, blood pressure, temperature, full blood cell count, and clotting screen are checked regularly. Lysis is withheld if the fibrinogen level falls below 100 mg/dL. We have found that it is easy to perform bedside angiography using a portable x-ray unit when it is also possible to advance the catheter within a sterile plastic sleeve.[18] In this way, progress of thrombolysis can be monitored without taking the patient back to the operating room.

The patient is also examined for clinical signs of improvement or distal embolization of thrombus. Distal embolization can be dramatic and alarming. The patient experiences sudden pain and numbness in the foot or leg. Although small emboli are clinically silent, large fragments of a partially lysed clot from the aortoiliac segment can acutely occlude the profunda femoris, popliteal, or tibial arteries. Repositioning the infusion catheter more distally, increasing the dose, giving new boluses of thrombolytics, and thromboaspiration are all helpful treatment options in this situation.[19]

ILLUSTRATIVE CASE EXAMPLES

Case Illustration 1

A 65-year-old man underwent bilateral iliac stenting for intermittent claudication with use of two Smart stents (Cordis, a Johnson & Johnson Company, Miami Lakes, FL) (Figure 23-1). The stents were deployed in the common iliac arteries, which were both calcified. Two weeks later, he was readmitted as an emergency with an acutely ischemic left leg. He was immediately given 10,000 international units of heparin and an intravenous heparin infusion commenced. Because thrombolysis was considered likely, a noninvasive multislice CT angiogram was performed. This showed thrombus occluding the left iliac stent from the aortic bifurcation to the level of the hypogastric artery. Because the patient's leg was not severely ischemic, it was thought appropriate to treat him by using a combination of the AngioJet catheter (Possis Medical, Minneapolis, MN) and thrombolysis, rather than by open surgery. Access was gained from bilateral retrograde femoral approaches with use of 6F sheaths. Initially, the AngioJet catheter was used followed by placement of a Unifuse lytic catheter (Angiodynamics). Subsequent angiography showed restoration of blood flow through the common iliac artery; however, it was evident there was disease present proximal and distal to the Smart stent. Therefore two kissing stents were deployed proximally and one further Smart stent deployed distally into the left external iliac artery. Completion angiography confirmed satisfactory improvement. The patient was discharged 2 days later with no subsequent problems.

Case Illustration 2

A 72-year-old man with a symptomatic 5-cm abdominal aortic aneurysm was treated by endoluminal grafting with use of an Anaconda device (Vascutek Terumo, Ann Arbor, MI) (Figure 23-2). This is a modular endograft composed of thin woven polyester and hoop stent rings. One month later, the patient was seen with a sudden onset of left-sided intermittent claudication. CT angiography demonstrated occlusion of the left limb of the endograft. In the operating room, access was gained from a retrograde femoral artery approach. Aortography was used as a road map to place the lytic catheter, which allowed complete recanalization of the left limb of the endograft. Because no apparent cause for this thrombosis was found, no further intervention was performed. The patient was discharged the following day with no sequelae.

DISCUSSION

The greatest advantage of aortoiliac thrombolysis is that it is much less invasive for the patient than open vascular surgery. The greatest disadvantages are the time required to achieve recanalization in this arterial segment and the potential for bleeding complications. The best results are seen in recent occlusions.[20] Yet, successful lysis simply restores the artery to its prethrombotic state, and the underlying cause of the thrombus, for example, atheromatous stenosis, needs to be corrected.

Evidence supporting thrombolysis as an alternative to surgery comes from three large randomized controlled trials. The Rochester Trial randomly assigned

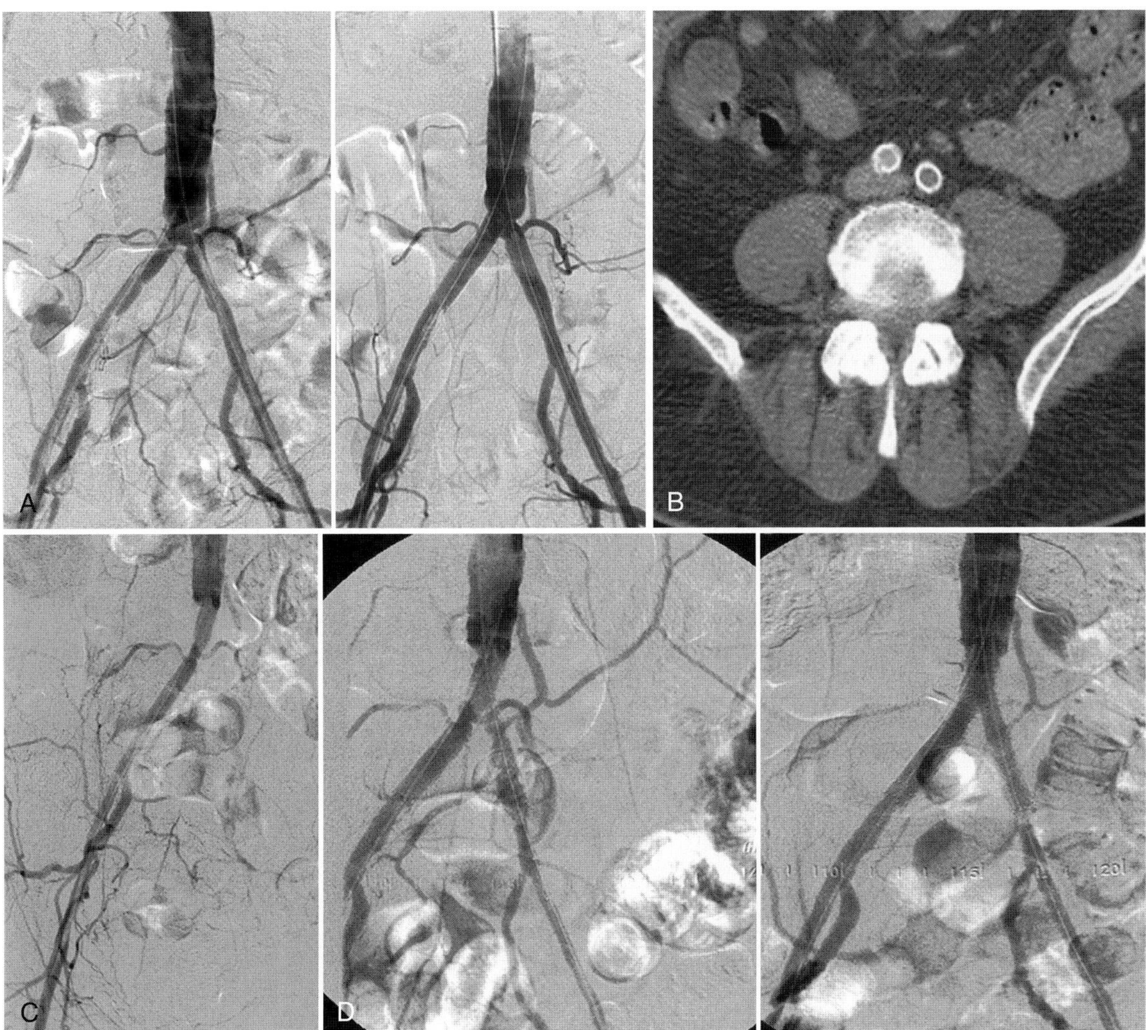

FIGURE 23-1 **A,** Digital subtraction aortography shows stenoses at the origin of both common iliac arteries, which are treated by bilateral iliac stents. **B,** Two weeks later, CT scanning demonstrates occlusion of the left common iliac artery, which is otherwise well deployed. **C,** Operative angiography shows occlusion of the left iliac artery before treatment. **D,** Thrombolysis and the AngioJet device successfully restore patency. Kissing stents are then placed across the aortic bifurcation together with a further iliac stent, which is deployed into the origin of the external iliac artery.

114 patients with ischemia of less than 7 days to surgery or thrombolysis with urokinase. Although the amputation rate was identical in both groups, the survival at 12 months was significantly better in the thrombolysis group (84% vs. 58%).[21]

The STILE Trial randomly assigned 393 patients from 31 centers to receive surgery or a thrombolysis therapy. Although the study was terminated prematurely, a post-hoc analysis showed the patients who presented within 14 days had a lower death and/or amputation rate at 6 months in the lysis group compared with the surgery group (15.3% vs. 37.5%). A reverse trend was seen in patients who presented at over 14 days.[20]

The TOPAS Trial randomly assigned 548 patients from 113 centers worldwide and compared catheter-directed thrombolysis using recombinant urokinase versus surgery in patients presenting within 14 days of an acute arterial occlusion. There was no significant difference in either amputation rate or mortality.[22]

Although meta-analysis of these three trials showed no significant difference in limb salvage or mortality, the complications of stroke and hemorrhage were significantly higher in the thrombolytic groups.[23] The overall risk of hemorrhagic stroke in another meta-analysis of more than 1400 patients undergoing peripheral thrombolysis was 1%; major and minor bleeding occurred in 5% and 15%, respectively.[24] Therefore although thrombolysis is lighter on the patient than surgery, careful selection of patients is required. A recent study has provided some indication of which patients *not* to consider for thrombolysis.[25] In a study in 195 patients undergoing treatment by catheter-directed t-PA for

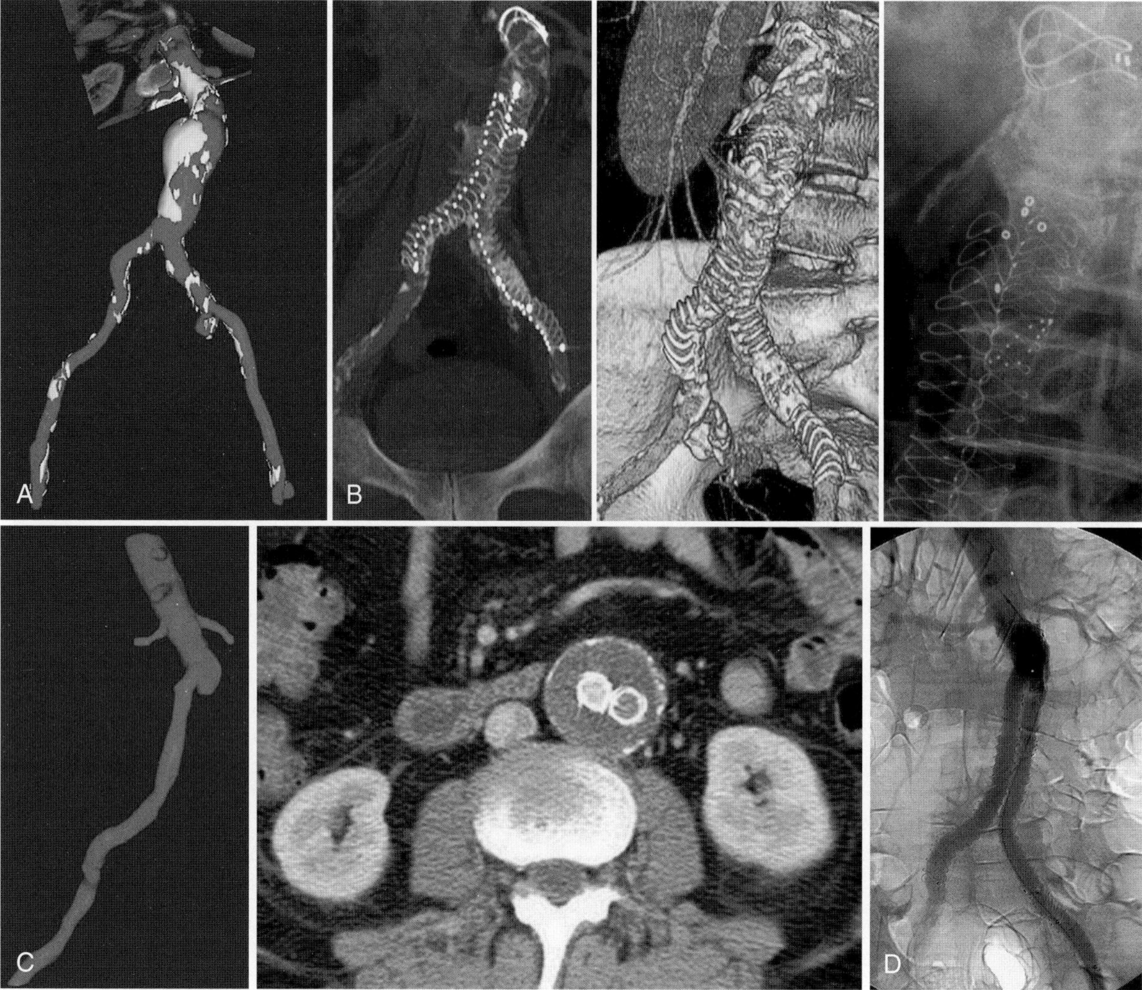

FIGURE 23-2 **A,** A reconstructed three-dimensional (3-D) CT angiogram showing an abdominal aortic aneurysm before endoluminal grafting. **B,** 3-D CT angiography and plain x-ray scan show exclusion of the aneurysm with use of an Anaconda endoluminal graft (Vascutek Terumo, Ann Arbor, MI) with good positioning. **C,** Axial and 3-D CT angiograms demonstrate occlusion of the left limb of the device. **D,** Operative aortogram after successful thrombolysis.

peripheral arterial disease, those with ischemic heart disease and foot ulcers were found to be at higher long-term risk for both amputation and death. A lesser degree of lysis and the presence of a neurologic motor deficit were both associated with higher amputation rates. Renal insufficiency, cerebrovascular disease, and acute lower limb ischemia were associated with increased mortality.

Recently, other percutaneous endovascular devices have been developed that either mechanically disrupt thrombus, aspirate clot, or assist thrombolysis.[26-30] We have more recently used the EKOS ultrasound device (EKOS Corporation, Bothell, WA) to assist thrombolysis because there are indications that this method achieves thrombolysis more rapidly than conventional infusion.[28] Intraluminal high-frequency, low-power ultrasound separates clot fibrin, allowing a better delivery of the lytic agent without fragmenting the clot and causing emboli. The EKOS system is compatible with a 6F sheath (Figure 23-3).

CONCLUSION

In conclusion, thrombolysis is of value in selected cases of aortoiliac thrombosis. Although we have only rarely performed thrombolysis of a completely occluded aorta, we have found great benefit in being able to use thrombolysis to treat iliac artery occlusions, thrombosed iliac stents, and endoluminal grafts. Randomized controlled trials have found that thrombolysis has similar limb salvage and mortality rates compared with open surgery. Although lysis is less invasive for the patient, it needs to be remembered that bleeding complications, including stroke, are more common than with surgery.

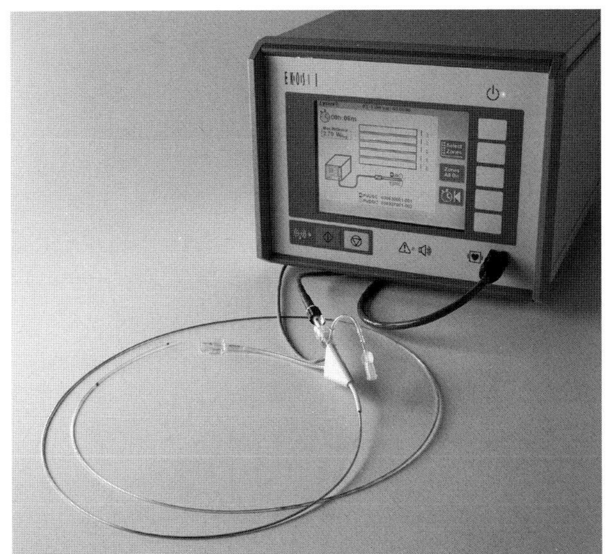

FIGURE 23-3 The EKOS (EKOS Corporation, Bothell, WA) ultrasound-enhanced thrombolytic system.

It is preferable to perform thrombolysis in a dedicated endovascular suite, where any underlying cause for thrombosis can be treated. Thrombolysis works best in cases of recent thrombosis, preferably within a few days of presentation. Careful patient selection, a thorough and detailed workup, and good clinical judgment are required to successfully use thrombolysis in aortoiliac disease.

References

1. Tillett WS, Garner RL: The fibrinolytic activity of haemolytic streptococci, *J Exp Med* 58:485–502, 1933.
2. Tillett WS, Sherry S: The effect in patients of streptococcal fibrinolysin (streptokinase) and streptococcal desoxyribo-nuclease on fibrinous, purulent and sanguinous pleural exudations, *J Clin Invest* 28:173, 1949.
3. Cliffton EE: The use of plasmin in humans, *Ann NY Acad Sci* 68:209–229, 1957.
4. McNicol GP, Reid W, Bain WH, et al: Treatment of peripheral arterial occlusion by streptokinase infusion, *BMJ* 1:1508–1502, 1963.
5. Fogarty TJ, Cranley JJ, Crause RJ, Hafenr CD: A method for extraction of arterial emboli and thrombi, *Surg Gynec Obstet* 116:241–244, 1963.
6. Reid W: Anticoagulants. In Reid W, Pollock JG, editors: *A surgeon's management of gangrene*, London, 1978, Pitman Medical, pp 220–225.
7. Bachmann F: The plasminogen-plasmin enzyme system. In Colman RW, Hirsh J, Marder VJ, Salzman EW, editors: *Haemostasis and Thrombosis: basic principles and clinical practice*, Philadelphia, 1994, Lippincott, pp 1592–1622.
8. Razavi MK, Lee DS, Hofmann LV: Catheter-directed thrombolytic therapy for limb ischemia: current status and controversies, *J Vasc Interv Radiol* 15:13–23, 2004.
9. Van Breda A, Katzen BT, Deutsch AS: Urokinase versus streptokinase in local thrombolysis, *Radiology* 165:109–111, 1987.
10. Sasahara AA, St Martin CC, Henkin J, Barker WM: Approach to the patient with venous thromboembolism: treatment of thrombolytic agents, *Hematol Oncol Clin North Am* 6:1141–1159, 1992.
11. Macfarlane RG, Pinot JJ: Fibrinolytic activity of normal urine, *Nature* 159:779, 1947.
12. Credo RB, Burk SE, Barker WM, et al: Recombinant urokinase (r-UK): biochemistry, pharmacology, and clinical experience. In Sasahara AA, Loscalzo J, editors: *New therapeutic agents in thrombosis and thrombolysis*, New York, 1997, Marcel Dekker, pp 513–537.
13. Ouriel K, Kandarpa K, Schuerr DM, et al: Pro-urokinase versus urokinase for re-canalization of peripheral occlusions, safety and efficacy: the PURPOSE trial, *J Vasc Interv Radiol* 10:1083–1091, 1999.
14. Semba CP, Murphy TP, Bakal CW, et al: Thrombolytic therapy with use of alteplase (rt-PA) in peripheral arterial occlusive disease: review of the clinical literature, *J Vasc Interv Radiol* 11:149–151, 2000.
15. Keyt BA, Paoni NF, Refino CJ, et al: A faster-acting and more potent form of tissue plasminogen activator, *Proc Natl Acad Sci USA* 91:3670–3674, 1994.
16. ASSENT-2 Investigators: Single-bolus tenecteplase compared with front-loaded alteplase in acute myocardial infarction: the ASSENT-2 double blind randomised trial, *Lancet* 354:716–722, 1999.
17. Mesa A, Villareal R, Krajcer Z: Endoluminal treatment of acute aortoiliac thrombosis, *Cathet Cardiovasc Intervent* 50:78–82, 2000.
18. Diethrich EB: Thrombolysis in aorto iliac arterial occlusive disease. In Moore WS, Ahn S, editors: *Endovascular Surgery*, Philadelphia, 2001, W B Saunders, pp 213–220.
19. Khanna NN, Kasliwal RR: Catheter-directed intra-arterial thrombolytic therapy. In Heuser RR, Henry M, editors: *Textbook of peripheral vascular interventions*, London, 2008, Informa UK, pp 99–110.
20. Results of a prospective randomized trial evaluating surgery versus thrombolysis for ischemia of the lower extremity: the STILE Trial, *Ann Surg* 220:251–268, 1994.
21. Ouriel K, Shortell CK, DeWeese JA, et al: A comparison of thrombolytic therapy with operative revascularization in the initial treatment of acute peripheral arterial ischemia, *J Vasc Surg* 19:1021–1030, 1994.
22. Ouriel K, Veith FJ, Sasahara AA, et al: A comparison of recombinant urokinase with vascular surgery as initial treatment for acute arterial occlusion of the legs. Thrombolysis or Peripheral Arterial Surgery (TOPAS) investigators, *N Engl J Med* 338:1105–1111, 1998.
23. Palfreyman SJ, Michaels JA, Booth A: A systematic review of intra-arterial thrombolytic therapy for peripheral vascular occlusions, *Eur J Vasc Endovasc Surg* 19:143–157
24. Berridge D, Niakin GS, Hopkinson BR: Local low-dose intra-arterial thrombolytic therapy, the risk of major stroke and haemorrhage, *Br J Surg* 76:1230–1232, 1989.
25. Kuoppala M, Franzen S, Lindblad B, Acosta S: Long-term prognostic factors after thrombolysis for lower limb ischemia, *J Vasc Surg* 47:1243–1250, 2008.
26. Lutsep HL: Mechanical endovascular recanalization therapies, *Curr Opin Neurol* 21:70–75, 2008.
27. Rogers JH, Laird JR: Overview of new technologies for lower extremity revascularization, *Circulation* 116:2072–2085, 2007.
28. Wissgott C, Richter A, Camusella P, Steinkamp HJ: Treatment of critical limb ischemia using ultrasound-enhanced thrombolysis (PARES Trial): final results, *J Endovasc Ther* 14:438–443, 2007.
29. Yusuf SW, Whitaker SC, Gregson RHS, et al: Prospective randomised comparative study of pulse spray and conventional local thrombolysis, *Eur J Vasc Endovasc Surg* 10:136–141, 1995.
30. Motarjeme A: Ultrasound-enhanced thrombolysis, *J Endovasc Ther* 14:251–256, 2007.

CHAPTER

24

Balloon Angioplasty in Aortoiliac Arterial Occlusive Disease

Kristofer M. Charlton-Ouw, Mark G. Davies, Alan B. Lumsden

Peripheral arterial occlusive disease (PAD) is one manifestation of systemic atherosclerosis. According to the National Health and Nutritional Examination Survey, 2.5% of adults between the ages of 50 and 59 years and 14.5% of adults older than age 70 years have evidence of PAD.[1] However, most patients have no symptoms, despite evidence of major arterial occlusions.[2] The most common symptom of PAD is intermittent claudication (IC). Patients with isolated aortoiliac disease tend to be younger and have a lower likelihood of preexisting coronary arterial disease. Those with femoropopliteal disease, infragenicular disease, or multilevel disease tend to have the lowest ankle-brachial indices (ABI) and the highest likelihood of coronary artery disease. Aortoiliac stenosis and occlusion can lead to symptoms in several tissue beds such as buttock and lower-extremity muscle ischemia and erectile dysfunction. More severe manifestations include rest pain and gangrene, which are more often seen with multilevel disease such as combined aortoiliac and femoropopliteal/tibial disease. Women are more likely to have isolated aortic lesions whereas men are more likely to have multilevel disease.[3] Before the availability of endovascular techniques, open surgery was the mainstay of treatment for severe symptomatic PAD. For lesions of the aorta and short proximal iliac artery lesions, percutaneous transluminal angioplasty with or without stenting has emerged as an excellent alternative with good technical success rates and durable results. Stenting of the aortoiliac region will be dealt with in Chapter 25; here we discuss the merits and techniques of balloon angioplasty as a stand-alone procedure in the aortoiliac segment and as an adjunct to stenting.

INDICATIONS

The primary indication of aortoiliac balloon angioplasty is for symptomatic arterial occlusive disease in the aortoiliac segment caused by atherosclerosis and restenosis at sites of previous intervention or bypass. Other indications discussed elsewhere include fibromuscular dysplasia and certain vasculitides. There has been a perceptible shift to lower the threshold for intervention with the spread of endovascular techniques. Traditional surgical teaching was medical management for patients with IC because most never progressed to limb loss and surgical bypass results did not show a clear benefit in this group.[4] However, many authors now accept that patients with IC have decreased quality of life (QoL) and the inability to perform routine daily activities.[5] In patients with aortoiliac arterial occlusive disease, both hemodynamic and QoL measures significantly improved after endovascular and surgical intervention.[6,7] Therefore it is increasingly acceptable to intervene in patients with so-called disabling claudication (Rutherford grade III, Fontaine stage II). The results of the Claudication: Exercise Vs. Endoluminal Revascularization (CLEVER) study should help provide guidance on optimal treatment for patients with IC.[8]

The TransAtlantic Inter-Society Consensus (TASC) classification scheme was recently updated[9,10] and provides guidelines on optimal treatment strategies based on the anatomic features of the arterial occlusive lesion (Table 24-1). The American College of Cardiology and the American Heart Association also have published practice guidelines created in collaboration with the Society for Vascular Surgery and endorsed by TASC.[11] The Society of Interventional Radiology has separate classification and practice guidelines.[12] If endovascular treatment is indicated, controversy exists between primary stenting versus angioplasty with *selective* stenting. Suffice it to say that angioplasty alone (with stenting reserved for complications or residual stenosis) can be an effective and cost-efficient treatment strategy.[6,13,14] Nevertheless, many authors advocate

TABLE 24-1 TASC Classification of Aortoiliac Disease

TASC lesion	Consensus therapy	Lesion description
A	Data support primary endovascular approach.	• Unilateral or bilateral stenosis of CIA • Unilateral or bilateral single short (≤3 cm) stenosis of EIA
B	Data support primary endovascular approach but support a secondary open approach.	• Short (≤3 cm) stenosis of infrarenal aorta • Unilateral CIA occlusion • Single or multiple stenosis totaling 3-10 cm involving the EIA but not extending into the CFA • Unilateral EIA occlusion not involving the origins of the internal iliac or CFA
C	Data support primary open approach but support a secondary endovascular approach for high-risk patients.	• Bilateral CIA occlusions • Bilateral EIA stenosis 3-10 cm long but not extending into the CFA • Unilateral EIA stenosis extending into the CFA • Unilateral EIA occlusion involving the origin of the internal iliac and/or CFA • Heavily calcified unilateral EIA occlusion with/without involvement of origins or internal iliac and/or CFA
D	Data support primary open approach.	• Intrarenal aortoiliac occlusion • Diffuse disease involving the aorta and both iliac arteries requiring treatment • Diffuse multiple stenosis involving the unilateral CIA, EIA, and CFA • Unilateral occlusions of both CIA and EIA • Bilateral occlusions of EIA • Iliac stenosis in patients with AAA requiring treatment and not amenable to endograft placement or other lesions requiring open aortic or iliac surgery

Norgren L, Hiatt WR, Dormandy JA, et al: Inter-Society Consensus for the Management of Peripheral Arterial Disease (TASC II), *J Vasc Surg* 45 (suppl S):S5-67,2007.
AAA, Abdominal aortic aneurysm; *CFA,* common femoral artery; *CIA,* common iliac artery; *EIA,* external iliac artery; *TASC,* TransAtlantic Inter-Society Consensus.

primary[15-19] or direct stenting,[20,21] and between 20% and 50% of patients in trials of angioplasty with selective stenting have a stent implanted.[6,22-24]

ASSESSMENT

The assessment of patients with suspected aortoiliac occlusive disease includes the usual history and physical examination with special attention to the pain-free and maximal walking distance and notation of QoL impairments. Pulse examination and inspection for the presence of ulcers should be performed. An ABI of ≤0.9 is 95% sensitive and 100% specific in detecting PAD.[10] Specifically for aortoiliac disease, femoral pulses will be diminished and segmental pressures will be lower in the thigh than in the arm. Continuous-wave Doppler signals in the common femoral artery (CFA) will show delayed systolic upstroke. B-mode ultrasound will show decreased amplitudes, and waveforms will be low resistance and monophasic with loss of reverse flow. In the presence of aortoiliac disease, CFA peak systolic flow velocities distal to the stenosis will be decreased to <80 cm/s (Figure 24-1). Within the stenosis, peak systolic velocities will be increased >100% compared with adjacent segments.[25] Other modalities commonly used to quantify location and severity of disease are computed tomographic (CT) angiography, magnetic resonance (MR) angiography, and invasive diagnostic angiography. However, if the ABI or duplex ultrasound examinations do not reveal arterial disease, other etiologies should be considered such as thromboembolism, venous disease, orthopedic disease, or spinal stenosis.

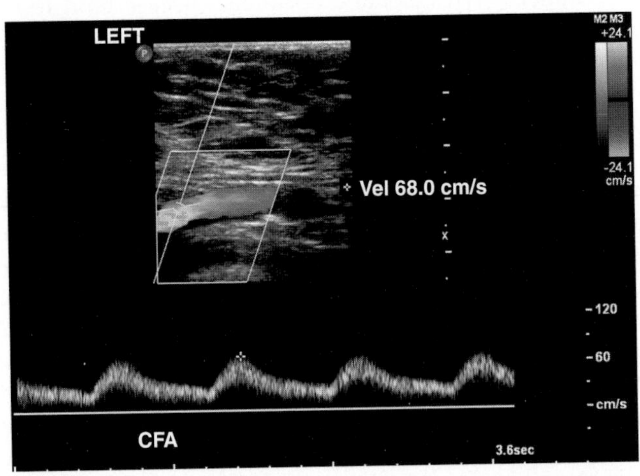

FIGURE 24-1 Lower-extremity arterial duplex examination in a patient with aortoiliac occlusive disease. The peak systolic velocity distal to the stenosis is <80 cm/s with monophasic waveforms.

Once aortoiliac arterial disease is confirmed, revascularization strategies should be based on the presenting symptoms coupled with the severity and location of disease. The TASC II classification (see Table 24-1)

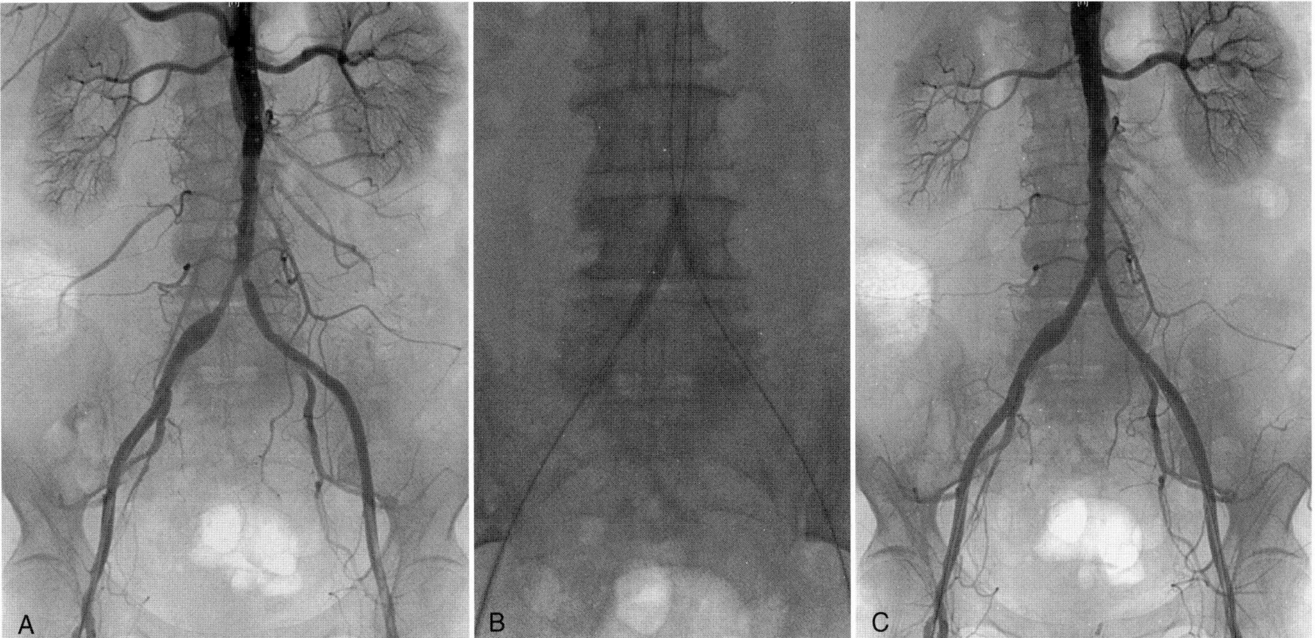

FIGURE 24-2 **A,** Angiogram of a patient with diffuse aortic and proximal iliac occlusive disease. There are bilateral common iliac stenoses with poststenotic dilatation of the right common iliac artery. *(Image courtesy K. Charlton-Ouw and A. Azizzadeh.)* **B,** Kissing-balloon technique. **C,** Poststent angiogram.

requires a morphologic description of the lesions, and treatment recommendations are evidence or consensus based. Stenoses in the common iliac artery (CIA) or single short lesions in the external iliac artery (EIA) ≤3 cm are considered type A, and an endovascular stratagem is recommended. TASC II recommends open surgical treatment for type D lesions, which include infrarenal aortic occlusions, greater than 10 cm aortoiliac stenoses, EIA occlusion, and any iliac stenoses in a patient with abdominal aortic aneurysm not suitable for endovascular exclusion. Types B and C (stenosis or occlusions 3-10 cm in length) can be treated by either endovascular or open surgical approaches.[10] TASC II does not specify the mode of endovascular intervention.

TECHNIQUE

Patients undergoing endovascular aortoiliac intervention often can be treated with local anesthesia and sedation. The general guidelines for selecting wires, catheters, and angioplasty balloons are discussed elsewhere in this text. For aortoiliac lesions, it is helpful to size the aortic diameter by preprocedural axial imaging. Depending on the location of the lesion, ipsilateral femoral access using a retrograde approach can be used for iliac stenosis. Lesions near the CFA may require contralateral access. Uncommonly, arm access may be required when the angle of the aortic bifurcation is acute. If the kissing-balloon technique is being used, bilateral femoral access is usually obtained. Intravenous anticoagulation is given (e.g., heparin) to raise the activated clotting time to greater than 200 to 250 seconds (but <400 seconds),[26-28] or bivalirudin can be used without monitoring the clotting time. The lesion is crossed with a hydrophilic guidewire, and angiographic views are obtained. Once access is gained across a lesion, the correct balloon will need to be selected. Sizing is based on the healthy arterial segment proximal and distal to the lesion. Because contrast angiography provides only luminal detail, especially for diffuse lesions, optimal sizing is based on noninvasive imaging of the native vessel such as ultrasound, CT, or MR.[29] In practice, however, sizing is often performed by measuring luminal diameter in arterial segments relatively free of disease that are adjacent to the lesion. Patient discomfort or pain can limit overexpansion.

The example in Figure 24-2 shows the angiogram of a 72-year-old woman with disabling claudication. She has diffuse infrarenal aortic disease, 70% stenosis in the right CIA, and 80% stenosis in the left CIA. Poststenotic dilatation is noted in the distal right CIA (see Figure 24-2, *A*). Mean arterial pressures were measured, and there was no gradient from the visceral aorta to the bifurcation. There was a greater than 10 mm Hg gradient across the iliac lesions. Figure 24-2, *B*, shows the kissing-balloon technique with use of a 6- × 29-mm balloon on the right and a 6- × 24-mm balloon on the left iliac artery. Postangioplasty angiography showed a right iliac dissection and a residual greater than 30% stenosis in the left CIA. A stainless steel balloon-expanded stent was deployed in each CIA with the results shown in Figure 24-2, C.

In addition to selecting the type of balloon (e.g., standard polyethylene, cryoplasty, or cutting), the balloon brand and size should be tailored to the lesion and native vessel wall. Normally, the balloon should not be oversized past the diameter of the native vessel wall.[30] There are a myriad of brands to choose from, some with hydrophilic coatings and low profiles, and each has a slightly different deployment mechanism.

Iliac Angioplasty

Oblique views expose the common and external iliac bifurcations. Unless coming from the arm, a 75- or 80-cm–shaft balloon angioplasty catheter is usually appropriate. Most devices track over a 0.018- or 0.035-inch wire and fit through a 5F to 6F sheath. After sizing, the correct balloon diameter (usually 5-10 mm) and length (usually 2-4 cm) should be selected. Inflation pressures vary by the balloon manufacturer and degree of calcification. There are no universal guidelines on the duration or number of balloon inflations and no evidence that this affects outcome. Some animal studies indicate that prolonged balloon inflation times lead to increased intimal hyperplasia,[31] but the optimal inflation duration has not yet been determined in humans. Because sudden iliac artery distension may cause pain in the awake patient, some recommend using an undersized balloon first and then upsizing.

The Dutch Iliac Stent Trial Study Group defined the success of angioplasty alone as an intra-arterial pressure gradient across the lesion of less than 10 mm Hg. In equivocal cases, additional gradient measurements were obtained after vasodilatation.[6] TASC II defined hemodynamic significance in aortoiliac disease as a pressure gradient of 5 to 10 mm Hg and 10 to 15 mm Hg after vasodilatation.[10] The U.S. Food and Drug Administration defined residual stenosis after angioplasty as a pressure gradient $\geq$5 mm Hg or greater than 30% stenosis by angiography. In cases of postangioplasty residual stenosis, stent placement is indicated.

Aortic Angioplasty

Lateral angiographic views are helpful to note posterior plaque and to visualize visceral vessels. The location of the inferior mesenteric artery (IMA) should be noted if patent. Angioplasty, postballoon dissections, and stents can impinge on the IMA origin, although it can usually be sacrificed without sequelae. The selected balloon size should be sized on the basis of normal adjacent aortic segments.[29,32] When the lesion involves the CIA origins, bilateral simultaneous balloons are deployed in each iliac extending into the distal aorta. This so-called kissing-balloon technique prevents plaque redistribution or embolization into the contralateral artery.[33] For more proximal lesions, a single balloon is used. Balloon sizes can now accommodate a variety of aortic diameters up to 26 mm. Similar to the iliac arteries, suboptimal angioplasty results are an indication for stent placement.

PATHOPHYSIOLOGY AND GENERAL PRINCIPLES OF BALLOON ANGIOPLASTY

Atherosclerosis is an inflammatory-mediated process that leads to deposition of lipoproteins and other plasma components within the arterial wall. Although the exact mechanism is not completely understood, endothelial adhesion molecules and cytokines facilitate the migration and proliferation of leukocytes, especially macrophages, into the vessel wall.[34] The root cause of the increased endothelial permeability is unknown, but the clustering of atherosclerotic plaques at branch vessels and bifurcations indicates that increased turbulence and decreased shear stress play a major role.[35] Mature atherosclerotic lesions form a fibrous cap over a necrotic- and lipid-filled core. Calcification of lesions leads to reduced elasticity and is mediated by the intimal-medial smooth muscle cells.[36] The degree of lesion calcification affects angioplasty results[37] and was found to be associated with the presence of diabetes in a study of amputated extremities.[38]

Angioplasty of atherosclerotic lesions is a controlled dissection of the vessel wall as a result of the crush and stretch injury. The response within the vessel wall is dependent on the composition of the plaque and the nature of the injury. The degree of injury is proportional to the balloon length, dilating force, and duration of inflation. After balloon expansion, the vessel wall is stretched, the plaque is fractured, and its components are redistributed. Intravascular ultrasound (IVUS) with radiofrequency analysis showed that the fibrous and fibrofatty components of the plaque were pushed into adjacent vessel wall segments outside of the balloon length.[37] Thus the increased luminal diameter after angioplasty is due to a combination of plaque redistribution and wall stretch. Some portion of the plaque volume may also be lost to embolization.[37,39,40] Small dissections and plaque separations are common but generally do not lead to clinically significant adverse events. The vessel can recoil after angioplasty, which may be one cause of a technically poor result.

On a cellular level, the endothelium is denuded and there is injury and activation to the underlying smooth muscle cells and adventitial fibroblasts. In animal models, apoptosis or programmed cell death within the wall occurs at 1 to 2 hours after angioplasty and wanes by 4 hours.[41] The body mounts an inflammatory response in response to the angioplasty injury with infiltration of both neutrophils and monocytes and the creation of a milieu of cytokines. Within 48 hours after angioplasty, smooth muscle cells proliferate within the media and eventually migrate to the intima.[42] A second phase of smooth muscle cell proliferation occurs within the intima after 7 days and continues for several weeks. In addition, myofibroblasts are activated within the adventitia and may contribute to chronic elastic recoil or negative remodeling. The response of smooth muscle cells and production of extracellular matrix leads to the development of the intimal hyperplastic lesion. Intimal hyperplasia can result in positive remodeling, which allows the lumen to remain open; in contrast, negative remodeling narrows the lumen, which results from constriction of the intimal hyperplastic lesion. In the longer term, intimal hyperplastic lesions developed a variant of atherosclerosis termed accelerated atherosclerosis. The original atherosclerotic lesion is histologically different from restenosis because of intimal hyperplasia and is the vascular equivalent of scar tissue. Intimal hyperplasia, elastic recoil, negative remodeling, and atherosclerotic progression all contribute to restenosis after balloon angioplasty.

OUTCOMES

A recent Cochrane Review identified four prospective randomized trials comparing aortoiliac bypass surgery with angioplasty.[4] Only the Veterans Administration Cooperative Study[43] specifically segregated lesions into either proximal or distal. Primary patency was greater in the surgery group at 1 year but was equivalent at 4 years. Longer follow-up also showed increased mortality in the surgery group (odds ratio 1.74). Both groups showed significant but equivalent improvements in QoL measurements. The authors concluded that angioplasty produced equivalent outcomes compared with open bypass surgery. Subsequently, reports stated that patency rates of aortobifemoral bypass grafts differ depending on the indication and severity of disease.[10] A meta-analysis reported 5-year patency rates ranging from 72% to 94%.[44] Results are worse for extra-anatomic bypass.[45] Given the good outcomes and the lower morbidity and mortality, endovascular therapy is recommended for anatomically suitable aortoiliac lesions in reasonable-risk patients.

Another meta-analysis of case series from the early 1990s comparing angioplasty with selective stenting versus primary stenting of iliac lesions showed a slight benefit for primary stenting in terms of initial technical success and primary patency.[46] Although Richter et al.[47] published an earlier randomized trial of iliac angioplasty versus stenting in German, the Dutch Iliac Stent Trial Study Group later published the only significant multicenter, prospective, randomized trial in the English literature.[6] Two hundred seventy-nine patients with IC were randomly assigned to either direct stenting or angioplasty with selective stenting. In the selective stent group, stents were placed only if a residual pressure gradient of greater than 10 mm Hg existed regardless of the lesion's postangioplasty appearance. Initial procedural success, complications (81% vs. 82%), QoL improvements, 2-year clinical success (78% vs. 77%), 2-year cumulative patency (71% vs. 70%), and reintervention rates were all statistically similar between the two groups. In separate publications, the authors confirmed that angioplasty with selective stenting is more cost-effective than direct stenting.[13] Long-term follow-up supported the group's initial results with a 5-year freedom from reintervention rate at about 80% of patients in both groups.[48] Although patients in the selective stent group had slightly better improvement in symptoms 5 to 8 years after treatment, there was no statistical difference in ABI, patency, or QoL.[14] Since the initial randomized trials, several studies have been

TABLE 24-2 Results of Selected Series of Balloon Angioplasty in Symptomatic Infrarenal Aortic or Aortoiliac Stenosis Published After 1995

	Initial technical success (%)	Stent implanted (%)	1-Yr primary patency (%)	5-Yr primary patency (%)	Complications (%)	30-Day mortality (%)
Audet et al., 1998[32]	85	13	88	88	0.05	0
Elkouri et al., 1999[50]	96	0	80	64*	0	0
de Vries et al., 2004[51]	98	35	75	75	0.07	0
Rosset et al., 2001[49]	100	58	94†	NA	0	0

**83% 4-Year primary patency for isolated aortic stenosis and 55% for aortoiliac disease.*
†2-Year primary patency.
NA, Not available.

TABLE 24-3 Results of Selected Series of Balloon Angioplasty in Symptomatic Iliac Stenosis Published After 1995

	Initial technical success (%)	Stent implanted (%)	1-Yr primary patency (%)	5-Yr primary patency (%)	Complications (%)	30-Day mortality (%)
Johnston, 1993[†56]	96.5	0	77.2	54.0	3.9	0.3
Tetteroo et al., 1998[6]	81	43	80	NA*	4	0
Becquemin et al., 1999[23]	93.5	23.8	86.5	75.4	8.1	0
Kudo et al., 2005[22]	99.3	23	76	49	0.7	0
Galaria et al., 2005[24]	98	51	85	53	7	1.8
AbuRahma et al., 2007[54]	100	Unknown	83	69	24	0

**Long-term results available from Klein WM, van der Graff Y, Seegers J, et al. Dutch Iliac Stent Trial: long-term results in patients randomized for primary or selective stent placement, Radiology 2006, 238:734-744,2006.*

†Number of patients with critical limb ischemia presented as percentage of 667 procedures: claudicants (91.3%), salvage (8.8%), and other (3.1%). Note that percentages total over 100%. Results are for iliac stenosis "success rates" as defined by the authors. Success rates for iliac occlusions are 59.8% and 48.0% at 1 and 3 years, respectively.

NA, Not available.

published that support angioplasty (often with selective stenting) of both aortic[32,49-52] and iliac[22,23,53] arterial occlusive lesions (Tables 24-2 and 24-3). However, many of these studies are nearly 10 years old, and it may be that improvements in stent design and technology will move more practitioners to primary or direct stenting. Chapter 25 makes a comparison of various aortoiliac revascularization techniques.

In general, long-term results from angioplasty with selective stenting show excellent 1-year primary patency rates exceeding 80% with high technical success and low morbidity and mortality. Five-year primary patency rates are >70% for isolated aortic lesions[32,50,51] but can drop to as low as 49% to 54%[22,50] for distal or diffuse aortoiliac disease (see Tables 24-2 and 24-3). Results from the previously mentioned meta-analysis of 1300 patients (33% with critical limb ischemia [CLI]) show an initial technical success of aortoiliac angioplasty alone of 91% (range 81.9%-98.6%); a 4-year pooled primary patency of 64% (range 58%-87%, excluding technical failures); and a 4-year pooled secondary patency of 80%.

Angioplasty-alone results are best for short, proximal lesions such as in isolated infrarenal aortic or CIA lesions, but outcomes become less favorable for more distal lesions involving the internal iliac artery or CFA. These results are reflected in the TASC II classification where diffuse lesions or disease involving the CFA are listed as types C or D (see Table 24-1).[10] AbuRahma and colleagues[54] used angioplasty with selective stenting in 41 patients from 1994 to 1999, then used primary stenting in 110 patients from 2000 to 2005. They showed equivalent short-term and midterm results between selective and primary stenting groups for TASC A and B lesions. However, the 3-year primary patency rates in TASC C and D lesions were 28% for selective stenting versus 72% for primary stenting.

The indication for intervention—claudication versus CLI—reflects severity of disease and also predicts long-term outcome. Five-year patency rates are much better for patients with IC than with CLI.[55] Because the Dutch Iliac Stent Trial Study Group mostly included patients with IC and excluded patients with aortic stenosis or any stenosis greater than 10 cm (equivalent to TASC II type D), their conclusions may not apply to patients with CLI or more severe disease. The greater the proportion of patients with CLI, the worse the patency rate becomes,[56] but not all authors have found this association.[24,46]

Several other factors appear to negatively affect the outcome of aortoiliac angioplasty including the distal extent of disease,[50,57] long-segment stenosis, multilevel disease,[50,54,58] smoking history, and renal failure.[22,24,48] Galaria and Davies[24] retrospectively reviewed 276 patients with TASC A and B iliac lesions who had angioplasty with selective stenting (see Table 24-3). The presence of distal disease, hypertension, hypercholesterolemia, and renal insufficiency predicted decreased primary patency. These data indicate that primary stenting may be favorable in certain patients.[22,54,59] Female gender may also adversely affect endovascular interventions[48,60] possibly because of the smaller vessel caliber, but not all groups have found this association. These factors make comparison between different study results difficult because the reporting is not uniform.

Follow-up is commonly with clinical assessment and ABI measurements. A return of symptoms or a drop in ABI of greater than 0.1 prompts further imaging. Clinical decline is often the result of restenosis at the previous intervention site or progression of atherosclerotic disease. Repeated endovascular or open surgical bypass can be safely performed in cases of restenosis.[61]

OTHER ANGIOPLASTY-RELATED TECHNIQUES

Recanalization

Since Reekers and Bolia first introduced subintimal angioplasty techniques in 1998,[62] a number of case reports and small series have shown promise in recanalizing calcified, chronically occluded vessels. Lipsitz and et al[63] treated chronic arterial occlusions by subintimal angioplasty in 39 patients (only 2 had occluded external iliac arteries). Technical success was achieved in 87%, and 2 patients had distal embolization requiring treatment. Hemodynamic patency rates were 74% at 1 year and 59% at 2 years. All technical failures were due to an inability to reenter the true lumen. Several devices have since been developed for luminal reentry after subintimal angioplasty, such as the Outback (Cordis Endovascular, Warren, NJ) and the Pioneer (Medtronic, Santa Rosa, CA) reentry catheters. The Pioneer requires a 6F sheath and uses IVUS to orient the reentry tip into the lumen. The Outback also requires a 6F sheath and uses radiopaque makers to guide the reentry tip. Jacobs et al.[64] reviewed their experience using reentry devices in 24 chronic occlusions after failure of standard reentry techniques. With use of the reentry devices, all lesions were successfully crossed and the true lumen reentered. All lesions were stented after angioplasty, and two perforations were treated with deployment of a covered stent. Several other devices are marketed for crossing chronic occlusions including use of radiofrequency ablation (e.g., PowerWire, Baylis, Mississauga, Ontario, Canada), high-frequency vibration (e.g., Crosser, FlowCardia, Sunnyvale, CA), and "dilatable"-tip guidewires (e.g., Voletek, Ovalum Vascular, Asheville, NC). Use of thrombolysis in aortoiliac arterial occlusive disease was dealt with in Chapter 23.

Cryoplasty

Cryoplasty combines balloon angioplasty with delivery of cold thermal energy to the vessel wall. Cryoplasty balloons are currently available in diameters from 2 to 8 mm and in lengths from 2 to 10 cm (PolarCath, Boston Scientific, Natick, MA). Animal studies have shown that application of cold thermal energy to the vessel wall inhibits intimal hyperplasia by inducing apoptosis.[65] No randomized clinical trials exist that evaluate cryoplasty compared with other conventional interventions. A recent Cochrane review identified several case series, but no study looked specifically into cryoplasty in the native aortoiliac arteries.[66] Karthik et al.[67] treated 10 patients with iliofemoral restenosis with percutaneous transluminal cryoplasty balloons. All patients had restenosis of the treated lesions by 1 year, and the authors concluded that cryoplasty does not have a role in treating restenosis in the iliofemoral arteries.[67] More encouraging results have been reported in infrainguinal unintervened de novo lesions.[68] Given the lack of randomized data and case series with only small patient numbers, cryoplasty for aortoiliac disease cannot be properly evaluated at this time.

Cutting Balloon Angioplasty

Given that intimal hyperplastic stenoses are tough, collagen-filled lesions, cutting balloon angioplasty (CBA) has been proposed to treat these restenotic lesions. Cutting balloons are currently available in over-the-wire and monorail systems in diameters ranging from 2 to 8 mm and in lengths from 1.5 to 2 cm (Peripheral Cutting Balloons, Boston Scientific). Ahmed et al.[69] used IVUS before and after CBA and surmised that the blades anchor the balloon in place and increase luminal dimension by extrusion of cut intimal hyperplastic material through the stent struts and by redistribution inside the vessel wall. Unlike conventional angioplasty, CBA does not significantly increase the diameter of the stent within the vessel. This was confirmed by subsequent studies.[70] A randomized clinical trial showed that in-stent restenosis treated with CBA required fewer adjunctive devices, such as additional stents and balloons, than conventional angioplasty.[71] The authors also noted that conventional angioplasty had a higher incidence of balloon slippage out of the stenotic area when inflated as compared with CBA. However, the 7-month restenosis rate at about 30% was the same for both groups.[71]

In addition to restenosis of angioplasty and stents, CBA has also found application in intimal hyperplasia complicating hemodialysis access,[72,73] vein bypass grafts,[74] and prosthetic bypass grafts.[75] CBA appears to improve procedural angiographic success in cases where conventional angioplasty is unable to dilate the intimal hyperplastic lesion. Nevertheless, recurrent restenosis is still a problem.

COMPLICATIONS

General complications in treating aortoiliac disease will be discussed in depth in Chapter 27. In brief, early complications include procedural mishaps, thromboembolism, and access problems. Periprocedural cardiovascular and cerebrovascular incidents after aortoiliac angioplasty are uncommon. Most series report no or very low perioperative mortality. Complication rates in older studies for iliac angioplasty range from 2.3% to 13.4% with a major complication rate of about 2.7%.[30] Given that the largest angioplasty balloons require up to a 12F sheath, it is no surprise that bleeding is one of the most common complications. Most can be managed conservatively, but those that require blood transfusions portend a worse outcome.[76] Suspicion for retroperitoneal bleeding prompts a CT scan. Indications for groin exploration and hematoma evacuation are evidence of ongoing bleeding, severe pain, progressive enlargement, skin compromise, femoral nerve compression, and wound infection. Other access site complications include pseudoaneurysm, arteriovenous fistula, acute arterial occlusion, and symptomatic distal embolization.

Arterial dissection may not be listed as a complication in the literature,[77] because some authors listed dissection as an indication for stenting.[29] The Dutch Iliac Stent Study Trial Group proposed to stent only hemodynamically significant dissections producing a gradient of greater than 10 mm Hg but in practice reported several protocol deviations of stent placement without meeting the pressure gradient threshold.[6] Advocates of direct stenting cite avoidance of dissection as an advantage of stenting without first performing angioplasty.[15,18]

Arterial rupture complicates iliac angioplasty in 0.3% of patients.[30] In one report of more than 1100 patients with PAD, 46% of whom underwent endovascular iliac artery revascularization, perforation occurred in only 2 patients.[77] Rupture occurs more often in heavily calcified lesions or during high-pressure inflation.[78] Suspicion for rupture during the procedure prompts contrast injection. Serial CT scans can be used to diagnose and evaluate progression. Treatment of perforation or rupture entails reversal of anticoagulation, balloon tamponade, and blood transfusions when appropriate. Bleeding control with deployment of covered stents is advocated by several authors.[78-80] Yeo et al.[79] recommend balloon tamponade for up to 15 to 20 minutes during which time a covered stent should be selected in case bleeding recommences after balloon deflation.

CONCLUSION

Existing randomized controlled trials of symptomatic aortoiliac atherosclerotic disease indicate that aortoiliac balloon angioplasty with selective stenting is efficacious and cost-effective. Restenosis after angioplasty is due to intimal hyperplasia, elastic recoil, and negative remodeling. In properly selected patients, patency rates of angioplasty approach those of aortobifemoral bypass grafts with less morbidity. The TASC II classification can be used to segregate those patients best served by endovascular therapy from those best suited to surgery. Angioplasty with selective stenting is best reserved for short, proximal lesions corresponding to TASC II types A and B. Iliac lesions that are distal, long (>3 cm), and multilevel appear to do better with primary or direct stenting. Certain lesions and patient characteristics coupled with improved stent design appear to be leading to greater use of primary and direct stenting.

References

1. Selvin E, Erlinger TP: Prevalence of and risk factors for peripheral arterial disease in the United States: results from the National Health and Nutrition Examination Survey, 1999-2000, *Circulation* 110(6):738–743, 2004.
2. Fowkes FG, Housley E, Cawood EH, et al: Edinburgh Artery Study: prevalence of asymptomatic and symptomatic peripheral arterial disease in the general population, *Int J Epidemiol* 20 (2):384–392, 1991.
3. Staple TW: The solitary aortoliliac lesion, *Surgery* 64(3):569–576, 1968.
4. Fowkes F, Leng G: Bypass surgery for chronic lower limb ischaemia, *Cochrane Database Syst Rev* (2):CD002000, 2008.
5. Breek JC, Hamming JF, De Vries J, et al: The impact of walking impairment, cardiovascular risk factors, and comorbidity on quality of life in patients with intermittent claudication, *J Vasc Surg* 36(1):94–99, 2002.
6. Tetteroo E, van der Graaf Y, Bosch JL, et al: Randomised comparison of primary stent placement versus primary angioplasty followed by selective stent placement in patients with iliac-artery occlusive disease. Dutch Iliac Stent Trial Study Group, *Lancet* 351(9110):1153–1159. 18, 1998.
7. Bosch JL, van der Graaf Y, Hunink MG: Health-related quality of life after angioplasty and stent placement in patients with iliac artery occlusive disease: results of a randomized controlled clinical trial. The Dutch Iliac Stent Trial Study Group, *Circulation* 99(24):3155–3160, 1999.
8. Murphy TP, Hirsch AT, Ricotta JJ, et al: The Claudication: Exercise Vs. Endoluminal Revascularization (CLEVER) study: Rationale and methods, *J Vasc Surg* 47(6):1356–1363, 2008.
9. Dormandy JA, Rutherford RB: Management of peripheral arterial disease (PAD). TASC Working Group. TransAtlantic Inter-Society Consensus (TASC), *J Vasc Surg* 31(1 Pt 2):S1–S296, 2000.
10. Norgren L, Hiatt WR, Dormandy JA, et al: Inter-Society Consensus for the Management of Peripheral Arterial Disease (TASC II), *J Vasc Surg* 45(suppl S):S5–67, 2007.
11. Hirsch AT, Haskal ZJ, Hertzer NR, et al: ACC/AHA 2005 practice guidelines for the management of patients with peripheral arterial disease (lower extremity, renal, mesenteric, and abdominal aortic): a collaborative report from the American Association for Vascular Surgery/Society for Vascular Surgery, Society for Cardiovascular Angiography and Interventions, Society for Vascular Medicine and Biology, Society of Interventional Radiology, and the ACC/AHA Task Force on Practice Guidelines (Writing Committee to Develop Guidelines for the Management of Patients With Peripheral Arterial Disease): endorsed by the American Association of Cardiovascular and Pulmonary Rehabilitation; National Heart, Lung, and Blood Institute; Society for Vascular Nursing; TransAtlantic Inter-Society Consensus; and Vascular Disease Foundation, *Circulation* 113(11):e463–e654, 2006.
12. Guidelines for percutaneous transluminal angioplasty, *J Vasc Interv Radiol* 14(9 Pt 2):S209–217, 2003 Sep.
13. Bosch JL, Tetteroo E, Mali WP, et al: Iliac arterial occlusive disease: cost-effectiveness analysis of stent placement versus percutaneous transluminal angioplasty. Dutch Iliac Stent Trial Study Group, *Radiology* 208(3):641–648, 1998.
14. Klein WM, van der Graaf Y, Seegers J, et al: Dutch iliac stent trial: long-term results in patients randomized for primary or selective stent placement, *Radiology* 238(2):734–744, 2006.

15. Onal B, Ilgit ET, Yucel C, et al: Primary stenting for complex atherosclerotic plaques in aortic and iliac stenoses, *Cardiovasc Intervent Radiol* 21(5):386–392, 1998.
16. Yilmaz S, Sindel T, Yegin A, et al: Primary stenting of focal atherosclerotic infrarenal aortic stenoses: long-term results in 13 patients and a literature review, *Cardiovasc Intervent Radiol* 27 (2):121–128, 2004.
17. Ansel GM: Primary stenting of the iliac artery, *Endovascular Today*, May 2005, pp. 43–44.
18. Poncyljusz W, Falkowski A, Garncarek J, et al: Primary stenting in the treatment of focal atherosclerotic abdominal aortic stenoses, *Clin Radiol* 61(8):691–695, 2006.
19. Klonaris C, Katsargyris A, Tsekouras N, et al: Primary stenting for aortic lesions: from single stenoses to total aortoiliac occlusions, *J Vasc Surg* 47(2):310–317, 2008.
20. Lagana D, Carrafiello G, Mangini M, et al: Endovascular treatment of steno-occlusions of the infrarenal abdominal aorta, *Radiol Med (Torino)* 111(7):949–958, 2006.
21. Cuisset T, Hamilos M, Melikian N, et al: Direct stenting for stable angina pectoris is associated with reduced periprocedural microcirculatory injury compared with stenting after predilation, *J Am Coll Cardiol* 51(11):1060–1065, 2008.
22. Kudo T, Chandra FA, Ahn SS: Long-term outcomes and predictors of iliac angioplasty with selective stenting, *J Vasc Surg* 42(3):466–475, 2005.
23. Becquemin JP, Allaire E, Qvarfordt P, et al: Surgical transluminal iliac angioplasty with selective stenting: long-term results assessed by means of duplex scanning, *J Vasc Surg* 29(3):422–429, 1999.
24. Galaria II, Davies MG: Percutaneous transluminal revascularization for iliac occlusive disease: long-term outcomes in Trans-Atlantic Inter-Society Consensus A and B lesions, *Ann Vasc Surg* 19(3):352–360, 2005.
25. Zierler RE: Ultrasound assessment of lower extremity arteries. In Zwiebel WJ, Pellerito JS, editors: *Introduction to vascular ultrasonography*, 5th ed, Philadelphia, 2000, Saunders.
26. Chew DP, Bhatt DL, Lincoff AM, et al: Defining the optimal activated clotting time during percutaneous coronary intervention: aggregate results from 6 randomized, controlled trials, *Circulation* 103(7):961–966, 2001.
27. Tolleson TR, O'Shea JC, Bittl JA, et al: Relationship between heparin anticoagulation and clinical outcomes in coronary stent intervention: observations from the ESPRIT trial, *J Am Coll Cardiol* 41(3):386–393, 2003.
28. Brener SJ, Moliterno DJ, Lincoff AM, et al: Relationship between activated clotting time and ischemic or hemorrhagic complications: analysis of 4 recent randomized clinical trials of percutaneous coronary intervention, *Circulation* 110(8):994–998, 2004 Aug 24.
29. Uberoi R, Tsetis D: Standards for the endovascular management of aortic occlusive disease, *Cardiovasc Intervent Radiol* 30(5): 814–819, 2007.
30. Tsetis D, Uberoi R: Quality improvement guidelines for endovascular treatment of iliac artery occlusive disease, *Cardiovasc Intervent Radiol* 31(2):238–245, 2008.
31. Hehrlein C, Weinschenk I, Metz J: Long period of balloon inflation and the implantation of stents potentiate smooth muscle cell death: possible role of chronic vascular injury in restenosis, *Int J Cardiovasc Intervent* 2(1):21–26, 1999.
32. Audet P, Therasse E, Oliva VL, et al: Infrarenal aortic stenosis: long-term clinical and hemodynamic results of percutaneous transluminal angioplasty, *Radiology* 209(2):357–363, 1998.
33. Tegtmeyer CJ, Kellum CD, Kron IL, et al: Percutaneous transluminal angioplasty in the region of the aortic bifurcation. The two-balloon technique with results and long-term follow-up study, *Radiology* 157(3):661–665, 1985.
34. Rosenfeld ME, Ross R: Macrophage and smooth muscle cell proliferation in atherosclerotic lesions of WHHL and comparably hypercholesterolemic fat-fed rabbits, *Arteriosclerosis* 10(5):680–687, 1990.
35. Tsou JK, Gower RM, Ting HJ, et al: Spatial regulation of inflammation by human aortic endothelial cells in a linear gradient of shear stress, *Microcirculation* 15(4):311–323, 2008.
36. Trion A, van der Laarse A: Vascular smooth muscle cells and calcification in atherosclerosis, *Am Heart J* 147(5):808–814, 2004.
37. Wei H, Schiele F, Descotes-Genon V, et al: Changes in unstable coronary atherosclerotic plaque composition after balloon angioplasty as determined by analysis of intravascular ultrasound radiofrequency, *Am J Cardiol* 101(2):173–178, 2008.
38. Soor GS, Vukin I, Leong SW, Oreopoulos G, Butany J: Peripheral vascular disease: who gets it and why? A histomorphological analysis of 261 arterial segments from 58 cases, *Pathology* 40 (4):385–391, 2008.
39. Karnabatidis D, Katsanos K, Kagadis GC, et al: Distal embolism during percutaneous revascularization of infra-aortic arterial occlusive disease: an underestimated phenomenon, *J Endovasc Ther* 13(3):269–280, 2006.
40. Lam RC, Shah S, Faries PL, et al: Incidence and clinical significance of distal embolization during percutaneous interventions involving the superficial femoral artery, *J Vasc Surg* 46(6): 1155–1159, 2007.
41. Perlman H, Maillard L, Krasinski K, et al: Evidence for the rapid onset of apoptosis in medial smooth muscle cells after balloon injury, *Circulation* 95(4):981–987, 1997.
42. Ferns GA, Raines EW, Sprugel KH, et al: Inhibition of neointimal smooth muscle accumulation after angioplasty by an antibody to PDGF, *Science* 253(5024):1129–1132, 1991.
43. Wolf GL, Wilson SE, Cross AP, et al: Surgery or balloon angioplasty for peripheral vascular disease: a randomized clinical trial. Principal investigators and their Associates of Veterans Administration Cooperative Study Number 199, *J Vasc Interv Radiol* 4(5):639–648, 1993.
44. de Vries SO, Hunink MG: Results of aortic bifurcation grafts for aortoiliac occlusive disease: a meta-analysis, *J Vasc Surg* 26 (4):558–569, 1997.
45. Ricco JB, Probst H: Long-term results of a multicenter randomized study on direct versus crossover bypass for unilateral iliac artery occlusive disease, *J Vasc Surg* 47(1):45–53, 2008, discussion 4.
46. Bosch JL, Hunink MG: Meta-analysis of the results of percutaneous transluminal angioplasty and stent placement for aortoiliac occlusive disease, *Radiology* 204(1):87–96, 1997.
47. Richter GM, Roeren T, Noeldge G, et al: [Initial long-term results of a randomized 5-year study: iliac stent implantation versus PTA], *Vasa* 35:192–193, 1992.
48. Klein WM, van der Graaf Y, Seegers J, et al: Long-term cardiovascular morbidity, mortality, and reintervention after endovascular treatment in patients with iliac artery disease: the Dutch Iliac Stent Trial Study, *Radiology* 232(2):491–498, 2004.
49. Rosset E, Malikov S, Magnan PE, et al: Endovascular treatment of occlusive lesions in the distal aorta: mid-term results in a series of 31 consecutive patients, *Ann Vasc Surg* 15(2):140–147, 2001.
50. Elkouri S, Hudon G, Demers P, et al: Early and long-term results of percutaneous transluminal angioplasty of the lower abdominal aorta, *J Vasc Surg* 30(4):679–692, 1999.
51. de Vries JP, van Den Heuvel DA, Vos JA, et al: Freedom from secondary interventions to treat stenotic disease after percutaneous transluminal angioplasty of infrarenal aorta: long-term results, *J Vasc Surg* 39(2):427–431, 2004.

52. Westcott MA, Bonn J: Comparison of conventional angioplasty with the Palmaz stent in the treatment of abdominal aortic stenoses from the STAR registry. SCVIR Transluminal Angioplasty and Revascularization, *J Vasc Interv Radiol* 9(2):225–231, 1998.
53. Cambria RA, Farooq MM, Mewissen MW, et al: Endovascular therapy of iliac arteries: routine application of intraluminal stents does not improve clinical patency, *Ann Vasc Surg* 13(6):599–605, 1999.
54. AbuRahma AF, Hayes JD, Flaherty SK, et al: Primary iliac stenting versus transluminal angioplasty with selective stenting, *J Vasc Surg* 46(5):965–970, 2007.
55. Becker GJ, Katzen BT, Dake MD: Noncoronary angioplasty, *Radiology* 170(3 Pt 2):921–940, 1989.
56. Johnston KW: Iliac arteries: reanalysis of results of balloon angioplasty, *Radiology* 186(1):207–212, 1993.
57. Powell RJ, Fillinger M, Walsh DB, et al: Predicting outcome of angioplasty and selective stenting of multisegment iliac artery occlusive disease, *J Vasc Surg* 32(3):564–569, 2000.
58. Johnston KW, Rae M, Hogg-Johnston SA, et al: 5-year results of a prospective study of percutaneous transluminal angioplasty, *Ann Surg* 206(4):403–413, 1987.
59. Tsetis D, Belli AM, Morgan R, et al: Preliminary experience with cutting balloon angioplasty for iliac artery in-stent restenosis, *J Endovasc Ther* 15(2):193–202, 2008.
60. Timaran CH, Stevens SL, Freeman MB, et al: External iliac and common iliac artery angioplasty and stenting in men and women, *J Vasc Surg* 34(3):440–446, 2001.
61. Schurmann K, Mahnken A, Meyer J, et al: Long-term results 10 years after iliac arterial stent placement, *Radiology* 224(3):731–738, 2002.
62. Reekers JA, Bolia A: Percutaneous intentional extraluminal (subintimal) recanalization: how to do it yourself, *Eur J Radiol* 28(3): 192–198, 1998.
63. Lipsitz EC, Ohki T, Veith FJ, et al: Does subintimal angioplasty have a role in the treatment of severe lower extremity ischemia? *J Vasc Surg* 37(2):386–391, 2003.
64. Jacobs DL, Motaganahalli RL, Cox DE, et al: True lumen re-entry devices facilitate subintimal angioplasty and stenting of total chronic occlusions: Initial report, *J Vasc Surg* 43(6):1291–1296, 2006.
65. Grassl ED, Bischof JC: In vitro model systems for evaluation of smooth muscle cell response to cryoplasty, *Cryobiology* 50(2):162–173, 2005.
66. McCaslin JE, Macdonald S, Stansby G: Cryoplasty for peripheral vascular disease, *Cochrane Database Syst Rev* (4):CD005507, 2007.
67. Karthik S, Tuite DJ, Nicholson AA, et al: Cryoplasty for arterial restenosis, *Eur J Vasc Endovasc Surg* 33(1):40–43, 2007.
68. Samson RH, Showalter DP, Lepore MR Jr, et al: CryoPlasty therapy of the superficial femoral and popliteal arteries: a single center experience, *Vasc Endovascular Surg* 40(6):446–450, 2006.
69. Ahmed JM, Mintz GS, Castagna M, et al: Intravascular ultrasound assessment of the mechanism of lumen enlargement during cutting balloon angioplasty treatment of in-stent restenosis, *Am J Cardiol* 88(9):1032–1034, 2001.
70. Montorsi P, Galli S, Fabbiocchi F, et al: Mechanism of cutting balloon angioplasty for in-stent restenosis: an intravascular ultrasound study, *Catheter Cardiovasc Interv* 56(2):166–173, 2002.
71. Albiero R, Silber S, Di Mario C, et al: Cutting balloon versus conventional balloon angioplasty for the treatment of in-stent restenosis: results of the restenosis cutting balloon evaluation trial (RESCUT), *J Am Coll Cardiol* 43(6):943–949, 2004.
72. Vorwerk D, Adam G, Muller-Leisse C, et al: Hemodialysis fistulas and grafts: use of cutting balloons to dilate venous stenoses, *Radiology* 201(3):864–867, 1996.
73. Song HH, Kim KT, Chung SK, et al: Cutting balloon angioplasty for resistant venous stenoses of Brescia-Cimino fistulas, *J Vasc Interv Radiol* 15(12):1463–1467, 2004.
74. Garvin R, Reifsnyder T: Cutting balloon angioplasty of autogenous infrainguinal bypasses: short-term safety and efficacy, *J Vasc Surg* 46(4):724–730, 2007.
75. Engelke C, Morgan RA, Belli AM: Cutting balloon percutaneous transluminal angioplasty for salvage of lower limb arterial bypass grafts: feasibility, *Radiology* 223(1):106–114, 2002.
76. Yatskar L, Selzer F, Feit F, et al: Access site hematoma requiring blood transfusion predicts mortality in patients undergoing percutaneous coronary intervention: data from the National Heart, Lung, and Blood Institute Dynamic Registry, *Catheter Cardiovasc Interv* 69(7):961–966, 2007.
77. Belli AM, Cumberland DC, Knox AM, et al: The complication rate of percutaneous peripheral balloon angioplasty, *Clin Radiol* 41(6):380–383, 1990.
78. Allaire E, Melliere D, Poussier B, et al: Iliac artery rupture during balloon dilatation: what treatment? *Ann Vasc Surg* 17(3):306–314, 2003.
79. Yeo KK, Rogers JH, Laird JR: Use of stent grafts and coils in vessel rupture and perforation, *J Interv Cardiol* 21(1):86–99, 2008.
80. Chatziioannou A, Mourikis D, Katsimilis J, et al: Acute iliac artery rupture: endovascular treatment, *Cardiovasc Intervent Radiol* 30(2):281–285, 2007.

CHAPTER

25

Intravascular Stenting in Aortoiliac Arterial Occlusive Disease

Kristofer M. Charlton-Ouw, Mark G. Davies, Alan B. Lumsden

Intravascular stent placement evolved in an attempt to recover failed angioplasty outcomes. Poor immediate technical results stem from heavy plaque burden, calcification, and dissection. Early restenosis after angioplasty is often due to elastic recoil, whereas late restenosis stems from negative remodeling and intimal hyperplasia. Percutaneous transluminal angioplasty is a durable procedure (see Chapter 24), and intravascular stenting was developed as an adjunct to the procedure. There is some evidence that stenting reduces complications, such as thromboembolism and dissection, and leads to increased patency in the patients with the most severe disease and in those that have certain disease patterns and comorbidities. Nevertheless, there remains controversy among authors who prefer angioplasty with *selective* stenting, primary stenting (after predilatation with angioplasty), and direct stenting (without predilatation). An additional debate exists over open- and closed-cell stent designs and covered and uncovered stents. Drug-eluting and biodegradable stents are under development. Furthermore, the long-term results of endovascular techniques must be compared with those of open bypass surgery.

No prospective randomized trials have compared the results of aortoiliac stenting and open bypass surgery. The Veterans Administration Cooperative Study showed no statistically significant difference between angioplasty and open bypass surgery, but only men were enrolled and no stents were used.[1] Ballard and colleagues[2] prospectively compared the nonrandomized outcomes of open surgery and primary stenting. At 3.5 years the cumulative primary patency of bypass grafts was 93% versus 68% for the stent group. However, the surgery group had more extensive lesions, and although more patients in the stent group had single-vessel runoff, more patients in the surgery group had triple-vessel runoff. Timaran et al.[3] conducted a similar, more recent study and confirmed the better 5-year primary patency of surgical bypass versus stenting (86% vs. 64%). Neither of these studies used the newer nitinol stents.

The Dutch Iliac Stent Trial Study Group conducted the only randomized trial published in English that compares selective stent use versus direct stenting[4]; however, it was published before the first TransAtlantic Inter-Society Consensus (TASC) classification in 2000.[5] Although the quality of the study was high and the authors concluded that angioplasty with selective stenting produces slightly improved symptomatic success rates and equivalent patency at more than 5 years, the treated lesions were not classified and mostly patients with intermittent claudication (IC) were enrolled (94%).[6] Because mostly patients with IC were included in the study and no anatomic details of the lesions were provided, comparison with patients with critical limb ischemia or more severe disease is difficult. In the Dutch trial, only a balloon-expanded Palmaz stent was used. Practitioners today have a wider choice of self- and balloon-expandable stents and stent grafts with newer materials such as nitinol.

The U.S. Food and Drug Administration (FDA) has so far approved seven stents for use in the iliac arteries (http://www.fda.gov). All other stents have regulatory approval for use in other vascular beds or organs. For example, many stents approved for use in the biliary tree have been implanted off-label in the aortoiliac vasculature. In the European Union, intravascular stents must obtain the CE mark that signifies compliance with European Directives (http://ec.europa.eu). Stents with CE marking for iliac use may not have FDA approval, so that many studies in the literature involve the use of stents that are unavailable or unapproved for iliac use in the United States.

Unfortunately, stent design is often driven by market considerations rather than scientific evidence of improved efficacy.[7] Stent selection can be divided into material, and design, as well as balloon versus self-expandable. Self-expanding stents are made of either Elgiloy or nitinol, whereas balloon-expandable stents are made of stainless steel, cobalt alloy, or platinum. Each of the stent materials has different structural properties and biocompatibility. The approved and marketed iliac stents are (Table 25-1) the E-Luminexx (Bard Peripheral Vascular, Tempe, AZ), the Wallstent and Express LD Iliac (Boston Scientific, Natick, MA), the Zilver (Cook Medical, Bloomington, IN), and the SMART and the Palmaz stents (Cordis Corporation, Warren, NJ). The IntraStent (ev3, Redwood City, CA), a stainless steel, unmounted, balloon-expandable stent similar to the Palmaz, is also approved for iliac artery use but is marketed mostly for biliary use by the company. In addition, several covered stents are available, but so far only the Gore Viabahn (W. L. Gore & Associates, Inc., Flagstaff, AZ) is approved for use in iliac arteries. The Viabahn is also available with and without the company's proprietary heparin-bonded luminal surface.

INDICATIONS

The epidemiology, symptoms, and assessment of aortoiliac disease are discussed in Chapter 24. Medical management is the mainstay of treatment for symptomatic and mild–moderately symptomatic patients with peripheral arterial disease. More severe presentations (Rutherford grade I-III; Fontaine stage IIb-IV) often require more invasive intervention, but results from randomized trials comparing optimal medical therapy with endovascular therapy for patients with IC are pending.[8] Table 25-2 compares patency and complication rates of different revascularization techniques. As discussed in Chapter 24, published guidelines, such as the updated TASC classification,[9] help determine the most appropriate intervention on the basis of the lesion characteristics. Type A lesions should be treated primarily with endovascular therapy, whereas type D lesions should be offered open surgery primarily. Types B and C lesions can be treated with either modality depending on patient- and practitioner-specific circumstances. Box 25-1 lists absolute and relative indications for open surgery.

TABLE 25-1 Features of the Currently Marketed and Approved Iliac Artery Stents

Product name (company)	Type	Material	Introducer size (F)	Stent diameters (mm)	Stent lengths (mm)
E-Luminexx (Bard)	SE, open-cell	Nitinol	6	7-10	20-100
Wallstent (Boston Scientific)	SE, closed cell	Elgiloy	6	6-10	27-100
Zilver 518 and 635 (Cook)	SE, open cell	Nitinol	5-6	6-10	20-80
SMART (Cordis)	SE, open cell	Nitinol	6	6-10	20-100
Express LD Iliac (Boston Scientific)	BE, open cell	Stainless steel	6-7	6-11	17-57
Palmaz— premounted (Cordis)	BE, closed cell	Stainless steel	6-7	4-8	10-29
Palmaz—unmounted (Cordis)	BE, closed cell	Stainless steel	10	8-12	30
Viabahn (W. L. Gore)	Stent graft	ePTFE/nitinol	7-12	5-13	25-150

BE, Balloon-expanding; *ePTFE,* expanded polytetrafluoroethylene; *SE,* self-expanding.

TABLE 25-2 Comparison of Selected Revascularization Results in Iliac Disease

Intervention	Technical success (%)	1-Yr primary patency (%)	5-Yr primary patency (%)	10-Yr primary patency (%)	Complications (%)	30-Day mortality (%)
Angioplasty with selective stenting*[4,14,20,60]	82-100	76-87	49-75	27	1-24	0-2
Direct or primary stenting*[4,107]	72-100	78-95	54-72	NA	2-11	0-2.7
Aortobifemoral or direct bypass†[108,109]	>99	>90	80-95	72-87	11	1-3
Aortoiliac endarterectomy[109-111]	>99	>90	72-95	88	≈2	1-7
Axillofemoral bypass[111-114]	>99	74-86	58-79	NA	9.2	<1-5

* *Includes long-segment and chronic total occlusions.*
†*Data from meta-analysis; complication and mortality rates from studies starting after 1975.*
NA, Not available.

There is debate whether a stent *need not* be placed in all lesions deemed appropriate for endovascular repair. Several authors favor stent implantation in all cases,[10-12] and others favor a more selective approach.[13-15] However, in certain situations primary or direct stenting is appropriate and the practice standard. The absolute and relative indications for iliac stent implantation are listed in Box 25-2. Stents are placed (1) for aortoiliac lesions *without* predilatation angioplasty (direct stenting), (2) for aortoiliac lesions *with* predilatation angioplasty (primary stenting), or (3) only after suboptimal angioplasty results (selective stenting). Several reports indicate that covered stents are useful in dealing with complications, such as perforation or rupture, fistulae, and heavy thrombus burden. Although no long-term data are yet available, use of covered stents for uncomplicated aortoiliac atherosclerotic disease is still under investigation.[16-18]

There is no evidence from randomized controlled trials indicating superiority of direct or primary stenting over selective stenting. Selective stenting is more cost-effective[19] but is more cumbersome for the treating physician and may produce lower technical success rates and higher complication rates, especially dissection.[20] Klein et al.[6] reported long-term follow-up data on the Dutch Iliac Stent Trial and found no benefit to primary stenting. However, that trial began enrolling in the early 1990s and only used a balloon-expandable stainless steel stent (Palmaz) for all stented lesions.[4] In addition, as stated previously, the trial mostly enrolled patients with IC and excluded patients with any occlusions greater than 5 cm or inability to pass a wire intraluminally. There is increasing evidence that subintimal angioplasty with primary stenting produces good results even in occlusions greater than 5 cm.[21] Such techniques are challenging the current TASC guidelines, which will undoubtedly require more frequent updates in the future. Newer self-expanding nitinol stents may produce better long-term results, and drug-eluting stents may improve long-term patency rates even further.

TECHNIQUE AND STENT SELECTION

Techniques for aortoiliac stenting generally follow those of angioplasty as described in Chapter 24. Once the lesion is crossed with a wire, angioplasty is often performed to predilate the lesion and facilitate stent passage. An angioplasty balloon is generally selected to match the size of the native vessel wall (e.g., 8-10 mm) except in cases of severe calcification. Proponents of the direct stenting technique do not routinely predilate and deploy the stent first. Caution needs to be taken to ensure that the stents do not become dislodged while attempting passage through a tight stenosis. Another technique, especially with balloon-mounted stents, is to advance the device catheter and sheath over the stenotic lesion. The sheath can then be withdrawn to expose the stent and avoids accidental stent dislodgment. Stents may be slightly oversized by 10%

BOX 25-1

INDICATIONS FOR OPEN SURGICAL BYPASS IN AORTOILIAC ARTERIAL OCCLUSIVE DISEASE

- Infrarenal aortoiliac occlusion
- Associated abdominal aortic aneurysm not amenable to endovascular treatment
- Diffuse aortoiliac disease extending into the external iliac artery
- Multiple failed endovascular attempts

BOX 25-2

ABSOLUTE AND RELATIVE INDICATIONS FAVORING PRIMARY OR DIRECT ILIAC STENT IMPLANTATION VERSUS ANGIOPLASTY ALONE

- Suboptimal results after aortoiliac angioplasty
  - ≥30 stenosis
  - Residual pressure gradient ≥5-10 mm Hg
  - Unstable subintimal dissection
- Chronic total occlusions >5 cm and after subintimal angioplasty
- Stenotic lesions with increase risk of thromboembolism such as in ulcerated plaques

with respect to the luminal diameter. Angioplasty after stent deployment is used to eliminate residual stenoses greater than 30% of the lumen. Patient discomfort is a good indication of the limit of postdilatation ballooning.

The angiogram in Figure 25-1 demonstrates a case of acute on chronic lower-extremity ischemia. There is diffuse, calcified aortoiliac disease with occlusion of the left iliac artery (see Figure 25-1, *A*). After balloon thrombectomy, calcified plaque is noted in the left common iliac artery (CIA) causing high-grade stenosis with residual thrombus (see Figure 25-1, *B*). A 10- × 39-mm stainless steel, balloon-expandable stent was deployed in the right CIA. A 9- × 59-mm stainless steel, balloon-expandable, covered stent was used in the left CIA. Poststent angiography shows restoration of luminal patency (see Figure 25-1, *C*).

Balloon-Expandable Stents

The Palmaz and the Express LD Iliac are the only approved and marketed balloon-expandable stents available in the United States (Figure 25-2). However, many biliary stents are used off-label in the aortoiliac arteries. Both the IntraStent and the larger-sized Palmaz stents come unmounted and must be compressed and deployed on an angioplasty balloon. The Palmaz is available in a premounted state in the smaller stent diameters (4-8 mm). It has a closed-cell design and is made from stainless steel. This design, although inflexible, provides considerable radial stiffness. The Express LD is an open-cell design and is available premounted in all sizes. Balloon-expandable stents can be dilated beyond the listed diameter by dilating them with larger balloons but cannot be resheathed or repositioned once deployed. As mentioned previously, the radial stiffness is advantageous when treating calcified lesions. However, after the critical external force is reached, balloon-expandable stents are subject to crush deformities. Because most balloon-expandable stents are usually made of stainless steel, they do not have the superelastic recoil properties of nitinol. Other balloon-expandable stent materials include platinum and cobalt alloy.

Although early self-expandable stent systems suffered from foreshortening or jumping forward on delivery, balloon-expandable stents can be deployed with precision. They are often used by proponents of direct stenting and are ideal for the stenting of focal lesions in relatively straight vessels. Because of their inherent rigidity, balloon-expandable stents are generally not placed in tortuous vessels or across joints.

Self-Expandable Stents

Self-expanding stents are constrained within a delivery catheter until positioned and deployed. Because no balloon is needed to deploy the stent, the delivery devices are generally smaller than balloon-expandable stent systems. The prototype is the Wallstent, which is constructed from Elgiloy, a cobalt-alloy stainless steel (Figure 25-3). Elgiloy was originally made as a tough, anticorrosive material for watches.

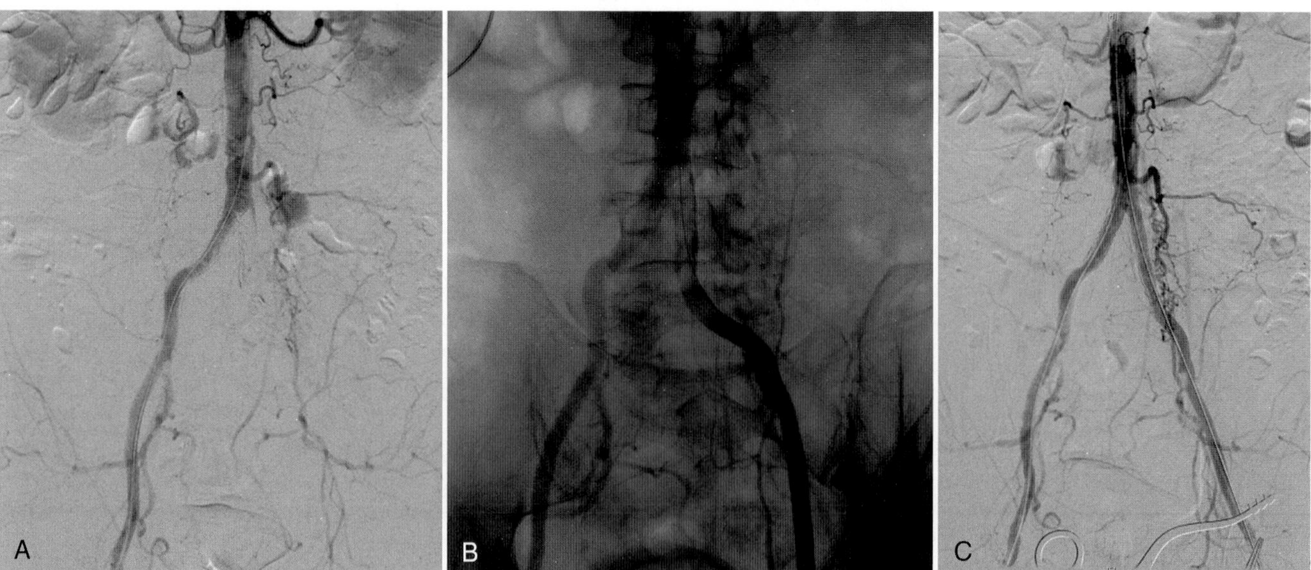

FIGURE 25-1 **A,** Angiogram showing diffuse, calcified aortoiliac disease with occluded left iliac artery. **B,** Repeat angiogram after open balloon thrombectomy showing residual left common iliac stenosis and thrombus. **C,** Poststent angiogram. A 10- × 39-mm stainless steel, balloon-expandable stent was deployed in the right common iliac artery. A 9- × 59-mm stainless steel, balloon-expandable, covered stent was used in the left common iliac artery. *(Courtesy K. Charlton-Ouw and A. Azizzadeh.)*

The Wallstent is made from braided wires that are not soldered together so that it expands spontaneously when released from the constraining device. The flexibility of its braided design comes at the cost of significant foreshortening as it expands, making positioning difficult. Depending on the vessel and stent size, the foreshortening can be more than 20% of the undeployed length.[22] However, the company claims that the stent can be resheathed and repositioned even after 87% deployment. Unlike nitinol superelastic self-expanding stents, the radial or hoop strength of the Wallstent is dependent on its axial endpoint fixation because of its woven design.[7] In general, the Wallstent has less radial force than nitinol stents. Like nitinol stents, the cobalt-alloy stents can reform after crush injuries.[22] It has a closed-cell design and is available as a covered stent that is approved for use in the biliary system.

New iliac-approved, self-expanding, open-cell iliac stent designs, such as the Cordis SMART stent and the Cook Zilver stent, use nitinol wire. Nitinol is a nickel-titanium "shape-memory alloy," the shape of which is temperature dependent. At high temperature, the nitinol wires are shaped into the stent configuration. As the metal cools, it assumes a linear shape and is constrained within the delivery catheter. After exposure to body temperature, the stent resumes its original shape after deployment. This means that nitinol stents can withstand external crush deformities and offer high radial strength.[23] Nevertheless, prospective, randomized trials did not show a difference in 1-year patency or overall complication rates between the Elgiloy and nitinol stents.[24] All self-expanding stents buckle at a lower external pressure than balloon-expandable stents but revert to their original shape after that force is removed. In addition, the nitinol stents tend to spring forward on deployment leading to misplacement and incomplete lesion coverage.[25] These nitinol stents cannot be resheathed and redeployed after exposure to body temperature, unlike the Wallstent.

For tortuous vessels, a flexible stent and deployment system is needed. The most flexible and conformable stent systems are self-expanding Wallstent and nitinol stents.[22,23] For direct stenting techniques self-expanding stents do not have the radial stiffness sometimes needed to overcome calcified lesions so that postdilatation ballooning is often necessary.[23]

Covered Stents

Chapter 26 addresses stent grafts in arterial occlusive disease in detail. In brief, several authors have used stent grafts or covered stents in treating aortoiliac and iliofemoral occlusive disease. No covered stents have FDA approval for use in arterial occlusive disease

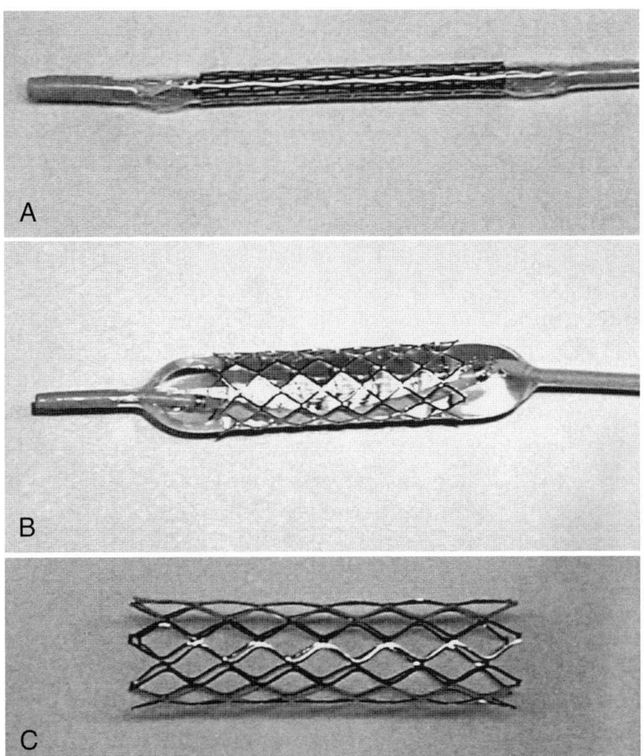
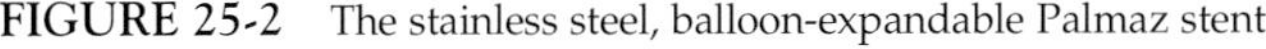

FIGURE 25-2 The stainless steel, balloon-expandable Palmaz stent.

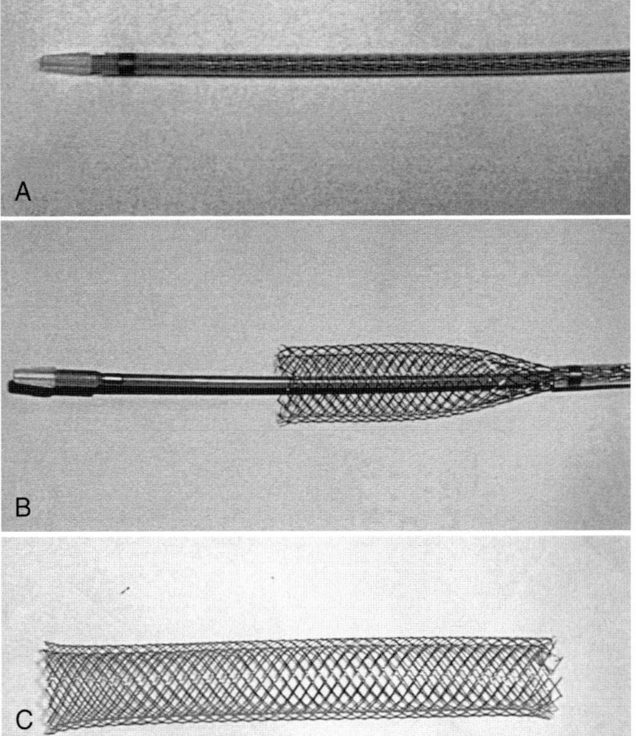

FIGURE 25-3 The cobalt alloy, self-expandable Wallstent.

TABLE 25-3 Outcomes of Selected Bare Metal Stent Studies in Iliac Artery Stenosis

	Technical success (%)	1-Yr primary patency (%)	5-Yr primary patency (%)	Major complications (%)	30-Day mortality(%)
De Roeck et al., 2006[56]	97.4	94	77	5.4	2.7
Leville et al., 2006[57]	91	~80	NA*	10	3.4
Murphy et al., 2004[58]	98	89	75	7	0.5
Vorwerk et al., 1996[115]	NA	95	72	3.4	NA

**Five-year patency rates not available, but 3-year primary patency was 76%.*
NA, Not available.

BOX 25-3

CLASSIFICATION OF IN-STENT RESTENOSIS[32]

1. Focal (≤10 mm)
2. Diffuse (>10 mm)
3. Proliferative (>10 mm and extending outside the stent)
4. Occlusion

in the iliac arteries, but several studies have shown promise. Most reports outside of investigational series have used covered stents to treat iliac perforation or rupture.[26-28] The Gore Viabahn is currently the only stent graft approved for iliac use. Several other balloon- and self-expanding stents have approval in the tracheobronchial or biliary systems but have frequently been used off-label in the aortoiliac arteries. Cynamon and colleagues[29] used covered stainless steel stents to treat aortoiliac stenosis in 18 patients with concomitant femoral artery disease. Primary patency was 81% at 2 years.[29] Rzucidlo et al.[16] performed stent grafting in 34 patients with aortoiliac occlusions or diffuse disease using covered Elgiloy stents. One-year primary patency was 70%, but they also had a high percentage of patients undergoing a concomitant common femoral endarterectomy. Weisinger et al.[18] deployed covered nitinol stents in 60 iliac arteries with a 1-year primary patency rate of 91%, which is comparable with patency rates of bare metal stents (Table 25-3). Nevertheless, no randomized trials exist at this time showing that covered stents are superior to bare metal stents.

VESSEL REACTION TO STENTING

Although the initial response to injury of the vessel is similar for angioplasty and stenting with balloon angioplasty, the vessel long-term reaction to the presence of intravascular stents is different.[30] Several factors—mostly derived from the coronary literature—influence the vessel reaction to stenting: stent design, length, composition, delivery system, and deployment technique.[31] In-stent restenosis (ISR) is classified on the basis of length of restenosis in relation to overall stent length. Four categories of ISR have been defined (Box 25-3).[32] After balloon angioplasty, there is intimal hyperplasia development, elastic recoil, and negative remodeling. In contrast, after stent placement, elastic recoil and negative remodeling are eliminated by the stent scaffold.[33] Thrombus formation followed by intimal hyperplasia development are the main contributors to ISR.[34,35]

Stent placement in a vessel results in a generalized injury to the vessel but, in addition, causes focal injures at the areas of strut placement. Intravascular ultrasound scanning has demonstrated that stents do not always completely oppose the vessel wall along its entire length thus resulting in uneven injury along its length.[33] After 1 minute the surface is covered by fine layers of proteins, predominantly fibrinogen. After stent placement, the surface of the metal implanted into the vessel is covered by a strongly adherent monolayer of protein within 5 seconds.[36] The holes between the stent wires are filled with thrombus, and the adherence of platelets and leukocytes is enhanced by disturbance of electrostatic equilibrium.[37,38] The basic mechanisms of smooth muscle cell proliferation and migration after stent placement are the same as those after balloon injury.[39] However, the intimal hyperplastic process in a stent is more prolonged and robust than in a balloon-injured artery and is proportional to the depth of injury the recipient vessel sustains[40] and the inflammatory response induced.[41] The injury can often be much more significant at the ends than in the body of the stent. Early after stenting in humans (≤11 days), fibrin, platelets, and acute inflammatory cells are always present in association with stent struts.[42] In addition, the adventitial response is prolonged with adventitial giant cell body formation being noted. Stents prevent chronic elastic recoil but cause progressive atrophy of the media.[43]

The degree of stent–arterial wall interface influences the severity of associated inflammation. Increased numbers of inflammatory cells were seen when the stent struts were adjacent to injured media or lipid core rather than fibrous plaque. Chronic inflammation occurs adjacent to stent struts at all time points, especially greater than 12 days after stenting. Plaque compressed by stent struts is seen in 91% of vessel sections with penetration of the stent struts into the lipid core a common event.[42] A neointima containing smooth muscle cells develops within 2 weeks, and histologic success or failure of the stent is determined by neointimal growth within the stent and is not influenced by artery or stent size. Neointimal thickness was increased when medial damage was present compared with struts in contact with atherosclerotic plaque or an intact media. Furthermore, increased intrastent neointimal growth was present in histologic failures, and increased neointimal area correlated with increased stent size relative to the proximal reference artery lumen. Therefore stent oversizing relative to the reference lumen appears to be an undesirable goal in deployment. Despite these histologic changes neointimal cell density and the composition of the proteoglycan deposition in coronary stents were similar to those in matched angioplastied coronary vessels.[42,44]

Risk factors for ISR include diabetes and prior restenosis,[45] and there is a correlation with prolonged in-stent thrombus and hyperglycemia.[46] Other risk factors for thrombosis include penetration of necrotic core, malapposition, overlapping stent placement, excessive stent length, stent fracture, and bifurcation lesions.

OUTCOMES

Isolated atherosclerotic, infrarenal, aortic lesions in the absence of iliac stenosis are uncommon. No randomized trials exist for isolated aortic lesions such as the Dutch Iliac Stent Trial. Most series show 5-year primary patency rates of more than 75% for angioplasty with selective stenting. Klonaris et al.[47] published a small series of 12 patients treated with direct stenting. Technical hemodynamic success was achieved in 92%, and primary patency during a mean follow-up of 18 months was also 92%. Unfortunately, this retrospective series used different recanalization techniques and different stent types. In addition, the range of follow-up was wide (6-37 months). Other studies of direct stenting suffer from similar shortcomings but nevertheless show excellent primary patency rates greater than 85%.[11,48-50] One reason the patency rates for isolated aortic lesions may be better for primary or direct stenting instead of angioplasty and selective stenting is that the effects of ISR caused by intimal hyperplasia may not be as significant in such a large vessel.

Aortic lesions that extend distally into the iliac arteries require special techniques when stenting because of the risk of contralateral luminal compromise. The kissing-stent techniques were published by Kuffer[51] and Palmaz[52] in the early 1990s. The stents are deployed with the distal ends within the iliac arteries, and the proximal ends are often within the distal aorta. This attempts to reconstruct the aortic bifurcation and prevents a unilateral stent from impinging on the contralateral iliac artery. However, this technique has somewhat lower patency rates than iliac-only implantation. Midterm primary patency rates in the literature range from 58% to 80%.[53,54] Mohammed et al.[54] found few sequelae resulting from stenting nondiseased limbs using the kissing-stent technique. Grenier and colleagues[55] found that crossover of more than half the stent width of the aortic portion of the stents is a risk factor for decreased patency. Nevertheless, this technique is widely used and is critical for stenting lesions at the aortic bifurcation.

For stenotic lesions in the iliac arteries, stenting has a durable and proved track record that compares well with that of open surgical techniques (see Tables 25-2 and 25-3). Many recent reports show 3-year secondary patency rates ≥90% with limb salvage rates >95% even in TASC C and D et al.[56,57] At 8 years of follow-up, Murphy et al.[58] had primary, assisted, and secondary patency rates of 74%, 81%, and 84% with an overall limb-salvage rate of 98% using multiple different stent types. Similarly, Reyes et al.[59] had cumulative primary and secondary patency rates of 65% and 87% at 7 years after iliac Wallstent implantation. Galaria and Davies[60] retrospectively reviewed data from two Veterans Affairs Medical Centers that used a selective stenting approach to TASC A and B iliac lesions and found 10-year primary assisted and secondary patency rates of 71% and 72%. Limb salvage rates in this difficult population were 87% at 10 years. Other reports of treatment of more severe disease showed less favorable long-term results.[61] Factors affecting patency rates from different studies are listed in Box 25-4.

The fate of side branches, such as the internal iliac artery, the origins of which are covered by stents, is unclear. Sapoval et al.[62] followed by angiography 22 of 29 patients whose Wallstent covered the internal iliac artery origin. After a mean follow-up of about 2 years, 41% had occlusion or severe stenosis greater than 70% at the ostium. To our knowledge, there is no evidence

BOX 25-4

RISK FACTORS FOR IN-STENT RESTENOSIS AND DIMINISHED PATENCY IN ILIAC STENTS*

- Longer lesions (and longer stent lengths)
- Occlusions
- Critical limb ischemia
- Diabetes
- Chronic renal insufficiency
- Dyslipidemia
- Distal stenosis or poor runoff
- Current tobacco use
- Female sex (?)
- Smaller vessel diameter (?)
- External iliac artery stents (?)

*References 3, 57, 58, 60, 62, 115.

supporting increased side-branch patency with open-cell versus closed-cell stents in the iliac arteries.

Endovascular treatment of chronic iliac artery occlusions was first described by Tegtmeyer in 1979.[63] Since then, techniques to cross chronic occlusions of the iliac artery have been reported by several authors.[21,64,65] Vorwerk et al.[13] reported a 1-year primary patency rate of 87% and 78% after 4 years using Wallstents in more than 100 patients. More recently, using Elgiloy and nitinol self-expanding stents, Carnevale et al.[66] reported a 97% initial success rate with 1- and 3-year primary patency rates of 91% and 84%. Uher and colleagues[67] used a variety of both self- and balloon-expanding stents to treat iliac occlusions. Their initial technical success was 97% with 1- and 3-year primary patency rates of 79% and 69%. Funovics et al.[68] found 1- and 4-year primary patency rates of 74.5% and 64%. Multivariate Cox regression analysis found that longer lesions, incomplete stent coverage, and distal stenosis were risk factors for poor patency (see Box 25-4). These reports indicate that stenting of iliac occlusions have slightly lower but acceptable short-term and midterm patency rates. Yilmaz et al.[21] found no difference in outcomes between lesions crossed with an intraluminal versus a subintimal technique. Distal embolization may be more of a problem in certain patients with chronic occlusion because nearly every report had at least one case. Some authors prefer direct stenting (without predilatation) in cases of occlusion and hypothesize that the stent struts help prevent release of thrombus during recanalization.[62]

IN-STENT RESTENOSIS

Although negative remodeling and elastic recoil are successfully dealt with by stenting, intimal hyperplasia is the main cause of ISR. Treatment of restenosis generally entails conventional balloon angioplasty with or without additional stent placement. However, placement of another stent within an artery prone to intimal hyperplasia may exacerbate the process.[69] Other techniques for dealing with ISR include cutting balloon angioplasty[70,71] (discussed in Chapter 24) and debulking techniques, such as atherectomy.

Schurmann et al.[61] found that the majority of patients undergoing treatment for iliac restenosis by balloon angioplasty or additional stent placement had recurrent restenosis. Many of these patients required multiple reinterventions, including open bypass surgery. Many of the data on repeated stenting of ISR come from the coronary literature, and most studies show a high rate of restenosis.[72,73] Biodegradable stents offer useful luminal scaffolding and high procedural success rates but allow vessel remodeling and limit intimal hyperplasia because they provoke a more limited inflammatory response. Unfortunately, although animal studies have shown a reduction in intimal hyperplasia, biodegradable coronary stents have not resulted in improved luminal diameter.[74,75] Drug-eluting stents seem likely to be the most promising future development to reduce restenosis but have not yet been extensively studied outside the coronary vasculature.

Given the effects of intimal hyperplasia and progression of atherosclerotic disease, a regular poststent surveillance program is customary. Commonly, patients are seen within a month after stenting for clinical examination, arm-thigh indices, and duplex ultrasound examination. Follow-up is more frequent in the first 2 years, and intervals lengthen thereafter. Long-term follow-up examinations occur annually and sooner if symptoms recur. If patients are without recurrent symptoms, some authors report biannual follow-up.[58]

MAGNETIC RESONANCE IMAGING COMPATIBILITY

Patients may require magnetic resonance imaging (MRI) for a variety of reasons after stent implantation. Recent American Heart Association guidelines affirmed the general safety of MRI after intravascular stent implantation.[76] Nitinol and titanium alloy stents are considered MRI safe and may be imaged in at least a 1.5-tesla (T)–strength magnet immediately after implantation.[77] For example, the Cook Zilver stents are rated safe in a 3-T magnet as per manufacturer's safety instructions. The Wallstent's Elgiloy contains only small amounts of iron and is considered nonferromagnetic.[78] The Palmaz is made of stainless steel and is ferromagnetic. An MRI should not be immediately obtained after stainless steel stent implantation. After 8 weeks, the stainless steel stent is completely endothelialized with sufficient ingrowth and is considered safe to undergo MRI. It is believed that contact with the vessel wall and ingrowth between the struts provide anchoring of stents. It is unclear how fine vibrations and heating of ferromagnetic stents affect restenosis.[76]

SPECIAL CIRCUMSTANCES

Radiation-Induced Arteritis

Radiation-induced arteritis leading to symptomatic ischemic symptoms in the lower extremities is rare. The lesions are angiographically indistinguishable from atherosclerotic disease but are limited to the irradiated bed. Histologically, the lesions are different from atherosclerosis and include vessel wall fibrosis, hyalinization, and thickening. Vasa vasorum and vessel wall necrosis may lead to thrombus or ulcer formation and eventual luminal narrowing and occlusion.[79] With the growth of radiation therapy for pelvic and gynecologic malignancy, the iliac arteries seem especially at risk. This entity may be more common in the carotid arteries after treatment for head and neck malignancy. Himmel and colleagues[80] reviewed 162 cases and found that doses between 40 and 80 Gy are associated with arteritis of the iliofemoral arteries. Several case reports describe successful treatment of these lesions with percutaneous techniques including stenting.[81] Some authors favor primary or direct stenting to counteract the chronic fibrosis and inflammatory effects of radiation-induced arteritis.[82] The long-term durability of angioplasty and stenting in these patients is unknown.

Renal Transplantation

A stenosis in the iliac artery proximal to the transplanted renal artery anastomosis has the same systemic effect of transplant renal artery stenosis, such as hypertension and poor graft function. Symptoms of claudication and decreased femoral or distal pulses increase the suspicion for iliac artery stenosis.[83] Once suspected, ultrasound examination can help to further define the lesion.[84] Becker and colleagues[85] found that 92 out of 819 patients were suspected of having transplant renal artery stenosis (11.2%). Actual transplant renal artery stenosis was found in 24 (2.9%), proximal iliac stenosis was found in 15 (1.8%), and 5 (0.6%) had both. Factors found to be associated with proximal iliac artery stenosis after renal transplantation were type 1 diabetes in the recipient, panel reactive antibodies, increasing recipient weight at time of transplantation, and donor age.[85] Several reports indicate that angioplasty and/or stenting improve graft function, hypertension, and symptoms.[83,84]

Hybrid Cases

To treat multilevel or bilateral disease, specialists have combined endovascular techniques with open surgical techniques. Proximal surgical inflow procedures can be combined with distal endoluminal revascularization. Conversely, endovascular aortoiliac procedures can be combined with femoropopliteal or femorodistal open bypass. Because of the different stent types, lesion characteristics, and surgical target revascularizations, a comparison of hybrid techniques is impossible. Imaginative hybrid techniques have been tailored to patient anatomy in treating both occlusive and aneurysmal disease.

AbuRahma et al.[86] treated 41 patients with bilateral iliac stenoses using combined femorofemoral bypass and iliac angioplasty with selective stenting. Initial success, patency, and limb salvage and complication rates were significantly different depending on the length of the treated iliac lesion. For iliac stenoses <5 cm 1- and 3- year patency rates were 96% and 85%, whereas for iliac stenoses >5 cm patency rates dropped to 46% and 31%, respectively.

Kudo et al[14] reviewed 104 consecutive patients after iliac angioplasty with selective stenting, and Cox regression analysis showed that femoral artery stenosis was one of the predictors of failure. However, Timaran et al.[87] looked at patients with iliac disease and poor distal runoff and found that open infrainguinal revascularization did not improve iliac stent patency. Nevertheless, endovascular inflow procedures such as iliac stenting *do* improve infrainguinal bypass graft patency.[88] From these studies, it appears that establishing inflow is critical to the patency of distal surgical revascularization but that it is safe to deploy iliac artery stents without concomitant infrainguinal revascularization.

COMPLICATIONS

Chapter 27 discusses endovascular aortoiliac complications in detail. However, it is worth emphasizing several stent complications here. In brief, complications

BOX 25-5

PROCEDURE-RELATED COMPLICATIONS OF AORTOILIAC STENTING

- **I.** Access site
  - **A.** Bleeding: hematoma, retroperitoneal hematoma
  - **B.** Pseudoaneurysm
  - **C.** Arteriovenous fistula
  - **D.** Acute arterial thrombosis
  - **E.** Infection
  - **F.** Neuropathic pain
- **II.** Wire or catheter passage
  - **A.** Vessel disruption or perforation
  - **B.** Intimal dissection
  - **C.** Stent dislodgment
  - **D.** Distal embolization
- **III.** Other
  - **A.** Stent deployment: misplacement, migration, embolization
  - **B.** Device infection
  - **C.** Contrast: allergic reaction, nephropathy
  - **D.** Thrombosis: in-stent, side branch, extrinsic compression
  - **E.** Cardiopulmonary and cerebrovascular

can be divided into major versus minor and early versus late. Early complications can be further separated into (1) access site, (2) related to the passage of catheters and devices, and (3) others (Box 25-5). Overall complication rates in selected series are listed in Tables 25-2 and 25-3. In general, 30-day mortality and the major complication rates are acceptable. The range in complication rates reflects the disease severity, lesion characteristics, and reporting differences, but occlusions and longer lesions appear to have higher complication rates.[86]

The most common complication for all percutaneous techniques is access site bleeding. Some studies in the coronary literature cite the incidence of groin hematoma as high as 11%.[89] Hematomas requiring blood transfusions are much less common but portend higher mortality.[90] Several risk factors have been identified that predispose patients to groin hematoma including the use of an implanted device, sheath size greater than 6F, female sex, emergency procedure, renal sufficiency, aspirin use, obesity, and age older than 65 years.[90,91] Improperly sealed arterial punctures can lead to pseudoaneurysm. However, the most feared access site complication is retroperitoneal hematoma. Thigh or lower abdominal pain, numbness or quadriceps weakness, falling hematocrit, hypotension, and tachycardia should raise the suspicion of retroperitoneal hematoma and should prompt early pelvic computed tomographic scanning. It is hoped that, with the introduction of smaller-diameter devices, the incidence of access site bleeding will decrease. The role of arteriotomy closure devices in affecting access site bleeding is unclear.[92-96] New closure devices and modifications to older devices are frequently introduced, which makes comparison difficult.

Arterial rupture causing retroperitoneal hematoma can also occur as a result at the site of angioplasty or stenting. Some authors recommend balloon tamponade, reversal of anticoagulation, and, if anatomically appropriate, use of a covered stent.[28] Balloon-expandable covered stents can be used for more precise deployment, whereas self-expanding covered stents are recommended in tortuous iliac vessels.

Small intimal dissections, even those that are hemodynamically significant, are often not listed in the literature after angioplasty because stenting stabilizes the dissection and scaffolds the flap against the vessel wall. Some dissections are intentional such as in crossing chronic occlusions via a subintimal plane. Despite stenting, significant, flow-limited dissections were found to occur in about 7% of cases.[97] Most cases can be corrected with the deployment of additional stents.

Distal embolization and thrombosis are particularly concerning in cases of chronic occlusions but occur in 1.6% of iliac interventions overall.[98] Endovascular recanalization techniques can be attempted, but larger emboli not responsive to catheter thrombolysis or aspiration may consist of atheroma and require surgical thromboembolectomy. Smaller atheromatous emboli are a cause of livedo reticularis or blue toe syndrome.[99] Recent retrospective reviews of iliac stenting in chronic occlusions cite a thromboembolic event rate between 4% and 9%.[66,68] Stent fracture can precipitate occlusion,[100] although this occurs less frequently than with femoropopliteal stents. Even the stents themselves can migrate or embolize.[97,101]

Device infection typically presents between 1 and 2 weeks after implantation, and even bare metal stents are susceptible.[102] Symptoms include the usual systemic manifestations such as fever. Immunologic compromise and long procedure times are probable risk factors. Most infections are due to gram-positive bacteria, implicating skin contamination. Other causes are due to enteric and ureteral fistulas.[103] Many, including our group, advocate preprocedure antibiotics, although there is little direct evidence to support it.

Stent fracture is distinctly rare in the iliac arteries but can occur even in nitinol stents without evidence of external compression.[100] Studies on stent fracture in the femoropopliteal arteries have shown that longer stents and stents-within-stents are more prone to fracture and that stent fracture is associated with a higher incidence of ISR and occlusion.[104] Iliac artery stent fractures have been reported in both balloon- and self-expanding stents.[100,105]

CONCLUSION

No prospective randomized studies have confirmed the suspicion of many practitioners that primary or direct stenting of aortoiliac atherosclerotic lesions offers a long-term outcome benefit. Proponents cite higher technical success rates and lower rates of hemodynamically significant dissection that favor stenting. Stent deployment offers several theoretic benefits over angioplasty alone, and, in the Dutch Iliac Stent Trial, >40% of patients in the selective stent group received a stent to improve the hemodynamic outcome.[4] Application of stents beyond TASC A and B lesions and in occlusions shows excellent results. Widespread use of antiplatelet and procedural anticoagulant agents has decreased the acute thrombosis rate.[98,106] However, the main shortcoming of stenting is restenosis caused by intimal hyperplasia. Control of systemic factors, such as hyperlipidemia, and the development of drug-eluting or biodegradable stents[75] may mitigate the undesirable smooth muscle cell proliferation and intimal hyperplasia. Aortoiliac stenting has good long-term outcomes but often requires reintervention to achieve patency outcomes comparable with those of open bypass surgery.

References

1. Wolf GL, Wilson SE, Cross AP, et al: Surgery or balloon angioplasty for peripheral vascular disease: a randomized clinical trial: principal investigators and their Associates of Veterans Administration Cooperative Study Number 199, *J Vasc Interv Radiol* 4(5):639–648, 1993 Sep-Oct.
2. Ballard JL, Bergan JJ, Singh P, et al: Aortoiliac stent deployment versus surgical reconstruction: analysis of outcome and cost, *J Vasc Surg* 28(1):94–101; discussion 101–3, 1998.
3. Timaran CH, Prault TL, Stevens SL, et al: Iliac artery stenting versus surgical reconstruction for TASC (TransAtlantic Inter-Society Consensus) type B and type C iliac lesions, *J Vasc Surg* 38(2):272–278, 2003 Aug.
4. Tetteroo E, van der Graaf Y, Bosch JL, et al: Randomised comparison of primary stent placement versus primary angioplasty followed by selective stent placement in patients with iliac-artery occlusive disease: Dutch Iliac Stent Trial Study Group., *Lancet* 351(9110):1153–1159, 1998.
5. Dormandy JA, Rutherford RB: Management of peripheral arterial disease (PAD). TASC Working Group. TransAtlantic Inter-Society Consensus (TASC), *J Vasc Surg* 31(1 Pt 2):S1–S296, 2000.
6. Klein WM, van der Graaf Y, Seegers J, et al: Dutch iliac stent trial: long-term results in patients randomized for primary or selective stent placement, *Radiology* 238(2):734–744, 2006.
7. Stoeckel D, Bonsignore C, Duda SH: A survey of stent designs, *Minim Invasive Ther Allied Technol* 11(4):137–147, 2002.
8. Murphy TP, Hirsch AT, Ricotta JJ, et al: The Claudication: Exercise Vs. Endoluminal Revascularization (CLEVER) study: rationale and methods, *J Vasc Surg* 47(6):1356–1363, 2008.
9. Norgren L, Hiatt WR, Dormandy JA, et al: Inter-Society Consensus for the Management of Peripheral Arterial Disease (TASC II), *J Vasc Surg* 45(Suppl S):S5–S67, 2007.
10. Sullivan TM, Childs MB, Bacharach JM, et al: Percutaneous transluminal angioplasty and primary stenting of the iliac arteries in 288 patients, *J Vasc Surg* 25(5):829–838, discussion 38–9, 1997.
11. Yilmaz S, Sindel T, Yegin A, et al: Primary stenting of focal atherosclerotic infrarenal aortic stenoses: long-term results in 13 patients and a literature review, *Cardiovasc Intervent Radiol* 27 (2):121–128, 2004.
12. Ansel GM: Primary stenting of the iliac artery, *Endovasc Today* 43–44, 2005.
13. Vorwerk D, Guenther RW, Schurmann K, et al: Primary stent placement for chronic iliac artery occlusions: follow-up results in 103 patients, *Radiology* 194(3):745–749, 1995.
14. Kudo T, Chandra FA, Ahn SS: Long-term outcomes and predictors of iliac angioplasty with selective stenting, *J Vasc Surg* 42(3):466–475, 2005.
15. Rundback JH: Provisional stenting of the iliac arteries, *Endovascular Today* 45–47, 2005.
16. Rzucidlo EM, Powell RJ, Zwolak RM, et al: Early results of stent-grafting to treat diffuse aortoiliac occlusive disease, *J Vasc Surg* 37(6):1175–1180, 2003.
17. Maynar M, Zander T, Qian Z, et al: Bifurcated endoprosthesis for treatment of aortoiliac occlusive lesions, *J Endovasc Ther* 12 (1):22–27, 2005.
18. Wiesinger B, Beregi JP, Oliva VL, et al: PTFE-covered self-expanding nitinol stents for the treatment of severe iliac and femoral artery stenoses and occlusions: final results from a prospective study, *J Endovasc Ther* 12(2):240–246, 2005.
19. Bosch JL, Tetteroo E, Mali WP, et al: Iliac arterial occlusive disease: cost-effectiveness analysis of stent placement versus percutaneous transluminal angioplasty. Dutch Iliac Stent Trial Study Group, *Radiology* 208(3):641–648, 1998.
20. AbuRahma AF, Hayes JD, Flaherty SK, et al: Primary iliac stenting versus transluminal angioplasty with selective stenting, *J Vasc Surg* 46(5):965–970, 2007.
21. Yilmaz S, Sindel T, Luleci E: Subintimal versus intraluminal recanalization of chronic iliac occlusions, *J Endovasc Ther* 11 (2):107–118, 2004.
22. Bosiers M, Deloose K, Verbist J, et al: Review of stents for the carotid artery, *J Cardiovasc Surg* 47(2):107–113, 2006.
23. Duerig TW, Wholey M: A comparison of balloon- and self-expanding stents, *Minim Invasive Ther Allied Technol* 11(4): 173–178, 2002.
24. Ponec D, Jaff MR, Swischuk J, et al: The Nitinol SMART stent vs Wallstent for suboptimal iliac artery angioplasty: CRISP-US trial results, *J Vasc Interv Radiol* 15(9):911–918, 2004.

25. Ahmed MH, Nanjundappa A, Laird JR: Complications after iliac artery interventions, *Endovasc Today* 55–57, 2005.
26. Bierdrager E, Lohle PN, Schoemaker CM, et al: Successful emergency stenting of acute ruptured false iliac aneurysm, *Cardiovasc Intervent Radiol* 25(1):72–73, 2002.
27. Sanada J, Matsui O, Arakawa F, et al: Endovascular stent-grafting for infected iliac artery pseudoaneurysms, *Cardiovasc Intervent Radiol* 28(1):83–86, 2005.
28. Yeo KK, Rogers JH, Laird JR: Use of stent grafts and coils in vessel rupture and perforation, *J Interv Cardiol* 21(1):86–99, 2008.
29. Cynamon J, Marin ML, Veith FJ, et al: Stent-graft repair of aorto-iliac occlusive disease coexisting with common femoral artery disease, *J Vasc Interv Radiol* 8(1 Pt 1):19–26, 1997.
30. Cwikiel W: Restenosis after balloon angioplasty and/or stent insertion origin and prevention, *Acta Radiol* 43(5):442–454, 2002.
31. Lowe HC, Oesterle SN, Khachigian LM: Coronary in-stent restenosis: current status and future strategies, *J Am Coll Cardiol* 39(2):183–193, 2002.
32. Mehran R, Dangas G, Abizaid AS, et al: Angiographic patterns of in-stent restenosis: classification and implications for long-term outcome, *Circulation* 100(18):1872–1878, 1999.
33. Hoffmann R, Mintz GS, Dussaillant GR, et al: Patterns and mechanisms of in-stent restenosis. A serial intravascular ultrasound study, *Circulation* 94(6):1247–1254, 1996.
34. Moreno PR, Palacios IF, Leon MN, et al: Histopathologic comparison of human coronary in-stent and post-balloon angioplasty restenotic tissue, *Am J Cardiol* 84(4):462–466, A9, 1999.
35. Virmani R, Farb A: Pathology of in-stent restenosis, *Curr Opin Lipidol* 10(6):499–506, 1999.
36. Baier RE, Dutton RC: Initial events in interactions of blood with a foreign surface, *J Biomed Mater Res* 3(1):191–206, 1969.
37. Emneus H, Stenram U: Metal implants in the human body: a histopathological study, *Acta Orthop Scand* 36(2):115–126, 1965.
38. Parsson H, Cwikiel W, Johansson K, et al: Deposition of platelets and neutrophils in porcine iliac arteries after angioplasty and Wallstent placement compared with angioplasty alone, *Cardiovasc Intervent Radiol* 17(4):190–196, 1994.
39. Bai H, Masuda J, Sawa Y, et al: Neointima formation after vascular stent implantation. Spatial and chronological distribution of smooth muscle cell proliferation and phenotypic modulation, *Arterioscler Thromb* 14(11):1846–1853, 1994.
40. Schwartz RS, Huber KC, Murphy JG, et al: Restenosis and the proportional neointimal response to coronary artery injury: results in a porcine model, *J Am Coll Cardiol* 19(2):267–274, 1992.
41. Kornowski R, Hong MK, Tio FO, et al: In-stent restenosis: contributions of inflammatory responses and arterial injury to neointimal hyperplasia, *J Am Coll Cardiol* 31(1):224–230, 1998.
42. Farb A, Sangiorgi G, Carter AJ, et al: Pathology of acute and chronic coronary stenting in humans, *Circulation* 99(1):44–52, 1999 Jan 5-12.
43. Sanada JI, Matsui O, Yoshikawa J, et al: An experimental study of endovascular stenting with special reference to the effects on the aortic vasa vasorum, *Cardiovasc Intervent Radiol* 21(1): 45–49, 1998.
44. Farb A, Kolodgie FD, Hwang JY, et al: Extracellular matrix changes in stented human coronary arteries, *Circulation* 110 (8):940–947, 2004.
45. Abizaid A, Kornowski R, Mintz GS, et al: The influence of diabetes mellitus on acute and late clinical outcomes following coronary stent implantation, *J Am Coll Cardiol* 32(3):584–589, 1998.
46. Carter AJ, Bailey L, Devries J, Hubbard B: The effects of uncontrolled hyperglycemia on thrombosis and formation of neointima after coronary stent placement in a novel diabetic porcine model of restenosis, *Coron Artery Dis* 11(6):473–479, 2000.
47. Klonaris C, Katsargyris A, Tsekouras N, et al: Primary stenting for aortic lesions: from single stenoses to total aortoiliac occlusions, *J Vasc Surg* 47(2):310–317, 2008.
48. Nyman U, Uher P, Lindh M, et al: Primary stenting in infrarenal aortic occlusive disease, *Cardiovasc Intervent Radiol* 23(2):97–108, 2000.
49. Schedel H, Wissgott C, Rademaker J, et al: Primary stent placement for infrarenal aortic stenosis: immediate and midterm results, *J Vasc Interv Radiol* 15(4):353–359, 2004.
50. Poncyljusz W, Falkowski A, Garncarek J, et al: Primary stenting in the treatment of focal atherosclerotic abdominal aortic stenoses, *Clin Radiol* 61(8):691–695, 2006.
51. Kuffer G, Spengel F, Steckmeier B: Percutaneous reconstruction of the aortic bifurcation with Palmaz stents: case report, *Cardiovasc Intervent Radiol* 14(3):170–172, 1991.
52. Palmaz JC, Encarnacion CE, Garcia OJ, et al: Aortic bifurcation stenosis: treatment with intravascular stents, *J Vasc Interv Radiol* 2(3):319–323, 1991.
53. Haulon S, Mounier-Vehier C, Gaxotte V, et al: Percutaneous reconstruction of the aortoiliac bifurcation with the "kissing stents" technique: long-term follow-up in 106 patients, *J Endovasc Ther* 9(3):363–368, 2002.
54. Mohamed F, Sarkar B, Timmons G, et al: Outcome of "kissing stents" for aortoiliac atherosclerotic disease, including the effect on the non-diseased contralateral iliac limb, *Cardiovasc Intervent Radiol* 25(6):472–475, 2002.
55. Greiner A, Muhlthaler H, Neuhauser B, et al: Does stent overlap influence the patency rate of aortoiliac kissing stents? *J Endovasc Ther* 12(6):696–703, 2005.
56. De Roeck A, Hendriks JM, Delrue F, et al: Long-term results of primary stenting for long and complex iliac artery occlusions, *Acta Chir Belg* 106(2):187–192, 2006.
57. Leville CD, Kashyap VS, Clair DG, et al: Endovascular management of iliac artery occlusions: extending treatment to TransAtlantic Inter-Society Consensus class C and D patients, *J Vasc Surg* 43(1):32–39, 2006.
58. Murphy TP, Ariaratnam NS, Carney WI Jr, et al: Aortoiliac insufficiency: long-term experience with stent placement for treatment, *Radiology* 231(1):243–249, 2004.
59. Reyes R, Carreira JM, Gude F, et al: Long-term follow-up of iliac Wallstents, *Cardiovasc Intervent Radiol* 27(6):624–631, 2004 Nov-Dec.
60. Galaria II, Davies MG: Percutaneous transluminal revascularization for iliac occlusive disease: long-term outcomes in TransAtlantic Inter-Society Consensus A and B lesions, *Ann Vasc Surg* 19(3):352–360, 2005.
61. Schurmann K, Mahnken A, Meyer J, et al: Long-term results 10 years after iliac arterial stent placement, *Radiology* 224 (3):731–738, 2002.
62. Sapoval MR, Chatellier G, Long AL, et al: Self-expandable stents for the treatment of iliac artery obstructive lesions: long-term success and prognostic factors, *AJR Am J Roentgenol* 166 (5):1173–1179, 1996.
63. Tegtmeyer CJ, Moore TS, Chandler JG, et al: Percutaneous transluminal dilatation of a complete block in the right iliac artery, *AJR Am J Roentgenol* 133(3):532–535, 1979.
64. Amankwah KS, Costanza MJ, Gahtan V: Percutaneous recanalization of the occluded iliac artery: examples, techniques, and complications, *Vasc Endovascular Surg* 41(5):440–447, 2007.
65. Cho JR, Kim JS, Cho YH, et al: Subintimal angioplasty of an aortoiliac occlusion: re-entry site created using a transseptal needle under intravascular ultrasound guidance, *J Endovasc Ther* 14(6):816–822, 2007.
66. Carnevale FC, De Blas M, Merino S, et al: Percutaneous endovascular treatment of chronic iliac artery occlusion, *Cardiovasc Intervent Radiol* 27(5):447–452, 2004.

67. Uher P, Nyman U, Lindh M, et al: Long-term results of stenting for chronic iliac artery occlusion, *J Endovasc Ther* 9(1):67–75, 2002.
68. Funovics MA, Lackner B, Cejna M, et al: Predictors of long-term results after treatment of iliac artery obliteration by transluminal angioplasty and stent deployment, *Cardiovasc Intervent Radiol* 25(5):397–402, 2002.
69. Di Mario C, Marsico F, Adamian M, et al: New recipes for in-stent restenosis: cut, grate, roast, or sandwich the neointima? *Heart* 84(5):471–475, 2000.
70. Engelke C, Morgan RA, Belli AM: Cutting balloon percutaneous transluminal angioplasty for salvage of lower limb arterial bypass grafts: feasibility, *Radiology* 223(1):106–114, 2002.
71. Tsetis D, Belli AM, Morgan R, et al: Preliminary experience with cutting balloon angioplasty for iliac artery in-stent restenosis, *J Endovasc Ther* 15(2):193–202, 2008.
72. Alfonso F, Cequier A, Zueco J, et al: Stenting the stent: initial results and long-term clinical and angiographic outcome of coronary stenting for patients with in-stent restenosis, *Am J Cardiol* 85(3):327–332, 2000.
73. Al-Sergani HS, Ho PC, Nesto RW, et al: Stenting for in-stent restenosis: A long-term clinical follow-up, *Catheter Cardiovasc Interv* 48(2):143–148, 1999.
74. Waksman R, Pakala R, Kuchulakanti PK, et al: Safety and efficacy of bioabsorbable magnesium alloy stents in porcine coronary arteries, *Catheter Cardiovasc Interv* 68(4):607–617. discussion 18–9, 2006.
75. Di Mario C, Ferrante G: Biodegradable drug-eluting stents: promises and pitfalls, *Lancet* 371(9616):873–874, 2008.
76. Levine GN, Gomes AS, Arai AE, et al: Safety of magnetic resonance imaging in patients with cardiovascular devices: an American Heart Association scientific statement from the Committee on Diagnostic and Interventional Cardiac Catheterization, Council on Clinical Cardiology, and the Council on Cardiovascular Radiology and Intervention: endorsed by the American College of Cardiology Foundation, the North American Society for Cardiac Imaging, and the Society for Cardiovascular Magnetic Resonance, *Circulation* 116(24):2878–2891, 2007.
77. Shellock FG, Crues JV III: MR Safety and the American College of Radiology White Paper, *AJR Am J Roentgenol* 178 (6):1349–1352, 2002.
78. Spinoza DJ, Angle JF, Hagspiel KD, et al: Iliac artery stenting: a review of devices and technical considerations, *Applied Radiology* 10–24. July, 1998.
79. Chuang VP: Radiation-induced arteritis, *Semin Roentgenol* 29 (1):64–69, 1994.
80. Himmel PD, Hassett JM: Radiation-induced chronic arterial injury, *Semin Surg Oncol* 2(4):225–247, 1986.
81. Baerlocher MO, Rajan DK, Ing DJ, et al: Primary stenting of bilateral radiation-induced external iliac stenoses, *J Vasc Surg* 40 (5):1028–1031, 2004.
82. Lorenzi G, Rolli A, Domanin M, et al: Regarding "percutaneous transluminal angioplasty for emboligenic arterial lesions after radiotherapy of axillary arteries." *J Vasc Surg* 24(2): 297–298, 1996.
83. Aikimbaev K, Akgul E, Aksungur E, et al: Iliac artery stenosis as a cause of posttransplant renal failure and claudication, *Int Urol Nephrol* 39(4):1273–1276, 2007.
84. Voiculescu A, Hollenbeck M, Plum J, et al: Iliac artery stenosis proximal to a kidney transplant: clinical findings, duplex-sonographic criteria, treatment, and outcome, *Transplantation* 76 (2):332–339, 2003.
85. Becker BN, Odorico JS, Becker YT, et al: Peripheral vascular disease and renal transplant artery stenosis: a reappraisal of transplant renovascular disease, *Clin Transplant* 13(4):349–355, 1999.
86. AbuRahma AF, Robinson PA, Cook CC, et al: Selecting patients for combined femorofemoral bypass grafting and iliac balloon angioplasty and stenting for bilateral iliac disease, *J Vasc Surg* 33 (Suppl 2):S93–S99, 2001.
87. Timaran CH, Ohki T, Gargiulio NJ III, et al: Iliac artery stenting in patients with poor distal runoff: Influence of concomitant infrainguinal arterial reconstruction, *J Vasc Surg* 38(3):479–484. discussion 84–5, 2003.
88. Timaran CH, Stevens SL, Freeman MB, et al: Infrainguinal arterial reconstructions in patients with aortoiliac occlusive disease: the influence of iliac stenting, *J Vasc Surg* 34(6):971–978, 2001.
89. Berry C, Kelly J, Cobbe SM, et al: Comparison of femoral bleeding complications after coronary angiography versus percutaneous coronary intervention, *Am J Cardiol* 94(3):361–363, 2004.
90. Yatskar L, Selzer F, Feit F, et al: Access site hematoma requiring blood transfusion predicts mortality in patients undergoing percutaneous coronary intervention: data from the National Heart, Lung, and Blood Institute Dynamic Registry, *Catheter Cardiovasc Interv* 69(7):961–966, 2007.
91. Konstance R, Tcheng JE, Wightman MB, et al: Incidence and predictors of major vascular complications after percutaneous coronary intervention in the glycoprotein IIb/IIIa platelet inhibitor era, *J Intervent Cardiol* 17(2):65–70, 2004.
92. Resnic FS, Blake GJ, Ohno-Machado L, et al: Vascular closure devices and the risk of vascular complications after percutaneous coronary intervention in patients receiving glycoprotein IIb-IIIa inhibitors, *Am J Cardiol* 88(5):493–496, 2001.
93. Meyerson SL, Feldman T, Desai TR, et al: Angiographic access site complications in the era of arterial closure devices, *Vasc Endovascular Surg* 36(2):137–144, 2002.
94. Nikolsky E, Mehran R, Halkin A, et al: Vascular complications associated with arteriotomy closure devices in patients undergoing percutaneous coronary procedures: a meta-analysis, *J Am Coll Cardiol* 44(6):1200–1209, 2004.
95. Koreny M, Riedmuller E, Nikfardjam M, et al: Arterial puncture closing devices compared with standard manual compression after cardiac catheterization: systematic review and meta-analysis, *JAMA* 291(3):350–357, 2004.
96. Arora N, Matheny ME, Sepke C, et al: A propensity analysis of the risk of vascular complications after cardiac catheterization procedures with the use of vascular closure devices, *Am Heart J* 153(4):606–611, 2007.
97. Ballard JL, Sparks SR, Taylor FC, et al: Complications of iliac artery stent deployment, *J Vasc Surg* 24(4):545–553, discussion 53–5, 1996.
98. Tsetis D, Uberoi R: Quality improvement guidelines for endovascular treatment of iliac artery occlusive disease, *Cardiovasc Intervent Radiol* 31(2):238–245, 2008.
99. Sarwar S, Al-Absi A, Wall BM: Catastrophic cholesterol crystal embolization after endovascular stent placement for peripheral vascular disease, *Am J Med Sci* 335(5):403–406, 2008.
100. Higashiura W, Sakaguchi S, Morimoto K, et al: Stent Fracture and Reocclusion After Placement of a Single Self-Expanding Stent in the Common Iliac Artery and Endovascular Treatment, *Cardiovasc Intervent Radiol* 31:1013–1017, 2008.
101. Lam RC, Rhee SJ, Morrissey NJ, et al: Minimally invasive retrieval of a dislodged Wallstent endoprosthesis after an endovascular abdominal aortic aneurysm repair, *J Vasc Surg* 47 (2):450–453, 2008.
102. Hogg ME, Peterson BG, Pearce WH, et al: Bare metal stent infections: case report and review of the literature, *J Vasc Surg* 46 (4):813–820, 2007.

103. Aarvold A, Wales L, Papadakos N, et al: Arterio-Ureteric Fistula Following Iliac Angioplasty, *Cardiovasc Intervent Radiol*, 2008.
104. Scheinert D, Scheinert S, Sax J, et al: Prevalence and clinical impact of stent fractures after femoropopliteal stenting, *J Am Coll Cardiol* 45(2):312–315, 2005.
105. Sacks BA, Miller A, Gottlieb M: Fracture of an iliac artery Palmaz stent, *J Vasc Interv Radiol* 7(1):53–55, 1996.
106. Rousseau HP, Raillat CR, Joffre FG, et al: Treatment of femoropopliteal stenoses by means of self-expandable endoprostheses: midterm results, *Radiology* 172(3 Pt 2):961–964, 1989.
107. Bosch JL, Hunink MG: Meta-analysis of the results of percutaneous transluminal angioplasty and stent placement for aortoiliac occlusive disease, *Radiology* 204(1):87–96, 1997.
108. de Vries SO, Hunink MG: Results of aortic bifurcation grafts for aortoiliac occlusive disease: a meta-analysis, *J Vasc Surg* 26 (4):558–569, 1997.
109. Brewster DC: Current controversies in the management of aortoiliac occlusive disease, *J Vasc Surg* 25:365–379, 1997.
110. Connolly JE, Price T: Aortoiliac endarterectomy: a lost art? *Ann Vasc Surg* 20(1):56–62, 2006.
111. Urayama H, Ohtake H, Yokoi K, et al: Long-term results of endarterectomy, anatomic bypass and extraanatomic bypass for aortoiliac occlusive disease, *Surg Today* 28(2):151–155, 1998.
112. Onohara T, Komori K, Kume M, et al: Multivariate analysis of long-term results after an axillobifemoral and aortobifemoral bypass in patients with aortoiliac occlusive disease, *J Cardiovasc Surg (Torino)* 41(6):905–910, 2000.
113. Martin D, Katz SG: Axillofemoral bypass for aortoiliac occlusive disease, *Am J Surg* 180(2):100–103, 2000.
114. Passman MA, Taylor LM, Moneta GL, et al: Comparison of axillofemoral and aortofemoral bypass for aortoiliac occlusive disease, *J Vasc Surg* 23(2):263–269, discussion 269–271, 1996.
115. Vorwerk D, Gunther RW, Schurmann K, et al: Aortic and iliac stenoses: follow-up results of stent placement after insufficient balloon angioplasty in 118 cases, *Radiology* 198(1):45–48, 1996.

CHAPTER

26

Endovascular Grafting in Aortoiliac Arterial Occlusive Disease

Daniel Silverberg, Michael L. Marin

Aortoiliac occlusive disease may be a significant cause of lower-extremity ischemic symptoms. In the past, most patients have been treated with a variety of open surgical procedures, including aortobifemoral and extra-anatomic bypasses. In select disease, aortobifemoral bypass is still considered a treatment standard with patency rates reported of 85% to 90% at 5 years and 70% to 75% at 10 years.[1] Aortobifemoral bypass has demonstrated the best long-term durability but is associated with a perioperative complication rate of up to 30%.[2] Perioperative morbidity and mortality and late graft limb failures may compromise the long-term results of these procedures. In addition, patients with severe comorbid medical illnesses including cardiac, pulmonary, and renal insufficiency may not be suitable candidates for extensive aortoiliac reconstruction.

Over the past several years, endovascular modalities have emerged as attractive alternatives to the open procedures and provide a wide array of additional therapeutic modalities for the treatment of aortoiliac occlusive disease. A recent TransAtlantic Inter-Society Consensus (TASC) document on the treatment of peripheral vascular disease stated that patients with TASC A and TASC B iliac lesions may undergo endovascular treatment.[3] Patients with TASC C iliac disease with involvement of multiple iliac segments and TASC D iliac disease are best treated with open revascularization.[3]

Angioplasty with selective stenting and primary stenting of the iliac arteries has been performed with varying degrees of long-term success. Four-year primary patency rate of 50% to 80% can be expected after angioplasty with selective stent placement, depending on lesion length, location, and severity. Best results have been observed with short, nonocclusive lesions of the common iliac artery (CIA). In spite of the encouraging results of short isolated stenoses, long-segment or multilevel disease involving the CIA and external iliac artery (EIA) does not appear to be effectively treated with angioplasty and stenting alone. These patients frequently have multilevel disease, the lesions of which extend beyond the EIA into the common femoral artery (CFA). These lesions are less suitable for angioplasty and stenting, because they do not have a clear healthy "endpoint" in which to land the stent, and stenting across the inguinal ligament with bare metal stents has been associated with stent fracture, compression, and thrombosis. The results of endovascular treatment of diffuse, multilevel iliac occlusive disease involving the EIAs have been disappointing with primary and secondary patency rates after stent treatment only 30% and 53%, respectively. EIA disease has been reported to be a powerful predictor of decreased primary and primary assisted iliac patency rates.[2,4,5] In one study, EIA disease had a relative risk of 3.1 for predicting failure of iliac primary patency.[5] These patients frequently require more extensive revascularization methods, such as aortobifemoral or extra-anatomic bypasses.

The role of stent grafts of the iliac arteries for the treatment of iliac occlusive disease has evolved slowly over the years, and its current role is not well defined. This chapter focuses on the role of iliac artery stent grafting for aortoiliac occlusive disease. In addition, its role as an adjunctive procedure in facilitating delivery of devices for aortic aneurysm repair in the presence of iliac artery occlusive disease as conduits is also discussed.

STENT GRAFTS: HISTORICAL PERSPECTIVES AND DEVICES

Endovascular grafting for long-segment iliac occlusive disease was first described in 1986 by Volodos

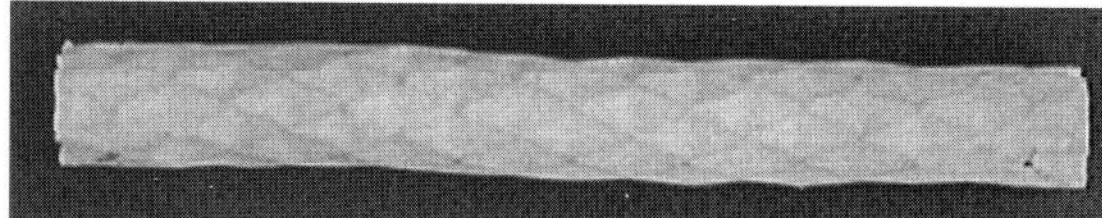

FIGURE 26-1 The Passager stent graft fabricated from an ultrathin woven polyester fabric and supported by a nitinol self-expandable stent.

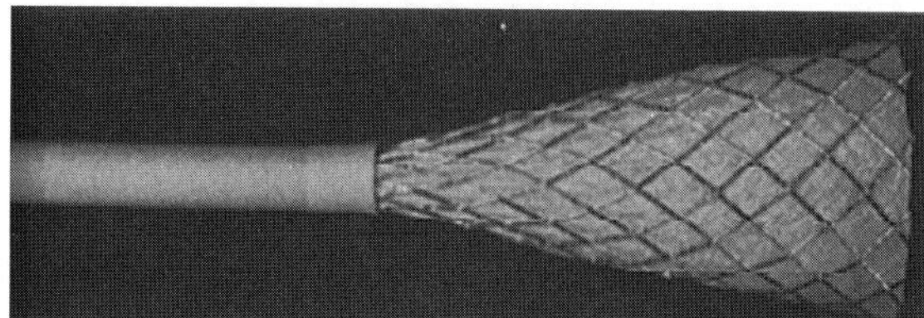

FIGURE 26-2 The Cortiva endovascular stent graft is a small-profile device (7F to 9F) constructed of braided steel wire and wrapped with a fine polyurethane fiber.

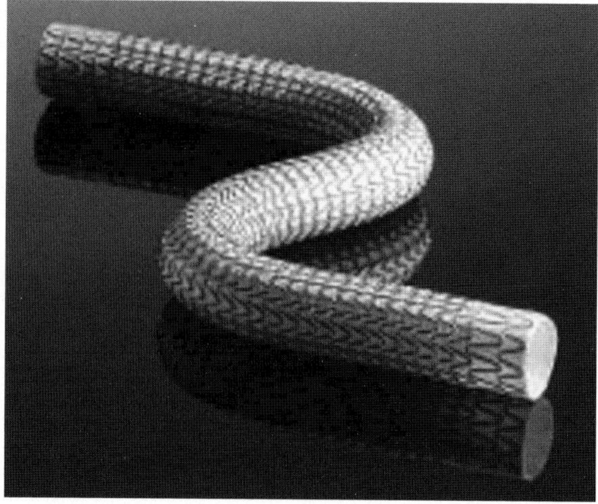

FIGURE 26-3 The Viabahn endovascular stent graft is constructed with a reinforced, ePTFE liner attached to an external self-expandable nitinol stent structure.

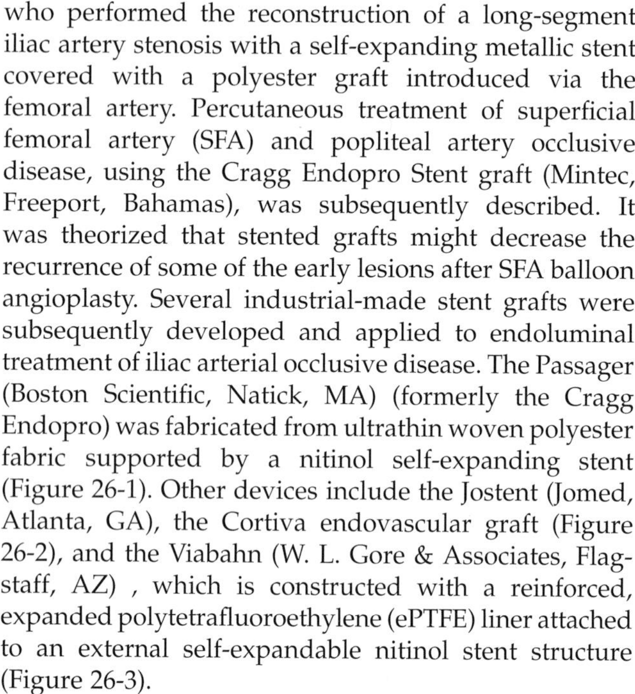

who performed the reconstruction of a long-segment iliac artery stenosis with a self-expanding metallic stent covered with a polyester graft introduced via the femoral artery. Percutaneous treatment of superficial femoral artery (SFA) and popliteal artery occlusive disease, using the Cragg Endopro Stent graft (Mintec, Freeport, Bahamas), was subsequently described. It was theorized that stented grafts might decrease the recurrence of some of the early lesions after SFA balloon angioplasty. Several industrial-made stent grafts were subsequently developed and applied to endoluminal treatment of iliac arterial occlusive disease. The Passager (Boston Scientific, Natick, MA) (formerly the Cragg Endopro) was fabricated from ultrathin woven polyester fabric supported by a nitinol self-expanding stent (Figure 26-1). Other devices include the Jostent (Jomed, Atlanta, GA), the Cortiva endovascular graft (Figure 26-2), and the Viabahn (W. L. Gore & Associates, Flagstaff, AZ) , which is constructed with a reinforced, expanded polytetrafluoroethylene (ePTFE) liner attached to an external self-expandable nitinol stent structure (Figure 26-3).

A homemade endovascular device composed of a balloon-expandable Palmaz stent (Cordis, Endovascular, Warren, NJ) and an ePTFE graft was first used for the treatment of aortoiliac occlusive disease in 1993 at Montefiore and Mount Sinai Medical Centers in New York.[6,7] Since then it has continued to accrue clinical experience. This device, described below, requires exposure of the femoral artery for delivery and reconstruction of coexisting femoral artery disease. Its significant advantage, however, is that it provides the option of performing adjunctive outflow procedures with the graft below the inguinal ligament. This is beneficial when the occlusive disease extends distal to the EIA.

METHODS

Endovascular grafting of the iliac arteries is performed in the operating room with exposure and control of the CFA, deep femoral artery, and SFA on the affected side. The type of anesthetic used (general, local, or epidural) is generally determined by the patient's overall condition, as well as by the need for other adjunctive procedures, such as infrainguinal bypasses for outflow disease.

Recanalization of the occluded or the stenosed iliac segment is achieved in either an antegrade or a retrograde manner with the use of directional catheters and guidewires. Antegrade recanalization is possible in the presence of a patent contralateral system. After achieving percutaneous access to the contralateral iliac artery, a guidewire is advanced "up and over" the aortic bifurcation and in a prograde fashion is guided across the diseased iliac artery on the affected side (Figure 26-4). This technique allows for maximal control of arterial inflow and ensures that the recanalization process begins proximally within the native arterial lumen. After recanalization of the diseased iliac artery, the guidewire is retrieved through an arteriotomy site of the exposed CFA on the diseased artery side. When the up-and-over technique is not feasible, retrograde recanalization may be used. This may be accomplished with a 0.035-inch hydrophilic guidewire and an angled directional catheter. After successful wire recanalization, the diseased iliac artery is predilated along the length of the disease with an 8-mm–diameter angioplasty balloon. This allows uninterrupted delivery of the stent graft within its sheath.

The endovascular stent graft consists of a balloon-expandable stent sewn to a thin-walled 6- or 8-mm

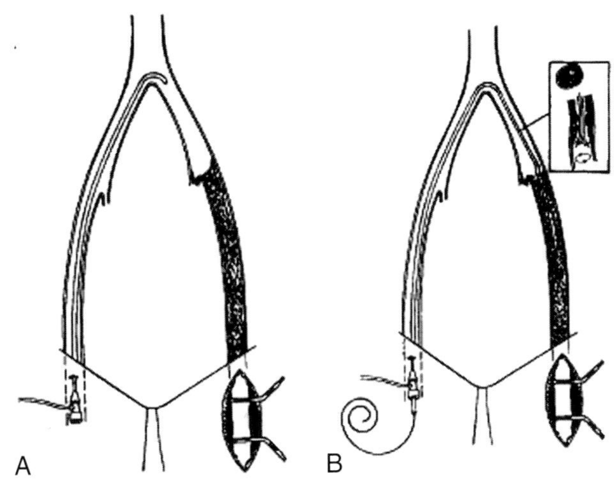

FIGURE 26-4 Contralateral CFA puncture and placement of an up-and-over sheath before recanalization of the diseased iliac segment **(A)**. A wire is advanced in a prograde fashion through the occlusion **(B)**.

FIGURE 26-5 Endovascular stented graft. A PTFE graft's proximal end is sewn to a balloon-expandable stent.

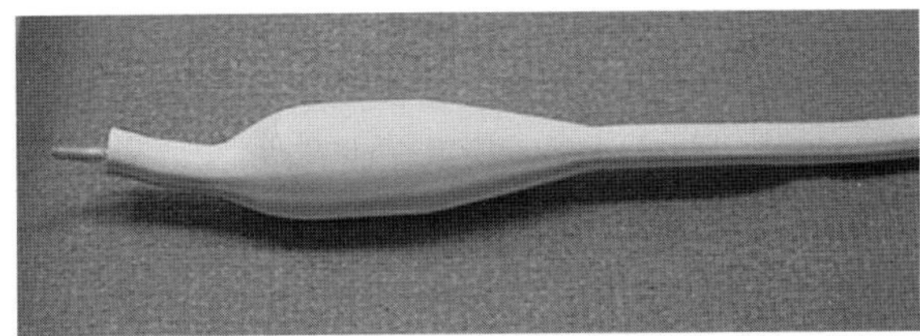

FIGURE 26-6 The PTFE is predilated at the tip to an appropriate diameter.

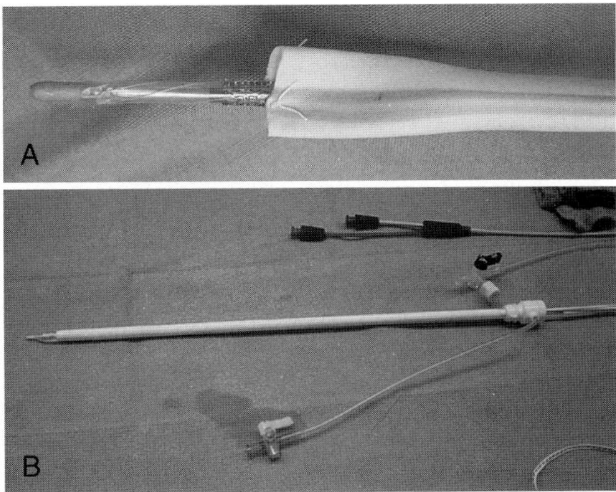

FIGURE 26-7 **A,** The stent and PTFE graft are loaded onto an angioplasty balloon. **B,** The balloon, stent, and PTFE graft are then back-loaded into a sheath (typically 16F).

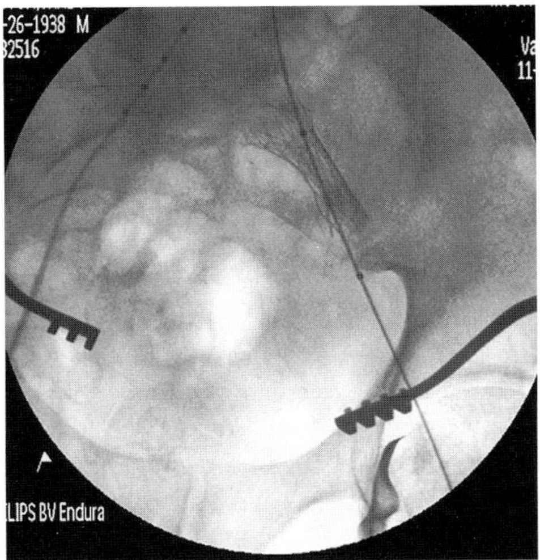

FIGURE 26-8 The Palmaz stent is deployed in the iliac artery.

ePTFE Impra (Impra, Tempe, AZ) graft or Gore PTFE graft (Figure 26-5). The ePTFE is predilated at the tip to an appropriate diameter (the diameter of the CIA at the seal zone) (Figure 26-6), sewn to the stent, and then crimped onto an angioplasty balloon sized for the iliac artery (Figure 26-7, *A*). The balloon, stent, and PTFE graft are then back-loaded into a sheath (typically 16F) (see Figure 26-7, *B*). A 6-mm by 2-cm angioplasty balloon is positioned at the proximal end of the sheath and serves as a tapered tip for the delivery system. The fabricated delivery system is then inserted transfemorally under fluoroscopy over the guidewire. When the device is positioned adequately in the proximal iliac artery, the leading balloon is deflated and withdrawn. The 16F sheath is withdrawn, exposing the Palmaz stent and the proximal segment of the PTFE graft. The stent is expanded, and the remainder of the PTFE graft is deployed (Figure 26-8). The distal end of the PTFE graft is brought out through the common femoral arteriotomy (Figure 26-9) and is inserted into a suitable outflow vessel (Figure 26-10). Should outflow disease necessitate a concomitant infrainguinal operation, Figure 26-11 shows the options available to achieve this. Figure 26-12 demonstrates angiographic images after successful treatment of an EIA occlusion using a stent graft.

RESULTS

Nevelsteen et al.[8] reported on their experience on the treatment of occlusive iliac disease using a Palmaz stent sewn to a PTFE graft, similar to the one described above. Twenty-nine iliac arteries in 24 patients were treated. Outflow procedures were performed in all cases and consisted of profundoplasties and/or femorodistal grafting. The overall success for graft placement was

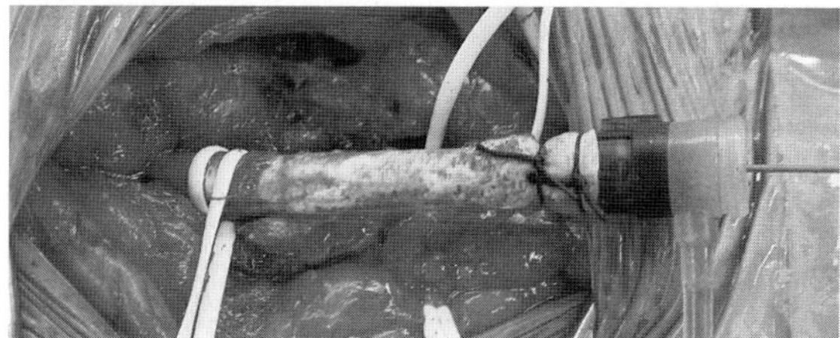

FIGURE 26-9 The distal end of the PTFE graft is brought out through the common femoral arteriotomy.

93%. The procedure-related mortality was 9% (2 patients) with one death caused by bowel infarction and the other by cardiac failure. The primary and secondary patency rates after a mean follow-up of 12.9 months were 85% and 95%, respectively. The corresponding limb salvage rate was 95%. Occlusion of the endovascular graft was reported in 2 cases.

Rzucidlo et al.[2] reported their experience with treating 34 patients with self-expanding stent grafts. Indications included rest pain (65%) and tissue loss (35%). TASC C or D lesions were present in 85% of the patients. Stents used were Wallgrafts (Boston Scientific, Natick, MA) in 88% of patients and Viabahn grafts in 12% of patients. Concomitant common femoral endarterectomy was performed in 53% of patients. Technical success was achieved in all patients. At 12 months primary patency was 70%, and primary assisted patency was 88%. Four stent grafts became occluded because of distal EIA or proximal CFA disease. These required subsequent common femoral endarterectomy and either EIA stent grafting or extra-anatomic bypass grafting. Eighty percent of primary failures were in patients who did not undergo concomitant CFA endarterectomy during the initial stent graft placement. They concluded that concomitant common femoral endarterectomy in patients with multilevel iliac disease may improve durability of the stent graft repair.

Marin et al.[7] reported their experience with 17 patients who underwent treatment with endovascular iliac stent grafts in combination with conventional infrainguinal bypasses. All patients had limb-threatening ischemia caused by aortoiliac and femoral popliteal occlusive disease. The stent grafts were composed of a Palmaz balloon-expandable stent sutured to the proximal end of a 6-mm thin-walled PTFE graft and delivered in a fashion similar to that described earlier. The distal end of the graft was anastomosed to a patent distal arterial vessel (CFA, SFA, or deep femoral artery). Conventional surgical bypasses were then constructed from PTFE (15) or saphenous vein (2) and extended to the popliteal artery (12), tibial (2), or contralateral femoral artery (3). Technical success was achieved in 94% of the patients. The 1-year primary and secondary patency rates were 94% and 100%, respectively. Three grafts

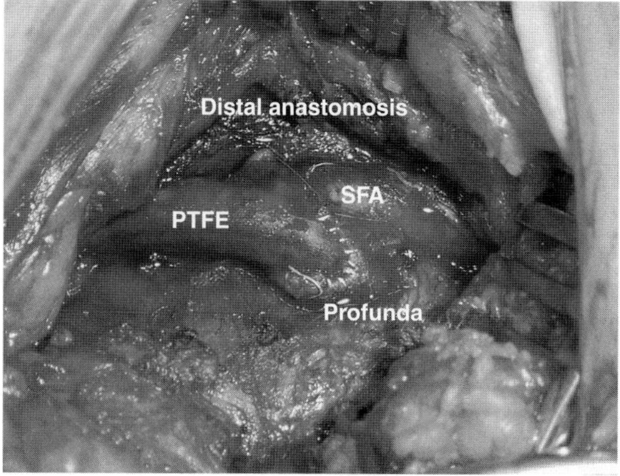

FIGURE 26-10 The distal end of the graft is sewn into an appropriate outflow vessel.

required a thrombectomy during a 24-month follow-up period. One graft failed because of progression of distal disease, one because of proximal embolic disease, and one because of a proximal CIA stenosis. All were successfully revised. Minor complications occurred in 23% of patients.

Wain et al.[6] reported midterm results of stent grafts for treatment of aortoiliac disease in 52 patients. Entry criteria included chronic, long-segmental occlusions, eccentrically calcified stenoses, diffuse segmental disease (>10 cm in length), and disadvantaged runoff. Indications for surgery were gangrene (81%) and rest pain (19%). All endovascular grafts were "homemade," as described previously. The 4-year primary and secondary endovascular graft patency was 66.1% and 72.3%, respectively, and limb salvage rate was 88.7%. Fifteen grafts failed primarily after an average of 7 months after surgery. Patency was restored by open thrombectomy and graft revision in 7 grafts and with thrombolytic therapy with or without angioplasty in 4 patients. Four other grafts remained closed and required conventional bypass procedures.

THE USE OF STENT GRAFTS AS CONDUITS FOR ENDOVASCULAR ANEURYSM REPAIR

Iliac occlusive disease and tortuosity may limit the ability to safely treat abdominal aortic aneurysms and thoracic aortic aneurysms by endovascular methods. Challenges related to the access vessels may result in significant perioperative morbidity and potentially mortality. Access-related complications have been reported with a frequency of up to 28% in some series.[9] The outer diameters of current delivery systems range from 18F to 24F for infrarenal endografts and 21F to 25F for thoracic endografts. As such, adjunctive measures to

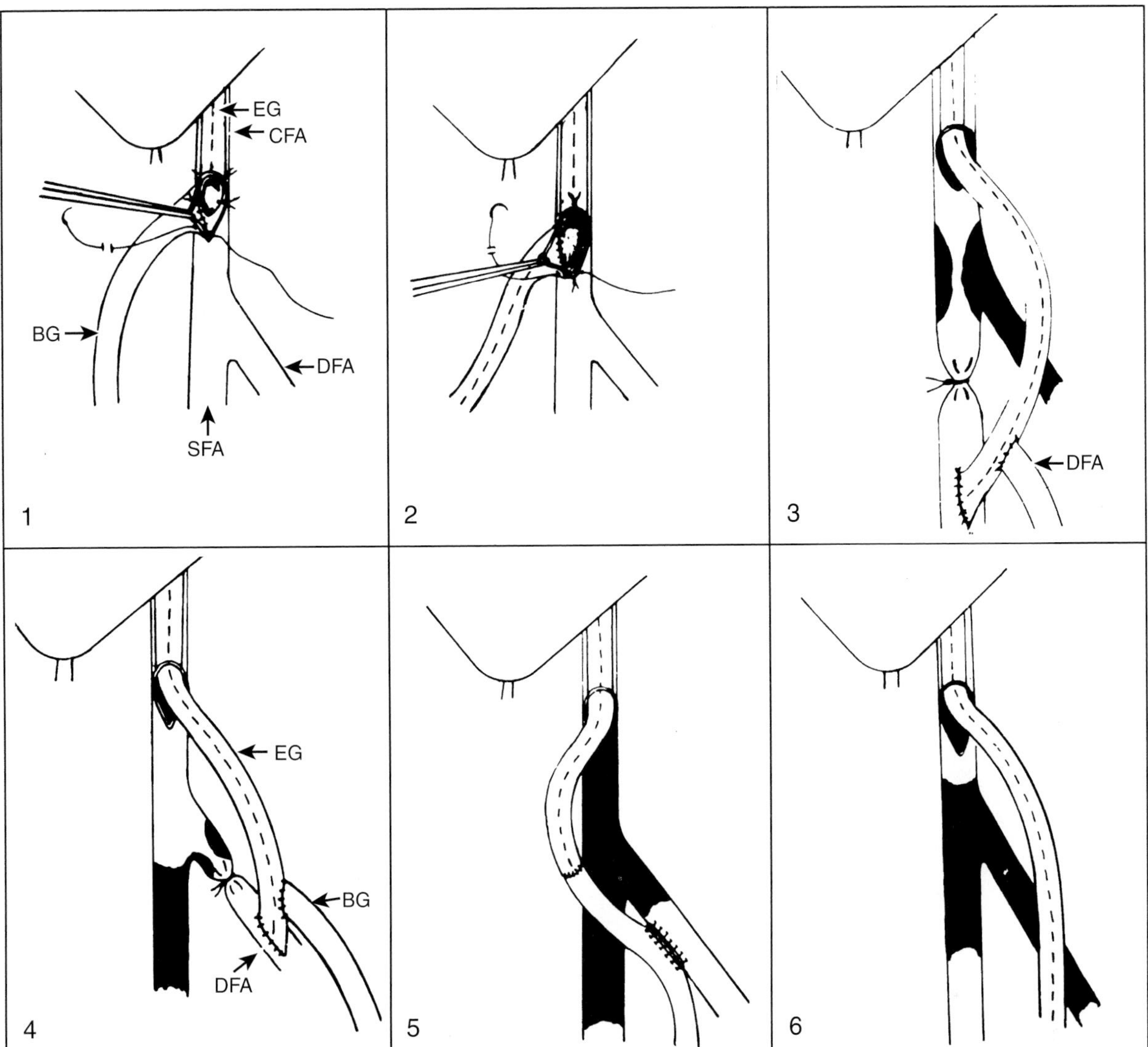

FIGURE 26-11 Different options for outflow procedures. Distal end of endovascular graft can be anastomosed to patent distal arterial tree in several ways. *1,* Type 1, endoluminal anastomosis to femoral artery is performed and separate proximal anastomosis of distal extravascular graft is performed to femoral arteriotomy. *2,* Type 2, intravascular anastomosis and proximal anastomosis of distal extravascular graft are included in single anastomotic closure. *3,* Type 3, stented graft is brought out through femoral arteriotomy and anastomosed to patent distal SFA. From this site distal extension or crossover femorofemoral extension can be performed if necessary. *4,* Type 4, endovascular graft is brought out through femoral arteriotomy and anastomosed to patent distal deep femoral artery. Extension to distal arterial tree or to contralateral femoral artery can be performed from this graft if necessary. *5,* Type 5, end of endovascular graft is brought out through femoral arteriotomy and distal graft extension is anastomosed end-to-end to this graft and side-to-side to patent distal deep femoral artery and extended further to distal arterial tree; *6,* type 6, endovascular graft is brought out through femoral arteriotomy and can bypass multiple levels of occlusive disease and be anastomosed distally to popliteal or tibial arteries if all femoral vessels are occluded. *BG,* Distal bypass graft; *DFA,* deep femoral artery;*EG,* endovascular graft.

compensate for diseased access vessels are frequently necessary. The adjunctive use of iliac conduits extends the pool of patients to which this technology can be applied.

In certain patients with challenging iliac artery anatomy requiring stent grafting for aortic aneurysms, we use homemade stent grafts to facilitate delivery of the stent grafts. Those patients with circumferentially calcified CIAs that would be technically challenging for conventional external iliac conduits may be more appropriate for stent grafting. The conduit is constructed as described previously. The endoluminal conduit is delivered transfemorally after judicious predilatation of the iliac artery as necessary. Once the stent is in the CIA, the sheath is withdrawn, the stent is expanded, and the PTFE is then dilated to at least 10 mm throughout its entire length down to the groin (Figure 26-13). At this point, the endoluminal conduit can be accessed in a similar fashion to a native vessel to allow for delivery of the device. On completion of

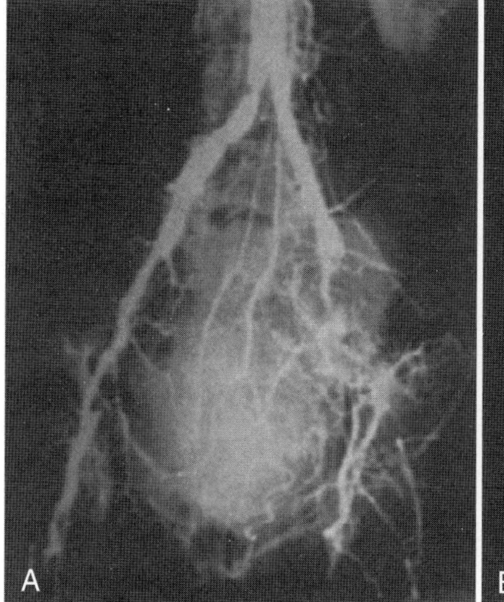

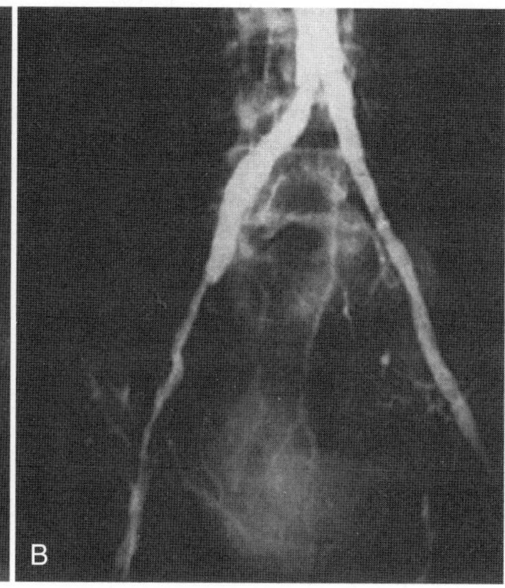

FIGURE 26-12 Angiogram of a 62-year-old woman with critical left lower-extremity ischemia. **A,** Complete occlusion of her left EIA. **B,** Angiogram after successful recanalization and deployment of a stented graft extending from her CIA to her CFA. This stent graft was combined with a conventional femoral popliteal bypass.

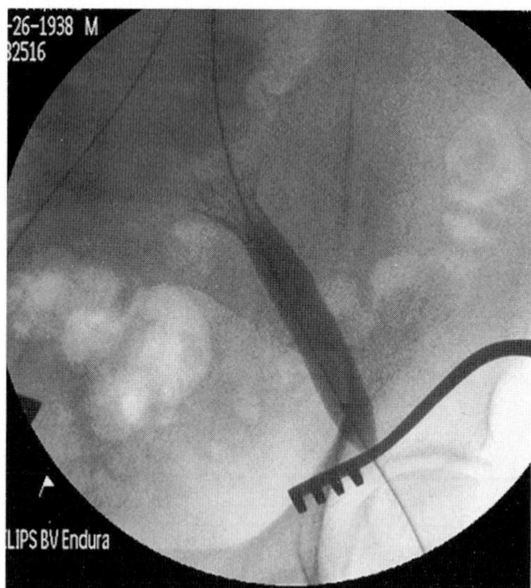

FIGURE 26-13 Endoluminal conduit: aggressive dilatation of the PTFE to accommodate delivery of EVAR stent grafts.

the procedure, the PTFE is anastomosed to the femoral artery.

We recently reviewed our 5-year experience using endoluminal conduits for facilitation of endovascular aneurysm repair (unpublished data). Of 20 endoluminal conduits placed over this period, technical success, defined as the ability to place a conduit and to deliver the stent graft, was achieved in 18 of the 20 patients. Two patients had iliac artery rupture during the deployment of the conduit. Mean follow-up was 10 months. Late morbidity related to the conduits occurred in 2 patients. In 1 patient a stenosis developed in the conduit, and the patient was seen with claudication and given treatment with a graft extension. In the other patient occlusion of the graft developed and required an axillo-bifemoral bypass.

SUMMARY

Endovascular grafting for occlusive arterial disease is a technically feasible and potentially safe option for treatment of aortoiliac occlusive disease and demonstrates encouraging short-term and midterm patency. The technology is particularly useful in high-risk patients who are otherwise unfit for major surgical reconstruction. Similar technology may be applied to facilitate delivery of stent grafts for aneurysm repair in patients with iliac occlusive disease.

References

1. Poulias GE, Doundoulakis N, Prombonas E, et al: Aorto-femoral bypass and determinants of early success and late favourable outcome: experience with 1000 consecutive cases, *J Cardiovasc Surg (Torino)* 33(6):664–678, 1992.
2. Rzucidlo EM, Powell RJ, Zwolak RM, et al: Early results of stent-grafting to treat diffuse aortoiliac occlusive disease, *J Vasc Surg* 37 (6):1175–1180, 2003.
3. Norgren L, Hiatt WR, Dormandy JA, et al: TASC II Working Group. Inter-Society Consensus for the Management of Peripheral Arterial Disease (TASC II), *J Vasc Surg* 45(Suppl S):S5–67, 2007.
4. Carlos H, Timaran MD, Scott L, et al: External iliac and common iliac artery angioplasty and stenting in men and women, *J Vasc Surg* 34:440–446, 2001.
5. Powell RJ, Fillinger M, Bettmann M, et al: The durability of endovascular treatment of multisegment iliac occlusive disease, *J Vasc Surg* 31(6):1178–1184, 2000.
6. Wain RA, Veith FJ, Marin ML, et al: Analysis of endovascular graft treatment for aortoiliac occlusive disease: what is its role based on midterm results? *Ann Surg* 230(2):145–151, 1999.

7. Marin ML, Veith FJ, Sanchez LA, et al: Endovascular aortoiliac grafts in combination with standard infrainguinal arterial bypasses in the management of limb-threatening ischemia: preliminary report, *J Vasc Surg* 22(3):316–324; discussion 324–5, 1995.
8. Nevelsteen A, Lacroix H, Stockx L, et al: Stent grafts for iliofemoral occlusive disease, *Cardiovasc Surg* 5(4):393–397, 1997.
9. Fairman RM, Velazquez O, Baum R, et al: Endovascular repair of aortic aneurysms: critical events and adjunctive procedures, *J Vasc Surg* 33(6):1226–1232, 2001.

CHAPTER

27

Complications Associated With Endovascular Management of Aortoiliac Arterial Occlusive Disease

Juan Carlos Jimenez

Angioplasty and stenting of the aorta and iliac arteries provide an excellent alternative to aortofemoral bypass for atherosclerotic occlusive disease, and excellent patency rates can be achieved with minimal patient morbidity. Despite excellent safety and efficacy, complications arising from these procedures require prompt identification and may require urgent treatment. Common complications after endovascular therapy for aortoiliac arterial occlusive disease are presented, as well as appropriate management strategies.

ARTERIAL WALL DISSECTION

Arterial wall dissection is one of the more frequently encountered complications after balloon angioplasty (Figure 27-1). Diagnosis is usually made at the time of the initial procedure during completion angiography. Intravascular ultrasound can also be used to establish the diagnosis and delineate the anatomy of the true vessel lumen. Circumferential plaques with heavy calcification are particularly at risk for acute dissection after angioplasty, especially at branch points (i.e., aortic bifurcation, external iliac artery [EIA]). However, balloon overinflation can cause dissection in any vessel even in the presence of minimal calcification. Ballard et al.[1] reviewed a series of 147 iliac stents placed in 98 limbs (72 patients) and reported 13 iliac artery dissections (13.3%). Three dissections (3.1%) resulted in complete occlusions, and these arteries were all salvaged by deployment of an additional stent. Seven (7.1%) resulted in hemodynamically significant stenoses and were successfully treated with placement of an additional stent. Three dissections did not require treatment because of a widely patent iliac artery and the absence of a systolic pressure gradient (<5 mm Hg).[1]

Timaran et al.[2] noted four arterial dissections (4.7%) in a series of 85 iliac angioplasty and stent procedures. One required aortofemoral grafting for revascularization. In a later study from the same institution comparing iliac artery stenting versus surgical reconstruction for Trans-Atlantic Inter-Society Consensus (TASC) type B and C iliac lesions, 18 arterial dissections were reported out of 188 patients (9.6%).[3] Four patients required subsequent aortofemoral bypass grafting for arterial reconstruction.

Arterial access site dissection can also cause significant postprocedural morbidity and lead to outflow obstruction and limb ischemia. Lesions in the common femoral artery (CFA) are less amenable to endovascular repair compared with dissections of the common iliac artery (CIA) and EIA. The use of percutaneous closure devices, especially in calcified vessels, can lead to separation of arterial wall layers and subsequent occlusion. The incidence of access site dissection was 0.42% in a series of 3062 consecutive patients who underwent cardiac catheterization.[4] Six dissections were located in the EIA, and six were in the CFA. Fifty percent of the CFA lesions were treated with self-expanding stents, and 50% were treated surgically. Seven-month follow-up yielded no further significant complication in these patients. Of the six EIA dissections, five were treated with self-expanding stents and one was treated conservatively. At a mean follow-up of 9.6 months, all patients given treatment for EIA dissections were symptom free.

The development of improved stent technology now allows the majority of acute arterial dissections after balloon angioplasty and stent deployment to be

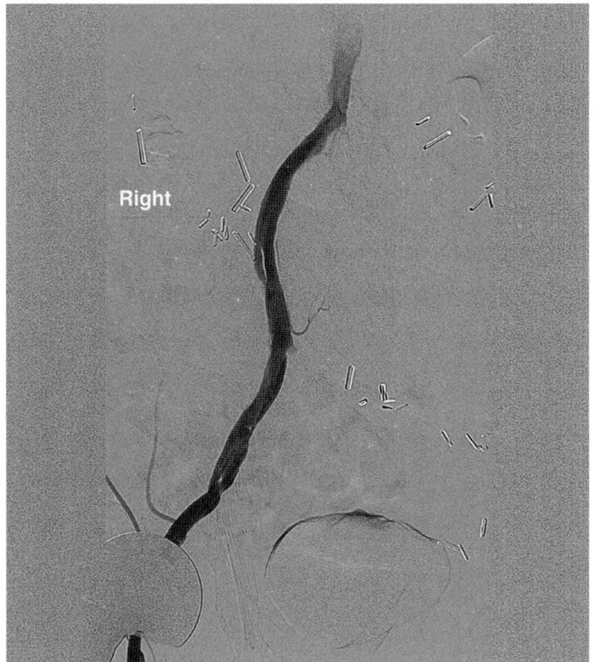

FIGURE 27-1 Acute dissection in the right CIA after guidewire placement and manipulation.

managed with endovascular techniques. Maintenance of guidewire access across the lesion within the true lumen is critical because balloon inflation and/or deployment of a stent in the false lumen likely requires open surgical repair. Angiography usually demonstrates the presence of retained contrast within the arterial wall. Intravascular ultrasound can also be used to determine the lead point and location of the true lumen if they are not clear.

All acute procedure-related dissections after angioplasty and/or stenting require urgent treatment. Because it is difficult to predict which lesions may heal with conservative treatment, benign angiographic appearance and/or the lack of a pressure gradient should not deter immediate stent placement. The stent should be extended to adjacent uninvolved segments of artery and secured with balloon insufflation. If a balloon-expandable stent is used, care must be taken to avoid overinflation and oversizing because of the risk of further extending the dissection. Dissections located close to the aortic bifurcation or extending into the contralateral CIA require the use of bilateral "kissing stents."

ACUTE ARTERIAL THROMBOSIS

Acute thrombosis after balloon angioplasty and stenting within the aorta and iliac arteries usually occurs because of an unrecognized technical problem such as dissection or residual stenosis. Transmural injury to the arterial wall during balloon inflation can lead to platelet aggregation and subsequent thrombosis. Inadequate anticoagulation while traversing occlusive lesions may also result in thrombus formation; however, this is more common in smaller arteries with lower flow rates. Most large series reviewing outcomes after endovascular aortoiliac interventions report rates of occurrence under 1%.[5-8]

Management of acute arterial thrombosis depends on the extent and severity of the occlusion. Balloon angioplasty alone is inadequate to treat this condition and has a high likelihood of distal embolization. Maintenance of guidewire access is again of critical importance. If no contraindications exist, pulse thrombolysis with 1 to 2 mg of alteplase can be performed if the thrombus is angiographically visualized. Overnight thrombolytic infusion can be maintained if persistent thrombus is present with arterial outflow beds after completion angiography. If a dissection flap is visualized, placement of a stent across the intimal defect is the appropriate method of treatment. Antiaggregate therapy (i.e., aspirin, clopidogrel) inhibits platelet adherence to affected arterial segments during the postprocedural period and may prevent late thrombosis.

DISTAL ARTERIAL EMBOLIZATION

Distal embolization after catheterization and angioplasty of the aorta and iliac arteries remains a rare but potentially limb-threatening condition when clinical manifestations occur. This complication can also occur as a consequence of intra-arterial thrombolytic therapy after clot lysis. In a contemporary review of 493 patients treated with stents for aortoiliac occlusive disease by Lin et al.,[9] the incidence of atheroembolization was 1.6%. Ballard et al.[1] noted one patient in whom distal embolization developed requiring operative thrombectomy in a series of 98 iliac arteries after stenting (1.0%).

Patients with diffusely irregular plaques in the distal aorta and iliac arteries with visible thrombus are particularly at risk for dislodgment of particles during wire and catheter passage and balloon angioplasty. Aneurysms with extensive mural thrombus also are at risk for atheroembolization and outflow vessel obstruction. Emboli are usually of mixed consistency composed of cholesterol crystals and preexisting thrombus. These particles induce platelet aggregation, thrombosis, and an endothelial inflammatory response, which may result in luminal obstruction and tissue ischemia.[10] Patients can present with a wide array of symptoms ranging from mild pain to distal gangrene and tissue loss. This process is commonly referred to as blue toe syndrome and may require subsequent distal amputation. Cholesterol embolization leading to diffuse skin and myonecrosis, compartment syndrome, and systemic rhabdomyolysis has also been reported.[10]

Studies suggest that the majority of patients who have distal microembolization after aortoiliac intervention remain asymptomatic.[11,12] Kudo et al.[12] measured distal microembolic signals during 10 iliac stenting procedures at the level of the tibioperoneal trunk in patients without infrainguinal occlusive disease. Although no distal embolic complications were observed, 541 microembolic signals were detected. The highest incidence and intensity of microembolic signals were observed at the time of stent deployment.

There is evidence to suggest that iliac angioplasty may result in prolonged distal embolization even hours after the termination of the intervention.[11] Al-Hamali et al.[11] monitored embolic signals in the CFA using a 2-MHz Doppler probe before and after percutaneous transluminal angioplasty in 10 patients. Before iliac angioplasty, asymptomatic embolic signals were detected in 4 of 10 patients in the CFA. After percutaneous transluminal angioplasty, emboli were detected in 9 of 10 patients at 30 minutes and in 8 of 10 patients at 2 hours after the procedure. All patients remained asymptomatic. The presence of emboli was detected in 50% of patients even 24 hours after the procedure but at a lower frequency of occurrence.

Although the majority of distal emboli after iliac angioplasty remain clinically silent, severe cases can be challenging to manage, and they can put the patient at high risk for subsequent limb loss. Episodes of "new-onset" or acute pain after an endovascular intervention or clinical signs of worsening ischemia should prompt the surgeon to perform a runoff angiogram. Wire access across the area of occlusion should be maintained if possible. Intravenous heparin should be administered to maintain an activated clotting time of greater than 250 seconds to prevent further thrombosis and clot propagation at the site of occlusion. The source of acute embolus is frequently the angioplasty site; however, clot formation within the access sheath can also be the main cause. The sheath should be aspirated and flushed aggressively with heparinized saline solution. A continuous heparin saline infusion can also be initiated. If the angioplasty site is implicated as the source of the problem, placement of a stent across the embolizing arterial segment should be performed.

Additional endovascular maneuvers to treat an acute embolus include passage of a catheter to the affected artery and local administration of papaverine and/or nitroglycerin to vasodilate the distal peripheral arterial bed and relieve spasm. If possible, a multi–side-port infusion catheter such as a Cragg-McNamara infusion catheter (ev3 Endovascular, Plymouth, MN) or a multiple side-hole infusion wire should be positioned across the area of occlusion, and pulse thrombolysis with 1 to 2 mg alteplase should be performed. If persistent filling defects are present, an overnight thrombolytic infusion should be administered. Extraction catheters can also assist in removal of acute embolic debris with use of aspiration thrombectomy.

If endovascular maneuvers fail to restore patency to the arterial outflow, cutdown of the femoral, popliteal, and tibial arteries can be performed and surgical embolectomy attempted. Arterial bypass may be performed if these less-invasive treatment modalities fail.

ARTERIAL PERFORATION

Acute perforation after balloon angioplasty of the aorta and iliac arteries is a potentially fatal complication (Figure 27-2). It can lead to rapid hemodynamic instability and blood loss, even when recognized early and treated promptly. The incidence of acute perforation was 0.9% in a multicenter series of 587 iliac angioplasty procedures with Palmaz stent placement.[13] Allaire et al.[14] found the incidence to be 0.8% in a series of 657 iliac dilatations over a 19-year period. Arterial rupture after balloon angioplasty often occurs when spiculated intimal calcium is disrupted and penetrates the vessel wall after intervention. Balloon oversizing and overinflation both predispose to acute vessel perforation, especially in heavily calcified vessels with high-grade stenoses.

Complaints by the patient of acute, severe back and/or abdominal pain are usually the first sign that vessel perforation has occurred. Maintenance of guidewire access across the area of perforation is important, and rapid tamponade can be achieved with reinflation of the angioplasty balloon across the area of extravasation. Care must be taken not to overinflate and enlarge the vessel wall defect. Contralateral femoral access can also be used to place a compliant balloon in the aorta for temporary proximal control.

Temporary balloon occlusion allows mobilization of additional supplies (i.e., sheaths, covered stents) that may or may not be readily available. It also allows for fluid resuscitation and/or administration of blood products if necessary. Deployment of a covered stent (i.e., Viabahn, W. L. Gore & Associates, Flagstaff, AZ; Wallgraft, Boston Scientific, Natick, MA) can avoid the need for surgical conversion in most cases. Rapid exchange to a larger-diameter sheath for introduction of the covered stent is invariably required. This should be performed carefully with guidewire access maintained across the perforation.

Failed attempts to definitively control acute bleeding with a covered stent require urgent laparotomy and surgical repair. Hemostasis with digital compression of

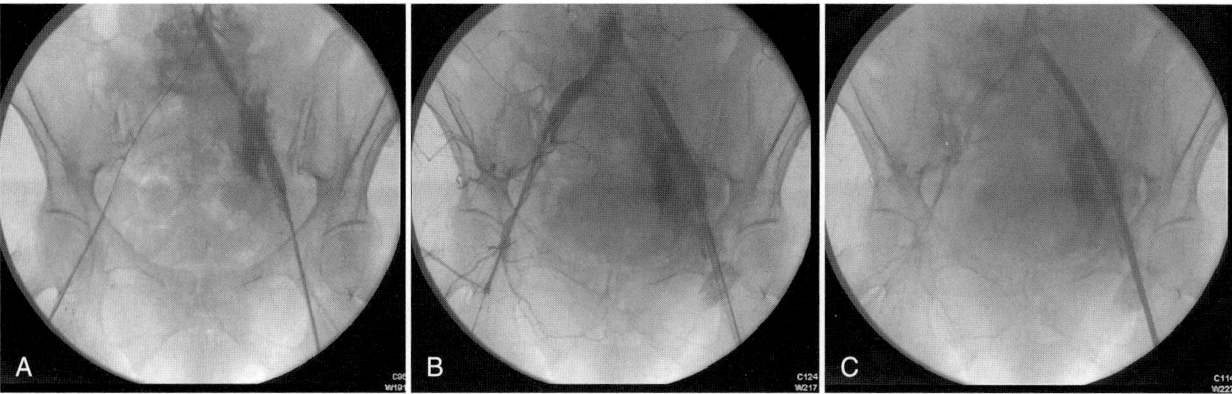

FIGURE 27-2 **A,** Acute perforation of the left CIA after balloon angioplasty. Note free extravasation of contrast into the retroperitoneum. The patient had acute left-sided flank pain and hypotension. **B,** Balloon tamponade at the area of perforation with a noncompliant angioplasty. **C,** Treatment of acute iliac perforation with deployment of a stent graft across the area of perforation.

the distal aorta or proximal iliac artery is effective and allows intravenous resuscitation with fluids and blood products. Balloon angioplasty leads to increased friability of the arterial wall, and adequate exposure of untreated proximal arterial segments should be performed. Interposition grafting or aortofemoral bypass may be required to reestablish adequate lower-extremity perfusion.

INFECTION

Although rare, infections of the arterial wall have been reported after balloon angioplasty and placement of both bare metal and covered stents[15-17] (Figure 27-3, *A* and *B*). The true incidence is unknown, and reports in the literature are limited to case studies. Subsequent development of infected pseudoaneurysms at the site of angioplasty and stent deployment, as well as femoral artery access sites, has also been reported.[18,19]

Hearn et al.[20] examined the effects of a delayed bacterial challenge administered after stent placement in the iliac arteries in a swine model. Balloon-expandable metallic stents were implanted in 14 iliac arteries. An angioplasty without stent placement was also performed in the contralateral iliac artery at the same setting. Four weeks later, an intravenous *Staphylococcus aureus* bacterial challenge was administered, and the iliac arteries were harvested and sent for microbiologic and pathologic analysis.[20] Fifty percent of stent/artery complexes were culture positive for *S. aureus*, and only one of the 14 angioplastied arteries was positive. Inflammatory changes associated with the stent infections included transmural neutrophil infiltration and focal areas of necrosis within the adjacent arterial wall. The authors suggested that stent infection may occur after delayed bacterial challenge and the administration of prophylactic antibiotics at the time of stent implantation

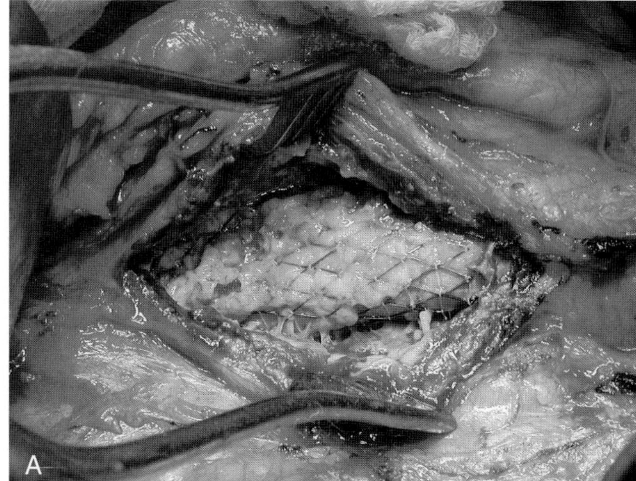

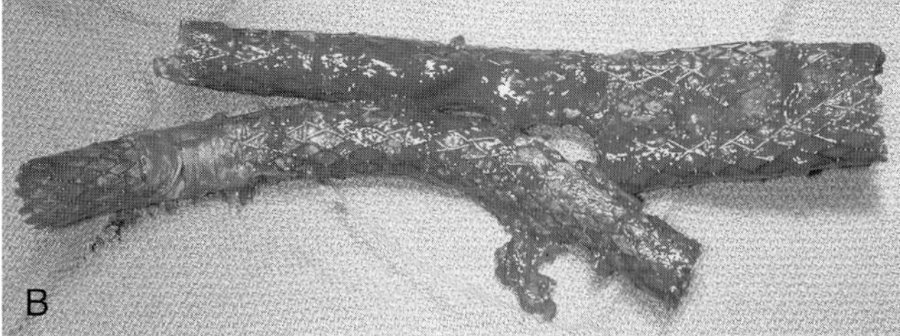

FIGURE 27-3 **A** and **B,** Infection of an aortoiliac stent graft with subsequent removal. Note the necrotizing inflammatory changes within the arterial wall and the poor incorporation of the stent within the arterial lumen. Cultures of the stent and arterial wall were positive for *S. aureus*.

should be strongly considered. Patients undergoing subsequent procedures with risk of bacterial seeding (i.e., dental procedures) should also be administered antibiotics for prophylaxis.

Although cases of infected covered stent grafts have been described more frequently, bare metal stent infections are traditionally believed to be less common.[21-24] A recent review of bare metal stent infections by Hogg et al.[25] found 35 cases reported since 1966. The most common presenting symptoms are fever, chills, malaise, pain, and petechiae. Progression of the infection can lead to arterial septic endarteritis and vessel wall destruction. This can lead to stent thrombosis, formation of pseudoaneurysms, formation of septic emboli, and vessel wall perforation and bleeding.[25]

Bacteria commonly found in skin flora such as *S. aureus* and *Staphylococcus epidermidis* commonly cause most aortoiliac stent infections.[26,27] Gram-negative rods, *Enterococcus faecalis, Pasteurella multocida,* diphtheroids, and anaerobes have also been implicated.[24,27] Severe fungal infections in immunocompromised patients have also been described with significant patient morbidity.[28]

Diagnosis of these infections is frequently delayed after exclusion of various other sources of bacteremia, and a high index of suspicion should be maintained for prompt diagnosis. Appropriate imaging studies include ultrasonography, computed tomography, angiography, and tagged white blood cell scans. Multiple radiographic modalities are often required before the diagnosis is established. Treatment includes removal of all infected stent material and aggressive debridement of the infected vessel wall. Revascularization is frequently necessary and should be performed with autogenous tissue conduits. Extra-anatomic bypass (i.e., axillobifemoral bypass) can also be used if infection of the aortoiliac system necessitates operative stent removal and vessel débridement. Staged extra-anatomic revascularization and abdominal exploration have been described in the literature with comparable results to simultaneous repair, and they remain the preferred approach at our institution.[29]

Access site infections can also be a major source of morbidity for patients undergoing aortoiliac interventions for occlusive disease, especially when associated with closure devices. The true incidence of this complication is not clearly known and likely underreported. In a review of 2680 femoral artery closures performed with three different closure devices (VasoSeal, Datascope, Montvale, NJ; Angio-Seal, St. Jude Medical, Minnetonka, MN; and Techstar, Perclose, Redwood City, CA), the incidence of infection was 1.5%.[30] Appropriate treatment includes administration of intravenous antibiotics, operative exploration, removal of all infected prosthetic material, vessel wall débridement, and arterial reconstruction. Frequently, patch angioplasty of the EIA and CFA with autogenous conduit is required for maintenance of arterial continuity. Saphenous vein remains an excellent choice if available. In cases of ipsilateral superficial femoral artery occlusion, endarterectomy of the occluded vessel can be performed and an autogenous arterial patch can be constructed.

OTHER ASSOCIATED COMPLICATIONS

Antegrade and retrograde stent migration has been described after deployment in the aorta and iliac arteries for occlusive disease.[31,32] The true incidence is not known and is likely underreported. Treatment varies depending on the extent of stent migration, and both endovascular and open approaches have been described.[1,31]

Secondary aortoenteric fistula after placement of aortic stent grafts has also been described.[33,34] Although it has been reported primarily after endovascular treatment for aneurysmal disease, it can occur after deployment of covered stents in the aortoiliac segment for occlusive disease.[35] This complication is rare and limited to case reports. Berqvist et al.[33] conducted a review of the literature and found 16 cases. The most common presenting symptoms were gastrointestinal bleeding, abdominal pain, sepsis, and anemia. The overall operative mortality rate was 7%. The most common treatment was extra-anatomic bypass followed by abdominal exploration and stent graft removal.

Arterioureteric fistula has also been described after angioplasty and stenting of the EIA for occlusive disease.[36] The patient underwent extensive prior pelvis surgery and irradiation for malignancy. Present symptoms included abdominal pain, hematuria, and the presence of brisk contrast extravasation into the ureter and bladder. Successful endovascular treatment using a covered stent has been described.[36]

CONCLUSION

A high index of suspicion and prompt diagnosis are required to manage acute complications after endovascular treatment of the aorta and iliac arteries for occlusive disease. Although the majority may be treated with minimally invasive techniques, physicians performing these interventions will likely encounter complications requiring surgical intervention. Periprocedural patient morbidity and mortality can be decreased with increased awareness and appropriate management of these potential complications.

References

1. Ballard JL, Sparks SR, Taylor FC, et al: Complications of iliac artery stent deployment, *J Vasc Surg* 24:545–555, 1996.
2. Timaran CH, Stevens SL, Freeman MB, et al: Predictors for adverse outcome after iliac angioplasty and stenting for limb threatening ischemia, *J Vasc Surg* 36:507–513, 2002.
3. Timaran CH, Prault TL, Stevens SL, et al: Iliac artery stenting versus surgical reconstruction for TASC (TransAtlantic Inter-Society Consensus) type B and type C iliac lesions, *J Vasc Surg* 38:272–278, 2003.

4. Prasad A, Compton A, Prasad A, et al: Incidence and treatment of arterial access dissections occurring during cardiac catheterization, *J Interv Cardiol* 21:61–66, 2008.
5. Kudo T, Chandra FA, Ahn SS: Long-term outcomes and predictors of iliac angioplasty with selective stenting, *J Vasc Surg* 42:466–475, 2005.
6. Tetteroo E, van der Graaf Y, Bosch JL, et al: Randomised comparison of primary stent placement versus primary angioplasty followed by selective stent placement in patients with iliac-artery occlusive disease, *Lancet* 351:1153–1159, 1998.
7. Murphy TP, Ariaratnam NS, Carney WI, et al: Aortoiliac insufficiency: Long-term experience with stent placement for treatment, *Radiology* 231:243–249, 2004.
8. Klonaris C, Katsargyris A, Tsekouras N, et al: Primary stenting for aortic lesions: From single stenoses to total aortoiliac occlusions, *J Vasc Surg* 47:310–317, 2008.
9. Lin PH, Bush RL, Conklin BS, et al: Late complication of aortoiliac stent placement—atheroembolization of the lower extremities, *J Surg Res* 103:153–159, 2002.
10. Sarwar S, Al-Absi A, Wall BM: Catastrophic cholesterol crystal embolization after endovascular stent placement for peripheral vascular disease, *Am J Med Sci* 335:403–406, 2008.
11. Al-Hamali A, Baskerville P, Fraser S, et al: Detection of distal emboli in patients with peripheral arterial stenosis before and after iliac angioplasty: A prospective study, *J Vasc Surg* 29:345–351, 1999.
12. Kudo T, Inoue Y, Nakamura H, et al: Characteristics of peripheral microembolization during iliac stenting: Doppler ultrasound monitoring, *Eur J Vasc Endovasc Surg* 30:311–314, 2005.
13. Palmaz JC, Laborde JC, Rivera FJ, et al: Stenting of the iliac arteries with the Palmaz stent: Experience from a multicenter trial, *Cardiovasc Intervent Radiol* 15:291–297, 1992.
14. Allaire E, Melliere D, Poussier B, et al: Iliac artery rupture during balloon dilatation: What treatment? *Ann Vasc Surg* 17:306–314, 2003.
15. Krupski WC, Pogany A, Effeney DJ: Septic endarteritis after percutaneous transluminal angioplasty, *Surgery* 98:359–362, 1985.
16. Schachtrupp A, Chalabi K, Fischer U, et al: Septic endarteritis and fatal iliac wall rupture after endovascular stenting of the common iliac artery, *Cardiovasc Surg* 7:183–186, 1999.
17. Cleveland KO, Gelfand MS: Invasive staphylococcal infections complicating percutaneous transluminal coronary angioplasty: three cases and review, *Clin Infect Dis* 21:93–96, 1995.
18. Kondo Y, Muto A, Ando M, et al: Late infected pseudoaneurysm formation after uneventful iliac artery stent placement, *Ann Vasc Surg* 21:222–224, 2007.
19. Scheinert D, Ludwig J, Schroder M, et al: Pseudoaneurysm formation at the site of external iliac artery stents: Percutaneous stent-graft treatment, *J Endovasc Ther* 8:303–307, 2001.
20. Hearn AT, James KV, Lohr JM, et al: Endovascular stent infection with delayed bacterial challenge, *Am J Surg* 174:157–159, 1997.
21. Hulin SJ, Morris GE: Aortic endograft infection: Open surgical management with endograft preservation, *Eur J Vasc Endovasc Surg* 34:191–193, 2007.
22. Sharif MA, Lee B, Lau LL, et al: Prosthetic stent graft infection after endovascular abdominal aneurysm repair, *J Vasc Surg* 46:442–448, 2007.
23. Hart JP, Eginton MT, Brown KR, et al: Operative strategies in aortic graft infections: Is complete graft excision always necessary? *Ann Vasc Surg* 19:154–160, 2005.
24. Sternbergh WC, Conners MS, Money SR: Explantation of an infected endograft with suprarenal barb fixation, *J Vasc Surg* 38:1136, 2003.
25. Hogg ME, Peterson BG, Pearce WH, et al: Bare metal stent infections: Case report and review of the literature, *J Vasc Surg* 46:813–820, 2007.
26. Swain TW 3rd, Calligaro KD, Dougherty MD: Management of infected aortic prosthetic grafts, *Vasc Endovascular Surg* 38:75–82, 2004.
27. Silberfein EJ, Lin PH, Bush RL, et al: Aortic endograft infection due to *Pasteurella multicoda* following a rabbit bite, *J Vasc Surg* 43:393–395, 2006.
28. Liapis CD, Petrikkos GL, Paraskevas KI, et al: External iliac artery mucormycosis in a renal transplant patient, *Ann Vasc Surg* 20:253–257, 2006.
29. Seeger JM, Preter HA, Welborn MB, et al: Long-term outcome after treatment of aortic graft infection with staged extra-anatomic bypass grafting and aortic graft removal, *J Vasc Surg* 32:451–459, 2000.
30. Carey D, Martin JR, Moore CA, et al: Complications of femoral artery closure devices, *Catheter Cardiovasc Interv* 52:3–7, 2001.
31. Civillini E, Melissano G, Baccellieri D, et al: Delayed upstream migration of an iliac stent, *Eur J Vasc Endovasc Surg* 34:214–216, 2007.
32. Slonim SM, Dake MD, Razavi MK, et al: Management of misplaced or migrated endovascular stents, *J Vasc Interv Radiol* 10:851–859, 1999.
33. Bergqvist D, Bjorck M, Nyman R: Secondary aortoenteric fistula after endovascular aortic interventions: A systematic literature review, *J Vasc Interv Radiol* 19:163–165, 2008.
34. Saratzis N, Saratzis A, Melas N, et al: Aortoduodenal fistulas after endovascular stent-graft repair of abdominal aortic aneurysms: Single center experience and review of the literature, *J Endovasc Ther* 15:441–448, 2008.
35. Kahlke V, Brossman J, Klomp HJ: Lethal hemorrhage caused by aortoenteric fistula following endovascular stent implantation, *Cardiovasc Intervent Radiol* 25:205–207, 2002.
36. Aarvold A, Wales L, Papadakos N, et al: Arterio-ureteric fistula following iliac angioplasty, *Cardiovasc Interven Radiol* 31:821–823, 2008.

SECTION IV

INFRAINGUINAL ARTERIAL OCCLUSIVE DISEASE

CHAPTER

28

Balloon Angioplasty and Stenting for Femoral-Popliteal Occlusive Disease

Brian G. DeRubertis

Chronic lower-extremity arterial occlusive disease is a common problem encountered by vascular surgeons, resulting in claudication in 6 of every 1000 persons in the United States and contributing to thousands of amputations yearly.[1,2] Atherosclerotic stenoses and occlusions of the superficial femoral artery (SFA) are common patterns of arterial disease both in patients with claudication and in those with limb-threatening ischemia. Although endovascular therapy for lower-extremity peripheral arterial disease is still evolving, considerable progress has been made in this area, in terms of both technologic advances and outcome evaluations. Balloons and stent delivery systems of increasingly low profile have been developed, allowing easier lesion crossing. Self-expanding nitinol stents with increased flexibility and resistance to kinking show promise over balloon-expandable stainless steel stents used in earlier reports.[3,4] Although outcomes after percutaneous intervention have yet to prove equivalent to those of open surgical revascularization, specific groups of patients may receive sufficient symptom relief to warrant avoidance of the risk of complications that accompanies surgical bypass.

ROLE OF ENDOVASCULAR THERAPY

Lifestyle modification, risk factor reduction, exercise programs, and pharmacologic therapy continue to play an important role in the management of patients with chronic lower-extremity disease and remain the first line of therapy for patients with claudication. However, persistent disabling symptoms or progression of vascular disease to limb-threat will ultimately require more invasive therapy in some patients. For these patients, open surgical bypass has resulted in excellent outcomes for both claudication and limb-threatening conditions for many years and remains the gold standard today.[5-8] Although 5-year secondary patency rates are commonly quoted at greater than 80% in many single-institutional series, not all patients have acceptable conduit, and results diminish considerably in patients who require the use of suboptimal conduit. Five-year patency rates below 25% are sometimes seen in patients with prosthetic graft material.[9]

Furthermore, another potential drawback of open surgical reconstruction is the morbidity and mortality associated with the operation. Patients with chronic lower-extremity disease often have a number of associated comorbidities that put them at risk for major perioperative complications with open surgery. Overall mortality can even exceed 10% in some series of surgical reconstruction for patients with limb-threat, and major complication rates in this group can range from 20% to 50%.[10-12] In addition, because many patients requiring lower extremity revascularization already have functional limitations attributable to other comorbidities, the recovery period for patients undergoing open surgical revascularization can be considerable. This remains true even in the absence of significant perioperative complications. It has even been demonstrated in one study that fewer than 50% of patients return to their preoperative functional status by 6 months after surgery.[13]

Considering these drawbacks of open surgical revascularization, the past decade has brought growing enthusiasm for the use of percutaneous intervention for occlusive disease of the femoropopliteal arterial circulation. Percutaneous revascularization has multiple advantages, including the ability to perform the procedure with the patient under local anesthesia without the use of general or spinal anesthesia. Perioperative complications rates are considerably reduced compared with series of open surgical bypass. Although arterial access complications can occur in 5% to 10% of percutaneous

TABLE 28-1

Rutherford category	Clinical description
0	Asymptomatic
1	Mild claudication
2	Moderate claudication
3	Severe claudication
4	Rest pain
5	Minor tissue loss, nonhealing ulcer, or focal gangrene
6	Major tissue loss or gangrene, extending above the transmetatarsal level

Modified from Rutherford RB, Flanigan DP, et al: Suggested standards for reports dealing with lower extremity ischemia, J Vasc Surg *4:80-94, 1986.*

BOX 28-1

GENERAL TECHNIQUE FOR FERMOROPOPOLITEAL BALLON ANGIOPLASTY AND STENTING

1. Percutaneous arterial access
2. Diagnostic angiography
3. Lesion and re-entry point identification
4. Working sheath placement and anticoagulation
5. Lesion crossing with wire/catheter
6. Confirmation of luminal re-entry
7. Reposition of guide-wire
8. Balloon angioplasty and repeat angiography
9. Stent deployment and postdilation
10. Completion angiography

procedures, the avoidance of lower-extremity incisions eliminates most serious wound complications. Among the most important benefits for most patients are the earlier ambulation and return to the preoperative functional status. Percutaneous procedures can be performed regardless of availability of acceptable conduit. Finally, restenosis or recurrence of symptoms can often be treated with reintervention, without the need to move to open surgical bypass in most patients.

EVALUATION OF PATIENTS WITH FEMOROPOPLITEAL OCCLUSIVE DISEASE

Patients with femoropopliteal occlusive disease can present with either lifestyle-altering claudication or limb-threatening ischemia. Initial evaluation of these patients requires a thorough history and physical examination followed by appropriate vascular laboratory studies. In patients with claudication, the severity and duration of symptoms must be assessed, because patients with recent or acute onset of claudication may have a thrombotic or embolic component to their disease that would obviously be managed differently than chronic occlusive disease. Response to prior conservative measures should be documented. Despite the reduced morbidity of percutaneous interventions relative to open surgery, these procedures are not free from risks, and first-line therapy for patients with claudication remains conservative measures including exercise programs, smoking cessation, and pharmacotherapy. Patients with claudication often have disease limited to the femoropopliteal circulation with sparing of distal runoff, and this disease pattern should be demonstrable through appropriate vascular laboratory studies. Patients with limb-threat, on the other hand, often have multilevel disease. The multiple medical comorbidities that tend to accompany this latter group make them ideal candidates for the minimally invasive nature of percutaneous revascularization, but the potential need for multilevel intervention with several endovascular modalities must be anticipated. In patients with ulceration or gangrene, an assessment of the degree of tissue loss must be made. Severity of ischemia should be determined by Rutherford grades for both claudicants and patients with limb-threat for the purpose of preoperative risk stratification and postoperative evaluation of outcomes (Table 28-1).[14]

Preoperative computed tomographic and magnetic resonance angiography can be used to evaluate the arterial system before intervention. These imaging modalities can help to evaluate inflow, identify stenoses or occlusions, and identify luminal reentry targets. Many interventionalists, however, forgo routine preoperative axial imaging and instead rely primarily on vascular laboratory studies for preoperative planning. The combination of ankle-brachial indices, segmental pressures, and pulse-volume waveform tracings can provide a quantitative measure of the degree of ischemia and can accurately localize the disease in most patients. Arterial duplex ultrasound can help to further localize the lesions and accurately determine the severity of stenoses or presence of occlusions.

TECHNIQUE OF SUPERFICIAL FEMORAL ARTERY ANGIOPLASTY AND STENTING

Regardless of the device or platform chosen for lesion treatment, there are several important principles common to all percutaneous interventions. These steps are outlined in Box 28-1 and described in detail in the following sections.

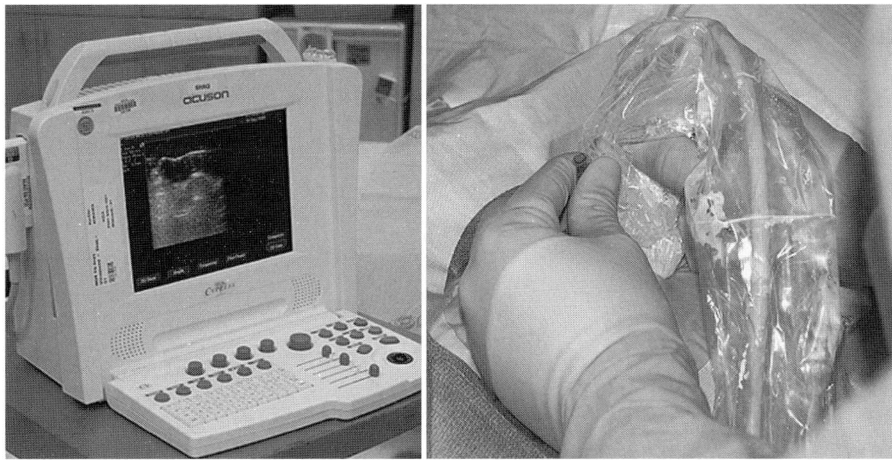

FIGURE 28-1 Duplex-guided puncture of the CFA can reduce the incidence of improperly placed arterial punctures and thereby reduce bleeding or closure-device–related complications.

Access

Arterial access can be obtained either with a 4F micropuncture kit or with a standard 18-gauge arterial access needle. If the procedure is performed with use of fluoroscopic guidance, the puncture site should be centered over the femoral head but below the inguinal ligament, because the bifurcation of the common femoral artery (CFA) occurs below this bony landmark in most patients, and this structure also provides support for compression of the artery after sheath removal. Alternatively, duplex ultrasound can be used to guide and visualize arterial puncture, thus ensuring appropriate puncture placement in the CFA and avoiding areas of atherosclerotic plaque (Figure 28-1). Duplex ultrasound guidance of the arterial puncture is especially helpful in antegrade punctures, because it helps avoid puncturing the artery close to the bifurcation and can be used to visualize placement of the wire directly toward the SFA. Although antegrade punctures can be useful for distal tibial interventions or when extra support is required for traversing chronic total occlusions of the femoropopliteal circulation, most interventions in the femoropopliteal vessels can be performed from the contralateral approach, which is generally preferred for logistic reasons. Patients with orificial disease or flush occlusions of the SFA are never appropriate candidates for antegrade punctures.

Imaging

After arterial access and placement of a short 5F sheath in the contralateral femoral artery, a flush catheter is positioned at the level of the renal arteries for aortoiliac angiography. After assessment of inflow, the bifurcation is crossed with use of the flush catheter and a 0.035-inch Stiff Angled Glidewire (Terumo, Somerset, NJ), the flush catheter is exchanged for a 5F Angled Glide Catheter (AngioDynamics, Queensbury, NY), and this catheter is then positioned at the inguinal ligament for selective lower-extremity angiograms. With the tip of the Glide Catheter in the proximal CFA, 3- to 5-mL injections of 50% iso-osmolar nonionic contrast are used to evaluate the SFA and infrapopliteal runoff. This volume and strength of contrast are generally sufficient to obtain the necessary visualization for lesion evaluation and often allow the entire study and intervention to be performed with a volume of less than 50 to 75 mL for SFA disease. Although there are multiple strategies to avoid contrast-induced nephropathy during these interventions,[15,16] this attention to contrast volume may well be the most important factor. Imaging should be done in at least two obliquities to fully evaluate for areas of hemodynamically significant stenoses, and proper obliquities are required in specific areas to visualize bifurcations. For example, one view of the right CFA should be performed in a 30- to 45-degree right anterior oblique to separate the SFA from the profunda femoris artery and allow assessment of the origins of these two vessels. When the SFA is stenotic but patent throughout its entire course, then image quality can be improved and contrast volume can be reduced by selectively catheterizing the SFA for subsequent views, thereby preventing contrast from being injected into the profunda femoris circulation. However, in cases of medium- to long-segment total SFA occlusions, the profunda femoris artery is a source of important collaterals, and injection of contrast into this artery is required for opacification and identification of the distal reconstitution that will serve as the target reentry point. Once the lesions have been delineated, the Stiff Angled Glidewire is reinserted and positioned in the SFA or profunda femoris artery and used to exchange the short 5F sheath for a 6F Balkin 45-cm sheath (Cook Medical, Bloomington, IN), which is positioned

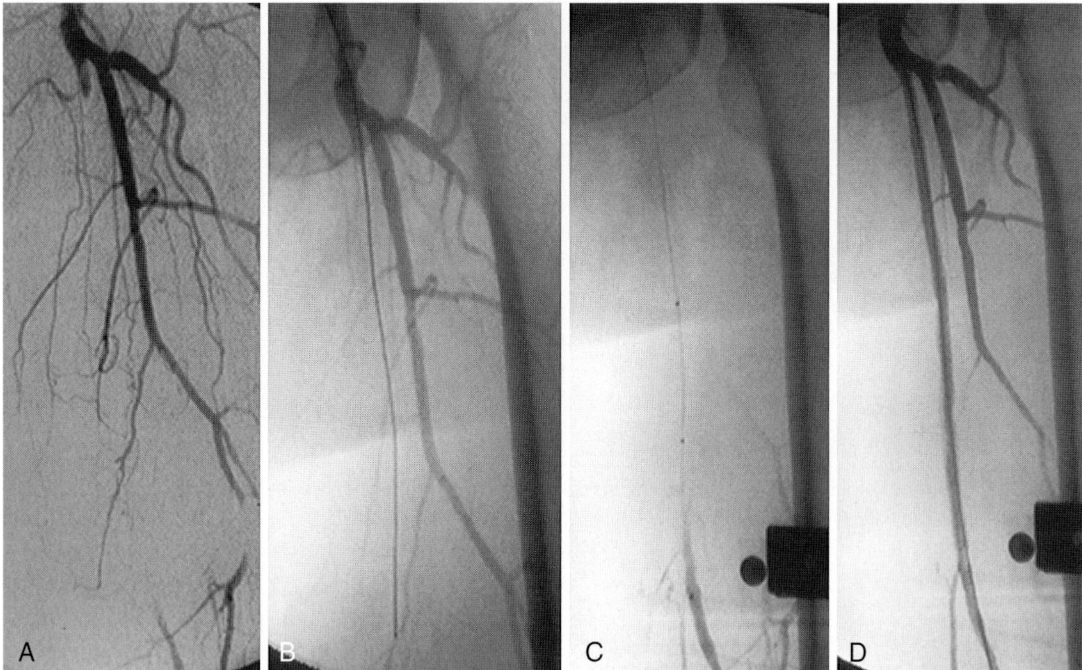

FIGURE 28-2 Technique for subintimal recanalization of a chronic total occlusion. Selective left lower-extremity angiogram **(A)** demonstrates a complete occlusion of the SFA with reconstitution at the level of the adductor hiatus. A stiff guidewire is advanced in the subintimal plane, using caution to avoid dissecting beyond the first several millimeters of the area of reconstitution **(B)**. A Quick Cross catheter (Spectranetics, Colorado Springs, CO) is then brought to this level, and, on wire removal, blood return through the catheter demonstrates that reentry into the true lumen has been achieved. This is confirmed by angiography through the catheter, demonstrating the distal outflow vessel **(C)**. The guidewire is then readvanced **(D)**, and balloon angioplasty and stenting result in continuous inline arterial flow without residual stenoses.

with the tip in the contralateral CFA. This sheath provides support for lesion crossing and allows contrast injection for subsequent angiography. After successful sheath placement, the patient is anticoagulated with 100 units/kg of intravenous heparin to maintain an activated clotting time of greater than 250 seconds.

Lesion Crossing

The two most important factors to delineate before attempting lesion crossing are (1) presence of a total occlusion (vs. high-grade stenosis) and (2) reconstitution point of the target vessel. In patients with hemodynamically significant stenoses of the SFA without complete occlusions, every attempt is made to maintain luminal position and avoid dissection into the subintimal plane, because a subintimal dissection will ultimately require successful luminal reentry, can extend the length of the artery requiring treatment, and may increase the complexity of the procedure. This is done by using a steerable angled wire, such as a 0.035-inch Angled Glidewire (Terumo), which is a hydrophilic wire that has a floppy tip to prevent dissecting the artery but still has sufficient support throughout the body of the wire to allow for maneuvering the tip. With use of a torque device attached to the wire at all times, the tip of the wire is steered around the stenoses while the advancement of the wire is visualized at all times. When the tip of the wire encounters an obstacle and deforms, the wire is immediately retracted and turned in a different orientation to seek the true lumen. Directional advancement of the wire is facilitated by supporting the wire with a 5F Angled Glide Catheter (AngioDynamics). If the lesion is nearly occlusive, luminal position may be more easily maintained by changing to a smaller wire, such as the 0.014-inch ASAHI Grand Slam (Abbott Vascular, Abbott Park, IL), which has a shapable floppy tip and is well suited to traversing high-grade stenoses. The body of this wire is supportive enough to allow passage of a larger catheter, such as a 0.035-inch Quick Cross catheter (Spectranetics, Colorado Springs, CO), after lesion crossing (Figure 28-2).

Chronic total occlusions often require more supportive wires and catheters, and it is generally difficult or impossible to ascertain whether the occlusion is being traversed in a "luminal" or subintimal plane. However, one should attempt to keep the wire positioned in the center of the occluded vessel and prevent excessive spiraling of the wire that suggests a "deep subintimal" plane. A 0.035-inch Stiff Angled Glidewire (Terumo) in conjunction with a 0.035-inch Angled Glide Catheter (AngioDynamics) or 0.035-inch Quick Cross catheter has sufficient support to cross most chronic occlusions. Unlike the technique described for crossing stenoses, the technique for traversing chronic total occlusions often requires a J conformation of the wire in which the floppy portion of the hydrophilic wire folds onto itself and creates a loop, thus allowing the more rigid body of the wire to be used to enter a subintimal plane. This J-loop is then extended the length of the occlusion, followed and supported by the catheter until reaching the previously identified target of reentry. Once this area is reached, one assesses for luminal reentry.

Early identification of the most proximal site of target vessel reconstitution is essential during recanalization of total occlusions (see Figure 28-1). Extension of a subintimal dissection plane beyond this area of reconstitution jeopardizes future surgical bypass targets and violates the principle of preserving bypass options during percutaneous intervention. Therefore, once the identified reconstitution point is reached with the guidewire, the catheter should be advanced to this position and the guidewire removed. Back-bleeding through the catheter typically indicates reentry into the true lumen of the reconstituted vessel and then can be followed with a gentle injection of 1 to 2 mL of 50% contrast through the catheter to confirm reentry. If no back-bleeding is appreciated, then injecting through the catheter will only result in increasing the size of the dissection plane and make reentry attempts more difficult. Instead, the catheter should be withdrawn into the region of the occlusion and redirected to find a different route through the lesion and into the true lumen. If multiple attempts at luminal reentry are unsuccessful, then a reentry device such as the Pioneer Catheter (Medtronic, Minneapolis, MN) may be used to obtain luminal access without compromising the distal vasculature. Alternatively, patients in whom reentry into the true lumen has proved unsuccessful or patients with lesions that are heavily calcified or otherwise difficult to cross may be better served with surgical bypass.

Lesion Treatment With Balloon Angioplasty and Stenting

After lesion crossing and confirmation of luminal reentry, the guidewire is reinserted into the distal outflow vessel as a guide for the balloon catheter and stent delivery systems. Treatment generally begins with balloon angioplasty either as a primary treatment or for predilatation before stent deployment. Balloon size can be estimated on the basis of angiographic images or rarely through the use of intravascular ultrasound, and length assessment can be facilitated by the use of a radiopaque marker tape affixed to the patient's leg. Balloon and stent diameters typically range from 5 to 7 mm in the SFA and 4 to 5 mm in the popliteal artery. The balloon is inflated to nominal pressure as indicated on the specific catheter's instructions to reach full profile, and the lesion is observed fluoroscopically during inflation to ensure that all stenoses or "waists" on the balloon have been dilated effectively. After removal of the catheter repeated angiography in multiple planes is performed to assess the result. The majority of interventionalists practice selective stenting, in which stents are placed for residual stenoses of greater than 30%, flow-limiting dissections, or large spiral dissections.

Balloon catheters are commercially available from a variety of manufacturers for 0.014-inch, 0.018-inch, and 0.035-inch guidewire platforms. Although the smaller-profile balloons can go through sheaths as small as 4F, most interventions are performed through 6F sheaths to accommodate a stent when required. Early reports of stent implantation in the SFA were plagued with stent fractures and occlusions because these procedures were performed with stainless steel balloon-expandable stents.[3,4] More recently, the use of self-expanding nitinol stents has largely replaced the use of stainless steel stents in the femoropopliteal circulation because these offer excellent radial force with increased flexibility and resistance to kinking and fracturing. With the exception of the IntraCoil bare metal stent (ev3 Endovascular, Plymouth, MN), all other stainless steel and nitinol stents are designed for use in the biliary tree and used routinely in the vascular system as an off-label indication. More recently, the Viabahn (W. L. Gore & Associates, Flagstaff, AZ) polytetrafluoroethylene-covered stent has gained the Food and Drug Administration approval for use in the SFA. Although this covered stent graft has the potential for reduced myointimal hyperplasia by preventing tissue ingrowth between stent interstices, a disadvantage is the loss of collateral blood vessels along the course of the stented region and increased potential for acute ischemia in cases of stent graft failure.

OUTCOMES AFTER BALLOON ANGIOPLASTY AND STENTING

Although open surgical bypass remains the gold standard by which all percutaneous interventions must be judged, a considerable amount of literature has accumulated to support the use of balloon angioplasty and stenting of the femoropopliteal arteries. These data have led to the adoption of endovascular therapy as a first-line modality for claudication and limb-threatening ischemia in many centers.

Data regarding the effectiveness of balloon angioplasty alone have been accumulating for approximately 30 years and include both single-center trials and multiple large meta-analyses.[17-19] Results of these studies have generally shown balloon angioplasty alone to be a safe and reliable procedure with a high rate of technical success, albeit with patency rates below that of surgical bypass. Johnston[17] reported the outcomes of 254 angioplasty procedures of the femoropopliteal circulation, which included an 88% technical success rate and 6-year clinical success rate of 36%. As in most studies examining percutaneous revascularization, he found that patency rates varied with indication (claudication > occlusions) and adequacy of distal runoff. Krepel et al.[18] also reported a high technical success rate of 84% in 164 limbs, with outcomes out to 7 years. The long-term patency rates of lesions treated with angioplasty alone in this study were 70% at 5 years and 60% at 7 years.[18] A meta-analysis of 923 angioplasty procedures from 1993 to 2000 revealed 3-year patency rates that varied considerably by indication and lesion type.[19] Three-year patency was 61% for patients presenting with claudication and stenotic lesions, 48% for claudication and occlusive lesions, 41% for limb-threatening ischemia and stenotic lesions, and 30% for limb-threatening ischemia and occlusions.

Because of the vastly different recovery periods and associated morbidity between percutaneous revascularization and open surgical bypass, level I evidence from randomized controlled trials is sparse for these interventions. However, balloon angioplasty alone compared with open surgical bypass has been evaluated in a randomized controlled manner in the Bypass Versus Angioplasty in Severe Ischemia of the Leg (BASIL) Trial.[20] This was a multicenter trial in the United Kingdom that randomly assigned 452 patients over a 5-year period beginning in 1999. Two hundred twenty-eight patients were randomly assigned to bypass surgery and 224 to angioplasty for the treatment of limb-threatening ischemia. Amputation-free survival at 12 and 36 months was 68% and 57%, respectively, for those assigned to surgery first and 71% and 52%, respectively, for those randomly assigned to angioplasty first, demonstrating no significant benefit of surgery over angioplasty.

Despite the findings of the BASIL Trial regarding short-term amputation-free survival, primary patency rates have universally been shown to be lower after angioplasty than after open surgical bypass, and the implantation of stents in the SFA has been performed for many years with the hope of improving outcomes. Initial reports evaluated the use of balloon-expandable stents compared with angioplasty alone. Cejna et al.[3] randomly assigned 141 patients to angioplasty alone versus angioplasty with implantation of a balloon-expandable Palmaz stent and found no difference in 1- and 2-year angiographically determined patency rates between these groups. Because stainless steel stents have been demonstrated to develop stent fractures and associated thrombosis when placed in the SFA, the use of flexible nitinol stents has largely supplanted the use of stainless steel stents. Although data regarding the benefit of nitinol stents are somewhat conflicting, there is evidence that stent implantation may be beneficial, especially in long lesions. In the Femoral Artery Stenting Trial (FAST), 244 patients with chronic limb ischemia and lesions of length less than 10 cm were randomly assigned to percutaneous angioplasty alone or angioplasty plus nitinol stent implantation.[21] At 12-month follow-up, duplex-determined restenosis rate was 39% in the angioplasty group compared with 31% in the stent group ($p = 0.377$, not significant), nor was there a difference in Rutherford grade. However, another recent randomized trial by Schillinger et al.[22] examining the same topic offered different results. This study randomly assigned 104 patients with claudication or limb-threatening ischemia to balloon angioplasty with selective stenting versus primary stenting. At 12-month follow-up, the rates of restenosis on duplex ultrasonography were 37% and 63%, for the angioplasty group and primary stenting group, respectively ($p = 0.01$). Furthermore, the primary stenting group demonstrated significantly longer treadmill distances at 6 and 12 months than the angioplasty group. Worth noting is the difference in lesion length between these two trials. Although the FAST allowed for patients with lesions up to 100 mm in length, the average lesion length in this trial was only 45 mm, whereas the average length in the Schillinger trial was over 130 mm. When considering these results in conjunction with the lesion lengths, one may hypothesize that stenting may have increased utility in long-segment lesions, though further study will ultimately be required to determine this.

Although the benefit of stenting over angioplasty alone is not yet fully defined, it is clear that percutaneous revascularization for femoropopliteal occlusive disease can be performed with a low morbidity and achieve reasonable intermediate-term patency rates. This fact has allowed percutaneous revascularization to evolve into a first-line therapy at many centers and even to compare favorably with surgical bypass in selected patients with appropriate anatomy. There are multiple large retrospective series detailing the contemporary outcomes for balloon angioplasty and stenting with currently available devices from these centers. Conrad et al.[23] examined the results of angioplasty with or without stenting for claudication and limb-threatening ischemia in 238 consecutive limbs over a period from 2002 to 2004. The procedures included angioplasty alone in 78% and stenting in 22%. Technical success rate was 97%, major morbidity was 3%, and there were no deaths. Thirty-six–month primary patency was 54%, and limb salvage in patients with limb-threatening ischemia was

89%. These results are similar to those reported by this author in a review of 1000 percutaneous interventions over a 5-year time period from 2001 to 2006.[24] This report included 528 procedures involving angioplasty with or without stenting limited to the femoropopliteal circulation. For this subset of interventions, mortality was 1%, major complication rate was 3.2%, and technical success rate was 92%. Thirty-six–month primary patency rate was 51%, with secondary patency rate reaching 69%. Limb-salvage rate in those with limb-threatening ischemia was 80%.

CONCLUSION

The evolution of devices and techniques for balloon angioplasty and stenting of the femoropopliteal circulation has allowed percutaneous intervention to become a mainstay of therapy for occlusive disease of this region. These procedures can be accomplished with minimal morbidity and mortality in patients with either claudication or limb-threatening ischemia. Future study should be directed at determining the causes of failure after percutaneous intervention and comparing the outcomes in patients treated by balloon angioplasty and stenting with those of other minimally invasive modalities, such as atherectomy.

References

1. Centers for Disease Control and Prevention: Hospital discharge rates for nontraumatic lower extremity amputation by diabetes status—United States, 1997, *MMWR Morb Mortal Wkly Rep* 50 (43):954–958, 2001.
2. Centers for Disease Control and Prevention: Diabetes-related amputations of lower extremities in the Medicare population—Minnesota, 1993-1995, *MMWR Morb Mortal Wkly Rep* 47 (31):649–652, 1998.
3. Cejna M, Turnher S, et al: PTA versus Palmaz stent in femoropopliteal artery obstructions: a multicenter prospective randomized study, *J Vasc Interv Radiol* 12:23–31, 2001.
4. Grimm J, Muller-Hulsbeck S, et al: Randomized study to compare PTA alone versus Palmaz stent placement for femoropopliteal lesions, *J Vasc Interv Radiol* 12:935–942, 2001.
5. Klinkert P, Schepers A, Burger DH, et al: Vein versus polytetrafluoroethylene in above-knee femoropopliteal bypass grafting: five-year results of a randomized controlled trial, *J Vasc Surg* 37 (1):149–155, 2003.
6. Zannetti S, L'Italien GJ, Cambria RP: Functional outcome after surgical treatment for intermittent claudication, *J Vasc Surg* 24 (1):65–73, 1996.
7. Abbott WM, Green RM, Matsumoto T, et al: Prosthetic above-knee femoropopliteal bypass grafting: results of a multicenter randomized prospective trial. Above-Knee Femoropopliteal Study Group, *J Vasc Surg* 25(1):19–28, 1997.
8. Veith FJ, Gupta SK, Ascer E, et al: Six-year prospective multicenter randomized comparison of autologous saphenous vein and expanded polytetrafluoroethylene grafts in infrainguinal arterial reconstructions, *J Vasc Surg* 3(1):104–114, 1986.
9. Klinkert P, van Dijk PJ, Breslau PJ: Polytetrafluoroethylene femorotibial bypass grafting: 5-year patency and limb salvage, *Ann Vasc Surg* 17(5):486–491, 2003.
10. Goshima KR, Sr Mills JL, Hughes JD: A new look at outcomes after infrainguinal bypass surgery: traditional reporting standards systematically underestimate the expenditure of effort required to attain limb salvage, *J Vasc Surg* 39(2):330–335, 2004.
11. Schepers A, Klinkert P, Vrancken Peeters MP, et al: Complication registration in patients after peripheral arterial bypass surgery, *Ann Vasc Surg* 17(2):198–202, 2003.
12. L'Italien GJ, Cambria RP, Cutler BS, et al: Comparative early and late cardiac morbidity among patients requiring different vascular surgery procedures, *J Vasc Surg* 21(6):935–944, 1995.
13. Gibbons GW, Burgess AM, Guadagnoli E, et al: Return to well-being and function after infrainguinal revascularization, *J Vasc Surg* 21(1):35–44, 1995.
14. Rutherford RB, Flanigan DP, et al: Suggested standards for reports dealing with lower extremity ischemia, *J Vasc Surg* 4:80–94, 1986.
15. Brar SS, Shen AY, Jorgensen MB, et al: Sodium bicarbonate vs sodium chloride for the prevention of contrast medium–induced nephropathy in patients undergoing coronary angiography: a randomized trial, *JAMA* 300(9):1038–1046, 2008.
16. Duong MH, MacKenzie TA, Malenka DJ: *N*-acetylcysteine prophylaxis significantly reduces the risk of radiocontrast-induced nephropathy: comprehensive meta-analysis, *Catheter Cardiovasc Interv* 64(4):471–479, 2005.
17. Johnston KW: Femoral and popliteal arteries: reanalysis of results of balloon angioplasty, *Radiology* 183(3):767–771, 1992.
18. Krepel VM, van Andel GJ, van Erp WF, Breslau PJ: Percutaneous transluminal angioplasty of the femoropopliteal artery: initial and long-term results, *Radiology* 156(2):325–328, 1985.
19. Muradin GS, Bosch JL, Stijnen T, et al: Balloon dilation and stent implantation for treatment of femoropopliteal arterial disease: meta-analysis, *Radiology* 221(1):137–145, 2001.
20. Adam DJ, Beard JD, Cleveland T, et al: BASIL trial participants. Bypass versus angioplasty in severe ischaemia of the leg (BASIL): multicentre, randomised controlled trial, *Lancet* 366 (9501):1925–1934, 2005.
21. Krankenberg H, Schlüter M, Steinkamp HJ, et al: Nitinol stent implantation versus percutaneous transluminal angioplasty in superficial femoral artery lesions up to 10 cm in length: the femoral artery stenting trial (FAST), *Circulation* 116(3):285–292, 2007.
22. Schillinger M, Sabeti S, Loewe C, Dick P, et al: Balloon angioplasty versus implantation of nitinol stents in the superficial femoral artery, *N Engl J Med* 354(18):1879–1888, 2006.
23. Conrad MF, Cambria RP, Stone DH, et al: Intermediate results of percutaneous endovascular therapy of femoropopliteal occlusive disease: a contemporary series, *J Vasc Surg* 44(4):762–769, 2006.
24. DeRubertis BG, Faries PL, McKinsey JF, et al: Shifting paradigms in the treatment of lower extremity vascular disease: a report of 1000 percutaneous interventions, *Ann Surg* 246(3):415–423, 2007, discussion 422-424.

CHAPTER

29

Peripheral Arterial Atherectomy for Infrainguinal Arterial Occlusive Disease

Jacob Buth, Alexander V. Tielbeek

Peripheral arterial occlusive disease of the arteries to the leg has an age-adjusted prevalence of 12%.[1,2] The major symptoms for this localization of peripheral arterial occlusive disease are intermittent claudication (IC) and critical leg ischemia (CLI). The goals for treatment in these patients are to relieve symptoms at exercise, ischemic pain at rest, and ulceration and to prevent limb loss.[3]

The treatment of femoropopliteal and infrapopliteal arteries has been among the least effective of all endovascular procedures. These arteries are much longer than elsewhere in the human body, usually have a high plaque burden and a relatively low flow, and are exposed to excessive forces from compression by the adductor tendon and flexion in the hip and knee joints. These stresses make these vessel segments prone to atherosclerotic disease.

In patients with IC exercise treatment usually is prescribed as a first step. However, angioplasty, where feasible, is more effective in increasing walking distance than exercise, and the cost-effectiveness ratio is within the generally accepted range.[4] Traditional surgical treatment of infrainguinal vascular disease consists of a femoropopliteal bypass. Although bypass surgery provides superior long-term patency, clinical relief of claudication, and limb-salvage rates, it is associated with a high morbidity and mortality.[5,6] Lamuraglia[6] provided statistics on 2404 bypass grafts. Overall results were a 30-day mortality/major morbidity rate of 19.5% and 2.7%, 11.7% wound infection, and major systemic complications in 5.9%.[6] This nontrivial complication rate explains the continued interest in the development of effective endovascular techniques. In addition, from a cost-effectiveness point of view, balloon angioplasty is the preferred initial strategy over bypass in patients with disabling intermittent claudication and femoropopliteal stenoses or occlusions.[7]

ENDOVASCULAR PROCEDURES FOR FEMOROPOPLITEAL AND INFRAPOPLITEAL DISEASE

Although balloon angioplasty can be an effective treatment for short lesions in the iliac arteries, the results of percutaneous transluminal angioplasty for more complex or longer lesions in the femoropopliteal segment had been disappointing. Factors that negatively affect long-term outcome of treatment include lesion length, total occlusion, diabetes mellitus, poor crural artery runoff, CLI, and the "normal" diameter of the target artery.[8,9] The TransAtlantic Inter-Society Consensus (TASC) document states that there are insufficient data to recommend endovascular treatment in TASC C lesions, that is, single stenoses or occlusions longer than 5 cm and multiple stenoses or occlusions, each 3 to 5 cm, with or without heavy calcification.[10] TASC A and B lesions are established indications for endovascular treatment. Transluminal balloon angioplasty of femoropopliteal stenoses in claudicants demonstrated primary patency rates after 1 year of 47% to 86%. The negative effect of lesion length on patency was primarily caused by failed initial crossings in longer lesions and in total occlusions. Newer studies had better outcomes caused by improvements in guidewires and catheters. The representatives at TASC of the Cardiovascular and Interventional Radiology Society of Europe found this a reason to increase the threshold for endovascular treatment of single stenoses and occlusions to 10 cm. Femoropopliteal stents have been applied for eccentric stenoses, long-segment lesions, and stenoses caused by intimal hyperplasia at graft anastomoses. In addition, stents have proved to be useful as a bailout when balloon angioplasty failed because of extensive dissection. However, restenosis in the stented segment caused by intimal hyperplasia is quite frequent in the first 9 months. The primary patency after 1 year following stenting of femoropopliteal stenoses or occlusions ranged from 22% to 81%.[11]

Stent implantation and balloon dilatation for the treatment of femoropopliteal artery arterial disease have been compared in a number of older and more recent randomized studies and meta-analyses. Patients with IC and short (<10 mm) lesions dominated these studies. Both techniques yielded similar midterm and long-term patency rates.[12,13] For more severe femoropopliteal lesions, the results of stent implantation seem more favorable.[14] The make of the stent may present a difference. In a recent, as-yet-unpublished study (RESILIENT trial), new-technology nitinol self-expanding stents were compared with balloon dilatation alone and demonstrated residual/recurrent stenoses at 12 months in only 13% of the stent group compared with 54% in patients with percutaneous transluminal angioplasty alone.[15]

Patients with CLI and femoropopliteal disease may be treated with use of a comparable algorithm as in claudication. Obviously, effectiveness of endovascular treatment in this patient category is affected by longer lesions, higher incidence of total occlusions, and poor runoff. In addition, the prevalence of diabetes is significantly higher and limb loss is more likely when treatment fails. The ability of endovascular techniques to alleviate arterial disease, either alone or in conjunction with catheter treatment or bypass of proximal disease, is appealing.[16] The recent application of bioabsorbable stents including poly-L-lactic and magnesium alloy in the infrapopliteal segment is the newest development. Bosiers et al.[17] showed that these stents had a primary patency of 72% at 12-month follow-up. Restenosis rates in femoropopliteal vessels were higher than with balloon angioplasty.

The application of the sirolimus-coated SMART nitinol self-expanding stent (Cordis, Bridgewater, NJ) has been assessed in femoropopliteal arteries in the SIROCCO trials.[18] These studies failed to document a significantly lower in-stent restenosis rate in patients receiving the drug-eluting stents compared with noncoated SMART stents at 6 months. In the sirolimus group as well as in the noncoated stents, stent fractures were observed in some patients. No other studies have reported any proof of advantage of drug-eluting stents either.

PERIPHERAL ARTERIAL ATHERECTOMY

Of the various atherectomy methods that were developed in the 1990s, two broad categories can be distinguished: extirpative and ablative. In the first, atheroma is removed by means of shaving or cutting and is subsequently collected for removal. The second method includes pulverization of atheroma into particles that can traverse the capillary system or are resolved by a chemical reaction. Atherectomy is performed in the catheterization laboratory or in the operating room. Procedural monitoring is most often by means of fluoroscopic angiography, although intravascular ultrasonography (IVUS) and angioscopy are sometimes used.[19,20]

The primary target area of atherectomy is the femoropopliteal segment, but application in the iliac, tibioperoneal, subclavian, and renal arteries has been reported as well. The Simpson AtheroCath, Transluminal Extraction Catheter (TEC), and Pullback Atherectomy Catheter (PAC) are extirpative devices; the Rotablator and Kensey catheter are ablative devices.[21-25] Most of these devices have been withdrawn from the market for several years.

Directional Atherectomy

Atherectomy was considered a major advance in percutaneous coronary intervention in the early 1990s. However, larger randomized clinical trials demonstrated relatively higher rates of restenoses, and short- and long-term outcomes were not improved over balloon angioplasty.[26] The Simpson AtheroCath was the original atherectomy device for coronary vessels. Use of this device in peripheral arteries has been extensively assessed in the author's institution. Technical limitations and inferior long-term results as opposed to balloon angioplasty were observed.[27,28] The atherectomy catheter combined a "cutting and retrieval" mechanism. A balloon was inflated to push the cutter against the atheromatous arterial wall. By this, the obstructing plaque protrudes into the cylindric housing of the device. A high-speed rotating cutter shaves off the plaque and pushes it into a collection chamber at the tip. The size of the atherectomy catheter is chosen so that it is slightly greater than the arterial target segment. The rotating cutter (2000 rpm) is driven by a battery-powered motor. Multiple passes with the rotary knife switched on are made. During the procedure the collection chamber has to be emptied several times, and the process is repeated until a satisfactory angiographic result is obtained (Figure 29-1). The initial results with this apparatus were favorable with technical success rates varying from 86% to 97%.[22,29-31] Technical success is defined as absence of residual stenosis of greater than 30% diameter reduction.[28] Complications were infrequent.

The basis for the use of all atherectomy devices is the potential advantage of debulking plaque, which theoretically reduces the risk of reocclusion or restenosis compared with use of balloon dilatation. Overall, initial outcome and complication rates appeared to be acceptable, but intermediate and long-term efficacy of Simpson's atherectomy has generally been disappointing. Restenosis has been explained in the literature in various

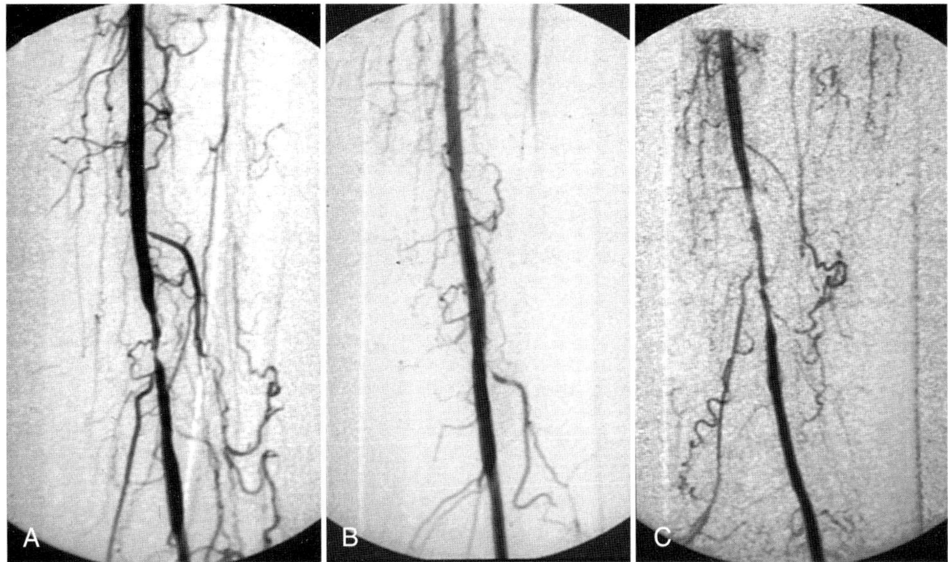

FIGURE 29-1 **A,** Initial stenosis. **B,** Results of initial atherectomy with the Simpson Atherotome. **C,** Arteriography demonstrating restenosis after 6 months. It is thought that the barotrauma, caused by balloon inflation, may be responsible for the relatively high restenosis rate with this device.

ways.[32,33] Insufficient tissue removal, luminal enlargement partially caused by the distending effect of the low-pressure balloon with the Simpson catheter, and a higher rate of myointimal hyperplasia resulting from a greater arterial trauma caused by the device have all been proposed as causes of late luminal loss.

The ability of any devices to influence the restenosis pattern depends on initial lumen gain during the procedure and on the process of myointimal hyperplasia, which causes restenosis. The net result depends on which effect is stronger. Vroegindeweij et al.,[28] in a serial follow-up of treated arterial segments using color duplex scanning, assessed the pattern of restenosis in patients who had undergone either directional atherectomy or balloon dilatation. It appears that early after treatment there is little difference between atherectomy and balloon angioplasty with regard to lumen width. After an average period of 8 months, however, substantially more restenoses were observed in patients who had undergone atherectomy (58% vs. 34%) with balloon angioplasty, whereas in the subgroup of patients with lesions of 2 cm or greater length the difference was statistically significant. The duration of the interval suggested that increased myointimal hyperplasia is the primary factor responsible for the decline in patency. The difference observed between results of balloon angioplasty and those of atherectomy may be explained by the stronger simulation of the smooth muscle cells in the media achieved via the latter method (Figure 29-2).

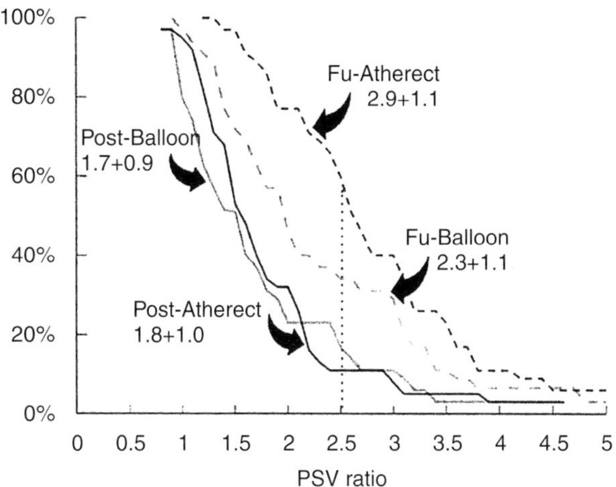

FIGURE 29-2 Cumulative frequency distribution curves showing the percentage of patients with given peak systolic velocity (PSV) ratios within the first 3 months *(Post-Atherect, Post-Balloon)* and at the time of the highest observed PSV ratio during late follow-up *(Fu-Atherect, Fu-Balloon).* The value on the ordinate represents the percentage of patients with PSV ratios greater than the corresponding value at the abscissa. Starting at a normal level of approximately 0.0, 100% of patients have a greater PSV ratio. The 3-month curves reflect a similar distribution of luminal dimensions among the two treatment groups. At late follow-up the curve for atherectomy lies to the right of the curve for balloon angioplasty, reflecting an increased restenosis rate in atherectomy-treated patients. The percentage of patients with a PSV ratio of 2.5 or greater is 58% in atherectomy-treated patients and 34% in balloon angioplasty–treated patients (see *dotted vertical line*).

IVUS has been used to enhance the procedural luminal gain of plaque excision. Tielbeek et al.[19] demonstrated the efficacy of this adjunct in that the minimal transverse lumen diameter and free luminal area increased substantially after IVUS-directed additional atherectomy passes (Figure 29-3). However, the improved luminal enlargement did not result in a better 1-year patency. It is likely that arterial wall overstretch and Dotter effect may have been responsible for the observed favorable

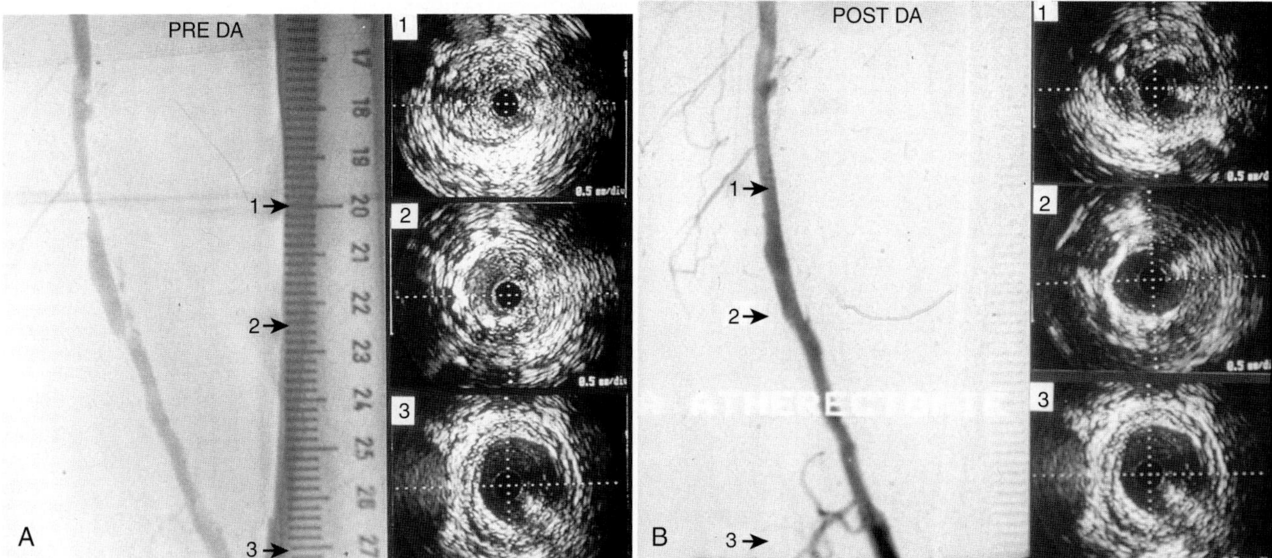

FIGURE 29-3 Arteriography and IVUS cross-sectional images at stenotic sides of the superficial femoral artery (corresponding with *upper arrow* and *middle arrow* in arteriogram) were subsequently treated with atherectomy. The *lower arrow* in arteriogram demonstrates a normal reference arterial segment. **A,** IVUS findings correspond to arteriographic findings. **B,** Similar segments illustrated after atherectomy demonstrated satisfactory lumen enlargement after multiple atherectomy passages.

FIGURE 29-4 Artist's drawing of the SilverHawk Plaque Excision System. The mode of apposition of the rotating cutter to the atheroma is by activation of a hinge system (different from the balloon action in the old Simpson system).

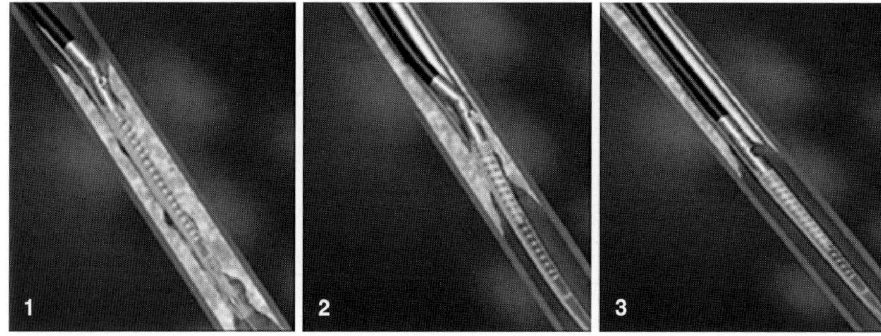

initial result. A further reduction in plaque volume than obtained with the Simpson device may result in better midterm outcome. These and other observations caused the Simpson atherectomy device to be withdrawn from the market some years ago.

CURRENT ATHERECTOMY METHODS

Excisional Atherectomy

More recently, excisional atherectomy has gained interest. The SilverHawk Plaque Excision System (FoxHollow Technologies, Redwood City, CA) was approved in 2003 by the U.S. Food and Drug Administration for the treatment of peripheral arterial occlusive disease and has become the dominant current directional atherectomy device in use for lower-extremity peripheral arterial disease.

The SilverHawk device debulks without balloon inflation for apposition, and it apposes the atheroma through a hinge system (Figure 29-4). The working segment of the apparatus contains a rotating carbide cutter, with variable height depending on the device used, which rotates at a speed of 8000 rpm. It shaves atherosclerotic material from the arterial wall to compress it within a distal storage chamber. This chamber is in the nose cone and acts as a large container for atherosclerotic debris. Multiple catheter passes are made through the diseased segment, during which the blade is rotationally directed sequentially toward all quadrants of the vessel lumen (Figure 29-5). Significant debulking of the lesion can be achieved without barotrauma as no balloon compression is involved. Meanwhile, the cutter can be used in adjunction with balloon angioplasty. The cutter is powered by a palm-sized drive unit. The SilverHawk comes in seven different sizes to allow treatment from the femoral to the tibial or pedal vessels. Of the femoropopliteal catheters,

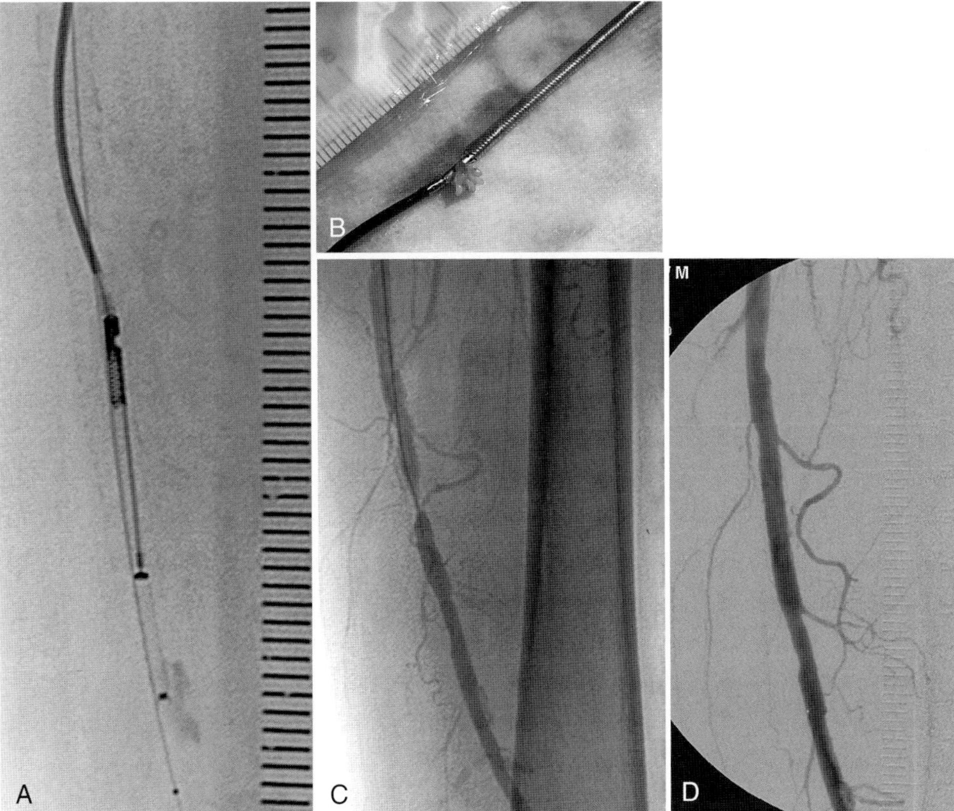

FIGURE 29-5 **A,** Arteriogram of SilverHawk device within the superficial femoral artery. **B,** Excised atheromatous material after one directional passage. **C,** Arteriogram of the initial stenotic lesion treated in this patient. **D,** Satisfactory end result after multiple passages in four directional quadrants of the vessel lumen.

the MS (for vessel diameters of 3.5-5.0 mm) design has a somewhat lower-profile cutter than the standard large LS (for vessel diameters of 4.5-7.0 mm) design, which is intended to be used in calcified lesions. In-stent restenoses can be treated as well.

Peer-reviewed literature regarding outcome of SilverHawk's excisional atherectomy accumulates slowly. At a search of the recent literature (from January 2006 until June 2008) we found five studies on excisional atherectomy in the femoropopliteal[34-38] and one in the infrapopliteal[39] vessels that met the accepted Society for Vascular Surgery/International Society for Cardiovascular Surgery criteria of reporting. However, not in all studies were life-table methods used to present primary and secondary patency (i.e., freedom from recurrent or new stenoses in the target vessel) and not all studies used routine duplex surveillance to identify restenosis or new disease (Table 29-1). The primary patency ranged from 10% to 84% after 1 year. The highest primary patency was observed by Zeller et al.[35] in a subgroup of de novo lesions. These investigators observed worse results in restenotic lesions and in in-stent restenoses. Secondary patency was in some studies markedly higher because of the use of secondary surgical interventions. Target vessel revascularization rates were between 4% and 70%. The amputation rate ranged from nil to 25%. Zeller et al.[39] also reported on the use of excisional atherectomy in the infrapopliteal arteries and observed a 58% primary and 88% secondary patency after 1 year. The concluding comments in the reviewed reports on the SilverHawk atherectomy performance ranged from "safe and effective for use in lesions causing CLI," to "poor midterm outcome." For use in the femoropopliteal segment two of the investigator groups had a relatively positive judgment, whereas two were primarily negative and one commented that the performance was similar to that of other endovascular techniques. The experience with the treatment of infrapopliteal lesions was described as "encouraging."[39] One study reported on the risks and consequences of macroembolization as assessed by using embolic filter devices. Compared with angioplasty and stenting, SilverHawk atherectomy was associated with a higher incidence of embolization. In all patients in this device category group macro-debris was found in the filter. The clinical significance of this finding, however, needs to be determined in future studies.[40]

TABLE 29-1 Peer-Reviewed Publications 2006 to 2008 on Experience With the Silverhawk Excisional Atherectomy Device

Study	No. patients	No. limbs	No. lesions	Lesion severity	Lesion length	Symptom severity (%)	Procedural success (%)
Kandzari, et al.[34]	69	76	159	34% had vessel occlusion	65 millimeter	CLI	99
Zeller, et al.[35,*]	84	100	131	—	31-43 millimeter	IC or CLI	86-100
Yancey, et al.[36]	16	17	18	TASC-C	TASC-C	CLI	88
Keeling, et al.[37]	60	66	70	TASC-C,D	88 millimeter	CLI in 67	87
Chung SW, et al.[38]							
Zeller, et al.[39†]	20	20	40	TASC-A,B,C	—	CLI in 60	90
	36	—	49	22% occlusion	46 millimeter	CLI in 53	98

	Early adverse events	Late adverse events	Follow-up method	Primary patency	Secondary patency or other main outcome	Target vessel/lesion revascularization	Conclusion of study
Kandzari, et al.[34]	1%	23% at 6 months	Clinical	—	82% limbsalvage at 6 months	4% at 6 months	Safe and effective in CLI
Zeller, et al,[35,*]	—	—	Duplex US	54%-84% at 12 months	91%-100% at 12 months	16%-47% at 12 months	Favorable results in de novo lesions but not in restenoses
Yancey, et al.[36]	17 events including 3 amputations	2 amputations	Duplex US	22% at 12 months	70% limb salvage	19% including surgical revascularization	High rate of restenosis at midterm
Keeling, et al.[37]	—	17% restenosis 33% reocclusions 1.7% amputations	Duplex US	62% at 12 months	76% at 12 months	14% incl. surgical revascularzation	Outcome similar to other endovascular treatments. TASC CD: Higher rate of restenosis
Chung SW, et al.[38]	15%	25% amputations	Duplex US	10%	70% including surgical reinterventions in most patients	70% including surgical revasculation	Poor midterm outcome
Zeller et al. 39[†]	3%	No amputations	Duplex US	58% at 12 months	88% at 12 months	24%	Midterm results encouraging

*This article used subgroups: de novo lesions, restenosis, in-stent restenosis.
†This study included only treatments of infrapopliteal lesions.
CLI, Critical limb ischemia; *IC*, intermittent claudication; *duplex US*, duplex ultrasound; *amputation*, limb amputation.

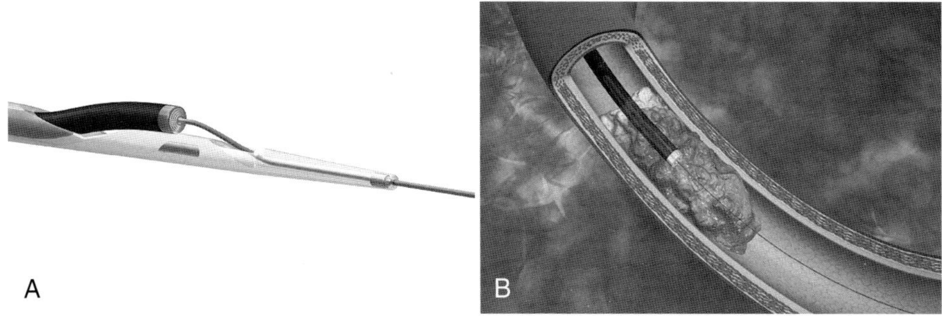

FIGURE 29-6 A, The Spectranetics excimer laser system adapted for eccentric recanalization, that is, the Turbo-Booster system. B, Artist rendering of the laser atherectomy recanalization of a complete occlusion of a peripheral artery.

Rotational Atherectomy

Since the heyday of the different rotational atherectomy devices in the 1990s, two new systems have been assessed in recent years. The principle of the Diamond 360 degrees Orbital Atherectomy System was described by Heuser.[41] An eccentrically mounted diamond-coated crown rotates at high speed to sand away plaque as the crown is slowly advanced through narrowed or occluded sections of an artery. As crown rotations increase centrifugal force presses the crown against the stenotic lesion to enhance plaque removal. Clinical experience with this system has not been published yet.

The Pathway PV atherectomy system (Pathway Medical Technologies, Redmond, WA) was assessed by Zeller et al.[42] This system is a rotating, aspirating, expandable catheter for removal of atherosclerotic debris and thrombus. The catheter tip remains at a defined nominal diameter (2.1 mm) when spinning clockwise but expands to a maximum diameter (3.0 mm) when rotating counterclockwise. Saline solution is infused into the treatment area through ports located at the distal segment of the catheter. The excised material is aspirated via ports into the catheter lumen and transported to a collection bag. Two pumps are used, one for aspiration and one for infusion. This atherectomy device was used in 15 patients with lower limb ischemia of Rutherford stages 2 to 5. The interventional success was 100%. Adjunctive balloon angioplasty was used in 47% and stenting in 13%. The severe adverse event rate at 30 days was 20%, including one vessel wall perforation, one false aneurysm at the access site, and one dissection and embolization (resolved by aspiration thrombectomy). Further treatment data will be collected in a European multicenter registry.[42]

Excimer Laser Atherectomy

Laser-assisted balloon angioplasty was initially introduced in the 1980s. The original laser systems, most frequently neodymium:yttrium-aluminum-garnet lasers, were associated with considerable vessel wall damage from thermal energy, which resulted in a high incidence of vessel spasm, thrombosis, and failure of the revascularization. The excimer laser does not seem to have the technical shortcomings of "hot lasers" and has been introduced as a vascular atherectomy device. The advantage of ultraviolet light lies in its short penetration depth of 50 μm and its ability to break molecular bonds by a photochemical rather than a thermal process. Lower-energy photons cause less thermal damage, and the risk of vessel wall perforation is minimized by the use of more flexible catheters. Laser atherectomy has the potential to treat patients at high surgical risk because of their medical condition or complex anatomic lesions (Figure 29-6). Despite the treatment of long occlusions, Scheinert et al.[43] observed a high technical success rate (90.5%). The primary patency rate at 1 year was disappointing, although a secondary patency rate of 75% was achieved because of intensive surveillance and frequent reintervention. A limiting factor of laser atherectomy has been the inability to create a channel much larger than the diameter of the laser wire. Although technical improvements have been developed and are subject of clinical investigation, clinical outcomes of laser-assisted balloon angioplasty constitute the majority of current reported experience.[44] Midterm outcomes were published by Stoner et al.[45] of a patient group with a mixed severity of symptoms (65% CLI and 35% claudication), treated lesions in 72% in the femoropopliteal segment, in 35% infrapopliteal, and lesion severity varying from TASC A to D. This study demonstrated a technical success rate (<50% residual stenoses) of 88%.[45] Adjunctive angioplasty was used in 75% and stenting in 13% of cases. Laser-assisted revascularization was the definitive treatment for 58% of patients, and the overall primary patency rate at 12 months was 44%. The limb salvage rate at 1 year of patients with CLI was 55%. Risk factors for amputation included renal failure, diabetes mellitus, poor tibial runoff, and failed primary patency. These surgeons concluded that laser atherectomy can be used with a high initial success rate. Systemic factors known to severely compromise outcome of endovascular therapy affected midterm results of laser atherectomy including the chance of limb salvage. In summary, the overall results tend to mirror other contemporary percutaneous revascularization reports.[45]

CONCLUSION

The last decade is characterized by the development of a series of new devices that merely are updates of atherectomy devices and other endovascular systems used in the 1990s. Advancements are modest; however, they seem real. Initial procedural success has improved in the currently available technologies. The diffuse nature of vascular occlusive disease continued to compromise midterm endovascular outcome. In addition to active treatment of systemic risk factors, careful surveillance at follow-up and frequent use of secondary procedures including surgical revascularization are effective to improve outcome. These observations do not alter the preferred strategy of "endovascular treatment first" in the integral interventional approach to the patient with vascular obstructive lower-limb disease.

References

1. Crigui MH, Fronek A, Barrett-Connor E, et al: The prevalence of peripheral arterial disease in a defined population, *Circulation* 71:510–515, 1985.
2. Hiatt WR, Hoag S, Hamman RF: Effect of diagnostic criteria on the prevalence of peripheral arterial disease: the San Luis Valley Diabetes Study, *Circulation* 91:1472–1479, 1995.
3. Hiatt WR: Medical treatment of peripheral arterial disease and claudication, *N Engl J Med* 21:1608–1621, 2001.
4. de Vries SO, Visser K, de Vries JA, et al: Intermittent claudication: cost-effectiveness of revascularization versus exercise therapy, *Radiology* 222:25–36, 2002.
5. Adam JD, Beard JD, Cleveland T, et al: Bypass versus angioplasty in severe ischaemia of the leg (BASIL): multicentre, randomised controlled trial, *Lancet* 366:1925–1934, 2005.
6. Lamuraglia G: Data from the National Surgical Quality Improvement Programme, presented at the Vascular Annual Meeting, June 6-8, San Diego, CA.
7. Hunink MGM, Wong JB, Donaldson MC, et al: Revascularization for femoropopliteal disease: a decision and cost-effectiveness analysis, *JAMA* 274:165–171, 1995.
8. Henriksen LO, Jorgensen B, Holstein BE, et al: Percutaneous transluminal angioplasty of infrarenal arteries in intermittent claudication, *Acta Chir Scand* 154:573–576, 1988.
9. Jeans WD, Armstrong S, Cole SE, et al: Fate of patients undergoing transluminal angioplasty for lower-limb ischemia, *Radiology* 177:559–564, 1990.
10. TransAtlantic Inter-Society Consensus (TASC) document on management of peripheral arterial disease (PAD), *J Vasc Surg* 31:S104, 2000.
11. Gray BH, Olin JW: Limitations of percutaneous transluminal angioplasty with stenting for femoropopliteal disease, *Semin Vasc Surg* 10:8–16, 1997.
12. Vroegindeweij D, Vos LD, Tielbeek AV, et al: Balloon angioplasty combined with primary stenting versus balloon angioplasty alone in femoropopliteal obstructions: a comparative randomized study, *Cardiovasc Intervent Radiol* 20:420–425, 1997.
13. Krankenberg H, Schlüter M, Steinkamp HJ, et al: Nitinol stent implantation versus percutaneous transluminal angioplasty in superficial femoral artery lesions up to 10 cm in length: the femoral artery stenting trial (FAST), *Circulation* 116:285–292, 2007.
14. Muradin GS, Bosch JL, Stijnen T, et al: Balloon dilatation and stent implantation for treatment of femoropopliteal arterial disease: meta-analysis, *Radiology* 221:137–145, 2001.
15. Katzen BT, Laird JR, et al: For the Resilient study participants: the Resilient trial, *Intervent News* 28(1): 2007.
16. Varty K, Bolia A, Naylor AR, Bell PR, London NJ: Infrapopliteal percutaneous transluminal angioplasty by safe and successful procedure, *Eur J Vasc Endovasc Surg* 9:341–345, 1995.
17. Bosiers M, et al: BEST BKT trial, *Intervent News* (30):10, 2008.
18. Duda SH, Bosiers M, Lammer J, et al: Sirolimus-eluting versus bare nitinol stent for obstructive superficial femoral artery disease. The SIROCCO II trial, *J Vasc Interv Radiol* 16:331–338, 2005.
19. Tielbeek AV, Vroegindeweij D, Buth J, et al: Comparison of intravascular sonography and intra-arterial digital subtraction angiography after directional atherectomy of short lesions in femoropopliteal arteries, *J Vasc Surg* 23:436–445, 1996.
20. Marzelle J: Angioscopy in the operating room, *J Cardiovasc Surg (Torino)* 37(suppl 3):11–16, 1996.
21. Schwarten DE, Katzen PT, Simpson JB, et al: Simpson catheter for percutaneous transluminal removal of atheroma, *Am J Radiol* 150:799–801, 1998.
22. Simpson JB, Zimmerman JJ, Selmon RM: Transluminal artherectomy. Initial clinical results in 27 patients, *Circulation* 74 (suppl 2). II-203, 1986.
23. Wholey MH, Jarmolowski CR: New reperfusion devices. The Kensey catheter, the atherolytic reperfusion wire device and the transluminal extractor catheter, *Radiology* 172:947–952, 1989.
24. White CJ: Peripheral atherectomy with the pullback atherectomy catheter: procedural safety and efficacy in a multicenter trial, *J Endovasc Surg* 5:9–17, 1998.
25. Myers KA, Denton MJ: Infrainguinal atherectomy using the Auth Rotablator. Patency rates and clinical success for 36 procedures, *J Endovasc Surg* 2:67–73, 1995.
26. Adelman AG, Cohen EA, Kinball BP, et al: A comparison of directional atherectomy with balloon angioplasty for lesions of the left anterior descending coronary artery, *N Engl J Med* 329:228–233, 1993.
27. Tielbeek AV, Vroegindeweij D, Buth J, et al: Comparison of balloon angioplasty and Simpson atherectomy for lesions in the femoropopliteal artery: angiographic and clinical results of a prospective randomised trial, *J Vasc Interv Radiol* 7:837–844, 1996.
28. Vroegindeweij D, Tielbeek AV, Buth J, et al: Directional atherectomy versus balloon angioplasty in segmental femoropopliteal artery disease: two-year follow-up using color-flow duplex, *J Vasc Surg* 21:235–269, 1995.
29. von Pölnitz A, Merligh A, Berger H, et al: Percutaneous peripheral atherectomy: angiographic and clinical follow-up of 60 patients, *J Am Coll Cardiol* 15:682–688, 1990.
30. Dorros G, Iyer S, Lewin R: Angiographic follow-up and clinical outcome of 126 patients after percutaneous directional atherectomy Simpson AtheroCath for occlusive peripheral vascular disease, *Cathet Cardiovasc Diagn* 22:79–84, 1991.

31. Graor RA, Withlow P: Atherectomy for peripheral vascular disease: two-year patency and factors influencing patency, *J Am Coll Cardiol* 17(suppl):106A, 1991.
32. McLean GK: Percutaneous peripheral atherectomy, *J Vasc Interv Radiol* 4:465–480, 1993.
33. Waller BF, Pinkerton CA: Cutters, shavers and scrapers. The importance of atherectomy devices and clinical relevance of tissue removal, *J Am Coll Cardiol* 15:426–428, 1990.
34. Kandzari DE, Kiesz RS, Allie D, et al: Procedural and clinical outcomes with catheter-based plaque excision in critical limb ischemia, *J Endovasc Ther* 13:12–22, 2006.
35. Zeller T, Rastan A, Sixt S, et al: Long-term results after directional atherectomy of femoropopliteal lesions, *J Am Coll Cardiol* 48:1573–1578, 2006.
36. Yancey AE, Minion DJ, Rodriguez C, et al: Peripheral atherectomy in TransAtlantic Inter-Society Consensus type C femoropopliteal lesions for limb salvage, *J Vasc Surg* 44:503–509, 2006.
37. Keeling BW, Shames ML, Stone PA, et al: Plaque excision with the SilverHawk catheter: early results in patients with claudication or critical limb ischemia, *J Vasc Surg* 45:25–31, 2007.
38. Chung SW, Sharafuddin J, Chigurupati R, et al: Midterm patency following atherectomy for infrainguinal occlusive disease: a word of caution, *Ann Vasc Surg* 22:358–365, 2008.
39. Zeller T, Sixt S, Schwarzwälder U, Schwarz T, et al: Two-year results after directional atherectomy of infrapopliteal arteries with the SilverHawk device, *J Endovasc Ther* 14:232–240, 2007.
40. Shammas N, Dippel EJ, Coiner D, et al: Preventing lower extremity distal embolization using embolic filter protection: results of the PROTECT Registry, *J Endovasc Ther* 15:270–276, 2008.
41. Heuser RR: Treatment of lower extremity vascular disease: the Diamondback 360 degrees Orbital Atherectomy System, *J Cardiovasc Surg (Torino)* 49:167–177, 2008.
42. Zeller T, Krankenberg H, Rastan A, et al: Percutaneous rotational and aspiration atherectomy in infrainguinal peripheral arterial occlusive disease: a multicenter pilot study, *J Endovasc Ther* 14:357–364, 2007.
43. Scheinert D, Laird JR Jr, Schroder M, et al: Excimer laser–assisted recanalization of long, chronic superficial femoral artery occlusions, *J Endovasc Ther* 8:156–166, 2001.
44. Laird JR, Zeler T, Gray BH, et al: Limb salvage following laser-assisted angioplasty for critical limb ischemia: results of the LACI multicenter trial, *J Endovasc Ther* 13:1–11, 2006.
45. Stoner MC, deFreitas DJ, Phade SV, et al: Mid-term results with laser atherectomy in the treatment of infrainguinal occlusive disease, *J Vasc Surg* 46:289–295, 2007.

CHAPTER

30

Endarterectomy in Infrainguinal Arterial Occlusive Disease

Suzanne S. Gisbertz, Jean-Paul de Vries, Frans L. Moll

The first semiclosed removal of an arterial obstruction was done in 1894, by the surgeon Sévéréanu, who called the procedure "desobliteration par catheterisme artériel." He passed a urethral catheter through the crural arteries at the site of a below-knee amputation incision and restored blood flow. This resulted in a below-knee amputation instead of an above-knee amputation that was originally planned. Guinard, in 1901, attempted in a similar case to remove thrombus in an artery with a long clamp, and Martin noted the restoration of collateral circulation in those cases. Lejars, in 1902, was probably the first to deobstruct occluded arteries by passing catheters through one or more arteriotomy sites. Delbet, in 1911, knowing about these attempts, stated that thrombectomy alone in cases of "arteriitis" had little chance for prolonged success because uncorrected vascular wall disease would cause rethrombosis in the vessel in a short time.[1] The clinical application of these anecdotal reports did not occur until 1947, when the first successful semiclosed endarterectomy by Dos Santos of Lisbon, Portugal, was presented by René Leriche to the Academy of Surgery.[2] This procedure may be considered the precursor of semiclosed endarterectomy with the use of a ring stripper, described by De Bakey and Cooley[3] in 1954 for the aorta and iliac arteries, and by Cannon and Barker[4] in 1955 for the superficial femoral artery (SFA). The first intimal ring stripper consisted of a metal shaft with a metal ring at the end, at a 90-degree angle to the shaft. Cannon and Barker positioned the ring with sharp edges at a 105-degree angle to the shaft. Some of the first strippers were made of flexible piano strings. Barker preferred a heavier design in which the edges of the ring were blunt to minimize the risk of perforation. Vollmar modified the ring stripper in the late 1960s by placing the ring at a 135-degree angle and by using a smooth elliptical ring instead of a circular one (Figure 30-1). This model supposedly causes the least shear stress when the intimal core is loosened from the adherent adventitial arterial wall. The Cannon and Vollmar ring loops are still being used today. Van der Heijden et al.[5] prospectively followed 231 successfully performed semiclosed endarterectomies. A 5-year overall cumulative primary patency rate of 71% was achieved at a single institution.[5]

REMOTE ENDARTERECTOMY

The operative strategy of semiclosed endarterectomy was largely abandoned in the 1970s, as bypass surgery superseded it. A variation on semiclosed endarterectomy is the less-invasive remote SFA endarterectomy (RSFAE) developed in 1994. Short-term and midterm patency rates of retrospective studies so far are promising, with reported primary patency rates of 61% to 69% at 18 to 33 months.[6,7] Besides promising patency rates this procedure has the benefits of minimally invasive surgery because only one groin incision is needed; there are possibly fewer wound-related problems and prosthetic material can be avoided. In addition, hospital stay will likely be shorter. Furthermore, this procedure does not compromise future surgical interventions, including venous or prosthetic bypass grafting. When reocclusion occurs, the consequences are generally less severe compared with bypass grafting: amputation is rarely necessary. Smeets et al.[8] evaluated a group of 239 patients after successful remote endarterectomy. Seventy-nine (33%) SFAs reoccluded; however, 80% of patients still had improved or unchanged symptoms. Only two below-knee amputations were performed.[8]

Technique

The common femoral artery, SFA, and profunda femoris artery are exposed through a single groin

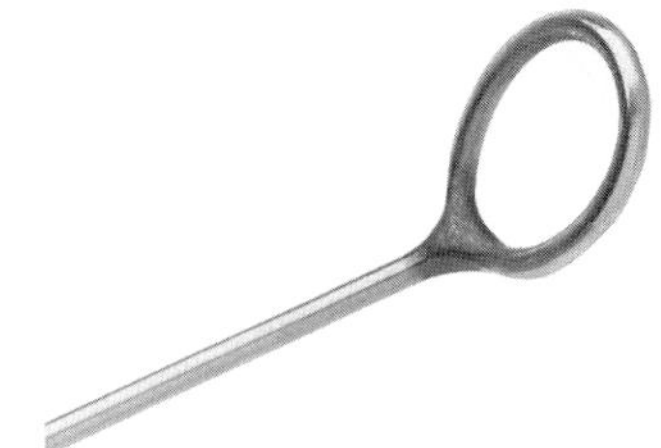

FIGURE 30-1 The Vollmar Dissector.

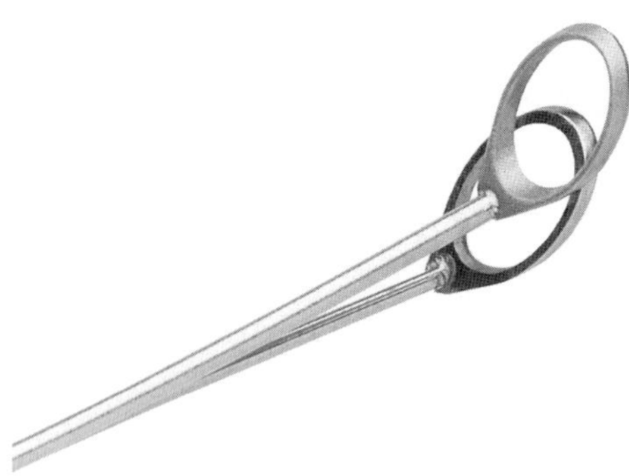

FIGURE 30-2 The Mollring Cutter.

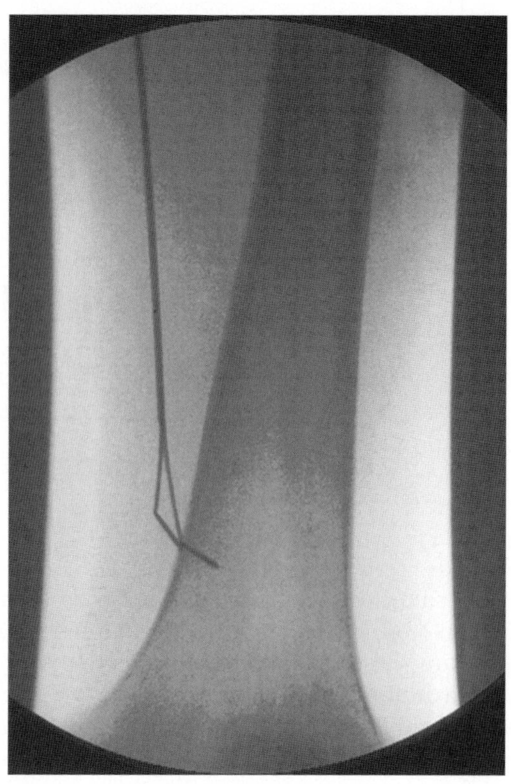

FIGURE 30-3 The Mollring Cutter transecting the intima core under fluoroscopic guidance.

incision. Arteriotomy in the proximal SFA is followed by dissection of the intima core beyond the occluded SFA segment with use of the Vollmar ring stripper (Vollmar Dissector, Aesculap, South San Francisco, CA) under fluoroscopic guidance. The ring stripper is exchanged for a Mollring Cutter (LeMaitre Vascular, Burlington, MA) to remotely transect the intima core (Figures 30-2 and 30-3). After removal of the intima core, the transection zone is passed by a 0.035-inch Terumo guidewire (Terumo Somerset, NJ) and secured with a stent. A stent that is eligible for use in proximity of the knee joint with its torsion and flexion forces is the aSpire stent (LeMaitre Vascular). This stent has a polytetrafluoroethylene (PTFE)-covered nitinol framework with a DNA helical structure, offering the possibility of preserving collaterals (Figure 30-4). It is flexible and has a high radial strength. By means of a completion arteriography, eventual distal thromboembolic load can be verified and embolectomy can be done with a Fogarty Graft Thrombectomy Catheter (Baxter Vascular Systems, Irvine, CA) if necessary. A common femoral and profunda femoris endarterectomy can be performed, and the arteriotomy may be closed with or without patch.

There is a learning curve for this procedure: approximately five to 10 operations are needed to master the technique.

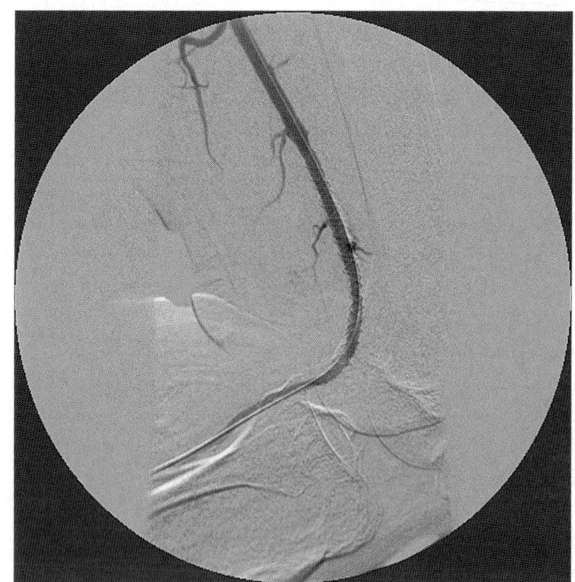

FIGURE 30-4 aSpire stent with knee in flexion. Collaterals are being preserved.

Results

So far, only retrospective studies have been published. A summary of selected literature will be given in this chapter. Recently, the authors performed a multicenter trial randomizing between RSFAE and above-knee femoropopliteal bypass, to prove the value of this operation as a durable procedure compared with bypass surgery. Short-term results have been analyzed and will be discussed here (unpublished data).

Ho et al.[9,10] were the first to describe the results of RSFAE. The primary patency rate of their first 101 procedures at 30 months follow-up was 55%.[9,10] Eighty-three percent of restenoses were detected within the first postprocedural year, presumably caused by aggressive neointimal hyperplasia. After the first year, the restenosis rate declined and was thought to be caused by progression of atherosclerotic disease rather than neointimal hyperplasia. These results showed that revision of early recurrent stenoses improves patency rates, whereas late restenoses do not seem to progress to reocclusion and may be treated conservatively. They found that the restenoses were equally distributed throughout the SFA and not limited to the region of the stent. Smeets et al.[11] continued follow-up of this cohort, extending it to 183 procedures. The 5-year cumulative primary patency rate was 38%.[11] They observed a continued development of a preserved collateral network.

Rosenthal et al.[7] showed improving patency rates after introduction of the aSpire stent at the distal transaction zone. In a multinational retrospective trial, studying 210 patients, primary and assisted primary patency rates were 60.6% and 70.2%, respectively, at 3-year follow-up.[7] Like Smeets et al. they described mild symptoms only after reocclusion of the SFA.[8]

The authors randomized 116 patients in a multicenter, prospective trial to compare patency rates of RSFAE (n = 61) and supragenicular bypass surgery (n = 55) for long occlusions of the SFA (unpublished data). Indications for surgery were severe claudication (n = 77), rest pain (n = 21), or tissue loss (n = 18). Initial technical success was 92% in the endarterectomy group versus 100% in the bypass group. Reasons for conversion in the endarterectomy group were perforation (n = 3), dissection (n = 1), or heavy calcification (n = 1). Only 25 patients (45%) in the bypass group had a sufficient saphenous vein suitable for bypass grafting. The other 30 patients received a PTFE graft (PTFE bypass; W. L. Gore & Associates, Flagstaff, AZ). Hospital stay was significantly shorter in the endarterectomy group, with a median of 4 days compared with 6 days in the bypass group ($p = 0.004$). Primary patency rates after 1-year follow-up were 61% for remote endarterectomy and 73% for femoropopliteal bypass ($p = 0.094$). Secondary patency was 79% for both groups. Subdividing between venous and prosthetic grafts showed superiority for vein with a primary patency rate of 89% compared with 63% for PTFE and a secondary patency rate of 94% versus 63% at 1-year follow-up. Compared with endarterectomy these differences are not significant. Limb salvage was 98% in both groups. Multivariate analysis in the RSFAE subgroup showed female gender as a significant predictor of reocclusion and restenosis concerning the primary patency rate, with a hazard ratio of 3.47 (95% confidence interval 1.17-10.35; $p = 0.025$) and assisted primary patency rate with a hazard ratio of 3.12 (95% confidence interval 1.34-7.28; $p = 0.008$). An explanation could be the smaller diameter of the SFA in women, although we have no data to support this.

This trial demonstrated that RSFAE is a minimally invasive adjunct in the treatment of chronic long occlusions of the SFA, with significantly shorter hospital stay and comparable assisted primary and secondary patency rates to bypass surgery. There is, however, a (nonsignificant) difference in primary patency, in favor of bypass. The venous bypass is superior, but only 45% of patients had a sufficient saphenous vein available. For patients lacking the saphenous vein, RSFAE could be the procedure of choice because prosthetic material can thus be avoided.

SURVEILLANCE AND MEDICATION

Routine postoperative surveillance of the deobstructed SFA has proved its value after RSFAE.[9] All patients enter a duplex scanning surveillance program consisting of duplex scanning after 6 weeks and 3, 6, 9, and 12 months after surgery. The first postprocedural year even asymptomatic restenoses are treated, because, as stated before, previous studies have shown that revision of early restenoses will improve long-term patency rates.[10] Usually, the restenoses can be treated by endovascular means: percutaneous transluminal angioplasty with or without additional stent placement.

All patients are given antiplatelet therapy before the procedure consisting of acetylsalicylic acid (100 mg daily) or coumarin derivatives (dose is according to the international normalized ratio [INR], with a target INR between 2.5 and 3.5 in most patients) on indication (e.g., cardiac disease). This regimen is continued after the operation. Whether clopidogrel should be standard treatment for patients after RSFAE remains uncertain. The CAPRIE study has shown an additional protective effect of clopidogrel over aspirin on adverse cardiovascular events; however, the TransAtlantic Inter-Society Consensus II document does not recommend standard treatment with clopidogrel for patients with peripheral arterial occlusive disease.[12,13] Two recent trials did add clopidogrel to aspirin in the postoperative management of patients after RSFAE. Martin et al.[14] showed a marked primary patency rate of 70%, whereas Lenti et al.[15] provided results similar to our patency rate: 64% at 1-year follow-up. Independent of their lipid spectrum, patients are given statin therapy, before surgery. Statins prevent restenosis by inhibition of inflammation and thrombosis besides their lipid-lowering effects.[16]

FUTURE PERSPECTIVES

RSFAE is a valuable adjunct in the revascularization of chronic long-segment occlusions of the SFA, especially in the absence of the greater saphenous vein.

Early restenosis within 1 year after RSFAE caused by presumed aggressive neointimal hyperplasia remains the Achilles heel of the RSFAE procedure. Therefore future prevention of neointimal hyperplasia seems to be the key to successfully preventing restenosis progressing to reocclusion. Recent research is focusing on this subject, with the development of gene and drug therapy, cryotherapy, drug-eluting stents, endothelial cell seeding, and laser, radiation, or brachytherapy. Different stents have been tested since the development of RSFAE, facing demanding forces close to the knee joint. The first series describing RSFAE placed a Palmaz stent at the distal transaction zone, resulting in a primary patency of 55% at 24 months.[9] More recently, the aSpire stent was introduced, a PTFE-covered nitinol frame with an open structure, offering the possibility of preserving collaterals. Patency rates of 69% at 18 months were shown.[6] Although restenosis does not seem to be restricted to the stent, there might be additional gain in the development of different stents or methods to secure the intima at the transection zone. Drug-eluting stents are being evolved, such as the sirolimus-eluting SMART stent. A difference in restenosis could not be demonstrated in a recent randomized trial, with for both bare and coated stents a restenosis rate of 22% 24 months after PTA.[17] Perhaps results will improve after surgically debulking the SFA, which leaves the proliferative cells bare and therefore possibly more sensitive to drug treatment. The recently developed nitric oxide–eluting aSpire should reduce platelet adhesion, platelet aggregation, leukocyte adhesion, and smooth muscle cell proliferation, but no trials (besides animal models) confirm its effectiveness yet.[18] Bioabsorbable stents offer the advantage of removing the stimulus for neointimal hyperplasia and are currently in experimental trials. A recent randomized trial by Tepe et al.[19] showed promising results with balloon catheters for percutaneous transluminal angioplasty coated with paclitaxel. Paclitaxel might inhibit the proliferation of vascular smooth muscle cells because of the exposure to a chemotaxis substance. They found significantly less lumen reduction at 6 months and a remarkably lower reintervention rate at 6 and 24 months of 4% and 15%, respectively, for the paclitaxel group versus 37% and 52% for the control group.[19] Again, results might improve after surgically removing the intima core. The role of cryoplasty is not yet defined, with conflicting results and no randomized trials performed so far.[20] But this could be a promising new method to secure the intima at the transection zone.

Combinations of these new endovascular techniques with remote endarterectomy of the SFA are currently investigated. Results will be published in the near future.

SUMMARY

- RSFAE has the benefits of minimally invasive surgery without compromise of future (surgical) interventions.
- Restenoses can usually be treated by endovascular means.
- The consequences are generally less severe after reocclusion compared with bypass surgery.
- Remote endarterectomy is a true alternative to femoropopliteal bypass grafting with comparable assisted primary patency rates.
- For patients lacking the greater saphenous vein, prosthetic material can be avoided.

References

1. Reboul H, Laubry P: Endarterectomy in the treatment of chronic endarteriitis obliterans of the limbs and abdominal aorta, *Proc R Soc Med* 43:547–552, 1950.
2. Dos Santos JC: [Sur la desobstruction des thromboses arterielles anciennes], *Mem Acad Chir* 73:409–411, 1947.
3. De Bakey ME, Cooley DA: Surgical considerations of acquired diseases of the aorta, *Ann Surg* 139:763–777, 1954.
4. Cannon JA, Barker WF: Successful management of obstructive femoral arteriosclerosis by endarterectomy: experience with a semi-closed technique in selected cases, *Surgery* 38:48–60, 1955.
5. Van der Heijden FH, Eikelboom BC, van Reedt Dortland RW, et al: Long-term results of semiclosed endarterectomy of the superficial femoral artery and the outcome of failed reconstructions, *J Vasc Surg* 18(2):271–279, 1993.
6. Rosenthal D, Martin JD, Schubart PJ, et al: Remote superficial femoral artery endarterectomy and distal aSpire stenting: multicenter medium-term results, *J Vasc Surg* 40(1):67–72, 2004.
7. Rosenthal D, Martin JD, Smeets L, et al: Remote superficial femoral artery endarterectomy and distal aSpire stenting: results of a multinational study at three-year follow-up, *J Cardiovasc Surg (Torino)* 47(4):385–391, 2006.
8. Smeets L, Huijbregts HJ, Ho GH, et al: Clinical outcome after reocclusion of initially successful remote endarterectomy of the superficial femoral artery, *J Cardiovasc Surg (Torino)* 48 (3):309–314, 2007.
9. Ho GH, van Buren PA, Moll FL, et al: Incidence, time-of-onset, and anatomical distribution of recurrent stenoses after remote endarterectomy in superficial femoral artery occlusive disease, *J Vasc Surg* 30(1):106–113, 1999.
10. Ho GH, van Buren PA, Moll FL, et al: The importance of revision of early restenosis after endovascular remote endarterectomy in SFA occlusive disease, *Eur J Vasc Endovasc Surg* 19(1):35–42, 2000.

11. Smeets L, Ho GH, Hagenaars T, et al: Remote endarterectomy: first choice in surgical treatment of long segmental SFA occlusive disease? *Eur J Vasc Endovasc Surg* 25:583–589, 2003.
12. A randomised, blinded, trial of clopidogrel versus aspirin in patients at risk of ischaemic events (CAPRIE) CAPRIE Steering Committee, *Lancet* 348(9038):1329–1339, 1996.
13. Norgren L, Hiatt WR, Dormandy JA, et al: TASC II Working Group. Inter-society consensus for the management of peripheral arterial disease, *Int Angiol* 26(2):81–157, 2007.
14. Martin JD, Hupp JA, Peeler MO, et al: Remote endarterectomy: lessons learned after more than 100 cases, *J Vasc Surg* 43(2):320–326, 2006.
15. Lenti M, Cieri E, De Rango P, et al: Endovascular treatment of long lesions of the superficial femoral artery: results from a multicenter registry of a spiral, covered polytetrafluoroethylene stent, *J Vasc Surg* 45(1):32–39, 2007.
16. Lumsden AB, Rice TW, Chen C, et al: Peripheral arterial occlusive disease: magnetic resonance imaging and the role of aggressive medical management, *World J Surg* 31(4):695–704, 2007.
17. Duda SH, Bosiers M, Lammer J, et al: Drug-eluting and bare nitinol stents for the treatment of atherosclerotic lesions in the superficial femoral artery: long-term results from the SIROCCO trial, *J Endovasc Ther* 13(6):701–710, 2006.
18. Hou D, Narciso H, Kamdar K, et al: Stent-based nitric oxide delivery reducing neointimal proliferation in a porcine carotid overstretch injury model, *Cardiovasc Intervent Radiol* 28(1):60–65, 2005.
19. Tepe G, Zeller T, Albrecht T, et al: Local delivery of paclitaxel to inhibit restenosis during angioplasty of the leg, *N Engl J Med* 358(7):689–699, 2008.
20. McCaslin JE, MacDonald S, Stansby G: Cryoplasty for peripheral vascular disease, *Cochrane Database Syst Rev* (4):CD005507, 2007.

CHAPTER

31

Stent Grafting for Infrainguinal Arterial Occlusive Disease

Brian G. DeRubertis

Although open surgical vascular reconstruction remains the "gold standard" for patients with symptomatic arterial occlusive disease of the lower extremities, these operations can exact a heavy price in terms of morbidity and mortality. Complication rates between 20% and 50% and mortality rates of up to 10% have commonly been reported after femoropopliteal or femorotibial bypass.[1-3] In addition, postoperative recovery from these operations can be prolonged, and many patients have not returned to baseline level of functioning even months after surgery.[4] Percutaneous revascularization has emerged as an alternative to open surgical reconstruction and has been applied to both patients with claudication and those with limb-threat. Percutaneous therapy offers significantly lower morbidity and mortality rates, as well as reduced recovery periods.

The primary clinical limitation with endovascular therapy is the reduced patency compared with open surgical bypass. All series reporting the outcomes of lower-extremity percutaneous interventions have demonstrated a reduced patency and higher reintervention rates than comparable series of open surgical reconstruction. In recent years, there has been a proliferation of devices capable of treating femoropopliteal occlusive disease, including self-expanding nitinol stents, laser and excisional atherectomy devices, cryoplasty angioplasty balloons, and others. These devices have been applied to patients with lower-extremity arterial occlusive disease with the hope of increased patency and decreased restenosis rates. Although different devices have demonstrated advantages in specific disease patterns or patient populations and initial results have been promising, intermediate and long-term data suggest that restenosis remains an important limitation common to all of these percutaneous modalities. Rates of restenosis and failure of percutaneous therapy appear to be related to a number of risk factors, including lesion length, lesion type (occlusion vs. stenosis), TransAtlantic Inter-Society Consensus classification, quality of distal runoff, and systemic factors such as presence of diabetes and end-stage renal disease.[5-7]

RATIONALE AND IMPORTANT CONSIDERATIONS REGARDING STENT GRAFT USE

The primary modes of failure in following percutaneous treatment of the femoropopliteal circulation include acute (early) thrombosis or restenosis as a result of intimal hyperplasia or progression of atherosclerotic disease. Luckily, acute thrombosis after balloon angioplasty, stenting, or atherectomy is relatively rare with the use of current antiplatelet regimens. In terms of restenosis, many of the clinical failures after percutaneous interventions occur in the first 12 to 24 months after intervention, suggesting that intimal hyperplasia is the predominant mode of restenosis rather than progression of atherosclerotic disease (Figure 31-1). Support for this observation has been provided in experimental animal models that have demonstrated that development of intimal hyperplasia and increased neointimal thickness is associated with balloon angioplasty and stent implantation.[8]

One of the techniques proposed to combat the effects of intimal hyperplasia within the percutaneously treated femoropopliteal circulation involves the implantation of covered stent grafts, or "endovascular femoropopliteal bypass grafting." Early reports of stent graft use in the femoropopliteal circulation for aneurysmal and occlusive disease originated in the early 1990s and involved the use of Dacron-covered endografts. Considerable improvements on these earlier devices have occurred

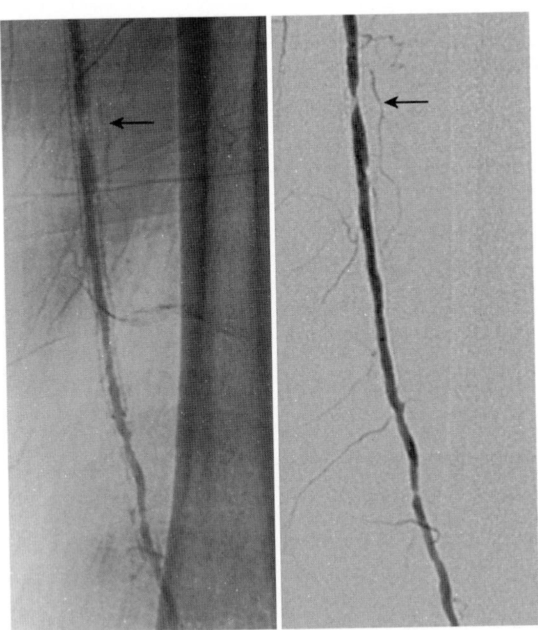

FIGURE 31-1 Patient with previous angioplasty and stenting of the SFA with a bare-metal nitinol stent. Note the smooth stenosis in the midportion of the stent *(arrows)* consistent with intimal hyperplasia secondary to ingrowth of hyperplastic tissue through the interstices of the stent.

in the last 15 years, and currently there are several commercially produced endografts that are available in sizes appropriate for femoropopliteal use. These modern devices are composed of self-expanding nitinol or balloon-expandable stainless steel stents covered by expanded polytetrafluoroethylene (ePTFE) material. The delivery systems for these devices have become increasingly lower in profile and allow for percutaneous delivery in many cases. Currently available stents include ePTFE-covered nitinol self-expanding stents (aSpire, Vascular Architects, San Jose, CA; Hemobahn/Viabahn Endoprosthesis, W. L. Gore & Associates, Flagstaff, AZ; and Fluency, Bard, Murray Hill, NJ), and balloon-expandable stainless steel stents (iCast, Atrium Medical Group, Hudson, NH; and Jostent, Abbott Vascular (Abott Park, IL)).

The primary advantage of covered stents in the femoropopliteal circulation is the exclusion of ingrowth of intimal hyperplasia in the native artery or between the interstices of bare-metal stents. The exclusion of intimal hyperplasia and other thrombogenic components of the treated arterial wall and the development of a more uniform flow surface provided by the covered stent graft has the potential to translate into improved patency and extended relief of symptoms compared with other endovascular modalities.

An important consideration when using stent grafts in the femoral and popliteal arteries involves the loss of collateral vessels from the diseased segment. With both open surgical bypass and endovascular interventions other than stent grafting, collateral vessels are not necessarily disturbed and can ultimately maintain perfusion in the event of graft or stent failure. After balloon angioplasty or atherectomy in particular, restenosis is often associated with a return to preintervention level of perfusion, and maintenance of collaterals can be demonstrated angiographically (Figure 31-2). Conversely, the use of stent grafts results in loss of collaterals along the region requiring treatment, and subsequent thrombosis or restenosis of the stent graft may result in significantly worse limb perfusion than before the operation, and potentially even acute limb-threatening ischemia.

Because of the potential for development of acute limb-threat after occlusions of stent grafts placed in the femoropopliteal circulation, proper patient selection is crucial to ensure good outcomes. Most authors recommend adherence to the following basic principles when performing stent grafting of the infrainguinal circulation: (1) ensure adequate inflow, (2) cover entire diseased segment, (3) ensure adequate tibial runoff (ideally two or more nondiseased tibial runoff vessels), (4) preserve collaterals whenever feasible, (5) never compromise the origin of the profunda femoris artery, and (6) maintain full anticoagulation during the intervention to avoid periprocedure thrombosis. In addition, one should consider alternative therapy if the patient has a contraindication to antiplatelet therapy, the profunda femoris artery is heavily diseased, there is extensive calcification that could preclude full expansion of the endograft, or there is multilevel disease from the femoral to the tibial circulation. Although stent grafting of the infrainguinal circulation has been applied successfully to patients with chronic limb-threatening ischemia, the anatomic constraints listed previously generally limit their use in those with rest pain and tissue loss and instead favor use of this modality in patients with claudication whose disease is often limited to the femoropopliteal segments.

TECHNIQUE OF INFRAINGUINAL STENT GRAFTING

Access, Sheath Placement, and Initial Diagnostic Imaging

Appropriate placement of the common femoral artery (CFA) puncture is an important first step in treating lower-extremity arterial occlusive disease with stent grafts, because the patients require full anticoagulation during the procedure and sheath sizes can range between 7F and 9F. Therefore, misplaced punctures in the superficial femoral artery (SFA) or close to the

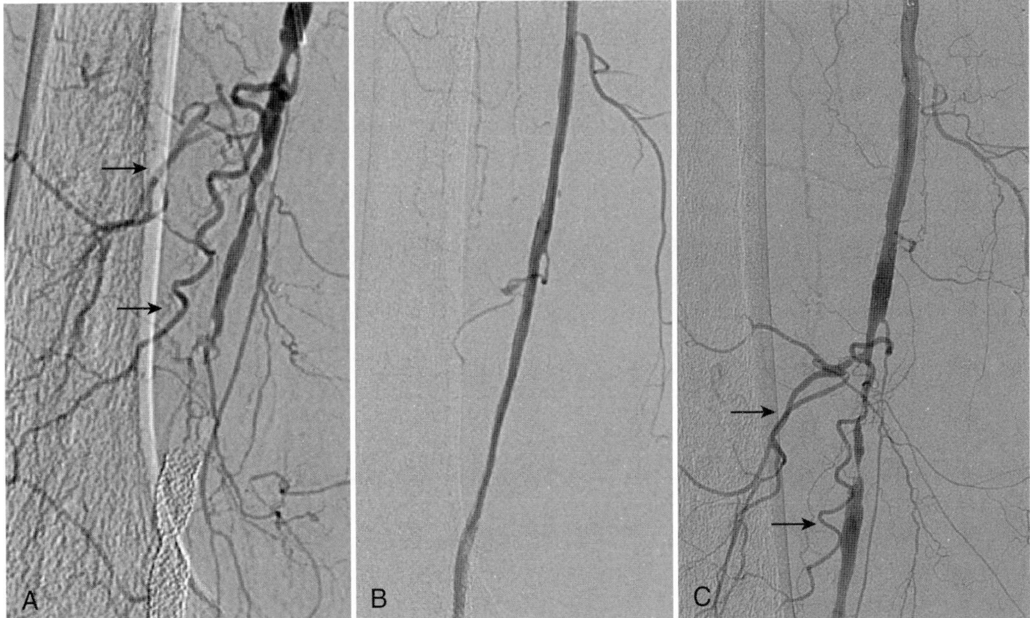

FIGURE 31-2 **A,** This panel illustrates the importance of collateral preservation in patients treated with percutaneous methods of revascularization. After several prior failed percutaneous and open surgical revascularization attempts, the patient's below-knee circulation is largely perfused through large collaterals emanating from the distal SFA *(arrows).* **B,** After atherectomy, these collaterals are no longer visualized because of the brisk antegrade flow through the native femoropopliteal circulation. **C,** However, on development of restenosis 8 months later, the lower leg is again perfused largely by these same collaterals *(arrows)* that were spared during the initial percutaneous intervention.

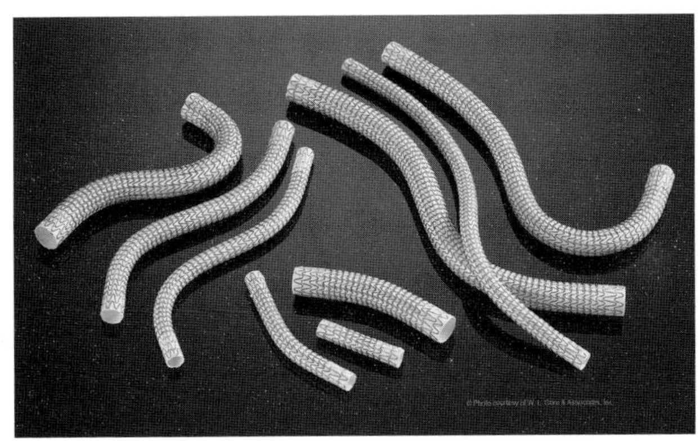

FIGURE 31-3 The Viabahn Endoprosthesis (W. L. Gore & Associates, Inc.) is composed of a helical nitinol stent that supports a heparin-bonded ePTFE graft. It is available for use in the SFA in diameters ranging from 5 to 8 mm and is delivered through sheath sizes of 7F to 8F.

common femoral bifurcation that preclude use of closure devices can significantly complicate access site management at the conclusion of the case. Duplex-guided puncture of the CFA with a 4F micropuncture kit allows exact puncture placement and confirmation of such before introduction of a larger working sheath.

After initial contralateral femoral access, selective lower-extremity diagnostic angiography is performed to assess the degree of disease in the infrainguinal circulation, determine the distal superficial femoral or popliteal reconstitution point (in the case of total occlusions), and evaluate distal runoff. At this time, a decision is made regarding the appropriateness of the patient's anatomy for stent graft use. Factors that are associated with poor outcomes after stent graft placement for infrainguinal occlusive disease are listed in Box 31-1, and patients with these characteristics may be best treated with other percutaneous modalities or surgical bypass.

Lesion Crossing, Stent Graft Selection, and Device Deployment

Once the target lesion is identified, an appropriately sized contralateral sheath is placed (generally 7F-8F), and the patient is systemically anticoagulated with 100 units/kg of intravenous heparin. Activated clotting time is maintained above 250 seconds with additional heparin boluses as needed. The lesion is traversed in standard fashion with a glide catheter and hydrophilic guidewire, and then an angiogram is performed to confirm luminal position in the reconstituted target vessel. The distally reconstituted vessel should be free from atherosclerotic disease and composed of a healthy arterial segment. All diseased segments should be covered by the stent graft, though one should avoid coverage of large collaterals unnecessarily. Accurate measurements should then be taken of the artery diameter at the proximal and distal landing zones, as well as

BOX 31-1

RELATIVE CONTRAINDICATIONS TO STENT GRAFT USE IN THE SUPERFICIAL FEMORAL ARTERY

- Heavily or circumferentially calcified lesions
- Severe multilevel (femoropopliteal and tibial) disease
- Inadequate arterial inflow or significant CFA disease
- Reduced tibial runoff (less than one continuous nondiseased vessel)
- Severe disease of the profunda femoris
- Multiple large collaterals in target lesion region
- Contraindication to antiplatelet therapy (absolute contraindication to stent graft use)

CFA, Common femoral artery.

BOX 31-2

TIPS FOR AVOIDING COMPLICATIONS WITH INFRAINGUINAL STENT GRAFTING

- Avoid unnecessary coverage of large collaterals.
- Maintain full anticoagulation during the procedure and antiplatelet therapy after surgery.
- Avoid significant oversizing to prevent graft infolding.
- Confine postdilatation to the covered portion of the vessel.
- Do not encroach on profunda femoris artery.
- Follow patients closely for symptom recurrence or duplex-detected restenosis.
- Intervene promptly for hemodynamically significant restenosis.

the total treatment length. Oversizing of the stent graft to the vessel diameter should be limited to approximately 5% to 10%, because excessive oversizing can lead to infolding or invagination of the graft and ultimately stent graft thrombosis.

Before stent graft deployment, lesions must be predilated with balloon angioplasty or debulked with laser or excisional atherectomy to ensure full stent graft expansion. After deployment of self-expanding covered stents, the stent should be postdilated with an appropriately sized noncompliant angioplasty balloon to correct any surface irregularities. Caution should be exercised not to extend beyond the device to avoid barotrauma to the normal arterial wall.

Completion angiography is then performed to ensure full expansion of the stent graft, assess for infolding or kinking, and confirm preservation of distal runoff and absence of embolic complications (Figure 31-4). The working sheath is then removed over a wire, and a closure device can be used to manage the puncture site. Use of closure devices not only allows earlier mobilization but also eliminates the need for reversal of anticoagulation and allows immediate use of antiplatelet therapy. Dual antiplatelet therapy with aspirin 325 mg and clopidogrel (Plavix) 75 mg daily is recommended immediately after the procedure and then continued indefinitely if no contraindications exist.

Postoperative surveillance for recurrent symptoms, change in pulse examination results, or deterioration in noninvasive vascular laboratory study parameters is crucial to ensuring good outcomes with stent graft use in the femoropopliteal circulation. Duplex ultrasound is used routinely to evaluate the treated region and assess for "edge-stenosis." Any hemodynamically significant lesions detected on duplex ultrasound should prompt percutaneous reintervention to avoid sudden stent graft thrombosis. Reintervention can include balloon angioplasty alone, atherectomy, or extension of the stent graft if necessary. Tips for optimal outcome after stent graft use in the femoropopliteal circulation are emphasized in Box 31-2.

RESULTS OF INFRAINGUINAL STENT GRAFTING FOR OCCLUSIVE DISEASE

The first reported use of a covered stent graft described a "homemade" device comprising a Palmaz stent (Cordis Endovascular, Warren, NJ) covered with a PTFE membrane.[9] This was followed shortly thereafter

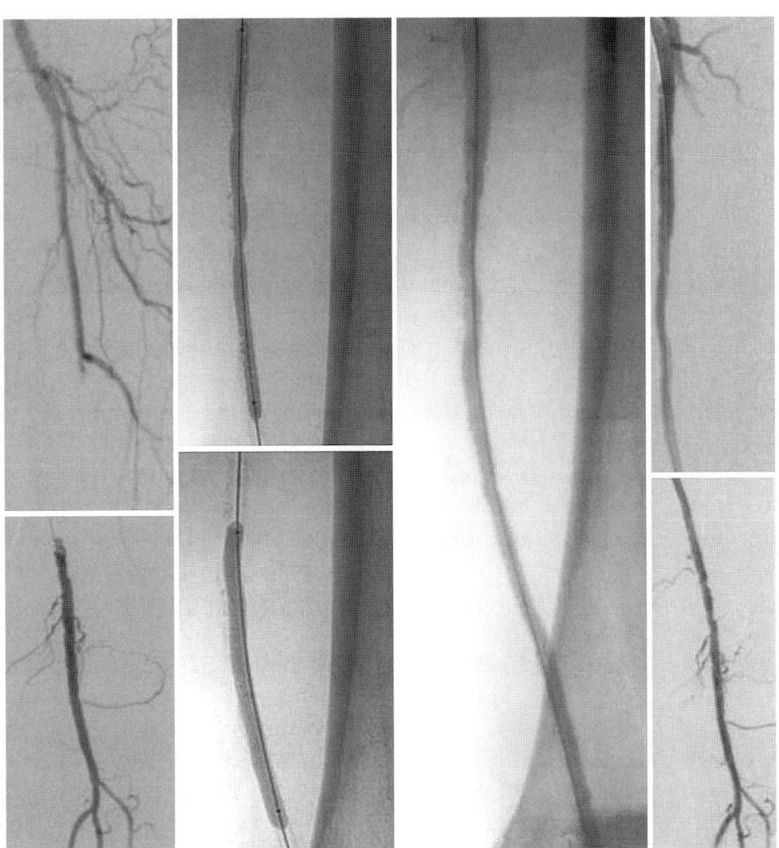

FIGURE 31-4 Recanalization and angioplasty of an occluded SFA, with subsequent implantation of a Viabahn Endoprosthesis. Optimal results depend on adequate inflow and outflow, appropriate sizing of the target vessel, postimplantation balloon angioplasty limited to the treated region, and maintenance of antiplatelet therapy after surgery.

by the development of the nitinol stents covered in Dacron fabric.[10-12] The Cragg Endopro System (Minimally Invasive Technologies SARL, Le Ciotat, France) was a low-molecular-weight, heparin-coated, Dacron-covered nitinol stent developed for use in the iliac and femoral circulation. The earliest publication on this device was a report of 40 patients with symptomatic stenoses or occlusions of the iliac and femoropopliteal circulation treated by balloon angioplasty followed by implantation of the Cragg Endopro System stent graft.[11] Although technical success rate was high at 98%, 2 of 21 femoropopliteal stents were occluded at 4 months, and a third patient required reintervention for inflow stenosis. Complications included distal embolization and acute thromboses. Patients with femoropopliteal stents were more likely to have complications and restenosis than patients with iliac stents.

Another study that evaluated the safety and efficacy of the Cragg Endopro System assessed outcomes in 11 patients treated for claudication in the face of SFA stenoses or occlusions.[12] Mean ankle-brachial indices increased significantly from 0.65 before treatment to 0.87 after treatment, and stent implantation was successful in all patients. Overall primary patency was 45%, and secondary patency was 56% at a mean follow-up of 17.2 months. Unfortunately, complication rates were high, including thrombosis of the stent graft in 5 of 11 patients. In addition, these authors noted a high rate of fever and pain at the operative site, eventually referred to as postimplantation syndrome.

Postimplantation syndrome was also noted in a later study, in which up to 40% of patients had pain at the treated site accompanied by fever and leukocytosis.[10] This report described 30 consecutive patients undergoing Dacron-covered nitinol stent placement for femoropopliteal occlusive disease. Restenosis was a common entity in these patients, with primary and secondary patency rates of 23% and 60%, respectively, at 12 months. Furthermore, a pattern of edge-stenosis was described in which intimal hyperplasia ingrowth affected the proximal and distal aspects of the stent, a phenomenon that continues to plague these interventions with today's current devices.

Since these earlier Dacron-covered devices, several manufacturers have developed ePTFE-coated nitinol stents with applicability for the femoropopliteal circulation. The lower crossing profiles of these newer devices have allowed percutaneous delivery and have likely contributed to reduced periprocedural complications. Several groups have now reported outcomes following the use of these covered stent grafts in the SFA with follow-up periods of up to 4 years.

The largest of these studies describes the results from the aSpire Registry, which included 166 limbs (150 patients) enrolled at 16 centers and treated with the self-expanding aSpire ePTFE-covered stent graft in the SFA (51 limbs) and popliteal artery (115 limbs). These procedures were performed for claudication in 91 limbs and limb-threat in 74 limbs. Periprocedural complication rate was 13%, and technical success was achieved in 97%. Primary and secondary patency rates were 64% and 74%, respectively, at 12 months and 59% and 67%, respectively, at 24 months. Limb salvage for limb-threat patients was 86% during the study period.[13]

The most commonly used ePTFE-covered device in current practice is the Hemobahn/Viabahn Endoprosthesis. This device is an ePTFE graft externally supported by a helical nitinol stent (see Figure 31-3). It is available for use in the SFA in diameters ranging from 5 to 8 mm and is offered in lengths of 2.5 cm, 5 cm, 10 cm, and 15 cm. Viabahn grafts of these diameters can be delivered through sheath sizes ranging from 7F to 8F.

Experience with the Hemobahn/Viabahn Endoprosthesis for the treatment of iliac and femoral occlusive disease was first published by Lammer et al.[14] This report included SFA stent graft placement in 80 limbs. Overall complication rate was 17%, and stent graft thrombosis within 30 days was seen in three (3.7%) patients with use of an anticoagulation strategy of daily aspirin and systemic heparin for 48 hours after the procedure. Primary patency of the femoral arteries was 90% and 79% at 6 months and 12 months, respectively, and secondary patency was 93% at 12 months.

These early studies have been further substantiated with midterm results from prospectively acquired data. Jahnke et al.[15] reported on 52 patients treated with the Hemobahn stent graft for relatively long occlusions and stenoses (mean coverage length of 10.9 cm) of the SFA. Technical success rate was 100%. Overall complication rate was 23% and included four patients (7.7%) with distal embolization. Mean ankle–brachial index improved significantly, from 0.54 to 0.89, and primary patency rate was 78% and 74% at 12 and 24 months, respectively. Secondary patency rate was 88% and 83% at 12 and 24 months, respectively.

The use of stent grafts for the femoropopliteal circulation has recently been compared with angioplasty and surgical bypass in several randomized controlled clinical trials.[16-18] A multicenter trial published in 2008 compared the use of the Viabahn endoprosthesis with percutaneous transluminal angioplasty alone in the treatment of SFA lesions up to 13 cm in length.[16] The study included patients with disabling claudication or chronic limb-threatening ischemia and excluded those with contraindication to antiplatelet therapy, previous stent placement in the target lesion, lesions within 5 mm of the profunda origin, and less than one continuous tibial runoff vessel. Patients were randomly assigned to treatment with a Viabahn Endoprosthesis or balloon angioplasty with selective bare-metal stents for a residual stenosis of greater than 30%. Although this study was terminated early because of the need for design modifications on the delivery system and because of problems with the original study outcome definitions, analysis of enrolled patients did demonstrate a 1-year primary patency benefit for those randomly assigned to treatment with a stent graft (65% vs. 40% for angioplasty alone). Patency benefit, as well as improved technical success rate, for those randomly assigned to the stent graft arm was seen in patients with lesion lengths of greater than 3 cm. There were no observed differences between the stent graft arm and the angioplasty arm in terms of early or late major adverse events.

A recent publication compared the use of stent grafts in the SFA versus surgical femoral-to-above-knee prosthetic bypass.[18] One hundred limbs in 86 patients with femoropopliteal occlusive disease and at least single-vessel tibial runoff were randomly assigned to endovascular treatment with the Viabahn Endoprosthesis or open surgical bypass to the above-knee popliteal artery with prosthetic graft (either Dacron or ePTFE). Procedures were performed for patients with claudication or chronic limb-threatening ischemia. Mean coverage length in patients randomly assigned to the Viabahn treatment arm was 25.6 cm, with a mean of 2.3 stent grafts per limb. After surgery, patients in this arm were managed with aspirin 325 mg and clopidogrel 75 mg daily. At a median follow-up of 18 months, there was no statistical difference in primary and secondary patency between the two treatment arms. Primary and secondary patency at 12 months was 73.5% and 83.9%, respectively, for the stent graft group and 74.2% and 83.7%, respectively, for the bypass group. During the follow-up period, graft thrombosis was seen in 13 patients in the stent graft arm and 10 patients in the surgical bypass arm. Of the 13 stent grafts, one occurred immediately after surgery, a second occurred within 30 days of intervention, and the remainder occurred an average of 5.4 months after surgery. Of the thrombosed stent grafts, one patient required amputation, five were reopened with thrombectomy or thrombolysis, and six required open surgical bypass. Limb salvage between the two treatment arms was not significantly different (98% in the stent graft arm, 89% in the surgical bypass arm).

Each of the prospective studies and randomized trials evaluating the use ePTFE-covered nitinol stents in the femoropopliteal circulation has shown substantial improvements in patency outcomes compared with Dacron-

TABLE 31-1 Primary Patency Rates After Stent Grafting for Infrainguinal Occlusive Disease

Author	Device	No. limbs	1-Yr patency (%)	2-Yr patency (%)
Maynar et al. (1997)[12]	Cragg Endopro (Dacron-nitinol)	11	45 (17 mo)	NA
Ahmadi et al. (2002)[10]	Cragg Endopro (Dacron-nitinol)	30	23	NA
Lenti et al. (2007)[13]	aSpire (spiral PTFE-nitinol)	166	64	59
Lammer et al. (2000)[14]	Hemobahn (ePTFE-nitinol)	80	79	NA
Jahnke et al. (2003)[15]	Hemobahn (ePTFE-nitinol)	52	78	74
Saxon et al. (2008)[16]	Viabahn (ePTFE-nitinol)	97	65	NA
McQuade et al. (2009)[18]	Viabahn (ePTFE-nitinol)	50	73.5	NA

ePTFE, Expanded polytetrafluoroethylene; *NA*, not available.

covered stents (Table 31-1). In addition, complication rates appear much lower, and the pain, fever, and leukocytosis comprising postimplantation syndrome do not appear to be an issue with the ePTFE-covered stents. Furthermore, the preceding studies regarding the Hemobahn/Viabahn stent grafts were performed with the original device, which has since been modified by adding heparin bonding to the graft, and this may ultimately serve to reduce thrombosis rate and further improve patency rates.

CONCLUSION

Stent grafting for infrainguinal occlusive disease has become a viable treatment option for patients with claudication and chronic limb-threatening ischemia. Improvements in graft design and delivery systems have likely contributed to the improved outcomes seen with contemporary devices compared with initial reports of use of Dacron-covered stents. Graft thrombosis remains a vexing problem and can result in development of acute ischemia requiring emergent reintervention. Proper patient selection is important to optimize results and avoid complications. Mounting evidence from randomized clinical trials suggests that outcome after stent grafting for femoropopliteal occlusive disease may be equivalent to that of surgical bypass with prosthetic grafts.

References

1. Goshima KR, Mills JL Sr, Hughes JD: A new look at outcomes after infrainguinal bypass surgery: traditional reporting standards systematically underestimate the expenditure of effort required to attain limb salvage, *J Vasc Surg* 39(2):330–335, 2004.
2. Schepers A, Klinkert P, Vrancken Peeters MP, et al: Complication registration in patients after peripheral arterial bypass surgery, *Ann Vasc Surg* 17(2):198–202, 2003.
3. L'Italien GJ, Cambria RP, Cutler BS, et al: Comparative early and late cardiac morbidity among patients requiring different vascular surgery procedures, *J Vasc Surg* 21(6):935–944, 1995.
4. Gibbons GW, Burgess AM, Guadagnoli E, et al: Return to well-being and function after infrainguinal revascularization, *J Vasc Surg* 21(1):35–44, 1995.
5. Conrad MF, Cambria RP, Stone DH, et al: Intermediate results of percutaneous endovascular therapy of femoropopliteal occlusive disease: a contemporary series, *J Vasc Surg* 44 (4):762–769, 2006.
6. Clark TW, Groffsky JL, Soulen MC: Predictors of long-term patency after femoropopliteal angioplasty: results from the STAR registry, *J Vasc Interv Radiol* 12(8):923–933, 2001.
7. Ihnat DM, Duong ST, Taylor ZC, et al: Contemporary outcomes after superficial femoral artery angioplasty and stenting: the influence of TASC classification and runoff score, *J Vasc Surg* 47 (5):967–974, 2008.
8. Salam TA, Taylor B, Suggs WD, et al: Reaction to injury following balloon angioplasty and intravascular stent placement in the canine femoral artery, *Am Surg* 60(5):353–357, 1994.
9. Cragg AH, Dake MD: Percutaneous femoropopliteal graft placement, *Radiology* 187:643–648, 1993.
10. Ahmadi R, Schillinger M, Maca T, et al: Femoropopliteal arteries: immediate and long-term results with a Dacron-covered stent-graft, *Radiology* 223(2):345–350, 2002.
11. Henry M, Amor M, Ethevenot G, et al: Initial experience with the Cragg Endopro System 1 for intraluminal treatment of peripheral vascular disease, *J Endovasc Surg* 1:31–43, 1994.
12. Maynar M, Reyes R, Ferral H, et al: Cragg Endopro System I: early experience. I. Femoral arteries, *J Vasc Interv Radiol* 8 (2):203–207, 1997.
13. Lenti M, Cieri E, De Rango P, et al: Endovascular treatment of long lesions of the superficial femoral artery: results from a multicenter registry of a spiral, covered polytetrafluoroethylene stent, *J Vasc Surg* 45(1):32–39, 2007.
14. Lammer J, Dake MD, Bleyn J, et al: Peripheral arterial obstruction: prospective study of treatment with a transluminally placed self-expanding stent-graft. International Trial Study Group, *Radiology* 217(1):95–104, 2000.
15. Jahnke T, Andresen R, Müller-Hülsbeck S, et al: Hemobahn stent-grafts for treatment of femoropopliteal arterial obstructions: midterm results of a prospective trial, *J Vasc Interv Radiol* 14 (1):41–51, 2003.

16. Saxon RR, Dake MD, Volgelzang RL, et al: Randomized, multicenter study comparing expanded polytetrafluoroethylene–covered endoprosthesis placement with percutaneous transluminal angioplasty in the treatment of superficial femoral artery occlusive disease, *J Vasc Interv Radiol* 19(6):823–832, 2008.
17. Saxon RR, Coffman JM, Gooding JM, et al: Long-term results of ePTFE stent-graft versus angioplasty in the femoropopliteal artery: single center experience from a prospective, randomized trial, *J Vasc Interv Radiol* 14(3):303–311, 2003.
18. McQuade K, Gable D, Hohman S, et al: Randomized comparison of ePTFE/nitinol self-expanding stent graft vs prosthetic femoral-popliteal bypass in the treatment of superficial femoral artery occlusive disease, *J Vasc Surg* 49(1):109–115, 2009.

CHAPTER

32

Endovascular Management of Infrapopliteal Occlusive Disease

Daniel M. Ihnat, Joseph L. Mills, Sr.

As technology continues to rapidly advance, increasingly complex arterial occlusive disease that was once treated solely by open surgical techniques is now being treated by endovascular therapy. This is especially true for infrapopliteal arterial disease. In 2005, the Bypass Versus Angioplasty in Severe Ischaemia of the Leg (BASIL) trial[1] was published, a prospective, randomized trial comparing endovascular versus open surgical revascularization as a first-line treatment for patients with severe limb ischemia. The trial demonstrated equivalent amputation-free survival between both groups, implying that treating all patients with endoluminal techniques as a first-line treatment does not preclude future bypass options. Because endoluminal techniques are significantly less invasive than open treatments, most physicians treating peripheral arterial disease have adopted an "endoluminal attempt first" policy for the majority of patients requiring revascularization. Unfortunately, scientific analysis has not been able to keep pace with rapidly evolving technology; we still need to quantify the durability of the various endoluminal techniques used to treat infrapopliteal disease and determine which patient subgroups might benefit from open bypass first.

Interpretation of the existing literature on infrapopliteal endoluminal interventions is challenging because of lack of standardized reporting criteria among various reports, inadequate definition of study groups, limited follow-up duration, small numbers, and the heterogeneity of the patterns of peripheral arterial disease treated. Study end points have also varied significantly. Different authors report binary restenosis rates of 50% or 75%, some note patency rates, and still others use the somewhat obscure end points of target lesion revascularization or target extremity revascularization. The latter end points were adopted from the percutaneous coronary revascularization literature but do not conform to published Society for Vascular Surgery reporting standards[2] for treatment of lower-extremity ischemia and provide no meaningful data on patency or restenosis rates. Furthermore, many studies fail to use life table or Kaplan-Meier analysis when reporting restenosis, patency, or target extremity revascularization rates. In addition to the lack of standardized end points, many reports combine the treatment of patients with variable degrees of ischemia and several levels of arterial occlusive disease when reporting patency rates. Because larger arteries have more favorable results with endoluminal therapy, the inclusion of femoropopliteal or iliac arterial treatments improves the overall outcome compared with studies limited to tibial interventions. This is especially common for infrapopliteal interventions, because the overwhelming majority of patients requiring such procedures have critical limb ischemia (CLI), and many have multilevel arterial occlusive disease. Similarly, authors who include patients with claudication who underwent tibial interventions to "improve the outflow" of femoropopliteal interventions will have superior results compared with series restricted to tibial interventions performed only for CLI. Furthermore, reports that perform objective tests such as duplex ultrasound or angiographic surveillance to determine patency are more reliable than those that only report "clinical patency." This is especially true for reports that include tibial interventions for claudication. Finally, the TransAtlantic Inter-Society Consensus (TASC) statement[3,4] summarized the importance of lesion length; treatment of longer lesions results in poorer patency rates. Despite this, many authors fail to define either the mean lesion treatment length or TASC classification, making comparisons with other studies impossible.

APPROACHES FOR TREATMENT OF INFRAPOPLITEAL ARTERIAL OCCLUSIVE DISEASE

Given the variable quality of reports in the literature on endoluminal tibial interventions, comparing and contrasting the efficacy of different treatment modalities remain challenging. Some general conclusions, however, can be reached. First, technical failures are more common when treating infrapopliteal lesions compared with more proximal occlusive disease.[5] Although the percentage of technical failures is significantly impacted by the complexity of the lesions treated, experienced interventionalists typically report[6-9] 10% to 20% incidence of technical failures for infrapopliteal arterial interventions, compared with 5% to 10% for femoropopliteal endovascular procedures.[10,11] This is not surprising, because the infrapopliteal arteries are smaller and more easily perforated, and reentry into the true lumen is more difficult. Second, patients treated for infrapopliteal disease more often have CLI than those undergoing more proximal interventions; patients with CLI in general fare more poorly than claudicants after endoluminal therapy.

In addition to the standard antegrade recanalization techniques, authors have reported approaches using retrograde tibial or pedal artery access. With use of the latter technique, the guidewire is used to cross the tibial artery occlusion in a retrograde fashion and is snared through a proximal catheter placed from an antegrade approach. The occlusive lesion is subsequently treated through a larger-caliber femoral sheath, thus limiting the arterial puncture size in the smaller pedal artery. By using this retrograde access, authors[12] have successfully treated infrapopliteal artery occlusive disease that had previously been unsuccessfully treated with standard endoluminal techniques. A further extension of this technique is the Subintimal Arterial Flossing with Antegrade-Retrograde Intervention (SAFARI) technique.[13] In this technique, when the true lumen cannot be reentered by guidewires passed from both antegrade and retrograde directions, the distal wire is snared inside the subintimal space with use of the proximal access, and the lesion is subsequently treated.

When determining whether or not to treat infrapopliteal occlusive disease with endoluminal, open, or a combined technique, one must weigh various factors, such as degree of ischemia (e.g., rest pain or minor or major tissue loss), patient comorbidities, the skill level of the interventionalist, the quality of available conduit, the expected durability of the revascularization, and the patient's expected longevity. Although a prolific body of patency data exists for open infrapopliteal bypass, the data for endoluminal therapy are quite limited and still lack long-term follow-up[6-9,14-20] (Table 32-1). A recent meta-analysis[14] of infrapopliteal angioplasty demonstrated a technical success rate of 89% ± 2.2%. The primary and secondary patency rates were 58% and 68% at 1 year and 49% and 63% at 3 years (Table 32-2). These patency rates are generally inferior to the reported rates for open bypass to infrapopliteal arteries with use of vein grafts[21] but equivalent to or better than polytetrafluoroethylene[22] (PTFE) bypass; the primary and secondary patency rates are 82% and 86% at 1 year and 72% and 77% at 3 years for vein grafts, compared with 59% and 66% at 1 year and 41% and 51% at 3 years for PTFE grafts.

Trying to elucidate which endoluminal treatment modality is best suited for the range of atherosclerotic lesions encountered remains unclear (Table 32-3). Requisite randomized studies comparing two different endoluminal treatment techniques for infrapopliteal arterial occlusive disease have not been performed. Several prospective nonrandomized trials have been reported; one such study[15] found angioplasty alone to be equivalent to nitinol stent placement, with 82% versus 78% patency rates at 1 year, respectively. These results are similar to those of single-center studies, which reported 1-year patency rates of 67% with excisional atherectomy[19] and 86% for sirolimus-eluting stents.[17] All of these studies lack intermediate and long-term follow-up, clouding the assessment of whether nitinol stents, drug-eluting stents, or endoluminal treatment in general will create long-term problems in the runoff vessels. Data from femoropopliteal endovascular interventions[23] indicate that stent failure is associated with a significant deterioration of the tibial runoff vessels in up to 35% of patients; deterioration in the runoff vessels has not been described after endoluminal treatment of infrapopliteal arteries. Currently, modalities such as cryoplasty and laser atherectomy lack published 1-year data for infrapopliteal arterial interventions. Despite the lack of a clearly superior treatment modality, several authors have described risk factors for poor outcomes. Occlusions longer than 10 cm,[6,7] TASC D lesions,[9] lack of a suitable distal bypass target,[9] balloon-expandable stents,[17] paclitaxel-eluting stents,[18] and the presence of diabetes mellitus or end-stage renal failure[24] are all factors associated with diminished patency rates.

TREATMENT OUTCOMES: OPEN BYPASS VERSUS ENDOVASCULAR THERAPY

Interestingly, despite generally poorer reported patency rates, limb salvage rates appear similar for endoluminal treatments compared with open surgical bypass for patients with CLI. In a meta-analysis of the endoluminal treatment of infrapopliteal arterial

TABLE 32-1 Comparative Results of Published Series on Endoluminal Therapy for Infrapopliteal Artery Occlusive Disease

Series	No. treated	Average lesion length (cm)	Lesion/patient characteristics	Primary patency	Technical failures included (%)	Factors affecting patency (RR)
PERCUTANEOUS TRANSLUMINAL ANGIOPLASTY ONLY						
Vraux et al., 2000[6]	40	NR	All CLI, all tibial occlusions	56% 1 yr	22	>10 cm occlusion
Vraux and Bertoncello, 2006[7]	50	NR	All CLI, all tibial occlusions	46% 1 yr	18	>10 cm occlusion Extension into popliteal artery
Tartari et al., 2004[8]	20	NR	All CLI, all tibials	70% 6 mo	No (15)	
Romiti et al., 2008,[14] meta-analysis	2653	NR	94.7% CLI, all tibials	65% 6 mo 58% 1 yr 49% 3 yr	11	
SELECTIVE STENTING						
Giles et al., 2008[9]	176	NR	93% CLI, 8% stented	53% 1 yr 51% 2 yr	7	TASC D (2.8) No target (2.2)
Peregrin et al., 2008[15]	66 PTA 16 stent	NR NR	All CLI, all tibials	82% 1 yr 78% 1 yr	0	
NITINOL STENTS						
Bosiers et al., 2007[16]	51	3.2	All CLI, all tibials	76% 1 yr	0	
DRUG-ELUTING STENTS						
Siablis et al., 2007[17]	58	1.35	All CLI, all tibials DES vs. BMS	40% 1 yr (BMS) 86% 1 yr (DES)	1.7	Sirolimus-eluting stents
Siablis et al., 2007[18]	32	2.6	All CLI, all tibials, 24% occlusions	30% 1 yr	0	Paclitaxel-eluting stents
ATHERECTOMY						
Zeller et al., 2007[19]	36	4.6 ± 4.1	53% CLI, 88% tibials	67% 1 yr 60% 2 yr		
MULTIPLE TREATMENT TECHNIQUES						
Bosiers et al., 2006[20]	443	NR	All CLI, 80% patients with rest pain; all tibials, 21% occlusions	69% 1 yr PTA 76% 1 yr stent 75% 1 yr Athx	0	18% PTA 68% stent 14% Athx

Athx, Atherectomy; *BMS,* bare metal stents; *CLI,* critical limb ischemia; *DES,* drug-eluting stents; *NR,* not reported; *PTA,* percutaneous transluminal angioplasty; *RR*, *relative risk; TASC,* TransAtlantic Inter-Society Consensus.

TABLE 32-2 Meta-Analysis of Infrapopliteal Angioplasty[14] Compared With Popliteal-Tibial Bypass[21]

	Primary patency (%)		Secondary patency (%)		Limb salvage (%)		Patient survival (%)	
Time (yr)	PTA	Bypass	PTA	Bypass	PTA	Bypass	PTA	Bypass*
1	58.1 ± 4.6	81.5 ± 2	68.2 ± 5.9	85.9 ± 1.9	86 ± 2.7	88.5 ± 2.2	87 ± 2.1	87-95
3	48.6 ± 8	72.3 ± 2.7	62.9 ± 11	76.7 ± 2.9	82.4 ± 3.4	82.3 ± 3	68.4 ± 5.5	70-82
5		63.1 ± 4.3		70.7 ± 4.6		77.7 ± 4.3		68-72

**Selected literature[24-26] reporting patient survival after popliteal-tibial bypass.*
PTA, Percutaneous transluminal angioplasty.

TABLE 32-3 Endoluminal Treatment Options for Infrapopliteal Arterial Occlusive Disease

Modality	Treatment option
Angioplasty	Standard balloon angioplasty
	Subintimal angioplasty
	Cutting balloon angioplasty
	Cryoplasty
Debulking	Excisional atherectomy
	Laser atherectomy
	Rotational atherectomy
Stents	Self-expanding (nitinol)
	Balloon-expandable
	Drug-eluting (sirolimus; paclitaxel)
	Absorbable (not currently FDA approved)

FDA, Food and Drug Administration.

occlusive disease,[14] the 1- and 3-year limb salvage rates were 86% and 82%, respectively. These are nearly identical to limb salvage rates for open surgical bypass of infrapopliteal arteries,[21] 89% and 82%. Given the lower patency rates of endoluminal therapy, the similarity of limb salvage rates compared with open bypass most likely reflects a combination of factors. First, many patients with CLI require only that the revascularization remain patent long enough to allow healing of the index ischemic wound. Thus angioplasty may suffice for a patient with a life expectancy less than 2 years who has a small noninfected ischemic ulcer. Second, most endoluminal treatments do not preclude future bypass, particularly if the endoluminal treatment fails in the short term. In fact, the BASIL trial[1] reported that 22% of the patients randomly assigned to endoluminal therapy eventually underwent open bypass. If, despite an angiographically successful endoluminal intervention, a patient fails to obtain adequate arterial perfusion for wound healing, open surgical bypass should be performed whenever feasible. This concept may be especially applicable when treating patients with large ischemic foot wounds, lateral foot wounds, and heel ulcers (Figures 32-1 and 32-2).

CLI is associated with significant intermediate mortality rates. In fact, the 5-year mortality for CLI is worse than that of many malignancies and ranges from 40% to 60%. True comparative data for patient survival with endovascular or open surgical treatment currently do not exist. Survival rates after endovascular treatments are somewhat difficult to reconcile, however, reflecting not only significant variability in the definitions of CLI but also marked differences in the duration

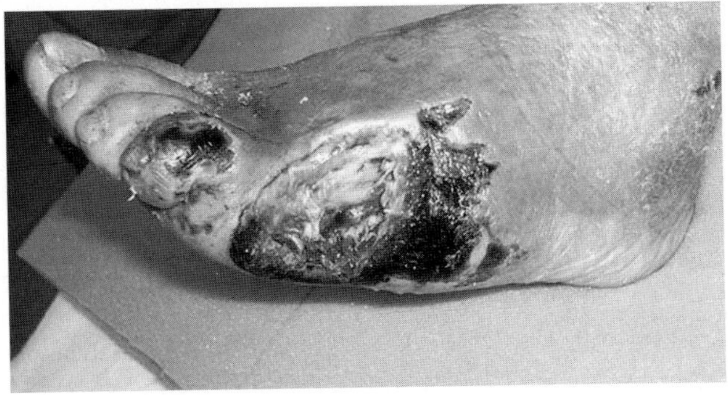

FIGURE 32-1 Photograph of a nonhealing ischemic fifth toe amputation site in a patient with severe tibial artery occlusive disease and type 2 diabetes mellitus.

of follow-up among available reports. In the largest meta-analysis reported to date, Romiti et al.[14] found patient survival to be 68% at 3 years. Recent reports[25-27] of popliteal to tibial artery surgical bypasses describe patient survival rates ranging from 68% to 72% at 4 to 5 years. Interestingly, subset analysis of the BASIL trial[1] revealed that both amputation-free survival (hazard ratio = 0.37) and all-cause mortality (hazard ratio = 0.34) were significantly better in the period 2 years after randomization for patients undergoing bypass surgery first. These findings imply that patients expected to live longer than 2 years may benefit from an initial surgical bypass. Health-related quality of life data comparing open and endoluminal techniques are sparse. In the BASIL trial,[1] health-related quality of life was not significantly different between bypass surgery and endoluminal therapy in the first 12 months after randomization.

Reported complication rates after endoluminal therapy typically range from 8% to 17% in the literature.[5] The most common complications include hematoma, perforation, and distal embolization. A meta-analysis of infrapopliteal endoluminal interventions[14] found an overall complication rate of 7.8%, with hematoma (3.1%), thrombosis (2.1%), embolization (1%), and perforation (0.7%) being the most common.

PATIENT SELECTION AND TECHNICAL CONSIDERATIONS

At our institution, we prefer to use an antegrade, ipsilateral femoral artery access in patients with isolated infrapopliteal occlusive disease. Although this can create challenges in patients with a large pannus and in positioning the sterile table used to stabilize the guidewire, it facilitates access to the pedal arteries, especially in tall patients and patients with a narrow aortic bifurcation angle. We routinely use periprocedural clopidogrel (extending to at least 6 weeks after

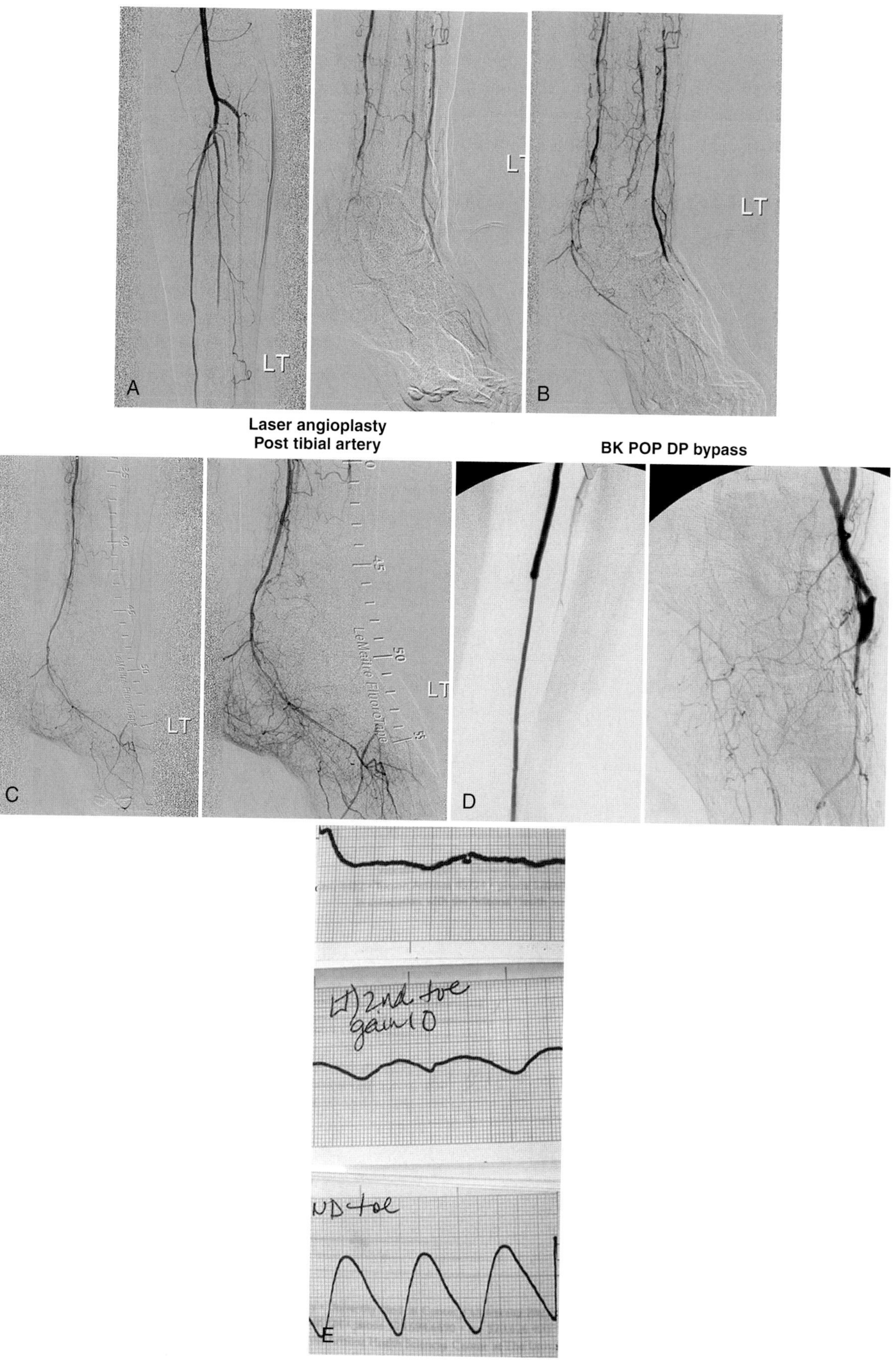

FIGURE 32-2 **A,** Initial diagnostic angiogram demonstrating three-vessel tibial occlusive disease. **B,** Lateral foot angiogram before intervention. **C,** Lateral foot angiogram form after laser-assisted a angioplasty of the posterior tibial and plantar arteries. **D,** Complete angiogram form after a below-the-knee poplilteal artery to dorsalis pedis artery bypass. **E,** Three representative second toe Doppler arterial waveforms: flat digital waveform before intervention; mildly improved waveform after laser-assisted angioplasty; and markedly improved, highly pulsatile waveform after dorsalis pedis bypass.

intervention, if not indefinitely) and intraprocedural systemic anticoagulation with unfractionated heparin. In fact, we monitor heparin dosage more strictly for tibial compared with other more proximal endoluminal interventions, striving to maintain an activated clotting time of more than 300 seconds. We use both 0.035-inch hydrophilic wires and 0.014-inch wires to cross the target lesion. Once reentry into the true lumen of the distal target is confirmed with angiography with use of dilute contrast, we typically exchange the initial short sheath for a long sheath so that its tip can be placed near the area of concern. The sheath segment that remains outside the patient is formed into a gentle, 180-degree curve, allowing the wires, catheters, and devices to remain securely on the mobile fluoroscopy table. Early placement of a long sheath, with the tip advanced close to the treatment area, also facilitates crossing the lesion by improving wire and catheter pushability and allows periodic angiography via the sheath port without having to exchange catheters and use a Tuohy-Borst adapter.

In general, we prefer over-the-wire balloons for longer lesions because of superior pushability and occlusion-crossing characteristics, as compared with rapid-exchange monorail systems. We find over-the-wire balloons especially helpful in patients with diabetes and renal failure, who tend to have severely and diffusely calcified tibial arteries. For shorter lesions, monorail systems work well, and we typically use either a cutting balloon, or plain old balloon angioplasty (POBA) (Figure 32-3). Cutting balloons are useful for focal fibrotic or heavily calcified lesions (Figure 32-4). In patients with long segment disease, we frequently rely on a combination of angioplasty and atherectomy to debulk occlusive lesions (Figure 32-5). With this approach, we find the need to stent exceedingly rare. We do not think debulking before planned stent placement yields a patency benefit. We reserve the use of bare tibial stents as a bailout procedure to address flow-limiting dissections and use covered stents to treat the rare instance of major bleeding from vessel perforation. We liberally infuse intra-arterial vasodilators (papaverine in 10- to 30-mg aliquots) and thrombolytics (alteplase in 2- to 4-mg aliquots) to resolve areas of possible spasm or early thrombus formation. Obtaining preintervention angiograms of the runoff vessels remains important, to allow comparison with the completion angiogram and rule out distal embolization. Distal embolization can most often be treated with catheter aspiration.

The most critical role of the vascular and endovascular surgeon is to ensure that the circulation has been improved sufficiently to allow healing of the ischemic wound. Objective preoperative and postoperative, noninvasive assessment of the limb hemodynamics is therefore an essential component of both open and endovascular therapy. Postintervention ankle–brachial index and toe pressure measurements are mandatory to quantify the improvement in arterial circulation and to confirm that the circulation has sufficiently improved for wound healing. Some authors have advocated the endoluminal revascularization of multiple tibial arteries in patients with CLI to maximize foot perfusion and minimize the adverse impact of restenosis; current data are insufficient to support or refute this strategy. If we think we have obtained a satisfactory

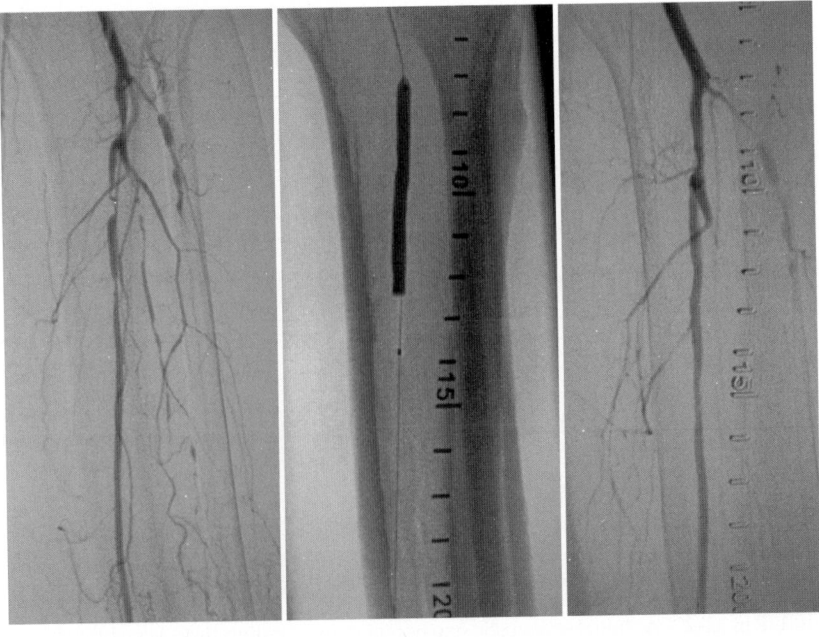

FIGURE 32-3 Angiogram demonstrating tibioperoneal trunk and proximal peroneal artery occlusive disease successfully treated with plain old balloon angioplasty (POBA), and a completion angiogram demonstrating the result.

endoluminal result and still have not achieved adequate arterial perfusion, we proceed immediately to open bypass whenever feasible. This is especially important in patients with large ischemic or recently infected wounds. We have found pedal bypass to be superior to endoluminal therapy in restoring arterial circulation in certain subsets of patients, especially those with extensive tissue loss.

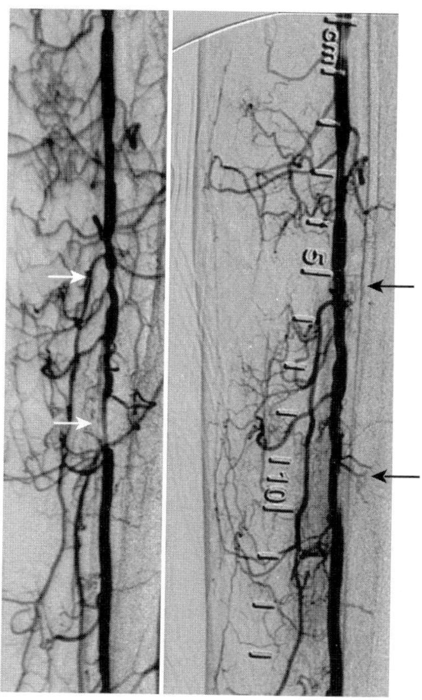

FIGURE 32-4 Angiogram of a patient with a 4-cm–long segment of occlusive disease in the anterior tibial artery, successfully treated with a 2.5-cm cutting balloon.

On balance, endovascular techniques are increasingly being applied in patients with CLI. The endovascular literature on infrapopliteal arterial occlusive disease is predominantly composed of ill-defined patient groups with short follow-up and a general failure to use Society for Vascular Surgery reporting standards. Despite these limitations, endovascular therapy appears to be more broadly applicable to patients with CLI than previously thought. Endovascular therapy is especially suited for focal tibial lesions. Treating even longer segment disease is quite reasonable if the patient with CLI is treated earlier in his or her course (rest pain or small ischemic ulcer), compared with patients presenting with failed toe amputations, extensive tissue loss, or tissue loss extending to the midfoot or heel. A general lack of long-term follow-up exists in the literature; yet, the paradigm shift toward endovascular surgery does not appear to have significantly impacted limb salvage rates either positively or negatively. Although endovascular therapy is less morbid in the short term, it is more likely to require reintervention than bypass, and its long-term potential adverse impact on outflow remains unclear. In fact, intermediate follow-up of the BASIL trial suggests improved survival in patients having bypass first for CLI if they live beyond 2 years after their first intervention. A multitude of alternative endoluminal treatment techniques currently exist. Besides the notably poor results with balloon-expandable stents and paclitaxel-eluting stents, no one technique appears to offer a significant advantage with regard to patency. The rapidly evolving endoluminal technology and its application to the infrapopliteal arteries make this one of the most exciting areas in vascular surgery.

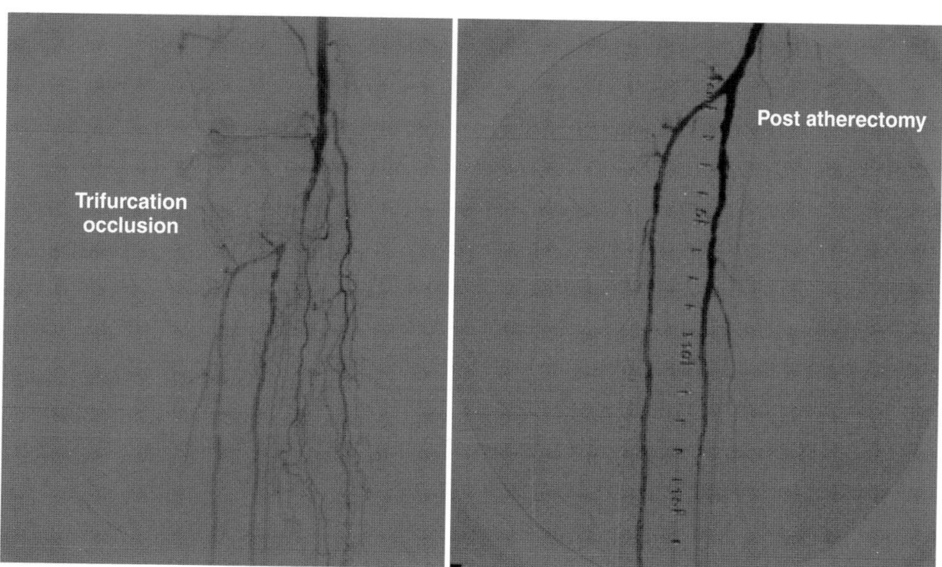

FIGURE 32-5 Angiogram of a patient with an ischemic heel ulcer, and trifurcation occlusive disease successfully treated with excisional atherectomy.

References

1. Adam DJ, Beard JD, Cleveland T, et al: Bypass versus angioplasty in severe ischaemia of the leg (BASIL): multicenter, randomized controlled trial, *Lancet* 366:1925–1934, 2005.
2. Rutherford RB, Baker D, Ernst C, et al: Recommended standards for reports dealing with lower extremity ischemia: revised version, *J Vasc Surg* 26:517–538, 1997.
3. Management of peripheral arterial disease (PAD): TASC Working Group. Trans-Atlantic Inter-Society Consensus (TASC), *J Vasc Surg* 31:S1–S296, 2000.
4. Trans-Atlantic Inter-Society Consensus for the management of PAD, *J Vasc Surg* 43(suppl):S33–S36, 2007 Jan.
5. Met R, Van Lienden KP, Koelemay MJW, et al: Subintimal angioplasty for peripheral arterial occlusive disease: a systematic review, *Cardiovasc Intervent Radiol* 31:687–697, 2008.
6. Vraux H, Hammer F, Verheist R, et al: Subintimal angioplasty of tibial occlusions in the treatment of critical limb ischemia: mid-term results, *Eur J Vasc Endovasc Surg* 20:441–446, 2000.
7. Vraux H, Bertoncello N: Subintimal angioplasty of tibial vessel occlusions in critical limb ischemia: a good opportunity? *Eur J Vasc Endovasc Surg* 32:663–667, 2006.
8. Tartari S, Zattoni L, Rolma G, et al: Subintimal angioplasty of infrapopliteal artery occlusions in the treatment of critical limb ischemia. short-term results, *Radiol Med* 108:265–274, 2004.
9. Giles KA, Pomposelli FB, Hamdan AD, et al: Infrapopliteal angioplasty for critical limb ischemia: relation of TransAtlantic Intersociety consensus class to outcome in 176 limbs, *J Vasc Surg* 48:128–136, 2008.
10. Kamiya C, Sakamoto S, Tamori Y, et al: Long-term outcome after percutaneous peripheral intervention vs. medical therapy for patients with superficial femoral artery occlusive disease, *Circulation* 72:734–739, 2008.
11. Schillinger M, Sabeti S, Loewe C, et al: Balloon angioplasty versus implantation of nitinol stents in the superficial femoral artery, *N Engl J Med* 354:1879–1888, 2006.
12. Botti CF, Ansel GM, Silver MJ, et al: Percutaneous retrograde tibial access in limb salvage, *J Endovasc Ther* 10:614–618, 2003.
13. Spinosa DJ, Leung DA, Harthun NL, et al: Simultaneous antegrade and retrograde access for subintimal recanalization of peripheral arterial occlusion, *J Vasc Interv Radiol* 14:1449–1454, 2003.
14. Romiti M, Albers M, Brochado-Neto FC, et al: Meta-analysis of infrapopliteal angioplasty for chronic critical limb ischemia, *J Vasc Surg* 47:975–981, 2008.
15. Peregrin JH, Smirova S, Koznar B, et al: Self-expandable stent placement in infrapopliteal arteries after unsuccessful angioplasty failure: one-year follow-up, *Cardiovasc Intervent Radiol* 31:860–864, 2008.
16. Bosiers M, Deloose K, Verbist J, et al: Nitinol stenting for treatment of 'below-the-knee' critical limb ischemia: 1-year angiographic outcome after Xpert stent implantation, *J Cardiovasc Surg* 48:455–461, 2007.
17. Siablis D, Karnabatidis Katsanos K, et al: Sirolimus-eluting versus bare stents after suboptimal infrapopliteal angioplasty for critical limb ischemia: enduring 1-year angiographic and clinical benefit, *J Endovasc Therapy* 14:241–250, 2007.
18. Siablis D, Karnabatidis D, Katsanos K, et al: Infrapopliteal application of paclitaxel-eluting stents for critical limb ischemia: midterm angiographic and clinical results, *J Vasc Interv Radiol* 18:1351–1361, 2007.
19. Zeller T, Sixt S, Schwarzwälder U, et al: Two-year results after directional atherectomy of infrapopliteal arteries with the SilverHawk device, *J Endovasc Ther* 14:232–240, 2007.
20. Bosiers M, Hart JP, Deloose K, et al: Endovascular therapy as the primary approach for limb salvage in patients with critical limb ischemia: experience with 443 infrapopliteal procedures, *Vascular* 14:63–69, 2006.
21. Albers M, Romiti M, Brochado-Neto FC, et al: Meta-analysis of popliteal-to-distal vein bypass grafts for critical ischemia, *J Vasc Surg* 43:498–503, 2006.
22. Albers M, Battistella VM, Romiti M, et al: Meta-analysis of polytetrafluoroethylene bypass grafts to infrapopliteal arteries, *J Vasc Surg* 37:1263–1269, 2003.
23. Ihnat DM, Duong ST, Taylor ZC, et al: Contemporary outcomes after superficial femoral artery angioplasty and stenting: the influence of TASC classification and runoff score, *J Vasc Surg* 47:967–974, 2008.
24. Aulivola B, Gargiulo M, Bessoni M, et al: Infrapopliteal angioplasty for limb salvage in the setting of renal failure: do results justify its use? *Ann Vasc Surg* 19:762–768, 2005.
25. Mills JL, Gahtan V, Fujitani RM, et al: The utility of vein bypass grafts originating from the popliteal artery for limb salvage, *Am J Surg* 68:646–651, 1994.
26. Brown PS, McCarthy WJ, Yao JS, et al: The popliteal artery as inflow for distal bypass grafting, *Arch Surg* 129:596–602, 1994.
27. Ballotta E, Da Giau G, Gruppo M, et al: Infrapopliteal arterial revascularization for critical limb ischemia: is the peroneal artery at the distal third a suitable outflow vessel? *J Vasc Surg* 47:952–959, 2008.

CHAPTER

33

Complications and Their Management After Endovascular Intervention in Infrainguinal Arterial Occlusive Disease

Evan C. Lipsitz, Brian N. King

Over a decade ago it was estimated that in the near future 40% to 70% of all vascular interventions would be performed with use of an endovascular method.[1] At many centers a majority of interventions for infrainguinal occlusive disease are performed with use of an endovascular approach. It cannot be overstated that the most effective way of method of dealing with procedural complications is to avoid them altogether. In every case, a diagnostic or therapeutic procedure should be undertaken only when a thoughtful analysis of the risk/benefits and options has been performed and an informed discussion held with the patient. Similarly, the earlier a complication is recognized the more likely it is to be successfully treated. This is especially true in the endovascular realm where treatment options may be limited by the available tools and the remote nature of the access site. Operators must develop and pay special attention to tactile feedback from wires and catheters and not simply follow the procedure visually on the monitor. If complications of an endovascular procedure are not recognized in a timely manner, access across the treatment site may be lost, leading to further difficulty in treating the complication.

The incidence and severity of complications after infrainguinal endovascular procedures depend on the type of procedure and the access site that is chosen. Therapeutic, as opposed to diagnostic, procedures have a higher incidence of complications because of the use of larger sheath sizes, the need for intraprocedural and sometimes postprocedural anticoagulation, overall procedural time, and the complexity of the manipulations required.[2] Prograde punctures may be associated with a higher incidence of local complications than retrograde punctures, especially in obese patients. The incidence of complications also depends on the status of the access vessels in terms of atherosclerosis and tortuosity, as well as the patient's body habitus and general medical condition.

ACCESS COMPLICATIONS

The vast majority of percutaneous infrainguinal diagnostic and therapeutic interventions are performed via a common femoral arterial puncture. Proper aseptic technique, as with all invasive procedures, is required to reduce the risk of infection. Local anesthetic (without epinephrine) is infiltrated into the skin and subcutaneous tissues. Ideally, the femoral sheath is also anesthetized. Adequate anesthesia will keep the patient comfortable and reduce the chances of the patient moving suddenly in response to pain, which can lead to a complication at either the access or the treatment site. Care should be taken not to inject excessive local anesthetic because this may cause tissue plane dissection and increase the risk of pseudoaneurysm formation by enlarging the potential space around the vessel. The ideal puncture is a single-pass, anterior wall—only cannulation at a 45-degree angle to the vessel with the bevel of the needle facing upward. On entering the vessel there should be brisk, pulsatile bleeding, and the guidewire should pass easily without resistance or buckling. Occasionally, after pulsatile flow is established it may be necessary to bring the needle closer to an approximately 30-degree angle to facilitate passage of the wire. If careful planning is exercised before puncture, the complication rate after femoral cannulation should be low.

Complications of Arterial Puncture

The most frequent complications after femoral puncture are groin hematoma and pseudoaneurysm formation.[2,3] Additional complications include arteriovenous fistulae (AVFs), retroperitoneal hemorrhage, arterial dissection, arterial thrombosis, septic sequelae, and injury to adjacent structures (femoral neuropathy and deep venous thrombosis). The Society of Interventional Radiology has published reported rates and thresholds for complications after diagnostic angiography (Table 33-1).[4]

Oweida and colleagues[3] reported the Emory group's experience with postcatheterization vascular complications and found pseudoaneurysm to be the most common complication requiring operative repair, occurring in nearly two thirds of patients requiring repair. In their retrospective review of nearly 5000 patients undergoing coronary angioplasty, the authors identified 55 complications requiring operative repair, for an overall rate of 1%.[3] Excluded from the study were patients who had a diagnostic catheterization or those who had an uncomplicated groin or retroperitoneal hematoma. Advanced age and postprocedural anticoagulation independently correlated with an increased risk of postcatheterization vascular complication. McCann et al.[5] found a similar incidence of hemorrhagic and ischemic complications in a study of 16,350 patients undergoing diagnostic or therapeutic cardiac catheterization. Vascular complications requiring repair occurred in 146 patients (0.89%) and included repair of pseudoaneurysm (n = 64) or AVF (n = 8) in the hemorrhagic group and thromboembolectomy (n = 56) or vascular reconstruction (n = 18) in the ischemic group. In a multivariate analysis, congestive heart failure, female gender, and therapeutic catheterization were found to be significantly associated with vascular injury.

Groin hematomas can vary in presentation, from mild to massive. Clinically significant hematomas are often associated with overlying ecchymosis and can progress to include skin ulceration, breakdown, and infection in severe cases. Most hematomas can be safely observed; however, those that continue to expand, that involve skin necrosis or infection, or that cause a compressive femoral neuropathy should be promptly evacuated. Operative intervention is associated with high wound morbidity, likely because of the obliteration of subcutaneous tissues by the hematoma. Also, injury to adjacent neurovascular structures can occur during dissection in these patients who often have distorted anatomy from the hemorrhage and hematoma.[6]

As uncomplicated groin hematomas resolve there may be tracking of the ecchymosis inferiorly and posteriorly onto the thigh down to or below the knee, occasionally involving the scrotum or labia. Patients may express concern as to whether this represents ongoing bleeding but, in the absence of other findings, can be reassured that it is only superficial and represents the normal process of resolution and resorption of the hematoma.

TABLE 33-1 Indicators and Thresholds for Complications in Diagnostic Arteriography

	Reported rates (%)	Major adverse event threshold (%)
PUNCTURE SITE COMPLICATIONS		
Hematoma (requiring transfusion, surgery, or delayed discharge)	0.0-0.68	0.5
Occlusion	0.0-0.76	0.2
Pseudoaneurysm/ arteriovenous fistula	0.04-0.2	0.2
CATHETER-INDUCED COMPLICATIONS (OTHER THAN PUNCTURE SITE)		
Distal emboli	0.0-0.1	0.5
Arterial dissection/ subintimal passage	0.43	0.5
Subintimal injection of contrast	0.0-0.44	0.5
Major contrast reactions	0.0-3.58	0.5
Contrast-associated nephrotoxicity	0.2-1.4	0.2

From Singh H, Cardella JF, Cole PE, et al. Quality improvement guidelines for diagnostic arteriography, J Vasc Interv Radiol, *14:S283, 2003.*

NOTE: All values supported by the weight of literature evidence and panel consensus.

Pseudoaneurysm formation occurs when the puncture site fails to seal and blood flows into the potential space outside the artery, resulting in formation of a pressurized cavity adjacent to the artery (Figure 33-1). Blood may flow both into and out of the cavity. With time, a thick pseudocapsule may develop and have the appearance of a true aneurysm. The diagnosis may be suspected when there is a tender, pulsatile mass in the groin or when a bruit is appreciated. Pseudoaneurysms are most frequently diagnosed by duplex ultrasound evaluation. They may also be detected as an incidental finding on computed tomographic (CT) scans that have been obtained for other reasons in patients without groin symptoms. Treatment options include observation, ultrasound-guided techniques, and surgical repair.

Asymptomatic pseudoaneurysms less than 3 cm in size can often safely be observed with serial clinical and duplex examinations, because many will thrombose spontaneously.[7,8] Toursarkissian and colleagues[8] followed patients with pseudoaneurysm less than 3 cm

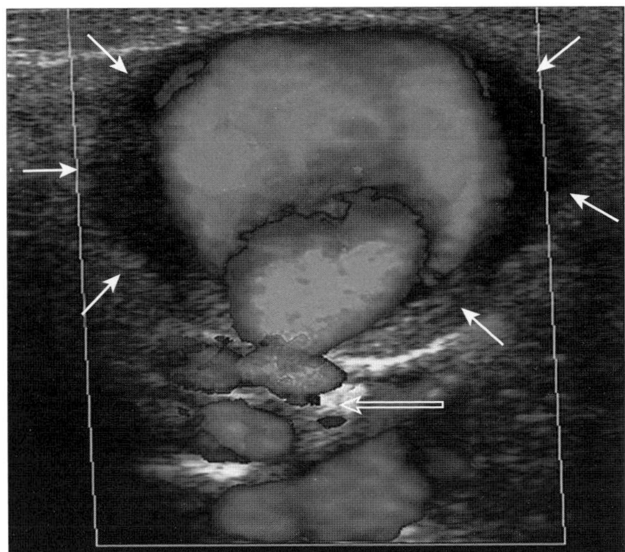

FIGURE 33-1 Large pseudoaneurysm seen on duplex originating from the CFA *(white arrows)*. Location of the neck is indicated by the *open arrow*.

and observed spontaneous closure in 72 of 82 patients (87.8%). Patients receiving anticoagulation were excluded. In general, nonoperative results are less favorable in patients receiving anticoagulation. Repeated imaging after spontaneous thrombosis should be performed to confirm persistent pseudoaneurysm thrombosis.

Ultrasound-guided compression is an effective, noninvasive method for the treatment of pseudoaneurysms. In our experience approximately 70% to 80% of all groin pseudoaneurysms can be successfully compressed. The technique involves direct visualization and compression with use of the ultrasound probe to confirm cessation of blood flow within the sac. The goal is to compress the neck, not simply the sac, preventing flow into the sac and allowing blood within the sac to thrombose. The technique requires skill and persistence on the part of the operator performing the compression. Care should be taken not to compress the underlying artery completely. Major advantages of this method are that it is noninvasive, involves no contrast, and can easily be repeated if necessary. However, it can be uncomfortable for patients and time-consuming for vascular laboratory staff. Patients may require the use of analgesics and/or sedatives for successful compression.

Ultrasound-guided thrombin injection can take just minutes, offers a high success rate, and avoids many of the risks associated with surgical exploration. Advantages of this approach are that it is minimally invasive, is relatively painless, and achieves rapid thrombosis. A major potential disadvantage is embolization of thrombin via flow into the artery from a nonoccluded neck. Other disadvantages include inadvertent injection of the artery and/or vein. This technique should not be used in patients with short, wide pseudoaneurysm necks, given the risk of thrombin embolization and subsequent arterial thrombosis. Ultrasound-guided thrombin injection is an off-label use of thrombin.

Surgical repair is the most definitive therapy and is indicated for infection, rapid expansion, rupture, large hematoma with overlying skin necrosis, femoral neuropathy resulting from compression, need for prolonged anticoagulation, inability to follow up with serial duplex examinations, and failure of ultrasound-guided techniques. There are two main approaches for operative repair: (1) proximal and distal arterial control followed by pseudoaneurysm débridement with primary suture repair and (2) direct pseudoaneurysm exploration, débridement, and primary suture repair. In the first approach proximal arterial control may be obtained via a separate retroperitoneal incision approximately one to two fingerbreadths above the inguinal ligament with exposure of the external iliac artery such that a clamp may be applied. It is not necessary to obtain circumferential control, but care must be taken to establish a plane between the artery and surrounding structures, especially the external iliac vein. If this is not accomplished, injury to the vein can occur during clamp placement, which can be difficult to repair. The groin incision is then made and exploration begun at the most inferior aspect of the incision. Control of the distal common femoral artery (CFA) or, in the case of large inferiorly extending pseudoaneurysms, of the proximal superficial femoral artery (SFA) and profunda femoris artery is then obtained. Again, circumferential control is not required but the same principles of careful dissection apply. Clamps may then be positioned but not secured, and exploration of the arterial defect is undertaken. When bleeding is encountered, clamps are applied and the defect repaired as described. In the second method the pseudoaneurysm is approached directly through a single groin incision. Arterial control is obtained either by proximal and distal exposure of the vessel or by control with finger pressure. In both cases there must be adequate exposure, suction, and lighting to facilitate repair.

In either case, the surgeon must be certain to identify the true arterial wall and its defect, because it is easy to misidentify the overlying fascia as a contused arterial wall. This is best accomplished by identifying the anterior wall of the artery proximal and/or distal to the puncture site because inflammation often obscures the anatomy directly over the puncture site. The femoral sheath is then opened at a site remote from the injury, and the dissection proceeds toward the puncture site. Suture placement in the overlying fascial layer instead of the arterial wall can lead to recurrent pseudoaneurysm formation.

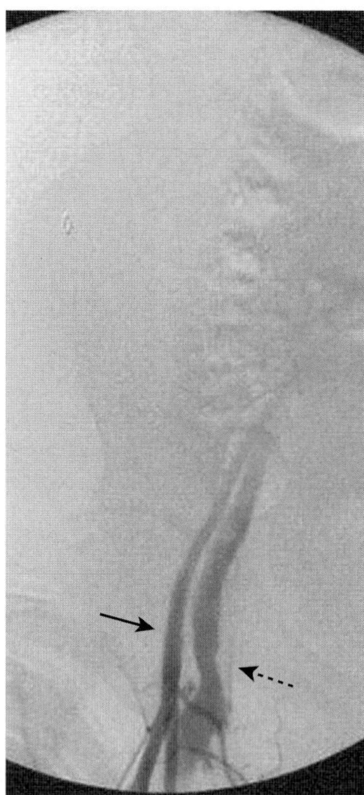

FIGURE 33-2 Angiography of an AVF between the CFA *(solid arrow)* at its bifurcation and the common femoral vein *(dashed arrow).*

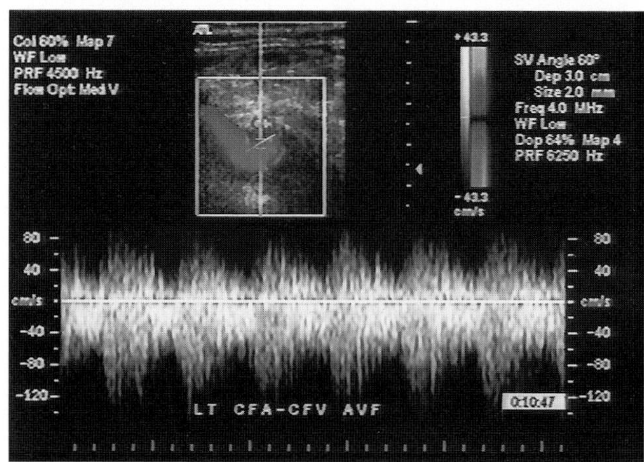

FIGURE 33-3 Duplex ultrasonogram indicating alternating flow patterns within an AVF between the CFA and common femoral vein.

Repair may be accomplished by using local, regional, or general anesthesia depending on the size and location of the cavity and the medical condition of the patient. Although surgical repair provides a definitive result, there are several potential complications including those related to anesthesia, wound infection, neuralgia, swelling, lymphatic leak, and scarring, which may complicate any subsequent interventions. Patients with large hematomas and skin necrosis have a higher incidence of wound complications and frequently require the placement of drains.

Pseudoaneurysms may infrequently develop days or even weeks after a procedure. Patients requiring long-term anticoagulation are at greater risk for this complication. The onset of symptoms is generally acute and may be associated with exercise, straining, or coughing. Patients may report feeling a "pop" at the puncture site and frequently thereafter may complain of groin pain. There may or may not be associated ecchymosis or obvious hematoma. Duplex evaluation or other imaging study is warranted in such a situation.

AVFs most commonly arise from a low puncture, with cannulation of both the profunda femoris vein and artery (Figure 33-2). The profunda femoris vein crosses between the bifurcation of the SFA and the profunda femoris artery, then courses posteriorly to the profunda femoris artery. The presence of a continuous femoral murmur is suggestive of the diagnosis. Diagnosis is best confirmed with duplex ultrasonography, which shows turbulent flow in the fistula tract, arterial flow signals in the vein proximal to the AVF, and decreased arterial flow distal to the AVF compared with the contralateral artery (Figure 33-3).[6] Treatment options include observation, ultrasound-guided compression, endovascular stenting, and surgical repair. Toursarkissian and associates[8] followed patients with iatrogenic femoral AVFs with serial duplex examinations and documented spontaneous resolution in 46 of 57 patients (80.7%). The average time to spontaneous closure was 28 days, and 90% were closed at 4 months. The study excluded patients who required long-term anticoagulation. As with pseudoaneurysms, ultrasound-guided compression has been used to treat AVFs. Patients with an AVF arising from the body of the SFA or profunda femoris artery distal to the bifurcation may be considered candidates for placement of a covered stent across the AVF. Care must be exercised to avoid stent positioning across the orifice of the SFA or profunda femoris artery. Currently, such an endovascular approach should rarely be considered. Its greatest potential benefit would be in patients with large, chronic fistulas. We do not recommend covered stent placement in the CFA, because the site is surgically accessible and future transfemoral arteriography and revascularization operations will be jeopardized. Any endovascular option must take into account the development of intimal hyperplasia and subsequent therapeutic options required to treat it. Last, surgical repair should be considered in patients with large fistulas or those in whom symptoms develop, for example, those with leg edema or venous ulcerations caused by venous hypertension. Operative repair may include proximal and distal arterial control (with or

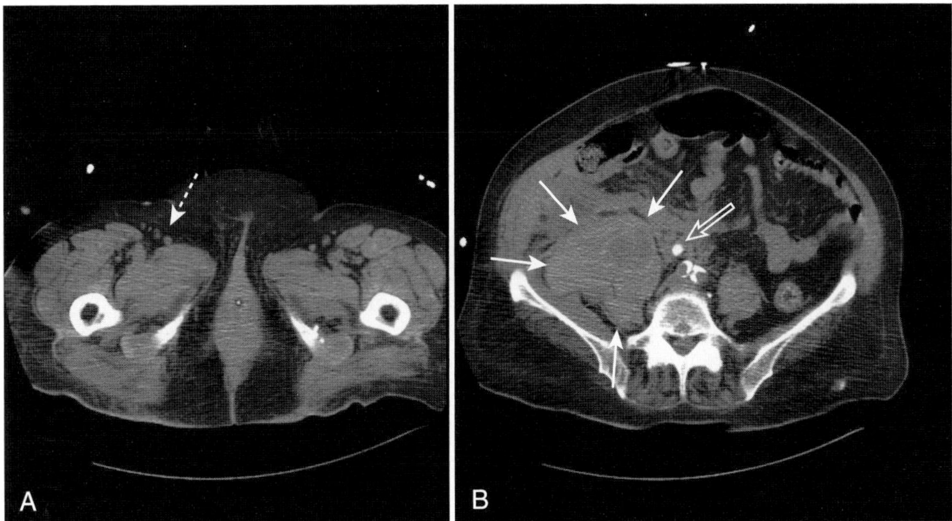

FIGURE 33-4 Large retroperitoneal hematoma after cardiac catheterization. **A,** Note the absence of a groin hematoma *(dashed arrow)*. **B,** The hematoma is seen *(solid arrows)*, as well as an ipsilateral contrast-filled hydroureter resulting from compression *(open arrow)*. Also note calcification at the aortic bifurcation.

without venous control), suture ligation and division for small AVFs, and patch angioplasty for larger tracts. Rare complications of iatrogenic AVFs include congestive heart failure and aneurysmal degeneration of the proximal artery.

Retroperitoneal hemorrhage is one of the most serious complications that may follow groin puncture, because of its attendant morbidity and mortality (Figure 33-4). Bleeding and retroperitoneal hematoma formation can have differing etiologies. In addition to nonsealing of the puncture site after sheath removal, bleeding around the sheath may occur during the course of the procedure. This is particularly true in patients who receive anticoagulation. Retroperitoneal hemorrhage may also be a result of bleeding from an abandoned puncture site. Vigilance and timely diagnosis are the key components to successfully managing patients with this potentially devastating complication. Any patient with postprocedural abdominal, back, flank, or pelvic pain, with or without hypotension, should be suspected of having the diagnosis and undergo a prompt evaluation. Risk factors include high arterial puncture (above the inguinal ligament), postcatheterization anticoagulation, female sex, and thrombocytopenia.[9] Two-wall (through and through anterior and posterior) arterial wall puncture may increase the risk as well, because of bleeding arising from the posterior wall. Clinical manifestations may vary, making the diagnosis difficult, and include the asymptomatic patient with unremarkable results of physical examination, to those with development of abdominal or back pain, femoral neuropathy, a falling hematocrit, and in severe cases hypotension, hemorrhagic shock, and abdominal compartment syndrome.

The diagnosis is best confirmed with a CT scan of the abdomen and pelvis, though bedside ultrasonography may be used in a patient in unstable condition. If there is no evidence of ongoing hemorrhage, nonoperative treatment is often successful and includes reversal of anticoagulation, aggressive volume resuscitation (often requiring transfusion), intensive care unit monitoring, and repeated imaging. Endovascular techniques including use of covered stents to treat iliac injuries can be used particularly when identified in the intraoperative period during completion femoral angiography. Sealing of an external iliac puncture site with balloon tamponade has also been described.[10] Operative exploration with hematoma evacuation and arterial repair (if ongoing bleeding is present) should be performed in patients who are unresponsive to resuscitation, who have a compression femoral neuropathy, or in whom an abdominal compartment syndrome develops. Exploration can be achieved through a groin incision, retroperitoneal flank incision, midline laparotomy, or combination of incisions depending on the etiology and location of the bleeding. In this setting it is more likely that retroperitoneal exposure will be required.

The use of an antegrade (prograde) femoral artery puncture provides several advantages for the performance of infrainguinal endovascular interventions, including greater guidewire and catheter control because of improved pushability, trackability, and torque when compared with procedures performed via a contralateral approach over the aortic bifurcation. This approach may be associated with a greater incidence of access site complications, including inability to pass the sheath, pseudoaneurysm, and vessel injury. This is especially true in obese patients where the working area may be limited by a large pannus. There are several techniques that can help reduce the incidence of these complications. The puncture should be initiated just above the pelvic brim where the external iliac artery courses anteriorly, then dives slightly posteriorly, becoming the CFA as it passes below the inguinal ligament. It is advantageous to use a relatively stiff wire when placing the sheath so as to avoid kinking of the sheath in the subcutaneous tissues. A small cutaneous incision and the use of manual support while advancing the sheath over the wire through the subcutaneous tissues are also effective measures.

There is a tendency to selectively cannulate the profunda femoris artery when performing a prograde puncture because of the angle of the superficial femoral deep femoral bifurcation. When this situation occurs the use of a "buddy" wire technique reduces the risk of losing access while attempting to cannulate the SFA. In this technique the wire that passed into the profunda femoris artery is left in place and a second wire, preferably an angled hydrophilic wire, is placed through the sheath. Contrast injections are performed and allowed to reflux into the CFA showing the position of the femoral bifurcation. In all likelihood, the common femoral puncture site will be within approximately 1 cm of the femoral bifurcation. The sheath can then be withdrawn into the CFA and the second wire directed into the SFA. The first wire can then be withdrawn from the profunda femoral artery and the sheath advanced with its dilator over the second wire into the SFA. If the sheath is inadvertently completely withdrawn from the artery during the course of the maneuver, it can be replaced over the original wire located in the profunda femoris artery. If the puncture is directly over, distal, or into the profunda femoris, the sheath will likely need to be withdrawn and a new puncture attempted.

Other access sites including direct puncture of the popliteal or tibial vessels for the retrograde treatment of lesions have been described. Each has its own particular challenges based on its location, although the principles of gaining access remain the same.

Occasionally the nature of a procedure will call for access to be obtained with direct exposure of the vessel. In this instance many of the complications listed above, as well as those resulting from sheath withdrawal and closure devices, can be nearly eliminated. Such may be the case in a patient who requires an iliac angioplasty and stent in conjunction with a distal bypass. There is some potential morbidity from the surgical cutdown, and the approach must be individualized on the basis of patient anatomy.

The most effective way to avoid access site complications is careful preoperative planning. In an effort to reduce these complications, there are a number of factors to consider before gaining CFA access. First, puncture the CFA directly over the femoral head. To accurately do so, place this bony landmark in the center of the fluoroscopic image to avoid parallax error. In obese patients, introducer needle passage under fluoroscopy can be done to avoid high or low punctures. Second, employ a 45-degree angle of approach. Too acute of an angle may result in a "high stick," which can lead to hematoma or pseudoaneurysm formation caused by inadequate hemostasis at the time of sheath removal. In contrast, too steep of an angle may lead to a low puncture, making sheath placement difficult and potentially leading to guidewire kinking. Also, low punctures carry a risk of AVF creation between the deep femoral artery and vein. Third, perform access site arteriography liberally. If guidewire passage proves to be difficult, remove the guidewire, and, if pulsatile bleeding is still present, perform local angiography through the introducer needle. This step will reliably confirm an intraluminal, rather than intramural, needle tip position, and will readily identify any adjacent occlusive disease or arterial dissection. Last, try to avoid placement of hydrophilic, highly flexible wires through the introducer needle. To-and-fro movement of this type of wire in an introducer needle can lead to lacerations of the wire coating or even wire transection.

Injury to Adjacent Structures (Vessels, Nerves, Viscera)

Injury to adjacent structures generally results from hematoma formation and compression rather than direct injury. These injuries, including femoral neuropathy, may present in a delayed fashion, especially in patients receiving anticoagulation (Figure 33-5). When identified acutely, compression femoral neuropathy resulting from a groin hematoma or pseudoaneurysm should be

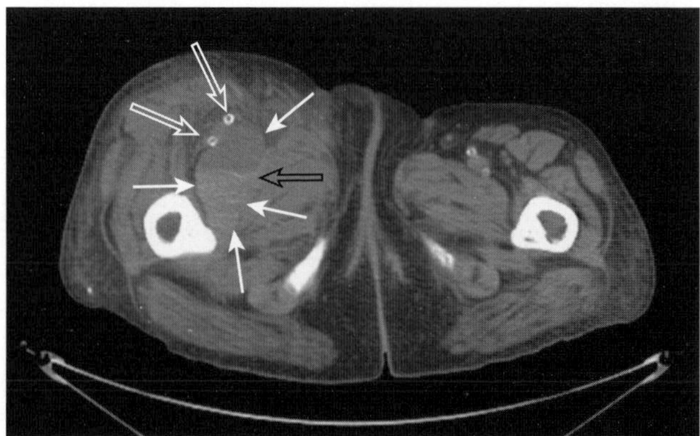

FIGURE 33-5 Moderate-sized hematoma in the intramuscular space adjacent to and compressing the femoral sheath *(solid arrows)* in patient receiving anticoagulation. Contrast layering is seen within the hematoma *(black open arrow)*. A calcified SFA and deep femoral artery are seen *(white open arrows)*.

evacuated to decrease the risk of long-term neurologic sequelae. When a chronic compression is identified, elective decompression is performed although the neurologic impairment may not be affected. Direct puncture of the femoral vein may result in bleeding or even deep vein thrombosis. Deep vein thrombosis may also arise from misdirected or excessive manual pressure at the time of sheath removal, or from the use of a device that applies nonfocal pressure, for example, sandbags. Injury to the intra-abdominal or pelvic viscera may occur in the setting of a high puncture, or when a groin hernia containing visceral contents is present. This may be especially true when there is a femoral hernia.

Complications of Wire and Sheath Placement

Femoral and/or iliac artery dissection may occur during guidewire passage or sheath or catheter exchanges. Care must be exercised when initial guidewire passage is met with resistance. The tendency to forcefully push the wire may lead to creation of a dissection plane, plaque elevation, and potentially arterial thrombosis. In this circumstance, introducer needle manipulations (gentle changes in angle of approach and repositioning of the needle bevel) and guidewire movement under fluoroscopy should be employed. Confirm intraluminal positioning via angiography with a gentle hand injection of a low volume, low pressure of contrast. If contrast appears to be intravascular but fails to empty, persisting on subsequent imaging, a dissection has likely occurred. If the dissection is not flow limiting, in the vast majority of cases treatment is not required. However, if flow is impaired, balloon angioplasty is warranted, with stent placement for lesions resistant to angioplasty. If the injury is in immediate proximity to the puncture site, exploration and repair of the artery may be required. When advancing an introducer sheath, one must be sure that the tapered dilator is locked into place, because pushing a sheath without its tapered dilator can lead to significant endoluminal trauma ("snowplowing"). Finally, communicate with the patient during sheath placement, because sudden patient movement in response to unexpected pressure and/or pain can distort the artery leading to injury. Some dissections may not be evident on angiography and may be detected by other imaging modalities, such as duplex or CT. In this situation treatment may also be performed under duplex guidance.

Injury to the aortic bifurcation can occur when working from a contralateral puncture. This type of injury is more likely to occur when there is a steep bifurcation with calcified and diseased distal aorta and iliac arteries. Kinking of the sheath can also occur when working over the top of a steep bifurcation. A wire or catheter should be maintained through the sheath at all times to minimize this complication. If these are withdrawn the sheath may kink, prohibiting passage of guidewires and catheters. In this case it may become necessary to reposition the sheath in the ipsilateral iliac artery and to reestablish contralateral access. If the bifurcation is deemed too steep, or if there is disease of either or both iliac arteries that may be compromised by the placement of wires, sheaths, or catheters, a prograde puncture may be advisable to effectively treat a contralateral lesion.

Femoral artery thrombosis after transfemoral angiography is relatively rare but can occur in a number of situations. In the setting of diffuse disease, access site thrombosis may not be readily apparent. This complication usually arises in the patient with a small-caliber, heavily diseased CFA. In these circumstances, the introducer sheath may occlude the vessel lumen leading to subsequent thrombosis, particularly if adequate procedural anticoagulation is not achieved. Another frequent cause is elevation of a large posterior plaque with resultant obstruction of the native lumen. Plaque elevation can also lead to an obstructive process when the free edge is proximal to the hinged portion, causing an occlusion with removal of the sheath and plaque movement with forward blood flow. Although dissections that are created against the direction of flow are generally asymptomatic, they may cause occlusion if they are flow limiting. Careful planning, including puncture of the larger, less-diseased femoral artery, as well as use of a micropuncture set, can reduce these types of complications. Finally, overzealous manual compression of the femoral artery after sheath removal can lead to arterial thrombosis (discussed later in this chapter).

If wires and catheters are passed blindly, that is, without fluoroscopic or ultrasound guidance, they may enter large or small side branches. If the wire is continuously advanced without imaging, wire perforation may occur and can lead to potentially significant intramuscular or visceral hemorrhage. This complication is exacerbated when a subsequent intervention is performed during which anticoagulation is administered. To prevent such an occurrence, the lead end of the guidewire should be visualized along its course until the final destination is reached.

Embolization, which is discussed in greater detail below, may also result simply from the passage of wires and catheters. The occurrence of cholesterol emboli is far more likely in patients with diffuse atherosclerotic disease, especially of the aortoiliac segment. Care must be taken when manipulating catheters and guidewires in such diseased vessels. If diffuse atherosclerotic changes with extensive plaque or intraluminal thrombus are seen on a preprocedural study, such as a CT scan, careful consideration of the planned intervention should be undertaken to minimize or avoid manipulations within the diseased segment. Livedo reticularis may result from microembolization to the dermal vessels of the buttocks, thighs, legs, and trunk. It presents as a purple irregular mottling of the skin in all or some of these areas. Microembolization to the renal vessels may also occur and present with compromised renal function or poorly controlled hypertension. This situation must be distinguished from that of contrast nephropathy. Treatment may include anticoagulation to limit progression of small-vessel thrombosis.

Arterial spasm may develop, particularly in noncalcified vessels. This may lead to compromised outflow and to indwelling catheters becoming occlusive, predisposing to thrombosis. Vasodilators such as papaverine or nitroglycerin may be administered, preferably in a catheter-directed manner to treat this occurrence.

COMPLICATIONS CROSSING LESIONS

In many cases the most dangerous part of an endovascular intervention is crossing the lesion, be it stenotic or occlusive. This step begins with manipulation of a highly diseased portion of the artery. In the case of stenotic lesions, attempts to cross the lesion may result in dissection, creation of an in situ thrombosis, embolization, or perforation. Dissection or in situ thrombosis may convert a stenosis into an occlusion and require a change in treatment plan. Although it does not rule out endovascular treatment, it may complicate or delay therapy. Guidewire perforations may be safely observed in many cases and are generally self-limited. Microembolization may result from the dislodging of multiple, small cholesterol particles, frequently from the aorta or iliacs, that travel and embed in small arterioles or capillaries resulting in trash foot or blue toe syndrome. It may also result from embolization of small fragments of clot that form in situ and embolize. In this situation particles are not amenable to embolectomy, and supportive treatment with anticoagulation is the treatment required. In the case of larger emboli, suction embolectomy via an endovascular approach may be performed through the existing access. In cases where an embolus cannot be retrieved via endovascular techniques, surgical embolectomy may be required to restore patency. In the most severe cases, embolization to a heavily diseased segment may occur and require reconstruction with a bypass to achieve limb salvage. Thrombolysis may also be employed in combination with these other methods. Ideally, difficult lesions are identified before surgery, and caution is exercised when crossing the stenosis or occlusion. If multiple attempts to cross a lesion prove unsuccessful, subsequent attempts are best limited in an effort to prevent or minimize these potential complications.

COMPLICATIONS OF TREATING LESIONS

Although lower-extremity endovascular interventions for occlusive disease are "minimally invasive" procedures, they are nonetheless invasive procedures with an effectiveness that is predicated on the creation of a controlled arterial injury.

When performing an intervention operators should be cognizant of the location of the distal end of the wire. If the wire is allowed to advance too far, injury such as dissection, perforation, or thrombosis may result and may go unrecognized until a completion angiogram is taken. If possible, the end of the wire should be kept within the field of view or at least located fluoroscopically and the appropriate position relative to the table marked.

Embolization, Dissection, and Thrombosis

Embolization may occur as discussed earlier. In this case embolization occurs as a result of the intervention with rates that differ depending on the method used. Angioplasty results in "controlled trauma" to a given narrowed area of the affected vessel. During balloon dilatation the plaque is split, and the media is stretched. This results in an increased luminal diameter and cross-sectional area of the artery. There are several negative effects that result from angioplasty, including the creation of an irregularly fractured plaque, damage to the media as a result of barotrauma, and desquamation of endothelium. In addition, longitudinal dissection planes are created, and plaque fracture may extend some distance proximal and/or distal to the actual angioplasty site.

Embolization of atheromatous debris, acute thrombus, or cholesterol material into the arterial circulation can occur at any step in an endovascular procedure. Although macroemboli can significantly alter outflow anatomy, more often than not the process involves microemboli, which may result in a clinically silent course. Some endovascular surgeons use distal protection devices to attenuate the risk of downstream embolization, particularly in cases where the perceived risk is high (e.g., atherectomy). Using continuous transcutaneous Doppler ultrasound, Lam and colleagues[11] quantified the rate of embolization at various phases in 60 patients undergoing percutaneous interventions of the SFA. Embolic signals were detected in every patient during wire crossing, balloon angioplasty, stent deployment, and atherectomy, in order of increasing embolic signal frequency. However, clinically and angiographically significant distal embolization occurred in only one patient (1.6%). On the basis of these results, the authors concluded that the routine use of distal protection devices during SFA interventions was not warranted.

In addition to the atheromatous lesion itself, the introducer sheath may be a source of embolic matter. Acute thrombus can form within an introducer sheath or on its tip. Intermittent flushing with heparin-saline can reduce the risk of this complication. Furthermore, anticoagulation should routinely be instituted during therapeutic interventions, including angioplasty, stenting, and atherectomy. The adequacy of anticoagulation should be verified with serial coagulation parameters.

The clinical impact of distal embolization varies from the asymptomatic patient to those in whom focal cutaneous gangrenous lesions, blue toe syndrome, trash foot, and even limb loss develop. In the patient with severe infrageniculate occlusive disease, embolization and subsequent loss of a single tibial runoff vessel can be disastrous. Completion angiography after percutaneous interventions confirms the status of the outflow anatomy. If such a process is identified, treatment options include local lytic therapy, suction embolectomy, thrombectomy, or fluoroscopically assisted thromboembolectomy. Last, the importance of preprocedural and postprocedural bilateral lower-extremity pulse examinations cannot be overemphasized, particularly when an intervention is performed from the contralateral femoral artery. An obvious change in the pulse examination results should prompt an evaluation to exclude a local (puncture-related) or distal (embolic) complication.

Newer technologies have been developed that aim to reduce some of the negative effects of traditional angioplasty. Cutting balloons contain several longitudinally mounted circumferential microtomes that are designed to cut the plaque in multiple planes before it ruptures. This is thought to lead to more uniform vessel wall dilatation, less plaque fracture, and reduced arterial dissection. Cryoplasty balloons freeze the plaque before dilatation leading to the development of microfractures, again allowing for a more uniform dilatation without large plaque fracture or dissection.

Atherectomy involves the longitudinal shaving of plaque from the vessel wall and, because of this, may be especially prone to embolization. Higher rates of embolization have been demonstrated with this technique when compared with balloon angiopolasty.[11]

Subintimal angioplasty may result in embolization of plaque from the distal end point or other debris from the subintimal plane. Embolization may occur either during dissection or with balloon angioplasty but will likely not become apparent until a flow lumen has been restored.

Perforation, Rupture, and Reentry Devices

Perforation and/or rupture may occur within native arteries, vein grafts, or at anastomotic sites of previously placed autogenous or prosthetic bypass grafts. Perforation may occur as a result of penetration of the vessel with a wire, as a result of balloon dilatation, or from treatment with a debulking device, such as an atherectomy catheter. Perforation at the distal endpoint of native arteries resulting from the treatment of occlusive lesions may or may not be of clinical significance. This is especially true if recanalization is not achieved. In this setting there is not an increase in the flow or pressure in the affected segment, and the perforation may seal spontaneously. Perforation in the setting of stenotic lesions, including vein grafts, may require treatment with covered stent placement or open repair. Patients are almost uniformly anticoagulated during interventions, which must be taken into consideration in the treatment plan for these perforations.

In the course of crossing occlusive lesions with techniques such as subintimal angioplasty, perforation of the vessel may occur (Figure 33-6). In this scenario the perforation may appear severe, but in general simply removing the wire will allow the occluded segment to recoil, sealing the site without sequelae. This is provided that the occluded segment has not been balloon dilated or otherwise instrumented. The resulting hematoma can then be managed accordingly.

During the treatment of bypass graft stenoses, anastomotic disruption may result from balloon angioplasty at either the proximal or distal anastomoses of failing vein or prosthetic grafts. In the case of vein grafts, rupture of the graft itself may occur requiring the placement of a covered stent or an open repair. If the vein cannot be repaired, an interposition graft may be required.

Fluoroscopically assisted thromboembolectomy may also result in anastomotic disruption when attempting to remove adherent clot from the proximal anastomosis of a prosthetic graft with use of a ringed thrombectomy catheter. This device has an adjustable-pitch corkscrew wire at its distal tip. The pitch of the wire is controlled by a sliding switch on the handle. Because this device is considerably stiffer than a standard balloon catheter, it is able to dislodge thrombus that the balloon catheter cannot. However, the risk of damage to the artery is proportionally increased. The scenario of anastomotic disruption requires that proximal control be obtained either with an intraluminal balloon catheter or via an open approach. In this scenario an open repair is usually required.

Occlusion of Collateral Vessels

A major concern regarding recanalization techniques that are of uncertain durability is whether or not patients will be clinically worse in the event of target site restenosis or occlusion. In the event of such a procedural failure the patients' clinical status will be dependent on the quality and quantity of the collateral vessels supplying

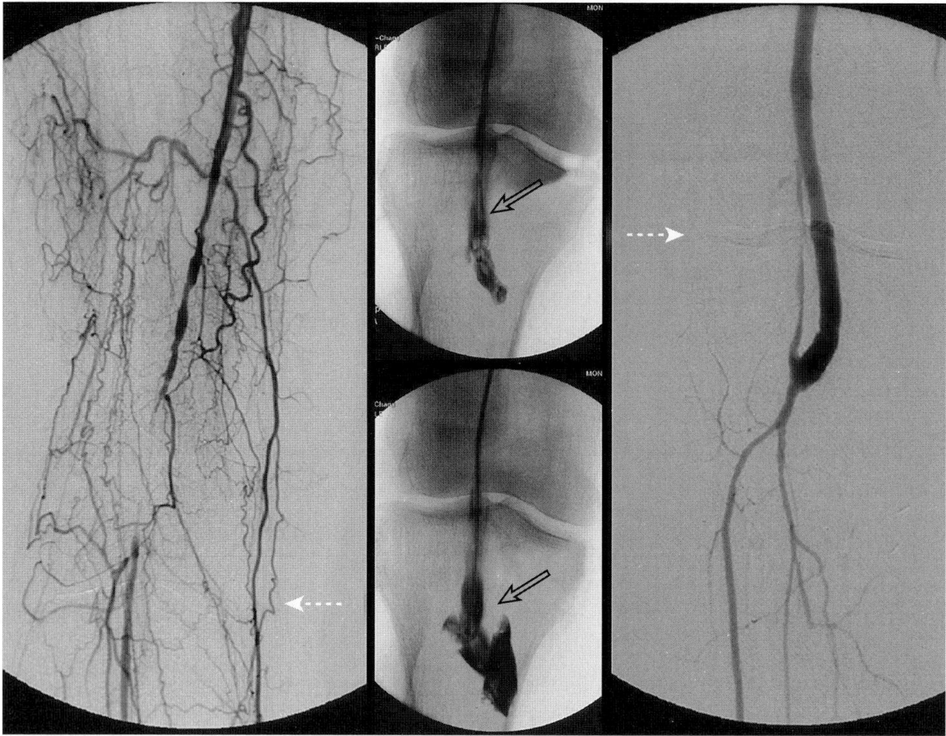

FIGURE 33-6 *Left panel,* Occlusion of the popliteal artery. *Middle panels,* Perforation of the popliteal artery after attempt at subintimal angioplasty with extravasation of contrast. *Right panel,* After removal of wires a popliteal bypass was performed. Note no further extravasation of contrast. The knee joint is indicated by the *dashed arrows* in the *left* and *right panels.*

the area distal to the occlusion. Although perhaps not classically considered a complication, a basic principle in the treatment of lower-extremity occlusive disease is that the patient should be clinically no worse off in the event of target lesion restenosis or occlusion than he or she was before the procedure. The clinical status is therefore dependent on the preservation of collateral vessels. This principle applies to both traditional open surgical procedures and endovascular procedures. It may not always be possible to preserve all collateral vessels, but every attempt should be made to do so for the long-term benefit of the patient. In some cases subintimal angioplasty may actually open collateral vessels that were not filling before the procedure.[12]

The most effective method for avoiding injury to collateral vessels is to avoid including them in the treated segment. When large collateral vessels are visualized in a position that may be jeopardized by the planned intervention, alternative approaches must be carefully considered. When this is not possible, all attempts to avoid injury to the vessel should be carried out. For example, when a large collateral is located at the origin of an occlusion and subintimal angioplasty is planned, the wire and catheter should be directed specifically at the wall of the artery opposite the origin of the collateral vessel to minimize the chances of injury (Figure 33-7).

COMPLICATIONS OF STENT PLACEMENT

Independent of a successful angioplasty the placement of intraluminal stents may have its own unique set of complications.

Failure to Deploy

Failure of a stent to deploy is an unusual complication that may occur when there is significant tortuosity or angulation in the approach to the lesion, causing the delivery system to distort or deform. In the case of self-expanding stents, which are unsheathed for deployment, failure is usually due to difficulties with the delivery system as a result of the anatomic factors mentioned above. Balloon-expandable stents, which are premounted on the balloon catheter, may fail to deploy as a result of inability to inflate the balloon. Alternatively, the stent may become dislodged from the balloon during passage to the treatment site. Stents that fail to deploy, or deploy only partially, generally can be retrieved. If the stent is partially deployed such that it cannot be recaptured, options include completing the deployment and accepting an ineffective or misplaced stent in a relatively normal segment of artery, attempting to snare and recapture the stent via an endovascular approach

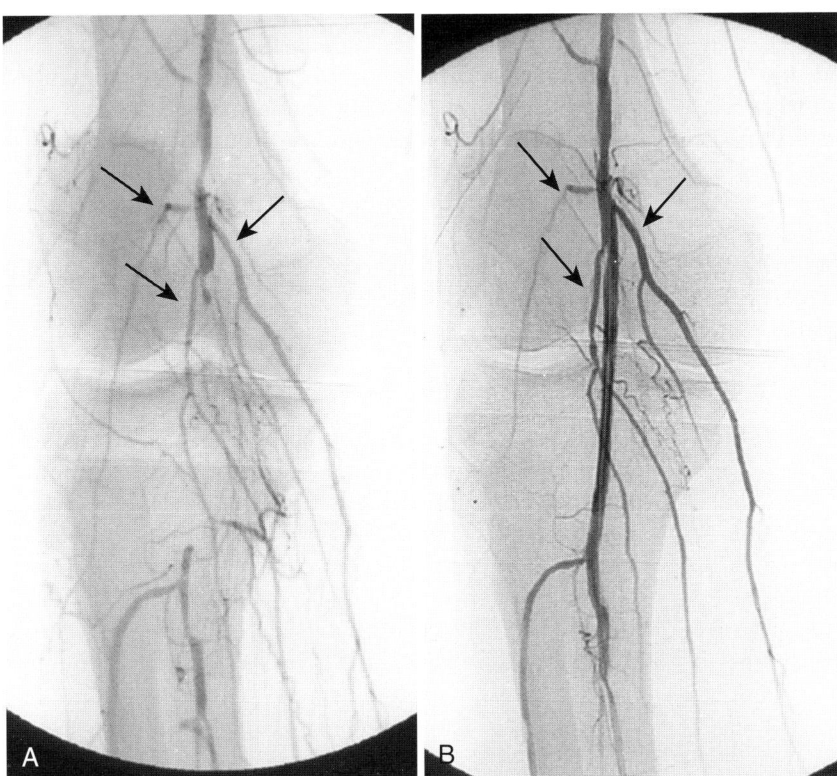

FIGURE 33-7 Collateral vessels identified **(A)** and preserved **(B)** following subintimal angioplasty.

from either the same or a new access site, or open stent retrieval.

Maldeployment/Inappropriate Sizing

Occasionally stents may be deployed such that they are kinked or incompletely opposed to the arterial wall. This situation becomes more likely in tortuous vessels or when there is diffuse, irregular, calcified plaque. In many cases no intervention is required, but manipulations with selective balloon inflation within the stent can remedy the situation.

Stent Embolization

Stents may be incompletely or prematurely deployed with resulting embolization. Snaring and resheathing of these stents may be possible in some cases but may require upsizing of the sheath. Depending on the type of stent it may also be "trapped" and stented against the arterial wall with the use of a second stent.

Jailing of Collateral Vessels

Studies have shown that "jailing," or covering collateral vessels with bare stents, may result in the loss of these collaterals.[13] In many cases, covering these vessels is unavoidable to achieve successful treatment. Whenever possible, however, the shortest possible stent that avoids coverage of collaterals should be used. When using self-expanding stents, it should be remembered that if the stent is oversized, it may not foreshorten to its designed length, covering more of the vessel than planned. Not only may the collaterals be covered at the time of deployment, but the development of intimal hyperplasia and stent occlusion will almost certainly lead to the loss of all collaterals in the treated segment. Careful preprocedural and intraprocedural planning is the best method for avoiding unwanted collateral coverage.

Stretching of Stent With Resultant Stent Fracture

An underappreciated complication of arterial stenting is stent fracture. Stent fracture may occur late as a result of mechanical fatigue or early in association with suboptimal deployment. When it occurs during deployment it is generally due to excessive tension on the stent with resultant stretching of the device. It should be suspected when a stent seems to have deployed at longer than its anticipated length. When this occurs it is often associated with a less-favorable clinical outcome. In a comprehensive review, Rits and associates[14] reported a wide range in the incidence of stent fracture (2%-65% in the superficial artery). The authors reported higher fracture rates when long femoral segments were treated and in the setting of multiple stent deployment with overlap. Stents placed in arteries that traverse the hip or knee joint are exposed to a great degree and variety of mechanical stresses and are at increased risk for fracture. Ideally, stent fractures should be detected with ultrasound or plain films and treated before symptoms develop. However, these lesions may be difficult to appreciate with these modalities in routine practice. Treatment may require placement of additional stents.

SYSTEMIC COMPLICATIONS

The complications of endovascular intervention are not limited only to the access and treatment sites but may be systemic in nature. Once again, although they are minimally invasive procedures, as with all interventions the systemic effects of treatment must also be considered. Radiation exposure is discussed in Chapters 4 and 5.

Complications of Anticoagulation

Complications related to the use of anticoagulation may be due to excessive or inadequate anticoagulation. Most interventionalists are familiar with the risks of overanticoagulation including pseudoaneurysm formation, bleeding around the sheath, bleeding at the treatment site, and bleeding from remote sites including retroperitoneal hemorrhage and stroke. Partial or complete reversal of anticoagulation is frequently required in this situation. Inadequate anticoagulation may also lead to complications such as thrombosis at the treatment site, embolization of clot formed on the catheters and guidewires, and thrombosis of the access vessel. Finally, derangements in coagulation may occur as a result of underlying or hypercoagulable states. Heparin-induced thrombocytopenia is an acquired hypercoagulable state that should be suspected in the setting of falling platelet count and that requires discontinuation of all heparin and treatment with an alternative agent such as argatroban or lepirudin.

Complications can also result from the reversal of anticoagulation with protamine sulfate. Although such reactions are rare and occur most commonly in patients with diabetes taking neutral protamine Hagedorn (NPH) insulin, they can result in significant hypotension and require aggressive resuscitation. When given, protamine should be administered slowly over several minutes with a small initial dose to prevent reaction and to facilitate successful treatment should a reaction occur.

Complications of Thrombolysis

The complications of thrombolysis are similar to those of overanticoagulation, and many cases are more attributable to the effects of the adjunctive anticoagulation than the thrombolytic agent itself. This may be especially true for intracerebral bleeding where uncontrolled hypertension also plays a major role. Patients may also have allergic reactions to these agents requiring discontinuation and treatment.

Contrast Toxicity

Adverse reactions to contrast agents may vary widely in their severity and clinical presentation from minimal transient elevations in serum creatinine level to major anaphylactic reactions. These reactions may be systemic or affect only a single organ system. Systemic reactions to contrast agents may be mild (pain, itching), moderate (hypotension, wheezing), or severe (unresponsiveness, arrhythmias, cardiac arrest). Minor reactions are frequently related to the osmolality of the agent. For example, pain can be greatly reduced with the use of low-osmolality agents.

There are several risk factors associated with the development of systemic reactions including severe allergies, active asthma, and cardiac disease. Shellfish allergies have traditionally been thought to be closely associated with contrast sensitivity, but this has not been shown to be a stronger risk factor than the presence of any other severe allergy.[15] In addition, although a prior contrast reaction does increase the likelihood of a subsequent reaction, it does not help to predict the severity of such a reaction.[16]

The treatment of systemic contrast reactions is dictated by the nature and severity of the episode. Vasovagal reactions can be treated with Trendelenburg position and fluids. Respiratory reactions may resolve spontaneously but should be treated to prevent progression to a more severe reaction. Adrenergic inhalers are the first line of treatment, which can be followed by intramuscular or intravenous epinephrine if these local measures fail. Cardiopulmonary reactions may require full cardiopulmonary resuscitation.

Contrast nephrotoxicity is the third leading cause of acute renal failure in hospitalized patients and may occur in up to 6% of unselected patient populations and up to 50% of high-risk populations. Nearly all patients receiving radiographic contrast have a small, transient decrease in glomerular filtration. However, the exact definition of contrast nephropathy is variable. Contrast nephropathy is generally defined as a rise in the serum creatinine level to greater than 25% or more than 0.5 mg/dL above baseline in the absence of other inciting events.[17] The elevation in creatinine typically occurs within 24 to 48 hours of contrast administration. The peak increase occurs between 3 and 5 days with a return to baseline by 7 to 10 days. In the majority of cases the renal failure is nonoliguric and entirely reversible. Lactic acidosis resulting from contrast nephropathy in patients with diabetes who take the oral hypoglycemic medication metformin is a rare complication.[18] It has been recommended by some that patients discontinue this medication 24 hours before any contrast study whereas others have suggested that patients not restart the medication until 48 hours after the procedure only if there is no evidence of nephrotoxicity.[17]

Preexisting renal insufficiency is the single most important risk factor for the development of contrast nephrotoxicity. Patients with a creatinine level of above 1.5 mg/dL have up to a 21-fold increased risk of contrast nephropathy compared with patients with a normal creatinine level.[19] There are several other important factors that may increase the risk for the development of contrast nephropathy including dehydration, diabetes mellitus, contrast volume, congestive heart failure, and concurrent exposure to other nephrotoxic agents, factors that may act synergistically.

Principles for the prevention of contrast nephrotoxicity include selection of the appropriate diagnostic and/or therapeutic modality, preprocedural correction of risk factors, ensuring adequate hydration, eliminating or reducing any additional nephrotoxic agents, limiting the amount of contrast administered, and close follow-up of serum creatinine level after the procedure. All patients undergoing contrast procedures should receive adequate hydration either orally or intravenously at the time of the procedure such that positive fluid balance and high urine output are achieved. Patients with preexisting renal insufficiency should be hydrated well before and after these procedures. Patients with cardiopulmonary dysfunction must be monitored closely while receiving hydration. Because of their cost, low-osmolality, nonionic contrast agents are generally reserved for use in patients with underlying renal dysfunction, especially patients with diabetes and patients with potential hemodynamic instability, where the demonstrated benefit has been greatest.

Agents that increase renal blood flow have been proposed as a method to reduce contrast nephropathy. In the case of diuretics, this is based on the theoretic advantage that loop diuretics (e.g., furosemide) might decrease medullary oxygen consumption and hence the potential for ischemic injury during contrast studies. Mannitol, alone or in conjunction with loop diuretics, has also been proposed to reduce contrast nephropathy. Finally, low-dose dopamine and agents that selectively increase renal blood flow have been trailed. Presently there is no evidence to suggest that the use of mannitol, diuretics, or low-dose dopamine reduces the risks of contrast nephropathy, and they may in fact increase the risk by their tendency to produce negative fluid balance and dehydration. On the basis of studies suggesting that reactive oxygen species may play a major role in the pathogenesis of contrast nephropathy, the antioxidant *N*-acetylcysteine has been evaluated for a potential protective effect. Recent studies, in patients undergoing contrast CT scanning and cardiac catheterization, have showed some reduction of contrast nephropathy.[20] Studies with the selective dopamine-1 (DA-1) receptor agonist fenoldopam have shown significant reductions in the incidence of contrast nephropathy.[21] Fenoldopam is given parenterally but has no stimulatory effect on dopamine-2 (DA-2) or adrenergic receptors (both cause vasoconstriction) as does dopamine at higher doses. Fenoldopam has been found to increase renal blood flow and improve glomerular filtration rates, while reducing both systolic and diastolic blood pressures in patients with hypertension (mild blood pressure reductions were seen in normotensive patients).[21]

As is the case with any medication and/or imaging modality the best way to reduce toxicity is use the lowest volume and concentration of the agent possible. Presently, maintenance of adequate hydration is the most important factor in preventing contrast nephropathy.

Infectious Complications

Septic complications after infrainguinal endovascular procedures are rare and include endocarditis, arteritis, mycotic aneurysm formation, and stent infections. We routinely administer prophylactic antibiotics against gram-positive organisms as part of our angiography protocol. Treatment of any concurrent infections, such as infected wounds, should be maintained during treatment. Infections of the access site are rare, but their occurrence is increased when prosthetic materials, for example, sheaths or catheters, are left in place. The use of careful aseptic technique and avoidance of access sites that may have recent infection reduce the chance of access site infection.

COMPLICATIONS AT CLOSURE

Vessel Occlusion After Manual Pressure

As mentioned earlier in this chapter, overzealous manual compression of the femoral artery after sheath removal can lead to arterial thrombosis. This may occur in normal, as well as small and diseased, arteries. Proper technique for sheath removal involves the use of firm, direct, manual pressure directly over the site of arterial entry. The operator must remember that the puncture is located proximal (in the case of retrograde puncture) or distal (in the case of prograde puncture) to the skin entry site with a distance that varies depending on the angle of approach and body habitus of the patient. Whoever is performing this task must have an appreciation of these facts, as well as any procedural details that may be relevant. When removing a sheath and holding manual pressure, the operator should be able to appreciate the pulse of the underlying vessel directly under the fingers, ensuring adequate flow through the vessel at the level of the puncture site. This point emphasizes the importance of the preprocedural and postprocedural pulse examinations of both lower extremities, preferably by the same clinician. The occurrence of this complication should prompt correction of the thrombosis and evaluation of the inflow and outflow vessels for the presence of any lesions. The balance between prevention of postprocedural hemorrhage and thrombosis must be kept in mind when removing access.

There are several points to be kept in mind that may help avoid a complication when removing arterial sheaths. The operator should be cognizant of the dose of anticoagulant (and reversal agent) given during the procedure. Clotting parameters are assessed before sheath removal (e.g., activated clotting time). The activated clotting time should be in the range of the preprocedural baseline or more arbitrarily have a value of less than 150 seconds. When applying manual pressure, the pressure should be centered on the location of the arterial puncture and not the skin entry site. A larger sheath size may necessitate a longer period of manual compression. Twenty minutes of pressure should suffice for 5F sheaths, whereas up to 40 minutes may be required for 7F sheaths. We do not use sandbags or other devices because they tend to be anatomically imprecise. If using a closure device, one should familiar with its characteristics and indications.

It is essential to document the patient's preoperative pulse examination results in both extremities. If after sheath removal the previously present pedal pulse is absent, one must exclude the possibility of a thromboembolic complication or arterial dissection. If hypotension ensues after sheath removal, aggressive measures should be taken to rule out the possibility of ongoing bleeding (e.g., retroperitoneal hemorrhage). An agitated, moving patient will increase the risk of a bleeding complication. The use of sedation must be titrated to allow the patient to cooperate with any instructions and not to a degree that the patient moves excessively. Finally, patients must cooperate with the prescribed length of bed rest after the procedure.

Complications of Closure Devices

The use of vascular closure devices (VCDs) to seal the femoral arteriotomy site after angiography has become increasingly popular on the basis of the purported advantages of earlier patient ambulation, shorter recovery room stays, and the ability to continue or not reverse anticoagulation. Vascular closure devices are of two basic types, those that plug the puncture site from either inside the lumen or outside the lumen and those that suture or clip the puncture site closed. Complications with these devices can be divided into failure to close the puncture site, partially or completely, and occlusion of the access vessel, again partial or complete. If the puncture site is not sealed, management options include the use of manual compression or open exploration. Maldeployment of a closure device may require primary arterial repair or patch angioplasty. When access vessel occlusion occurs, surgery is usually required to correct the problem. If the occlusion is partial, patients may have no symptoms or may have new-onset or worsening claudication. In the setting of a complete occlusion, urgent vessel exploration and thromboendarterectomy are the required treatment. Infection and pseudoaneurysm formation can also result from the use of closure devices and are discussed elsewhere in this chapter.

A number of studies comparing manual compression with VCD use have demonstrated similar hemorrhagic complication rates.[22] Ischemic complications, however, seem to occur more frequently with VCD use, particularly in female patients.[23] New-onset claudication after transfemoral angiography in which a VCD was used should alert the clinician that an ischemic sequela may be present. Complex arterial repairs are often required, including thromboendarterectomy, embolectomy, and even interposition grafting. Dissection is generally difficult when a closure device has been used, because of the extensive inflammation and scarring that occurs with these devices. Selective use of VCD should be exercised, avoiding deployment in a patient with a small CFA (<5 mm), severe peripheral vascular disease, or suboptimal puncture.[23]

LATE COMPLICATIONS

All interventions, both open and endovascular, are finite. The durability of an endovascular intervention depends on several factors, including technique, medical adjuncts, and patient biology. In general, early failures (<30 days) after endovascular intervention are usually due to technical failures resulting from the presence of residual or newly created defects or to a thrombogenic state. These technical failures may be due to incomplete angioplasty, recoil of the vessel, the presence of a residual flow-limiting lesion, or failure to debulk the lesion and create an adequate flow channel. The negative effects of angioplasty have been discussed above, and, because of these, an already diseased vessel may be at increased risk for restenosis or occlusion along an even greater length than was encompassed by the original lesion. Thus, the entire arterial segment may be considered somewhat vulnerable and must be closely monitored. Midterm failures (30 days–18 months) are generally due to the development of intimal hyperplasia and/or pathologic remodeling, whereas late failures (>18 months) are frequently due to progression of the underlying atherosclerotic disease process.

There are several negative effects resulting from endovascular intervention itself that impact the durability of an endovascular intervention. Angioplasty leads to irregularly fractured plaque, damage to the media that occurs from stretching, and desquamation of endothelium. There is also the potential for embolization and the creation of intimal flaps. In addition, longitudinal dissection planes are created, and plaque fracture can extend a good distance proximal and/or distal to the actual angioplasty site. Because of these negative effects, the already diseased vessel may be at increased risk for restenosis or occlusion along an even greater length than was encompassed by the original lesion. In the case of atherectomy, an irregular, raw surface, at least partially denuded of endothelium, is left after the flow channel diameter is improved. Therefore, the entire treated arterial segment may be considered somewhat vulnerable and must be followed. A sound arterial duplex surveillance protocol permits early detection of recurrent or de novo lesions in most cases. Stent placement after angioplasty or atherectomy counteracts the effects of pathologic remodeling by preserving luminal diameter but exacerbates the degree of intimal hyperplasia.[24]

A rare and potentially morbid complication of stenting is aneurysm formation. Coronary artery aneurysms have been described after both angioplasty and stenting. It is possible that aggressive balloon angioplasty oversizing may cause a significant deep arterial injury. This injury may cause significant thinning or destruction of the media and lead to reduced wall thickness, increased wall stress, and subsequent development of an aneurysm.[25] Failure to completely cover an arterial dissection with a stent after balloon angioplasty may also lead to aneurysm formation. A perhaps more serious scenario arises when a pseudoaneurysm is detected in the presence of a stent infection. In addition to fever, leukocytosis, and bacteremia (*Staphylococcus aureus* most commonly), patients may present with a painful mass, or petechiae in the affected limb. Leaving an indwelling sheath for prolonged periods of time, repeated access or procedures, or remote sites of infection may predispose patients to septic arterial complications.[26] The sequelae can be devastating, including pseudoaneurysm rupture and death. Prompt treatment with intravenous antibiotics and a low threshold for operative intervention are recommended. Finally, as newer technologies such as the use of drug-eluting stents are applied to the periphery, other as yet unforeseen local and systemic complications may become apparent with their treatment dictated by the clinical scenario and available methods.

A surveillance protocol using duplex ultrasound can improve long-term patency of endovascular interventions and potentially delay or eliminate the need for additional, more invasive therapies. Such a protocol can also help identify other complications discussed in this chapter and thereby facilitate their management.

References

1. Veith FJ: Presidential address: Charles Darwin and vascular surgery, *J Vasc Surg* 25:8–18, 1997.
2. Messina LM, Brothers TE, Wakefield TW, et al: Clinical characteristics and surgical management of vascular complications in patients undergoing cardiac catheterization: interventional versus diagnostic procedure, *J Vasc Surg* 13:593, 1991.
3. Oweida SW, Roubin GS, Smith RB, et al: Postcatheterization vascular complications associated with percutaneous transluminal coronary angioplasty, *J Vasc Surg* 12:310, 1990.
4. Singh H, Cardella JF, Cole PE, et al: Quality improvement guidelines for diagnostic arteriography, *J Vasc Interv Radiol* 14:S283, 2003.
5. McCann RL, Schwartz LB, Pieper KS: Vascular complications of cardiac catheterization, *J Vasc Surg* 14:375, 1991.
6. Mukherjee D: Case 52. In Upchurch GR, Henke PK, editors: *Clinical scenarios in vascular surgery*, Philadelphia, 2005, Lippincott Williams & Williams, pp 259.
7. Allen BT, Munn JS, Stevens SL, et al: Selective non-operative management of pseudoaneurysms and arteriovenous fistulae complicating femoral artery catheterization, *J Cardiovasc Surg* 33:440, 1992.
8. Toursarkissian B, Allen BT, Petrinec D, et al: Spontaneous closure of selected iatrogenic pseudoaneurysms and arteriovenous fistulae, *J Vasc Surg* 25:803, 1997.
9. Kent KC, Moscucci M, Mansour KA, et al: Retroperitoneal hematoma after cardiac catheterization: prevalence, risk factors, and optimal management, *J Vasc Surg* 20:905, 1994.
10. Mak GY, Daly B, Chan W, et al: Percutaneous treatment of post catheterization massive retroperitoneal hemorrhage, *Cathet Cardiovasc Diagn* 29:40, 1993.
11. Lam RC, Shah S, Faries PL, et al: Incidence and clinical significance of distal embolization during percutaneous interventions involving the superficial femoral artery, *J Vasc Surg* 46:1155, 2007.
12. Lipsitz EC, Ohki T, Veith FJ, et al: Fate of collateral vessels following subintimal angioplasty, *J Endovasc Ther* 11:269, 2004.
13. Aliabadi D, Tilli FV, Bowers TR, et al: Incidence and angiographic predictors of side branch occlusion following high-pressure intracoronary stenting, *Am J Cardiol* 80:994, 1997.

14. Rits J, van Herwaarden JA, Jahrome AK, et al: The incidence of arterial stent fractures with exclusion of coronary, aortic, and non-arterial settings, *Eur J Vasc Endovasc Surg* 36:339, 2008.
15. Lasser EC, Berry CC, Talner LB, et al: Pre-treatment with corticosteroids to alleviate reactions to intravenous contrast material, *N Engl J Med* 317:845, 1987.
16. Bettmann MA: Physiologic Effects and Systemic Reactions. In Baum S, editor: *Abrams' angiography*, ed 4, Philadelphia PA, 1996, Lippincott Williams & Wilkins, pp 22.
17. Murphy SW, Barrett BJ, Parfrey PS: Contrast nephropathy, *J Am Soc Nephrol* 11:177, 2000.
18. Thomsen HS, Morcos SK: Contrast media and metformin: guidelines to diminish the risk of lactic acidosis in non-insulin-dependent diabetics after administration of contrast media. ESUR Contrast Media Safety Committee, *Eur Radiol* 9:738, 1999.
19. Rudnick MR, Berns JS, Cohen RM, et al: Contrast-media associated nephrotoxicity, *Semin Nephrol* 17:15–26, 1997.
20. Diaz-Sandoval LJ, Kosowsky BD, Losordo DW: Acetylcysteine to prevent angiography-related renal tissue injury (the APART Trial), *Am J Cardiol* 89:356, 2002.
21. Kini AS, Mitre CA, Kim M, et al: A protocol for prevention of radiologic contrast nephropathy during percutaneous coronary intervention: effect of selective dopamine receptor agonist fenoldopam, *Cathet Cardiovasc Intervent* 55:169, 2002.
22. Nikolsky E, Mehran R, Halkin A, et al: Vascular complications associated with arteriotomy closure devices in patients undergoing percutaneous coronary procedures: a meta-analysis, *J Am Coll Cardiol* 12:1200, 2004.
23. Schumacher PM, Ross CB, Wu YC, et al: Ischemic complications of percutaneous femoral artery catheterization, *Ann Vasc Surg* 21:704, 2007.
24. Mehran R, Dangas G, Mintz GS, et al: Patterns of in stent restenosis: angiographic classification and implications for long-term clinical outcome, *Circulation* 100:1999, 1872.
25. Berkalp B, Kervancioglu C, Oral D: Coronary artery aneurysm formation after balloon angioplasty and stent implantation, *Int J Cardiol* 69:65, 1999.
26. Pruitt A, Dodson TF, Najibi S, et al: Distal septic emboli and fatal brachiocephalic artery mycotic pseudoaneurysm as a complication of stenting, *J Vasc Surg* 36:625, 2002.

SECTION V

VISCERAL ARTERIAL OCCLUSIVE DISEASE

CHAPTER

34

Endovascular Treatment of Renovascular Disease

Douglas B. Hood, Kim J. Hodgson

Although surgical revascularization of renal artery occlusive disease was long ago demonstrated to be of benefit to patients with renovascular hypertension, as well as selected patients with renal insufficiency, the associated morbidity and mortality of these procedures have discouraged their use in all but the most severe cases. The first renal artery angioplasty was performed by Dr. Charles Tegtmeyer in 1976. Renal artery angioplasty was an appealing alternative to renal artery bypass, which was the standard revascularization procedure at that time. Endovascular renal revascularization offers the potential for gaining the therapeutic benefits of the surgical procedures with reduced periprocedural risk and recovery time, albeit with a potential reduction in durability. This has led to an explosion in renal artery interventions, often with little preprocedural evaluation and frequently for the perceived benefit of "renal salvage," though data to support this indication, as reviewed later, are not compelling. Nonetheless, knowledge of the indications for and technique of percutaneous renal revascularization should be part of the armamentarium of all endovascular surgeons, for clearly a good number of patients seen in the average vascular surgery practice will benefit from this procedure.

Renal artery stenosis (RAS) is the most common cause of secondary hypertension, with an estimated incidence of 5% in the hypertensive population. Congenital anomalies, arteritis, trauma, arterial dissection, fibromuscular dysplasia, and atherosclerosis are all recognized causes of RAS. Among these, atherosclerosis is by far the most common etiology, accounting for 60% to 80% of cases of clinically significant renal artery disease. This review will summarize the current status of endovascular management of atherosclerotic RAS, with a focus on recently reported technical and clinical results.

NATURAL HISTORY

Atherosclerosis affecting the renal arteries is a progressive disease that most often results from encroachment of aortic plaque across or into the renal artery orifice. Because of this characteristic pattern, most clinically relevant atherosclerotic renal artery lesions are ostial in location, located within the most proximal 5 mm of the vessel. Once RAS becomes hemodynamically significant (>60%), progression to renal artery occlusion is a very real possibility. Using sequential angiograms, Tollefson and Ernst[1] found that RAS progressed at approximately 5% per year irrespective of the level of stenosis and that occlusion was associated with greater degrees of stenosis. Caps et al.[2] reported that 49% of patients with more than 60% RAS measured by duplex ultrasonography showed disease progression over a 3-year period. Zierler et al.[3] reported that the cumulative progression to occlusion of renal arteries with a baseline stenosis greater than 60% was 5% at 1 year and 11% at 2 years. A more recent randomized trial of patients with hypertension with lesions greater than 50% demonstrated that 16% of the medical treatment group progressed to occlusion at 1 year.[4] Renal artery occlusion is associated with loss of nephrons and atrophy of the kidney parenchyma, with a mean decrease in kidney length of 1.8 cm in the report of Zierler et al.[3] Renal atrophy can also occur in association with stenotic but nonoccluded renal arteries.[2]

DIAGNOSIS

Despite the rapid advances in technology in recent years, the most important component in the diagnosis of RAS is a high clinical suspicion. The clinical clues suggestive of RAS include onset of hypertension younger than 30 or older than 55 years of age; accelerated, resistant, or malignant hypertension; sudden, unexplained pulmonary edema; multivessel coronary artery or peripheral arterial disease; and unexplained congestive heart failure (CHF) or refractory angina. Patients with atherosclerotic RAS more often are male, are over 60 years of age, and have the typical atherosclerotic risk factors of diabetes, hyperlipidemia, tobacco use, and hypertension. RAS may also be suspected in patients with unexplained renal dysfunction or with new or worsening azotemia after administration of an angiotensin-converting enzyme inhibitor or angiotensin receptor antagonist. The physical finding of an abdominal or flank bruit supports the diagnosis but is present in only 25% of patients. Laboratory findings consistent with RAS include refractory hypokalemia and an elevated peripheral renin assay, either of which is found in only an occasional patient. Any of the above clinical findings, alone or in combination, raises the index of suspicion and should prompt diagnostic imaging of the renal arteries.

IMAGING STUDIES

Renal artery imaging no longer requires invasive angiography that, in the past, dissuaded many practitioners from aggressively pursuing the diagnosis of RAS in patients who were medically compromised. The development of less-invasive imaging techniques that provide a thorough investigation of renal artery anatomy has increased the recognition of RAS.

Renal duplex ultrasonography has emerged as an excellent test to screen patients for RAS. Although it requires significant technical expertise, it is a safe and relatively inexpensive modality that provides information concerning kidney size, cortical thickness, renal artery hemodynamics, and velocity profiles, as well as nonvascular anatomic renal abnormalities such as cysts. Several authors have documented the accuracy of using renal artery peak systolic velocities (PSVs) to detect RAS. A PSV above 180 to 220 cm/s has a reported sensitivity and specificity of 84% to 91% and 85% to 99%, respectively. In the experience of the authors, a PSV above 220 cm/s identified RAS with a sensitivity and specificity of 91% and 85%, respectively.[5] Importantly, the negative predictive value of 95% of this threshold value essentially eliminated the possibility of RAS, making duplex ultrasonography a highly useful screening test. However, limitations of ultrasound imaging of the renal arteries include large body habitus and overlying bowel gas obscuring identification of the renal arteries.

Renal duplex ultrasonography to measure renal arterial resistance may also offer a method to predict outcomes after therapy for RAS.[6,7] In the 2001 study by Radermacher et al.,[7] color Doppler ultrasonography was used to measure the renal resistance index in 138 patients who had unilateral or bilateral RAS of more than 50% and who underwent renal angioplasty or surgery. The procedure was technically successful in 95%. Creatinine clearance and 24-hour ambulatory blood pressure were measured before RAS was corrected and at 3-, 6-, and 12-month intervals and yearly thereafter. Mean follow-up was 32 months. Patients with an elevated renal resistance index (27% of the cohort) did not realize an improvement in blood pressure, whereas those with a normal index had a statistically significant improvement in mean arterial pressure to 3 years. Creatinine clearance declined in 80% of patients with an elevated renal resistance index despite technically successful revascularization. Forty-six percent of patients with an elevated renal resistance index became dependent on dialysis during follow-up, and 29% died. Patients with a normal resistance index had a significant increase in creatinine clearance, followed out to 60 months.

Magnetic resonance arteriography (MRA) using gadolinium is also a useful tool for evaluating renal artery anatomy. It has a sensitivity of 90% to 100% and a specificity of 76% to 94% when compared with conventional arteriography.[8,9] As a screening modality, MRA is more expensive and less patient-friendly than duplex, but it has become a valuable tool and the first-line screening test in institutions without reliable results with duplex scanning. However, correlation with arteriography has varied on the basis of equipment, technique, and the skill of the interpreter. In patients who have undergone previous placement of renal stents, MRA cannot be used to evaluate stent patency because of signal interference from the metal. Be aware that administration of MRA contrast agents in patients with compromised renal function may result in nephrogenic systemic fibrosis, a potentially fatal complication.[10]

Advances in computed tomographic imaging, including multislice computed tomographic angiography, have provided very accurate reconstructions of abdominal vascular anatomy and pathology. The major limitations to widespread use of this modality for RAS screening are the need for iodinated contrast and cost.

With use of any of the above modalities, the diagnosis of RAS can be reliably excluded, but conventional angiography is required for confirmation of positive results and to guide endovascular interventions. In the presence of renal insufficiency, carbon dioxide (Figure 34-1) or small amounts of gadolinium can be used in lieu of iodinated contrast agents.[11-13] Although both carbon dioxide and gadolinium have limitations, and the image quality is inferior to that obtained with use of conventional iodinated contrast agents, renal artery imaging is possible and reproducible. These alternative agents are particularly valuable for patients with ischemic nephropathy, in whom even small amounts of iodinated contrast may be injurious.

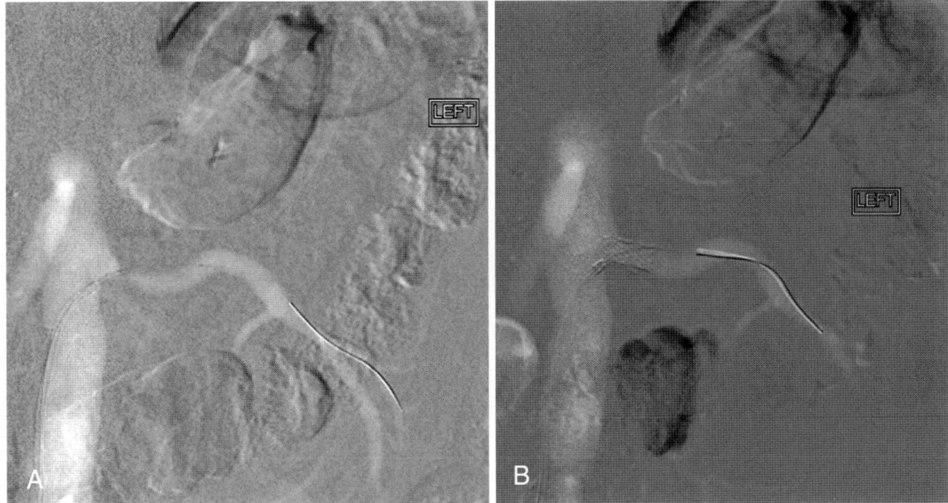

FIGURE 34-1 Selective CO_2 angiography before **(A)** and after **(B)** stent placement for a proximal left RAS.

When considering intervention for RAS, the clinician must recognize that the mere presence of anatomic RAS does not necessarily establish it as the pathophysiologic cause of hypertension or renal dysfunction. Consequently, the decision to intervene is ultimately a clinical judgment and can never be made with absolute certainty of benefit. In our opinion, physiologic tests such as peripheral or renal vein renin sampling and nuclear scanning are not sufficiently reliable to be of value in selecting patients for treatment. At our institution, intervention is considered when unilateral or bilateral RAS above 60% is documented and any of the following clinical parameters is present: poorly controlled blood pressure despite aggressive medical management, hypertension complicated by congestive heart failure or flash pulmonary edema, or progressive renal insufficiency.

ENDOVASCULAR MANAGEMENT

Following is a description of the techniques that we have used successfully for the endovascular management of renal artery lesions. It should be noted, however, that there are manifold variations on this technique, and each operator may find several other combinations of sheaths, guidewires, and other instruments that are equally efficacious.

Groin access via the femoral artery is used most commonly, although a brachial artery approach should be considered for renal arteries with significant caudal angulation or in patients with significant aortoiliac occlusive disease. For unilateral RAS we prefer to access the contralateral femoral artery, which usually provides a straighter path to the target lesion. After percutaneous arterial access and placement of a 6F sheath, a multi–side-hole catheter is placed in the abdominal aorta and positioned at approximately the level of the L1-2 vertebral interspace for flush aortography. Complete visualization of the renal artery origins may require anteroposterior and oblique views. With complicating anatomy, selective catheterization of one or both renal arteries may be required for better angiographic detail, but this is rarely necessary and increases the risk of embolization. Translesional pressure measurements may be performed for lesions of questionable hemodynamic significance, although we seldom find this necessary. A systolic pressure gradient of 20 mm Hg or greater is significant. Pressures should be measured simultaneously between the aorta and the renal artery beyond the stenosis with use of a 4F or smaller device (such as a 0.014-inch pressure-sensing guidewire) within the renal artery and a sheath or guiding catheter in the aorta at least 1F larger than the device in the renal artery.

Once the decision has been made to intervene on a stenosis, full heparinization is effected and the aortogram (Figure 34-2) reviewed to guide selection of an appropriately shaped guiding catheter. Guiding catheters are of braided construction, giving them column strength and "torque-ability," and their precurved tips serve to direct guidewires and other devices into the renal artery without actually projecting into the stenosis themselves. When selecting a guiding catheter shape, it is important to consider the shape the guiding catheter will have when it is constrained within the aorta, not just as it appears in the package, as the two can be very different. The guiding catheter can be advanced into the suprarenal position over a standard 0.035-inch angiographic guidewire, sealed at its hub with a Touhy-Borst adapter, and attached to a contrast-saline syringe manifold. The 0.035-inch guidewire is then withdrawn, allowing the guiding catheter to take its shape, and a 0.014-inch

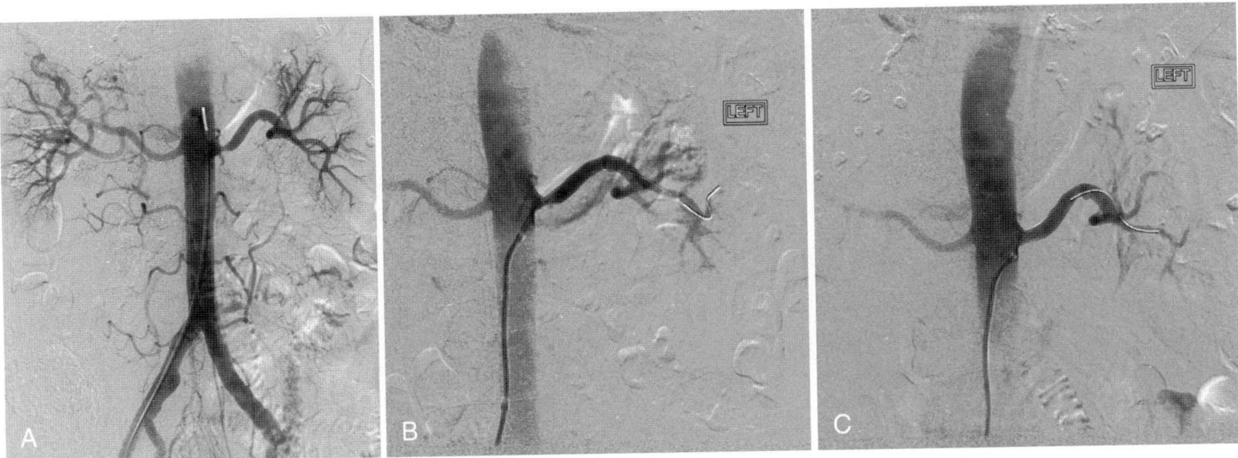

FIGURE 34-2 **A,** Nonselective aortogram showing proximal left RAS. **B,** Image after selective catheterization of the left renal artery, with placement of a guiding catheter near its orifice and guidewire crossing of the lesion. **C,** Completion angiogram after stenting.

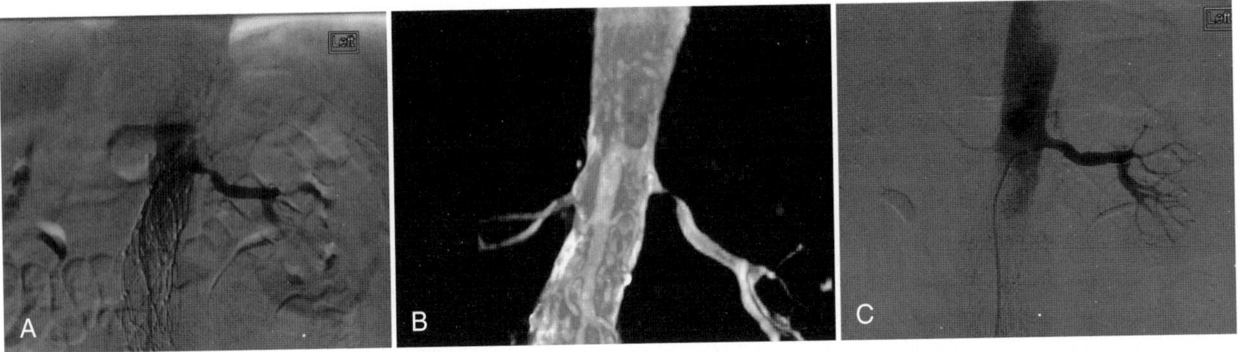

FIGURE 34-3 **A,** Left RAS in a patient with a previously placed aortic endograft. **B,** Rotational angiogram of same patient. **C,** Completion angiogram after stent placement.

guidewire is inserted into the guiding catheter and positioned just short of its tip. The guiding catheter is then retracted and rotated, as needed, to just engage the renal artery orifice, as confirmed by puffs of contrast injected through the manifold syringe. The prepositioned 0.014-inch guidewire is then manipulated through the lesion and positioned to provide adequate support without being too far into the renal hilar vessels, which could be traumatic to them. Angioplasty balloons and stents can now be advanced through the guiding catheter and over the guidewire to the site of intervention, with periprocedural imaging made possible by the guiding catheter positioned just proximal to the angioplasty balloon. If renal artery anatomy is otherwise suitable, an embolic protection device can be substituted for the guidewire, though the efficacy of this added expense has not yet been demonstrated.

Atherosclerotic lesions in the midportion of the main renal artery may be well treated with balloon angioplasty alone, but the more common ostial lesions generally require stent placement. We prefer premounted, balloon-expandable stents for their enhanced radial strength and accuracy of deployment. There are currently only three stents approved for use in the renal arteries (Genesis and Palmaz stents, Cordis Endovascular, Warren, NJ; AVE Bridge stent, Medtronic, Santa clara, CA) but there are several other commercially available stents of suitable sizes. Predilation is generally not required and may be undesirable because of potential microembolization of plaque fragments to the renal parenchyma. Most cases require a stent of 10 to 20 mm in length mounted on a 5 or 6 mm balloon. The stent is positioned across the lesion, with 2 to 3 mm of stent projecting into the aorta for ostial lesions. Once the stent is deployed, the balloon is deflated and withdrawn, being careful to maintain wire access across the lesion. Completion angiography is performed with contrast injected through the guiding catheter after retraction of the angioplasty balloon (Figure 34-3). The completion study should be critically assessed for technical success (<30% residual stenosis) and for the complications of renal artery dissection, thrombosis, emboli, or perforation of the renal parenchyma. With a satisfactory result, we generally use a closure device to seal the femoral puncture site after the sheath is removed.

RESULTS

Prospective trials comparing endovascular intervention with medical management or open surgical repair of RAS are few, but a substantial body of nonrandomized descriptive literature is available. Overall, the body of evidence is fragmented, often with varying definitions, inclusion and exclusion criteria, and the type of assessed endpoints. In general, published reports describe the results of endovascular treatment according to technical success, blood pressure response, renal function, and survival advantage.

Technical Success

Multiple series have analyzed the technical results of endovascular intervention. Interpretation of technical results in the various studies is sometimes challenging because of varying definitions of success and the lack of consistent use of postprocedural imaging. Technical success is most commonly defined as a residual stenosis of less than 30%, with no evidence of dissection, perforation, or branch vessel compromise. Inability to traverse the lesion is the most common cause of technical failure and occurs in 2% to 5% of cases.[14]

The use of stents has resulted in increased technical success and patency rates when compared with balloon angioplasty alone. In series published during the 1990s, technical success varied between 24% and 91% with use of primary angioplasty alone, with stenting reserved only for rescue indications.[14] In an effort to clarify the role of primary stenting in the treatment of atherosclerotic ostial stenosis, van de Ven et al.[15] performed a randomized prospective study that included 84 patients with hypertension. Ostial stenosis was defined as a reduction of 50% or more in luminal diameter within the first 10 mm of the aortic lumen. Immediate technical success was significantly better in the stent group than in the angioplasty group (88% vs. 57%, respectively), with equivalent complication rates. Analyzed on an intent-to-treat basis, primary patency (free of restenosis) at 6 months was only 29% in the angioplasty group and 75% in the stent group. Secondary patency (including treatment of restenosis) at 6 months was 51% and 80%, respectively. Clinical results at 6 months showed no difference between the groups in terms of blood pressure or serum creatinine level. In all, 12 patients in the angioplasty group received stents during follow-up, either for an unsuccessful initial result (5) or for recurrent stenosis (7). These authors concluded that by following a policy of selective stenting, with stent placement for technical failures and recurrent stenoses, stents could be avoided in about 40% of patients. However, because of the need for repeated interventions in those patients initially given treatment with angioplasty alone, primary stenting is probably more efficient for patients with ostial RAS caused by atherosclerosis. A meta-analysis of primary renal artery stenting by Isles et al.[16] documented a technical success of 96% to 100%. Restenosis rates after primary stenting were 9% and 39% at 6 and 12 months, respectively. Sivamurthy et al.[17] reported primary patency of 82% and primary assisted patency of 100% at 5 years.

The rate of procedural complications has also been evaluated. Alhadad et al.[18] found a 30-day mortality rate of 2% for renal artery interventions. Beutler et al.[19] reported an initial technical success in 61 of 63 patients with a 6% renovascular complication rate. More important, in the series of Beutler et al.,[19] 8% of patients showed clinical signs of cholesterol emboli with at least 20% of patients having a decrease in renal function. Martin et al.[20] reviewed complication rates from two large series and two meta-analyses to determine weighted complication rates. Periprocedural complication rates ranged from 12% to 36%. The most common complications were groin hematoma and puncture site trauma, both occurring in approximately 5%. The incidence of renal artery embolization varied from 1% to 8%, with renal artery occlusion rates between 0.8% and 2.5%.

Blood Pressure Response

Three randomized trials have compared the blood pressure response with endovascular intervention and pharmacologic therapy. Webster et al.[21] published the first randomized trial of angioplasty versus medical therapy in 1998, including 55 patients with hypertension and RAS in excess of 50%. Both medical and angioplasty groups demonstrated a significant reduction in blood pressure, with no significant difference between groups. Subgroup analysis, however, showed that patients with bilateral RAS had an improved blood pressure response with angioplasty. Plouin et al.[22] randomly assigned 49 patients to either angioplasty or medical therapy. No significant difference was found between the mean blood pressure of the two groups at 6 months, but significantly more patients were rendered free of pharmacologic treatment in the endovascular group.[22] Van Jaarsveld et al.[4] also prospectively compared the results of medical therapy versus angioplasty. This study also failed to show a compelling difference in blood pressure control between groups. Nevertheless, the number of antihypertensive medications was significantly lower in the angioplasty group. Of note, 44% of patients in the medical arm ultimately underwent angioplasty after 3 months because of poor blood pressure control.

The above prospective randomized trials compared renal artery angioplasty with or without selective stent placement with medical therapy. The benefit of routine primary stenting compared with medical therapy has not been evaluated. However, given the improved technical outcome with primary stenting compared with selective stenting, it would not be unreasonable to conclude that primary stenting may provide additional blood pressure benefit. A recent retrospective study of 100 patients with RAS by Pizzolo et al.[23] supports this assumption. In this study, primary stenting was performed in the majority of patients (67%) undergoing endovascular therapy. A significant improvement in blood pressure control was observed when compared with that of patients treated medically. Almost twice as many patients manifested an improvement in blood pressure control with endovascular intervention (57% vs. 29%). No patient in either group was cured.

A summary analysis of the above studies suggests that the endovascular management of RAS results in better blood pressure response compared with medical therapy, requiring fewer antihypertensive agents for control. Furthermore, it appears that this response can be enhanced by the use of stents.

Renal Function

The results of endovascular intervention for ischemic nephropathy have been less compelling. The above randomized trials also examined the renal response to intervention, and all failed to show consistent improvement in postintervention renal function compared with preintervention status. In the reports by Plouin et al.[22] and van Jaarsveld et al.,[4] mean serum creatinine level and creatinine clearance at 6 and 12 months were unchanged from pretreatment values. The study of Webster et al.[21] documented no change in serum creatinine; creatinine clearance was not evaluated.

However, in a retrospective study in patients with rapidly declining renal function, Beutler et al.[19] found that stent placement resulted in stabilization of renal function in 87% of patients. No effect on renal function was evident when patients with stable renal function were treated. Consistent with the findings of Beutler et al.[19] is a report by Ramos et al.,[24] in which patients with lower glomerular filtration rates (GFR) had larger improvements in GFR after endovascular intervention compared with patients with higher GFR before the procedure. In addition, when all patients were considered as a group, a significant increase in renal function was evident.[24] Burket et al.[25] reported that 43% of patients with baseline renal insufficiency showed significant improvement in renal function after intervention.

Surgical revascularization remains the one other option available for treatment of ischemic nephropathy caused by RAS. Randomized comparisons between surgical and endovascular therapy for ischemic nephropathy are not available. Reports by Marone et al.,[26] Hansen et al.,[27] and Hallet et al.[28,29] have all documented that surgical revascularization provides a substantial improvement in renal function, particularly if the RAS is bilateral or affects a solitary kidney. Furthermore, the proportion of patients that achieves benefit after surgical revascularizations is, in general, greater than that observed after endovascular therapy. Also, the more severe the renal insufficiency, the greater the benefit seen.

Two primary reasons have been proposed to explain why endovascular intervention has had less beneficial effect on renal function than expected despite excellent technical results. First, iodinated contrast agents may impart injury from which the compromised kidney cannot recover. The use of less-nephrotoxic contrast agents such as carbon dioxide in patients with compromised renal function (serum creatinine >1.8 mg/dL) may lessen the impact of this factor. Satisfactory renal artery imaging using carbon dioxide with digital imaging can be used to guide endovascular revascularization. At the very least, the use of carbon dioxide drastically reduces the amount of iodinated contrast required for renal interventions and thereby limits contrast-induced parenchymal injury.

The second reason given for the less-than-expected response after endovascular intervention is cholesterol embolization. This has led to the recent use of distal protection devices originally designed for coronary and carotid interventions. Recent studies suggest that embolic protection is associated with improved outcomes in terms of renal function when compared with historical controls.[30-32] However, these devices increase procedural complexity, and their effectiveness is not established.

In a recently published single-center prospective series, stenting with embolic protection was performed in 83 renal arteries.[33] All patients had baseline renal dysfunction with an estimated GFR of less than 60 mL/min and evidence of deterioration in renal function in the 6 months before intervention. Sixty percent of the filter baskets had gross evidence of macroscopic debris. Six months after intervention, 97% of patients had stabilization or improvement in renal function. If these improved results can be duplicated, the use of protection devices will certainly expand the indications for endovascular intervention in patients with renal dysfunction.

Survival

The expectation that improvement in blood pressure control and renal function after endovascular intervention will result in enhanced survival has yet to be conclusively documented. Only two studies have addressed this issue. Pillay et al.[34] found an overall mortality of 30% in 2 years in patients with either unilateral or bilateral RAS. No significant difference in survival was evident between patients who underwent endovascular treatment versus patients receiving optimal medical management.[34] However, patients in the endovascular group had a significantly higher baseline serum creatinine level. In contrast, Pizzolo et al.[23] found that 87% of patients receiving treatment with stent placement were alive at a median follow-up of 28 months, compared with 67% of patients who received medical treatment. Subsequent regression analysis, used in an effort to explain the observed benefit, found endovascular treatment to be the sole independent predictor of improved survival.

The Cardiovascular Outcomes in Renal Atherosclerotic Lesions (CORAL) study is an ongoing, National Institutes of Health–funded, clinical trial that may further clarify the ultimate outcome of renal artery stent placement with medical therapy compared with medical therapy alone.[35] This is a prospective, multicenter, randomized trial that is enrolling patients with RAS and systolic hypertension or renal dysfunction. The primary end point of this study is a composite of cardiovascular or renal outcomes, including death, stroke, myocardial infarction, CHF, progressive renal insufficiency, or need for permanent renal replacement therapy. Secondary outcomes include blood pressure response, longitudinal renal function, stent patency after stenting, quality of life, and cost-effectiveness. Results of this well-designed study are eagerly awaited.

Preliminary results of another large, prospective trial assessing the results of renal artery intervention have recently been reported but not yet published. The Angioplasty and Stenting for Renal Artery Lesions (ASTRAL) trial was designed to assess long-term effects of treatment in terms of preservation of renal function.[36] The trial enrolled 806 patients in the United Kingdom who were randomly assigned to catheter-based intervention (angioplasty and/or stent) plus medical therapy or to medical therapy alone. After 1 year of follow-up, there were no differences in serum creatinine level or the rates of renal events. There were also no differences in blood pressure or in the rates of myocardial infarction, stroke, CHF, or risk-adjusted mortality. More detailed publication of these results, including subgroup analyses, may provide additional clarification of the role of renal artery interventions for patients with significant RAS.

SUMMARY

The technical success of primary stenting, along with the low incidence of morbidity and mortality, has made endovascular management the primary therapy for atherosclerotic RAS in many institutions. Surgical revascularization of atherosclerotic RAS is now limited to patients with renal artery occlusions, multiple renal arteries, hilar or segmental renal artery lesions, or dissections or those in whom endovascular management fails.

The recent advances in stent technology and renal endovascular management have provided a technically reproducible method of percutaneously treating atherosclerotic RAS. In many centers, this has resulted in endovascular management being the primary therapy for atherosclerotic RAS. Although still controversial, it appears that endovascular management of RAS by primary stent deployment provides better blood pressure control than that afforded by best medical management. The impact on renal function is less than that found for hypertension, but there is evidence to suggest that the use of protection devices and primary stenting may enhance renal function outcomes. The ultimate benefit of enhanced survival after renal artery intervention remains an important question.

References

1. Tollefson DF, Ernst CB: Natural history of atherosclerotic renal artery stenosis associated with aortic disease, *J Vasc Surg* 14:327–331, 1991.
2. Caps MT, Perissinotto C, Zierler RE, et al: Prospective study of atherosclerotic disease progression in the renal artery, *Circulation* 98:2866–2872, 1998.
3. Zierler RE, Bergelin RO, Isaacson JA, et al: Natural history of atherosclerotic renal artery stenosis: a prospective study with duplex ultrasonography, *J Vasc Surg* 19:250–258, 1994.
4. van Jaarsveld BC, Krijnen P, Pieterman H, et al: The effect of balloon angioplasty on hypertension in atherosclerotic renal-artery stenosis, *N Engl J Med* 342:1007–1014, 2000.
5. Hua HT, Hood DB, Jensen CC, et al: The use of colorflow duplex scanning to detect significant renal artery stenosis, *Ann Vasc Surg* 14:118–124, 2000.
6. Cohn EJ, Benjamin ME, Sandager GP, et al: Can intrarenal duplex waveform analysis predict successful renal artery revascularization? *J Vasc Surg* 28:471–481, 1998.
7. Radermacher J, Chavan A, Bleck J, et al: Use of Doppler ultrasonography to predict the outcome of therapy for renal-artery stenosis, *N Engl J Med* 344:410–417, 2001.
8. Kent KC, Edelman RR, Kim D, et al: Magnetic resonance imaging: a reliable test for the evaluation of proximal atherosclerotic renal arterial stenosis, *J Vasc Surg* 13:311–318, 1991.
9. Schoenberg SO, Rieger J, Johannson LO, et al: Diagnosis of renal artery stenosis with magnetic resonance angiography: update 2003, *Nephrol Dial Transplant* 18:1252–1256, 2003.
10. Broome DR, Girguis MS, Baron PW, et al: Gadodiamide-associated nephrogenic systemic fibrosis: why radiologists should be concerned, *AJR Am J Roentgenol* 188:586–592, 2007.
11. Spinosa DJ, Matsumoto AH, Angle JF, et al: Safety of CO(2)- and gadodiamide-enhanced angiography for the evaluation and percutaneous treatment of renal artery stenosis in patients with chronic renal insufficiency, *AJR Am J Roentgenol* 176:1305–1311, 2001.
12. Sam AD 2nd, Morasch MD, Collins J, et al: Safety of gadolinium contrast angiography in patients with chronic renal insufficiency, *J Vasc Surg* 38:313–318, 2003.
13. Schreier DZ, Weaver FA, Frankhouse J, et al: A prospective study of carbon dioxide: digital subtraction vs standard contrast arteriography in the evaluation of the renal arteries, *Arch Surg* 131:503–508, 1996.

14. Leertouwer TC, Gussenhoven EJ, Bosch JL, et al: Stent placement for renal arterial stenosis: where do we stand? A meta-analysis, *Radiology* 216:78–85, 2000.
15. van de Ven PJ, Kaatee R, Beutler JJ, Beek FJ, et al: Arterial stenting and balloon angioplasty in ostial atherosclerotic renovascular disease: a randomized trial, *Lancet* 353:282–286, 1999.
16. Isles CG, Robertson S, Hill D: Management of renovascular disease: a review of renal artery stenting in ten studies, *Q J Med* 92:159–167, 1999.
17. Sivamurthy N, Surowiec SM, Culakova E, et al: Divergent outcomes after percutaneous therapy for symptomatic renal artery stenosis, *J Vasc Surg* 39:565–574, 2004.
18. Alhadad A, Ahle M, Ivancev K, et al: Percutaneous transluminal renal angioplasty (PTRA) and surgical revascularization in renovascular disease: a retrospective comparison of results, complications, and mortality, *Eur J Vasc Endovasc Surg* 27:151–156, 2004.
19. Beutler JJ, van Ampting JM, van de Ven PJ, et al: Long-term effects of arterial stenting on kidney function for patients with ostial atherosclerotic renal artery stenosis and renal insufficiency, *J Am Soc Nephrol* 12:1475–1481, 2001.
20. Martin LG, Rundback JH, Sacks D, et al: Quality improvement guidelines for angiography, angioplasty, and stent placement in the diagnosis and treatment of renal artery stenosis in adults, *J Vasc Intervent Radiol* 13:1069–1083, 2002.
21. Webster J, Marshall F, Abdalla M, et al: Randomised comparison of percutaneous angioplasty vs continued medical therapy for hypertensive patients with atheromatous renal artery stenosis. Scottish and Newcastle Renal Artery Stenosis Collaborative Group, *J Hum Hypertens* 12:329–335, 1998.
22. Plouin PF, Chatellier G, Darne B, et al: Blood pressure outcome of angioplasty in atherosclerotic renal artery stenosis: a randomized trial. Essai Multicentrique Medicaments vs Angioplastie (EMMA) Study Group, *Hypertension* 31:823–829, 1998.
23. Pizzolo F, Mansueto G, Minniti S, et al: Renovascular disease: effect of ACE gene deletion polymorphism and endovascular revascularization, *J Vasc Surg* 39:140–147, 2004.
24. Ramos F, Kotliar C, Alvarez D, et al: Renal function and outcome of PTRA and stenting for atherosclerotic renal artery stenosis, *Kidney Int* 63:276–282, 2003.
25. Burket MW, Cooper CJ, Kennedy DJ, et al: Renal artery angioplasty and stent placement: predictors of a favorable outcome, *Am Heart J* 139:64–71, 2000.
26. Marone LK, Clouse WD, Dorer DJ, et al: Preservation of renal function with surgical revascularization in patients with atherosclerotic renovascular disease, *J Vasc Surg* 39:322–329, 2004.
27. Hansen KJ, Starr SM, Sands RE, et al: Contemporary surgical management of renovascular disease, *J Vasc Surg* 16:319–331, 1992.
28. Hallett JW Jr, Fowl R, O'Brien PC, et al: Renovascular operations in patients with chronic renal insufficiency: do the benefits justify the risks? *J Vasc Surg* 5:622–627, 1987.
29. Hallett JW Jr, Textor SC, Kos PB, et al: Advanced renovascular hypertension and renal insufficiency: trends in medical comorbidity and surgical approach from 1970 to 1993, *J Vasc Surg* 21:750–760, 1995.
30. Henry M, Klonaris C, Henry I, et al: Protected renal stenting with the PercuSurge GuardWire device: a pilot study, *J Endovasc Ther* 8:227–237, 2001.
31. Holden A, Hill A: Renal angioplasty and stenting with distal protection of the main renal artery in ischemic nephropathy: early experience, *J Vasc Surg* 38:962–968, 2003.
32. Edwards MS, Craven BL, Stafford J, et al: Distal embolic protection during renal artery angioplasty and stenting, *J Vasc Surg* 44:128–135, 2006.
33. Holden A, Hill A, Jaff MR, et al: Renal artery stent revascularization with embolic protection in patients with ischemic nephropathy, *Kidney Int* 70:948–955, 2006.
34. Pillay WR, Kan YM, Crinnion JN, et al: Joint Vascular Research Group, UK. Prospective multicentre study of the natural history of atherosclerotic renal artery stenosis in patients with peripheral vascular disease, *Br J Surg* 89:737–740, 2002.
35. Cooper CJ, Murphy TP, Matsumoto A, et al: Stent revascularization for the prevention of cardiovascular and renal events among patients with renal artery stenosis and systolic hypertension: rationale and design of the CORAL trial, *Am Heart J* 152:59–66, 2006.
36. Mistry S, Ives N, Harding J, et al: Angioplasty and Stenting for Renal Artery Lesions (ASTRAL trial): rationale, methods, and results so far, *J Hum Hypertens* 21:511–515, 2007.

CHAPTER

35

Mesenteric Syndromes

Daniel Clair

Mesenteric ischemia accounts for only 0.1% of hospital admissions, but it is associated with a daunting mortality rate.[1] The mainstay of treatment has relied on prompt diagnosis and surgical treatment for the last 50 years; however, endovascular approaches have been increasingly used for mesenteric ischemia for the past two decades. Mesenteric angioplasty and stenting have become viable options for chronic mesenteric ischemia, and thrombolytic therapy has been used for acute superior mesenteric artery (SMA) occlusion.[2] The vast majority (95%) of patients with mesenteric ischemia present with acute ischemia.[3] Despite advances in treatment, morbidity and mortality for those presenting with acute mesenteric ischemia still remain high. Contemporary results report mortality ranges from 60% to 90%,[4] and the mortality rate has remained fairly constant over the past decade with little improvement in results.[5-7]

Securing a clinical diagnosis of both acute and chronic mesenteric ischemia can be challenging; hence many patients will undergo testing for a number of other potential etiologies for their abdominal pain. During this time, either an imaging study performed to assess for an alternative diagnosis identifies the diagnosis, the patient has systemic manifestations of frank ischemia, or the disease is not recognized. Autopsy data have demonstrated that the diagnosis was not identified in up to one third of patients before surgical exploration or death ensued, with a resultant mortality rate of 90%.[5,8] Patients with chronic mesenteric ischemia can tolerate several weeks of preoperative preparation. In contrast, patients with acute ischemia have only hours before irreversible gut ischemia ensues, followed by profound distributive shock, and resultant demise.

Treating mesenteric ischemia involves managing patients with a highly lethal condition, who often present beyond the point at which any intervention can improve survival. Although acute mesenteric thromboembolic occlusion is an infrequent event (8.6/100,000 person-years),[6] the opportunity to intervene demands a skilled clinician that can promptly diagnose mesenteric ischemia, and then these patients should be approached with the same vigilance with which one would approach a symptomatic abdominal aortic aneurysm. As soon as the diagnosis has been entertained, the surgical team must be prepared to rapidly implement diagnostic and therapeutic interventions to salvage the patient.

VASCULAR ANATOMY

In the abdomen, three main blood vessels supply the blood flow to the viscera. These vessels are interconnected in multiple areas to provide a collateral network for the foregut, midgut, and hindgut. The celiac trunk is the first of the three vessels arising from the anterior aorta (typically between the 11 o'clock and 1 o'clock positions) at the level of the twelfth thoracic vertebra and the first lumbar vertebra. The origin of this vessel arises at the interface of the thoracic and abdominal cavity between the muscular crura of the diaphragm, which attach to the lumbar vertebral bodies 1 to 3. After a short distance (approximately 1 cm), the celiac trunk branches into the common hepatic artery, the splenic artery, and the left gastric artery, supplying the foregut structures: liver, gallbladder, pancreas, duodenum, spleen, and stomach. There are several anatomic variants in this regional arterial supply. Both the left gastric artery and common hepatic artery can arise directly off the aorta near the celiac trunk (<2% of population). Rarely, the SMA can arise from a common celiomesenteric trunk (Figure 35-1). The most common anatomic variation surrounds the hepatic circulation. Ten percent of the population will have a replaced left hepatic artery arising from the left gastric artery, and 10% will have a replaced right hepatic artery arising from the SMA at the level of the middle colic artery.

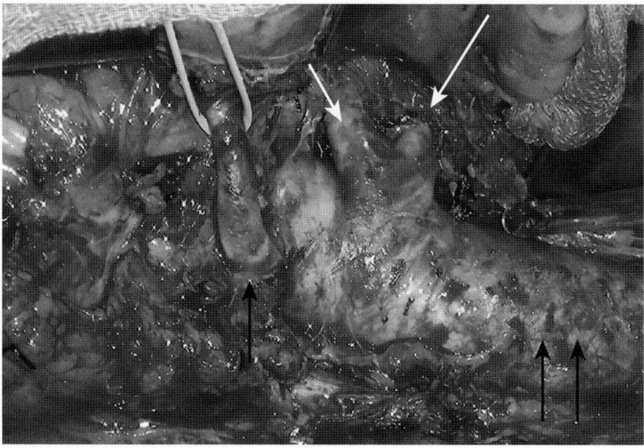

FIGURE 35-1 Retroperitoneal approach to the visceral segment of the aorta illustrating a celiomesenteric trunk. *Double black arrows* mark the supraceliac aorta. *Large white arrow* marks the celiac trunk, and *small white arrow* marks the SMA. Note the common celiomesenteric trunk. *Single black arrow* marks the left renal artery.

The celiac axis communicates to its partner visceral branches through several important anastomotic arcades. The gastroduodenal branch of the common hepatic artery and branches from the splenic artery communicate with the pancreaticoduodenal branches of the SMA, and a branch of the splenic artery communicates with the middle colic artery and the gastroepiploic arteries.[9]

Just distal to the origin of the celiac axis (usually about 1 cm), on the anterior surface of the aorta, the SMA arises. This artery feeds the entire midgut and terminates in the ileocolic artery. It lies posterior to the neck of the pancreas and crosses the uncus to the left of the superior mesenteric vein. In relationship to the duodenum, it passes anterior to the third portion of the duodenum and posterior to the fourth portion of the duodenum. The first branch of the SMA is the inferior pancreaticoduodenal artery followed shortly by short jejunal branches and the middle colic artery. Distal branches supply all of the small bowel, right colon, and the proximal two thirds of the transverse colon.

The ileocolic branch of the SMA communicates with the marginal artery of Drummond, a collateral running along the internal surface of the colon that allows communication between the SMA and the inferior mesenteric artery (IMA). This collateral vessel is also supplied by the middle colic artery, the source of blood supply for the hepatic flexure of the colon and the transverse colon. The middle colic artery will sometimes give rise to another alternate communication pathway from SMA (middle colic branch) to IMA (left colic branch) via a branch running parallel to the aorta in the transverse colon mesentery known commonly as the arc of Riolan (the meandering artery of Riolan).[9] The more proximal branches of the SMA provide arcades that supply the jejunum and ileum. There is a rich interconnected network within these arcades, and, although these branches do not communicate with the celiac axis or IMA, they provide an abundant source of collateralization within the SMA distribution itself.

From the lower portion of the abdominal aorta, the IMA arises off its anterior surface. The IMA communicates to the SMA via the marginal artery as outlined above, with the left colic artery providing the source of flow closest to the branches of the SMA into the marginal artery. This vessel supplies the distal portion of the splenic flexure, and there may be other direct connections between the colonic vessels in this region that allow further collateralization between the SMA and IMA. The IMA terminates in branches of the superior rectal artery, which through the hemorrhoidal vessels communicate with the internal iliac circulation, thus providing a mechanism to provide collateral blood supply to the distal colon and rectum from nonvisceral branches.[9] There are additional collateral pathways not outlined here that provide additional communications between these vessels.

The presence of multiple, redundant collaterals provides a network to limit the insult from obstruction of any single visceral vessel. It is therefore uncommon to have symptoms of chronic ischemia without obstruction of at least two visceral arteries; however, if collaterals are not developed, sudden occlusion of the celiac trunk may produce profound hepatic and foregut ischemia, and, similarly, sudden SMA occlusion may cause severe, acute, midgut ischemia. Understanding the anatomy and the collateral network is important in assessing and treating patients with mesenteric ischemia, whether chronic or acute in nature.

FORMS OF MESENTERIC ISCHEMIA

Chronic Mesenteric Ischemia

Inability to increase arterial blood flow to the viscera to meet postprandial demand results in chronic mesenteric ischemia. Unlike in acute mesenteric ischemia, visceral gangrene is rare. Atherosclerosis of the visceral vessel origins is the most common etiology. These patients typically have risk factors for atherosclerosis (diabetes, tobacco use, hypertension, and hyperlipidemia), as well as manifestations of atherosclerosis in other vascular territories (e.g., coronary artery disease, peripheral vascular disease). Nonatherosclerotic etiologies for chronic mesenteric ischemia are rare and include aneurysmal occlusion, chronic aortic dissection resulting in occlusion, stenosis or intermittent obstruction of arterial flow from the dissection flap, midabdominal coarctation, median arcuate ligament syndrome, fibromuscular dysplasia, Buerger's disease, and other vasculitides.

Acute Mesenteric Ischemia

The sudden loss of adequate arterial blood flow to the intestine results in acute mesenteric ischemia. This event is a surgical emergency that should initiate a medical system response (an institutional protocol) that parallels those already in place for symptomatic aneurysms. Patient salvage requires that the physician entertain the diagnosis early to either (1) activate an expedited diagnostic workup to an uncertain diagnosis or (2) initiate therapeutic intervention in a time frame that will restore bowel perfusion.

There are four fundamental etiologies of acute mesenteric ischemia: embolization (50%-60%), thrombosis (10%-20%), nonocclusive mesenteric ischemia (NOMI) (10%-20%), and mesenteric venous thrombosis (MVT) (10%).[10,11] Less common etiologies include thoracic aortic dissections (that extend to the visceral segment), hypercoagulable condition, fibromuscular dysplasia, and other vasculitides. Once the cycle of intestinal ischemia ensues, irreversible bowel ischemia may result in a situation that is incompatible with life. Small-bowel transplant is only performed in isolated centers with variable results, and often these patients have comorbidities that will preclude transplantation.

If the patient has no flow to ischemic tissue, he or she may not manifest systemic signs (or serologic derangements) until irrevocable damage has occurred. Once reperfusion occurs, ischemic tissues release tumor necrosis factor-α, interleukins, and cytokines that recruit polymorphonuclear neutrophils. Polymorphonuclear neutrophils compound tissue injury and amplify the inflammatory response by releasing destructive enzymes (myeloperoxidases, collagenases, and elastases). Once oxygen reaches inflamed tissue, the xanthine oxidase pathway converts oxygen to several oxygen free radicals that further exacerbate local tissue injury. When the inflammatory mediators and tissue breakdown products reach the hepatic circulation, the inflammatory cascade is amplified such that the systemic effects result in renal, pulmonary, and eventually cardiac failure.

Mesenteric arterial emboli are by far the most common mechanism for acute mesenteric ischemia, and the majority of emboli originate from cardiac lesions. Risk factors for cardiac emboli include atrial fibrillation (especially in patients with inadequate anticoagulation or left atrial dilation), valvular abnormalities (bicuspid aortic valve or valve prosthesis), and history of previous myocardial infarction (intracardiac thrombus, wall motion abnormality, or ventricular aneurysm). Arterial emboli most commonly embolize to the lower-extremity circulation (common femoral artery, aortic bifurcation, iliac bifurcation, and popliteal artery); however, 10% to 15% of emboli travel to the visceral vessels. Two thirds of patients with SMA embolization present with synchronous peripheral artery embolization, and the risk of this must be considered when treating these patients.[8]

The SMA is the most common site of visceral artery embolization for several reasons. It has a less acute angle off the aorta, has a higher basal flow rate compared with the celiac artery, and is much less resistant to acute ischemia. Typically, emboli enter the SMA orifice and lodge at the tapered segment (5-10 cm from the origin) near the middle colic artery. Because most collaterals from the foregut and the hindgut enter proximal to this location, the small bowel and right colon suffer immediate ischemia, but the first few centimeters of jejunum and the transverse colon may be spared. On exploration, the pattern of ischemia can determine the etiology of ischemia and localize the point of occlusion.

Acute mesenteric arterial thrombosis usually occurs in the setting of a preexisting atherosclerotic lesion (acute on chronic thrombosis). These patients typically have visceral atherosclerotic disease that has progressed over the course of several years, and, likewise, difficulties with food intolerance or weight loss may be elicited from the history. Unlike embolic occlusion, thrombotic occlusions typically occur flush with the aortic wall, where the atherosclerotic disease is most prevalent. Depending on the extent of collateralization, thrombotic occlusion of either the celiac artery or SMA produces a range of clinical symptoms varying from no symptoms to frank ischemia. It is particularly unusual for isolated celiac occlusion to produce symptoms of acute mesenteric ischemia; in contrast to this, SMA occlusion is more likely to produce ischemic symptoms. In the case of SMA occlusion, exploration often yields ischemia extending from the ligament of Treitz to the distal two thirds of the transverse colon, which is a clear difference in the extent of ischemic insult when compared with embolic occlusion.

NOMI occurs in the absence of arterial or venous occlusion but in the setting of low cardiac output. Originally described with the administration of digitalis, NOMI can occur in the setting of cardiac failure, after cardiac surgery, septic shock, hypovolemic shock, or other alpha constricting drugs (e.g., vasopressors, cocaine, amphetamines). Clinically, these patients are often admitted to the intensive care unit for critical conditions, and the process may take several days to develop, making it difficult to appreciate the cause of clinical deterioration and often difficult to diagnose. Frequently, these patients are hemodynamically unstable requiring pharmacologic cardiac support. Angiographic evaluation reveals patent macrovascular visceral circulation with distal arterial tapering because of vasoconstriction. After discontinuing any alpha-agonist vasoconstrictors and optimizing cardiac output, intra-arterial vasodilators are the treatments of choice in this setting (nitroglycerin or papaverine).

MVT refers to thrombosis of any visceral venous segment (portal vein, superior mesenteric vein, inferior mesenteric vein, or splenic vein); however, superior MVT accounts for the majority of cases resulting in mesenteric ischemia. These patients typically present with the severe abdominal pain similar to thromboembolic mesenteric ischemia, but MVT is more likely to present when the patient is younger and it has a slight female predominance. Primary MVT refers to spontaneous thrombosis without any underlying etiology, but, most commonly, MVT is due to a secondary etiology. Patients with portal hypertension or abdominal inflammation (diverticulitis, pancreatitis, bacterial peritonitis, inflammatory bowel disease, or trauma) are at high risk. One third of patients with MVT will have an underlying hypercoagulable syndrome, and they should be screened with a hypercoagulable profile.[12] Common syndromes include protein C and S deficiencies, factor V Leiden mutation, antithrombin III deficiency, antiphospholipid syndrome, hyperhomocysteinemia, and prothrombin 20210 mutation. Patients at risk for MVT also include those who are at higher risk for lower-extremity deep venous thrombosis (e.g., oral contraceptive use, pregnancy, tobacco use, dehydration, cirrhosis, nephrotic syndrome).

DIAGNOSIS

History and Physical Examination

The most important step in the management of patients with mesenteric ischemia is early recognition. The emergency department physician or primary care physician must recognize that the patient is at risk for mesenteric ischemia to prevent delays in management. Then the provider must determine from the history whether the patient has acute or chronic mesenteric ischemia.

Patients with chronic mesenteric ischemia are typically older and have a history of coronary artery disease, peripheral vascular disease, and risk factors for atherosclerosis. The classic presentation is "postprandial pain" that occurs in the epigastrium. Pain typically occurs 30 minutes after a meal and is described as dull, crampy, and vaguely localized. Some patients report the size of the meal to exacerbate symptoms and, in response, limit the size and frequency of meals (described as "food fear"). This food fear leads to weight loss, which can be significant, and most of these patients present thin and emaciated. These patients do have some malabsorption, but the nutritional derangements are more often due to poor intake.

The combination of postprandial abdominal pain and weight loss should prompt further diagnostic testing for mesenteric ischemia. Other constitutional symptoms such as diarrhea, constipation, nausea, and vomiting may also be present but are less specific. Based on the history alone, it is not possible to determine which visceral vessels are involved. Many of the symptoms can be confused with acute myocardial infarction, pulmonary embolism, pneumonia, gastroesophageal reflux disease, peptic ulcer disease, biliary colic, pancreatitis, irritable bowel disease, inflammatory bowel disease, and ischemic colitis. The patient may give a long history of laboratory studies, imaging studies, and even surgeries (cholecystectomy, appendectomy, and gynecologic procedures) without relief of their symptoms. In addition, on the basis of their weight loss and cachectic appearance, they may have undergone an exhaustive occult cancer evaluation. On examination, they will typically have temporalis muscle wasting and a scaphoid abdomen. An abdominal bruit may be heard in the epigastrium, but they typically have no tenderness to palpation. Signs of carotid artery stenosis (bruit) or peripheral vascular disease (decreased pulses) may be found, but the results of the remainder of their examination are typically normal.

The clinical presentation of acute mesenteric ischemia can be acute or subacute, over the course of days. The patient will often report a history suggestive of embolization (atrial fibrillation, prosthetic valve, recent admission for myocardial infarction, or possibly symptoms of an undiagnosed myocardial infarction in the recent history). The classic presenting feature of acute mesenteric ischemia is sudden onset of pain out of proportion to physical findings on abdominal examination. Of the symptoms those with acute mesenteric ischemia present with, the most common is abdominal pain (95%) followed by nausea (56%).[11] Other reported symptoms include acute gastrointestinal emptying (vomiting or diarrhea) and gastrointestinal bleeding. The presence or absence of bowel sounds is an unreliable finding. In the case of acute on chronic mesenteric ischemia, the patient may report classic symptoms of chronic mesenteric ischemia, that is, postprandial pain and weight loss for a period that has acutely progressed to intense, unrelenting, abdominal pain. The severity of symptoms correlates with clinical extent of ischemia. The mucosa of the bowel wall is the first layer to become ischemic, followed by the muscular layer, and serosa. Once the process has progressed to full-thickness wall necrosis, inflammation irritates the peritoneal lining correlating with the progression of examination results from no tenderness at all to findings of peritonitis.

Diagnostic Testing

The type of diagnostic tests and the order in which they are obtained are dictated by the patient's clinical condition. Once the clinician suspects the patient has chronic mesenteric ischemia on the basis of history and examination, the next screening study is typically duplex ultrasound, depending on its availability. This study is operator dependent and can be limited by the amount of bowel gas. If there is a high index of suspicion, these patients are typically very thin making the examination easier for the technologist. Velocity criteria for detecting lesions greater than 70% have been described for both the celiac trunk (>200 cm/s) and SMA (>275 cm/s).[13-15] For the SMA, this study detects greater than 70% stenosis with a sensitivity of 92%, a positive predictive value of 80%, and a negative predictive value of 99%; thus a negative study essentially excludes the diagnosis of mesenteric ischemia.[13]

Mesenteric ultrasound examinations are performed with the patient in a fasting state when visceral blood flow is relatively constant. Approximately 10 minutes after food enters the small bowel, both peak systolic and peak diastolic flow increase in response to vasodilation in the visceral bed, and additionally, reversal of flow is lost at the end of systole producing continuous flow. Authors have attempted to use the postprandial state as a means to establish a provocative test in patients with symptoms and a normal fasting ultrasound with varied results.[13,16] Using ultrasound as the first screening study avoids the risk for contrast agents and may rule out mesenteric vascular disease.

If the visceral ultrasound result is positive, or is inadequate or borderline, and in situations where it is not easily obtained and suspicion exists, then computed tomographic angiography (CTA) is now the most common imaging modality used to evaluate the mesenteric circulation. To be performed correctly, this study should involve axial imaging from the aortic arch through the common femoral arteries with use of intravenous contrast administration with reconstructions of the visceral component (coronal, sagittal, and three-dimensional views). CTA defines which vessels are involved, the character of the lesion(s) (calcified or noncalcified), the length of stenosis or occlusion, important collaterals that have developed, any aberrant vascular anatomy, and any incidental vascular pathology (abdominal aortic aneurysm or visceral aneurysm). CTA will also allow the clinician to assess the abdominal contents.[17] Including the arch and common femoral arteries allows the surgeon to assess the quality of access for endovascular planning and/or the quality of the aorta for open bypass.

CTA provides the surgeon with enough information to confirm the diagnosis and offer the patient treatment options. For the patient with renal insufficiency, repeating the duplex ultrasonography is a viable option for the patient with a low index of suspicion for chronic mesenteric ischemia, whereas proceeding directly with angiography (with either iodinated contrast or carbon dioxide) may be valid for the patient with a high index of suspicion. In the latter scenario, the surgeon should be prepared to intervene at the time of angiography.

In the setting of acute mesenteric ischemia, serum chemistry and hematologic studies usually do not aid in the diagnosis. Patients may have a subtle leukocytosis with a predominant neutrophilic shift or laboratory signs of dehydration (hemoconcentration or elevated blood urea nitrogen). It is important to understand that acidosis, hyperkalemia, and coagulopathy are late findings in acute mesenteric ischemia, and the lack of these findings should not reassure the clinician that there is time for further studies. Depending on the institutional availability, CTA can provide the operator with a wealth of information for both endovascular and open revascularization; however, not all institutions can obtain this study in a timely fashion. In a setting where these studies can not be obtained easily, if the clinician has a high clinical suspicion for acute mesenteric ischemia, the patient should proceed to treatment in an operative suite with fluoroscopic capabilities.

All other patients with a concern for acute mesenteric ischemia should undergo CTA as described above. Oral contrast agents should not be given because they are time consuming and obscure visualization of the distal mesenteric vasculature. CTA can delineate the mesenteric vessels and demonstrate the location of thrombosis or embolization. This is demonstrated by an acute cutoff of contrast and nonvisualization of contrast beyond the occlusion (Figures 35-2 and 35-3).[18,19] In the case of MVT, dilated mesenteric veins fill the abdomen, and the location of occlusion appears as a "target sign,"[20] where hypodense thrombus is surrounded by hyperdense vein wall. Subtle signs of bowel ischemia include edema and reactive ascites, whereas more extensive ischemia typically demonstrates bowel wall pneumatosis, pylephlebitis, and, in the setting of ischemic bowel perforation, free air (Figure 35-4).[17,18]

Mesenteric angiography remains the gold standard for diagnosis of acute mesenteric ischemia, but more commonly it is used as an adjunct to endovascular therapy of the visceral occlusion. The origin of the celiac and SMA are best visualized from a lateral projection, and typically selective injections are required of both the celiac and SMA to assess patency, degree of stenosis, and collateralization. Anterior-posterior views demonstrate the full extent of the celiac and SMA circulation. Thrombotic occlusion appears as flush aortic occlusion,

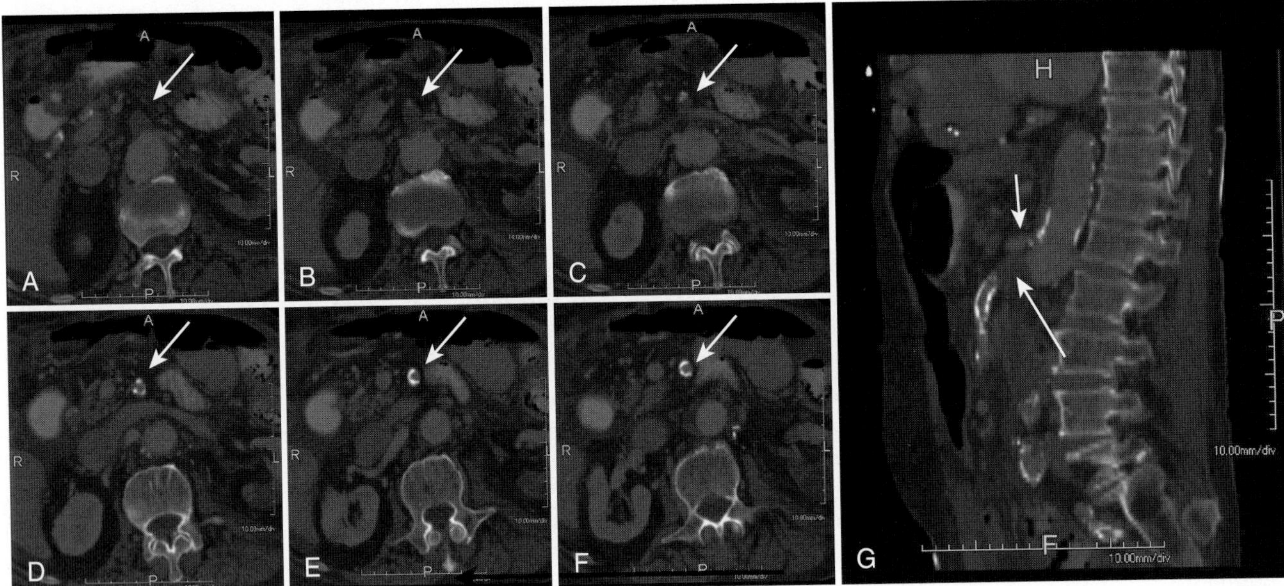

FIGURE 35-2 Example of acute SMA thrombosis. **A-F,** Contrasted axial images from cranial to caudal; *small white arrows* mark the SMA. **A** and **B,** Hypodense thrombus at the origin of the SMA. **D-F,** A calcified SMA can be seen with minimal contrast visualized, representing an acute occlusion. **G,** A sagittal reconstruction. The celiac is patent and marked with a *small white arrow.* The SMA occlusion is flush with the aorta and marked with the *large white arrow.*

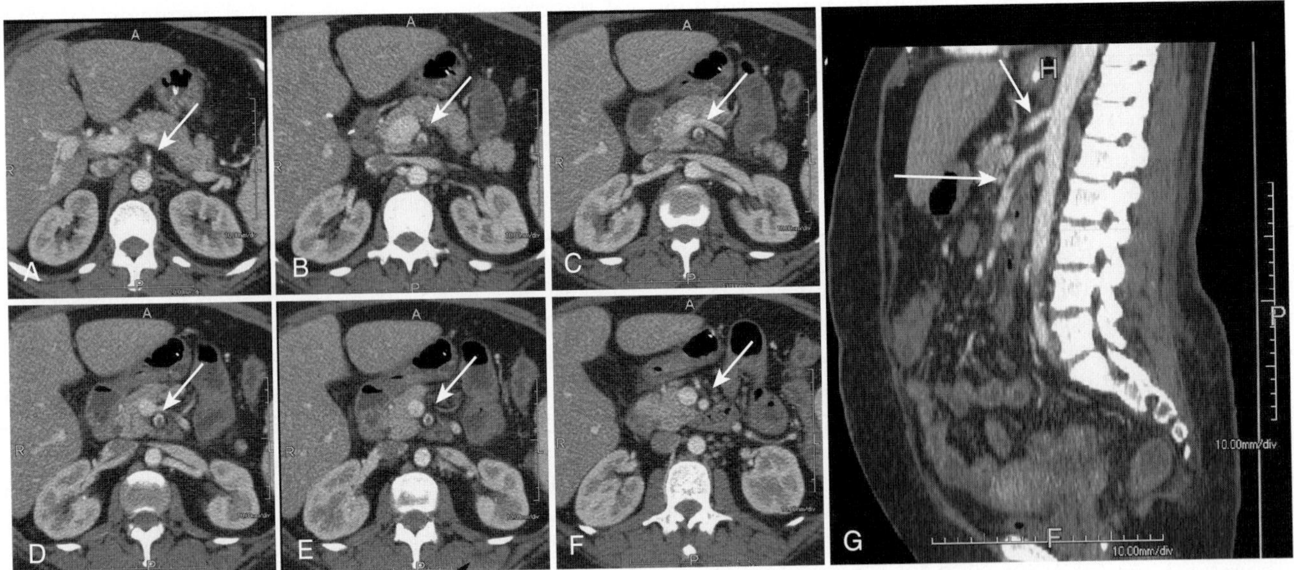

FIGURE 35-3 Example of acute SMA embolization. **A-F,** Contrasted axial images from cranial to caudal; *small white arrows* mark the SMA. **A,** A patent SMA origin. **B,** A partially occlusive filling defect begins and extends to **E. F,** There is a normal-caliber SMA, and contrast is beyond the partial occlusion. **G,** The sagittal reconstruction demonstrates the location and extent of embolization. *Small white arrow* marks the celiac artery, and *large white arrow* marks the SMA.

and embolus appears as an acute cutoff point, often with a proximal meniscus. In the case of NOMI, the macrovasculature is normal with progressive tapering and pruning of the distal mesenteric branches. In the setting of MVT, an arterial injection may demonstrate slow visceral flow, absent washout, and even aortic regurgitation of contrast.

ENDOVASCULAR THERAPY

Approach

In the case of chronic mesenteric ischemia, patients should undergo appropriate imaging assessment, duplex ultrasound examination, and CTA or MRA. CTA does not

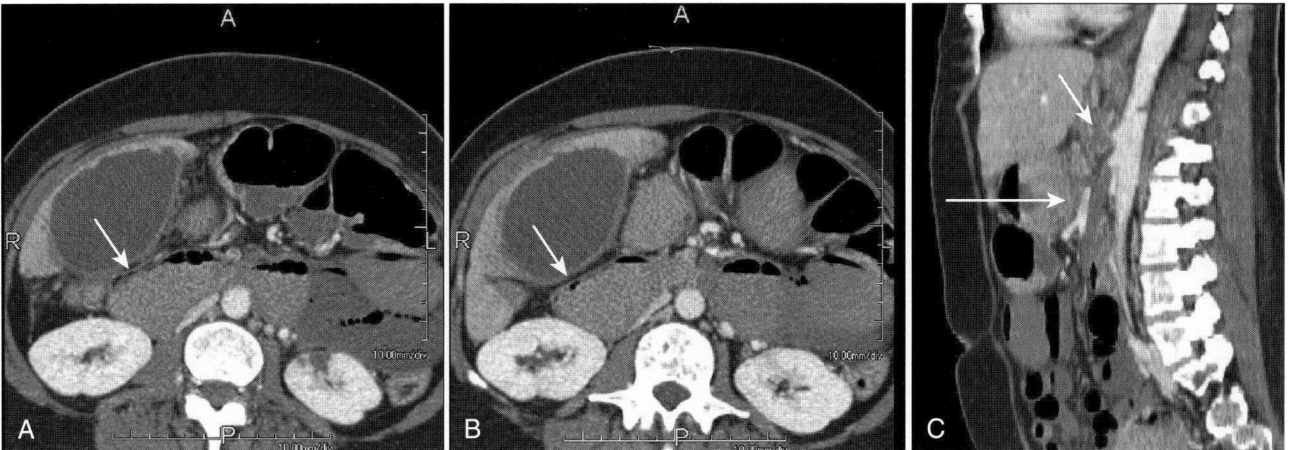

FIGURE 35-4 Example of bowel wall pneumatosis. This patient had a chronic celiac occlusion (**C**, *small white arrow*) and then presented with acute SMA occlusion (**C**, *large white arrow*). **A** and **B**, Representative axial images demonstrating pneumatosis within the proximal jejunum. Note the double wall appearance in the areas with pneumatosis.

obviate the need for duplex ultrasound because this will be compared with postintervention findings and can be used as a method for follow-up examinations. The utility of axial imaging for interventional planning cannot be overstated.

Preoperative medical optimization should be addressed in the elective setting. If the patient is not already receiving aspirin therapy, the use of aspirin in patients with peripheral vascular disease is paramount. Preoperative clopidogrel therapy is not necessary and can be reserved for those patients electively given endovascular therapy. The patient will receive a clopidogrel loading dose (typically 300 mg orally) before the procedure and then continue clopidogrel maintenance therapy (75 mg daily) for 1 to 3 months. Although no specific data exist regarding its benefit in visceral intervention, dual antiplatelet therapy with aspirin and clopidogrel reduces the embolic episodes after intervention in the cerebral circulation[21] and may also reduce stent thrombosis and restenosis rates.[22,23] This approach has thus become standard for all patients who do not have contraindications undergoing therapeutic mesenteric intervention. The patient is anticoagulated with intravenous heparin to a target activated clotting time of 250 to 300 seconds. The activated clotting time is monitored at intervals and maintained at this level throughout the procedure. Alternative anticoagulants (e.g., bivalirudin, argatroban) are reserved for patients with contraindications to heparin (heparin-induced thrombocytopenia) or occasionally when the patient has contraindications to protamine reversal.

In the setting of acute mesenteric ischemia, the patient's cardiac risk factors should be recognized, as well as other comorbidities and any history of prior surgical procedures. The patient should be immediately given treatment with a bolus of intravenous heparin (100 units/kg) in the emergency department to prevent thrombus propagation in the visceral bed.[24] Crystalloid resuscitation should be initiated to optimize cardiac performance and to reduce the intravenous contrast risk to the patient, and broad-spectrum antibiotics should also be given to combat the translocation of gut microbial flora. If CTA has been obtained in the acute setting, knowledge of the location of occlusion and the radiographic condition of the bowel will direct the operative plan. In the patient with late signs of bowel ischemia, axial imaging should be deferred, and the patient should be transferred to an endovascular operative suite. All other patients with acute mesenteric ischemia should receive axial imaging en route to the endovascular operative suite. Serologic markers, abdominal radiographs, and duplex ultrasound rarely alter the management of acute mesenteric ischemia.

Atherosclerotic mesenteric stenoses are usually focal aorto-ostial lesions, making them ideal for endovascular therapy. Balloon angioplasty in this region has resulted in significant elastic recoil, vessel dissection, and residual stenosis; therefore primary stenting has become routine. Endovascular treatment of the visceral vessels has been described via femoral, brachial, axillary, and retrograde approaches. With low-profile devices that are now available, the left brachial approach is the preferred approach for visceral interventions, although the femoral approach may be used depending on anatomic factors such as subclavian occlusion, severe proximal aortic tortuosity, and extensive atherosclerosis of the thoracic aorta. CTA before the procedure will provide information regarding these possibilities and can prove invaluable in assisting with approach selection.

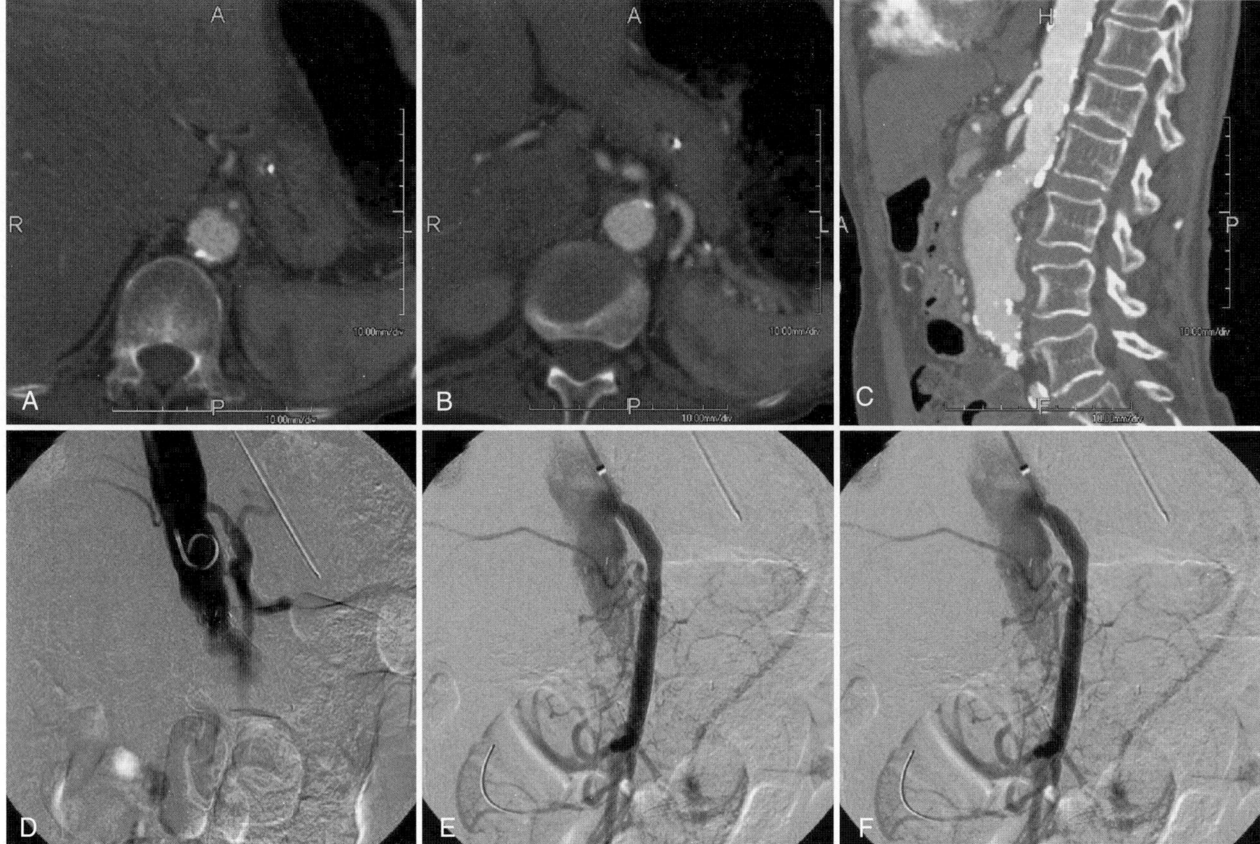

FIGURE 35-5 A patient with high-grade celiac and SMA stenosis. **A,** Preoperative axial imaging demonstrates high-grade stenosis of the celiac artery. **B,** The origin of the SMA is stenotic and calcified. **C,** Coronal view of the visceral segment of the aorta illustrating both the celiac artery and SMA stenosis. **D,** From a brachial approach, a lateral aortogram demonstrates both stenoses. **E,** The SMA has been selected, and a Palmaz stent is positioned across the stenosis. **F,** After stent deployment, an appropriately deployed stent with no residual stenosis is revealed.

Technique: Thrombolysis, Angioplasty, and Stenting

After wire access is obtained, typically a 5F sheath is placed in the access vessel. In the case of the brachial approach (used most commonly), a flush pigtail catheter or an angled selective catheter can be used to direct the wire into the descending thoracic aorta. An aortic flush catheter is placed at the body of T12/L1, and aortography is performed. An initial anterior-posterior projection will provide information about celiac and SMA patency, as well as reconstitution points in the setting of occlusion, and collateralization. The magnified lateral projection best illustrates the orifices of the celiac and SMA. These images are used to assess the locations of vessel origins, degree of stenosis, and the appropriate selective catheters for intervention.

Once nonselective imaging has been completed, selective access can be obtained to the visceral vessels for imaging and/or intervention. Selective imaging is most often obtained with a multipurpose, angled (MPA) catheter. The use of this catheter allows the tip of the catheter to be lodged in the orifice of the vessel with the back of the angle against the aortic wall and will keep the catheter from being forced out of the vessel origin during injections. With wire access across a stenosis, the catheter should be advanced to confirm that the lumen beyond the stenosis has been accessed. In many situations, once wire access across the lesion has been obtained, the hydrophilic wire can be exchanged for a medium-body curled-tip 0.035-inch wire (Rosen wire; Boston Scientific, Natick, MA) to be used to advance a longer interventional sheath to the origin of the vessel to be treated. After selective imaging, if the decision is made to perform intervention, a long 6F sheath is normally chosen for intervention (50-60 cm from the groin and 70-90 cm from the arm). Figures 35-5 and 35-6 illustrates SMA stent placement. If access across the lesion has not previously been obtained, then with this larger sheath in place from the brachial approach, typically an MPA catheter is used to gain selective vessel origin access. When access has been obtained from the groin, either a cobra catheter (Cook Medical, Bloomington, IN) or reverse-curved catheter

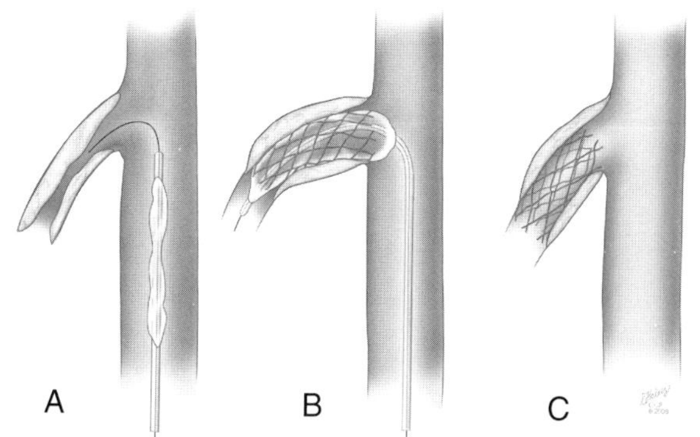

FIGURE 35-6 Illustration of potential stent displacement in SMA with intervention from the groin. **A,** Access into SMA. **B,** Balloon and stent in place in SMA with wire in position. Note how the interventional system raises the course of the SMA. **C,** with treatment system removed, the stent can lose the position proximally on the upper aspect of the vessel, potentially leading to early recurrence or residual narrowing. *(Reprinted with permission, cleveland clinic center for medical art & photography © 2009-2010. All rights reserved.)*

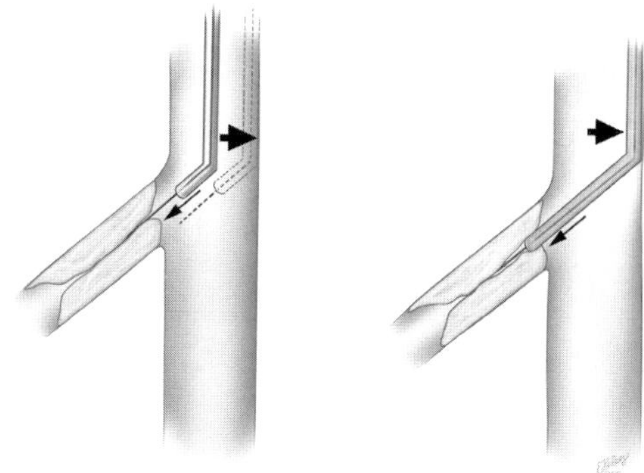

FIGURE 35-7 Catheters used during recanalization. Note that shorter-tipped catheters will be pushed away from vessel orifice, whereas catheters with a longer tip will allow forward pressure to be applied while the catheter gains support from posterior wall of the aorta. *(Reprinted with permission, cleveland clinic center for medical art & photography © 2009-2010. All rights reserved.)*

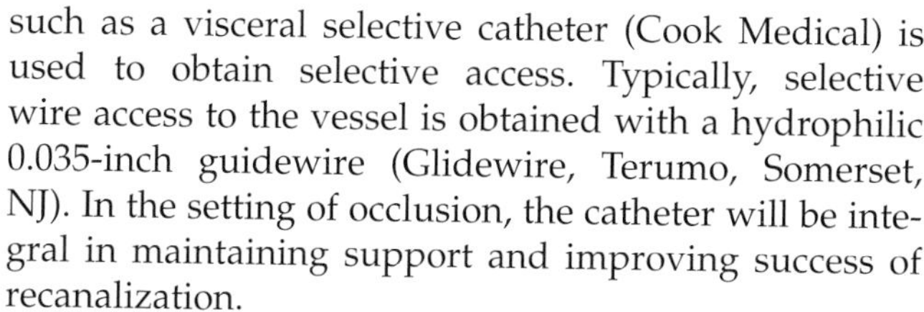

such as a visceral selective catheter (Cook Medical) is used to obtain selective access. Typically, selective wire access to the vessel is obtained with a hydrophilic 0.035-inch guidewire (Glidewire, Terumo, Somerset, NJ). In the setting of occlusion, the catheter will be integral in maintaining support and improving success of recanalization.

Achieving access across an origin occlusion into the patent distal vessel is, in the author's opinion, more easily achieved with brachial access. Again in this setting, the use of an angled catheter with a long tip is extremely helpful in maintaining forward pressure into the occlusion to allow wire passage. Shorter-tipped catheters will not allow forceful advancement of the wire and will result in failure of interventional therapy (Figure 35-7). Using access from above, the MPA can be positioned with its tip in the occluded origin of the branch and the "back" or angle of the catheter abutting the contralateral aortic wall. By advancing the catheter with the tip engaged at the vessel orifice, the angle can be lodged against the aortic wall. This method allows the interventionalist to direct significant caudal and anterior force on the wire without the catheter "bouncing out" of the origin of the vessel. Rapid rotation of the hydrophilic guidewire with minimal steady but forceful advancement should allow access across the majority of visceral occlusions. In some instances, the use of a "stiff" Glidewire (Terumo) may prove helpful, as may the use of a 0.014-inch wire. In some situations, with severe proximal aortic and arch tortuosity, it can be difficult to maintain access with the sheath in the area near the visceral segment because it will tend to "buckle" into the ascending aorta when exerting significant antegrade pressure. The use of a through-and-through wire down to the groin allows the interventionalist's assistant to maintain tension and keep the sheath in the necessary position, while attempts are made with the catheter to gain access across the lesion (Figure 35-8).

Once wire access across the occlusion has been obtained, the catheter should be advanced into the vessel. Then, confirmation of access across the lesion and into the patent distal vessel should be achieved. This is performed by advancing the catheter over the wire into the vessel. In some instances, a more tapered catheter (Quick-Cross catheter, Spectranetics, Colorado Springs, CO) may need to be exchanged for this purpose, to overcome the resistance of the occlusion, or, if a braided catheter has been used for selective vessel origin access, sometimes rotation and advancement of the catheter will allow passage across the occlusion. Once the catheter has been placed distally into the area of patent distal vessel, the wire should be removed and aspiration for the return of blood is performed. If blood return is achieved, one is likely in the distal vessel and a small dose of contrast is injected to ensure this is the case. If there is no return of blood through the catheter, it should be withdrawn a small amount (1-2 cm) to assess whether blood flow returns at this point. If blood flow is obtained, then contrast should be used to establish the position of the catheter in relation to the vessel itself. If there is no return of blood, one should replace the catheter at the origin of the occlusion and reattempt access across the occlusion attempting to gain access at the origin in a different plane. With experience, in 80% to 90% of cases, one should be able to achieve access across the lesion.

If the upper extremity cannot be used to obtain access, then attempts can be made from the groin. In this situation, a reverse-curve catheter must be used to access the origin of the vessel. It is easier to use a reverse-curve

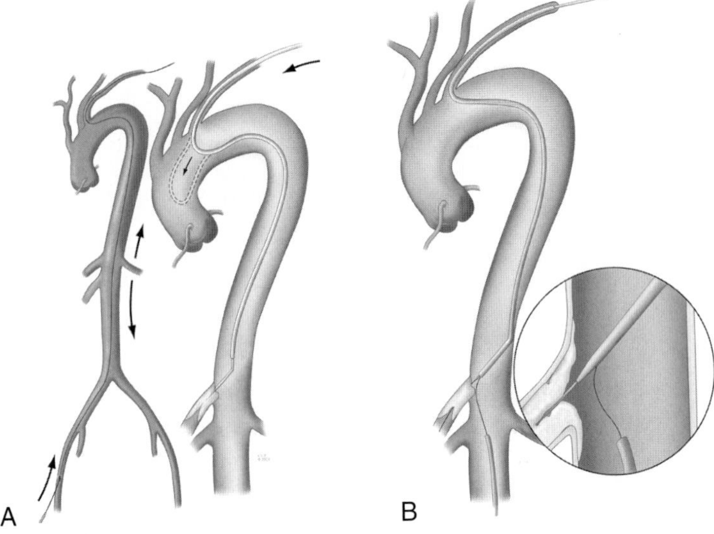

FIGURE 35-8 Tortuosity in the arch can be overcome with through-and-through wire access. **A,** Note the sheath "buckling" in the ascending aorta as force is applied to advance catheter or device forward into the superior mesenteric artery. **B,** Through-and-through wire access allows the sheath to be "held in place" and force to be applied advance catheter or device without "buckling" in the ascending aorta. *(Reprinted with permission, cleveland clinic center for medical art & photography © 2009-2010. All rights reserved.)*

catheter with a wide radius of curvature so that the catheter can be lodged into the origin occlusion while the back of the catheter is forced against the opposite arterial wall. In some circumstances, the use of a reverse-curve guide such as an internal mammary artery guide or a renal double-curve guide will allow this same maneuver and provide excellent stability of the system within the aorta. Similar maneuvers are used with the wire to gain access across the lesion, and either the reverse-curve catheter is "pulled" through the lesion or the guide is used to direct a catheter through the obstruction, again confirming position across the lesion and into a patent distal vessel by assessing blood return and injection of contrast.

When attempting to select an appropriately placed celiac or SMA stent, care must be made to ensure that the wire enters the lumen of the stent and does not traverse the interstices of the 2- to 3-mm of stent positioned into the aorta. A J-tipped glide wire may be useful in this situation to avoid crossing the interstices; however, in the setting of stenosis within a stent or occlusion of a stent, this may be impractical and the interventionalist needs to ensure that the tip of the catheter is within the origin of the stent before traversing with the wire. When the wire has traversed the interstices, it will typically pass easily, but catheters and balloons used for treatment will not pass through with ease. It is important to use a magnified view as a catheter traverses the stent. If there is any resistance, the wire is through the interstices; with enough force, the catheter and possibly even the sheath will pass through the stent interstices, but on magnified views this should be able to be determined. If this is unrecognized, angioplasty or additional stent placement will deform the previous stent and place the patient at risk for embolization and stent thrombosis.

Once the visceral vessel has been selected, returning to anterior-posterior projection can confirm placement of the wire tip. In the case of the celiac artery, it is import to confirm whether the wire is in the splenic or common hepatic artery. A wire exchange is performed for a J-tipped medium-weight wire, which can often be used for an intervention. Embolic protection wires have been used in this location; however, they are not routinely used. In the setting of chronic occlusion, or stenosis of the vessel, the therapeutic intervention most often undertaken at this point is stent placement. If the stenosis is high grade, predilation will often be necessary. A balloon-expandable stent is chosen on the basis of the size of the distal normal artery and length of lesion, ensuring there is enough stent length to position 2 to 3 mm in the aorta. Typically, a 6- to 8-mm–diameter stent is chosen. After the stent is in position, the stent is deployed, and the proximal stent is flared with a larger 8- to 10-mm balloon. Completion films are performed through the sheath and repeated in an anterior-posterior projection to assess for distal embolization or dissection.

Stent positioning and deployment are, in the authors' opinion, best performed from proximal (brachial) access. Intervening from this approach allows the vessel to assume its normal position during the intervention and ensures that an adequate portion of the stent can be positioned within the aorta proximally. Wire access from the groin will deform the origin of the vessel and may lead to malpositioning of the proximal aspect of the stent (Figure 35-9).

There are several options for endovascular management of thrombotic or embolic mesenteric occlusion in the setting of acute mesenteric ischemia. Here, rapid restoration of blood flow is imperative. Aspiration catheters can be attempted as a first-line therapy,[25,26] and several percutaneous mechanical thrombectomy devices (AngioJet, Possis Medical, Minneapolis, MN; Trellis; Bacchus Vascular, Santa Clara, CA) are available. Aspiration and mechanical thrombectomy have the advantages

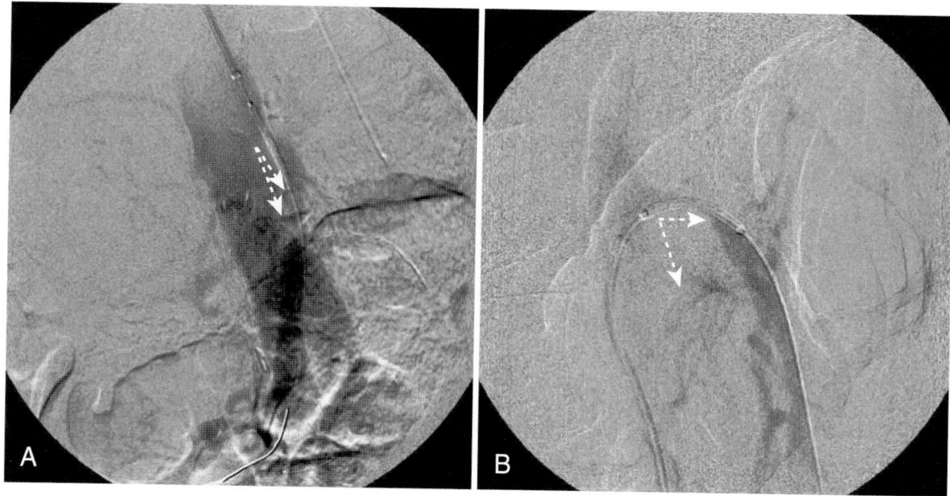

FIGURE 35-9 A comparison of the brachial and femoral approach for visceral angioplasty and stenting. **A,** From the brachial approach, the SMA has been selected, the sheath is in place, and a Palmaz stent is in position across the lesion. NOTE: The angle between the aorta and SMA *(white dashed arrows)* is unchanged from its normal position. **B,** From the femoral approach, a renal double-curved guide catheter is in position with a similar-sized Palmaz stent in position. The system has distorted the SMA origin such that the angle between the aorta and SMA is now nearly 90 degrees *(white dashed arrows)*. This may lead to malpositioning of the proximal aspect of the stent.

TABLE 35-1 Thrombolytic Regimens Used for Visceral Thrombolysis[29]

Medication	Bolus	Infusion	Half-life (min)	Comments
Tissue plasminogen activator	1-20 mg	1-4 mg/hr	2-6	Fibrin-bound plasminogen selective, most expensive
Urokinase	200,000 units	60,000-120,000 units/hr	15-20	Acts on both bound and free plasminogen
Streptokinase	250,000 units	5,000-10,000 units/hr	12-15	Risk of allergic reaction, may be neutralization with streptococcus antibodies, least expensive

Data from Kozuch PL, Brandt LJ: Review article: diagnosis and management of mesenteric ischaemia with an emphasis on pharmacotherapy, *Aliment Pharmacol Ther* 21(3):201–215, 2005.

of immediate return of perfusion limiting bowel ischemia,[27] and they theoretically could potentially either reduce the duration of thrombolytic therapy or eliminate the need for thrombolytic therapy altogether, although in most instances of acute occlusion, some duration of lytic therapy is necessary. All mechanical thrombectomy devices allow the instillation of heparin and thrombolytic agents at the time of thrombectomy. After instrumentation of the vessel, no matter what therapeutic device has been used, vasodilator should be given to counteract the vasoconstriction induced by the device, and, when treating for acute occlusion, continued lysis should be considered because it will be rare to have removed all thrombus or embolus with this initial intervention. Typically, thrombus has been generated beyond the origin occlusion or emboli are still lodged in the distal ileocolic segments. Assuming the patient is clinically stable, catheter-directed thrombolytic therapy should then be initiated.

Thrombolytic therapy has been used to treat acute mesenteric ischemia, but the patient's clinical status will dictate treatment. If it is clear the patient has complications of ischemic bowel such as perforation, and will require emergent resection, thrombolytic therapy is contraindicated. In addition, patients with very recent surgery (<7 days) or recent intracranial hemorrhagic event have absolute contraindications to thrombolysis, whereas patients with uncontrolled hypertension, a history of gastrointestinal bleeding, known cancer, and advanced age (age >80 years) have relative contraindications to this form of therapy.[28,29] To achieve the highest degree of success with lytic therapy, a wire must be placed across the thrombus into a distal patent target vessel. Typically, a hydrophilic-tipped guidewire is directed across the thrombus, followed by a diagnostic catheter that is used to confirm distal patency. At this time, the treatment length is determined for either an infusion catheter (10-20 cm), an infusion wire, or an infusion catheter and wire combination. For thrombotic/embolic occlusions near the origin of the vessel, a catheter is chosen; for those instances where the vessel is 4 mm or smaller in diameter, a wire alone is used. In the setting where there is both proximal and distal thrombus, the combination of catheter and wire is used. Thrombolytic regimens are listed in Table 35-1. The patient is given treatment with low-dose heparin through the access sheath, and the addition of vasodilator therapy with thrombolytic therapy offers the advantage of maintaining dilation of the distal visceral vasculature and is often used.

Visceral ischemia is compounded by vasoconstriction further limiting distal perfusion; therefore vasodilators have a role for improving perfusion in cases of thromboembolic mesenteric ischemia and more important those episodes caused by NOMI. With a selective catheter through the thrombus or embolus, papaverine, nitroglycerin, and α-antagonists have all been used, but papaverine has been reported most commonly. Papaverine is a cyclic adenosine monophosphate phosphodiesterase inhibitor, which leads to an increase in intracellular cyclic adenosine monophosphate, resulting in smooth muscle relaxation.[30] Because elimination occurs primarily via hepatic metabolism, the systemic effects are minimal.[30] Continuous infusion of papaverine can be performed at 30 to 60 mg/hr with minimal systemic side effects, and fluid resuscitation should be given to accommodate for volume shifts.[31] If the patient has a sudden drop in systemic blood pressure, the catheter has probably dislodged into the aorta.

In the setting of NOMI, vasodilator therapy alone is the treatment of choice, and surgery can be avoided if the patient does not have bowel infarction. In addition to optimizing cardiac performance in patients with NOMI, continuous papaverine instillation has been continued for as long as 5 days without adverse reactions.[32] Isolated papaverine instillation has improved mortality of acute NOMI to 40% to 50%.[31] Vasodilators alone do not address the underlying embolism or thrombosis, and therefore they should be used in conjunction with either mechanical or pharmacologic clot dissolution.

Once thrombolytic therapy has been initiated, it is imperative to closely monitor the patient in an intensive care unit for disseminated intravascular coagulopathy (prothrombin time, activated partial thrombin time, fibrinogen), signs of bleeding (hematocrit, gastrointestinal hemorrhage), and signs of progressive intestinal ischemia (worsening abdominal pain, persistent acidosis). Resolution of abdominal pain within 1 to 2 hours is the most important clinical sign that the patient is responding to thrombolytic therapy.[33] If the patient clinically improves, angiographic evaluation can be performed the following day, and, if the patient's condition worsens, repeated angiographic evaluation should be performed immediately. Even though the patient has resolution of pain, bowel ischemia can still occur.[2] In the case that the patient has persistent acidemia or peritonitis and requires surgical exploration, aminocaproic acid can be given to reverse the effects of TPA by binding reversibly to plasminogen. Aminocaproic acid is given intravenously with a loading dose of 5 g over an hour's time followed by 1 to 2 g over the subsequent 2- to 4-hour period; side effects include myopathy and necrosis.[12,31] Existing plasmin-activated fibrinogen will not be reversed; therefore it is prudent to also give fibrinogen replacement, as cryoprecipitate, during transfer to the operative suite.

After a period of 12 to 24 hours, repeated angiography should be performed to evaluate treatment. Not uncommonly there is still residual thrombus in distal jejunal or ileocolic branches. Depending on the size and extent of collateralization, efforts should be made to enter those vessels and either aspirate thrombus or continue thrombolytic therapy for another 12 to 24 hours. This process should be repeated until the bulk of thrombus has been removed. If there are still residual lumen abnormalities after 24 hours of therapy, balloon angioplasty can be performed. If the patient is found to have embolic disease, thrombolytic therapy can be discontinued with transition to long-term anticoagulation. Patients with acute thrombosis typically have a residual stenosis at the origin of the vessel and require angioplasty and stenting.

During endovascular treatment, the patient's clinical status may deteriorate requiring abdominal exploration, or, at the time of presentation, the patient's clinical status may mandate immediate exploration. Once acidosis and bowel necrosis are present, the patient is typically in clinical extremis. Performing open embolectomy and revascularization can involve 2 to 4 hours of operative time, and, in the setting of dead bowel, a vein conduit may further increase the duration of the procedure. An endovascular hybrid procedure involves exposing the SMA for a 3-cm segment, assessing the distribution of bowel ischemia, and then accessing the SMA in a retrograde fashion with a 6F sheath.[34] Access in this manner will allow performance of a retrograde angiogram to assess inflow. If there is an occlusion, the orifice can be treated with angioplasty and stented in a retrograde fashion to reestablish arterial inflow, which can then be assessed with completion angiography via the side arm of the sheath.[34] With inflow improved, proximal and distal control of the SMA is secured, and then the outflow is restored. Embolectomy catheters can be passed, vasodilators injected, and distal angiography performed from this location. At conclusion, the arteriotomy is closed, and the bowel is reassessed. Frankly necrotic segments are resected, and concerning areas are left in situ for a second-look operation in 12 to 24 hours. This technique avoids an aortic clamp and bypass graft and, most important, reduces the time for bowel reperfusion.

The primary treatment of MVT is broad-spectrum antibiotic therapy, volume resuscitation, and systemic anticoagulation. In the absence of clinical signs of bowel necrosis, medical management is sufficient, and abdominal exploration can be avoided. Using this management strategy, outcomes are better than those for thromboembolic acute mesenteric ischemia with mortality rates of 25% to 50%.[1,7] Regional thrombolytic therapy has been delivered via the mesenteric venous system (transjugular or percutaneous transhepatic approach) or via the mesenteric arterial system. The mesenteric arterial system is less complex and has the added advantage of clearing thrombus in the capillary circulation. There is not enough experience with thrombolytic therapy for MVT to determine which patients may benefit and should be treated.

After the treatment of acute mesenteric ischemia, anticoagulation should be initiated when the patient is safe from surgical bleeding, typically 12 to 24 hours after completion of therapy. There are no data on which to base anticoagulation management strategy in the postoperative period; patients should be anticoagulated with warfarin (Coumadin) to maintain an international normalized ratio two times normal for 3 to 6 months.[12] If the patient has atrial fibrillation, valvular abnormality, cancer, or known hypercoagulable condition, anticoagulation therapy should be instituted indefinitely. Unlike the treatment of thromboembolic acute mesenteric ischemia, it is imperative that patients with MVT continue to have anticoagulation immediately after any intervention. Long-term anticoagulation reduces subsequent morbidity and mortality from 50% to 20%.[12] Lifelong therapy is considered for all patients with an underlying hypercoagulable condition as the etiology for MVT; otherwise, 6 months of anticoagulation therapy is adequate.[12]

OUTCOMES

Asymptomatic Mesenteric Artery Stenosis

An incidental finding of mesenteric artery stenosis in an otherwise asymptomatic patient should simply be followed. It is a well-known fact that the incidence of asymptomatic mesenteric stenosis increases with increasing age (especially >70 years). Autopsy studies have documented rates as high as 29% for single-vessel mesenteric stenosis and 15% for two-vessel stenosis.[35] In a population of patients older than 65 years of age being monitored for cardiac risk factors, the incidence of asymptomatic celiac or SMA stenosis was found to be 17% by screening duplex examination.[36] After a full history and physical examination, none of these patients were found to have occult symptoms of chronic mesenteric ischemia. With a mean follow-up of 6 years, symptoms had not developed in any of the patients and none of the patients presented with acute mesenteric ischemia. During the same period the population had a 20% mortality rate because of cardiac events, illustrating the importance of aggressive medical management of atherosclerotic disease.[36]

In a more detailed review of asymptomatic mesenteric stenosis, patients were stratified on the basis of the number of vessels involved. Half the patients with two-vessel disease and three-vessel disease died during a follow-up period of 2.6 years.[37] Half of the deaths were attributed to mesenteric ischemia, whereas the remainder of deaths were attributed to coronary artery disease.[37] Therefore patients with asymptomatic visceral artery stenosis involving the celiac artery and SMA should be treated when possible. Treating isolated asymptomatic high-grade SMA stenosis is more controversial, and there is no current evidence to support observation or treatment. Endovascular treatment in good-risk patients avoids the devastating sequelae of acute mesenteric ischemia with low perioperative morbidity and mortality.

Chronic Mesenteric Ischemia

Endovascular stenting for chronic mesenteric ischemia demonstrates relief of symptoms in 72% to 90%, primary stent patency of 65%, primary assisted patency of 97%, and secondary patency of 99% (12 months of follow-up).[38,39] The 30-day morbidity rate varies from 3% to 30%, and mortality ranges from 0% to 7.7% (Table 35-2).[38,40] Symptoms recur in 21% of patients with visceral stents, and recurrence delineates patients with stent restenosis.[39] In addition, patients who have single-vessel treatment are more likely to demonstrate recurrent symptoms when stent restenosis occurs.[39] These findings mirror those of open surgical treatment. Evaluating outcomes when both the celiac and SMA were routinely bypassed compared with patients with single-vessel bypasses, those with limited revascularizations were more likely to have recurrent symptoms if that bypass occluded.[41] In addition, balloon-expandable stents are the most commonly used stent type for both celiac and SMA, but self-expanding stents have comparable patency rates.[38] Other factors such as the stent design and the number of stents deployed have little impact on clinical outcome. The majority of the morbidity of the endovascular procedure involves access-related complications (bleeding, pseudoaneurysms, and thrombosis), but in one series 4.6% of patients had bowel ischemia resulting from distal embolization requiring bowel resection.[38]

Occluded visceral vessels deserve special mention. Recanalization of visceral arteries has been avoided because of the perceived higher risk for periprocedural embolization, bowel necrosis, and higher stent restenosis

TABLE 35-2 Chronic Mesenteric Ischemia: a Literature Review of Outcomes Stratified by Open Versus Endovascular Treatment Modalities

Author	Yr	No.	Sx relief	Primary patency	In-hospital morbidity (%)	In-hospital mortality (%)
OPEN MESENTERIC REVASCULARIZATION						
McMillan et al.[45]	1995	25	75% 3 yr	89% 3 yr	12	6
Cho et al.[50]	2002	21	79% 5 yr	57% 5 yr	60	0
Park et al.[47]	2002	91	92% 5 yr	—	29	5
Kruger et al.[51]	2007	39	95% 5 yr	92% 5 yr	12	2.5
Biebl et al.[52]	2007	26	89% 2 yr	92% 2 yr	42	2.8
Atkins et al.[48]	2007	49	78% 1 yr	90% 1 yr 96% assisted	4	2
ENDOVASCULAR MESENTERIC REVASCULARIZATION						
Landis et al.[53]						
74% PTA 26% PTA/S	2005	29	90% 2 yr	70% 1 yr 88% assisted	10	0
Biebl et al.[52]						
4% PTA 96% PTA/S	2007	23	75% 1 yr	75% 1 yr	4	0
Atkins et al.[48]						
13% PTA 87% PTA/S	2007	31	77% 1 yr	58% 1 yr 65% assisted	13	3
Kougias et al.[11,*]						
PTA	2007	57	81% 2 yr	79% 2 yr	11	5
S	2007	122	72% 2 yr	65% 2 yr	3	2
PTA/S	2007	113	76% 2 yr	74% 2 yr	15	4
Sarac et al.[38]						
PTA/S	2008	65	75% 1 yr	65% 1 yr 97% assisted 99% 2° pat.	30.8	7.7

**Study represents a collective review of case series and case reports from 1995 to 2007.*

2° pat., Secondary patency; *PTA*, primary angioplasty, *PTA/S*, angioplasty and stenting; *S*, primary stenting; *Sx*, symptomatic.

rates caused by plaque burden; however, visceral recanalization is technically feasible and appears to have outcomes similar to those obtained in patients with stenotic lesions.[38,42]

Acute Mesenteric Ischemia

The outcomes for thrombolytic therapy in the setting of acute mesenteric ischemia are relegated to several small case series (Table 35-3). Patients' pathology consisted of both embolic and thrombotic occlusions. Urokinase was the most commonly used thrombolytic agent, adjunctive heparinization was used in most cases, and adjunctive papaverine was used in only three patients. Duration of thrombolytic therapy ranged from a single intraprocedural bolus to 48 hours of continued delivery, and technical resolution of thrombus was achieved in 83%.[2] There were five failures that required exploration, embolectomy, and bowel resection; four of the five patients survived. Technical failures did not correlate with duration of symptoms, location of thrombus (0-10 cm from the origin of SMA), or thrombolytic protocol.[2] Thrombolytic therapy with or without surgical intervention resulted in an in-hospital mortality of 17%.[2] Eight percent of patients had distal embolization with worsening abdominal pain prompting exploration. Minor

TABLE 35-3 Acute Mesenteric Ischemia: a Literature Review of Outcomes Stratified by Open Versus Endovascular Treatment Modalities

Author	Year	No.	In-hospital morbidity (%)	In-hospital mortality (%)
OPEN SURGICAL TREATMENT				
Cho et al.[50]	2002	23	60	52
Schoots et al.[1,*]	2004	3692	—	Thrombosis 70 Embolus 54
Kougias et al.[54]	2007	72	39	31
Kassahn et al.[7]	2008	60	—	60
ENDOVASCULAR TREATMENT				
Schoots et al.[2†]	2005	48	23	17

**Study represents a collective review from 1967 to 2002.*
†Study represents a collective review from 1979 to 2003.

gastrointestinal bleeding occurred in two patients, and 10% had minor access site bleeding.[2] These results are optimistic, but more experience is required to determine the true impact on outcomes.

Endovascular hybrid treatment for acute mesenteric ischemia has been reported in sporadic case reports, but theoretically it could improve overall outcomes. The largest series available for open retrograde stenting in the setting of acute mesenteric ischemia involved six patients.[43] The mortality in the hybrid group was 17% compared with 80% in the patients given treatment with open revascularization during the same period.[43] A selection bias exists, but there are clear advantages to minimizing the physiologic insult in this population.

FOLLOW-UP AND MONITORING

Patients with mesenteric artery stents should be followed with duplex ultrasound at regular intervals. Duplex ultrasound has been examined in patients both before and after visceral artery stent, and the peak systolic velocity does acutely drop to below 275 cm/s, and a follow-up increase correlates with stent restenosis.[44] It is important to note that patients may have elevated peak systolic velocities (still >275 cm/s) although the completion angiogram demonstrated a widely patent stent. Although the velocities are elevated, they are typically reduced compared with preprocedural values. In this setting, it is important to sample the SMA beyond the stent. Consistently high values in this setting could represent hyperdynamic flow caused by an occluded celiac axis.

Patients with recurrent symptoms or concern for stent restenosis should undergo CTA. CTA will determine whether there is progression of atherosclerosis in any untreated vessel, and it will provide an assessment of stent patency and stent malformation. Stent migration is typically an early phenomenon that can be seen with CTA, and intimal hyperplasia will appear as a hypodense ring lining the inside of the stent.[17] CTA also will allow the surgeon to plan for addition visceral vessel stenting or addressing stent restenosis.

After stent restenosis has been identified, a repeated intervention should be planned with correction of the underlying stenosis. If the restenosis occurred at the origin of the stent, then a second balloon-expandable stent could be deployed 2 to 3 mm into the aortic orifice, and this situation represents potential maldeployment of the first stent. For restenosis at the distal end of the stent, either a second balloon-expandable or self-expanding stent can be deployed to extend the treatment zone. In some patients, extension of balloon-expandable stents several centimeters into the SMA may cause kinking, and evaluation for this should be performed. The use of self-expanding stents to resolve this kinking should be considered. For in-stent restenosis, repeated balloon angioplasty with or without a second stent should be considered. Covered stents are only selectively used because of the concern of covering even small visceral branches; however, these can be used for proximal recurrent stenosis caused by intimal hyperplasia. If the patient returns with stent restenosis a second or third time, the patient should be considered for open surgical bypass if an operative candidate.

COMPARISON OF ENDOVASCULAR THERAPY AND OPEN REPAIR

There are no randomized controlled trials or prospective comparative studies comparing open surgery and endovascular therapy for the treatment of chronic mesenteric ischemia; however, there are several retrospective comparisons (see Table 35-1). Surgical bypass of the visceral vessels has a 5-year symptom-free survival of 79% to 90%,[40,42,44] and bypass grafts have 3-year primary patency of 89%.[40,42,44-46] On the contrary, endovascular stenting for chronic mesenteric ischemia demonstrates relief of symptoms in 72% to 90%, with primary stent patency of 65%, primary assisted patency of 97%, and secondary patency of 99% (12 months follow-up).[38,39] Endovascular therapy has similar results in regard to symptom resolution but with short follow-up periods, 1 to 2 years versus 3 to 5 years for open repair. In addition, the rate-limiting step of endovascular stents is the marked reduction in primary patency when compared with open repair. Endovascular therapy requires repeated interventions to obtain assisted patencies that rival those of open repair.

Factors associated with improved surgical visceral revascularization include younger age and the quality of aortic inflow and visceral outflow. In one series, all perioperative deaths occurred in patients older than 70 years old.[47] Surgical revascularization carries a contemporary 30-day operative morbidity of 4% to 60% and mortality of 2% to 6%; endovascular therapy carries a 30-day morbidity rate of 3% to 30% and mortality of 0% to 7.7% (see Table 35-2).[38,40] Given the studies listed, endovascular therapy appears to carry a lower mortality rate compared with open repair, with similar morbidity rates between the two approaches. It is important to understand that endovascular morbidity is often minor and related to access site complications, whereas perioperative morbidity tends to be more often systemic and more severe in the open surgical experience.

Surgical bypass is a valid initial option in young patients with good operative risk. With appropriate patient selection, their perioperative morbidity will be lowered and they will benefit from the durability of surgical bypass. Endovascular therapy should be the first line of treatment for elderly patients and those that are clearly at high operative risk. This is especially true for patients who have had significant weight loss and have significant malnutrition, who make up the majority of this patient population. The patients who do not have prohibitive risk factors for surgical bypass are less clearly defined; however, given the high rate of symptom relief, high primary-assisted patency, and lower mortality associated with endovascular therapy, most patients are probably best treated initially with endovascular therapy. This will be an ongoing debate with some centers reporting similar results of surgical bypass compared with endovascular therapy.[48] Ultimately, without better evidence, it will require the surgeon to make an individual risk assessment of the patient, determine the patient's periprocedural risk tolerance, and then proceed with the best treatment.

The outcomes of surgical revascularization of acute mesenteric ischemia are unacceptably high with perioperative mortality ranging from 31% to 70% (see Table 35-3), and, if no treatment is undertaken, mortality is 99.5%.[1,4,49] The etiology of acute mesenteric ischemia impacts survival; mortality for acute mesenteric thrombosis is higher than for embolic occlusion (77% and 54%, respectively) because of proximal occlusion causing more extensive bowel infarction.[1] NOMI carries a mortality rate of 75% because of the associated comorbidities leading to ischemia, and MVT has a mortality rate of 20% to 50%.[1] Patient and perioperative variables that increase mortality include age older than 70 years, acute renal insufficiency, metabolic acidosis, increased symptom duration, and need for bowel resection at repeat operations.[7,11] In a large collective review, patients who required both exploratory laparotomy and bowel resection performed poorly (mortality 70%-85%) regardless of etiology.[1]

Endovascular therapy has the potential to dramatically alter the clinical outcome of patients with acute mesenteric ischemia, but, given the relative infrequency of this disease, it is difficult for any one center to obtain a large experience. A compilation of series resulted in 48 patients that underwent endovascular and hybrid treatment for acute mesenteric ischemia. The in-hospital mortality of 17% is lower than that of any open surgical series. The technique described earlier offers a less-invasive method to address this critically ill population, and, with increased experience, endovascular therapy could dramatically improve the outcome of this condition.

CONCLUSION

Mesenteric ischemia remains one of the most lethal diseases treated by vascular surgeons. Although patients may not initially appear in extremis on presentation, patients with acute mesenteric ischemia have an extremely high mortality risk. The first priority should be restoration of flow to the bowel in a timely fashion, and endovascular therapy has the potential to improve that end point. If endovascular therapy is not readily available, immediate embolectomy or surgical revascularization is mandated to prevent death. The management of chronic mesenteric ischemia has evolved into several treatment options ranging from surgical bypass to endovascular therapy. Although restenosis rates are higher for visceral stents, periprocedural mortality is undeniably lower, and symptom relief is equivalent between the two techniques. Although restenosis rates remain a concern, primary-assisted and secondary patency rates are extremely high. Endovascular therapy will play an increasing role in management of this difficult patient population.

References

1. Schoots IG, Koffeman GI, Legemate DA, et al: Systematic review of survival after acute mesenteric ischaemia according to disease aetiology, *Br J Surg* 91(1):17–27, 2004.
2. Schoots IG, Levi MM, Reekers JA, et al: Thrombolytic therapy for acute superior mesenteric artery occlusion, *J Vasc Interv Radiol* 16(3):317–329, 2005.
3. Ozden N, Gurses B: Mesenteric ischemia in the elderly, *Clin Geriatr Med* 23(4):871–887, 2007, vii–viii.
4. Bradbury AW, Brittenden J, McBride K, et al: Mesenteric ischaemia: a multidisciplinary approach, *Br J Surg* 82(11):1446–1459, 1995.
5. Mamode N, Pickford I, Leiberman P: Failure to improve outcome in acute mesenteric ischaemia: seven-year review, *Eur J Surg* 165(3):203–208, 1999.
6. Acosta S, Ogren M, Sternby NH, et al: Incidence of acute thrombo-embolic occlusion of the superior mesenteric artery—a population-based study, *Eur J Vasc Endovasc Surg* 27(2):145–150, 2004.
7. Kassahun WT, Schulz T, Richter O, et al: Unchanged high mortality rates from acute occlusive intestinal ischemia: six year review, *Langenbecks Arch Surg* 393(2):163–171, 2008.
8. Acosta S, Ogren M, Sternby NH, et al: Clinical implications for the management of acute thromboembolic occlusion of the superior mesenteric artery: autopsy findings in 213 patients, *Ann Surg* 241(3):516–522, 2005.
9. Lin PH, Chaikof EL: Embryology, anatomy, and surgical exposure of the great abdominal vessels, *Surg Clin North Am* 80(1):417–433, 2000, xiv.
10. Lock G: Acute intestinal ischaemia, *Best Pract Res Clin Gastroenterol* 15(1):83–98, 2001.
11. Kougias P, El Sayed HF, Zhou W, et al: Management of chronic mesenteric ischemia. The role of endovascular therapy, *J Endovasc Ther* 14(3):395–405, 2007.
12. Frishman WH, Novak S, Brandt LJ, et al: Pharmacologic management of mesenteric occlusive disease, *Cardiol Rev* 16 (2):59–68, 2008.
13. Mitchell EL, Moneta GL: Mesenteric duplex scanning, *Perspect Vasc Surg Endovasc Ther* 18(2):175–183, 2006.
14. Moneta GL: Screening for mesenteric vascular insufficiency and follow-up of mesenteric artery bypass procedures, *Semin Vasc Surg* 14(3):186–192, 2001.
15. Moneta GL, Lee RW, Yeager RA, et al: Mesenteric duplex scanning: a blinded prospective study, *J Vasc Surg* 17(1):79–84; discussion 85-8, 1993.
16. Gentile AT, Moneta GL, Lee RW, et al: Usefulness of fasting and postprandial duplex ultrasound examinations for predicting high-grade superior mesenteric artery stenosis, *Am J Surg* 169 (5):476–479, 1995.
17. Shih MC, Hagspiel KD: CTA and MRA in mesenteric ischemia: part 1, Role in diagnosis and differential diagnosis, *AJR Am J Roentgenol* 188(2):452–461, 2007.
18. Furukawa A, Kanasaki S, Kono N, et al: CT diagnosis of acute mesenteric ischemia from various causes, *AJR Am J Roentgenol* 192(2):408–416, 2009.
19. Shih MC, Angle JF, Leung DA, et al: CTA and MRA in mesenteric ischemia: part 2, Normal findings and complications after surgical and endovascular treatment, *AJR Am J Roentgenol* 188 (2):462–471, 2007.
20. Bradbury MS, Kavanagh PV, Bechtold RE, et al: Mesenteric venous thrombosis: diagnosis and noninvasive imaging, *Radiographics* 22(3):527–541, 2002.
21. A randomised, blinded, trial of clopidogrel versus aspirin in patients at risk of ischaemic events (CAPRIE), *Lancet* 348 (9038):1329–1339. CAPRIE Steering Committee, 1996.
22. Atmaca Y, Dandachi R, Gulec S, et al: Comparison of clopidogrel versus ticlopidine for prevention of minor myocardial injury after elective coronary stenting, *Int J Cardiol* 87(2-3):143–149, 2003.
23. Bhatt DL, Topol EJ: Clopidogrel added to aspirin versus aspirin alone in secondary prevention and high-risk primary prevention: rationale and design of the Clopidogrel for High Atherothrombotic Risk and Ischemic Stabilization, Management, and Avoidance (CHARISMA) trial, *Am Heart J* 148 (2):263–268, 2004.
24. McKinsey JF, Gewertz BL: Acute mesenteric ischemia, *Surg Clin North Am* 77(2):307–318, 1997.
25. Kawarada O, Sonomura T, Yokoi Y: Direct aspiration using rapid-exchange and low-profile device for acute thrombo-embolic occlusion of the superior mesenteric artery, *Catheter Cardiovasc Interv* 68(6):862–866, 2006.
26. Sonoda K, Ikeda S, Koga S, et al: Successful treatment of acute occlusion in superior mesenteric artery of an elderly man by thrombus aspiration, *J Clin Gastroenterol* 41(10):933–934, 2007.
27. Tsuda M, Nakamura M, Yamada Y, et al: Acute superior mesenteric artery embolism: rapid reperfusion with hydrodynamic thrombectomy and pharmacological thrombolysis, *J Endovasc Ther* 10(5):1015–1018, 2003.
28. Soumerai SB, McLaughlin TJ, Ross-Degnan D, et al: Effectiveness of thrombolytic therapy for acute myocardial infarction in the elderly: cause for concern in the old-old, *Arch Intern Med* 162(5):561–568, 2002.
29. Kozuch PL, Brandt LJ: Review article: diagnosis and management of mesenteric ischaemia with an emphasis on pharmacotherapy, *Aliment Pharmacol Ther* 21(3):201–215, 2005.
30. Kukovetz WR, Poch G: Inhibition of cyclic-3′,5′-nucleotide-phosphodiesterase as a possible mode of action of papaverine and similarly acting drugs, *Naunyn Schmiedebergs Arch Pharmacol* 267(2):189–194, 1970.
31. Tabriziani H, Frishman WH, Brandt LJ: Drug therapies for mesenteric vascular disease, *Heart Dis* 4(5):306–314, 2002.
32. Kaleya RN, Boley SJ: Acute mesenteric ischemia: an aggressive diagnostic and therapeutic approach. 1991 Roussel Lecture, *Can J Surg* 35(6):613–623, 1992.
33. Simo G, Echenagusia AJ, Camunez F, et al: Superior mesenteric arterial embolism: local fibrinolytic treatment with urokinase, *Radiology* 204(3):775–779, 1997.
34. Milner R, Woo EY, Carpenter JP: Superior mesenteric artery angioplasty and stenting via a retrograde approach in a patient with bowel ischemia—a case report, *Vasc Endovascular Surg* 38(1):89–91, 2004.
35. Jarvinen O, Laurikka J, Sisto T, et al: Atherosclerosis of the visceral arteries, *Vasa* 24(1):9–14, 1995.
36. Wilson DB, Mostafavi K, Craven TE, et al: Clinical course of mesenteric artery stenosis in elderly Americans, *Arch Intern Med* 166(19):2095–2100, 2006.
37. Thomas JH, Blake K, Pierce GE, et al: The clinical course of asymptomatic mesenteric arterial stenosis, *J Vasc Surg* 27(5):840–844, 1998.
38. Sarac TP, Altinel O, Kashyap V, et al: Endovascular treatment of stenotic and occluded visceral arteries for chronic mesenteric ischemia, *J Vasc Surg* 47(3):485–491, 2008.
39. Silva JA, White CJ, Collins TJ, et al: Endovascular therapy for chronic mesenteric ischemia, *J Am Coll Cardiol* 47(5):944–950, 2006.
40. Kasirajan K, O'Hara PJ, Gray BH, et al: Chronic mesenteric ischemia: open surgery versus percutaneous angioplasty and stenting, *J Vasc Surg* 33(1):63–71, 2001.
41. McAfee MK, Cherry KJ Jr, Naessens JM, et al: Influence of complete revascularization on chronic mesenteric ischemia, *Am J Surg* 164(3):220–224, 1992.

42. Rose SC, Quigley TM, Raker EJ: Revascularization for chronic mesenteric ischemia: comparison of operative arterial bypass grafting and percutaneous transluminal angioplasty, *J Vasc Interv Radiol* 6(3):339–349, 1995.
43. Wyers MC, Powell RJ, Nolan BW, et al: Retrograde mesenteric stenting during laparotomy for acute occlusive mesenteric ischemia, *J Vasc Surg* 45(2):269–275, 2007.
44. Sharafuddin MJ, Olson CH, Sun S, et al: Endovascular treatment of celiac and mesenteric arteries stenoses: applications and results, *J Vasc Surg* 38(4):692–698, 2003.
45. McMillan WD, McCarthy WJ, Bresticker MR, et al: Mesenteric artery bypass: objective patency determination, *J Vasc Surg* 21 (5):729–740, 1995; discussion 740-741.
46. Mateo RB, O'Hara PJ, Hertzer NR, et al: Elective surgical treatment of symptomatic chronic mesenteric occlusive disease: early results and late outcomes, *J Vasc Surg* 29(5):821–831. discussion 832, 1999.
47. Park WM, Cherry KJ Jr, Chua HK, et al: Current results of open revascularization for chronic mesenteric ischemia: a standard for comparison, *J Vasc Surg* 35(5):853–859, 2002.
48. Atkins MD, Kwolek CJ, LaMuraglia GM, et al: Surgical revascularization versus endovascular therapy for chronic mesenteric ischemia: a comparative experience, *J Vasc Surg* 45(6):1162–1171, 2007.
49. Edwards MS, Cherr GS, Craven TE, et al: Acute occlusive mesenteric ischemia: surgical management and outcomes, *Ann Vasc Surg* 17(1):72–79, 2003.
50. Cho JS, Carr JA, Jacobsen G, et al: Long-term outcome after mesenteric artery reconstruction: a 37-year experience, *J Vasc Surg* 35(3):453–460, 2002.
51. Kruger AJ, Walker PJ, Foster WJ, et al: Open surgery for atherosclerotic chronic mesenteric ischemia, *J Vasc Surg* 46(5):941–945, 2007.
52. Biebl M, Oldenburg WA, Paz-Fumagalli R, et al: Surgical and interventional visceral revascularization for the treatment of chronic mesenteric ischemia—when to prefer which? *World J Surg* 31(3):562–568, 2007.
53. Landis MS, Rajan DK, Simons ME, et al: Percutaneous management of chronic mesenteric ischemia: outcomes after intervention, *J Vasc Interv Radiol* 16(10):1319–1325, 2005.
54. Kougias P, Lau D, El Sayed HF, et al: Determinants of mortality and treatment outcome following surgical interventions for acute mesenteric ischemia, *J Vasc Surg* 46(3):467–474, 2007.

SECTION VI

SUPRA-AORTIC TRUNK DISORDERS

CHAPTER

36

Subclavian and Vertebral Arteries: Angioplasty and Stents

Marc Bosiers, Koen Deloose, Jürgen Verbist, Patrick Peeters

Clinically significant atherosclerotic occlusive disease involving the supra-aortic vessels has traditionally been managed by surgical bypass or endarterectomy. A variety of extra-anatomic reconstructions have been described to treat each lesion depending on its specific location. Several series have documented that surgery is associated with a low complication rate along with an excellent patency rate and long-term symptomatic relief.[1-4]

Despite the success and durability of surgical revascularization, endovascular methods have gained popularity for the treatment of supra-aortic lesions involving the subclavian and vertebral arteries.[5-11] Several factors, including (1) the focal nature of the atherosclerotic plaque, (2) the high-flow state of the supra-aortic vessels, and (3) the significant reduction in morbidity compared with a major transthoracic reconstruction make percutaneous angioplasty (PTA) and stenting a particularly suitable alternative to surgery and explain why endovascular treatments have emerged as the first line of therapy in many centers.

INDICATIONS FOR INTERVENTION

The indications for endovascular therapy and open surgery are the same. In general, treatment is reserved for symptomatic lesions. The most commonly accepted indications for intervention in symptomatic patients are (1) subclavian disease with significant arm claudication, embolization, and/or vertebrobasilar insufficiency (VBI); (2) any lesion associated with transient ischemic attacks, and (3) recurrent angina after coronary artery bypass grafting (CABG) with the internal mammary artery (IMA) (coronary steal syndrome), amaurosis fugax, or stroke. The few exceptions in which treatment is indicated for asymptomatic patients are (1) vertebral artery stenosis greater than 80%, (2) subclavian disease before CABG with the IMA, and (3) subclavian lesions before arteriovenous fistula creation or to maintain arteriovenous fistula function.

Subclavian

The left subclavian artery is the most commonly involved artery in supra-aortic occlusive disease and is the target of therapy in more than 50% of the cases. Most subclavian lesions are asymptomatic and remain clinically insignificant. Most commonly, patients present with symptoms of decreased left brachial blood pressure or pulse along with vertigo or dizziness during arm exertion signifying VBI. This situation defines the subclavian steal syndrome,[7-9,12] in which vertebral artery flow is reversed and the posterior cerebral perfusion is compromised to maintain flow in the upper extremity.[12] Other patients with left subclavian disease may present with a coronary steal syndrome characterized by recurrent angina after CABG using the left IMA.[12-14] This also holds for the right side (Figure 36-1).

Vertebral

Occlusive lesions of the vertebral artery are usually not symptomatic, because an extensive network of cerebral collateralization is present to maintain cerebral perfusion. Revascularization may occasionally be required in the setting of a clearly defined VBI and diffuse atherosclerosis of the other cerebral vessels.[15] This is certainly the case if the contralateral vertebral is heavily diseased or occluded.

Also, in many patients one vertebral artery may be dominant, and this may lead to early symptoms of vertigo and dizziness when this vessel is involved with a hemodynamically significant lesion. However,

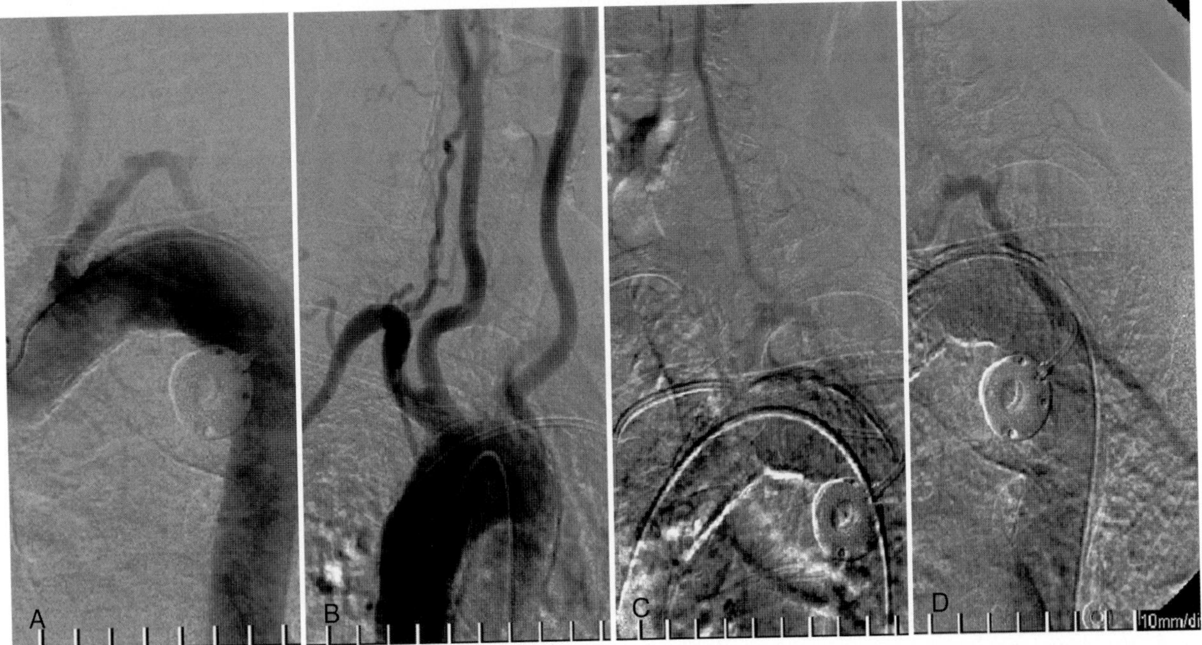

FIGURE 36-1 **A,** Arch aortogram demonstrating occlusion versus stenosis of left subclavian artery. **B,** Immediate filling of supra-aortic vessels except the left subclavian. **C,** Late filling of left vertebral artery with retrograde flow. **D,** Reconstitution of axillary artery via retrograde left vertebral flow.

when a significant internal carotid lesion is detected in the presence of a vertebral lesion and VBI, we elect to treat the carotid lesion first by either carotid endarterectomy or carotid artery stenting.

ENDOVASCULAR TREATMENT STRATEGY

Access

A properly positioned delivery sheath is extremely important and facilitates each step of the procedure. Access to supra-aortic vessels may be obtained from either a femoral, brachial, or combined approach. Occasionally, an open retrograde approach from the common carotid artery is necessary.

In treating stenotic lesions, for the femoral access either a 6F, 90-cm sheath or a guiding catheter is used. Preferred selective catheters for the femoral approach include the H-1, JB-2, vertebral, and Vitek catheters. Brachial access is done with a 35-cm sheath and a Berenstein or multipurpose catheter. Systemic heparin is given in all cases once access is obtained. With either approach a steerable, hydrophilic guidewire (Terumo Europe Leuven, Belgium) is used to cross the lesion. To stabilize the system during PTA and stent placement, the hydrophilic wire is replaced with a stiff Amplatz wire.

For the treatment of occlusions the brachial approach is usually preferred. A 35-cm sheath (5F or 6F) is used during brachial access. However, a femoral approach may be still be the best when there is a "nipple" at the ostium of the subclavian. In a few challenging cases, we have used a combined femoral and brachial approach. In this instance, the occlusion is crossed retrograde from the arm, and the guidewire is snared from a catheter inserted from the femoral approach. This "pull-through technique" provides dual access and may facilitate accurate stent placement in cases of severe vessel tortuosity and severely calcified occlusions (Figure 36-2).

Guidewires and Catheters

The choice of selective catheters is to some degree a matter of personal preference. For subclavian artery revascularization from a retrograde brachial approach, we like a multipurpose catheter, whereas from a femoral approach we prefer a vertebral or JB-2 catheter for the left subclavian and H-1 catheter for the right subclavian. Typically, a 0.035-inch hydrophilic-coated Terumo guidewire is used to cross the lesion. Sometimes a stiff 0.018-inch SV-guidewire can be very helpful for it allows us to use low-profile balloons and stents.

To cross vertebral lesions, which are typically located in the proximal one third of the artery, we generally prefer the femoral approach using a long sheath and 0.018-inch or 0.014-inch wires.

In the presence of severe tortuosity of the aortic arch and proximal subclavian artery, placement of the

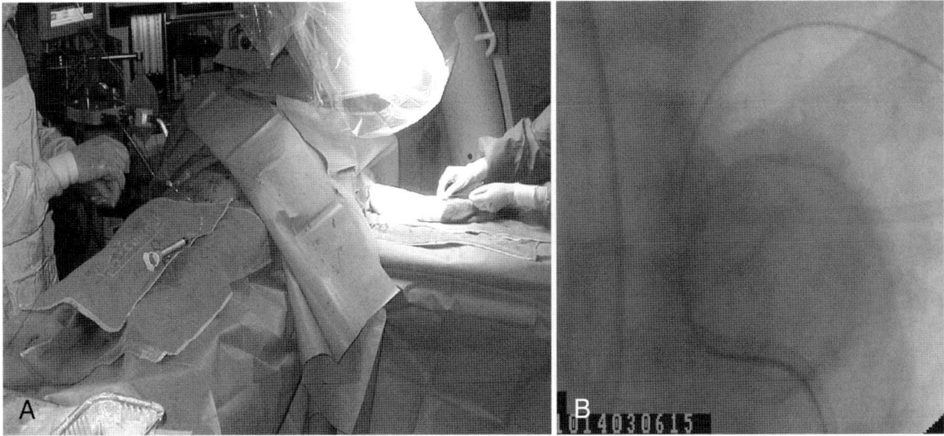

FIGURE 36-2 **A,** Combined femoral and brachial access. **B,** Sheath in aortic arch with wire exiting both accesses.

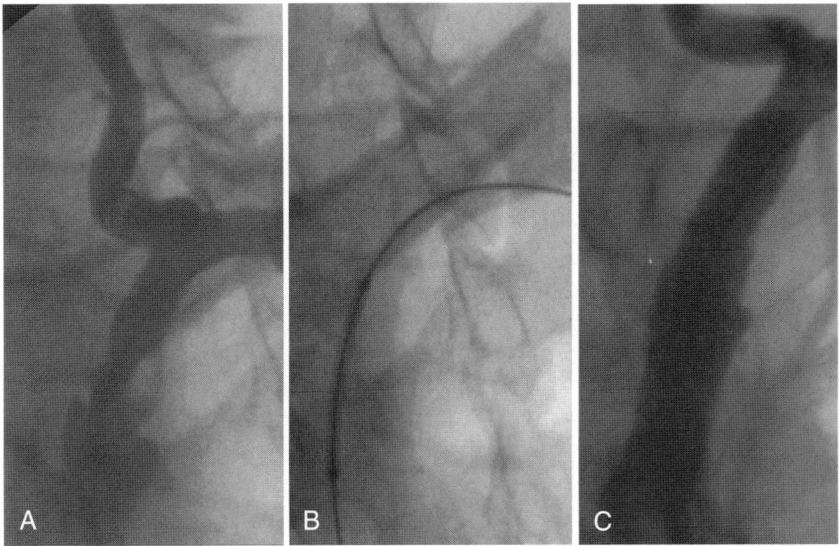

FIGURE 36-3 **A,** Prevertebral stenosis. **B,** Stent positioning. **C,** Final arteriogram.

guiding catheter may be difficult and yield poor backup support: using the buddy-wire technique stabilizes the guiding catheter in its proper position and allows stenting the vertebral artery origin stenosis in the complex anatomy.[16]

Angioplasty and Stents

Both balloon-expandable and self-expanding stents are used to treat subclavian lesions. Balloon-expandable stents are superior to self-expanding stents for ostial and prevertebral subclavian (proximal to vertebral artery origin) lesions (Figure 36-3). Deployment of balloon-expandable stents is more precise, and this is beneficial in ostial lesions where 1 to 2 mm of "overhang" of the stent into the aorta is desired. Also, for subclavian lesions, precise placement is critical so that the origin of the vertebral is not covered. In addition, balloon-expandable stents have more radial strength, and this may be beneficial because ostial lesions are generally more calcified. Nevertheless, recent case reports on balloon-expandable stent implantations cautioned about the occurrence of stent fractures leading the in-stent restenoses and even claimed the necessity of 6-month angiographic control to closely monitor stent behavior for the given indication.[17,18]

The increased flexibility of self-expanding stents makes them more suited for postvertebral (distal to vertebral artery origin) lesions because they may accommodate tortuous vessels better than balloon-expandable stents.

PTA may be performed before stent placement but is not recommended for ostial and prevertebral subclavian lesions because the risk of dissection from PTA is greater in these cases. Primary stenting reduces the risk for dissection and is commonly performed in this setting.

TABLE 36-1 Results of Subclavian Artery Treatment

Author	Period	Lesions (No.)	Technical success (%)	Restenosis rate (%)	Patency, 1-2 yr (%)	Patency, 3-5 yr (%)	Patency, 10 yr (%)
Sullivan et al.[9]	1993-1997	66	94	4.5	90	84	NA
Henry et al.[27]	1988-1998	135	94	14	90	85	NA
Agarwal et al.[28]	1994-2003	98	94	17	87	81	NA
Motarjeme[7]	1990-1995	151	93	NA	NA	80	NA
Eidlilidt et al.[29]	1994-2002	89	93	5	88	78	NA
Korner et al.[30]	1990-1998	43	84	24	NA	72	NA
Taha et al.[31]	1987-1997	47	89	7	NA	80	NA
Henry et al.[32]	1992-2006	237	94	12	NA	NA	78
Palchik et al.[33]	1992-2006	67	93	12	NA	81	80
AbuRahma et al.[34]	1993-2006	121	98	NA	93	70	NA

NA, Not available.

If PTA is deemed necessary, it is important not to oversize the balloon. We most commonly use a 4- to 6-mm balloon for predilation of subclavian lesions and use stents between 8 and 10 mm in diameter.

Historically, PTA alone is preferred for the treatment of vertebral lesions, and 2- or 3-mm–diameter coronary balloons are most commonly selected. However, the recurrence rate after vertebral PTA is 8% to 15%, and there is at least one report that suggests that restenosis may be reduced when stents are used to treat ostial lesions[19]; stent placement in the vertebral artery has been avoided, historically. Recently reports came available on the use of drug-eluting stents in the vertebral artery. Gupta et al.[20] reviewed data from 59 patients with either extracranial (n = 36) or intracranial stenoses (n = 29) treated with Cypher or Taxus stents. The majority of the extracranial stents were implanted in the vertebral artery (n = 31) or the internal carotid artery (n = 5). Most (95%) procedures were technically successful, and the periprocedural complication rate was 3% (one non–flow-limiting dissection and one stroke). Follow-up angiography (n = 41) or computed tomography (n = 7) performed at a median of 4 months after implantation revealed a restenosis rate of 6%.[20] These stent findings were confirmed by Ko et al.,[21] who did not observe any adverse neurologic event at 1 month after the implantation of balloon-expandable stents in 25 extracranial vertebral artery stenoses. On the basis of these data and our own experiences, we recommend coronary balloon-expandable stents for ostial lesions.

Cerebral Protection

Cerebral protection is routinely used for internal carotid artery stenting.[22-24] The benefit of cerebral protection during subclavian stenting is minimal, and the routine use of protection devices does not appear indicated in this case. Ringelstein and Zeumer[15] demonstrated that the risk of embolization to the posterior circulation is negligible during subclavian angioplasty, because protection is provided by reversal of flow in the vertebral artery. They demonstrated by duplex ultrasound that reversal of flow in the vertebral is maintained for a short period after angioplasty, and only after several minutes is antegrade flow restored. If protection is deemed necessary during a particular subclavian procedure, this can easily be accomplished by placing a 2- or 3-mm balloon at the origin of the vertebral artery or a carotid filter device.

ENDOVASCULAR RESULTS AND SURVEILLANCE

The long-term results after endovascular therapy in subclavian vessels are good (Table 36-1). One-year patency rates of greater than 85% are consistently reported in the literature.[5-11] More important, long-term symptomatic relief is achieved in a majority of cases. However, restenosis can occur and may be clinically significant in up to 40% of the cases at 4 years after intervention. A recent publication reporting on a single-center consecutive case series propagates the use of balloon-expandable drug-eluting stent systems, claiming they appear to decrease in-stent restenosis.[25] Although the idea seems reasonable, because of this limited evidence it is far too early to make any recommendation on the application of active coated stents.

Recurrences can be successfully treated by repeated angioplasty, preferably with a cutting balloon, and/or additional stent placement.

There is a clear distinction between the results achieved with endovascular therapy for subclavian stenoses versus subclavian occlusions. The procedure is a technical success in more than 90% when the vessel is stenotic compared with 60% to 80% when a total occlusion is present. Periprocedural complications are rare and most often minor when treating a stenosis. Primary stenting is the strategy to follow to decrease the risk of these devastating dissections. However, life-threatening complications such as aortic arch dissection can occur during recanalization of a subclavian occlusion. Last, long-term patency is better after the treatment of a stenosis versus an occlusion.[6-11] Because the recurrence rate after PTA alone for occlusions is unacceptable, stenting should be indicated after the revascularization of any occluded subclavian artery.[7-11]

In addition, several reports have documented the success of PTA with stent placement for the treatment of subclavian steal,[10-12,26] and recently a number of reports have confirmed the efficacy of endovascular therapy for treating left subclavian lesions before or after CABG with use of the left IMA.[12-14] A patency rate of 80% beyond 1 year has been reported in this situation.

At our institution, patients are followed closely for an extended period in an effort to detect recurrences early. History and physical examination are most often successful in detecting a recurrence, and duplex ultrasound is the best noninvasive test and is performed yearly. Further investigation with angiography is indicated if there is uncertainty about the status of the lesion or the clinical presentation remains unclear.

CONCLUSION

Percutaneous therapy has largely replaced surgical revascularization as the initial treatment of choice for patients with supra-aortic arterial occlusive disease. Several factors can make PTA and stenting a complex procedure that requires advanced endovascular skills for a successful outcome. The durability of PTA and stenting is excellent; however, in-line surgical reconstruction or extra-anatomic bypass is occasionally required for failure of endovascular techniques or if contraindications exist.

Acknowledgments

The authors thank the staff of Flanders Medical Research Program (http://www.fmrp.be), with special regards to Koen De Meester for performing the systematic review of the literature and providing substantial support to the data analysis and the writing of the article.

References

1. Kieffer E, Sabatier J, Koskas F, et al: Atherosclerotic innominate artery occlusive disease: early and long-term results of surgical reconstruction, *J Vasc Surg* 21:326–336, 1995.
2. Berguer R, Morasch MD, Kline RA: Transthoracic repair of innominate and common carotid artery disease: immediate and long-term outcome for 100 consecutive surgical reconstructions, *J Vasc Surg* 27:34–41, 1998.
3. Vitti M, Thompson B, Read R, et al: Carotid-subclavian bypass: a twenty-two–year experience, *J Vasc Surg* 20:411–417, 1994.
4. AbuRahma A, Robinson P, Jennings T: Carotid-subclavian bypass grafting with polytetrafluoroethylene grafts for symptomatic subclavian artery stenosis or occlusion: a 20-year experience, *J Vasc Surg* 32:411–418, 2000.
5. Reekers J: Subclavian artery stenosis is best managed by PTA and stent. In: *The evidence for vascular and endovascular reconstruction*, Philadelphia, 2002, Saunders, pp 101–105.
6. Insall R, Lambert D, Chamberlain J, et al: Percutaneous transluminal angioplasty of the innominate, subclavian, and axillary arteries, *Eur J Vasc Surg* 4:591–595, 1990.
7. Motarjeme A: Percutaneous transluminal angioplasty of supra-aortic vessels, *J Endovasc Surg* 3:171–181, 1996.
8. Criado F, Twena M: Techniques for endovascular recanalization of supra-aortic trunks, *J Endovasc Surg* 3:405–413, 1996.
9. Sullivan T, Gray B, Bacharach J, et al: Angioplasty and primary stenting of the subclavian, innominate, and common carotid arteries in 83 patients, *J Vasc Surg* 28:1059–1065, 1998.
10. Sheiban I, Dharmadhikari A, Melissano G, et al: Subclavian artery stenting: Immediate and mid term clinical follow-up results, *Int J Cardiovasc Intervent* 3:231–235, 2000.
11. Rodriguez-Lopez J, Werner A, Martinez R, et al: Stenting for atherosclerotic occlusive disease of the subclavian artery, *Ann Vasc Surg* 13:254–260, 1999.
12. Pollard H, Rigby S, Moritz G, et al: Subclavian steal syndrome: a review, *Australas Chiropr Osteopathy* 7:20–28, 1998.
13. Angle J, Matsumoto A, McGraw J, et al: Percutaneous angioplasty and stenting of left subclavian artery stenosis in patients with left internal mammary–coronary bypass grafts: clinical experience and long-term follow-up, *Vasc Endovascular Surg* 37:89–97, 2003.
14. Hallisey M, Rees J, Meranze S, et al: Use of angioplasty in the prevention and treatment of coronary: subclavian steal syndrome, *J Vasc Interv Radiol* 6:125–129, 1995.
15. Ringelstein EF, Zeumer H: Delayed reversal of vertebral artery blood flow following percutaneous transluminal angioplasty for subclavian steal syndrome, *Neuroradiology* 26:189–198, 1995.
16. Kizilkilic O: Vertebral artery origin stenting with buddy wire technique in tortuous subclavian artery, *Eur J Radiol* 61:120–123, 2007.
17. Kim SR, Baik MW, Yoo SH, et al: Stent fracture and restenosis after placement of a drug-eluting device in the vertebral artery origin and treatment with the stent-in-stent technique. Report of two cases, *J Neurosurg* 106:907–911, 2007.
18. Tsutsumi M, Kazekawa K, Onizuka M, et al: Stent fracture in revascularization for symptomatic ostial vertebral artery stenosis, *Neuroradiology* 49:253–257, 2007.
19. Piotin M, Spelle L, Martin J, et al: Percutaneous transluminal angioplasty and stenting of the proximal vertebral artery for symptomatic stenosis, *AJNR Am J Neuroradiol* 21:727–731, 2000.
20. Gupta R, Al-Ali F, Thomas AJ, et al: Safety, feasibility, and short-term follow-up of drug-eluting stent placement in the intracranial and extracranial circulation, *Stroke* 37:2562–2566, 2006.

21. Ko YG, Park S, Kim JY, et al: Percutaneous interventional treatment of extracranial vertebral artery stenosis with coronary stents, *Yonsei Med J* 45:629–634, 2004.
22. Iyer V, de Donato G, Deloose K, et al: The type of embolic protection does not influence the outcome in carotid artery stenting, *J Vasc Surg* 46:251–256, 2007.
23. Collaborative Group SPACE, Ringleb PA, Allenberg J, et al: 30 day results from the SPACE trial of stent-protected angioplasty versus carotid endarterectomy in symptomatic patients: a randomised non-inferiority trial, *Lancet* 368:1239–1247, 2006.
24. Setacci C, Cremonesi A: SPACE and EVA-3S Trials: The Need of Standards for Carotid Stenting, *Eur J Vasc Endovasc Surg* 33:48–49, 2007.
25. Akins PT, Kerber CW, Pakbaz RS: Stenting of vertebral artery origin atherosclerosis in high-risk patients: bare or coated? A single-center consecutive case series, *J Invasive Cardiol* 20:14–20, 2008.
26. Schillinger M, Haumer M, Schillinger S, et al: Outcome of conservative versus interventional treatment of subclavian artery stenosis, *J Endovasc Ther* 9:139–146, 2002.
27. Henry M, Amor M, Henry I, et al: Percutaneous transluminal angioplasty of the subclavian arteries, *J Endovasc Surg* 6:33–41, 1999.
28. Agarwal S, Chati M, Amor M: Endovascular therapy for subclavian artery lesions, Transcatheter Cardiovascular Therapeutics Presented at the conference, Washington, DC, 2003.
29. Eidlilidt G, Schnyder G, Chati Z: Subclavian artery stenting, Transcatheter Cardiovascular Therapeutics Presented at the conference, Washington, DC, 2002.
30. Körner M, Baumgartner I, Do D, et al: PTA of the subclavian and innominate arteries: long-term results, *Vasa* 28:117–122, 1999.
31. Taha A, Vahl A, de Jong S, et al: Reconstruction of the supra-aortic trunks, *Eur J Surg* 165:314–318, 1999.
32. Henry M, Henry I, Polydorou A, et al: Percutaneous transluminal angioplasty of the subclavian arteries, *Int Angiol* 26:324–340, 2007.
33. Palchik E, Bakken AM, Wolford HY, et al: Subclavian artery revascularization: an outcome analysis based on mode of therapy and presenting symptoms, *Ann Vasc Surg* 22:70–78, 2008.
34. AbuRahma AF, Bates MC, Stone PA, et al: Angioplasty and stenting versus carotid-subclavian bypass for the treatment of isolated subclavian artery disease, *J Endovasc Ther* 14:698–704, 2007.

CHAPTER

37

Innominate and Common Carotid Arteries: Angioplasty and Stents

Brian G. DeRubertis

The treatment of occlusive lesions of the innominate and common carotid arteries has undergone considerable evolution over the last several decades. The open surgical management of disorders of the supra-aortic trunks has become established as an effective and durable treatment option. However, the intra-thoracic location of most of these lesions and the resultant complexity of the operations required for correction of these lesions has prompted the development of endovascular solutions to this disease with the hope of achieving reduced morbidity and mortality. Overall experience with lesions of the innominate and common carotid arteries reported in the medical literature is significantly less than that with carotid bifurcation or subclavian artery disease, and this obviously carries implications for our understanding of the disease process, its natural history, and the outcome after open and endovascular interventions. In one of the larger series of surgical correction of carotid bifurcation, vertebral, and great-vessel disease, Wiley and Effeney[1] reported that only 7.5% were performed for innominate, common carotid, or subclavian disease. In several contemporary studies, innominate intervention comprised between 3% and 14% of all interventions for innominate and subclavian lesions.[2-4] However, a subset of patients exist who have isolated innominate or common carotid occlusive disease and a clear presentation with one of several clinical syndromes attributable to supra-aortic trunk disease. Furthermore, several centers have accumulated a significant experience with open surgical strategies for supra-aortic trunk revascularization, which is available for comparison with the results of the growing body of literature documenting results of endovascular revascularization.

In the absence of randomized clinical trials comparing open and endovascular approaches to treatment of innominate and common carotid disease, treatment choice must be individualized to the patient, with consideration given to the patient's overall medical condition, severity of symptoms, aortic arch anatomy (Figure 37-1), and number or severity of occlusive lesions in the supra-aortic trunk vessels. These factors should be considered in the context of the established results with open revascularization, as well as contemporary outcomes with current endovascular balloon and stent platforms and operator expertise. In many centers, endovascular treatment of these lesions has evolved into first-line therapy because of its relatively low morbidity and mortality.

General considerations during angioplasty and stenting of the innominate and common carotid arteries should include preoperative patient selection and risk stratification, minimization of risk of cerebral embolization, and technical issues involved in deployment of devices at vessel origins or bifurcations.

EVOLUTION OF THERAPY FOR LESIONS OF THE SUPRA-AORTIC TRUNK VESSELS

Open surgical revascularization of the supra-aortic trunks, including the innominate and common carotid arteries, was established as an effective and durable therapy for occlusive lesions of these vessels as a result of several large retrospective publications from centers with extensive experience with such procedures.[5-9] Wiley and Effeney[1] were among the first to report a large series of supra-aortic trunk revascularizations with their series of endarterectomies of the innominate artery in 1979. Subsequent studies reported the use of not only endarterectomy but also direct reconstruction with branched Dacron grafts from the nondiseased aortic arch to multiple supra-aortic vessels, generally through a median sternotomy. These studies ultimately

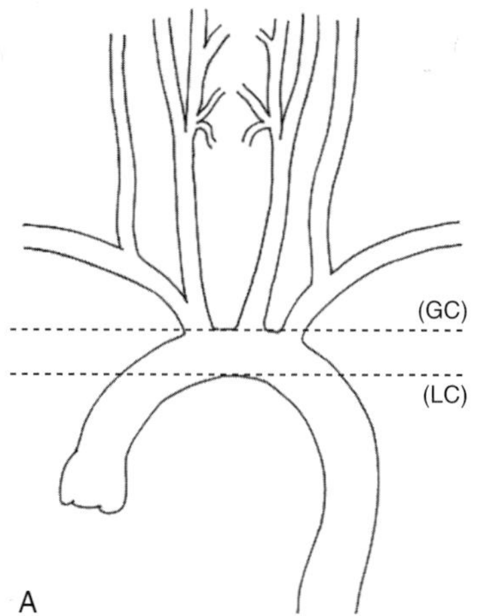

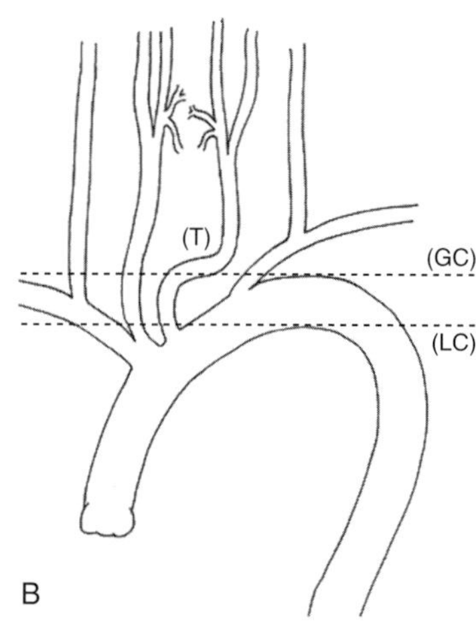

FIGURE 37-1 Aortic arch anatomy significantly impacts the difficulty of supra-aortic trunk interventions. A type I arch **(A)** in which the arch vessels originate above the greater curvature *(GC)* of the arch is more conducive to a femoral approach than an elongated type III arch **(B),** where the origins of the target vessels come off the aorta below the lesser curvature *(LC).* Type III anatomy, especially in conjunction with proximal vessel tortuosity *(T),* hinders stable sheath placement in target vessels.

demonstrated excellent long-term patency rates and acceptable morbidity and mortality rates with these operations.[6-10] Although extra-anatomic bypasses can be accomplished with lower morbidity, the patency of these grafts proved inferior to direct reconstruction by endarterectomy or bypass, and these later operations became the procedure of choice in those patients able to tolerate median sternotomy.

Endovascular therapy for arterial occlusive disease has made considerable progress in recent years, and this is true for intervention on the supra-aortic trunks as well. The development of balloon-expandable and self-expanding stents of multiple diameters and lengths that can be delivered through catheters of increasingly lower profile has improved the ability of interventionalists to treat these lesions. Obvious benefits of an endovascular approach to these lesions include the decreased morbidity and mortality, dramatically reduced hospital length of stay, and shorter overall recovery period. Although the literature regarding outcomes after endovascular interventions is not as robust as that of open repair, data on short- and intermediate-term patency have begun to accumulate and generally appear quite favorable.[2-4,11-14]

INNOMINATE ARTERY

Disease of the innominate artery is rare, occurring in a relatively small percentage of patients with brachiocephalic disease. Wiley and Effeney[1] found that patients with lesions of the innominate artery represented only 1.7% of those operated on for disease of the supra-aortic trunks. Because the innominate artery serves as a common origin for the right subclavian and right common carotid arteries, disease of this vessel can lead to both ischemic symptoms in the upper-extremity and neurologic symptoms. Furthermore, the large diameter and short length of this vessel can make percutaneous intervention challenging. Both the approach to this vessel and the selection of devices used for intervention must be considered carefully to avoid serious complications.

Clinical Presentation and Evaluation

The diagnosis of innominate artery stenosis or occlusion can largely be determined by the patient's presentation and physical examination results. Three clinical scenarios can generally be seen with innominate disease: (1) upper-extremity ischemia or embolization, (2) vertebral basilar symptoms, or (3) sequelae of cerebral embolization (Figure 37-2).

The severity of upper-extremity ischemia can range considerably because of the presence of collateral flow. Patients with innominate occlusions may have no symptoms or may present with symptoms ranging from effort-induced claudication to rest pain and ischemic ulceration. Although upper-extremity embolization is possible with innominate disease, the presence of isolated embolic lesions should also prompt consideration of vasculitis or central sources of embolic phenomenon. Neurologic symptoms can be the result of hemodynamic or embolic phenomenon in either the posterior or anterior cerebral circulation as a result of the innominate lesion. Posterior circulation symptoms, or vertebral basilar insufficiency, occur in conjunction with "subclavian steal" syndrome in which the contralateral cerebral circulation provides cross-filling of the ipsilateral hemisphere and ultimately of the ipsilateral upper extremity as a result of flow reversal in the vertebral artery. Symptoms of posterior circulation pathology typically include transient nonhemispheric motor or sensory deficits, bilateral visual loss, ataxia, and vertigo, diplopia, or

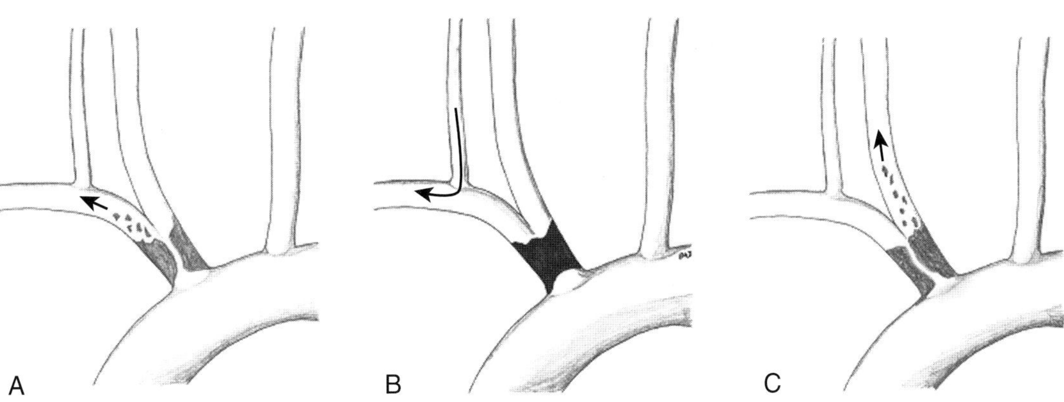

FIGURE 37-2 Innominate lesions can present with one of several clinical syndromes, including ipsilateral upper-extremity ischemia or embolization **(A)**, vertebrobasilar symptoms **(B)**, or embolization to the anterior cerebral circulation with resultant transient ischemic attacks, amaurosis, or cerebral infarction **(C)**.

dysarthria in conjunction with the aforementioned symptoms.[15] Symptoms attributable to the anterior cerebral circulation generally result from embolization and include transient ischemic attacks (TIAs), amaurosis fugax, or ipsilateral hemispheric stroke. Among series of open surgical and percutaneous interventions for innominate artery lesions, neurologic symptoms predominate. Cherry et al.[10] found that 77% of patients undergoing either endarterectomy or direct surgical reconstruction with prosthetic bypass for innominate disease had neurologic symptoms. Approximately 10% of these had both anterior and posterior cerebral circulation symptoms, 50% had isolated anterior circulation symptoms (amaurosis fugax and TIA), and 40% had isolated posterior symptoms.[10] In the same series, 54% had upper-extremity symptoms consisting of either claudication (64%) or embolization (36%). Almost 40% of patients had both neurologic and upper-extremity symptoms. Hüttl et al.[11] reported their experience with percutaneous revascularization of innominate artery lesions over a 19-year period and found a 70% incidence of neurologic symptoms (51% posterior circulation and 19% anterior circulation) and a 39% incidence of upper-extremity symptoms.[11]

The diagnosis of innominate stenosis or occlusion can be largely suspected by presentation with one of the clinical scenarios described earlier in the presence of characteristic physical signs. Evaluation of the patient with suspected supra-aortic trunk disease should begin with physical examination including evaluation of carotid, subclavian, brachial, and radial pulses. Auscultation of the carotid and subclavian arteries may reveal a bruit indicative of an occlusive lesion. Blood pressures from both arms should be obtained and compared, as should blood pressures from the lower extremities if bilateral supra-aortic trunk lesions are suspected. Duplex ultrasonography of the carotid arteries is useful for the evaluation of concomitant atherosclerotic disease of the carotid bulb and to determine directionality of flow in the vertebral arteries. The diagnosis can ultimately be confirmed by contrast angiography, which has long been the gold standard for evaluation of supra-aortic trunk lesions. However, in recent years axial imaging modalities with three-dimensional reconstructions have largely supplanted angiography for diagnostic purposes. Both computed tomographic and magnetic resonance angiography are useful tools not only for confirming occlusive lesions within the innominate artery but also for assessment of aortic arch type and variant anatomy, disease of the neighboring great vessels, and evaluation of the cerebral circulation. Noninvasive preprocedural imaging can assist in the decision between open and percutaneous revascularization and can aid in selecting the most effective approach for percutaneous revascularization.

Endovascular Approach to Innominate Artery Intervention

Treatment of innominate disease is undertaken primarily for symptomatic lesions, although intervention on an asymptomatic lesion is sometimes performed for patients with proximal subclavian or innominate stenoses who have had coronary bypass with internal mammary grafts. Options for interventional management of innominate lesions include (1) percutaneous transfemoral antegrade approach, (2) transbrachial retrograde approach, or (3) retrograde carotid access.

The most commonly used approach to innominate intervention is likely the antegrade transfemoral approach. Although this approach does not usually allow for embolic protection strategies while performing innominate interventions, the rate of clinically adverse events caused by emboli to the anterior cerebral

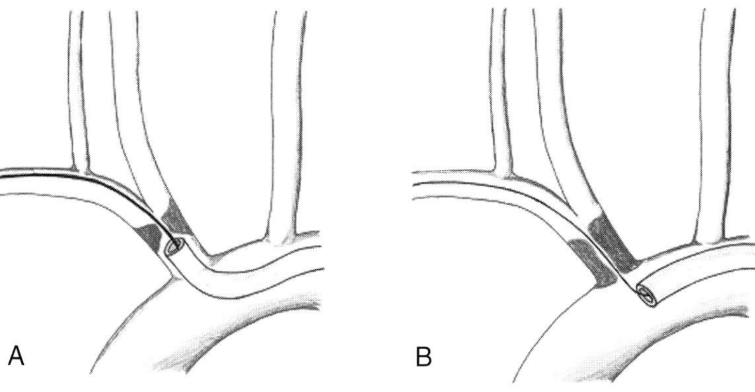

FIGURE 37-3 Even a short segment of patent innominate origin **(A)** can allow for placement of the sheath into this vessel and facilitate percutaneous intervention from a transfemoral approach. Flush occlusions of the innominate, however, generally prevent stable sheath placement from a femoral approach **(B)** and typically require brachial access for a retrograde approach.

circulation appears to be relatively low.[11,16] The femoral approach is preferred when a sufficient length of the proximal innominate artery origin exists before the stenosis or occlusion (Figure 37-3, *A*). Unlike percutaneous angioplasty of carotid bifurcation lesions where stable sheath placement is facilitated by advancing the tip of the sheath out of the aorta and into the distal common carotid, innominate interventions require treatment of lesions located at or just beyond the junction of the target vessel and the aortic arch. This prevents significant "purchase" of the sheath beyond the aortic arch and makes challenging anatomy, such as an elongated type III arch, prohibitively difficult to overcome through such an approach (see Figure 37-3, *B*). For innominate interventions with use of a femoral approach, femoral access is obtained via a common femoral puncture followed by placement of a short 5F sheath. A pigtail catheter is then advanced into the aortic arch, and unselected arch aortography is performed with use of the left anterior oblique orientation to open the aortic arch. After identification of the lesion and relevant arch anatomy, the patient is anticoagulated with 100 units/kg of intravenous heparin and maintained at an activated clotting time of >300 seconds. Oftentimes the innominate artery can be catheterized with a 5F simple angled catheter such as a Berenstein (AngioDynamics, Queensbury, NY), vertebral (AngioDynamics), or angled glide (Cook Medical, Bloomington, IN) catheter, although more elongated arches will sometimes require reverse-curve catheters such as a Vitek (Cook Medical) or a Simmons (AngioDynamics) catheter (Figure 37-4). Use of these reverse-curve catheters require re-forming of the catheter in the aortic arch and can increase the risk of embolization from aortic arch disease, and thus should be used cautiously. On cannulation of the innominate with a catheter and 0.035-inch guidewire, the catheter is advanced over the wire beyond the lesion and into the subclavian or external carotid artery. The guidewire is then exchanged for a supportive 0.035-inch exchange wire, such as a Stiff Shaft Angled Glidewire (Terumo

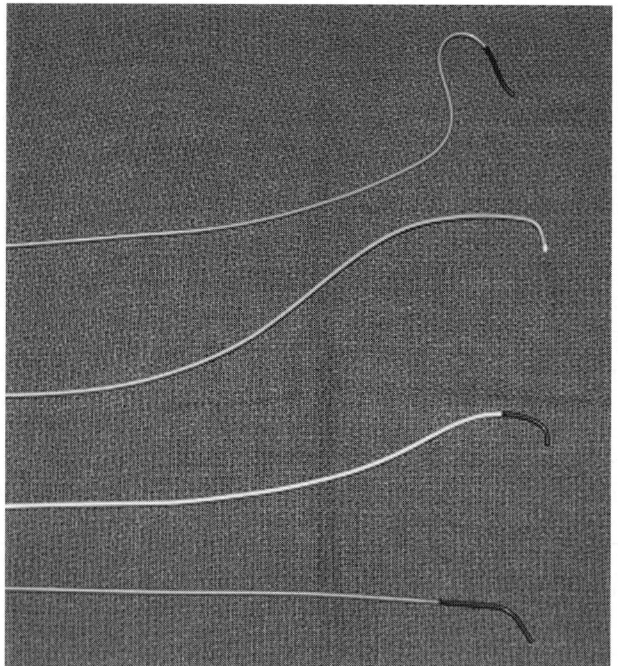

FIGURE 37-4 Most supra-aortic trunks can be catheterized with single-angled catheters such as a vertebral catheter *(bottom)*. Type III arch anatomy or bovine-variant of the left common carotid may require catheters with greater curvature, such as the JR2 or JR3 *(middle)* or a reverse-curve catheter, such as the Vitek *(top)*.

Somerset, NJ) or a Stiff Amplatz (AngioDynamics) to position a long (90 cm) 6F sheath (Shuttle select or Raabe; Cook Medical) into the origin of the innominate, or just beyond the lesion if difficulty crossing the lesion with a stent is anticipated. This sheath is then used for subsequent angiography and support for positioning of a stent. Although self-expanding nitinol stents can be used, premounted balloon-expandable stents are generally preferred in the innominate because of their increased radial force and accuracy in deployment even over short treatment lengths. Positioning of the stent is performed and confirmed by angiography; then the sheath is retracted if necessary to allow for deployment

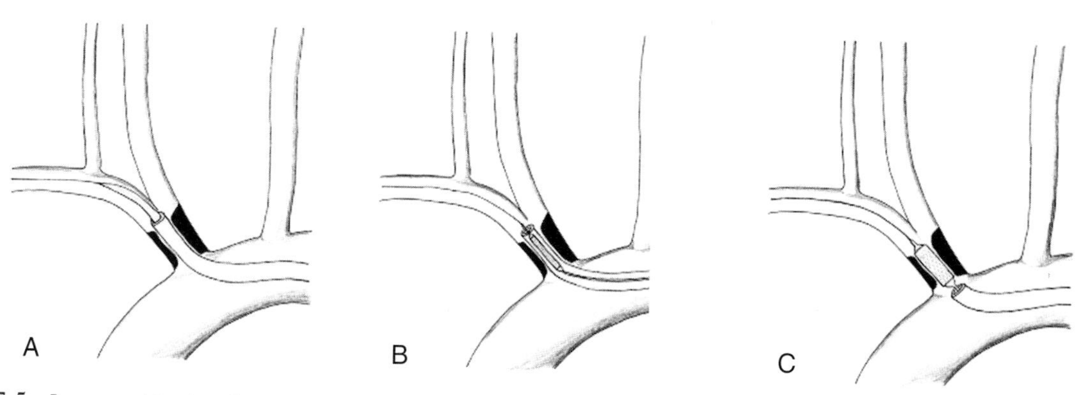

FIGURE 37-5 In cases of total occlusions or high-grade stenoses, positioning of the stent can be facilitated by first passing the sheath and dilator complex beyond the lesion **(A)**, followed by positioning the stent within the sheath **(B)** before retracting the sheath to allow for balloon expansion and stent placement **(C)**.

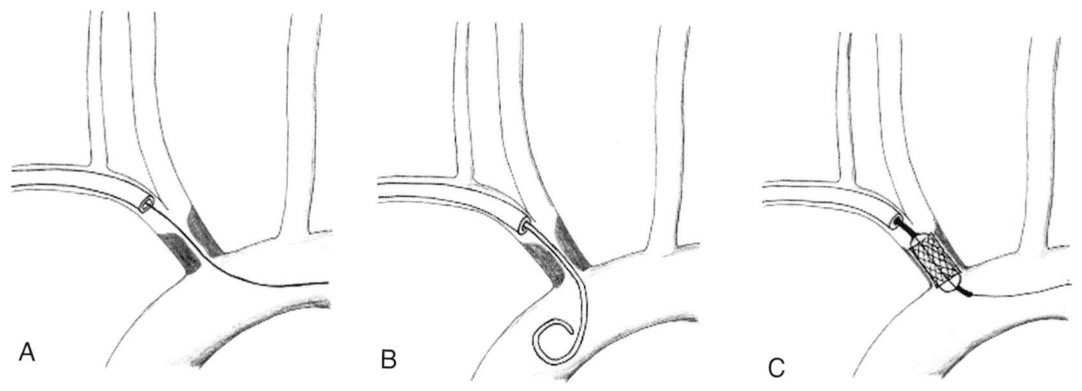

FIGURE 37-6 **A,** Technique for retrograde recanalization of an occluded innominate through a brachial approach includes placement of the sheath in close proximity to the occlusion to provide support for lesion crossing with a 0.035-inch guidewire. **B,** Once the lesion has been crossed, the catheter is exchanged for a pigtail catheter to perform angiography for the purpose of confirming intraluminal location and to delineate the extent of the lesion. **C,** Finally, the lesion is stented with a balloon-expandable stainless steel stent, which offers precise placement and excellent radial force.

(Figure 37-5). Because most innominate lesions occur at or close to the origin, the stent is often deployed with an overlap into the aorta of 1 to 2 mm. Stents for the innominate artery typically range from 8 to 12 mm in diameter and 2 to 3 cm in length.

Complete occlusions of the innominate artery, especially those that occur flush with the aorta, can be difficult to treat from an antegrade femoral approach and may be best approached from a retrograde ipsilateral brachial access. Brachial access can be obtained by either a brachial cutdown with proximal and distal control through a small incision near the antecubital fossa or through percutaneous brachial access. Although percutaneous brachial access has been associated with higher complication rates than femoral access,[17] several steps can be taken to reduce the risk of access site complications. Percutaneous access of the brachial artery should be performed directly over the medial epicondyle of the humerus to allow for effective manual compression against this bony prominence after sheath removal. The artery can be cannulated initially with a 4F micropuncture sheath under duplex guidance to ensure accurate sheath placement. This sheath is then exchanged over a stiff glide wire for a 25-cm 6F sheath that can be advanced such that the tip of the sheath is positioned in the proximal subclavian artery close to the occlusion. Positioning of the sheath in this fashion allows for considerable support when attempting to cross chronic occlusions (Figure 37-6, *A*), which can usually be achieved with the use of a stiff glide wire and an angled glide catheter or a more supportive catheter such as a Quick Cross catheter (Spectranetics, Colorado Springs, CO). Calcification around the origin of the innominate is often visible on fluoroscopy and can be used as a landmark to identify the aortic reentry point. Once reentry into the aortic arch is suspected, the wire is removed to assess for back-bleeding and allow for confirmatory angiography through the catheter (see Figure 37-6, *B*). When reentry has been confirmed, an appropriately sized balloon-expandable stent is brought into position and deployed (see Figure 37-6, *C*). For high-grade stenosis or total occlusions, crossing of the lesion with the stent can be aided by first advancing the sheath and dilator over the wire and beyond the lesion, then positioning the stent, followed by retraction of the sheath before stent deployment. Alternatively, predilation with a smaller balloon can be used before stent placement, and this technique can aid in vessel sizing as well.

Although most innominate lesions can be crossed and treated by either percutaneous femoral or brachial access, these approaches do not lend themselves well to the use of embolic protection techniques. Although deployment of embolic protection devices into the internal carotid artery is theoretically possible through a femoral approach, innominate lesions do not allow enough purchase beyond the aorta for the sheath to be left securely in position without a supportive guidewire stabilizing the system. Current embolic protection devices used in carotid bifurcation angioplasty and stenting are based on 0.014-inch platforms and do not provide sufficient support for a sheath positioned 1 to 2 cm into the innominate artery origin, nor are they sufficiently large to fit the common carotid artery in most cases. For those patients in whom there is a heightened risk of embolic complications (e.g., heavily diseased aortic arch, severe lesion calcification), a safer approach to endovascular treatment of an innominate lesion may by retrograde access through open surgical exposure of the common carotid artery in which the artery can be clamped distally to prevent cerebral embolization. This approach can also be used in conjunction with a standard carotid endarterectomy to simultaneously treat carotid bifurcation disease when present. The procedure is performed under electroencephalographic monitoring and begins with a short longitudinal incision made along the medial border of the sternocleidomastoid muscle to allow exposure of the common carotid artery. After the carotid is circumferentially dissected and ensnared with vessel loops, the patient is systemically heparinized, and an 18-gauge access needle is inserted retrograde into the common carotid artery. A short 6F sheath is placed over a wire into the proximal common carotid artery, and angiography is performed to delineate the extent of the lesion. A clamp is applied to the distal common carotid artery, and lesion crossing is performed in a similar manner as described for a retrograde brachial approach. After lesion crossing, a balloon-expandable stent is positioned so that the stent extends 1 to 2 mm into the aorta and spans the length of the lesion. After deployment, the delivery system is exchanged over the wire for a flush catheter that is positioned into the aorta and used for completion angiography. At this point, the sheath is removed as a clamp is applied to the common carotid proximal to the puncture site, and a Potts scissors is used to open the puncture site 1 to 2 mm as a transverse arteriotomy. This allows prograde and retrograde back-bleeding and flushing of the artery to wash out any embolic debris. The arteriotomy is then closed with several interrupted 6-0 Prolene sutures. Meticulous hemostasis must be ensured because these patients are given antiplatelet therapy with clopidogrel before surgery, although the risk of hematoma is not high with the limited incision and dissection that are necessary for exposing such a short segment of carotid artery required for this technique.

Embolic Sequelae During Innominate Intervention

Innominate interventions have the potential to produce embolic events as a result of showering particulate matter released during the procedure to either the upper extremity or the posterior or anterior cerebral circulation. Currently available embolic protection systems are generally not feasible for use during innominate interventions from either a transfemoral or transbrachial approach. Despite this fact, the results from published data regarding innominate angioplasty and stenting without embolic protection suggest that the risk of neurologic adverse events is actually quite low. Most studies combine the outcomes for subclavian and innominate artery stenting and thus prevent separate analysis of the innominate interventions; however, overall stroke rates in this aggregate group of patients are quite low, ranging from 0% to 2.1%.[2-4,11,16] The largest published series of percutaneous innominate interventions is a report from Hungary that included primary angioplasty of 89 innominate lesions over a 19-year period from a single institution.[11] This included intervention on 84 stenoses and 5 occlusions. The majority of patients were treated with a transfemoral approach (97%), and embolic protection devices or occlusion balloon maneuvers were not used in any patients. Only one stroke occurred (2%) from an occipital lobe infarction. There were four TIAs (6%), which resolved completely, and two access site complications (3%).

The low rate of neurologic events may be partially attributable to the reversal of flow that is present in the cerebral circulation in many patients with innominate occlusions or high-grade stenoses. Regardless of the apparent low risk, caution should always be exercised when performing interventions in the innominate artery because of the potentially devastating consequences of cerebral embolization. Patients who are considered to be at high risk for embolic events include those with such factors as severe lesion calcification or ulceration, a heavily diseased aortic arch, and antegrade right vertebral flow. These patients may be best served by performing the procedure via a retrograde technique in

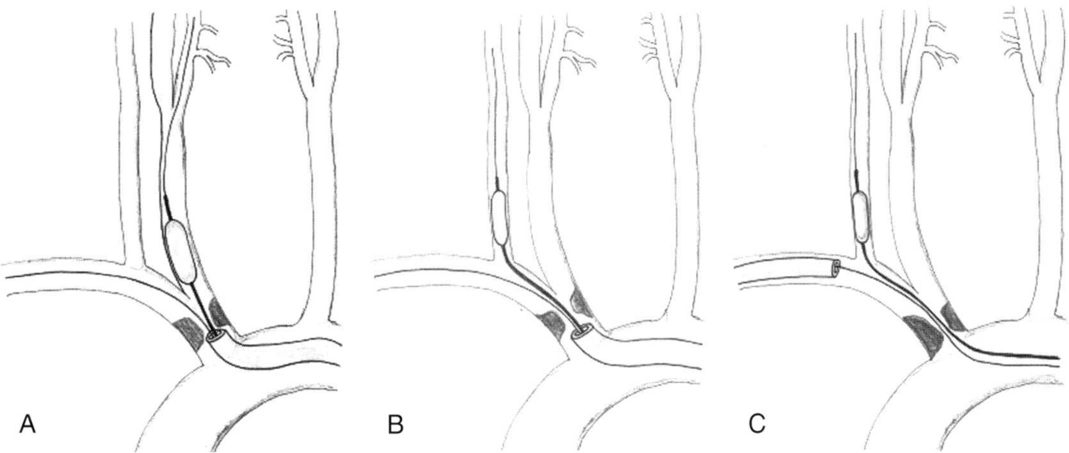

FIGURE 37-7 Currently available embolic protection systems are based on 0.014-inch platforms and do not generally provide sufficient support for intervention on the innominate artery. Alternative strategies for cerebral protection include the use of buddy wires to maintain access to or occlusion balloons to prevent flow through the common carotid **(A)** or vertebral **(B, C)** arteries.

TABLE 37-1 Complication Rates in Percutaneous Innominate and Subclavian Interventions

Study	No. of cases	All complications, No. (%)	TIA, No. (%)	Stroke, No. (%)	Death, No. (%)
Hüttl et al. (2002)[11]	89 innominate	7 (7.8)	4 (4.4)	1 (1.1)	0 (0)
Brountzos et al. (2004)[16]	10 innominate 39 subclavian	4 (8.3)	1 (2.1)	0 (0)	0 (0)
Woo et al. (2006)[4]	4 innominate 23 subclavian	0 (0)	0 (0)	0 (0)	0 (0)
Przewlocki et al. (2006)[3]	2 innominate 72 subclavian	7 (9.3)	0 (0)	0 (0)	0 (0)
Patel et al. (2008)[2]	11 innominate 166 subclavian	10 (5.9)	—	1 (0.6)	0 (0)

TIA, Transient ischemic attack.

TABLE 37-2 Patency Outcomes After Innominate and Subclavian Interventions

Study	Technical success rate (%)	Primary patency (%)	Secondary patency (%)	Mean follow-up (mo)
Hüttl et al. (2002)[11]	96.6	95 (at 33 mo)	98 (at 12 mo)	33.0
Brountzos et al. (2004)[16]	96.0	77 (at 24 mo)	92 (at 24 mo)	16.7
Przewlocki et al. (2006)[3]	93.3	77 (at 60 mo)	95 (at 36 mo)	24.4
Patel et al. (2008)[2]	98.3	83 (at 66 mo)	96 (at 54 mo)	35.2

conjunction with surgical exposure of the common carotid artery to enable distal control of the cerebral circulation and flushing of the carotid artery.

In addition to patient selection, other maneuvers that may be helpful in preventing cerebral embolization during angioplasty and stenting include primary stenting of the lesion without predilatation and manual external compression of the carotid artery during balloon angioplasty and stent deployment. More complex maneuvers include placement of a 0.014-inch buddy wire into the vertebral or internal carotid arteries to maintain access to these vessels in case of dissection or embolization

(Figure 37-7, *A*). Use of an occlusion balloon (2-3 mm in diameter) over this buddy wire and positioned at the origin of these vessels can further protect from embolization to the cerebral circulation (see Figure 37-7, *B*), but care must be taken to prevent dissection or intimal injury from oversized balloons. Finally, the use of adequate anticoagulation with intraoperative heparin administration, as well as preoperative antiplatelet therapy with aspirin and clopidogrel, is routine in these procedures to decrease the risk of thrombosis and minimize the neurologic sequelae from any microembolization that may occur.

Outcome After Innominate Intervention

There are no published reports comparing open surgical revascularization of lesions of the supra-aortic trunks with endovascular treatment in a prospective randomized fashion. Therefore outcomes after these procedures and comparisons between these two modalities must be determined from retrospective series. Although few publications have separately reported outcomes after revascularization of specific supra-aortic arch vessels, multiple retrospective studies have documented outcomes after open surgical reconstruction on these vessels as a group (Tables 37-1 and 37-2).[3,5,17] Direct surgical revascularization has been shown in these studies to be a durable and effective therapy, providing early symptom relief in approximately 95% of patients, with long-term relief of symptoms in 85% to 90%. These excellent outcomes, however, may come with significant morbidity and mortality, because stroke rates range from 0% to 8% and mortality ranges from 0% to 14.7% in these studies. A relatively recent publication by Berguer et al.[9] described 100 consecutive innominate and common carotid revascularizations in 98 patients over a 16-year period by either endarterectomy (n = 8) or transthoracic bypass (n = 92). This study demonstrated excellent primary patency rates of 98% and 88% at 5 and 10 years, respectively. However, there were eight strokes and eight deaths, for a combined stroke and death rate of 16%.

The potential for high complication rates in patients undergoing direct transthoracic revascularization of supra-aortic trunk lesions prompted the use of extra-anatomic bypasses (including axillary-axillary, carotid-subclavian, carotid-carotid) in many centers. There have been several retrospective single-center comparisons between these bypass and endovascular interventions for supra-aortic trunk occlusive disease, including a publication by Modarai et al.[14] This group retrospectively compared 35 extra-anatomic bypass procedures with 33 endovascular interventions (angioplasty without stenting) for lesions of the innominate, subclavian, and carotid arteries over a 20-year period. Similar complication rates were observed between the two groups whereas patency rates were higher in the surgical group (94% primary patency in surgical group at 5 years mean follow-up compared with 82% primary patency in endovascular group at 4 years), leading the authors to conclude that surgical revascularization with extra-anatomic bypass is superior to angioplasty for supra-aortic trunk disease. However, multiple other single-center retrospective reports have detailed quite acceptable outcomes for endovascular interventions, oftentimes citing results superior to those reported with extra-anatomic bypass.

Motarjeme[18] described 151 interventions (in 112 patients) on lesions of the innominate, vertebral, subclavian, and carotid arteries through a femoral approach with use of selective stenting over a 5-year period. Overall technical success rate was 93%. There was a single stroke (0.9%), and there were only five reocclusions over the 5-year study period. Patel et al.[2] reported their results with 177 lesions in 170 patients, including 166 subclavian lesions and 11 innominate lesions. Though the innominate lesions were not detailed separately, the overall outcomes were excellent. Procedures were performed with primary stenting through a femoral approach in the majority (86%) of cases, with a technical success rate of 98.3%. There were no deaths, and there was one stroke (0.6%). Primary and secondary patency rates were 83% and 96%, respectively, at a mean follow-up of 35 months. Hüttl et al.[11] reported the largest series of percutaneous interventions for isolated innominate lesions, including 89 lesions treated over a 19-year period at a single center in Hungary. These lesions included 84 stenoses and 5 occlusions, and all procedures were performed from the femoral approach with angioplasty alone. Mean follow-up was 33 months. Primary and secondary patency at 12 months was 93% and 98%, respectively, with only one stroke (1.1%) and four periprocedural TIAs (4.4%).

Direct surgical revascularization with endarterectomy or bypass through a transthoracic approach will likely remain the gold standard for a durable repair of these lesions in younger patients who can tolerate such an operation. However, the results described previously suggest that percutaneous intervention is an acceptable alternative to direct surgical reconstruction, especially in elderly patients or those with other significant comorbidities, and may ultimately replace both extra-anatomic bypass and direct transthoracic reconstruction as interventional techniques improve and long-term outcomes are better substantiated.

COMMON CAROTID ARTERY

The vast majority of extra-cranial carotid stenoses occur at the carotid bifurcation, and surgical and endovascular treatment of the carotid bifurcation has been well established by randomized trials supporting the use of endarterectomy and carotid bifurcation angioplasty and stenting in various patient subsets.[19,20] In contrast, lesions of the origin or proximal common carotid occur in fewer than 2% of patients with extracranial carotid disease,[1] and therefore data regarding percutaneous treatment of these lesions are scarce. Furthermore, the proximal location of these lesions within the course of the carotid artery leads to the same access issues as with innominate stenting with equivalent or perhaps higher risks in terms of cerebral embolization.

Clinical Presentation and Diagnostic Evaluation

Lesions of the common carotid artery present in an identical fashion as those of the carotid bifurcation. Patients may demonstrate TIAs or stroke or have no symptoms. Physical examination may reveal diminished or absent carotid pulses and a carotid bruit. Carotid duplex ultrasound can document degree of stenosis for extrathoracic lesions and determine flow directionality of the internal and common carotid artery, but lesions of the common carotid origin are often better imaged with computed tomographic angiography, magnetic resonance angiography, or conventional contrast angiography.

Although the natural history of common carotid lesions is less well characterized than those of the bifurcation, stenoses of greater than 70% in patients with symptoms and greater than 80% in patients without symptoms are generally thought to warrant treatment. Unlike patients with stenoses, patients without symptoms with common carotid occlusions are often observed without surgical or percutaneous intervention.

Endovascular Treatment of Common Carotid Disease

The two primary approaches to endoluminal therapy for common carotid disease include (1) retrograde approach through surgical exposure of the carotid artery and (2) antegrade transfemoral approach. As with innominate disease, selecting between these two approaches is determined by the location and severity of the occlusive lesions, the presence of concomitant disease in other arch vessels, and the perceived risk of cerebral emboli based on factors such as lesion type and arch anatomy.

Because common carotid disease often occurs in conjunction with bifurcation disease, the retrograde surgical access through a neck incision is a reasonable approach in selected patients because it allows for surgical treatment of the carotid bifurcation by an endarterectomy followed by retrograde angioplasty and stenting of common carotid disease. This may also be a favored approach in patients with high-grade lesions at the immediate origin of the common carotid in whom supportive sheath placement would be difficult or impossible. For this approach, a standard neck incision along the anterior border of the sternocleidomastoid muscle is made, and the procedure is begun with a carotid endarterectomy. Before completing the patch angioplasty, a 6F sheath is inserted under direct visualization in a retrograde orientation into the common carotid, and hemostatic control is achieved proximally by tightening a vessel loop around the sheath within the proximal common carotid. Through this sheath, retrograde recanalization and angioplasty/stenting is performed in a manner described earlier for lesions of the innominate artery. For left common carotid orificial lesions, a small overlap of the stent of 1 to 2 mm into the aorta is preferred. Although lesions of the mid-common carotid can be treated effectively with self-expanding nitinol stents, orificial lesions may be best treated with the more precise deployment of a stainless steel balloon-expandable stent. After stent placement, the sheath can be removed to allow flushing of debris from the artery before arteriotomy closure. With this approach, the larger incision and risk for neck hematoma make dual antiplatelet therapy before surgery less desirable, and therefore a safer alternative may be preoperative single antiplatelet therapy with aspirin, following by initiation of dual antiplatelet therapy with aspirin and clopidogrel in the postoperative period.

Patients whose common carotid stenoses are located in close proximity to the carotid bifurcation can be treated through a transfemoral access with embolic protection as is now routinely done for high-risk patients with symptomatic carotid bifurcation disease. This option becomes less feasible, however, with decreasing length or increasing tortuosity of the common carotid proximal to the first lesion. With a short or tortuous common carotid artery, sheath placement becomes less stable, and one risks losing sheath access to the carotid during the procedure. If sheath stability is a concern during treatment of tandem common and internal lesions, it may be more prudent to treat the internal carotid lesion first using embolic protection in the standard fashion, then remove the protection device and replace it with a 0.035-inch exchange wire (Stiff Shaft Angled Glidewire) positioned in the external carotid to support the sheath as it is withdrawn proximal to the common carotid lesion (Figure 37-8). The common lesion can then be treated in an unprotected fashion. Isolated lesions of the common carotid can also be treated with this technique, with consideration for the use of embolic protection positioned in the internal carotid artery based on the stability of the sheath within the proximal carotid.

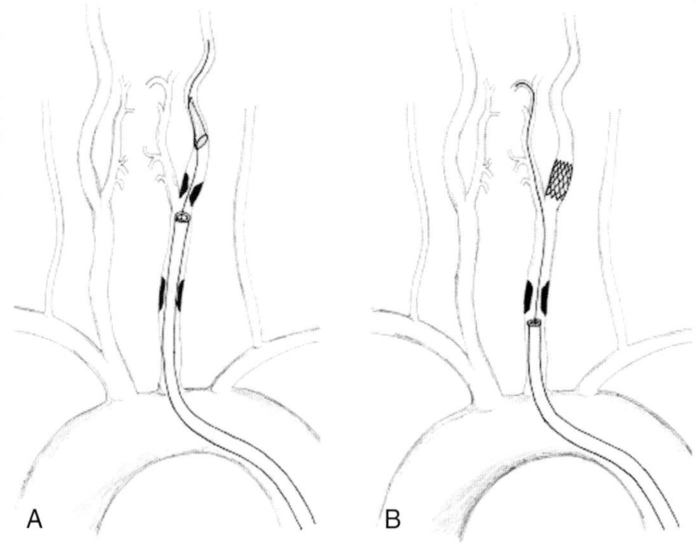

FIGURE 37-8 Tandem lesions of the common carotid and carotid bifurcation can be approached from the transfemoral route if arch anatomy is sufficiently favorable to allow stable placement. The bifurcation lesion can be treated by using embolic protection in the standard fashion **(A)**, followed by partially withdrawing the sheath to address the common carotid lesion. If sheath stability is of concern because of arch anatomy or a proximal lesion, it may be safer to remove the embolic protection device and perform the treatment of the common carotid lesion unprotected with a stabilizing guidewire in the external carotid **(B)** rather than risking the loss of sheath access with a fully deployed embolic protection device in the internal carotid.

Outcomes After Common Carotid Angioplasty and Stenting

There are few data regarding the outcome of common carotid endovascular interventions. Most reports are small retrospective series, and the majority report on the technique of surgical exposure of the carotid followed by retrograde endovascular treatment. The largest series of retrograde angioplasty procedures of the carotid was published in 2004 by Allie et al.[21] and included 23 patients who underwent stenting of the common carotid in conjunction with a carotid endarterectomy. The authors performed the angioplasty and stenting with an 8F sheath inserted into the common carotid before endarterectomy was performed, using predilation of the lesion followed by balloon-expandable stenting. Procedural success was 97%, mean follow-up was 34 months, and restenosis rate at 2 years was 8.7%. There are only two reports detailing the use of transfemoral stenting of the common carotid artery in the literature.[22,23] Chio et al.[22] reported the outcome of 42 proximal and orificial common carotid angioplasty and stenting procedures in 37 patients. Procedural success was 95%, and complications included two minor strokes (4.7%), no major strokes, and no periprocedural deaths. At 24 months mean follow-up, restenosis rate was only 5.1%. The largest series comes from Paukovits et al.[23] and details their results with percutaneous treatment of 153 proximal common carotid lesions in 147 patients over a 12-year period. All but one patient was treated through a femoral approach, and a single patient was treated by an axillary approach. The majority of patients were treated with stent placement after predilation (70.5%), generally over a 0.035-inch guidewire system. Embolic protection was used in 16 patients, 13 of which were done because of simultaneous treatment of a carotid bifurcation lesion. Technical success rate was 98.7%, and periprocedural neurologic complications included three (2.0%) ipsilateral major strokes and four (2.6%) TIAs. Nonneurologic complication rate was 6.4% and included primarily access site hematomas. There were no deaths. One-year and 4-year primary patency was 97.9% and 82.0%, respectively, whereas secondary patency at the same intervals was 100% and 88%, respectively. Although further supportive data with longer follow-up are required to be able to fully compare these procedures with direct surgical revascularization, these results are certainly encouraging and support the use of angioplasty and stenting of the proximal carotid artery in selected patients.

References

1. Wiley EF, Effeney DJ: Surgery of the aortic arch branches and vertebral arteries, *Surg Clin North Am* 59:669–680, 1979.
2. Patel SN, White CJ, Collins TJ, et al: Catheter-based treatment of the subclavian and innominate arteries, *Catheter Cardiovasc Interv* 71(7):963–968, 2008.
3. Przewlocki T, Kablak-Ziembicka A, Pieniazek P, et al: Determinants of immediate and long-term results of subclavian and innominate artery angioplasty, *Catheter Cardiovasc Interv* 67 (4):519–526, 2006.
4. Woo EY, Fairman RM, Velazquez OC, et al: Endovascular therapy of symptomatic innominate-subclavian arterial occlusive lesions, *Vasc Endovascular Surg* 40(1):27–33, 2006.
5. Carlson RE, Ehrenfeld WK, Stoney RJ, et al: Innominate artery endarterectomy: a 16-year experience, *Arch Surg* 112(11): 1389–1393, 1977.
6. Evans WE, Williams TE, Hayes JP: Aortobrachiocephalic reconstruction, *Am J Surg* 156(2):100–102, 1988.

7. Reul GJ, Jacobs MJ, Gregoric ID, et al: Innominate artery occlusive disease: surgical approach and long-term results, *J Vasc Surg* 14(3):405–412, 1991.
8. Kieffer E, Sabatier J, Koskas F, et al: Atherosclerotic innominate artery occlusive disease: early and long-term results of surgical reconstruction, *J Vasc Surg* 21(2):326–336, 1995.
9. Berguer R, Morasch MD, Kline RA: Transthoracic repair of innominate and common carotid artery disease: immediate and long-term outcome for 100 consecutive surgical reconstructions, *J Vasc Surg* 27(1):34–41, 1998.
10. Cherry KJ Jr, McCullough JL, Hallett JW Jr, et al: Technical principles of direct innominate artery revascularization: a comparison of endarterectomy and bypass grafts, *J Vasc Surg* 9(5): 718–723, 1989.
11. Hüttl K, Nemes B, Simonffy A, et al: Angioplasty of the innominate artery in 89 patients: experience over 19 years, *Cardiovasc Intervent Radiol* 25(2):109–114, 2002.
12. Zaytsev AY, Stoyda AY, Smirnov VE, et al: Endovascular treatment of supra-aortic extracranial stenoses in patients with vertebrobasilar insufficiency symptoms, *Cardiovasc Intervent Radiol* 29(5):731–738, 2006.
13. Payne DA, Hayes PD, Bolia A, et al: Cerebral protection during open retrograde angioplasty/stenting of common carotid and innominate artery stenoses, *Br J Surg* 93(2):187–190, 2006.
14. Modarai B, Ali T, Dourado R, et al: Comparison of extra-anatomic bypass grafting with angioplasty for atherosclerotic disease of the supra-aortic trunks, *Br J Surg* 91(11):1453–1457, 2004.
15. Ouriel K, May AG, Ricotta JJ, et al: Carotid endarterectomy for nonhemispheric symptoms: predictors of success, *J Vasc Surg* 1(2):339–345, 1984.
16. Brountzos EN, Petersen B, Binkert C, et al: Primary stenting of subclavian and innominate artery occlusive disease: a single center's experience, *Cardiovasc Intervent Radiol* 27(6):616–623, 2004.
17. Dorros G, Lewin RF, Jamnadas P, et al: Peripheral transluminal angioplasty of the subclavian and innominate arteries utilizing the brachial approach: acute outcome and follow-up, *Catheter Cardiovasc Diagn* 19(2):71–76, 1990 Feb.
18. Motarjeme A: Percutaneous transluminal angioplasty of supra-aortic vessels, *J Endovasc Surg* 3(2):171–181, 1996.
19. North American Symptomatic Carotid Endarterectomy Trial (NASCET) investigators: Clinical alert: benefit of carotid endarterectomy for patients with high-grade stenosis of the internal carotid artery, *Stroke* 22:816–817, 1991.
20. Gurm HS, Yadav JS, Fayad P, et al: SAPPHIRE Investigators. Long-term results of carotid stenting versus endarterectomy in high-risk patients, *N Engl J Med* 358(15):1572–1579, 2008.
21. Allie DE, Hebert CJ, Lirtzman MD, Wyatt CH, Khan MH, Khan MA, Fail PS, Chaisson GA, Keller VA, Vitrella DA, Allie SD, Allie AA, Mitran EV, Walker CM: Intraoperative innominate and common carotid intervention combined with carotid endarterectomy: a "true" endovascular surgical approach, *J Endovasc Ther* 11(3):258–262, 2004.
22. Chio FL Jr, Liu MW, Khan MA, et al: Effectiveness of elective stenting of common carotid artery lesions in preventing stroke, *Am J Cardiol* 92(9):1135–1137, 2003.
23. Paukovits TM, Haász J, Molnár A, et al: Transfemoral endovascular treatment of proximal common carotid artery lesions: a single-center experience on 153 lesions, *J Vasc Surg* 48(1):80–87, 2008.

CHAPTER

38

Carotid Bifurcation Stented Balloon Angioplasty With Cerebral Protection

Karthikeshwar Kasirajan, Peter A. Schneider

The purpose of this chapter is to describe the technique of carotid stent placement with embolic protection, provide current results of treatment, and offer an assessment of the overall role of carotid stenting in the management of carotid occlusive disease. Carotid angioplasty and stenting (CAS) is being evaluated as an alternative to carotid endarterectomy (CEA) for patients in need of mechanical repair of a clinically significant carotid artery stenosis. The technical challenges, the risk of cerebral embolization during CAS, and the current regulatory environment have tempered the use of CAS. Several carotid stent systems are approved for use in the United States for patients at high risk for CEA. These high-risk criteria are listed in Table 38-1. As data accumulate from CAS trials, the best role for CAS in the management of carotid bifurcation stenosis will be determined.

TECHNIQUE: CAROTID ANGIOPLASTY AND STENTING WITH DISTAL PROTECTION

The CAS procedure comprises the following steps: preprocedural evaluation, femoral access, aortic arch angiogram, selective common carotid cannulation and angiogram, carotid sheath access, crossing the carotid stenosis, filter placement, predilatation, stenting, postdilatation, completion angiogram, access site management, and postoperative care and follow-up. More detail is available regarding the technique of CAS.[1]

Preprocedural Evaluation

Patients are seen by a neurologist, and a National Institutes of Health Stroke Scale or other objective evaluation is completed before CAS. A computed tomographic (CT) scan or magnetic resonance (MR) imaging of the brain is obtained in patients with symptoms and in those older than 80 years of age to evaluate for preprocedural cerebral pathology. Initial duplex ultrasonographic evaluation is performed. Approved carotid stenting systems are limited to use in patients with symptomatic $\geq$50% stenosis or asymptomatic $\geq$80% stenosis. Patients are given antiplatelet therapy: aspirin daily and clopidogrel (Plavix) 75 mg per day for 5 days before the procedure. In all cases, patients should have received clopidogrel (total dose 300 mg) before the intervention. Patients are asked to discontinue antihypertensive medication on the day of the stent procedure, and these patients are best treated as the first case of the day (to avoid prolonged dehydration). Postoperative hypotension and/or bradycardia is more likely in patients with underlying cardiac disease. In patients with absent femoral pulses because of aortoiliac occlusion, a transbrachial approach may be considered. This approach is more challenging compared with the transfemoral approach, with need for a larger selection of reversed-angle catheters. The brachiocephalic anatomy should be studied before the procedure to assess candidacy for this approach. CAS in standard-risk patients and those at high risk for CEA but who have no symptoms are not currently approved for reimbursement under Medicare guidelines.

The procedure is performed with the patient under local anesthesia with minimal or no sedation to facilitate patient cooperation and continuous neurologic monitoring. An arterial line is placed for continuous blood pressure monitoring and electrocardiographic leads for cardiac monitoring. External pacer pads should be readily available. Patients with severe aortic stenosis undergo placement of a temporary venous pacemaker. Patients should have a detailed explanation of the need for continuous neurologic monitoring. Techniques such as squeezing a rubber toy aid in simple and effective neurologic monitoring during the procedure. Because of the minimal use of sedation, patients are often apprehensive and may have reactive systemic hypertension. Therefore it is important to document the patient's baseline blood pressure during the prior clinic visit. We avoid acutely reducing the blood pressure during the intervention with pharmacologic agents, because poststent hypotension/bradycardia is not uncommon. If an antihypertensive is required, it is best to use a short-acting agent. It is best to have a thorough understanding of the arch, carotid, and cerebral arterial anatomy before the procedure. This may be obtained by arteriogram or by CT angiography or MR angiography. This permits proper patient selection and procedural planning. Several anatomic factors may be considered relative contraindications to CAS, including severe arch atherosclerosis or tortuosity, diffuse common carotid artery (CCA) disease or tortuosity, severe angulation of the bifurcation, or kinking of the distal internal carotid artery (ICA).

Femoral Access

The right common femoral approach is the most convenient for catheter manipulations by the right-handed surgeon. A micropuncture set (21-gauge needle) may be used for the initial femoral access; this has significantly reduced the number of femoral access complications. After guidewire access an introducer sheath is placed in the common femoral artery that is the same size as that intended for the carotid stent placement.

Aortic Arch Angiogram

Arch manipulations with guidewires, catheters, and sheaths carry a risk of neurologic events. In several studies of CAS, especially early on in the experience, up to 1% of patients sustained a stroke in the contralateral hemisphere, suggesting that carotid access may be a contributor to morbidity.[2,3] Greater selectivity in patient selection has helped to improve this. It is also the authors' practice to administer systemic heparin before any aortic arch manipulation. A 260-cm angled Glidewire (Terumo, Somerset, NJ) is placed in the ascending aorta followed by a pigtail catheter. An initial arch angiogram is performed with the image intensifier in a left anterior oblique (LAO) position. The origins of the arch vessels are better exposed in this oblique projection. The pigtail catheter is subsequently withdrawn over a 260-cm angled Glidewire. Resist attempts to leave the Glidewire in place if inadvertent selective cannulation of the CCA is achieved while withdrawing the pigtail catheter from the aortic arch. It is almost impossible to withdraw the pigtail catheter from the aortic arch while maintaining Glidewire access in the CCA. As few manipulations are carried out in the aortic arch and great vessels as possible in hopes of lowering the risk of an embolic event.

Hypertension and advanced age are associated with increased tortuosity of the aortic arch. This makes no difference in the performance of CEA but directly influences the challenges posed for CAS. Negotiating the tortuous arch requires more manipulation for catheterization, a more embedded position of the exchange guidewire, and more maneuvers to achieve sheath placement. The tortuosity of the arch may be assessed very rapidly by drawing a horizontal line across the apex of the inner curvature of the arch.[4] Vessels that originate below the horizontal line at the apex of the aortic arch often are more difficult to selectively cannulate (Figure 38-1). The authors caution against carotid stenting in the setting of a "difficult arch" until the operator has become expert with selective cannulation of the CCAs in this situation. Training and credentialing

TABLE 38-1 Indications for Carotid Angioplasty and Stenting

General criteria	Anatomic criteria
Unstable angina	Lesions above C2 or lower than C6
MI within 30 days	Tandem carotid lesions requiring treatment
NYHA class 3 or 4 CHF	Restenosis after prior CEA
Multivessel coronary artery disease (nonrevascularizable)	Radical neck dissection or radiation
Left ventricular ejection fraction <30%	Tracheostomy
Cardiac or vascular surgery within 30 days	Bilateral high-grade carotid stenosis
COPD (FEV_1 < 30% of predicted)	Contralateral carotid occlusion
Age >75 yr	Contralateral CEA with cranial nerve injury

CEA, Carotid endarterectomy; *CHF,* congestive heart failure; *COPD,* chronic obstructive pulmonary disease; *FEV_1,* forced expiratory volume in the first second; *MI,* myocardial infarction; *NYHA,* New York Heart Association.

documents suggest varying numbers of carotid arteriograms as a prerequisite to initiating CAS training.[5,6]

Selective Common Carotid Cannulation

Selective cannulation of the arch vessels can be technically challenging and is a critical portion of CAS procedures. Most intent-to-treat failures are secondary to inability to selectively cannulate the CCAs. Catheterization can almost always be accomplished with use of one of two preshaped catheters: a simple curve catheter such as a vertebral catheter or a complex curve catheter such as the reversed-angle Vitek catheter (VTK, Cook Medical, Bloomington, IN). The image intensifier is maintained in its fixed position (LAO), and the bony landmarks may be used to guide vessel cannulation. Road-mapping techniques and simple marks made with a dry-erase pen on the screen may also help guide selective CCA cannulation. The catheter of first choice in most cases is a simple curve catheter such as a vertebral catheter. The angle formed by the vertebral catheter along with the tip angle on an angled Glidewire is adequate to cannulate the CCA in most patients. Once the Glidewire has accessed the CCA, the vertebral catheter is advanced over the Glidewire for selective angiograms of the CCA. Be careful to avoid inadvertently passing the guidewire into the carotid artery bifurcation. As the cerebral catheter rounds the turn from the arch into the CCA, it tends to straighten out and jump forward.

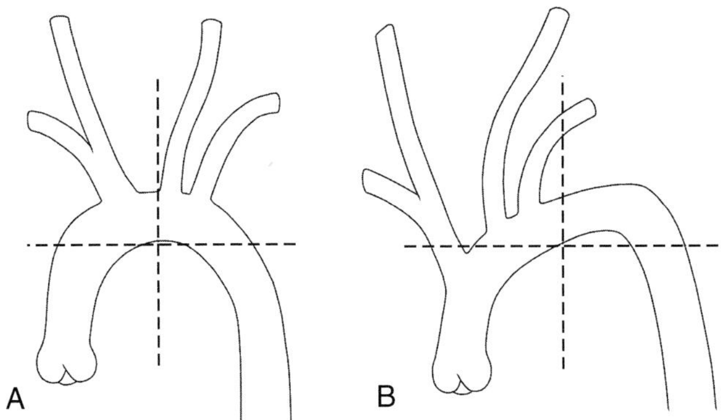

FIGURE 38-1 Arch configuration. **A,** The aortic arch is evaluated with the image intensifier in the left anterior oblique projection to separate the arch branches. A horizontal line is drawn across the apex of the arch on the inner curvature. The uppermost point of the arch acts as a fulcrum over which the catheter must work and the sheath must be placed. **B,** The arch often becomes more tortuous with age and with hypertension. The functional result is to lengthen the arch segment from which the branches arise and put them in a position such that the artery origins are to the right and inferior to the fulcrum. By drawing the horizontal line across the apex of the arch on the inner curve, it is readily apparent that working over the fulcrum will be more challenging. The further inferior to the horizontal line the branch origin is located, the more challenging the access for catheterization and also for sheath placement.

Reversed-angle catheters such as the VTK (Figure 38-2) are usually required when the aortic arch is tortuous or the CCAs are retroflexed toward the patient's left. Complex curve catheters, such as the VTK, are best re-formed in the proximal descending aorta and then pushed proximally, especially for cannulation of the left CCA. The VTK is the catheter of choice for cannulating the difficult arch with branch vessels arising in the ascending aorta. Reversed-angle catheters such as VTK and Simmons

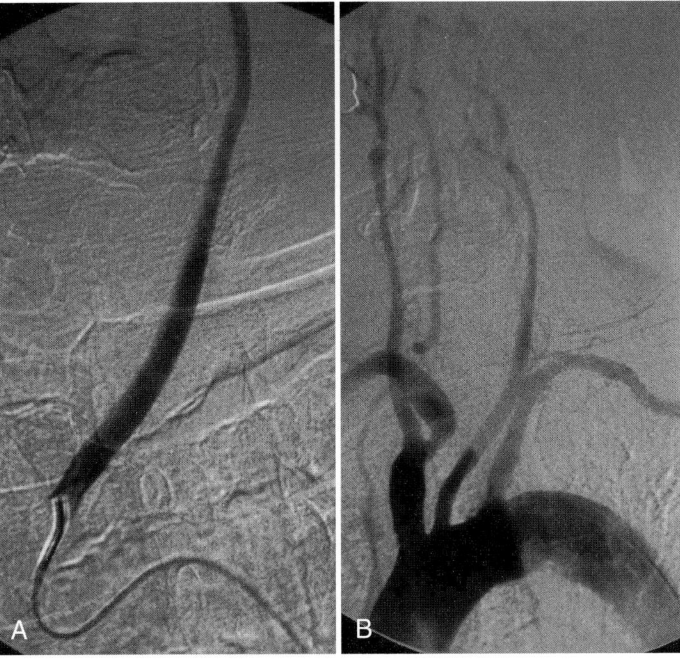

FIGURE 38-2 Complex curve catheter. The Vitek catheter is a complex curve catheter. It has an extra curve that allows the tip to be directed in a reversed fashion. This allows for cannulation of a difficult arch branch origin from a tortuous arch and to work over the fulcrum of the arch. **A,** In this arch configuration, the left CCA is somewhat retroflexed as the artery passes toward the patient's left. **B,** The Vitek catheter is advanced into the arch, and the tip of the catheter is used to cannulate the origin of the left CCA.

cannot be easily advanced into the branch vessels; they are used only to access the origin of the branch vessels for a selective angiogram of the carotid arteries. Because of the reverse angle, forward motion on these catheters will only advance the catheter further proximally in the aortic arch. Catheter access to the CCA after access with the reversed-angle catheter requires a subsequent catheter exchange. This requires the Glidewire to be placed in the CCA and the reversed angle catheter is withdrawn over the guidewire and replaced with the vertebral catheter. If the Glidewire cannot be maintained in the CCA while withdrawing the reversed-angle catheter, selective cannulation of the external carotid may be required with use of road-mapping techniques before catheter withdrawal. Reversed-angle catheters have a tendency to flip the guidewire as they exit the femoral sheath; hence the Glidewire needs to be grasped immediately after the tip of the reversed-angle catheter is seen exiting the femoral sheath.

Once selective cannulation of the CCA is performed, angiograms are performed with a 10-mL syringe filled with half-strength contrast. The carotid bifurcation is best visualized in the ipsilateral oblique position (approximately 60 degrees ipsilateral oblique). Multiple views may be needed to best open the carotid bifurcation, because the next step would involve selective cannulation of the external carotid artery (ECA). If an arteriogram or CT angiogram is performed before the CAS procedure, optimal angles for viewing the open carotid bifurcation can usually be derived from these studies. If a lateral view of the carotid bifurcation is required to open carotid bifurcation and cannulate the ECA, after the exchange guidewire is anchored in place, the sheath is best advanced by using an LAO view.

Lateral and craniocaudal anteroposterior intracranial images are obtained if they have not already been before CAS to identify any intracranial pathology and to document the intracranial circulation before CAS. A certain amount of experience must be gained in interpretation of intracranial images. Identifying small embolic events during or after CAS may be quite challenging.

Carotid Sheath Access

Carotid sheath access requires placement of an adequate length of exchange guidewire into the CCA. This sometimes can be accomplished by placing the tip of the exchange guidewire in the distal CCA but usually requires cannulation of the ECA and use of this vessel to anchor the stiff guidewire (Figure 38-3). Blind guidewire and catheter manipulation in the carotid artery must be avoided. Selective external carotid cannulation can be accomplished with a 260-cm angled Glidewire and the vertebral catheter. In case of a tight external stenosis a 3F catheter with a 0.018-inch wire (Tracker-18; Boston Scientific, Natick, MA) may be used, and the 0.018-inch wire is then exchanged for a stiffer 0.018-inch guidewire (Roadrunner; Cook Medical, Bloomington, IN) and predilated with a low-profile, monorail, 2-mm balloon. The balloon is withdrawn, and a vertebral catheter is passed into the ECA over the Roadrunner guidewire. An attempt should be made to reach as distally on the ECA as is possible. This allows adequate guidewire length for the subsequent placement of the carotid sheath. Passage of the stiff exchange guidewire into the small ECA branches must be done with caution to avoid injury or perforation to these small branches. CAS can usually be accomplished with a 6F or 7F sheath. The Glidewire is then withdrawn from the vertebral catheter and a 260-cm Amplatz (Terumo) super stiff wire is passed into the ECA. It is helpful to administer a little contrast into the catheter to confirm external carotid placement. Contrast injections into the carotid system should not be done unless free backflow of blood is present at the hub of the diagnostic catheter. Otherwise there is a risk of pushing microbubbles into the system. In the ECA, back-bleeding may at times be diminished by the tight fit of the catheter in the small ECA branches. In this event, the cerebral catheter is slowly withdrawn until adequate backflow is noted.

The vertebral catheter is withdrawn, leaving the Amplatz guidewire in the ECA. The groin sheath is removed. A 90-cm–long sheath (Pinnacle Destination or Shuttle Sheath [Terumo]) is advanced over the Amplatz guidewire into the CCA. Image the tip of the Amplatz guidewire in the ECA and the last turn from the arch into the CCA during sheath passage. If the tip of the advancing sheath hangs up at the turn into the CCA or the tip of the guidewire moves back, it indicates that the sheath is not advancing appropriately over the guidewire. Reassess the curvature in the system, and make sure that an adequate length of stiff exchange guidewire is present.

The dilator tip for the 90-cm carotid sheath is long and not well visualized during fluoroscopy. Identify the optimal length for the dilator to protrude from the sheath and to lock the Y-adaptor on the back end of the dilator in this position. After the dilator and sheath are advanced fully into the CCA, if a position closer to the bifurcation is needed, the dilator is held steady while the sheath is advanced over it. The stiff exchange guidewire and the dilator are withdrawn, and the carotid angiogram is repeated through the long 6F or 7F sheath with a road map of the carotid bifurcation stenosis.

Filter Placement and Stenting

This step may be performed with any one of a variety of distal protection devices that are available. The tip of the leading guidewire is hand shaped with a curve to provide directionality for crossing the lesion. Most

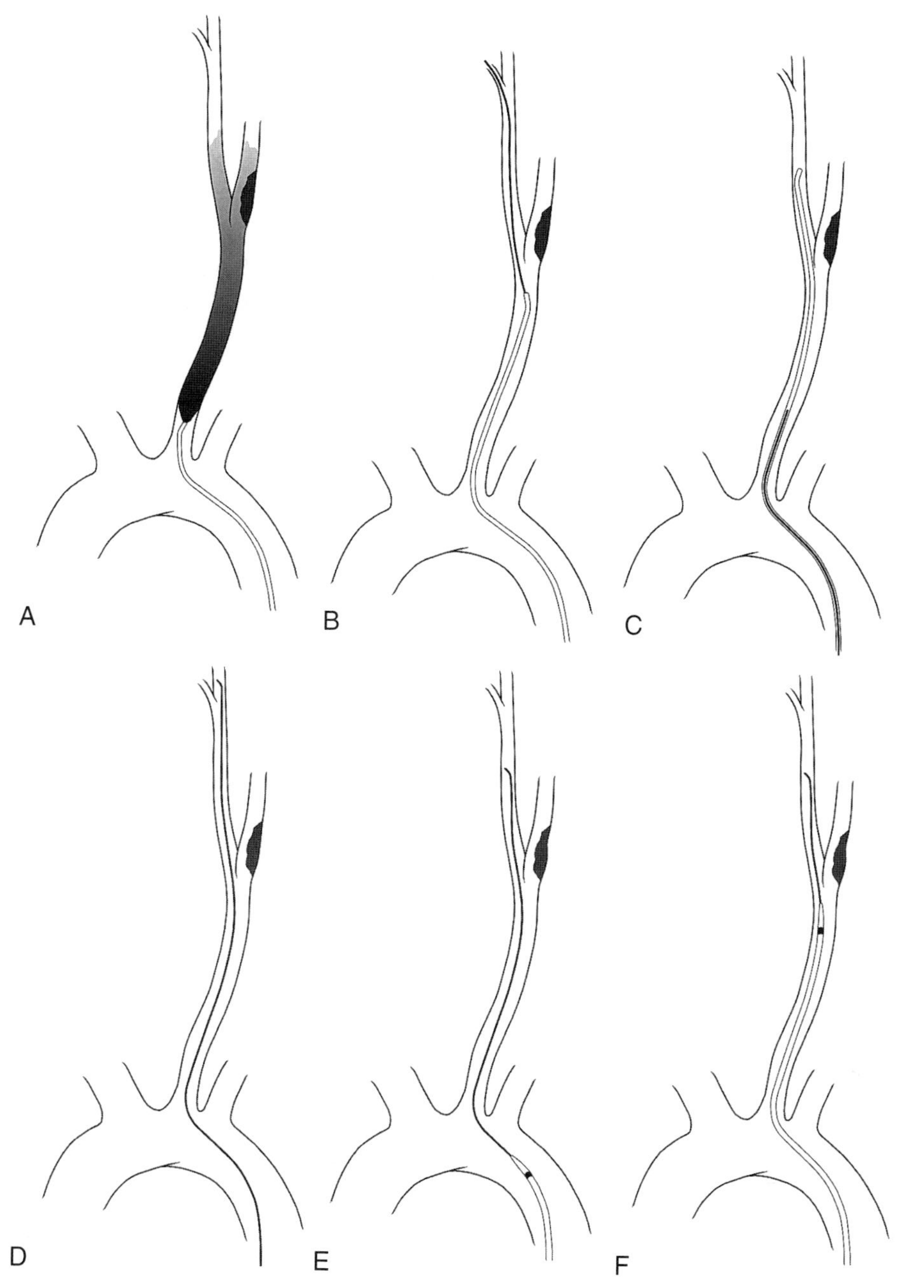

FIGURE 38-3 Sheath placement. **A,** The CCA is catheterized with a selective cerebral catheter. The carotid arteriogram is used as a road map to identify the bifurcation and the course of the ECA. **B,** The steerable Glidewire is advanced through the catheter and into the ECA. **C,** The cerebral catheter is advanced over the Glidewire so that the tip of the cerebral catheter is placed deep into the branches of the ECA. **D,** The Glidewire is removed, and a stiff exchange guidewire is placed. The cerebral catheter is then removed, leaving only the stiff exchange guidewire in place. **E,** The sheath is advanced over the stiff exchange guidewire. As the sheath rounds the turn from the arch into the CCA, there may be significant force on the system, and this is observed carefully. **F,** The sheath tip is advanced into the CCA into a position that is stable. Care must be taken to avoid placing the tip of the dilator into the bifurcation. After the sheath is in place, the dilator and stiff guidewire are removed.

lesions that are isolated to the proximal ICA are posterior wall plaques. In passing the guidewire tip to cross the lesion, the best pathway is usually anterior in the proximal ICA, just behind the flow divider. Bifurcation lesions that involve the distal CCA are usually more complex and less predictable. The key is to lead with the guidewire tip, do not make a loop, and be gentle in probing the lesion. After the lesion has been crossed, it is predilated with a 2- or 3-mm rapid exchange balloon (Figure 38-4). Some operators routinely administer small doses of atropine (0.25-0.5 mg) before balloon dilatation, except in patients with a recurrent stenosis. The pressure

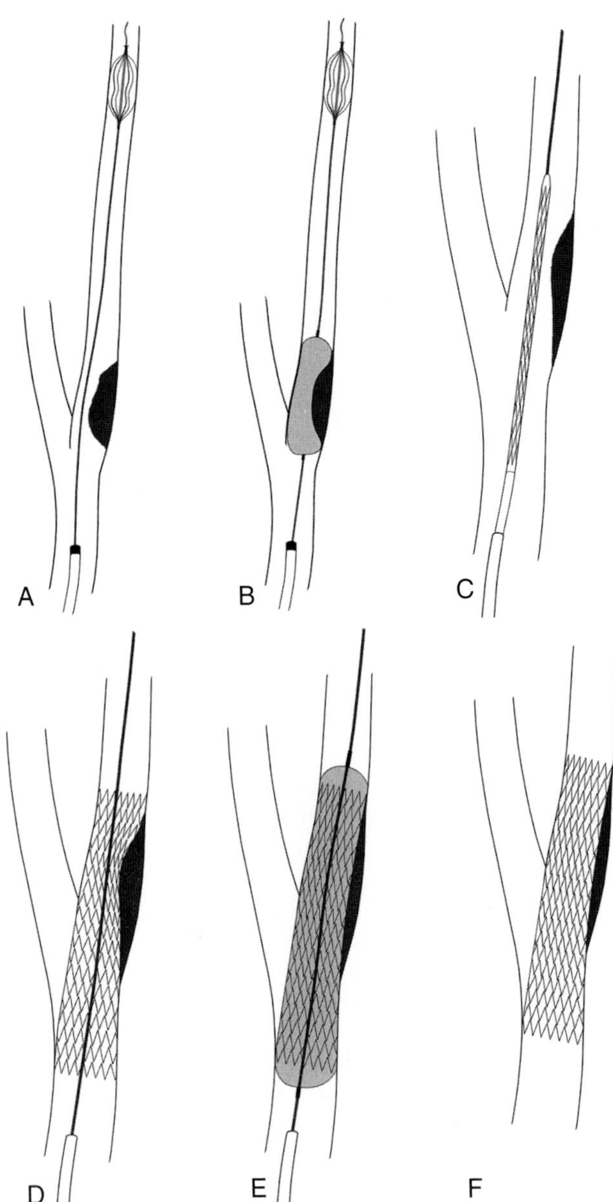

FIGURE 38-4 Stent of bifurcation lesion. **A,** An embolic protection filter is placed across the ICA lesion and deployed. **B,** Predilatation is performed after filter deployment and before stent placement. This is usually done with a 3- or 4-mm balloon. **C,** The stent delivery catheter is advanced across the lesion. **D,** The self-expanding stent is deployed from normal artery above the lesion to normal artery below the lesion. The stent extends from the internal to the CCA in most cases and goes across the origin of the ECA. **E,** Poststent dilatation is performed, usually with a 5- or 5.5-mm balloon. Overdilatation is not desirable. **F,** Completion angiography is performed showing prograde flow in the common and internal carotid arteries.

used for predilatation is nominal for the balloon used. Use higher pressure (14-16 atm) in heavily calcified stenoses. The duration of the predilatation depends on the appearance and behavior of the balloon. If the balloon immediately attains its full shape, the predilatation time is shorter. If the balloon attains its full shape slowly, the predilatation time is prolonged up to 120 seconds, especially in calcified lesions, which have a tendency for recoiling. Observe the monitor for bradycardia if a prolonged inflation is required.

A variety of self-expanding stents are available for use with the respective embolic protection devices. The self-expanding stent is deployed with use of landmarks, such as a bifurcation road map or the nearby vertebral bodies. The stent is placed from normal artery distal to the lesion to normal artery proximal to the lesion. The self-expanding stent is postdilated with a 5-mm balloon, or 6-mm rapid exchange balloon, depending on the size of the ICA. A 5-mm balloon percutaneous transluminal angioplasty (PTA) is often adequate; rarely is a 6-mm PTA required after stent deployment. The patient may again be pretreated with a small dose of atropine to blunt the carotid sinus response to stretching. A residual stenosis of less than 15% may be accepted, as the nitinol stents continue to expand with time. After stent deployment, shorter (2 cm) balloons are used to dilate the narrow portion of the stent where the residual stenosis is visible with use of fluoroscopy. The balloon used for poststent PTA is always maintained within the stent to avoid dissection. Nominal pressure is used to fully expand the balloon and the stent. In the majority of the cases, the stent is placed across the bifurcation into the CCA, crossing the origin of the ECA (Figure 38-5). To deploy the stent across the ECA has not resulted in adverse events; follow-up arteriograms and duplex ultrasound studies have demonstrated that the ECA remains patent in most patients.

Kinks and bends in the ICA may pose a problem with stent implants. Deploy stents across kinks only if they are isolated. Avoid placing the distal end of the stent into kinks and tortuosities of the ICA if more than a single bend is noted. Tortuosity cannot be eliminated, is displaced distally, and can become more exaggerated when a stent is placed and results in stiffening of a segment of artery. A tortuous ICA should be considered a relative contraindication for CAS, because acute occlusions are more common after stent placement in these tortuous vessels.

Completion Angiogram

After CAS, final angiograms are acquired in the projection that had demonstrated the maximum stenosis. Extra attention is paid to the ICA immediately distal to the stent. Spasm in this segment may be encountered. A small dose of intra-arterial nitroglycerin (100-200 mcg) is directly administered into the ICA, if significant spasm is encountered. Distal dissections are unusual and when present can be remedied with an additional stent of appropriate size. Reasonable prograde flow through the

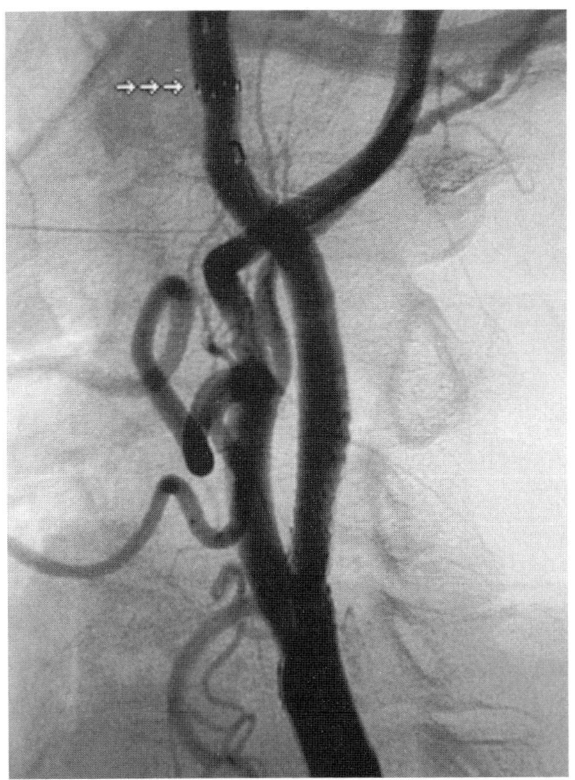

FIGURE 38-5 Carotid stent after placement. In this example, the embolic protection filter is in place in the distal extracranial ICA. The carotid stent has been placed across the bifurcation and passes across the origin of the ECA.

stented segment and the filter should be present. If there is slow flow or there is a filling defect with the filter, an aspiration catheter is used before filter removal. The filter retrieval catheter is passed carefully through the stent to capture the filter. Open cell stent designs have excellent contourability but also have diamond-shaped points in the lumen that can snag the retrieval catheter.

Post-CAS intracranial angiograms are obtained by most operators as a routine, and these may be compared with preoperative studies. The neurologic status of the patient is monitored during the procedure. The most common time for problems to develop is during or immediately after stent angioplasty.

Access Site Management

At the present time in suitable patients, access site hemostasis is achieved at the end of the procedure with use of one of several approved closure devices. If a calcified vessel is encountered during needle puncture, closure devices are not used. In this situation the long sheath is exchanged for a short sheath of the same caliber that is removed when the activated clotting time is less than 180 seconds, and manual pressure held for the appropriate time period.

Postoperative Care and Follow-up

Patients are monitored in the hospital overnight. It is not uncommon, especially in patients with a history of coronary artery disease, to have a heightened response to carotid sinus distension. Occasionally, 24 to 48 hours of inotropic support is required before the carotid sinus adapts to the radial force of the self-expanding stents. Avoiding extreme oversizing of the stents helps to decrease the incidence of post-CAS bradycardia and hypotension. The presence of significant hypotension in the absence of bradycardia is unusual in the immediate postprocedure period; it is worth emphasizing that other causes, for example, retroperitoneal bleeding related to access site problems, should also be excluded.

A neurologist is routinely involved in predischarge evaluation, and a National Institutes of Health stroke scale is completed before discharge. Carotid duplex scan is obtained if a patient has a neurologic event or if severe ICA spasm is seen on the completion angiogram, because this may influence postprocedure management. Medications include aspirin 325 mg/day indefinitely and clopidogrel 75 mg/day for 1 month. Follow-up includes 1-month, 6-month, and yearly clinical evaluation and duplex examination.

CEREBRAL PROTECTION DEVICES

Three methods of embolic protection are distal occlusion balloons, distal filter, and proximal occlusion (with or without flow reversal). Only distal filter devices have been approved in the United States.

Distal Embolic Protection Filters

Filter devices allow for continued flow into the intracranial ICA during intervention. These are 0.014-inch guidewire–based systems that have expandable and constrainable "baskets" or "umbrellas" near their distal ends; these baskets are intended to prevent particles of a certain diameter from passing into the brain (Figure 38-6). The filter is closed during placement, opened when located in the appropriate position distal to the carotid bifurcation lesion, and then closed before retrieval. Filter deployment mechanisms vary, but most are deployed by withdrawing an outer catheter that covers and restrains the filter, thus permitting self-expansion of the device. A filter may be fixed to the guidewire or may be separate from the initial guidewire. Examples of fixed-guidewire filters are the Accunet (Abbott Vascular Abbott Laboratories, Abbott Park, IL]) and the AngioGuard (Cordis Endovascular, Warren, NJ). The fixed-guidewire systems are simpler and require fewer steps. However, in the fixed-guidewire system,

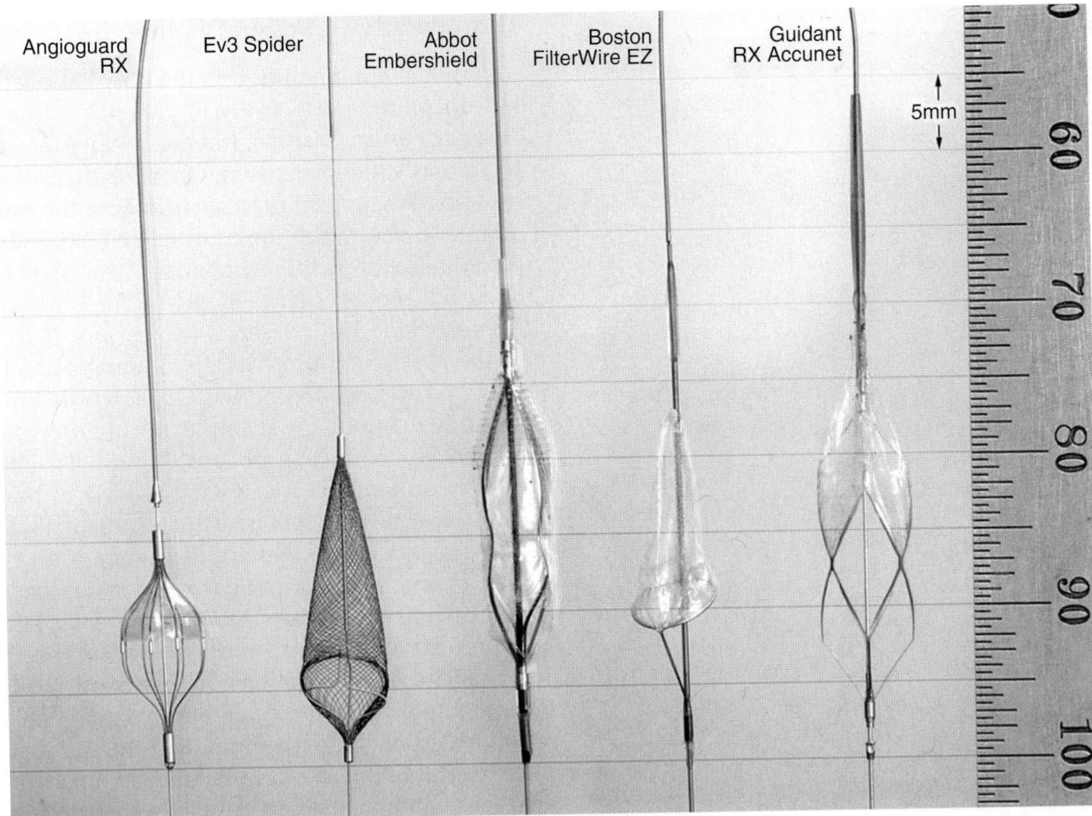

FIGURE 38-6 Embolic protection filters. These five filters have been approved for use in the United States during carotid stent placement. The Angioguard, Filterwire, and Accunet are fixed to the guidewire on which they are delivered. The Spider and the Emboshield are free wire systems. Each filter has a self-expanding element that promotes expansion in the distal ICA after deployment. Each filter has a different pore size in its catchment and also a specific landing zone required for placement.

any guidewire movement after the filter is deployed results in movement of the filter itself. In addition, the attachment of the filter to the guidewire limits the handling of the guidewire during lesion traversal. The free-guidewire systems permit usage of a choice of guidewires. When there is substantial tortuosity, a complex lesion, or other challenges, the free-guidewire systems have a substantial advantage. Examples of free-guidewire filters are the Emboshield (Abbott Vascular) and the Spider (ev3 Endovascular, Plymouth, MN).

Technique for Use of Distal Filters

1. Unlike balloon-occlusion devices, filter devices are designed to maintain flow into the distal ICA during the course of intervention. Do not place the filter until being certain that the sheath is in a stable position in the CCA because any movement of the sheath will also move the filter. After placement of a sheath into the CCA, the filter device is placed across the target lesion into a straight, normal segment of the distal extracranial ICA. Placing the device into a tortuous segment may be difficult and could impede filter function. An activated clotting time of 250 seconds or higher is required before placing filter devices.
2. The crossing profile of a filter is typically greater than standard guidewires. Occasionally, it may be difficult to cross extremely stenotic, tortuous, or calcified lesions. A "buddy wire" may be helpful in providing extra support during filter placement. A slightly larger sheath is needed to accommodate a buddy wire, such as a 7F sheath. If tortuosity is the issue, sometimes this can be improved by placing a stiff, but low-profile guidewire into the ECA. Occasionally, it is necessary to place a soft guidewire (0.010 or 0.014 inch) across the ICA lesion to permit filter passage.
3. Once deployed, and after each step of the intervention, flow of contrast through the device must be observed. If the device becomes filled with debris, it must be aspirated. When removing a full device, it is important not to recapture it completely, as debris may be extruded from it and embolize distally.

Distal Occlusion Devices

Balloon-occlusion devices cease flow in the ICA during the period of angioplasty and stenting. The

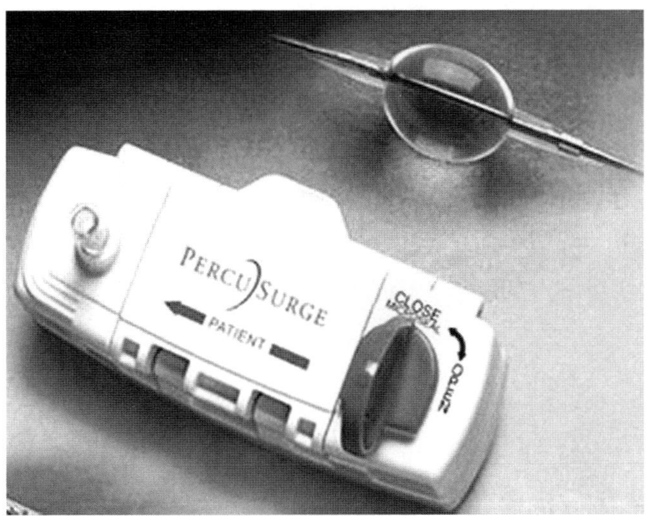

FIGURE 38-7 PercuSurge device. This device consists of a hypotube with a balloon on the end. After placement of the occlusion balloon distal to the carotid lesion, the lumen of the hypotube is used to inflate the balloon. Occlusion is achieved by the expanding balloon and is confirmed by arteriography. After stent placement, the ICA is evacuated by using an aspiration catheter. The balloon is deflated and removed.

PercuSurge Guard Wire (Medtronic AVE, Minneapolis, MN) is a compliant balloon housed on a 0.014-inch guidewire, with a rather ingenious valve (microseal adapter) that allows the balloon to remain inflated when the inflation device is removed (Figure 38-7). Angioplasty balloons, catheters, and stents can then be loaded onto the wire and removed while the balloon occludes the ICA. At the completion of the interventional procedure, the static column of blood in the ICA is aspirated by using a special catheter (Export catheter, Medtronic), to remove any embolic particles that may have accumulated. The balloon can be inflated from 3 to 6 mm in diameter, in 0.5-mm increments, depending on the size of the target artery. The device is approved for aortocoronary saphenous vein graft intervention and not for carotid use.

Proximal Occlusion and Flow-Reversal Devices

The Gore Neuro Protection System device is a proximal occlusion/flow reversal device in clinical trials in the United States. A large catheter (8F) is placed into the CCA (Figure 38-8). Flow is stopped by inflating a balloon surrounding the catheter and then placing an occlusion balloon in the ECA. The CCA catheter is connected to an external filter and then to the femoral vein, producing an arteriovenous fistula and reversal of flow in the ICA. At this point, intervention can be performed under complete protection, as antegrade flow in the ICA does not occur until after the procedure is terminated.

This technique has several advantages compared with standard CAS using distal filters. Surgeons experienced with CEA have long recognized the potential to dislodge the friable material present in carotid bifurcation plaques. Studies of carotid stenting with transcranial Doppler monitoring have demonstrated frequent embolic signals prevalent during several stages of the carotid stenting procedure including lesion crossing, predilation, stent placement, and postdilation. Diffusion-weighted MR imaging scans performed before and after CAS have shown evidence of lesions that are likely embolic. Most filters allow particles smaller than 100 μm to pass through, resulting in multiple small, usually asymptomatic, cerebral lesions in up to one third of patients with use of routine postprocedural diffusion-weighted MR studies of the brain. This type of distal microembolization, although not immediately associated with gross neurologic deficits, may lead to late cognitive impairment. Flow reversal permits CAS with the opportunity to diminish the high-intensity transits visible on transcranial Doppler examinations. Technically, the main challenges are the need for an 8F sheath and the need for ECA occlusion.

RESULTS OF CAROTID STENTING

During the late 1980s and early 1990s, a series of multicenter randomized controlled clinical trials (RCTs) conducted in Europe and North America demonstrated the superiority of CEA plus medical management versus medical management alone for the prevention of stroke among patients with atherosclerotic carotid bifurcation stenosis.[7-14] Coincident with the development of catheter-based technologies including stents, stent delivery systems, and cerebral protection devices, CAS has emerged as a potentially viable alternative, especially among patients who are at higher risk for perioperative complications after CEA.

CEA is an operation that has been exceedingly well studied. When performed by competent surgeons, the operation is safe and effective, providing durable protection against stroke with low rates of recurrent carotid stenosis.[15] The established guidelines derived from these studies in standard-risk patients for perioperative risk for stroke or death after CEA is 3% for patients without symptoms and 6% for patients with symptoms. In contrast, much of the published data on CAS consists of noncontrolled registries, most without independent verification of outcome events. The results of the prospective, randomized CREST Trial of CEA versus CAS in both asymptomatic and symptomatic patients, which concluded enrollment in July 2008, are awaited.[16]

The past several years have witnessed impressive technologic advancements in endoluminal stents, stent

Dilator
GORE
Balloon Sheath
GORE
Balloon Wire
Tear-Away
Sheath
GORE
External Filter
© Image courtesy of W. L. Gore & Associates, Inc.

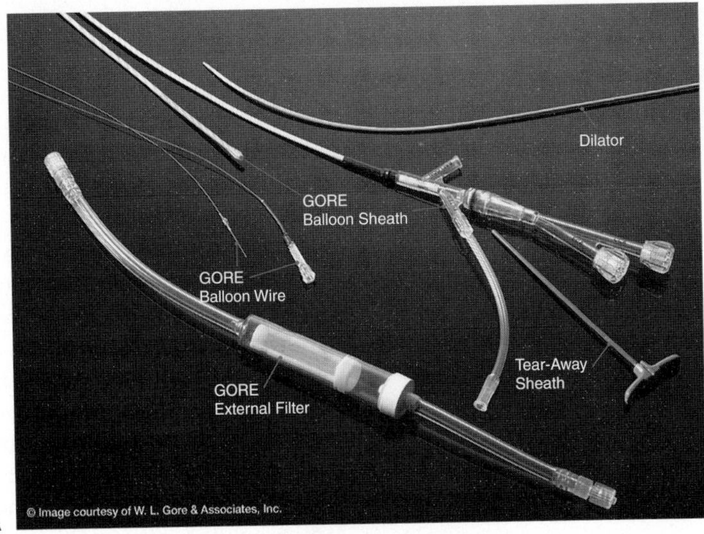

A

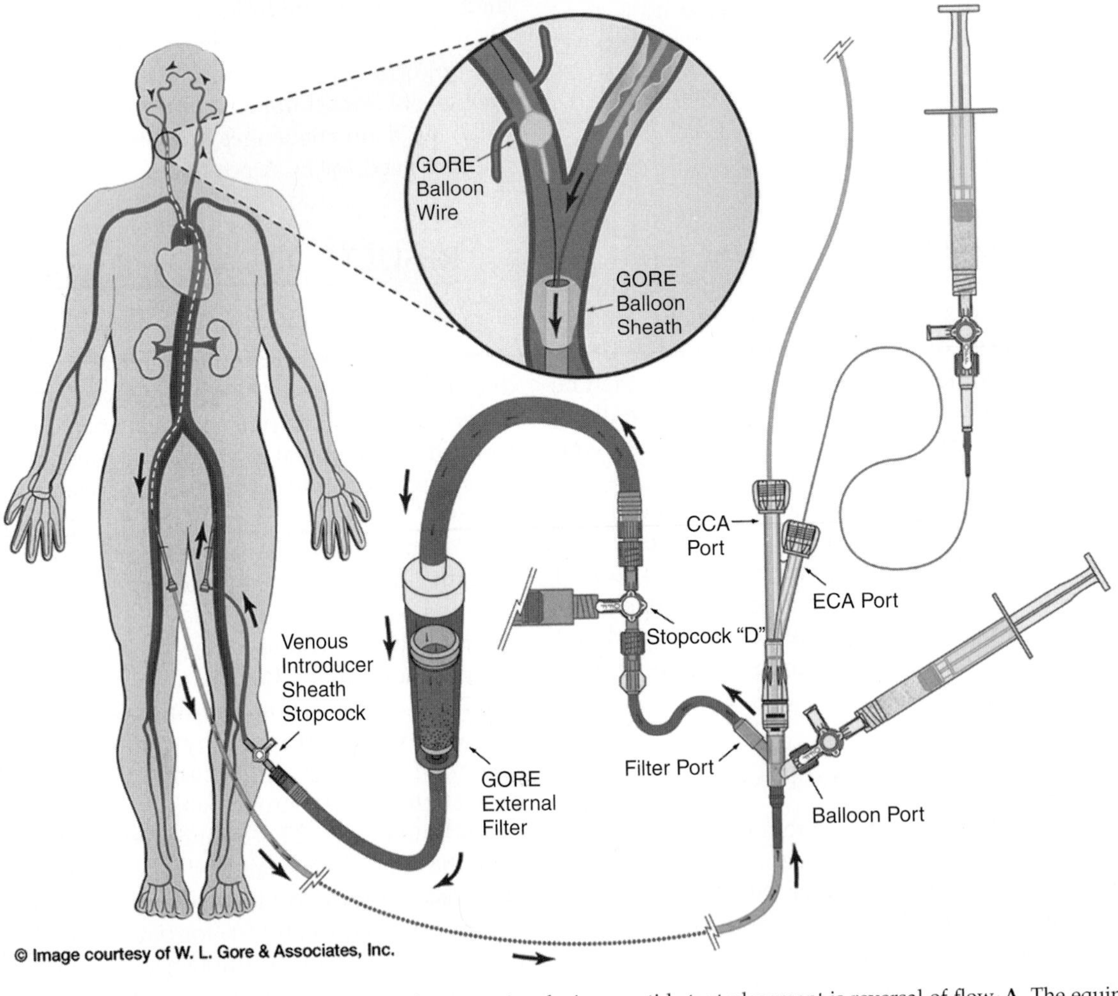

GORE
Balloon
Wire
GORE
Balloon
Sheath
CCA
Port
ECA Port
Stopcock "D"
Venous
Introducer
Sheath
Stopcock
Filter Port
GORE
External
Filter
Balloon Port
© Image courtesy of W. L. Gore & Associates, Inc.

B

FIGURE 38-8 Reversed-flow device. Another option for protection during carotid stent placement is reversal of flow. **A,** The equipment for this procedure. A sheath with an occlusion balloon is used to stop flow in the CCA while providing a conduit to reach the bifurcation. **B,** The circuit for reversed flow. Flow is reversed after placement of both an arterial sheath and a venous sheath. The ECA is occluded by using a balloon catheter. Flow through the carotid artery lesion is reversed during stent placement.

delivery systems, and cerebral protection devices. Together with these technologic improvements, growing familiarity and expertise with the technique of CAS have resulted in improved periprocedural complication rates that, in many institutions, appear to be nearly equivalent to those of CEA. The safety/efficacy data on CAS consist of several single-center case series and multicenter registries and three large published RCTs comparing CAS with CEA.

Observational Data

A summary of the largest observational studies of CAS, including single-center case series and multicenter registries, is shown in Table 38-2.[17-34] These studies demonstrated the feasibility of CAS and helped define indications, anatomic challenges, operating technique, and equipment development. The results of stent-supported angioplasty of the carotid arteries are superior to those of balloon angioplasty without stenting, presumably because of lower risks of distal embolization and recurrent stenosis with primary stent placement. Carotid angioplasty without stenting has no role in the management of carotid bifurcation atherosclerosis, and earlier studies of PTA without stenting are thus omitted from this analysis.

With use of data from Table 38-2, the weighted average of stroke rates from studies published from 1996 to 1998, 1999 to 2001, and 2002 to 2003 was 4.7%, 3.8%, and 2.6%, respectively. The explanation for this trend is almost certainly multifactorial. Technical success, defined as less than 30% residual arteriographic stenosis at the completion of the procedure, was reported in more than 95% of cases in all studies. The majority of these reports are notable for their poor documentation of the proportion of patients treated with prior neurologic symptoms and very limited long-term follow-up data.

High-Risk Registries of Carotid Angioplasty and Wtenting

Leading up to the forthcoming results of additional RCT data comparing CAS with CEA, there is much to be learned from a number of high-risk clinical registry data (Table 38-3).[3,35-37] Many of the clinical trials listed in Table 38-3 are nonrandomized registries of CAS in

TABLE 38-2 Summary of Published Results of Observational Studies of Carotid Angioplasty and Stenting

Study	Publication yr	Lesions (No.)	Cerebral protection (%)	30-Day outcome	
				Death (%)	Stroke (%)
Diethrich et al.[17]	1996	117	0	1.7	6.0
Wholey et al.[18]	1997	114	0	1.8	3.5
Yadav et al.[19]	1997	126	0	0.8	7.1
Henry et al.[25]	1998	174	18	0	2.9
Mathias et al.[29]	1999	799	NP		2.1
Shawl et al.[32]	2000	192	0	0	2.6
Wholey et al.[34]	2000	5210	Very low	1.9	3.9
d'Audiffret et al.[23]	2001	83	18		4.4
Reimers et al.[30]	2001	88	100		1.1
Roubin et al.[31]	2001	604	0	1.6	5.8
Al Mubarak et al.[20]	2002	164	100	1.2	1.2
Criado et al.[22]	2002	135	0	0	2.2
Guimaraens et al.[24]	2002	194	100	1.9	1.0
Henry et al.[25]	2002	184	100	0.5	2.2
Koch et al.[27]	2002	167	0		7.5
MacDonald et al.[28]	2002	150	50	1.3	6.0
Whitlow et al.[33]	2002	75	100	0	0
Cremonesi et al.[21]	2003	442	100		2.0
Hobson et al.[26]	2003	114	0	1.8	0.9

NP, Not published.

TABLE 38-3 High-Risk Prospective Registry Data

Name	Company	No. of patients	Stent	Embolic device	MAE (%)	Stroke (%)	Yr presented
ARCHeR 1	Guidant	158	Acculink	None	7.6	4.4	2003
ARCHeR 2	Guidant	278	Acculink	Accumet	8.6	6.8	2003
ARCHeR 3	Guidant	145	Acculink	Accunet	8.3	7.6	2003
BEACH	BSC	480	Wallstent	Filterwire	5.8	4.4	2005
CABERNET	BSC	454	Nexstent	Filterwire	3.9	3.4	2005
CREATE	ev3	160	Acculink	SpideRX	5.6	4.4	2005
SECuRITY	Abbott	305	Xactstent	Emboshield	7.5	6.2	2003
MAVErIC	Medtronic	399	Exponent	PercuSurge	5	3	2004

ARCHeR, The Acculink for Revascularization of Carotids in High-Risk patients; *BEACH,* Boston Scientific EPI: A Carotid stenting trial for High risk surgical patients; *BSC,* Boston Scientific Corporation; *CABERNET,* Carotid Artery revascularization using the Boston Scientific Filterwire EX system and the EndoTex NextStent Carotid Stent; *CREATE,* Carotid Revascularization with the ev3 Arterial Technology Evolution; *MAVErIC,* Evaluation of the Medtronic Self-Expanding Carotid Stent with Distal Protection of Carotid Artery Stenosis; *SECuRITY,* Registry Study to Evaluate the Neuroshield Bare Wire Cerebral Protection System and X-act Stent in Patients at High Risk for Carotid Endarterectomy.

high-risk patients organized in an attempt to gain Food and Drug Administration approval for stents and cerebral protection devices. The first carotid system to gain approval in the United States was the Acculink/Accunet, based on the results of the ARCHeR Trial.[3] The ARCHeR Trial (Acculink for Revascularization of Carotids in High-Risk Patients) is a registry of 513 patients treated with the Acculink stent and Accunet filter. This study included both symptomatic and asymptomatic high-risk patients, including patients with postendarterectomy restenosis. The periprocedural death and stroke rates were 2.3% and 5.3%, respectively.

Other findings from the high-risk registries include the following. The risk of contralateral events is persistent through several trials, reinforcing the importance of safe arch access.[2,3] Although distal embolic protection is widely accepted, and is in fact required to be reimbursed by Medicare, the efficacy of these devices in preventing perioperative events has been difficult to prove.[38,39] When CAS was rolled out to those with catheter skills, a high level of proficiency was obtained in performing CAS with fewer than 25 cases.[40] Octogenarians were found to have worse than expected outcomes than younger patients, with substantially rates of stroke after CAS.[16,40] Most of the high-risk registry data did not achieve the established benchmarks for perioperative stroke and death in standard-risk patients (3% for asymptomatic, 6% for symptomatic).

Randomized Trials Comparing Carotid Angioplasty and Stenting and Carotid Endarterectomy

The Stenting and Angioplasty with Protection in Patients at High Risk for Endarterectomy (SAPPHIRE) trial is the first large RCT completed in the United States, sponsored by Cordis Corporation, in which 307 (156 CAS, 151 CEA) patients were randomly assigned to receive CAS with use of the Precise stent together with the AngioGuard embolic protection device versus standard CEA.[2] Randomly assigned patients were considered high risk for CEA on the basis of medical or anatomic factors. Symptomatic patients with ≥50% stenosis and asymptomatic patients with ≥80% carotid stenosis were included. The perioperative stroke or death rates were 7/156 (4.5%) and 11/151 (7.3%) for the CAS and CEA groups, respectively ($p = 0.3$). When perioperative myocardial infarction is included in this composite end point (2.6% CAS, 7.3% CEA), the difference becomes statistically significant in favor of the CAS group, but the clinical significance of these myocardial infarctions is not clear. Although this is an underpowered trial with unexpectedly high periprocedural stroke rates in the CEA group (5.3%), especially when one considers that the majority of patients had no symptoms, the results indicate that, among high-risk patients, CAS appears to compare favorably with CEA. Given the low stroke risk for asymptomatic patients with carotid stenosis, the question of whether asymptomatic patients who are considered high risk should be considered for any type of carotid artery intervention should be addressed.

The Carotid Revascularization with Endarterectomy versus Stenting Systems (CARESS) study was a multicenter registry designed to study CAS in both symptomatic and asymptomatic patients who are not candidates for CREST and includes a concurrent nonrandomized CEA cohort.[41] Although it was a nonrandomized trial, it was designed to simulate standard community practice by taking all comers, mostly standard-risk patients. There was a 2:1 distribution of CEA to CAS. PercuSurge (Medtronic) with the Magic Wallstent (Boston Scientific)

TABLE 38-4 Summary of Results of Randomized Controlled Trials Comparing Carotid Angioplasty and Stenting With Carotid Endarterectomy

			MAEs (%)			
			30 days		1 yr	
Trial	Total No. of patients	Patient population	CAS	CEA	CAS	CEA
SAPPHIRE	334	Symptomatic and asymptomatic	5.8	12.6	12	20.1
CaRESS	397	Symptomatic and asymptomatic	2.1	4.4	10.9	14.3
CAVATAS	504	Symptomatic and asymptomatic	10	9.9		
SPACE	1214	Symptomatic only	6.84	6.34		
EVA-3S	527	Symptomatic only	9.6	3.9	6.1*	11.7

* *Six-month results.*

CaRESS, Carotid Revascularization with Endarterectomy versus Stenting Systems; *CAS,* Carotid Angioplasty and Stenting; *CAVATAS,* Carotid and Vertebral Artery Transluminal Angioplasty Study; *CEA,* carotid endarterectomy; *EVA-3S,* Endarterectomy Versus Stenting in Patients With Symptomatic Severe Carotid Stenosis; *MAE,* major adverse event; *SAPPHIRE,* Stenting and Angioplasty with Protection in Patients at High Risk for Endarterectomy; *SPACE,* Stent Supported Percutaneous Angioplasty Versus Endarterectomy.

comprised the system used for CAS. Overall, 32% had symptoms and 68% had no symptoms. There was no significant difference in the combined stroke or death rate at 30 days between CEA (3.6%) and CAS (2.1%) or at 1 year, CEA (13.6%) versus CAS (10%). This study demonstrated equivalence of CAS with CEA.

Two recently published trials from the European Union have had a significant effect on stenting in the United States, based on their publication in *The Lancet* and the *New England Journal of Medicine* (Table 38-4).[38,39,42] The Stent Supported Percutaneous Angioplasty versus Endarterectomy (SPACE) trial was a randomized trial in symptomatic standard-risk patients with carotid lesions greater than 70% by duplex examination conducted in Germany and Switzerland and was sponsored by several companies and institutions. A total of 1183 patients were randomly assigned within 180 days of carotid stenosis–related symptoms. Patients were to be treated within 14 days of randomization, and the primary outcome was ipsilateral stroke or death with 30 days of treatment. The results between both groups appeared similar with 42 primary events in the CAS group (6.9%) and 38 events in the CEA group (6.5%; $p = 0.09$). Despite a lack of distal protection in a significant number of stented patients the results appear to show near equivalence.

The Endarterectomy versus Stenting in Patients with Symptomatic Severe Carotid Stenosis (EVA-3S) was a French trial with national funding. Patients had to be suitable for both CEA and CAS, with greater than 60% stenosis and recently symptomatic. The study was stopped after 527 of the planned 872 patients were enrolled because of having reached a statistically significant difference between the treatment arms. The primary end point was seen in 9.6% of the CAS patients and in 3.9% of the CEA patients ($p = 0.01$). Unfortunately, the trial design was almost skewed to have a better result in the CEA arm. Surgeons had to have performed 25 CEAs in the year before enrollment, but a stent operator could have many fewer procedures. Additionally, first-time stent users were allowed to treat patients under the supervision of a qualified operator. Distal protection was only mandated after excess stroke risk in the stent arm during the protection-optional phase. Given the shortcomings in the design, it is difficult to reach definite conclusions that would change current practice patterns.

The Carotid Revascularization Endarterectomy versus Stent Trial (CREST) is a randomized trial designed to compare CAS and CEA among standard-risk asymptomatic and symptomatic patients with carotid stenosis. The trial is sponsored by the National Institutes of Health and employs the use of the Acculink stent and Accunet filter. Enrollment was recently completed.

The long-term durability of CAS appears to parallel that of CEA. The 3-year results of the SAPPHIRE trial show that the need for repeated revascularization after CAS is low and is similar to that of CEA.[43] This has also been shown in several postmarket studies.[44] These findings focus attention back to the perioperative risks of stroke and death with CAS and the need to achieve acceptable benchmarks to have broad acceptance of CAS.

CONCLUSION

Because of its less-invasive nature, percutaneous treatment of carotid bifurcation stenosis has several potential advantages over CEA including the elimination of local surgical complications, such as neck hematoma, infection, cranial nerve injury, and postoperative pain and scarring, in addition to reduced blood loss, and cardiopulmonary complications. However, optimum management of patients with carotid bifurcation stenosis requires thorough familiarity with the natural history of the disease process, as well as with *all* modes of therapy including medical management, CEA, and CAS.

RCTs comparing CEA with medical management have established CEA as the standard of care for the majority of patients with symptomatic and for highly selected patients with asymptomatic carotid bifurcation stenosis. These trials have established benchmark perioperative morbidity/mortality rates that can be achieved in standard-risk patients. The data on CAS consist of a limited number of RCTs in addition to a large number of case series and registries with inherent biases. These studies indicate that periprocedural complication rates after CAS have improved markedly over the past decade, probably because of many factors including improved technical skill and enhanced technology. Until additional large RCTs comparing CAS with CEA are completed, CEA should be considered the treatment of choice for standard-risk patients with carotid stenosis requiring intervention. For patients considered high risk for CEA, however, CAS is a viable alternative when performed in centers with established expertise and excellence.

References

1. Kasirajan K: Technique of carotid bifurcation angioplasty and stent placement: how I do it. In: Schneider PA, Bohannon WT, Silva MB, editors: *Carotid interventions*, New York, 2004, Marcel Dekker, pp 149–164.
2. Yadav JS, Wholey MH, Kuntz RE, et al: Stenting and angioplasty with protection in patients at high risk for endarterectomy investigators. Protected carotid-artery stenting versus endarterectomy in high-risk patients, *N Engl J Med* 351(15):1493–1501, 2004.
3. Gray WA, Hopkins LN, Yadav S, et al: ARCHeR Trial Collaborators: Protected carotid stenting in high-surgical-risk patients—the ARCHeR results, *J Vasc Surg* 44(2):258–268, 2006.
4. Bohannon WT, Schneider PA, Silva MB: Aortic arch classification into segments facilitates carotid stenting. In: Schneider PA, Bohannon WT, Silva MB, editors: *Carotid interventions*, New York, 2004, Marcel Dekker, pp 15–22.
5. Rosenfield KM, SCAI/SVMB/SVS: Writing Committee. Clinical competence statement on carotid stenting: training and credentialing for carotid stenting—multispecialty consensus recommendations, *J Vasc Surg* 41(1):160–168, 2005.
6. Connors JJ 3rd, Sacks D, Furlan AJ, et al: American Academy of Neurology; American Association of Neurological Surgeons; American Society of Interventional and Therapeutic Neuroradiology; American Society of Neuroradiology; Congress of Neurological Surgeons; AANS/CNS Cerebrovascular Section; Society of Interventional Radiology; NeuroVascular Coalition Writing Group. Training, competency, and credentialing standards for diagnostic cervicocerebral angiography, carotid stenting, and cerebrovascular intervention: a joint statement from the American Academy of Neurology, the American Association of Neurological Surgeons, the American Society of Interventional and Therapeutic Neuroradiology, the American Society of Neuroradiology, the Congress of Neurological Surgeons, the AANS/CNS Cerebrovascular Section, and the Society of Interventional Radiology, *Neurology* 64(2):190–198, 2005.
7. Beneficial effect of carotid endarterectomy in symptomatic patients with high-grade carotid stenosis, North American Symptomatic Carotid Endarterectomy Trial Collaborators, *N Engl J Med* 325(7):445–453, 1991.
8. Barnett HJ, Taylor DW, Eliasziw M, et al: Benefit of carotid endarterectomy in patients with symptomatic moderate or severe stenosis. North American Symptomatic Carotid Endarterectomy Trial Collaborators, *N Engl J Med* 339(20):1415–1425, 1998.
9. MRC European Carotid Surgery Trial: interim results for symptomatic patients with severe (70–99%) or with mild (0-29%) carotid stenosis: European Carotid Surgery Trialists' Collaborative Group, *Lancet* 337(8752):1235–1243, 1991.
10. Randomised trial of endarterectomy for recently symptomatic carotid stenosis: final results of the MRC European Carotid Surgery Trial (ECST)[comment], *Lancet* 351(9113):1379–1387, 1998.
11. Endarterectomy for asymptomatic carotid artery stenosis: Executive Committee for the Asymptomatic Carotid Atherosclerosis Study, *JAMA* 273(18):1421–1428, 1995.
12. Hobson RW, Weiss DG, Fields WS, et al: Efficacy of carotid endarterectomy for asymptomatic carotid stenosis. The Veterans Affairs Cooperative Study Group, *N Engl J Med* 328(4):221–227, 1993.
13. Mayberg MR, Wilson SE, Yatsu F, et al: Carotid endarterectomy and prevention of cerebral ischemia in symptomatic carotid stenosis. Veterans Affairs Cooperative Studies Program 309 Trialist Group, *JAMA* 266(23):3289–3294, 1991.
14. Halliday A, Mansfield A, Marro J, et al: MRC Asymptomatic Carotid Surgery Trial (ACST) Collaborative Group: prevention of disabling and fatal strokes by successful carotid endarterectomy in patients without recent neurological symptoms: randomised controlled trial, *Lancet* 363:1491–1502, 2004.
15. Hobson RW 2nd, Mackey WC, Ascher E, et al: Society for Vascular Surgery. Management of atherosclerotic carotid artery disease: clinical practice guidelines of the Society for Vascular Surgery, *J Vasc Surg* 48(2):480–486, 2008.
16. Hobson RW 2nd, Howard VJ, Roubin GS, et al: CREST Investigators. Carotid artery stenting is associated with increased complications in octogenarians: 30-day stroke and death rates in the CREST lead-in phase, *J Vasc Surg* 40(6):1106–1111, 2004.
17. Diethrich EB, Ndiaye M, Reid DB: Stenting in the carotid artery: initial experience in 110 patients, *J Endovasc Surg* 3(1):42–62, 1996.
18. Wholey MH, Wholey MH, Jarmolowski CR, et al: Endovascular stents for carotid artery occlusive disease, *J Endovasc Surg* 4 (4):326–338, 1997.
19. Yadav JS, Roubin GS, Iyer S, et al: Elective stenting of the extracranial carotid arteries, *Circulation* 95(2):376–381, 1997.
20. Al Mubarak N, Colombo A, Gaines PA, et al: Multicenter evaluation of carotid artery stenting with a filter protection system, *J Am Coll Cardiol* 39(5):841–846, 2002.
21. Cremonesi A, Manetti R, Setacci F, et al: Protected Carotid Stenting: clinical advantages and complications of embolic protection devices in 442 consecutive patients, *Stroke* 34(8): 1936–1941, 2003.
22. Criado FJ, Lingelbach JM, Ledesma DF, et al: Carotid artery stenting in a vascular surgery practice, *J Vasc Surg* 35(3):430–434, 2002.
23. d'Audiffret A, Desgranges P, Kobeiter H, et al: Technical aspects and current results of carotid stenting, *J Vasc Surg* 33 (5):1001–1007, 2001.

24. Guimaraens L, Sola MT, Matali A, et al: Carotid angioplasty with cerebral protection and stenting: report of 164 patients (194 carotid percutaneous transluminal angioplasties), *Cerebrovasc Dis* 13(2):114–119, 2002.
25. Henry M, Henry I, Klonaris C, et al: Benefits of cerebral protection during carotid stenting with the PercuSurge GuardWire system: midterm results, *J Endovasc Ther* 9(1):1–13, 2002.
26. Hobson RW, Lal BK, Chaktoura E, et al: Carotid artery stenting: analysis of data for 105 patients at high risk, *J Vasc Surg* 37 (6):1234–1239, 2003.
27. Koch C, Kucinski T, Eckert B, et al: [Endovascular therapy of high-degree stenoses of the neck vessels-stent-supported percutaneous angioplasty of the carotid artery without cerebral protection], *Rofo Fortschr Geb Rontgenstr Neuen Bildgeb Verfahr* 174(12): 1506–1510, 2002.
28. Macdonald S, McKevitt F, Venables GS, et al: Neurological outcomes after carotid stenting protected with the NeuroShield filter compared to unprotected stenting, *J Endovasc Ther* 9 (6):777–785, 2002.
29. Mathias K, Jager H, Sahl H, et al: [Interventional treatment of arteriosclerotic carotid stenosis], *Radiologe* 39(2):125–134, 1999.
30. Reimers B, Corvaja N, Moshiri S, et al: Cerebral protection with filter devices during carotid artery stenting, *Circulation* 104 (1):12–15, 2001.
31. Roubin GS, New G, Iyer SS, et al: Immediate and late clinical outcomes of carotid artery stenting in patients with symptomatic and asymptomatic carotid artery stenosis: a 5-year prospective analysis, *Circulation* 103(4):532–537, 2001.
32. Shawl F, Kadro W, Domanski MJ, et al: Safety and efficacy of elective carotid artery stenting in high-risk patients, *J Am Coll Cardiol* 35(7):1721–1728, 2000.
33. Whitlow PL, Lylyk P, Londero H, et al: Carotid artery stenting protected with an emboli containment system, *Stroke* 33(5):1308–1314, 2002.
34. Wholey MH, Wholey M, Mathias K, et al: Global experience in cervical carotid artery stent placement, *Catheter Cardiovasc Interv* 50(2):160–167, 2000.
35. Iyer SS, White CJ, Hopkins LN, et al: BEACH Investigators. Carotid artery revascularization in high-surgical-risk patients using the Carotid WALLSTENT and FilterWire EX/EZ: 1-year outcomes in the BEACH Pivotal Group, *J Am Coll Cardiol* 51 (4):427–434, 2008.
36. Hopkins LN, Myla S, Grube E, et al: Carotid artery revascularization in high surgical risk patients with the NexStent and the Filterwire EX/EZ: 1-year results in the CABERNET trial, *Catheter Cardiovasc Interv* 71(7):950–960, 2008.
37. Safian RD, Bresnahan JF, Jaff MR, et al: CREATE Pivotal Trial Investigators. Protected carotid stenting in high-risk patients with severe carotid artery stenosis, *J Am Coll Cardiol* 47 (12):2384–2389, 2006.
38. Mas JL, Chatellier G, Beyssen B, et al: Endarterectomy versus stenting in patients with symptomatic severe carotid stenosis, *N Engl J Med* 19(355):1660–1671, 2006.
39. Ringleb PA, Allenberg J, Bruckmann H, et al: 30 day results from the SPACE trial of stent protected angioplasty versus carotid endarterectomy in symptomatic patients: a randomized non-inferiority trial, *Lancet* 368:1239–1247, 2006.
40. Gray WA, Yadav JS, Verta P, et al: CAPTURE Trial Collaborators. The CAPTURE registry: predictors of outcomes in carotid artery stenting with embolic protection for high surgical risk patients in the early post-approval setting, *Catheter Cardiovasc Interv* 70 (7):1025–1033, 2007.
41. CARESS Steering committee: Carotid revascularization using endarterectomy or stenting systems (CARESS): phase I clinical trial, *J Endovasc Ther* 10:1021–1030, 2003.
42. Endovascular versus surgical treatment in patients with carotid stenosis in the Carotid and Vertebral Artery Transluminal Angioplasty Study (CAVATAS): a randomized trial, *Lancet* 357 (9270):1729–1737, 2001.
43. Gurm HS, Yadav JS, Fayad P, et al: Long-term results of carotid stenting versus endarterectomy in high-risk patients, *N Engl J Med* 358(15):1572–1579, 2008.
44. Katzen BT, Criado FJ, Ramee SR, et al: CASES-PMS Investigators. Carotid artery stenting with emboli protection surveillance study: thirty-day results of the CASES-PMS study, *Catheter Cardiovasc Interv* 70(2):316–323, 2007.

CHAPTER

39

Complication Management in Carotid Stenting

Kenneth V. Snyder, Sabareesh K. Natarajan, Adnan H. Siddiqui, Elad I. Levy, L. Nelson Hopkins

It is our choices . . . that show what we truly are, far more than our abilities.
—*JK Rowling:* Harry Potter and the Chamber of Secrets*

The above statement has special relevance to every aspect of carotid artery stenting (CAS), from patient selection, to the choice of approach (type of embolic protection), choice of devices, and choice of strategy for intraoperative complication management. The use of distal and proximal embolic protection in CAS for high-risk patients with extracranial internal carotid artery (ICA) stenosis has demonstrated a similar morbidity and mortality to carotid endarterectomy (CEA).[1-12] High-risk registries report a 30-day risk of myocardial infarction (MI), stroke, or death from 4.0% to 8.2%.[4-7,9,10,12] The Stenting and Angioplasty with Protection in Patients at High Risk for Endarterectomy (SAPPHIRE) trial reported a 5.8% 30-day and 12% 1-year combined morbidity and mortality.[11] Although the morbidity rates are relatively low, potential exists for devastating complications to occur at any stage of CAS.

CAS can be used to treat various arteriopathies that produce ICA stenosis, including atherosclerotic disease, dissection, fibromuscular dysplasia, pseudoaneurysm, and true aneurysm. This chapter focuses on specific technical approaches to prevent and manage complications and difficulties that may occur at each stage of CAS from puncture to closure of the femoral artery access site. The complications can be avoided or minimized and the patient's morbidity and mortality improved if the treating physician is aware of these nuances of complication avoidance and management. Although delayed neurologic, cardiac, and peripheral complications do occur, this chapter focuses on issues related to intraoperative complications that can be immediately identified and addressed, which in turn will minimize delayed morbidity.

SELECTING THE APPROPRIATE PATIENT FOR CAS

The most important factor for minimizing potential complications is selecting the appropriate patient for CAS.[13,14] Vascular anatomy that preempts difficult access (i.e., high degree of vessel tortuosity, circumferential calcification, type III arch, severe iliofemoral disease, string sign) and medical comorbidities (i.e., severe coronary artery disease [CAD]) should be considered. Patients with severe CAD have an increased risk for MI with hemodynamic changes associated with CAS. Therefore angioplasty after stenting is performed carefully to minimize any bradycardia or hypotensive episodes. Patients with recent large infarcts or crescendo transient ischemic attacks (TIAs) are at increased risk for neurologic perioperative complications, some of which may be attributed to reperfusion hemorrhage.[15,16] Waiting for 6 weeks after the ischemic event in patients with large infarcts before performing CAS may allow time for stabilization of cerebral collateralization and for infarct completion. Important to note is the fact that the greatest risk for stroke after TIAs and smaller infarcts is in the first 2 weeks after the event, so early treatment is warranted and newer technology along with careful technique will minimize risks. Although high-risk patients cannot be avoided entirely, identification of the high-risk criteria allows for appropriate perioperative planning minimizing complications. In addition, the circumstance may not allow a delay in treatment. Patients with a mobile thrombus or in urgent need of a coronary artery bypass graft (CABG) require prompt treatment; therefore perioperative blood pressure

*Rowling JK: *Harry Potter and the Chamber of Secrets*, New York, 1999, Scholastic Inc., page 333.

control is important to minimize complications. Patients with asymptomatic disease and severe medical comorbidities (ejection fraction less than 30%, active cardiac ischemia, severe chronic obstructive pulmonary disease, or severe peripheral vascular disease) may best be left alone if life expectancy appears less than 5 years. CEA remains a viable option for many of the high-risk CAS patients, and the two procedures appear complementary in most cases.

COMPLICATION MINIMIZATION AND MANAGEMENT

CAS is performed after the administration of mild sedation and local anesthesia. The patient is awake, which allows for rapid identification of neurologic changes and allows identification and management of potential problems that might otherwise not be identified until more serious sequelae are observed. Morbidity and mortality rates similar to those from published results have been achieved at our institute with the added benefit of a continuous neurologic examination.[17]

Preoperative Planning

Patients receive a loading dose of aspirin and clopidogrel 48 to 72 hours before CAS. Preferably, these patients should also receive aspirin and clopidogrel response tests because increasing numbers of aspirin nonresponders, as well as increased drug interactions with clopidogrel,[18] have been identified. The usual loading and daily doses used at our institution are a 650-mg loading dose with 320 mg daily for aspirin and a 600-mg loading dose with 75 mg daily for clopidogrel.

Arch type, determined by noninvasive imaging, should be reviewed,[19] and devices appropriate for the lesion should be chosen before treatment. Catheters should be on a continuous flush with normal saline solution with 5000 units of heparin at all times or, at minimum, should be flushed frequently. Air must be actively removed from each flush bag.

Femoral Artery Access

Femoral artery access is obtained with the goal being a single wall puncture and using Seldinger technique to place a 5F groin sheath. Brisk flow though the micropuncture needle will confirm arterial entry. Using the tip as a "sounding board" to transmit underlying pulsations of the artery and provide direction for access has worked well. Having a visual or audible recording of the patient's electrocardiogram can be helpful in cases of difficult access. In obese patients in whom palpation of a pulse is nearly impossible, the needle can be directed toward the superior medial quadrant of the femoral head under direct anteroposterior (AP) fluoroscopic guidance. Often, a 5F sheath is adequate to obtain initial runs, and a 6F Cook shuttle (Cook Medical, Bloomington, IN) can be used for stent deployment. A linear incision of approximately 0.5 cm is made to minimize soft-tissue hang-up when exchanging for the shuttle. This is best done before placement of the 5F sheath when the wire is in place. If proximal occlusion is needed, a 9F groin sheath is used for insertion of the necessary devices. A medium or long 9F sheath is used to minimize iliac injury. Whenever an 8F or larger groin sheath is used, a stiff exchange wire with its tip placed near the arch is recommended. An Amplatz J wire (Boston Scientific, Natick, MA) or a 0.038-inch wire can be used for this purpose. Appropriate dilation of the site is necessary, especially in patients with atherosclerosis. If any difficulty or resistance is observed, direct visualization of sheath placement under fluoroscopy is recommended. The case should be aborted if a dissection or significant hematoma develops, because subsequent heparinization may lead to worsening. Femoral artery runs should always be performed to confirm the absence of intimal injury, dissection, clot, or other complications. Entry approximately 1 cm above the inguinal fold or crease (approximately 3 cm below the inguinal line) usually yields arteriotomy entry above the bifurcation and below the inferior epigastric artery.

All team members should be aware of multiple puncture attempts or if access was difficult. Five to 10 minutes of manual compression may be sufficient before additional attempts are tried. If a sheath pass was attempted, either aborting an elective case or clamping the femoral arteriotomy in the groin and obtaining access via the femoral artery in the other groin is recommended. In either case, periodic assessment of the patient's groin for femoral pulses and development of a hematoma should be done throughout the case and if any hemodynamic instability occurs during the case. Careful review of the femoral artery run must be made in every case. Although bowel peristalsis can complicate some visualization, contrast extravasation cannot be missed.

At times, brachial or radial artery access can be used for stent delivery resulting from tortuosity or anatomic considerations. The same principles apply to access at these sites. The brachial site has a higher risk for direct nerve injury but is the only nonfemoral site that can tolerate a sheath larger than 6F.

Guide Catheter Placement

Vascular injury resulting in dissection or thrombotic occlusion, and thus stroke, can occur at any stage of wire or catheter manipulation. Therefore exquisite care must be taken to minimize direct catheter contact with the vascular luminal walls. A wire must always lead the catheter or a constant hemodynamic flux from the tip must be maintained to minimize this complication.

Multiple techniques are used to place the guide catheter into the common carotid artery (CCA). The most common technique involves the use of external carotid artery (ECA) branches as a support for device exchange. A diagnostic catheter is used to gain access to the CCA on the appropriate side. Under road map guidance, a relatively stiff exchange wire (0.035 stiff or 0.038-inch) is positioned into one of the distal ECA branches, ideally the occipital or posterior auricular branches. The biplane should be split so that the AP view can visualize the catheter around the arch, and the lateral view positioned at the neck can visualize the wire tip. Under direct visualization, an exchange is done. The diagnostic catheter is removed; the groin sheath is withdrawn. Direct pressure is maintained at the groin, while a 6F Cook shuttle (under flush) is exchanged over the wire. The insertion sheath of the shuttle must be held firmly in place so that there is a smooth transition from the tapered guide to the shuttle. Dry gauze should be available to aid with insertion of the shuttle at the groin. If there is difficultly going through soft tissue, the linear incision may need to be extended. If the shuttle inserts easily into the groin but there is difficulty at the femoral artery, the patient is asked to lift his or her hip on that side and this usually facilitates placement. In the event of any difficulty during placement, the shuttle should be placed under direct fluoroscopic visualization. Rarely, a 6F dilator can be used before insertion of the shuttle.

The patient can be heparinized for the procedure after the Cook shuttle is in the femoral artery and if there are no concerns with entry and the groin does not show any sign of hematoma. Glycopyrrolate is given at the same time as the heparin. With the AP plane in view of the arch and the lateral view showing the tip of the exchange wire in one of the external vessels, the shuttle is brought up into the CCA. Slight vibration of the shuttle, or "push-pull" of the catheter and wire, often yields manipulation of the catheter around difficult turns into the CCA. Once the shuttle is located approximately 5 cm from the carotid bifurcation, the insertion sheath and wire are pulled back as the shuttle is allowed to proceed further into the CCA, stopping approximately 3 cm before the bifurcation. The insertion sheath is not radiopaque and should not be kept in the shuttle close to the bifurcation because it might inadvertently cross the lesion. If the guide catheter will not navigate into the CCA, multiple attempts can cause the shuttle to herniate out of the CCA and back into the arch, and this can have deleterious consequences from an embolic standpoint. In such cases, the shuttle is left at the arch. The exchange wire is withdrawn, and a slip catheter is used for right-sided CAS or a Vitek catheter (Cook) is used for left-sided CAS. The insertion of an exchange wire through these bridging catheters can help to pass and stabilize the shuttle into the CCA. Rarely, a 6F or 7F Simmons 2 catheter (Codman Neurovascular, Raynham, MA) has to be used to obtain access.

Exchange from the ECA is safer than exchange in the CCA because there is less chance of inadvertently crossing the lesion. The rationale for placement into the occipital or greater auricular branch is that, in the rare instance of vessel perforation, a hematoma is more easily tolerated in these vessels than in the facial, lingual, or superficial temporal artery. The rare instance of ECA branch ruptures has been reported.[20] These events can be managed by intubation of the patient and direct tamponade of the hematoma. The procedure should be aborted and the heparin reversed. If massive swelling occurs as a result of rupture of the lingual artery, an emergent tracheostomy may be necessary. ECA vessel ruptures can be life threatening, and a tracheostomy set should always be available in the angiography suite. Once the airway has been secured, if the extravasation cannot be controlled by external pressure as documented on subsequent imaging, either temporary balloon occlusion or coil or glue (*N*-butyl cyanoacrylate) embolization of the vessel may be performed.

Rarely, exchange in the internal maxillary artery causes embolization into the ophthalmic collaterals, which may lead to visual loss. Embolization is also possible from superficial temporal artery collaterals. Once visual loss has occurred, angiography should be used to determine the location of the occlusion. Intra-arterial antiplatelet therapy into the ophthalmic artery can be used to sometimes open a central retinal artery occlusion. If a shower of emboli is suspected, a bolus dose of eptifibatide with or without a continuous infusion can be administered.

Embolic Protection

With the guide catheter safely in place, the next step is embolic protection. Distal filters are often used; however; proximal protection is now available and is preferred for recently symptomatic lesions, echolucent plaques, and other situations in which the embolic load is potentially large. Each time the lesion is crossed, there is a potential for embolic events to occur. According to a transcranial Doppler imaging study, the highest risk maneuver for embolic risk in unprotected stenting is postdilation angioplasty.[21] It is important to realize that microembolic phenomena occur at each stage of CAS and must be minimized. Distal embolic protection

(DEP) significantly lowers the risk of hits documented by transcranial Doppler imaging.[21]

Several DEP devices have been approved by the Food and Drug Administration for CAS: Accunet (Abbott Vascular, Santa Clara, CA), AngioGuard (Codman Neurovascular), Emboshield (Abbott), FiberNet (Lumen Biomedical, Plymouth, MN), Filterwire EZ (Boston Scientific), the Spider filter (ev3 Endovascular Plymouth, MN), and the PercuSurge balloon occlusion catheter (Medtronic AVE, Santa Rosa, CA). Proximal occlusion devices available are the MOMA (Invatec, Brescia, Italy) and the Gore flow reversal devices (W. L. Gore & Associates, Flagstaff, AZ). In our hands, a higher amount of embolic material seems to be recovered with use of proximal occlusion strategies; however, it is not clear whether this translates into less morbidity. In this section, we focus on complications with DEP devices.

A soft wire with slight curvature is used to cross the lesion under a highly magnified biplane road map. The ability to cross the lesion is the first critical step in stent deployment. Inability to cross the lesion after a few attempts should lead to reconsideration of CAS and possible abortion of the case, with CEA as an alternative. Rarely, the lesion can be crossed by the microwire, but the closed DEP cannot cross the lesion because of severe stenosis. In this rare instance, angioplasty with a small coronary balloon (Gateway [Boston Scientific] or Sprinter [Medtronic]) can facilitate DEP passage.

The filter should be sized to sufficiently oppose the carotid wall and deployed in a straight segment at the level of the arch of the C1 vertebra. Care should be taken to minimize wire tip placement intracranially. Operative complications with the filter can occur at any stage of exchange. The filter initially can be deployed inadvertently because of operator error. If the positioning is grossly in error, the filter can be captured and a new filter deployed. When unsheathing a filter or during device exchanges, the filter can be dragged along the ICA and even through the lesion. Extreme care must be taken with all exchanges. If significant DEP movement occurs during a procedure, carotid vasospasm may occur. This rarely requires treatment. However, improvement should be documented before removal of vascular access. If flow-limiting spasm persists, intra-arterial verapamil can be given.

If there is difficulty retrieving a device or if the retrieval catheter has been inadvertently misplaced or discarded, a 5F angled catheter can be used to recapture a DEP. In the extremely rare case of a free-floating filter, caused by shearing during recapture, a snare device or stenting the filter against the vessel lumen are options. Proximal occlusion should be considered during recovery maneuvers to minimize distal embolization. Alternatively, if the filter is thought to be full, a Penumbra suction catheter (Penumbra, Alameda, CA) can be positioned into a filter and the debris removed before recapture of the filter.

Predilation Angioplasty

Generally, a small balloon (3 × 30 mm) is used and underinflated. Blood pressure monitoring is critical at each dilational stage. Atropine may be necessary in the pre-CABG CAS patient. It is wise to have dopamine or phenylephrine infusions ready at the start of the case for rapid administration to avoid severe bradycardia and hypotension.

Stent Placement, Poststent Angioplasty, and Filter Capture

Stent placement complications usually involve deployment at the wrong site, in which case additional stents are usually deployed. Stenting along curvatures can be problematic, and forward energy is necessary to deliver the stent in the desired location. The use of intravascular ultrasound has aided in our choice of stent type, as well as judgment of the adequacy of apposition.

Another complication associated with stent deployment is subacute thrombosis. This has only been reported in two instances at our institute. Our practice is 4 weeks of dual antiplatelet therapy (aspirin and clopidogrel) and aspirin for life. The stent must be sized to the CCA, and the choice of stent cell size is dependent on plaque type and degree of tortuosity. Depending on how well the stent expands, poststent angioplasty is performed. The angioplasty balloon is chosen on the basis of the ICA dimensions.

Follow-up cervical carotid and intracranial runs are then performed and compared with previous imaging studies. If decreased ICA flow occurs after stent placement, severe spasm, dissection, plaque rupture, and a full filter must be considered as possible causes. Spasm should improve in subsequent runs. A dissection may need to be stented if it is flow limiting. Plaque rupture and a full filter must be carefully addressed. One option is to bring a Penumbra suction catheter into the filter to perform suction thrombectomy before filter capture. Another option is to drive the guide catheter (6F Cook) carefully through the stent to a position just proximal to the filter and then capture the filter with manual suction. The goal of these maneuvers is to prevent distal embolization of the embolic material within the full filter.

If filter capture proves difficult, turning the patient's head in a direction opposite to the vessel and asking him or her to inhale deeply can help straighten the vessel and facilitate recapture. If the sheath is impeded by the stent, rotation of the sheath as it is passed or repeated angioplasty with a larger balloon may help.

A 4F or 5F angled catheter can be used if all above maneuvers fail.

Femoral Closure

Review of the femoral artery angiogram will determine whether a percutaneous closure device can be used to close the arteriotomy and remove the groin sheath. Again, the sheath puncture should be above the carotid bifurcation and below the inferior epigastric artery. When in doubt, the sheath is left in place until the heparin wears off and then pressure is applied by hand and/or clamp. A clamp and hand pressure can be used to control any site bleeding, and rapid application of a clamp can be life saving when access through a 9F sheath is lost or a closure device has failed.

A Mynx device (Access Closure, Mountain View, CA) is used as our standard closure device for a 6F arteriotomy. This device causes minimum discomfort to the patient and can be used under direct fluoroscopic visualization in a patient with severely atherosclerotic iliofemoral disease. For a 7F or 8F arteriotomy, an 8F Angio-Seal (St. Jude Medical, St. Paul, MN) is used. For our 9F arteriotomies, two Perclose devices (Abbott Vascular) are used. Again, the importance of having extra hands and a clamp nearby cannot be overstated.

Intracranial Complications

Intracranial complications of CAS can be due to large-vessel occlusion, showering of emboli, or hemorrhage. In the acute phase, an intracranial angiogram should be performed and compared with preprocedure imaging studies to look for vessel cutoff, loss of capillary phase, or mass effect. If an acute occlusion is visualized, an immediate attempt to cross the lesion and recanalize the vessel with various modalities should be attempted. A Merci retriever (Concentric Medical, Mountain View, CA) or Penumbra can be used with or without intra-arterial thrombolysis. Intracranial stenting and angioplasty can also be attempted if necessary for large-vessel occlusion. A microcatheter run in conjunction with a guide catheter run should be performed to confirm the length of the occlusion and ensure that no contrast extravasation has occurred.

If a large area of loss of capillary phase is observed or if no obvious pathology is appreciated, the procedure should be completed as quickly and safely as possible, minimizing any further potential embolic risk. A non—contrast-enhanced computed tomographic (CT) scan should be obtained to exclude the presence of an intracranial hemorrhage. Protamine should be given immediately if a reperfusion hemorrhage is appreciated and systolic blood pressure maintained below 140 mm Hg. A repeated CT scan should be performed 2 to 3 hours later to ensure no further expansion or increase in the size of the hemorrhage. If the hemorrhage is expanding or life threatening, administration of recombinant factor VII and/or reversal of the antiplatelet agents may be necessary. If no intracranial hemorrhage is present, glycoprotein IIb/IIIa antiplatelet agents should be administered as a bolus dose plus a continuous infusion with a follow-up CT scan obtained 6 and 24 hours after the procedure to ensure absence of hemorrhagic conversion.

In-Stent Stenosis

The commonest complication after CAS is in-stent stenosis. Fortunately the need for re-treatment is not common. On long-term follow-up, in-stent narrowing of ≥40% diameter reduction has been observed in 42.7% of patients and of ≥60% diameter reduction in 16.4% at 5 years of follow-up.[22] Similarly, the SAPPHIRE investigators reported in-stent stenosis in 19.7% of patients at 1 year of follow-up.[23] Post-CAS in-stent stenosis is treated at a threshold of ≥80% diameter reduction or with neurologic symptoms.[24] Suggested predictors of in-stent restenosis after CAS are advanced age, female sex, implantation of multiple stents, previous carotid revascularization treatment, suboptimal result with residual stenosis, elevated postprocedural serum levels of acute-phase reactants, asymptomatic lesion, and use of balloon-expandable stents.[25] The treatment options for severe (>80%) in-stent stenosis are balloon angioplasty, repeated stenting, cutting balloon, and cutting balloon plus stent. In our series, in-stent stenosis was observed in 33 patients, and 12 of them were treated by endovascular means.

ILLUSTRATIVE CASE

Intraoperative Stroke Causing Neurologic Deficit (National Institutes of Health Stroke Scale 21)

This 75-year-old, right-handed, white man had a right hemispheric stroke in 2001 that resulted in mild left-upper extremity paresis. He had a chronic left ICA occlusion and had undergone two right CEAs (the site of the second CEA had been repaired with a patch graft). He presented with asymptomatic right ICA restenosis of greater than 80% identified on a preoperative evaluation for surgical biopsy and excision of a newly identified hilar mass. The cardiothoracic team requested a neurosurgical consultation regarding a treatment strategy for the patient's restenosis. The patient's history was also remarkable for MI, CAD, hypertension, dyslipidemia, type 2 diabetes, gastroesophageal reflux disease, and

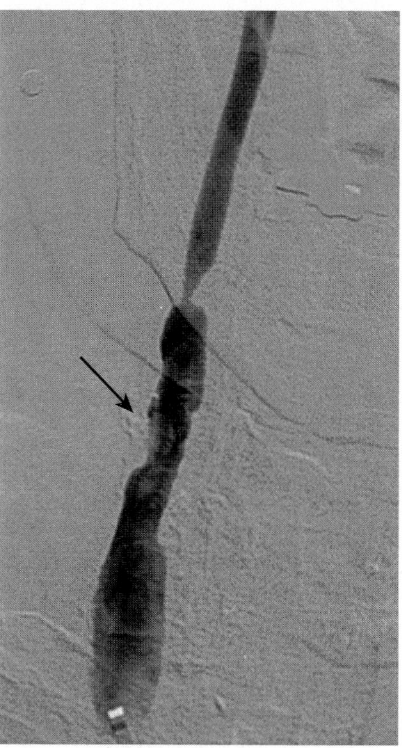

FIGURE 39-1 AP right carotid cervical angiogram shows long-segment, ulcerative stenosis. Notice the irregularity of the patch graft *(arrow)*.

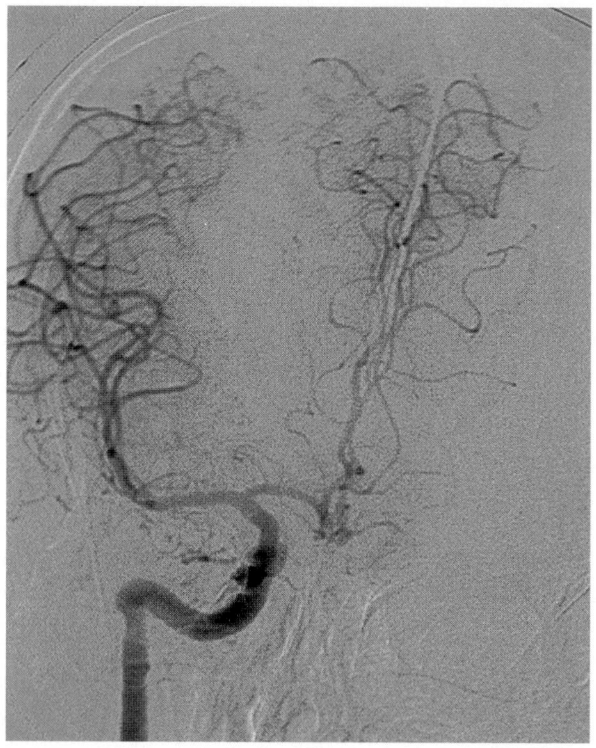

FIGURE 39-2 Right carotid injection, intracranial run, shows filling of both A2s from the right side (the patient had chronic left ICA occlusion).

chronic obstructive pulmonary disease. He was a smoker and had a family history of CAD and hypertension. He was taking aspirin and clopidogrel and had a mild left hemiparesis (grade 4/5) with a left pronator drift. His Karnofsky score was approximately 90.

On the basis of this information, the patient was scheduled for an angiogram and CAS with the expectation that he would be enrolled into the SAPPHIRE trial (AngioGuard embolic protection and Precise stent [Codman Neurovascular]). Femoral artery access was obtained without difficulty. Femoral artery runoff showed no contrast extravasation, no intimal injury, and no dissection or clot.

The angiogram showed a long-segment (65 mm), irregular, ulcerative stenosis of 81% in severity (Figure 39-1). Both A2s filled from the right side (consistent with the patient's history of chronic left ICA occlusion) (Figure 39-2). Figure 39-3 shows capillary filling throughout the right hemisphere despite the history of previous right-sided stroke with residual left-sided hemiparesis.

A 0.038-inch exchange wire was used to bring a 6F Cook shuttle into the top of the aortic arch. After removal of the Simmons 2 catheter and the groin sheath, a Vitek catheter was advanced through the shuttle and used as a bridge to advance the shuttle safely into the right CCA. The patient was given 5000 units of heparin, yielding an activated coagulation time of 230 seconds. The patient was then given an additional 1000 units of heparin plus glycopyrrolate. A 6-mm Angioguard was brought across the lesion and deployed at the level of the C1 arch. A Precise stent was brought up and deployed, covering the distal portion of the lesion. Because of the length of the lesion, the preoperative plan was to deploy two stents for adequate coverage. Contrast stasis could be visualized within the patch graft (Figure 39-4).

Soon after deployment of the first stent, the patient started to become restless and stopped speaking. Within minutes, a dense right hemiparesis had developed. The intracranial run showed flash filling of the anterior cerebral artery (Figure 39-5). Remembering that the patient had a chronic left ICA occlusion, it was thought that the new deficit was probably flow-related ischemia from spasm around the catheter or a full filter. Because the catheter was in the CCA, a full filter was more likely the cause.

The second stent was quickly deployed across the proximal portion of the lesion, overlapping the first stent. Another intracranial run after deployment of the second stent showed no changes (Figure 39-6). The patient's deficits remained unchanged. The filter capture

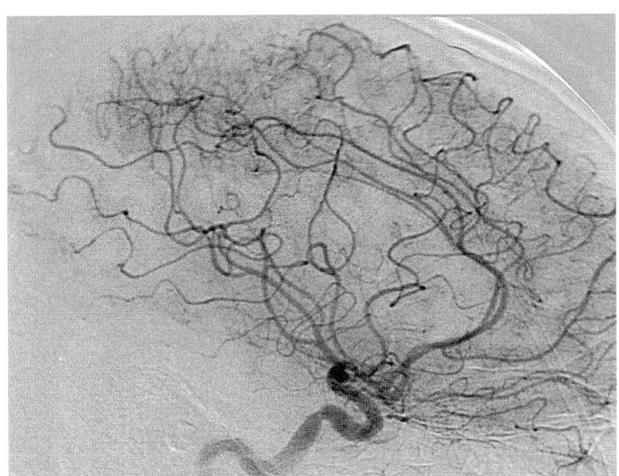

FIGURE 39-3 Right carotid injection, lateral intracranial view, shows full late arterial/early capillary phase throughout the hemisphere.

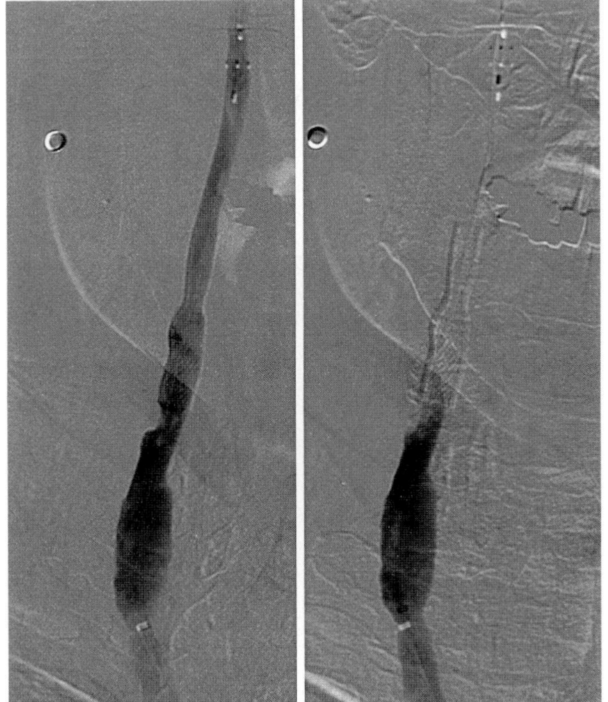

FIGURE 39-4 Right CCA injection, AP cervical view, after stent deployment. Notice the contrast stasis within the patch graft (*right*, delayed view).

device was quickly brought up and the filter recaptured. *Was the diagnosis of left hemispheric ischemia from a full filter correct? In this case, was directly capturing the filter the best maneuver?*

An intracranial run was obtained showing a wedge-shaped loss of late arterial/capillary phase (Figure 39-7). A large amount of debris and plaque was visualized

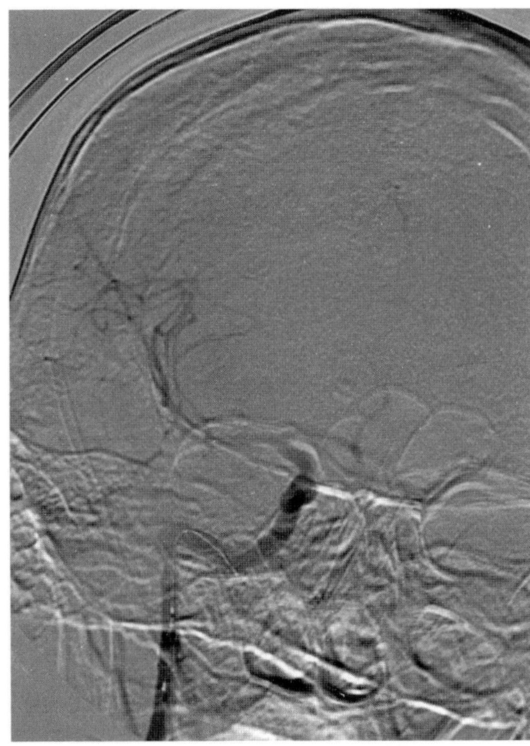

FIGURE 39-5 Right carotid injection, intracranial view, AP, shows trace anterior cerebral artery filling as compared with the prestent angiogram (see Figure 39-2).

within the filter. Intra-arterial eptifibatide was given. Catheters were removed, and a 7F groin sheath was left in place. The patient was taken for a CT scan on an emergency basis. On the way to the scanner, his right side returned to baseline strength and he regained some speech; however, he now developed left-sided hemiparesis.

The CT showed hypodensity consistent with the patient's old infarct (Figure 39-8). He continued to be given eptifibatide overnight, and a magnetic resonance imaging study was obtained in the morning (Figure 39-9). The diffusion-weighted imaging pattern was consistent with an embolic shower that was not present on the postoperative CT or CT perfusion images.

The patient's postprocedure National Institutes of Health Stroke Scale score was 21. His anticoagulation therapy was eventually bridged to warfarin. "Do-not-resuscitate" and "do-not-intubate" orders were placed. The remainder of his hospital course was complicated by MI and new-onset afibrillation. He was transferred to a rehabilitation facility with a National Institutes of Health Stroke Scale score of 14 but eventually died of complications of pneumonia.

There are several teaching points from this case. *Should this patient with an undiagnosed lung lesion have been treated? Should more preoperative imaging have been obtained instead of scheduling this patient for same-day*

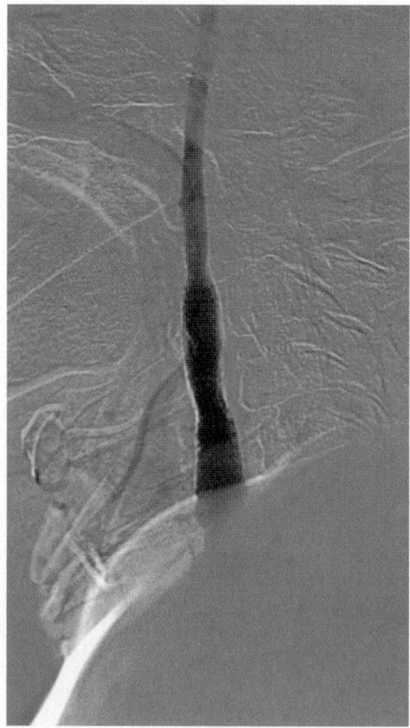

FIGURE 39-6 Right CCA injection, cervical lateral view, shows coverage of the stenosis with both stents with persistent contrast stasis.

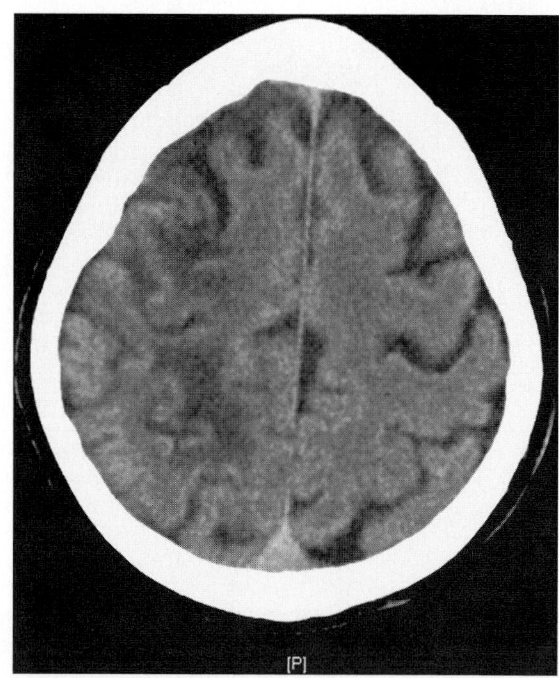

FIGURE 39-8 Postprocedure CT image does not show any new infarcts.

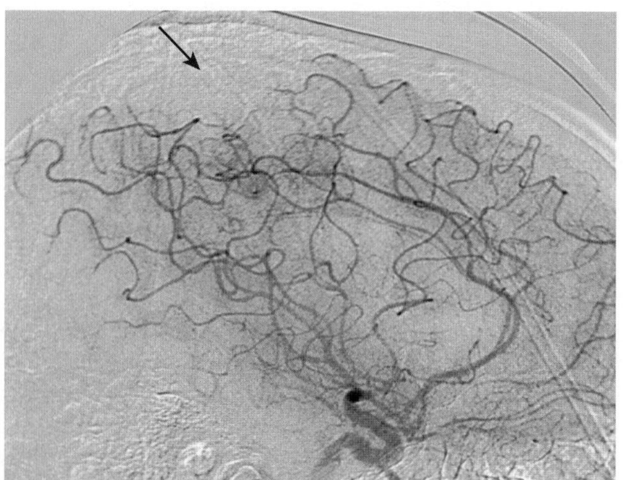

FIGURE 39-7 Loss of capillary phase when compared with Figure 39-3, as shown by *arrow.*

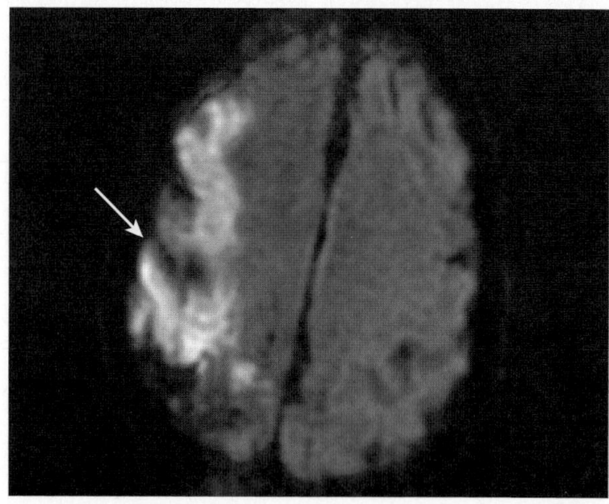

FIGURE 39-9 Diffusion-weighted magnetic resonance image shows new diffusion defects consistent with new stroke *(arrow).*

angiography and CAS? The patient was placed into a study that had devices that may not have been the best suited for his lesion. Imaging suggested the potential for large clot burden, and perhaps a different filter choice or proximal protection would have been a better option. As discussed in the previous section on full filters, a better method for the management of the full filter rather than direct capture might have minimized the patient's embolic risk. Use of a Penumbra catheter to perform suction thrombectomy or advancement of the Cook shuttle might have yielded a better clinical outcome.

SUMMARY

Patient selection is critical to minimizing CAS morbidity and mortality. Patients with asymptomatic disease and severe medical comorbidities (ejection fraction less than 30%, active cardiac ischemia, severe chronic obstructive pulmonary disease, or severe peripheral vascular disease) may be best left alone. Patients with difficult vascular anatomy may be best left to medical management if safe guide catheter placement would not be possible. Severely calcified, high lesions may be best treated by CEA.

Once an appropriate patient is chosen, adequate noninvasive preoperative imaging should be obtained, including aortic arch studies. Appropriate devices should be chosen. Medical optimization and preoperative dual platelet therapy and documentation of therapeutic response tests are necessary before intervention.

Technical problems with filters and stents can be minimized by a thorough understanding of the mechanism of deployment of each device before performing the procedure. Bailout techniques for various intraoperative complications have been reviewed. CAS can be performed with low morbidity and mortality. However, each stage of the procedure has the potential to be life threatening. An understanding of the implications of each stage of CAS, meticulous perioperative care, and careful patient selection will maximize the clinical benefit of the procedure. The pathogenesis and factors affecting in-stent stenosis have to be studied in further detail to modify our stent choices, patient selection, and technique that will reduce the incidence of in-stent stenosis.

References

1. CaRESS Steering Committee: Carotid revascularization using endarterectomy or stenting systems (CARESS): phase I clinical trial, *J Endovasc Ther* 10(6):1021–1030, 2003.
2. CaRESS Steering Committee: Carotid Revascularization Using Endarterectomy or Stenting Systems (CaRESS) phase I clinical trial: 1-year results, *J Vasc Surg* 42(2):213–219, 2005.
3. Bosiers M, Peeters P, Deloose K, Verbist J, Sievert H, Sugita J, Castriota F, Cremonesi A: Does carotid artery stenting work on the long run: 5-year results in high-volume centers (ELOCAS Registry), *J Cardiovasc Surg (Torino)* 46(3):241–247, 2005.
4. Das S, Bendok BR, Getch CC, et al: Update on current registries and trials of carotid artery angioplasty and stent placement, *Neurosurg Focus* 18(1):e2, 2005.
5. Gray WA, Hopkins LN, Yadav S, et al: Protected carotid stenting in high-surgical-risk patients: The ARCHeR results, *J Vasc Surg* 44(2):258–268, 2006.
6. Hopkins LN, Myla S, Grube E, Wehman JC, Levy EI, Bersin RM, Joye JD, Allocco DJ, Kelley L, Baim DS: Carotid artery revascularization in high surgical risk patients with the NexStent and the Filterwire EX/EZ: 1-year results in the CABERNET trial, *Catheter Cardiovasc Interv* 71(7):950–960, 2008.
7. Ramee S, for the Evaluation of the Medtronic AVE Self-expanding Carotid Stent System with Distal Protection in the Treatment of Carotid Stenosis (MAVEriC) Investigators: *Preliminary data from the MAVEriC I & II carotid stenting clinical trials (presentation)*, Washington DC, September 29, 2004, Presented at Transcatheter Cardiovascular Therapeutics (TCT) Meeting.
8. Safian RD, Bresnahan JF, Jaff MR, et al: Protected carotid stenting in high-risk patients with severe carotid artery stenosis, *J Am Coll Cardiol* 47(12):2384–2389, 2006.
9. White CJ, Iyer SS, Hopkins LN, et al: Carotid stenting with distal protection in high surgical risk patients: the BEACH trial 30 day results, *Catheter Cardiovasc Interv* 67(4):503–512, 2006.
10. Whitlow P: Registry Study to Evaluate the Neuroshield Bare Wire Cerebral Protection System and X-Act Stent in Patients at High Risk for Carotid Endarterectomy (SECuRITY): *Carotid artery stenting with a distal-protection device safe in high-risk patients*, Washington DC. 2003, September 17, 2003, Presented at Transcatheter Cardiovascular Therapeutics Meeting.
11. Yadav JS, Wholey MH, Kuntz RE, et al: Protected carotid-artery stenting versus endarterectomy in high-risk patients, *N Engl J Med* 351(15):1493–1501, 2004.
12. Anonymous. CAS: Clinical Trial Update, *Endovascular Today* 279. September 2004.
13. Goldstein LB, McCrory DC, Landsman PB, et al: Multicenter review of preoperative risk factors for carotid endarterectomy in patients with ipsilateral symptoms, *Stroke* 25(6):1116–1121, 1994.
14. Ouriel K, Hertzer NR, Beven EG, et al: Preprocedural risk stratification: identifying an appropriate population for carotid stenting, *J Vasc Surg* 33(4):728–732, 2001.
15. Meyer FB editor: *Sundt's occlusive cerebrovascular disease*, ed 2, Philadelphia (576 pages), 2004, W.B. Saunders.
16. Pritz MB: Timing of carotid endarterectomy after stroke, *Stroke* 28 (12):2563–2567, 1997.
17. Ecker RD, Sauvageau E, Levy EI, et al: Complications of carotid artery stenting at a high-volume teaching center: experience of University at Buffalo endovascular fellows from 2004 to 2006, *Neurosurgery* 62(4):812–816, 2008.
18. Ho PM, Maddox TM, Wang L, et al: Risk of adverse outcomes associated with concomitant use of clopidogrel and proton pump inhibitors following acute coronary syndrome, *JAMA* 301 (9):937–944, 2009.
19. Bates ER, Babb JD, Casey DE Jr, et al: ACCF/SCAI/SVMB/SIR/ASITN 2007 clinical expert consensus document on carotid stenting: a report of the American College of Cardiology Foundation Task Force on Clinical Expert Consensus Documents (ACCF/SCAI/SVMB/SIR/ASITN Clinical Expert Consensus Document Committee on Carotid Stenting), *J Am Coll Cardiol* 49 (1):126–170, 2007.
20. Ecker RD, Guidot CA, Hanel RA, et al: Perforation of external carotid artery branch arteries during endoluminal carotid revascularization procedures: consequences and management, *J Invasive Cardiol* 17(6):292–295, 2005.
21. Al-Mubarak N, Roubin GS, Vitek JJ, et al: Microembolization during carotid stenting with the distal-balloon antiemboli system, *Int Angiol* 21(4):344–348, 2002.
22. Lal BK, Hobson RW 2nd, Goldstein J, et al: In-stent recurrent stenosis after carotid artery stenting: life table analysis and clinical relevance, *J Vasc Surg* 38(6):1162–1168. discussion 1169, 2003.

23. Gurm HS, Yadav JS, Fayad P, et al: Long-term results of carotid stenting versus endarterectomy in high-risk patients, *N Engl J Med* 358(15):1572–1579, 2008.
24. Lal BK, Kaperonis EA, Cuadra S, et al: Patterns of in-stent restenosis after carotid artery stenting: classification and implications for long-term outcome, *J Vasc Surg* 46(5):833–840, 2007.
25. Van Laanen J, Hendriks JM, Van Sambeek MR: Factors influencing restenosis after carotid artery stenting, *J Cardiovasc Surg (Torino)* 49(6):743–747, 2008.

SECTION VII

VASCULAR GRAFT THROMBOSIS

CHAPTER

40

Aortoiliac Graft Limb Occlusion: Thrombolysis, Mechanical Thrombectomy

Ramyar Gilani, Vikram S. Kashyap

Aortoiliac occlusive disease (AIOD) and abdominal aortic aneurysms are common clinical problems in vascular surgery. In contemporary practice, endovascular treatment of AIOD has replaced many of the open reconstruction operations including aortobifemoral and aortoiliac bypass grafting.[1] Still, aortofemoral and aortoiliac bypass grafting remains an important treatment modality for AIOD, as well as aneurysm disease, for selected patients. Furthermore, many patients continue to survive with grafts placed before the 1990s when few endovascular options existed. In the properly selected patient, patency rates of aortoiliac grafts are excellent, approaching 85% to 90% at 5 years in a review of the literature.[2] Graft limb occlusion in grafts placed for aneurysm disease has been reported at 2%.[3] The main cause of limb failure in both aortoiliac and aortofemoral grafts is progression of atherosclerosis in the superficial or deep femoral artery or intimal hyperplasia at the distal graft-artery anastomosis. Progression of atherosclerosis at the proximal anastomosis of aortoiliac or aortofemoral grafts is rare unless the proximal anastomosis is placed far below the renal arteries where the aorta may be susceptible to further plaque development. Intimal hyperplasia, common at the distal site, is a rare cause of proximal anastomotic stenosis or occlusion because of the large caliber of both the aorta and the graft at that location. Dacron and polytetrafluoroethylene are the most common types of graft used for aortic reconstruction in this location. Graft type does not appear to be a factor in the incidence of limb graft failure.

Similar to AIOD treatment, endovascular therapy has supplanted open reconstruction for abdominal aortic aneurysm to a great extent. Endovascular aneurysm repair (EVAR) has dramatically changed treatment paradigms for aortic aneurysm disease. Stent grafts have been used to treat AIOD as well, although to a limited degree. These stent graft devices are a composed of a self-expanding stent exoskeleton that provides radial force while supporting a fabric-lined channel that aims to contain flow within the fabric lumen, thereby depressurizing the aneurysm sac and preventing rupture. As the experience with EVAR continues to grow, a set of complications unique to this procedure has been identified including endograft limb occlusion (ELO). Observed rates of iliac limb occlusion are less than 10%, making it a relatively uncommon event.[4] Reasons for ELO are numerous but include neck angulation, graft oversizing, external compression, change in aneurysm shape, as well as the other nonspecific causes, which are intimal hyperplasia, progressive atherosclerosis, and embolism. Technical risk factors associated with ELO include use of unibody unsupported endografts and extension of the iliac limb into the external iliac artery.[5] A contemporary vascular practice may see patients with aortoiliac graft limb occlusion in the setting of prior open or endovascular therapy. Of note, the restoration of patency for either graft or stent graft can be accomplished via similar techniques.

PRESENTATION

Regardless of previous aortoiliac intervention methodology, graft limb thrombosis in this arterial segment often manifests as acute limb ischemia (ALI). Classically, the findings associated with ALI are summarized by the 5 P's, including pulselessness, pain, pallor, paresthesia, and paralysis, listed in order of appearance from the original insult. The extent of ischemia is better categorized by using the modified Rutherford criteria for ALI.[6] Class I represents a viable limb that is not immediately threatened and limb salvage is possible with proper management. Class II limbs are severely ischemic and require expeditious workup and urgent intervention to preserve the limb. A distinction is made between class IIa and class IIb by which in the latter patients have progressive motor dysfunction. Class III ischemia describes an irreversibly ischemic foot in which limb salvage is usually not possible regardless of therapy and that would often require primary amputation.

In addition to findings localized to the ischemic bed, patients with acute arterial occlusion can often demonstrate systemic ischemic sequelae having a profound impact on the pulmonary, circulatory, and renal systems. However, not all patients with aortoiliac occlusion present with ALI. Depending on the degree of collateralization present, a wide spectrum of presentations is possible, including short-distance claudication and rest pain.

TREATMENT

Once a diagnosis of aortoiliac limb occlusion is established, then the focus is turned toward selecting the appropriate management. Initial maneuvers include systemic anticoagulation usually with heparin to inhibit clot propagation and prevent further clinical deterioration. Simultaneous resuscitation with intravenous fluids is also initiated to prepare a patient for surgery. Urgent evaluation for surgical therapy and/or thrombolysis is performed. Depending on the severity of the ischemia and condition of the patient, preoperative imaging may be obtained including computed tomographic angiography. Oftentimes, imaging data must be obtained by means available in the operating room. An endovascular suite allows high-quality angiography and on-table decision making for open versus endovascular therapies.

Traditionally, treatment of an occluded graft limb or stent graft would consist of open surgical intervention. Most commonly, this is a thromboembolectomy via an ipsilateral groin incision. Operative thromboembolectomy does allow one to examine the femoral anastomosis: the common "culprit" lesion for graft thrombosis. These lesions can be treated with patch angioplasty or revising the limb to the profunda femoris artery. Even though this usually is a straightforward procedure, there are multiple technical limitations. During ipsilateral thromboembolectomy, embolization to the contralateral leg can occur. Often robust inflow is not achieved with thromboembolectomy, necessitating extra-anatomic operations (i.e., femoral-to-femoral crossover, axillofemoral) that have inferior durability.[7] Thromboembolectomy without preoperative angiography precludes complete information regarding outflow, thrombus burden, distal embolization, and hemodynamics. Completion angiography after operative treatment is oftentimes cumbersome.

With recent advances in technology, a new spectrum of percutaneous methods is available to treat thromboembolism of aortoiliac grafts. These can be divided into two subcategories based on mechanism of action. First, and perhaps the more widely used of the two, is chemical thrombolysis. This technique relies on the delivery of a pharmacologic agent to the thrombus resulting in dissolution of the thrombus. Agents used for thrombolysis are classically plasminogen activators converting plasminogen into plasmin. Current agents preferentially cleave fibrin-bound plasminogen but have the potential to induce a systemic fibrinolytic state. A second category of percutaneous techniques is percutaneous mechanical thrombectomy (PMT), which is gaining more acceptance. PMT implies delivery of an intra-arterial device to the thrombus that fragments thrombus through mechanical forces. The selection of one treatment modality does not exclude the utilization of the other. Often the two techniques are used concurrently resulting in synergistic clot dissolution while striving to keep the complication rates minimized and limiting treatment times.

THROMBOLYSIS

Patient selection for thrombolysis is dependent on variables related to the patient, the disease process, and the likelihood that it will be successful. Questions to consider before starting thrombolysis include the following: (1) Can the patient tolerate the length of treatment? (2) Is the amount of thrombus burden suitable for thrombolysis? (3) Is the thrombus in an accessible location? (4) Will the potential benefit exceed the risks associated with thrombolysis? Candidates for treatment will predominately present with Rutherford class I and IIA ischemia. Some patients with class IIB ischemia can be considered solely for thrombolysis particularly if patient factors preclude open surgery and no other percutaneous methods are available. Of note, combining thrombolysis with PMT often lessens treatment time, allowing prompt restoration of some flow after initial treatment. Factors correlating with successful thrombolysis of an occluded bypass graft are (1) if the graft occlusion occurred within 14 days, (2) if a guidewire is able to traverse the area of occlusion, (3) if the graft has been in place for over a year, and (4) if a underlying causative lesion is discovered. Factors known to correlate with poor outcomes include diabetes, continued tobacco use, prosthetic graft material, and the inability to identify a "culprit" lesion.[8]

Before proceeding, details unveiled in the history and physical examination will aid in determining an access site. As mentioned before, preoperative imaging is often not available before intervention. Therefore the clinician must be attentive to details relating to prior interventions and pulse examination as guidance toward an appropriate access site. Patients with prior aortoiliac bypass grafting, iliac stenting, or EVAR have a narrow aortic neobifurcation that can be very challenging to gain access into from the contralateral side. It is prudent to avoid access sites in a region distal to the anticipated area of treatment. Along the same lines, multiple punctures at the access site must be avoided, and this is best done by gaining access with ultrasound imaging assistance. In the setting of aortoiliac graft occlusion, often the access site is the left brachial artery for reasons mentioned before (Figure 40-1). Via the left brachial artery, it is possible to reach a target area down to the level of the knees with currently available catheters. Sometimes, however, retrograde access is necessary to gain access across the affected area or perhaps to treat an underlying culprit lesion.

After access is established, an attempt is made to cross the length of thrombus with a wire before initiation of lysis, the so-called "guidewire traversal test" (Figure 40-2). If the wire is passed successfully, then success with lysis is thought to be more likely.[9] If the guidewire fails to pass, then regional thrombolysis can be used and reattempt performed in 6 hours. Once the infusion catheter is placed in the proper position (Figure 40-3), the thrombus is laced with the selected agent before lysis. Studies suggest that intrathrombus bolus of a lytic agent shortens the duration of lytic therapy.[10,11] Patients return for lysis checks every 12 to 24 hours and are monitored in the intensive care unit with special attention to complications of thrombolysis and response to therapy. Results of lytic therapy are quantified and graded according to definitions described in the National Audit of Thrombolysis for Acute Leg Ischemia (NATALI) database.[12] After an adequate level of clearance is achieved within the thrombosed vessel segment, an underlying causative lesion (Figure 40-4) may be identified and should be treated accordingly (Figure 40-5). The discovery of such culprit lesions weighs favorably on outcomes. Sullivan et al.[13] reported postthrombolysis 2-year patency rates of 79% in bypass graft where a flow-limiting lesion was identified in comparison with 9.8% when no such lesion was found.

PERCUTANEOUS MECHANICAL THROMBECTOMY

Despite tremendous success with thrombolysis, several aspects of the technique remain as disadvantageous limitations. First, thrombolysis requires time, at least 6 hours, to take effect, which is not always an abundant commodity when treating ALI. This fact restricts the

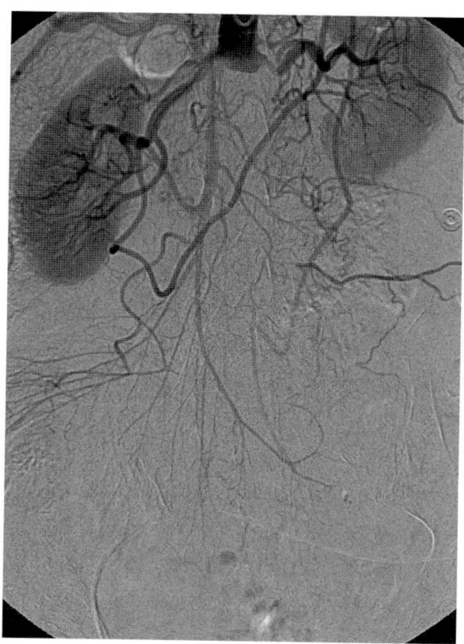

FIGURE 40-1 A 53-year-old woman presented with right leg acute limb ischemia. She had undergone aortic reconstruction in the early 1990s and a left hip disarticulation for ischemia and infection in 1998 at another institution. Aortography via a left brachial artery approach was performed and demonstrated an occluded aortobifemoral bypass graft.

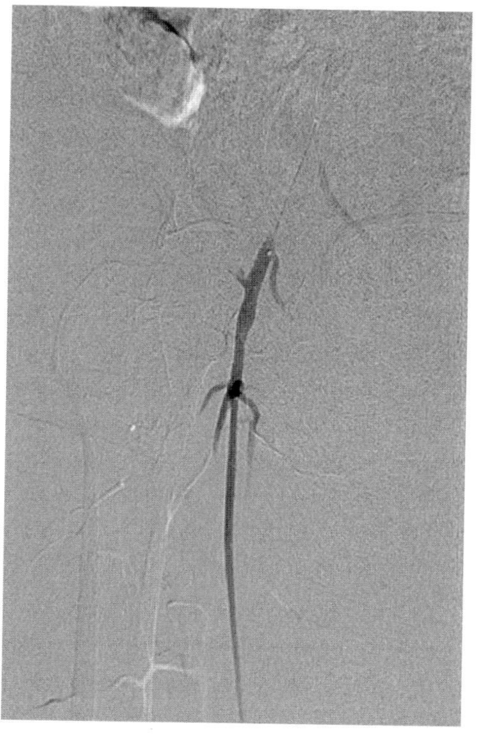

FIGURE 40-2 The right limb of the aortobifemoral bypass was crossed with use of a hydrophilic guidewire and catheter with relative ease indicating a fresh thrombus column ("guidewire traversal test"). Distal arteriography indicates patent common femoral and lower extremity arteries.

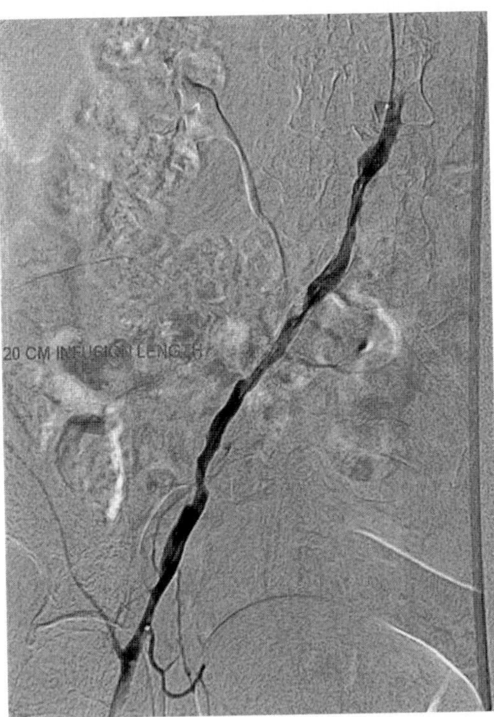

FIGURE 40-3 PMT allowed prograde perfusion soon after patient presentation. A long infusion catheter was used for catheter-directed thrombolysis with use of tissue plasminogen activator for the remnant thrombus.

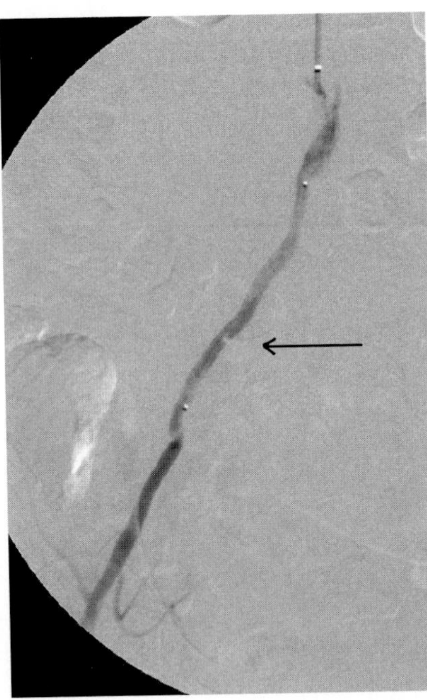

FIGURE 40-4 After 24 hours of thrombolysis, all of the thrombus burden was dissolved revealing the culprit lesion in the limb of the graft.

use of thrombolysis to Rutherford class I and IIA with certain exceptions. Second, greater thrombus burden along with longer infusion times impact the rate of complications. Hence the need to restore circulation in

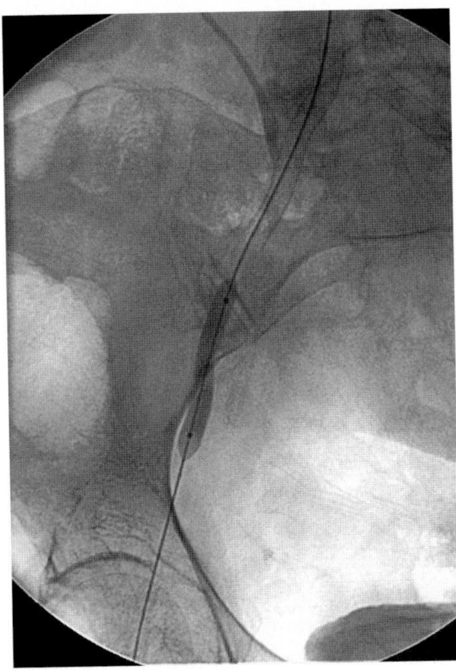

FIGURE 40-5 Percutaneous balloon angioplasty with a 7-mm semicompliant balloon was performed to treat the stenosis and restore normal perfusion to the leg.

a minimally invasive manner with the least amount of exposure to a lytic agent is created. This is the void filled by PMT. Current commercially available PMT devices are classified on the basis of mechanism of action as follows: clot aspiration devices, clot maceration devices, and acoustic energy disruption devices.[8] Because of the risk of embolization, clot maceration devices have little to no role in peripheral artery applications.

The AngioJet (Possis Medical, Inc., Minneapolis, MN) is an example of a clot aspiration device approved for peripheral artery interventions. The principle of the device surrounds employing the Venturi effect to aspirate thrombus. Furthermore, using the power-pulse spray technique, the catheter can be configured to infuse pressurized lytic agent into the thrombus thereby theoretically gaining better clot penetration. This bolused volume of agent is thought to be removed along with thrombus during aspiration and thought not to contribute toward systemic fibrinolysis.[14] When considering a patient with aortoiliac limb occlusion for PMT, those principles applicable to thrombolysis are adhered to once again. However, PMT enables the clinician to restore flow in a more expeditious manner than thrombolysis alone therefore expanding treatment not only to patients with class I and IIA ischemia but to patients with class IIB as well. Using PMT, it has been shown that flow can be reestablished within 72 minutes, which is comparable to results with traditional open techniques.[15]

The course for PMT follows in a similar manner to that of thrombolysis with a few key technical considerations. Once the catheter is properly positioned, clot aspiration is not immediately performed. Rather the clot is laced with a minimal amount of lytic agent (2 mg tissue plasminogen activator in 50 mL normal saline solution) with use of the power-pulse spray technique. After 20 minutes, clot aspiration commences with multiple antegrade and retrograde passes. The thrombus burden in an occluded aortoiliac graft can be large and cause hemolysis leading to renal dysfunction. This drawback can be avoided by limiting the volume of infusate to 500 mL.[8] In the setting of ELO, a theoretical disadvantage of PMT is the increased risk of graft dislodgment and creating type II endoleaks. This theoretical problem has not been seen clinically in our experience.

Despite numerous advantages with PMT, this remains mostly an adjunct to thrombolysis for ALI. PMT is quite effective at reestablishing flow in an expeditious manner and decreasing thrombus burden. In practice, PMT may be used as monotherapy in only 20% to 50% of cases, but in greater than 50% of cases further therapy with thrombolysis will be needed for remaining thrombus burden.[16] Therefore both therapies must be considered in a synergistic approach for the treatment of aortoiliac limb occlusion to potentiate quality outcome while striving to minimize adverse events.

References

1. Upchurch GR, Dimick JB, Wainess RM, et al: Diffusion of new technology in health care: the case of aorto-iliac occlusive disease, *Surgery* 136(4):812–818, 2004.
2. de Vries SO, Hunink MG: Results of aortic bifurcation grafts for aortoiliac occlusive disease: a meta-analysis, *J Vasc Surg* 26 (4):558–569, 1997.
3. Hallett JW Jr, Marshall DM, Petterson TM, et al: Graft-related complications after abdominal aortic aneurysm repair: reassurance from a 36-year population-based experience, *J Vasc Surg* 25 (2):277–284, 1997.
4. Bohannon WT, Hodgson KJ, Parra JR, et al: Endovascular management of iliac limb occlusion of bifurcated aortic endografts, *J Vasc Surg* 35(3):584–588, 2002.
5. Erzurum VZ, Sampram ES, Sarac TP, et al: Initial management and outcome of aortic endograft limb occlusion, *J Vasc Surg* 40(3):419–423, 2004.
6. Rutherford RB, Baker JD, Ernst C, et al: Recommended standards for reports dealing with lower extremity ischemia: revised version, *J Vasc Surg* 26(3):517–538, 1997.
7. Hertzer NR, Bena JF, Karafa MT: A personal experience with direct reconstruction and extra-anatomic bypass for aortoiliofemoral occlusive disease, *J Vasc Surg* 45(3):527–535, 2007.
8. Kashyap VS, Ouriel K: Thrombolysis and mechanical thrombectomy for acute arterial occlusions: current status and future directions, *Adv Vasc Surg* 12:41–57, 2006.
9. Patel N, Sacks D, Patel RI, et al: SCVIR reporting standards for the treatment of acute limb ischemia with use of transluminal removal of arterial thrombus, *J Vasc Interv Radiol* 12(5):559–570, 2001.
10. Thrombolysis in the management of lower limb peripheral arterial occlusion: a consensus document, *J Vasc Interv Radiol* 14 (9 Pt 2):S337–S349, 2003.
11. Valji K, Roberts AC, Davis GB, et al: Pulsed-spray thrombolysis of arterial and bypass graft occlusions, *AJR Am J Roentgenol* 156 (3):617–621, 1991.
12. Earnshaw JJ, Whitman B, Foy C: National Audit of Thrombolysis for Acute Leg Ischemia (NATALI): clinical factors associated with early outcome, *J Vasc Surg* 39(5):1018–1025, 2004.
13. Sullivan KL, Gardiner GA Jr, Kandarpa K, et al: Efficacy of thrombolysis in infrainguinal bypass grafts, *Circulation* 83(Suppl 2):I99–105, 1991.
14. Kasirajan K, Gray B, Beavers FP, et al: Rheolytic thrombectomy in the management of acute and subacute limb-threatening ischemia, *J Vasc Interv Radiol* 12(4):413–421, 2001.
15. Allie DE, Hebert CJ, Lirtzman MD, et al: Novel simultaneous combination chemical thrombolysis/rheolytic thrombectomy therapy for acute critical limb ischemia: the power-pulse spray technique, *Catheter Cardiovasc Interv* 63(4):512–522, 2004.
16. Ansel GM, George BS, Botti CF, et al: Rheolytic thrombectomy in the management of limb ischemia: 30-day results from a multicenter registry, *J Endovasc Ther* 9(4):395–402, 2002.

CHAPTER

41

Femoral-Popliteal-Tibial Graft Occlusion: Thrombolysis, Angioplasty, Atherectomy, and Stent

Paul M. Anain, Samuel S. Ahn

Because the number of infrainguinal grafts, both synthetic and autologous, has been increasing, the number of thrombosed grafts is increasing as well. This poses a difficult therapeutic dilemma for the clinician. With the consequences of thrombosed grafts being limb threatening, knowledge of diagnostic and therapeutic criteria must be in the armamentarium of the surgeon.

Immediate and early graft failures are primarily due to technical error, the most common being an imprecise suture line, and intimal flaps. Grafts may become twisted through tunnel sites or by kinking or entrapment. Vein grafts may become stenosed and may lead to immediate thrombosis (resulting from ligation of branches) or to unsuitable vein (resulting from varicosities or small veins). Inflow and outflow conditions and hypercoagulable states may also contribute to the early thrombosis of bypass grafts. Thrombosis after 1 month to 1 year is usually due to changes in the graft or at the suture line. In reversed saphenous vein grafts, thrombosis is usually due to fibrosis of a valve or fibrotic changes in the vein graft resulting from injury during saphenectomy. In situ vein graft defects commonly occur at the mobilized proximal and distal end of the vein graft. Thickening in the midportion of these grafts may be the result of fibrosis from the valve cuff. All arterial anastomoses at or just distal to the distal anastomosis are involved with some degree of intimal hyperplasia caused by turbulent flow. Thrombosis in 1 to 2 years is most often due to progressive atherosclerosis in the arteries proximal or distal to the arterial anastomosis.[1-3]

Thrombosis after vein grafting appears to level off after 2 years; however, with the use of prosthetic grafts, there is a continuous progressive failure.[2,4] The possible causes of the progressive failure are the absence of a true intima and the thrombotic potential of prosthetic grafts. Prosthetic grafts also have a higher incidence of intimal hyperplasia caused by the increased compliance mismatch.

Recent evidence indicates that traditional means of measuring successful infrainguinal bypass surgery outcomes underreport complications such as prolonged recovery and multiple interventions.[5] Nguyen et al.[6] found that 130 out of 188 vein grafts required a single revision, whereas 58 required more than one. Length of the graft and early revision were associated with development of subsequent lesions, indicating the need for vigilant surveillance after the first revision. Limb salvage may be more involved than originally thought, and revision may be the rule, rather than the exception.

The entire problem of occlusion can be circumvented if the progressive neointimal hyperplasia pathway can be disrupted. The PREVENT III trial tested inhibition of transcription factor E2F with edifoligide in vein grafts ex vivo. Although primary and primary assisted patency rates were not significantly different from those in the control group, secondary patency was significantly improved (83% vs. 78%). Though this treatment was not proved to be effective, the study, with 1404 subjects, is still valuable as the largest prospective, randomized study of vein bypass for advanced lower-extremity ischemia as of 2006,[7] as well as demonstrating successful genetic modulation of vein grafts ex vivo.[8] Inhibiting the growth of neointima remains a promising proactive approach to graft occlusion.

Evaluation of the patient presenting with an occluded infrainguinal graft is influenced by the clinical presentation. Patients showing signs of recurrent claudication can be evaluated on an elective basis, and those presenting with ischemic symptoms are evaluated on an urgent basis. Patients with indications for intervention, disabling claudication, or limb-threatening ischemia are best evaluated by means of arteriography. The indication for the original operation will predict the symptoms resulting from the occluded bypass graft. Patients who underwent surgery for disabling claudication usually present with recurrent symptoms, and those who presented initially for limb salvage present with limb-threatening ischemia. When the artery distal to the anastomosis becomes thrombosed along with the graft, however, the presenting symptoms are often more severe. At this point, a decision can be made regarding the best intervention for the occluded graft.

A ROLE FOR THROMBOLYSIS

Thrombolysis of grafts is best achieved by delivering the thrombolytic agent directly into the thrombus via a catheter. Thrombolysis alone rarely achieves long-term patency if the cause of the graft failure is not addressed. Progression of proximal or distal disease, anastomotic narrowing, or graft stenosis should be relieved after thrombolysis. Thrombolysis has the added benefit of opening collateral vessels that are not accessible to thrombectomy.[9-11]

Catheter-directed thrombolysis (CDT) of venous grafts in general has a disappointing 1-year patency rate of less than 30%. Synthetic grafts, on the other hand, have better results, presumably because the failure is due to reasons that are not related to the graft.[2,12] In the Surgery versus Thrombolysis for Ischemia of the Lower Extremity (STILE) study, both occluded arteries and grafts were studied. A subset included 124 patients who had a bypass graft occlusion of less than 6 months' duration. Of the 78 patients who were randomly assigned to undergo CDT, catheter placement failed in 39%. In the remaining 61% of successfully cannulated grafts, however, 82% of vein grafts and 85% of prosthetic grafts had patency restored. An underlying lesion was found in 81% of these grafts, with a reduction in the number of operative procedures in 42% of patients. There was a 19% amputation rate for both polytetrafluoroethylene (PTFE) and vein grafts within 30 days of occlusion. The overall outcome at 1, 6, and 12 months was similar for both the group undergoing thrombolysis and the group undergoing surgery. A subset analysis showed that bypass grafts that were occluded for more than 14 days were best treated with CDT and those that had chronic occlusion for more than 14 days were best treated with surgical intervention. Grafts to the popliteal artery had a better success rate than those to the distal tibial vessels.[13-15]

Technique

Tissue Plasminogen Activator

Tissue plasminogen activator (t-PA) is a direct activator of the fibrinolytic system, directly converting plasminogen to plasmin. Therefore t-PA has the theoretical advantage of being associated with a lower rate of hemorrhagic complications; however, this has never been shown clinically. Many people report a higher incidence of bleeding complications with t-PA than with UK. t-PA is easily delivered with our regimen of a 4-mg lacing dose administered directly into the clot, after which 1 mg/hr is given (irrespective of the patient's body weight) for 4 hours. The infusion is then stopped for 4 hours, during which time heparin is infused. The t-PA is begun again at the original dose for another 4 hours. We have found that this "sandwich" approach is effective in achieving thrombolysis and decreases the side effects of t-PA.

Nackman et al.[16] reported on 44 patients with thrombosed infrainguinal vein grafts who underwent thrombolysis with UK. The thrombolysis-related mortality rate was 2%, and nonfatal complications occurred in 16%. Thrombolysis was unable to restore graft patency in 25% of grafts (11 of 44). Of the 33 grafts that were successfully lysed, 88% required adjunctive intervention (surgery vs. angioplasty) after thrombolysis. The primary graft patency rate was 34% at 1 year and 25% at 2 years after thrombolysis. Multivariate analysis revealed better graft patency in patients without diabetes and in those with vein grafts that had been in place for longer than 12 months.

The indications for CDT of occluded graft have been described.[15] If the graft becomes thrombosed within 4 weeks of the original revascularization, surgical intervention and revision are recommended. If the graft is more than 4 weeks old, CDT can be used. Best results with CDT are achieved with vein grafts that have been occluded for less than 2 weeks (optimally less than 2 days) or with prosthetic grafts that have been occluded for less than 3 months.

After lysis of the occluded graft, to achieve the best long-term patency, the cause of the graft failure must be evaluated and treated. Proximal and distal vessels must be evaluated, and patency must be addressed. Likewise, anastomotic and graft lesions must be corrected, or ultimately the patency of the graft will be short-lived and rethromboses will be inevitable. If no identifiable cause of graft failure is found, other factors such as low-flow states, cardiac disease, or hypercoagulable states should be evaluated, and anticoagulation should be considered. Recently, a new recombinant t-PA drug similar to reteplase has been developed, with potential advantages over currently available agents. These newer agents may allow improved targeting of the agent to the fibrin clot, therefore decreasing both the amount of the fibrinolytic agent required and the frequency of hemorrhagic complications.

Glycoprotein IIb/IIIa Antagonists

Recent evidence in the literature has shown that the use of glycoprotein IIb/IIIa antagonists in conjunction with fibrinolytic agents allows for a reduced dose of the fibrinolytic agents and is able to overcome thrombolytic resistance.[17] Newer therapy has focused on the use of heparin and glycoprotein IIb/IIIa antagonists for acute thrombosis with dissolution of the clot. The role of glycoprotein IIb/IIIa inhibitors is evolving, and they will continue to be applied in conjunction with thrombolytics and in high-risk patients undergoing angioplasty.

A ROLE FOR ANGIOPLASTY

After an occluded bypass graft has been opened, by means of either thrombolysis or surgical thrombectomy, a correctable causative factor should be identified. If progression of disease in the iliac or the proximal femoral artery is noted, the inflow can be improved dramatically by percutaneous transluminal angioplasty (PTA), as described elsewhere in this text. Several studies have shown that long-term results are comparable with those achieved with reconstructive surgery.[18-20] If there is disease in the outflow vessels, angioplasty of the femoral and the popliteal vessels can also be used with reasonable success. Success rates have been between 40% and 70% at 5 years.[19,21,22] The results for femoropopliteal PTA are better for short (<3 cm) concentric lesions and when the runoff is at least fair.

Lesions intrinsic to the vein graft range between 5% and 45% of all vein graft failures.[23,24] PTA can be easily used in these lesions. The best results of PTA are seen in the treatment of short discrete lesions, particularly in the body of the grafts. Wilson et al.[25] performed PTA on 40 graft stenoses with good radiologic results. Twelve of the 40 had stenosis recurrence and required further intervention, 4 with surgery and the remaining 8 with repeated angioplasty; all 12 remained patent at 10 months. Greenspan et al.[26] showed good long-term patency of stenotic lesions of the deep vein–arterial bypass with good long-term results.

Other reports do not show such good results for vein bypass graft stenosis treated by means of angioplasty. Whittemore et al.[27] used balloon angioplasty to treat 30 patients with 54 stenotic lesions occurring in autogenous vein graft stenosis after infrainguinal reconstruction. The primary 5-year cumulative patency rate was 18%, with no significant difference observed in relation to indication, length of stenotic lesion, or requirement for preliminary thrombolytic therapy. The vein graft lesions requiring only a single angioplasty proved to have significantly higher patency rates (59%) than those requiring repeated dilatations (6%), however.

PTA works best in short-segment lesions in otherwise normal grafts. PTA of multiple long irregular stenoses can be performed with good initial success; rapid restenosis is the rule rather than the exception. In these circumstances, surgical revision with patch angioplasty or a jump graft is the best intervention. Berkowitz et al.[28] reported on PTA of 72 stenotic vein grafts that contained lesions less than 5 cm long and found the primary assisted patency rate to be 80%. Sanchez et al.[29] performed PTA on 44 vein grafts and reported a 66% patency rate at 2 years if the vein was at least 3 mm long and there was only a single lesion of less than 1.5 cm. Fifty-four grafts did not meet these criteria and had a patency rate of only 17%. Further reports describe better results when greater saphenous vein grafts are used rather than grafts from the lesser saphenous or the arm vein.[30]

Angioplasty for vein graft stenosis has best results when the lesions are single, concentric, and less than 3 cm in length and require only single angioplasty. Multiple long lesions that require angioplasty have a significantly higher restenosis and thrombosis rate. Angioplasty for prosthetic grafts is reserved for proximal and distal anastomotic intimal hyperplasia. Prosthetic infrainguinal bypass anastomosis is associated with an increased incidence of intimal hyperplasia compared with vein grafts because of the compliance mismatch between the prosthetic graft and the native artery. Stenosis within the body of prosthetic grafts is rare because of the intrinsic properties of the graft. Sanchez et al.[31] reported on 33 PTFE graft bypasses with anastomotic stenosis. The patency and the limb salvage rates were equivalent to those of their surgical interventions.

Cutting Balloon Angioplasty

A recent development in technology is cutting balloon angioplasty, where, instead of a smooth-sided balloon, an angioplasty balloon with three or four atherotomes arranged longitudinally is introduced and slowly inflated, cutting the vein intima. This potentially creates more predictable cleavage planes, avoiding unnecessary injury or inconsistent tearing of the occlusion.[32] However, early results have been mixed. Vikram et al.[33] found that in a limited number of patients (N = 38), cutting balloon angioplasty had higher percentages of patency at 4 to 6 weeks (82% vs. 74%), 6 months (80%

vs. 62%), and 12 months (50% vs. 36%) but could not justify the increase in patency over the additional cost of cutting balloons. However, results from other studies are contradictory, with varying rates of short-term and midterm success.[32,34] This indicates that cutting balloon angioplasty should be at least considered as a first-line treatment for infrainguinal vein graft occlusion, but more data are still needed, especially considering the range of success rates for normal PTA.

Technique

Multiple steps are required for angioplasty of a failed bypass graft. A sterile field is required in either an operating room or an angiography suite with imaging capability. After a sterile field has been obtained, vascular access is achieved, either via the proximal native artery or directly into the bypass graft. The lesion is first crossed with a floppy-tipped guidewire or a hydrophilic guidewire. After the lesion is crossed with a guidewire and the decision to perform angioplasty is reaffirmed, the patient should be adequately anticoagulated. An angiogram is obtained, and the lesion is identified by using either bony or externally placed landmarks or by using the road-mapping technique of fluoroscopy. After the appropriate-sized catheter is selected, it is placed over the guidewire and is directed to the lesion. The radiopaque markers are placed so that they will straddle the lesion. The balloon is then inflated to profile, preferably with an inflation device, which provides better control of the inflation pressures. The balloon catheter is inflated with a 50% contrast agent solution. This allows the expansion to be visualized but is not so highly concentrated as to inhibit deflation of the balloon. Inflation is carried out until the waist of the atherosclerotic lesion can be broken and the balloon is at full profile. The balloon should be inflated for 1 to 2 minutes at a time. Balloon inflation should be repeated until no further waist is seen on inflation. Higher pressures are required for lesions of intimal hyperplasia. Occasionally, the balloon catheter will not cross the lesion, and it will need to be predilated with a lower-profile balloon. After dilatation is completed, the balloon catheter is removed, leaving the guidewire traversing the lesion until completion angiography can be performed.

A ROLE FOR ATHERECTOMY

The development of anastomotic neointimal hyperplasia is a common occurrence in arterial bypass grafts. It occurs with increasing frequency in prosthetic grafts because of flow and compliance mismatch. Atherectomy physically removes plaque by cutting, pulverizing, or shaving it through a small arteriotomy site distant from the diseased site. There are many different atherectomy devices with various advantages and disadvantages. For example, the Simpson AtheroCath device (DVI, Redwood City, CA) offers both over-the-wire and fixed wire shaft design to facilitate its introduction to complex or simple stenotic lesions. The cutter device slices the plaque at 2000 rpm while simultaneously pushing the excised particles into a collection chamber.

Atherectomy offers the following advantages over PTA: it has greater immediate success with less dissection and acute occlusion, treats complex lesions, and reduces the restenosis rate.[35] Extirpative atherectomy is characterized by cutting or shaving of atheroma and directly removes the excised material from the vessel via a collection chamber. Ablative atherectomy uses high-speed rotational devices that pulverize atheroma into fragments small enough to be aspirated or removed through the reticuloendothelial system.[35] Rheolytic thrombectomy devices use high-velocity saline jets to create suction, macerate, and evacuate the thrombosis. The only rheolytic thrombosis device approved so far for use in peripheral infrainguinal arteries is the AngioJet RT catheter (Possis Medical, Minneapolis, MN).[36] It has been suggested that patients with stenosis of failing lower-extremity bypass grafts should be treated with atherectomy rather than PTA because the predominant lesion in graft failure is intimal hyperplasia, for which PTA has somewhat poor results, as discussed earlier. Directional atherectomy has been proved to be safe and effective in treating synthetic and vein graft stenosis at the anastomotic and intragraft areas.[37]

Porter et al.[37] reported the results of 52 directional procedures undertaken in 67 stenoses (28 anastomotic and 39 intragraft) in 44 vein grafts (atherectomy alone in 42 and atherectomy and angioplasty in 10). Forty-nine of 52 procedures (94%) were technically successful. At an average of 21 months, 82% of grafts remained patent without restenosis, whereas 11% failed (restenotic but patent) and 5% occluded. Clinically, 33 of 44 extremities (75%) were asymptomatic during follow-up. Life-table analysis of all 52 procedures revealed cumulative primary atherectomy patency rates for the 44 grafts of 82%, 78%, and 78% at 1, 2, and 3 years, respectively, after atherectomy.[37] Similarly, Dolmatch et al.[38] treated 17 patients with 23 areas of anastomotic stenosis in 18 lower-extremity bypass grafts (11 PTFE and 7 autologous saphenous vein). Lytic therapy was performed in 8 of the patients who presented with thrombosed bypass grafts. The technical success rate was 92%, with less than 50% restenosis at 74% of the areas of stenosis and an overall patency rate of 88%. Vinnicombe et al.[39] reported the early technical success rate in anastomotic neointimal hyperplasia associated with arterial grafts using the Transluminal Extraction Catheter (TEC). In a group of seven patients, they performed eight atherectomies at anastomotic sites and experienced a high technical success rate with good short-term results.

Misra[40] reported on the use of the TEC in 15 patients who presented with occluded infrainguinal bypass grafts. After all underwent successful lytic therapy, distal lesions that were thought to be the cause of the thrombus were found in all patients, and there was one concomitant proximal stenosis. The TEC was used to address the probable cause of the occlusion and the critically stenosed anastomotic lesions. An initial 100% success rate was immediately achieved with flow reestablished in the distal limb; 14 of the 15 patients remained well vascularized for more than 1 year.

The Simpson AtheroCath device is used for lesions in bypass grafts. As users of the other models began reporting their results with these devices in bypass grafts, comparison with the Simpson AtheroCath and balloon angioplasty was able to be made. Some early work suggests that atherectomy and angioplasty together result in better long-term patency than either balloon angioplasty or atherectomy alone. For eccentric calcified lesions smaller than 5 cm, directional atherectomy of vein graft stenosis is associated with a high technical and clinical success rate with low morbidity. The results of directional atherectomy appear long-lasting and are at least comparable with (if not surpassing) those of PTA. When combined with PTA, results approach the success rate of surgical intervention.

Technique

Atherectomy with the TEC is primarily performed percutaneously but can also be used adjunctively with open surgery. Predilatation of the artery may be required for passage of the TEC. Under fluoroscopic guidance, an appropriate-sized introducer catheter is placed, and a guidewire is passed through the lesion. An exchange catheter and a 0.014-inch TEC guidewire are then used. The catheter is advanced over the guidewire under fluoroscopic guidance until it meets resistance. The atherectomy catheter is activated, and the motor drive rotates the cutter while suction is applied. The cutter is passed over the guidewire until it reaches the obstructive lesion. Fluoroscopy documents the progress of the atherectomy and the size of the lumen. Multiple passages and cuts are made until the final lumen is less than 25% of the residual stenosis. If there is residual stenosis, adjunctive balloon angioplasty is performed to dilate the artery to a final adequate size.[41]

A ROLE FOR STENTING

The deployment of stents in failing bypass grafts is still controversial. The majority of the data are extrapolated from the literature on cardiac disease and dialysis access. Initial results show a high rate of technical success; however, restenosis as a result of intimal hyperplasia is common. At present, stenting of bypass grafts should be performed only in prospective trials or when all other interventions for graft survival have been attempted and failed.

SUMMARY

Although the vascular physician should be able to make the diagnosis and the proper management decisions for the patient with an occluded vascular graft, a team-oriented approach may be beneficial to the patient and the physicians involved. If the graft was placed less than 4 weeks before occluding, surgical intervention (revision or replacement) should be the main form of therapy. If the graft was placed more than 4

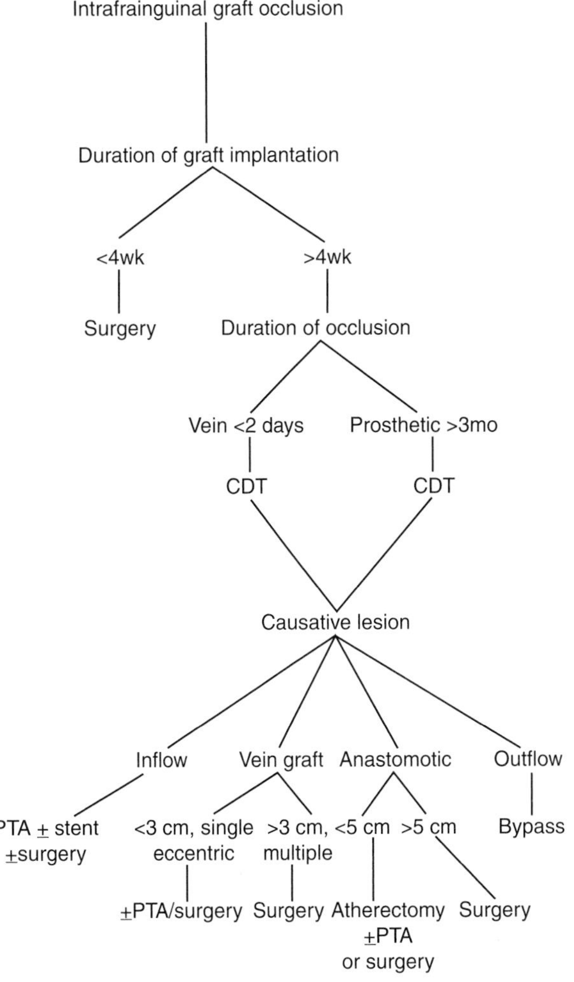

FIGURE 41-1 Algorithm for the treatment of infrainguinal graft occlusion. *CDT,* Catheter-directed thrombolysis; *PTA,* percutaneous transluminal angioplasty.

weeks before occlusion, the duration of the occlusion is an important factor. If a vein graft has been occluded for less than 2 weeks or a prosthetic graft for less than 3 months, CDT can be used. After lysis of the graft, inflow lesions can be addressed via PTA with or without stent placement or surgery, as the case may indicate. Intervention for outflow lesions can be bypass procedures, possible PTA, or atherectomy. For anastomotic lesions that are less than 5 cm in length and eccentric, PTA, atherectomy, or a combination of the two can be considered. Any intrinsic lesions of vein grafts unveiled by thrombolysis need intervention. If a single lesion less than 3 cm is found, PTA may be effective (Figure 41-1).

Any patient with graft thrombosis should be evaluated closely for the degree of ischemia, overall stability, and the ability to undergo possible interventions. These should be the prime indicators for the intervention rendered.

References

1. Licalzi LK, Stansel HC: Failure of autogenous reversed saphenous vein femoropopliteal grafting: pathophysiology and prevention, *Surgery* 91:352–358, 1982.
2. Whittemore AD, Clowes AW, Couch NP, et al: Secondary femoropopliteal reconstruction, *Ann Surg* 193:35–42, 1981.
3. Fuchs CA, Mitchener JS III, Hagen PO: Postoperative changes in autologous vein grafts, *Ann Surg* 188:1–11, 1978.
4. O'Donnell TF, Farber SP, Richmond DM, et al: Above-knee polytetrafluoroethylene femoropopliteal bypass graft: is it a reasonable alternative to the below-knee reversed autogenous vein graft? *Surgery* 94:26–31, 1983.
5. Goshima KR, Mills JL Sr, Hughes JD: A new look at outcomes after infrainguinal bypass surgery: traditional reporting standards systematically underestimate the expenditure of effort required to attain limb salvage, *J Vasc Surg* 39:330–335, 2004.
6. Nguyen LL, Conte MS, Menard MT: Infrainguinal vein bypass graft revision: Factors affecting long-term outcome, *J Vasc Surg* 40:916–923, 2004.
7. Conte MS, Bandyk DF, Clowes AW, et al: Results of PREVENT III: a multicenter, randomized trial of edifoligide for the prevention of vein graft failure in lower extremity bypass surgery, *J Vasc Surg* 43:742–751, 2006.
8. Morrisey NJ: Biological treatment of vein grafts and stents in lower-extremity arterial reconstruction, *Perspect Vasc Surg Endovasc Ther* 19:293–297, 2007.
9. Graor RA, Risius B, Young JR, et al: Thrombolysis of peripheral arterial bypass grafts: surgical thrombectomy compared with thrombolysis—a preliminary report, *J Vasc Surg* 7:347–355, 1988.
10. Belkin M, Donaldson MC, Whittemore AD, et al: Observations on the use of thrombolytic agents for thrombotic occlusions of infrainguinal vein grafts, *J Vasc Surg* 11:289–296, 1990.
11. Gardiner GA, Sullivan KL: Catheter directed thrombolysis for the failed lower extremity graft, *Semin Vasc Surg* 5:99–103, 1992.
12. Hye RJ, Turner C, Valji K, et al: Is thrombosis of occluded popliteal and tibial bypass grafts worthwhile? *J Vasc Surg* 20:588–597, 1994.
13. Results of a prospective randomized trial evaluating surgery versus thrombolysis for ischemia of the lower extremity. The STILE trial, *Ann Surg* 220:251–268, 1994.
14. Comerota AJ, Weaver FA, Hosking JD, et al: Results of a prospective, randomized trial of surgery versus thrombolysis for occluded lower extremity bypass grafts, *Am J Surg* 172:105–112, 1994.
15. Kroese A, Staxrud LE, Sandbaek G: When should we lyse an occluded femoropopliteal bypass? In Greenhalgh RM, editor: *Indications in vascular and endovascular surgery*, Philadelphia, 1998, W.B. Saunders.
16. Nackman GB, Walsh DM, Fillinger MF, et al: Thrombolysis of occluded infrainguinal vein grafts: predictors of outcome, *J Vasc Surg* 25:1023–1032, 1997.
17. Cannon CP: Rationale and initial clinical experience combining thrombolytic therapy and glycoprotein IIb/IIIa receptor inhibition for acute myocardial infarction, *J Am Coll Cardiol* 34:1395–1402, 1999.
18. Nieman HL, Bergan JJ, Yao JS: Hemodynamic assessment of transluminal angioplasty for lower extremity ischemia, *Radiology* 143:639–643, 1982.
19. Spence RK, Frieman DB, Gatenby R, et al: Long-term results of transluminal angioplasty of the iliac and femoral arteries, *Arch Surg* 116:1377–1386, 1981.
20. Kadir S, White RI, Kaufman SL, et al: Long term results of aortoiliac angioplasty, *Surgery* 94:10–14, 1983.
21. Krepel VM, van Andel GJ, van Erp WF, Breslau PJ: Percutaneous transluminal angioplasty of the femoropopliteal artery: initial and long-term results, *Radiology* 156:325–328, 1985.
22. Johnson KW, Rae H, Hogg-Johnston B, et al: 5 year results of a prospective study of a percutaneous transluminal angioplasty, *Ann Surg* 206:403–413, 1987.
23. Dunlop P, Varty K, Hartshorne T, et al: Percutaneous transluminal angioplasty of infrainguinal vein graft stenosis: long-term outcome, *Br J Surg* 82:204–206, 1995.
24. Ratliff D, Sayers R, Brennan JA, et al: Graft surveillance: the effect of intervention by angioplasty and surgery, *Br J Surg* 81:616, 1994.
25. Wilson YG, Davies AH, Currie IC, et al: Vein graft stenosis: incidence and intervention, *Eur J Vasc Endovasc Surg* 11:164–169, 1996.
26. Greenspan B, Pillari G, Schulman M, et al: Percutaneous transluminal angioplasty of stenotic deep vein arterial bypass grafts, *Arch Surg* 120:492–495, 1985.
27. Whittemore AD, Donaldson MC, Polak JF, et al: Limitations of balloon angioplasty for vein graft stenosis, *J Vasc Surg* 14:340–345, 1991.
28. Berkowitz HD, Fox AD, Deaton DH: Reversed vein graft stenosis: early diagnosis and management, *J Vasc Surg* 15:130–140, 1992.
29. Sanchez LA, Suggs WD, Marin ME: Is percutaneous balloon angioplasty appropriate in the treatment of graft and anastomotic lesions responsible for failing bypasses? *Am J Surg* 168:97–101, 1994.
30. Donaldson MC, Whittemore AD, Mannick JA, et al: Further experience with an all-autogenous tissue policy after infrainguinal reconstruction, *J Vasc Surg* 18:41–48, 1993.
31. Sanchez LA, Gupta SL, Veith FJ, et al: A ten year experience with one hundred fifty failing or threatened vein and polytetra-fluoroethylene arterial bypass grafts, *J Vasc Surg* 14:721–736, 1991.
32. Schneider PA, Caps MT, Nelken N: Infrainguinal vein graft stenosis: cutting balloon angioplasty as the first-line treatment of choice, *J Vasc Surg* 47:960–969, 2008.
33. Vikram R, Ross RA, Bhat R, et al: Cutting balloon angioplasty versus standard balloon angioplasty for failing infra-inguinal vein grafts: comparative study of short- and mid-term primary patency rates, *Cardiovasc Intervent Radiol* 30:607–610, 2007.
34. Garvin R, Reifsnyder T: Cutting balloon angioplasty of autogenous infrainguinal bypasses: Short term safety and efficacy, *J Vasc Surg* 46:724–730, 2007.

35. Ahn S, Concepcion B: Current status of atherectomy for peripheral arterial occlusive disease, *World J Surg* 20:635–643, 1996.
36. Ansel GM, George BS, Botti CF: Rheolytic thrombectomy in the management of limb ischemia: 30-day results from a multicenter registry, *J Endovasc Ther* 9:395–402, 2002.
37. Porter DH, Rosen MP, Skillman JJ, et al: Mid-term and long-term results with directional atherectomy of vein graft stenosis, *J Vasc Surg* 23:554–566, 1996.
38. Dolmatch BL, Gray RJ, Horton KM, et al: Treatment of anastomotic bypass graft stenosis with directional atherectomy: short-term and intermediate-term results, *J Vasc Interv Radiol* 6:105–113, 1995.
39. Vinnicombe SJ, Heenan SD, Belli AM, et al: Directional atherectomy in the treatment of anastomotic neointimal hyperplasia associated with prosthetic arterial grafts: technique and preliminary results, *Clin Radiol* 49:773–778, 1994.
40. Misra HP: Revascularization of the limbs with urokinase and TEC catheter endarterectomy for occluded bypass grafts, *Am J Surg* 166:756–759, 1993.
41. Ahn S, Concepcion B: Current status of atherectomy: options, patient selection and results. In Perler BA, Becker GJ, editors: *Vascular intervention: a clinical approach*, New York, 1997, Thieme.

CHAPTER

42

Brachiocephalic Graft Occlusion

Jon S. Matsumura, Colleen L. Jay

Revascularization of the brachiocephalic vessels is a challenging aspect of vascular surgery because of its many diverse etiologies, the complex anatomic background of brachiocephalic disease, and the varied symptoms with which these patients present. Fortunately, with timely recognition of the problem, appropriate selection of the procedure, and skillful execution of the reconstruction, most brachiocephalic revascularization procedures completely relieve symptoms and are relatively durable with excellent long-term patency. This chapter discusses the endovascular tools available to the surgeon faced with the uncommon problem of brachiocephalic graft occlusion.

DIAGNOSIS

Occlusion of carotid or subclavian bypass grafts may present with the original symptoms of cerebral ischemia or steal. Alternatively, graft occlusion may result in the obvious presentation of a cold hand. More often the presentation is less dramatic, and diagnosis of proximal brachiocephalic graft occlusion may not be immediately apparent when robust collateral pathways are present (Figure 42-1). Mild arm muscle cramps that are exercise dependent are often misinterpreted as generalized fatigue or musculoskeletal dysfunction. Also, dilation or frank aneurysm formation in brachiocephalic grafts can be asymptomatic in the early phases. Diagnosis of revascularization failure requires a high level of suspicion for any neurologic, arm, or hand symptoms or routine use of imaging surveillance (Figure 42-2).

Routine physical examination after brachiocephalic reconstruction includes inspection of both upper extremities for quality and symmetry of pulses and muscle strength and tone. The neck and periclavicular regions should be palpated and auscultated including examination under positional provocation when indicated. The fingertips and nail beds should be carefully examined for evidence of embolism or small-vessel occlusion. A detailed neurologic examination completes the physical assessment. Because failure of arch, carotid, subclavian, vertebral, and upper-extremity reconstructions is uncommon and often asymptomatic, the physician must be diligent to recognize the occasional graft occlusion.[1-3]

Noninvasive Testing

When clinical findings raise the suspicion of graft failure, noninvasive testing can be useful in confirming these findings and possibly preventing unnecessary use of conventional angiography. Segmental pressures may be assessed in the office and at the bedside and can objectively confirm hemodynamic failure of the reconstruction. Because of the superficial location of many brachiocephalic grafts, duplex ultrasonography can be used to assess most reconstructions. Additionally, duplex ultrasound may be useful for routine postoperative surveillance given its safety and relatively low cost. Magnetic resonance imaging is an excellent noninvasive test for imaging less-accessible arch and vertebral reconstructions. Plain radiographs can be used to monitor stent position and integrity. Finally, we have found helical computed tomography with three-dimensional reconstructions to be useful in the assessment of patients with thoracic outlet syndrome (Figure 42-3).

Angiography and Selection of Access Site

Endovascular therapy for brachiocephalic graft occlusion is almost always based on angiographic confirmation of the diagnosis and definition of the anatomy. Careful consideration should be given to selection of puncture sites especially if thrombolysis is being considered. Caliber of vessels, distance to the lesion, and anatomic turns are considered in making a decision regarding initial sheath placement. Often an initial

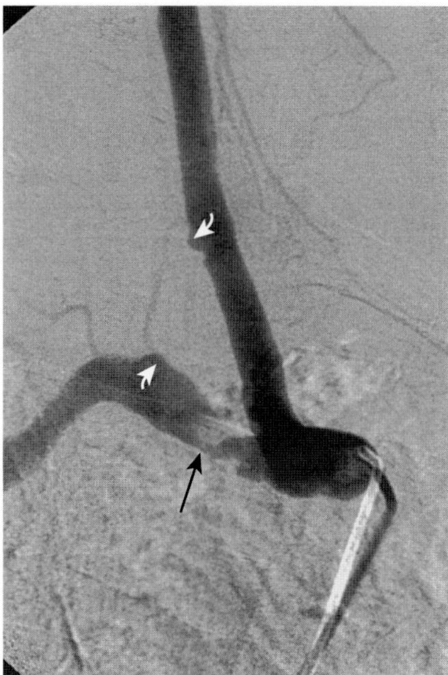

FIGURE 42-1 Patient who presented in late follow-up with occlusion of a right carotid subclavian bypass. (*Black arrow* points to proximal right subclavian stenosis. *White curved arrows* identify anastomotic sites of occluded graft.) The patient was successfully treated with subclavian angioplasty without stenting.

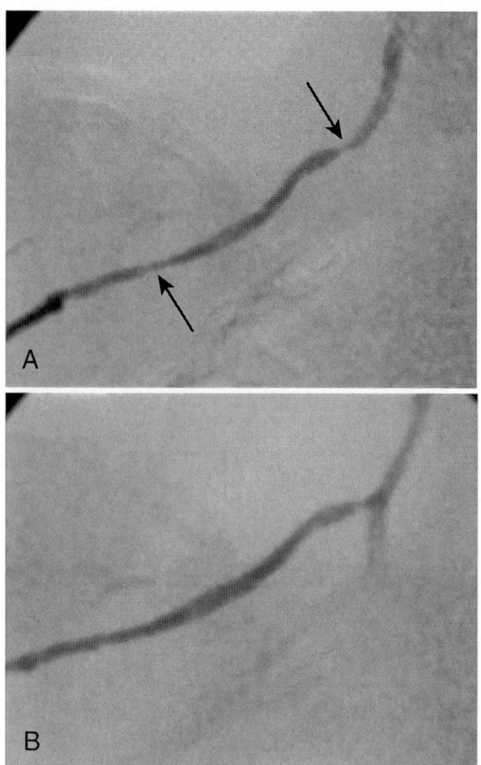

FIGURE 42-2 Patient who had two previous failed right-arm saphenous bypass grafts 20 and 10 years before most recent bypass. The current spliced arm vein graft developed two areas of duplex-detected restenosis (**A,** *black arrows*). Angioplasty resulted in good angiographic result **(B)** and improved duplex velocities.

femoral puncture for a diagnostic procedure is combined with a subsequent brachial puncture for endovascular therapy when difficult subclavian or innominate lesions are encountered, thus enabling performance of angiography from below simultaneous with balloon angioplasty or stent placement from the arm.

Many points may be stressed regarding what a "complete" diagnostic angiogram includes. For instance, in the assessment of upper-extremity ischemia, arch and bilateral selective injections are useful in assessing all potential inflow vessels for subsequent reoperation. Imaging of the subclavian and axillary arteries and distal branches with the arm in neutral and provocative positions is important in diagnosing recurrent compressive symptoms (Figure 42-4). When considering a bypass to the interosseous arteries, two views including an oblique view are useful to determine which branch is the more favorable target. This information is invaluable in planning the location of skin incisions. For patients with digital ischemia, magnified views of the hand with use of vasodilators are useful to assess different patterns of embolic disease on the basis of which digital vessels are affected.[4] When unilateral digital ischemia is present and no other obvious source is identified, oblique views of brachial branch vessel origins or post-thrombolysis views of the hand may reveal rare sources of embolism from circumflex humeral artery aneurysms or ulnar artery lesions. When there is suspicion of posterior circulation cerebral insufficiency, multiple views of the vertebral origins and intracranial images are essential.

ENDOVASCULAR INTERVENTIONS

There are many endovascular tools, developed primarily for use in the lower extremities, that have been applied to the brachiocephalic vessels. Thrombolysis, balloon angioplasty, and off-label stent placement are minimally invasive options for graft occlusion that avoid difficult reoperative dissections and offer less-morbid treatment of lesions within the confines of the chest or skull base. Often an endovascular procedure can be combined with a standard open technique to improve overall results and minimize the amount of exposure needed, reducing complication rates and shortening recovery time. The use of these hybrid procedures is frequently necessary when dealing with recurrent ischemia after an initial procedure has failed because multilevel disease may be present and the

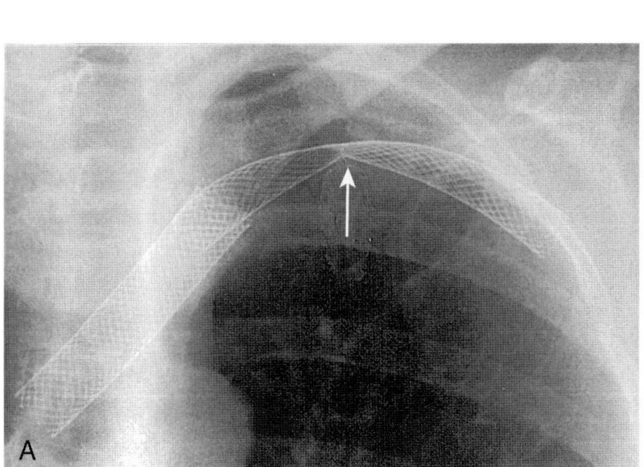

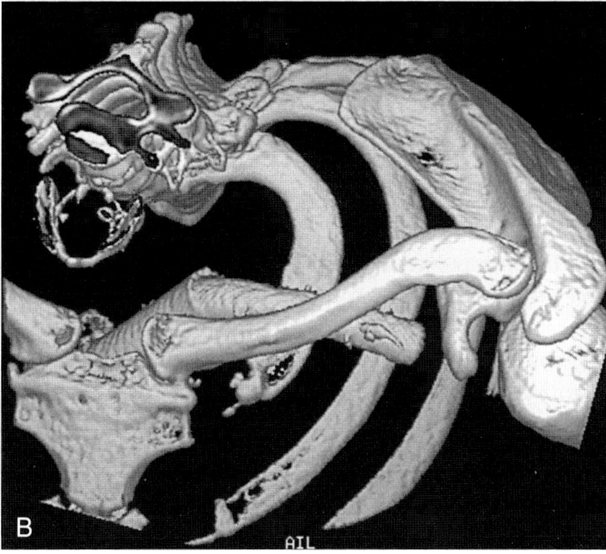

FIGURE 42-3 Radiographic studies demonstrating location of misplaced stents in left subclavian vein and innominate vein. **A,** Posteroanterior projection of stent with compression in costoclavicular space. (*White arrow* identifies area of compression.) **B,** Three-dimensional shaded-surface reconstruction of helical computed tomographic scan that depicts location of stent deep within the thoracic cavity, and relationship to adjacent bones.

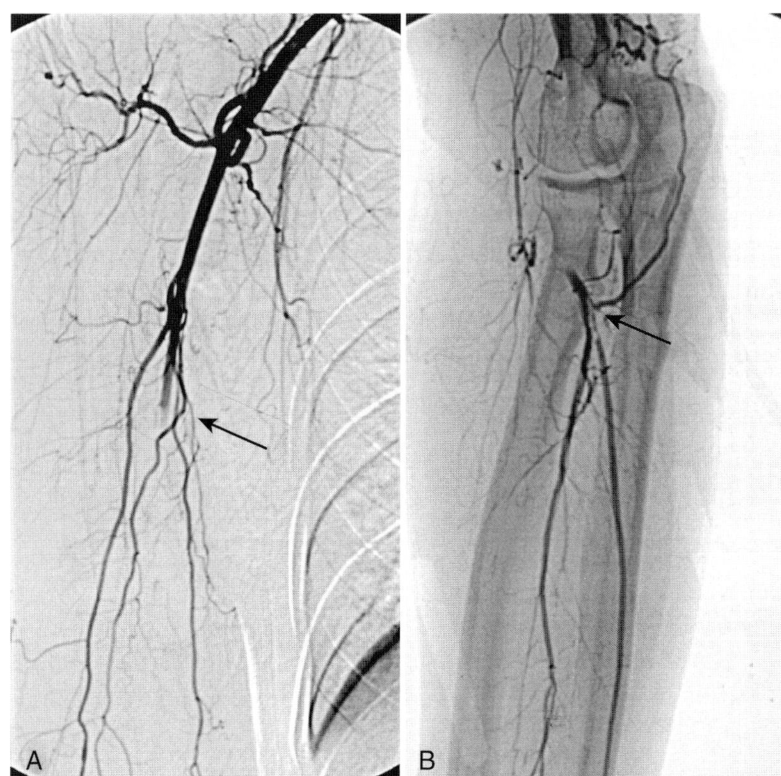

FIGURE 42-4 Arteriogram of a patient with recurrent right-hand ischemia after vein graft repair of right subclavian aneurysm. **A,** Brachial artery occlusion *(black arrow).* **B,** Distal reconstitution of forearm vessels with filling defect in proximal ulnar artery *(black arrow).* Emboli to the wrist and hand were also identified, and thrombolysis was used to improve the poor runoff.

simplest, most expedient procedure has already been performed and failed. It is important to note that most of the endovascular techniques described in this chapter are not approved for these specific uses by the U.S. Food and Drug Administration.

Thrombolysis

Catheter-directed thrombolysis has been evaluated extensively in comparison with open surgery in both the Thrombolysis or Peripheral Arterial Surgery (TOPAS) and Surgery versus Thrombolysis for Ischemia of the

Lower Extremity (STILE) trials.[5,6] Use of thrombolysis in the upper extremities is less frequent but can be effective in appropriately selected cases. Thrombolysis may be preferred in those patients with shorter duration of ischemia and in those with poor runoff, making it less likely to support a bypass on initial angiographic assessment (see Figure 42-4). Thrombolysis of the upper extremities often progresses rapidly, perhaps because of smaller thrombus burden. As such, more frequent angiographic assessment of progress should be considered. When ischemia is profound, the time needed for percutaneous thrombolysis to work may not be available. In these cases, intraoperative distal thrombolysis can be combined with proximal revascularization. Thrombolysis may also be rarely used for treatment of patent arteries with mobile thrombus proximal to the internal carotid or vertebral origins to reduce the risk of symptomatic embolization during endovascular manipulation. In the case of graft occlusion of carotid bypasses or bypasses proximal to patent vertebral vessels, we have not entertained thrombolysis because of concern about potential embolization of large amounts of thrombus when flow is restored. With all these techniques, concerns remain for hemorrhagic complications, and the use of thrombolytic agents should be avoided in patients with relative contraindications, such as uncontrolled hypertension and recent neurospinal injury or surgery.

Angioplasty

Angioplasty for recurrent symptomatic ischemia caused by graft failure is an attractive option, especially for lesions of the arch vessels[7,8] (see Figure 42-1). Balloon angioplasty of the primary native lesion can provide symptomatic relief while avoiding reoperative dissection in the neck and the attendant risks of cranial nerve, brachial plexus, phrenic nerve, and sympathetic chain injury (see Figure 42-2). Although embolism is always a concern with the brachiocephalic vessels, there seems to be transient protection from posterior circulation embolism when flow is reversed in the ipsilateral vertebral artery in subclavian steal syndrome.

Stenting

The use of stents in the off-label treatment of brachiocephalic disease has been evaluated less extensively than in the iliac circulation where selective stenting is common.[9] It is possible that arch vessel stent patency is similar to the iliac location because of the similar size of the arteries, but comprehensive trials have not been performed except for carotid bifurcation stenting. The reported primary patency of stenting for subclavian or innominate artery lesions is 91.7% and 77% at 1 and 2 years, respectively, in one review.[10] Another study found a primary patency rate of 87% with use of stents compared with 69% with angioplasty alone at 2.5 years and good long-term results with primary and secondary patency rates of 75% and 81% at 8 years.[11]

One promising area for endovascular stenting is in the treatment of recurrent symptomatic carotid stenosis.[12,13] Properly selected patients with anatomic risk factors that increase procedural risk for carotid endarterectomy appear to have the greatest relative benefit from the endovascular approach. These anatomic factors include inaccessible high lesions, restenosis after prior operations, cervical fusion, tracheostomy, previous ablative neck operations, and prior radiation therapy. In the Stenting and Angioplasty with Protection in Patients at High Risk for Endarterectomy (SAPPHIRE) trial, investigators showed the noninferiority of carotid artery stenting with the use of embolic protection device in high-risk patients and a slight decrease in cumulative incidence of death, stroke, and myocardial infarction at 30 days and ipsilateral stroke at 1 year.[14]

However, there are concerns regarding stent-associated branch artery occlusion including late restenosis and misdeployed devices; these concerns are accentuated when used in vessels supplying the brain. Furthermore, stent compression is possible in several areas of motion in the neck and arm and can result in stent fracture.[15-18] In fact, stent deformation in the costoclavicular space is frequently expected because of normal anatomic relationships during arm movement[19] (see Figure 42-3). Stent fracture can also be seen in brachiocephalic arteries outside the costoclavicular space (Figure 42-5). Finally, stent misplacement or migration constitutes a greater hazard in the central vessels than in the iliac arteries because flow patterns may carry a loose stent or embolus into a critical

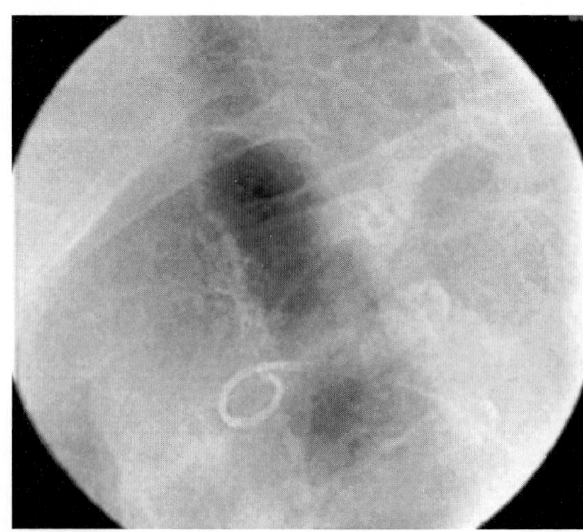

FIGURE 42-5 Off-label stent in innominate artery has fractured and deformed and migrated.

arterial bed. Occasionally, malpositioned stents may be retrieved from brachiocephalic arteries and veins by percutaneous or combined endovascular and open procedures. Remote disengagement of stents before removal is performed by constraining the devices radially (Figures 42-3, 42-6, and 42-7). Although stents may improve the patency of selected percutaneous treatments, it seems prudent to proceed cautiously with off-label use of these devices because the attendant risks of ischemia of the cerebral and upper-extremity vascular beds include significant morbidity.

Atherectomy

Atherectomy has limited use in the brachiocephalic circulation because of the relative fragility of the upper-extremity vessels and the greater clinical sequelae associated with embolization of debris to the brain. To date, there are no large reported series of percutaneous atherectomy of the brachiocephalic circulation, presumably because of the discouraging late patency rates reported in the infrainguinal position. Reported complications include intimal dissection, embolism, equipment breakage,

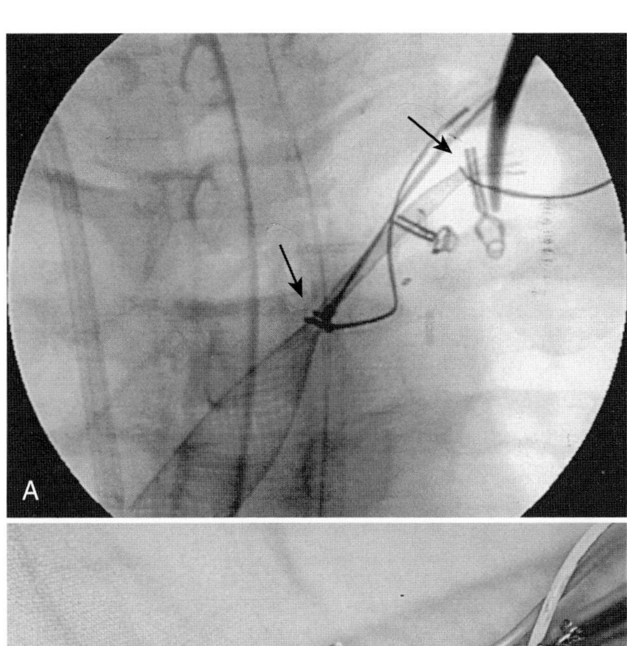

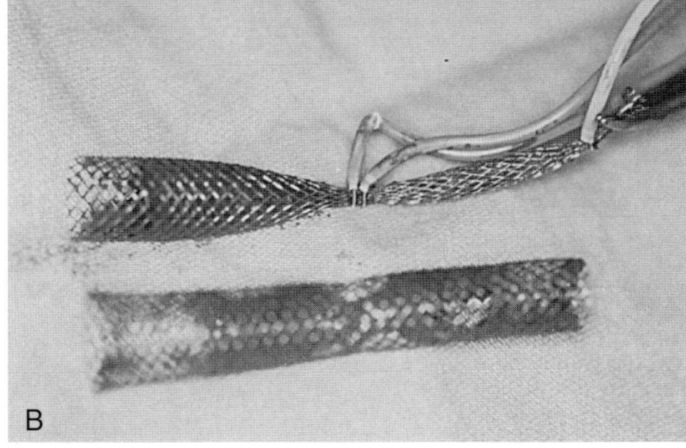

FIGURE 42-6 Combined use of open and endovascular techniques permits minimally invasive removal of the innominate stent in Figure 42-3. **A,** Fluoroscopic visualization of three separate snares, which are used to radially constrain the stent before removal, minimizing damage to the vascular tissues. With use of multiple snares, the end of the stent may be constrained with the first snare while the next snare is subsequently advanced a small increment. By sequentially reconstraining the stent, further advancement of the subsequent snare is permitted. (*Black arrows* identify tip of snares.) **B,** Intraoperative photograph of stents after removal.

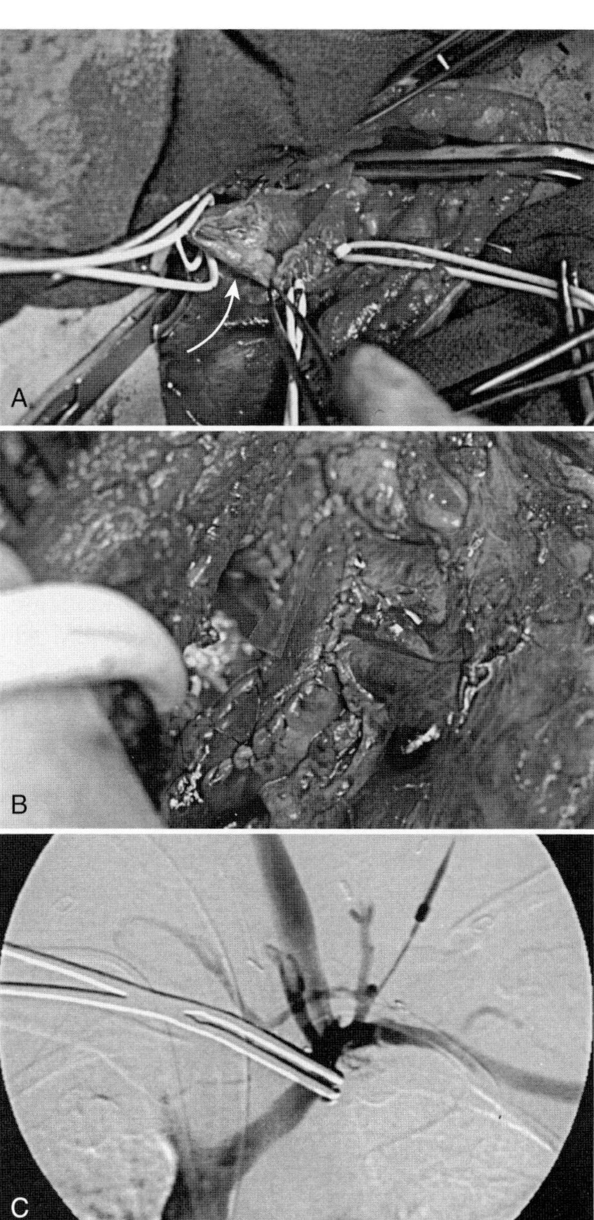

FIGURE 42-7 After removal of stents the standard decompressive procedure is performed, in this case claviculectomy, scalenectomy, and vein patch angioplasty. No thoracotomy or sternotomy was needed. **A,** Intraoperative photograph that demonstrates the native lesion located at the costoclavicular junction *(white curved arrow)* after stent removal (see Figure 42-6). **B,** Photograph of the subclavian vein after saphenous vein patch angioplasty. **C,** Intraoperative venogram showing widely patent subclavian vein.

transient hemoglobinuria, hematoma, wound infection, and limb loss in the infrainguinal series.[20] Percutaneous rotational atherectomy has been reported for recanalization of the brachial artery.[21] More experience with this and other alternative treatment options including cryoplasty, cutting balloons, and scoring balloons is needed before any definitive conclusions can be made.

AUGMENTING MANEUVERS

Endovascular procedures of the brachiocephalic vessels often require additional procedures, techniques, or pharmacologic adjuncts to improve their safety and effectiveness. Secondary procedures deserve greater meticulousness to prevent a third procedure from becoming necessary.

Decompression

A thorough search for the cause of graft occlusion commonly proceeds with assessment for inflow insufficiency, conduit problem, outflow insufficiency, and possible hypercoagulability. Compression of the vessel or conduit should always be considered in subclavian revascularization failure, especially when occurring in the costoclavicular region (see Figures 42-3 and 42-6). Compression may also occur in the scalene triangle, in the retropectoral tunnel, or at the humeral head. The latter two locations are more often seen in athletes who perform repetitive upper-extremity motions, such as baseball pitching.[22] The compressive element may be responsible for both the native disease and primary graft failure, and adequate decompression should improve the durability of the secondary procedure.

Cerebral Protection

Analogous with the cerebral monitoring and meticulous technical detail that attend carotid endarterectomy, endovascular treatment of brachiocephalic vessels deserves similar intense planning and monitoring and precise execution to minimize morbidity. A complication such as a stroke may be irreversible, unlike the usually correctable nature of leg ischemia. Diligent techniques to prevent iatrogenic air embolization, cautious endovascular manipulations, and monitoring of periprocedural blood pressure are all important. The use of temporary external or balloon occlusion of distal cerebral vessels may minimize the frequency of embolic complications. In addition to these maneuvers, reactive hyperemia induced by cuff deflation can be used to "sump" embolic debris into an arm rather than the ipsilateral cranial vessels during proximal arterial interventions.

Anticoagulation

Early failure of a primary brachiocephalic reconstruction that usually has very good patency suggests a very different natural history than that in a patient with continued primary graft function. If no obvious technical cause of failure is identified and rectified, it is reasonable to intensify antithrombotic regimens to improve secondary patency, and consideration should be given toward anticoagulation with vitamin K antagonists if there are no significant contraindications.

RESULTS

Complications of endovascular treatment of graft occlusion are similar to those of primary procedures and include inability to cross a target lesion with the guidewire, recoil after angioplasty (Figure 42-8), thrombosis, embolization, arterial injury, and puncture site complications. Patency of salvage procedures has not been well documented but is likely to be worse than in corresponding primary procedures. Patency of primary endovascular procedures ranges from 50% at 1 year for completely occluded subclavian arteries to 97% at 3.5 years for proximal subclavian stenosis.[23,24] Fortunately, limb salvage rates are still fairly good, possibly because of greater collateral development and intrinsic factors of the upper extremity that make it more tolerant of ischemia. Amputations are rare in long-term series.[25] However, when arm amputation is necessary, especially of the dominant hand, these patients have much greater loss of function than leg amputees.

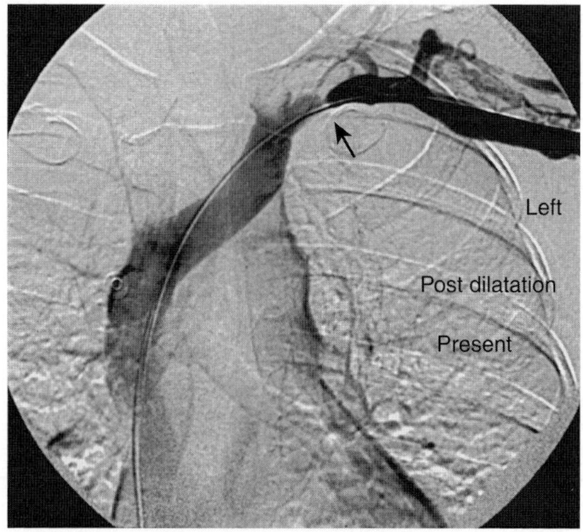

FIGURE 42-8 Angiogram from outside hospital demonstrating typical findings in primary subclavian vein thrombosis after thrombolysis and angioplasty. A lesion of the subclavian vein was identified that was resistant to balloon angioplasty *(black arrow).*

Comparison With Standard Management Options

Open approach to the patient with brachiocephalic graft occlusion includes observation when the patient is asymptomatic and the risks of symptomatic progression are minimal, direct surgical thrombectomy and revision of the bypass, native vessel endarterectomy, and redo bypass operations. Reoperative surgery carries increased risks of injury to adjacent structures, including the thoracic duct, major veins, and nerves.

Sometimes, alternative bypass grafts are possible through fresh tissue planes. This strategy alleviates some of the risks associated with a scarred field but usually involves a longer prosthetic bypass to a more distal, often smaller vessel with associated reduced patency rates compared with the original operation. Bypasses to the subclavian, axillary, and brachial vessels are possible with use of polytetrafluoroethylene (PTFE). Patency is 38% at 5 years when using PTFE compared with 71% with vein conduit, which is preferred when available.[25] Distal bypass to the forearm should be performed exclusively with use of autologous conduit because wrist bypass patency with PTFE is extremely poor (0% at 1 year).[25] Additionally, redo bypasses have distinctly decreased patency (48% at 5 years) compared with primary procedures (66%)[25] (see Figure 42-2). In contrast, proximal arch vessel reconstruction has durability approaching 100%, for both endarterectomy and arch bypass techniques.[26-29]

In comparison, endovascular surgery often provides revascularization via a short anatomic path, while avoiding dissection in the reoperative field. Patency of secondary procedures is not well studied, but primary endovascular treatment of large arch branches ranged from 77% to 87% at 2 years in reported series.[10,11] Because brachiocephalic bypass failure is often associated with multilevel disease caused by natural disease progression or distal embolization from the proximal lesion, combined endovascular and open operations may be the most optimal solution for these difficult problems. Care must also be exercised to avoid premature enthusiasm about applications of endovascular treatments until specifically designed devices and more data on safety and effectiveness are available.

References

1. Crawford ES, De Bakey ME, Morris GC Jr, Howell JF: Surgical treatment of occlusion of the innominate, common carotid, and subclavian arteries: a 10 year experience, *Surgery* 65(1):17–31, 1969.
2. McCarthy WJ, Flinn WR, Yao JS, et al: Result of bypass grafting for upper limb ischemia, *J Vasc Surg* 3(5):741–746, 1986.
3. Moore WS, Malone JM, Goldstone J: Extrathoracic repair of branch occlusions of the aortic arch, *Am J Surg* 132(2):249–257, 1976.
4. McNamara MF, Takaki HS, Yao JS, et al: A systematic approach to severe hand ischemia, *Surgery* 83(1):1–11, 1978.
5. Anonymous: Results of a prospective randomized trial evaluating surgery versus thrombolysis for ischemia of the lower extremity. The STILE trial, *Ann Surg* 220(3):251–266, discussion 266–8, 1994.
6. Ouriel K, Veith FJ, Sasahara AA: A comparison of recombinant urokinase with vascular surgery as initial treatment for acute arterial occlusion of the legs. Thrombolysis or Peripheral Arterial Surgery (TOPAS) Investigators [see comment], *N Engl J Med* 338 (16):1105–1111, 1998.
7. Criado FJ, Twena M: Techniques for endovascular recanalization of supra-aortic trunks, *J Endovasc Surg* 3(4):405–413, 1996.
8. Insall RL, Lambert D, Chamberlain J, et al: Percutaneous transluminal angioplasty of the innominate, subclavian, and axillary arteries, *Eur J Vasc Surg* 4(6):591–595, 1990.
9. Tetteroo E, van der Graaf Y, Bosch JL, et al: Randomised comparison of primary stent placement versus primary angioplasty followed by selective stent placement in patients with iliac-artery occlusive disease. Dutch Iliac Stent Trial Study Group, *Lancet* 351(9110):1153–1159, 1998.
10. Brountzos EN, Petersen B, Binkert C, et al: Primary stenting of subclavian and innominate artery occlusive disease: a single center's experience, *Cardiovasc Intervent Radiol* 27(6):616–623, 2004.
11. Henry M, Amor M, Henry I, et al: Percutaneous transluminal angioplasty of the subclavian arteries, *J Endovasc Surg* 6(1):33–41, 1999.
12. Diethrich EB, Ndiaye M, Reid DB: Stenting in the carotid artery: initial experience in 110 patients, *J Endovasc Surg* 3(1):42–62, 1996.
13. Dietrich E: Technique of carotid angioplasty. In Yao JS, Pearce WH, editors: *Techniques in Vascular and Endovascular Surgery*, Stamford, CT, 1998, Appleton and Lange, pp 475–488.
14. Yadav JS, Wholey MH, Kuntz RE, et al: Protected carotid-artery stenting versus endarterectomy in high-risk patients [see comment], *N Engl J Med* 351(15):1493–1501, 2004.
15. Johnson SP, Fujitani RM, Leyendecker JR, et al: Stent deformation and intimal hyperplasia complicating treatment of a post-carotid endarterectomy intimal flap with a Palmaz stent [see comment], *J Vasc Surg* 25(4):764–768, 1997.
16. Varcoe RL, Mah J, Young N, et al: Prevalence of carotid stent fractures in a single-center experience, *J Endovasc Ther* 15 (4):485–489, 2008.
17. Valibhoy AR, Mwipatayi BP, Sieunarine K, et al: Fracture of a carotid stent: an unexpected complication, *J Vasc Surg* 45(3): 603–606, 2007.
18. Surdell D, Shaibani A, Bendok B, et al: Fracture of a nitinol carotid artery stent that caused restenosis, *J Vasc Intervent Radiol* 18(10):1297–1299, 2007.
19. Matsumura JS, Rilling WS, Pearce WH, et al: Helical computed tomography of the normal thoracic outlet, *J Vasc Surg* 26 (5):776–783, 1997.
20. Ahn SS, Eton D, Yeatman LR, et al: Intraoperative peripheral rotary atherectomy: early and late clinical results, *Ann Vasc Surg* 6 (3):272–280, 1992.
21. Dorros G, Iyer S, Zaitoun R, et al: Acute angiographic and clinical outcome of high speed percutaneous rotational atherectomy (Rotablator), *Catheter Cardiovasc Diagnosis* 22(3):157–166, 1991.

22. Yao JS: Upper extremity ischemia in athletes, *Semin Vasc Surg* 11 (2):96–105, 1998.
23. Motarjeme A, Gordon GI: Percutaneous transluminal angioplasty of the brachiocephalic vessels: guidelines for therapy, *Int Angiol* 12(3):260–269, 1993.
24. Selby JB Jr, Matsumoto AH, Tegtmeyer CJ, et al: Balloon angioplasty above the aortic arch: immediate and long-term results, *AJR Am J Roentgenol* 160(3):631–635, 1993.
25. Mesh CL, McCarthy WJ, Pearce WH, et al: Upper extremity bypass grafting. A 15-year experience, *Arch Surg* 128(7):795–801, discussion 801–2, 1993.
26. Brewster DC, Moncure AC, Darling RC, et al: Innominate artery lesions: problems encountered and lessons learned, *J Vasc Surg* 2(1):99–112, 1985.
27. Cherry KJ Jr, McCullough JL, Hallett JW Jr, et al: Technical principles of direct innominate artery revascularization: a comparison of endarterectomy and bypass grafts, *J Vasc Surg* 9 (5):718–723, discussion 723–4, 1989.
28. Kieffer E, Sabatier J, Koskas F, Bahnini A: Atherosclerotic innominate artery occlusive disease: early and long-term results of surgical reconstruction, *J Vasc Surg* 21(2):326–336, discussion 336–7, 1995.
29. Van Damme H, Caudron D, Defraigne JO, et al: Brachiocephalic arterial reconstruction, *Acta Chir Belg* 92(1):37–45, 1992.

SECTION VIII

ANEURYSMAL DISEASE AND TRAUMATIC INJURIES

CHAPTER

43

Endovascular Repair of Thoracic Aortic Aneurysms

Joel E. Barbato, Jae S. Cho, Michel S. Makaroun

Open surgical replacement of the thoracic aorta has been the traditionally accepted means of addressing a number of thoracic pathologies for decades. In large series with experienced surgeons, operative mortality from open thoracic aortic repair can be as low as 3% to 8% with rates of paraplegia, the most feared complication of this operation, of 3% to 5%.[1,2] This operation, however, subjects the patient to significant hemodynamic shifts and is often limited by underlying chronic obstructive pulmonary disease and/or inability to tolerate single-lung ventilation. In addition, these operations are often associated with lengthy hospital stays and substantial patient discomfort.

With the advent of thoracic endografts that can be implanted through small groin incisions, sometimes with the patient under only local anesthetic, the overall risk to the patient has decreased and expanded the potential pool of patients who are candidates for repair. There are currently three devices—the Gore TAG, the Medtronic Talent, and the Cook TX2—that are commercially available in the United States. The Bolton Relay as well as the modified Medtronic Valiant devices are undergoing a phase II trial in the United States. This chapter will focus on the grafts that are either available or undergoing clinical trials in the United States and specific issues related to device deployment and follow-up of these patients.

DESCRIPTION OF DEVICES

Gore TAG

The TAG graft (W. L. Gore & Associates, Inc., Flagstaff, AZ) was the first thoracic endograft to gain Food and Drug Administration (FDA) approval in the United States for the treatment of descending thoracic aneurysms. Thus this is the most widely used device in the United States for both FDA-approved and off-label use. It is a nontapered tubular graft with expanded polytetrafluoroethylene (ePTFE) reinforced with fluorinated ethylene propylene (FEP) material and external nickel-titanium (nitinol) self-expanding stents (Figure 43-1). The stents are secured to the graft with ePTFE/FEP bonding tape. It has flared edges both proximally and distally to aid in seal apposition. The graft has an inlaid gold band that marks the proximal and distal edges although the flared ends protrude 7 to 9 mm beyond these. At each end of the graft is an additional ePTFE cuff that is external to the nitinol stents intended to aid in the ability of the graft to create a seal. The ePTFE fabric is a stronger variant introduced to replace the longitudinal deployment wire in the original device because of fractures. The new material also has a lower porosity intended to avoid a high incidence of sac enlargement discovered with the abdominal Gore Excluder device.[3]

The TAG device is constrained by a sleeve of ePTFE/FEP film that is held in place by a longitudinal seam that runs the entire length of the device. This seam is held together by an ePTFE line connected to a deployment knob located at the control end of the delivery catheter. Similar to the abdominal Excluder device, the device is deployed by pulling on the string, which opens the seam, thereby deploying the stent graft. Devices are available in 26- to 40-mm diameters and 10-, 15-, or 20-cm lengths, depending on the diameter. A 45-mm-diameter device is under clinical trial. The device requires a 20F to 24F sheath for delivery.

Landing zones of at least 2 cm are recommended although one must consider the quality of the aorta (presence of thrombus and/or calcification) and tortuosity of the landing zone and adjust the desired length accordingly, taking into account that the more aorta that is covered, the higher the potential for coverage of

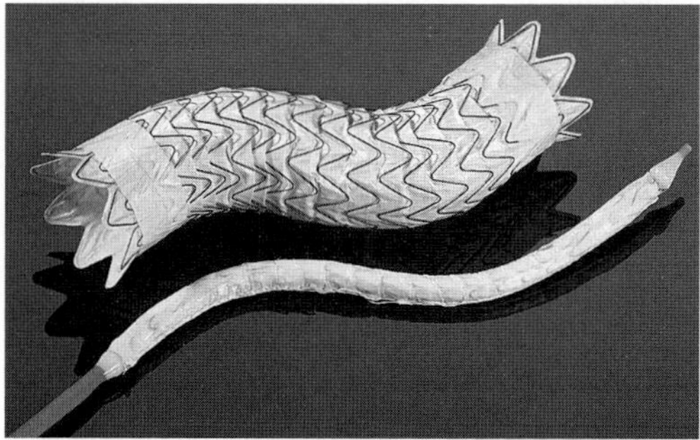

FIGURE 43-1 Gore TAG graft shown both deployed and while constrained on delivery system.

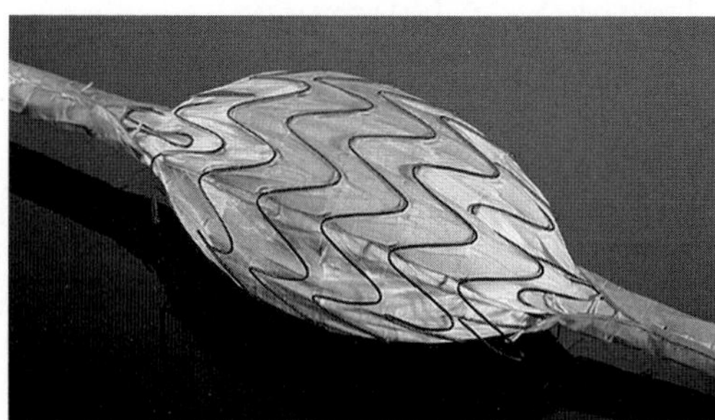

FIGURE 43-2 Deployment of the Gore TAG device showing initial opening at the middle of the graft.

intercostal vessels that may supply the spinal cord and affect paraplegia rates.

The TAG device does not require alignment with the aortic curvature and is deployed in a single step by pulling the deployment line. The endograft deploys from the middle of the graft out (Figure 43-2) to both ends. This is intended to avoid a "wind sock" effect that would occur with initial proximal release. The seal zones are subsequently ballooned with a trilobed balloon, which allows for continuous antegrade blood flow during ballooning.

The next generation C-TAG device is expected to enter a clinical trial in the United States for acute aortic dissections and traumatic aortic transections by the time this book is published. The device has several modifications including replacement of the covered scallops with bare metal without flares. This design, along with increased radial force, is intended to allow better conformability to angulated necks and improved apposition to the aortic wall. It will also have a broader range of diameters to allow treatment of smaller aortic diameters as is often seen in trauma patients.

The TAG underwent phase I trials in the United States in 1998 and 1999 and phase II trials from 1999 to 2001. The latter trial compared patients with a descending thoracic aneurysm treated with the TAG device with a nonrandomized open repair cohort. Successful implantation occurred in 139 of 142 patients. At 30 days, there were 3 deaths (2.1%) compared with 11 (11.7%) in the open surgical controls. The 5-year data have also been presented and will be summarized later in the chapter.[4]

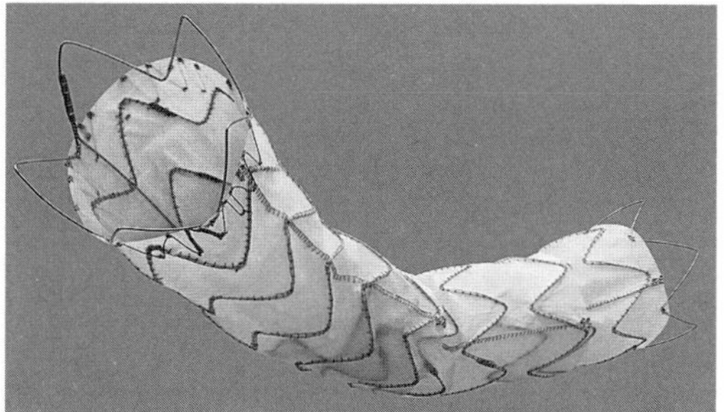

FIGURE 43-3 Medtronic Talent thoracic endograft.

Medtronic Talent

Medtronic's graft, Talent (Medtronic, Santa Rosa, CA), has been the most widely used thoracic endograft outside the United States and has been available worldwide since 1997. It just received FDA approval for commercial use in the United States in June 2008. The Talent has a nitinol skeleton that is attached to a woven polyester graft. The Talent has different configurations for proximal and distal use and is provided with cylindrical or tapered construction to accommodate the diameter differences along the length of the aorta (Figure 43-3). It is available in diameters ranging from 22 to 46 mm, but unfortunately available lengths are limited to 112 to 116 mm. It is delivered through a 22F to 25F delivery system. The proximal end has bare metal stents that aid in fixation and allow flow into covered branch vessels such as the left subclavian or the left carotid. A similar configuration is also available to aid in distal fixation with a bare stent component. The recommended graft oversizing is 10% to 20%. Because the device is available in only short lengths, most of the cases would require more than one device and multiple introduction of the devices through the iliac system. In the VALOR trial, an average of 2.7 devices were used per case.[5]

The Talent has a longitudinal support bar that runs the length of the graft and is intended to be aligned along the greater curvature of the aorta. The bar is marked with a "figure of 8" marker in the middle of the stent graft for identification and orientation. The sheath should be turned to locate the bar, which should be at the same side as the flushing port of the delivery system. This delivery system includes its own sheath, and the graft is deployed by a simple retraction of the outer sheath exposing the graft from proximal to distal and allowing the device to self-expand.

A newer version of the graft, the Valiant, is being used overseas and undergoing clinical trials in the United

States. This device has several changes from the Talent device. First, it uses the "Xcelerant" delivery system with a shortened tip for improved trackability, and the outer sheath has a hydrophilic coating to make it more stretch resistant and easier to deploy. Its bare stent design has also changed to eight peaks with less flare from its current five peaks to reduce pressure points and no longer has the longitudinal connecting bar for improved conformability. The device is also available in lengths up to 227 mm.

The 12-month pivotal results of the American trial studying the Talent graft (VALOR) are now available.[5] The study was a prospective, nonrandomized, multicenter trial of patients at low risk who were considered candidates for open repair. To be included, patients must have had a landing zone of at least 2 cm beyond the left common carotid and above the celiac artery. A total of 195 patients were enrolled between December 2003 and June 2005. The average maximal diameter of the aneurysms treated was 5.5 cm. Technical success occurred in 99.5% of cases with an average of 2.7 devices used per patient; 5.2% of patients underwent left subclavian artery (LSA) revascularization; and, similar to other trials, 21.1% of patients had an iliac conduit created for access. A third (33.5%) of patients had deployment of the proximal bare metal springs beyond the LSA. On average, the patients stayed in the intensive care unit for 2 days and total hospital stay averaged 6.4 days. At 30 days, all-cause mortality was 2.1% and, at 1 year, 16.1%. Aneurysm-related mortality at 1 year, however, was only 3.1%.

As with the other endografts, complication rates were relatively low. Spinal cord ischemia at 30 days, however, was somewhat higher than in other studies: paraplegia 1.5% and paraparesis 7.2% (another patient had paraplegia at 32 days). Major and minor stroke rates were 3.6% despite almost a third of patients having deployment of the bare stent fixation portion of the graft in the arch near the left carotid artery. Serious major adverse events were significantly less than in open surgery and occurred in 42.7% of patients although aneurysm rupture, and conversion to surgery at 1 year was only 0.5%. Persistent endoleaks were present in 12% of patients at 1 year with 6.5% of patients requiring a secondary endovascular procedure within the first year to treat an endoleak.

Cook TX2

The Cook TX2 stent graft (Cook Medical, Bloomington, IN) is a modular system consisting of a proximal and a distal component and was granted U.S. FDA approval for commercial use in May 2008. The graft is composed of stainless steel stents and woven Dacron. The graft is fully stented with the location of stents relative to the fabric varying along the length of the graft. At the ends of the device, the stents are on the inside of the graft; otherwise, the stents are on the outside. This is designed to optimize fabric apposition to the aortic wall and fabric-fabric interstent junctions. Visualization of the graft is enhanced by four gold radiopaque markers near the edge of the graft. The device is available in diameters from 28 to 42 mm in 2-mm increments and in lengths from 120 to 216 mm. There is also a tapered proximal graft that allows for a 4-mm difference between the proximal and distal necks. The delivery system is 20F to 22F.

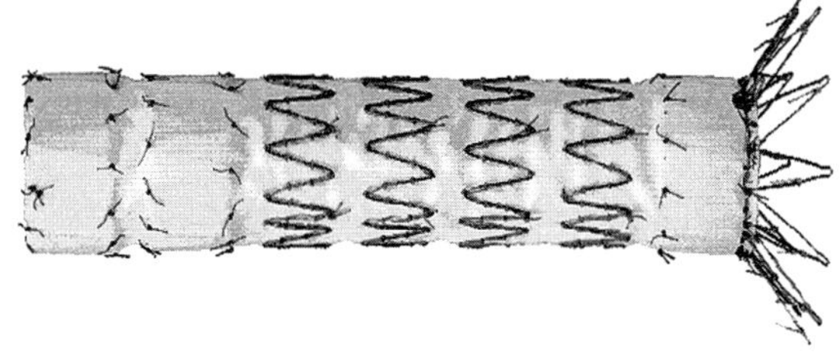

FIGURE 43-4 Cook TX2 thoracic endograft.

The TX2 system consists of a proximal (TX2P) and a distal (TX2D) component, with at least an intended two-stent overlap between them. This system is unique in using an active fixation system; the proximal end of TX2P is covered without bare stents and has caudally oriented barbs to prevent distal migration. The distal end of TX2D has bare stents with barbs directed cranially to prevent proximal migration (Figure 43-4). The bare stents in the distal end are designed to allow fixation of the device over the visceral vessels while maintaining patency of these vessels. However, this device requires a 3-cm landing zone both proximally and distally.

The TX2 device is deployed in a staged, controlled fashion, like its abdominal counterpart. The graft is first released by withdrawing the outer sheath with the proximal stent still constrained. Once position of the device is confirmed, deployment is completed by releasing the trigger wire. With use of a balloon, the device is secured in position.

The STARZ trial was a nonrandomized, controlled, multicenter, international trial designed to assess the safety and efficacy of this device conducted from March 2004 to July 2006.[6] It enrolled a total of 230 patients with 160 receiving endografts and 70 patients receiving open repair (51 of whom were collected retrospectively) to serve as controls. The trial allowed for penetrating aortic ulcers, as well as thoracic aneurysms. Ulcers constituted 14% of the patients in the thoracic endovascular aortic repair (TEVAR) arm and 10% in the open arm. Aneurysms were eligible for repair if they were $\geq$5 cm or if their growth rate was $\geq$5 mm per year. Because this trial was not randomized, there were some significant demographic differences between the two groups including a higher incidence of older and more obese patients in the TEVAR group, whereas those in the open group had a higher incidence of prior thoracic surgery or trauma.

Of the patients in the endovascular arm of the study, 29% underwent their procedure with a regional anesthetic. Conduits were used in 10% of cases. Thirty-day mortality was noninferior compared with the open cohort (98.1% vs. 94.3%; $p <0.01$). One-year aneurysm-related mortality was 94% in the TEVAR group and 88% in the open group. Overall morbidity was less at 30 days in the TEVAR group with significantly lower incidences of cardiovascular, pulmonary, and vascular complications.

Bolton Relay

The Bolton Relay thoracic graft (Bolton Medical, Sunrise, FL) is a self-expanding nitinol-based stent with a highly compliant polyester fabric (Figure 43-5). On the proximal portion of the product is a bare metal stent. This portion acts to anchor the device in place while maintaining patency of branch vessels. The Transport delivery system consists of coaxially arranged sheaths and catheters (primary introduction sheath, secondary delivery sheath with a preformed curve intended to conform to the arch, and thru lumen) and an apex release mechanism. The double-S configuration of the torsional longitudinal support bar is intended to naturally follow the anatomy of the aortic arch and to provide moderate columnar strength while maintaining flexibility and torque response.

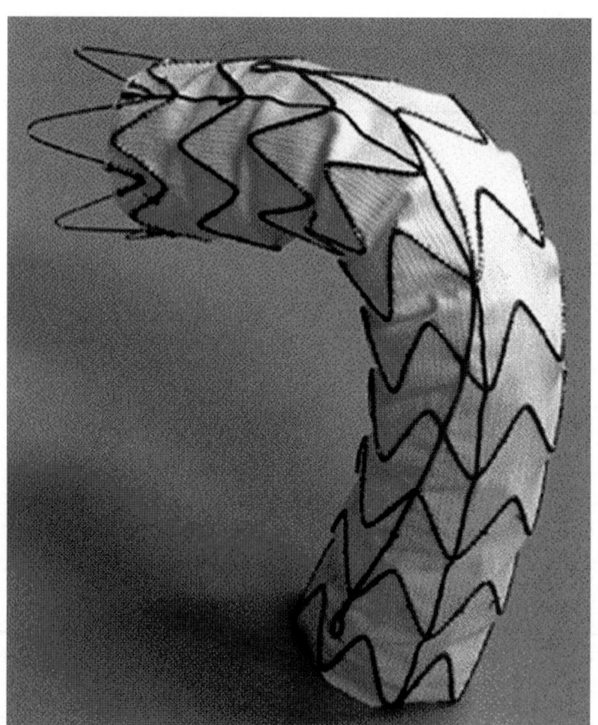

FIGURE 43-5 Bolton Relay thoracic graft demonstrating longitudinal stent and proximal bare stents for fixation.

Visualization of the device is enhanced by a series of radiopaque markers made of platinum and iridium attached to the endograft in various locations. The device is available in both tapered and nontapered configurations. Nontapered grafts are available in diameters from 22 to 46 mm in increments of 2 mm and in lengths from 100 to 250 mm in increments of 50 mm. The profile of the primary introducer sheath ranges from 22F to 26F. Tapered grafts taper in 4-mm increments from proximal to distal. The average recommended oversizing is 10% to 15%. A proximal landing zone of 25 mm is required, and the distal landing zone should be at least 30 mm. When using multiple grafts, a minimum of 50 mm of overlap is recommended.

The Relay device is deployed by first positioning the primary sheath in the abdominal aorta. The secondary sheath is then navigated through the thoracic aorta and positioned in the desired location. The device also uses a controlled-release mechanism like the TX2. The outer sheath is pulled to expand the endograft, and the proximal bare stents are released by a separate mechanism. Postdeployment ballooning is generally not required. No published data on this device currently exist.

PLANNING AND DEPLOYMENT

Access Issues/Conduits

Once the entry site is chosen on the basis of preoperative assessment, the ipsilateral common femoral artery is exposed in a standard fashion or accessed percutaneously by using a Preclose suture technique. The contralateral artery is accessed percutaneously for placement of a marker pigtail catheter. Alternative additional access can be obtained from the brachial for assistance with precise placement proximally or to aid in the delivery of devices in a very tortuous aorta. A stiff wire (Lunderquist [Cook Medical] or Meier [Boston Scientific, Natick, MA]) is placed into the ascending aorta. It is helpful to mark the back end of the wire on the table to detect any unintentional movement of the wire both proximally and distally.

On occasion, especially in women, who tend to have smaller iliac arteries, a conduit may be necessary for implantation of these thoracic grafts because of their rather large sheath requirements. This is effected by anastomosing a 10-mm Dacron graft onto the distal common iliac artery through a small retroperitoneal incision. The conduit can be used through that incision, or in obese individuals it can be brought out through the groin to allow a straight access to the iliac artery. The side of the conduit should be accessed through a small stab incision rather than the open end of it, to maximize stability of the sheath during later manipulations in the operation. On completion of the procedure, the conduit is divided at the base or converted to an iliofemoral bypass graft if the external iliac artery flow is compromised. This procedure can be done expeditiously without undue increase in operative time and is needed in 10% to 20% of patients.

Placement of a guidewire or a catheter into the celiac axis or superior mesenteric artery (when the celiac axis is to be covered) can serve as a guide. In the event imprecise deployment results in encroachment on the celiac axis or superior mesenteric artery, it can also provide a ready access to the vessel for retrograde stent placement. Similarly, the LSA can also be accessed via the left brachial artery and provide a ready access should restoration of flow to the LSA be required as mentioned earlier.

Management of the Left Subclavian Artery

As mentioned, the proximal seal zone is one of the significant challenges of thoracic endografting. The proximal aortic arch is divided into zones from proximal to distal labeled from zero to four. Typically an area of normal aorta of at least 20 to 30 mm is recommended to create a proper seal. Often this means impinging on or deploying proximal to the LSA, occurring in 15% to 33% of cases in the U.S. trials.

The LSA plays an important role in perfusion of both the brain and the spinal cord. In addition to well-documented perfusion of the brain via the left vertebral artery, the LSA also gives rise to the internal mammary artery and its anterior intercostal branches, as well as branches to the anterior spinal artery.[7] Branches from the costocervical trunk that arise from the subclavian artery can also provide important collateral branches to the spinal cord. When it is necessary to deploy the stent graft proximal to the LSA (Figure 43-6), careful preoperative assessment and planning can help identify patients who may be at risk for stroke if the LSA is covered without revascularization. In general, coverage of the LSA is well tolerated in the presence of normal arterial anatomy because of the presence of rich collateral networks.[8-10]

Selective LSA revascularization, either by a left common carotid artery to LSA bypass graft or LSA to left common carotid artery transposition, is, however, indicated in the presence of a dominant left vertebral artery, an aberrant right subclavian, a patent left internal mammary conduit to coronary arteries, or inadequate collaterals.[11,12] Revascularization should also be considered when an elevated risk of paraplegia exists with extensive coverage of the thoracic aorta combined with a previous infrarenal aortic replacement. The procedure is relatively simple and can be done with a modest increase in operative time, although it can be associated with recurrent laryngeal and phrenic nerve injuries and thoracic duct injuries.[12,13] Delayed revascularization can usually be performed in cases of arm ischemia without untoward effects.

Management of the Celiac Axis

The celiac artery marks the distal-most extent of TEVAR. Like the subclavian artery, however, the celiac artery can be covered in an attempt to extend the landing zone to create an appropriate seal when there is adequate collateral flow to the celiac bed via patent gastroduodenal artery. Criado et al.[14] observed no mesenteric ischemic complications with three cases of

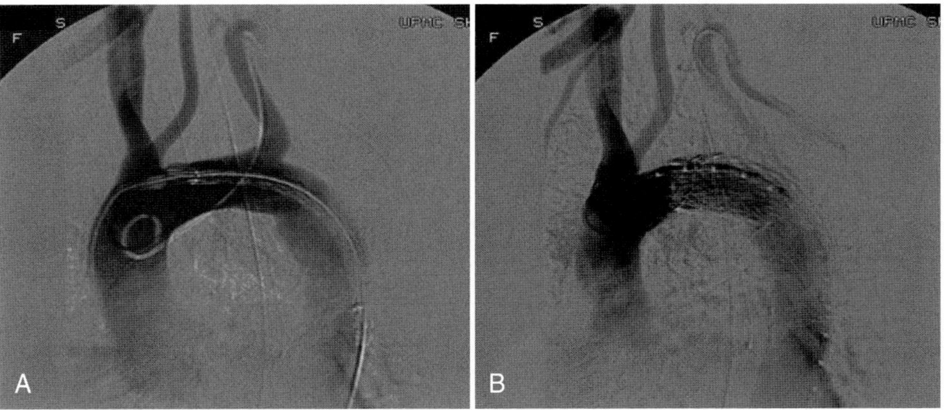

FIGURE 43-6 Angiogram of the aortic arch demonstrating predeployment **(A)** and postdeployment **(B)** runs with coverage of the LSA by the endograft.

celiac axis coverage. Vaddineni et al.[15] reported on their experience with planned celiac coverage. By extending beyond the celiac, they gained between 9 and 25 mm of extra seal zone. Only one patient had postoperative abdominal symptoms, which resolved without intervention. One must be prepared, however, to perform an open surgical bypass in these patients should collateral flow not be present.

Imaging

Aortography is obtained through a marker pigtail catheter with appropriate left anterior oblique (45 degrees or greater in some cases) projection of the image intensifier to widen the aortic arch and to separate the great vessels. For visualization of the distal landing zone, especially near the celiac axis, a full lateral projection may be necessary.

Delivery and Deployment

Once the landing zones are identified, the chosen stent graft is introduced via the delivery catheter/sheath, while visualizing the leading edge of the graft at all times as it is being introduced into the landing zone. There could be several areas of tortuosity that need to be negotiated during TEVAR: iliac, descending thoracic, and aortic arch. Most of the iliac tortuosity can be dealt with by using stiff wires and hydrophilic delivery systems, or use of a conduit through the common iliac artery if the tortuosity is excessive. For more proximal angulations, placement of a "buddy wire" or brachiofemoral wire can be used to help straighten the aorta. If the latter is used, a long catheter should be placed through the brachial artery across the origin of the subclavian artery to avoid possible injury at the subclavian ostium.

Instructions for use of each particular device dictate specific and unique procedural steps for deployment. However, certain general tips and rules apply. The device is placed beyond the target region and brought back to the target line to eliminate any stored forward energy. While this maneuver is being performed, constant forward pressure is applied on the wire to keep it pushed against the outer curvature of the aorta. This helps deploy the stent graft along the outer curvature of aorta and helps prevent distal migration during deployment.

At the time of deployment, temporary reduction of blood pressure helps minimize the wind sock effect, thereby reducing the risk of distal migration of the device. Complete cardiac arrest with adenosine is not necessary in most patients. Reducing aortic flow with rapid pacing can be used with devices that are deployed from the proximal end without controlled mechanism for release. The entire deployment procedure should be performed under fluoroscopic guidance. Avoiding excessively slow deployment and maintaining forward force on the wire may also be helpful to avoid a wind sock effect.

When more than one graft is needed, the smaller device should be deployed first to allow for adequate sealing at the junction. When more than two devices are used, the proximal and the distal landings zones may be treated first with the third larger device deployed between the two. Adequate overlap of at least 5 cm is necessary with all devices. For same-size devices longer overlap zones may be needed.

RESULTS

Analysis of TEVAR results is limited by the fact that there has not been a randomized trial comparing the efficacy of TEVAR with open repairs for the treatment of thoracic aortic aneurysm (TAA). Most series report either single-center or registry experience that consists of a mixture of anatomic locations, device types, and patient presentations rendering comparison between studies rather difficult. Furthermore, the available data do not reflect the early and late performance of currently available modified devices, as well as learning curves of both institutions and clinicians. Comparisons of open results are similarly limited. Thus the U.S. FDA trials of the three devices are the best sources of information on the safety and efficacy of TEVAR.

Early Results

Technical Success

Highly successful endograft deployment rates of 98% have been reported in all three U.S. FDA trials and in the Talent thoracic registry.[4-6,16] Access difficulties accounted for essentially all procedural failures in these studies. In EUROSTAR and the United Kingdom thoracic registry, a lower procedural success rate of 87% occurred, more reflective of current clinical practice outside of trial guidelines.

Mortality

A significant survival benefit was observed with TEVAR as compared with open repairs (2% vs. 6%) in the U.S. trials. When applied to a broad spectrum of pathologies, with 52% of its patients deemed at high risk for open repairs, EUROSTAR data reported a higher, but still favorable, mortality rate of 5.3% for TEVAR.[17] A meta-analysis of published literature shows clear survival benefits with TEVAR compared with the open procedure.[18]

Neurologic Complications

Neurologic complications are by far the most feared and devastating of all complications after TAA repairs, whether by endovascular or open means. TEVAR does not appear to confer any advantage over standard open repair in regard to stroke; the incidences of stroke ranged from 3% to 5% after both open repair and TEVAR.[5,6,12,19,20] Stroke occurs with TEVAR primarily because of instrumentation of the aortic arch and coverage of a critical source of blood to the brain.[14] Deployment of stent grafts proximal to the LSA has been associated with an increased risk of postoperative stroke. In the phase II TAG study, stroke occurred in 14% of patients with deployment of stent grafts proximal to the LSA compared with 1% when the stent graft was deployed distal to the LSA. Similarly, in the VALOR High-Risk trial, presented at the Society for Vascular Surgery meeting in Chicago in 2005, the incidence of stroke was 26% when the stent graft was deployed proximal to the LSA.[21] However, in the STARZ trial, all four strokes occurred with stent graft deployment distal to the LSA.[6] This finding is difficult to explain but may relate to the proximal deployment of the TX2, which normally starts more proximally and is then adjusted to its final position. Minimal manipulations and meticulous cleansing of wires, catheters, and delivery system and use of balloon molding only inside the stent graft cannot be overemphasized in minimizing the risk of stroke during TEVAR. Other independent predictors of stroke from the EUROSTAR data include female sex and prolonged procedure time (>2 hours 40 minutes).[20]

With respect to spinal cord injury (SCI), a combination of all three trials shows an advantage to TEVAR over open repair (6% vs. 10%). The incidence of paraplegia in the control group of these FDA trials was higher than what has been reported from centers of excellence, which have been as low as 3%.[1,2] However, it should be pointed out that paraparesis was included in SCI in these trials whereas most single-center series do not include it. In one study, when paraparesis was included the incidence of SCI after open repair was reported at 8.6%.[22] Conversely, if paraparesis is excluded in the TEVAR arms of the trials, paraplegia rate drops from 6% to 1.4%. The protective effects of TEVAR against SCI may be due to avoidance of thoracic aortic clamping and reduced hemodynamic disturbances at the spinal cord level because of lack of blood loss from intercostal back-bleeding. It should also be noted that SCI is not confined to the perioperative period. Delayed and recurrent SCI and paraplegia after TEVAR have been reported.[23]

Several factors have been linked to an increased risk of SCI after TEVAR: concomitant or previous open infrarenal aortic replacement, extensive thoracic aortic coverage, renal insufficiency, intraoperative hypotension (systolic blood pressure <80 mm Hg), and coverage of the hypogastric artery and LSA.[12,14,20,24,25] Some of these risk factors are beyond the clinician's control, but coverage of the LSA and hypogastric arteries can be averted by modifying the operative plan. Occlusion of the LSA has been shown to be associated with a significant increase in the incidence of paraplegia by the EUROSTAR collaborators, and recent reports suggest that LSA revascularization may be required more frequently than previously recognized for either left upper extremity ischemic symptoms or spinal cord protection.[11,12,20] It has been noted that lumbar and pelvic collaterals account for 25% of spinal cord blood supply, and a compromised hypogastric blood flow contributed to the development of SCI.[26] For this reason, preservation of internal iliac blood flow and a staged repair of synchronous TAA and abdominal aortic aneurysm to allow development of collateralization have been recommended.[27]

There is currently little uniformity over the use of spinal cord protective techniques in the use of thoracic endografts. Most of the clinical studies have allowed the individual practitioner to dictate which, if any, adjunctive measures are undertaken. One of the most commonly used adjuncts with TEVAR is cerebrospinal fluid (CSF) drainage. Although some use it routinely, most centers use it selectively on the basis of estimated risk of paraplegia of individual patients. The drain is inserted before surgery and maintained for 24 to 48 hours, keeping the CSF pressure under 10 mm Hg. Its efficacy has also been observed in reversal of delayed-onset paraplegia after TEVAR. Although it can be associated with hemorrhagic complications from catheter placement with reported incidence of 0% to 3%, CSF drainage should be used when an elevated potential for SCI exists such as extensive coverage of the thoracic aorta or with associated abdominal aortoiliac pathology.

Vascular Complications

Another complication that occurs commonly with TEVAR is access site injury. In the early TAG experience, a relatively high incidence of 14% was reported.[21] Introduction of a large sheath through relatively small iliac arteries accounts for this phenomenon. That women, who have smaller iliac arteries than men, constitute about 40% of TAA patients also contributes to this problem. With increased awareness of this complication its incidence has decreased to 6% in the confirmatory TAG trial.[19]

Endoleaks

The classification of endoleaks in thoracic grafts is the same as that for the infrarenal endografts. The incidence of endoleaks at 30 days was higher with the Talent device in the VALOR trial than with other devices. At

30 days, a nearly 26% incidence of endoleaks was reported with Talent as compared with 3.6% for TAG and 4.8% with TX2. A difference in reporting method may account for this difference. All endoleaks observed at any time before 30 days were included in the VALOR report whereas only those noted at the 30-day follow-up were reported in the other two studies.

Late Results

Late Survival

One-year data from all three U.S. trials have shown aneurysm-related survival benefit with TEVAR compared with open repairs, 95% vs. 89%, respectively. This survival advantage persisted at a 5-year follow-up in the TAG study. There were a total of 4 aneurysm-related deaths in the TAG group (2.8%) compared with 11 in the open cohort (11.7%; $p = 0.008$) showing a distinct aneurysm-related survival advantage for the TAG patients. This late aneurysm-related survival benefit with TEVAR was mostly due to perioperative survival benefit. Three of the 4 deaths in the TAG group occurred in hospital resulting from a stroke, a cardiac event, and sepsis. Only one late aneurysm-related death occurred at 2 months resulting from an aortoesophageal fistula. All of the open surgical deaths occurred within the first year and were related to respiratory failure (6), stroke (3), cardiac events (1), and aortoesophageal fistula (1). Major adverse events occurred in 28% of TAG patients and 70% of surgical controls ($p < 0.001$) in the postoperative period; this advantage for the TAG patient persisted at 12 months (42% vs. 77%; $p < 0.001$) and at 5 years (58% vs. 79%; $p = 0.001$). All-cause mortality between the two groups was similar: 68% for TEVAR and 67% for open groups.[4] This finding mirrors those of randomized endovascular repair of infrarenal abdominal aortic aneurysm (EVAR) trials in the abdominal aorta.[28]

For high-risk patient populations, studies from Stanford University have shown that late outcomes are poor with an actuarial survival rate of 31% at 5 years.[29] This observation is akin to the findings of the EVAR-2 trial and of EUROSTAR data for patients with abdominal aortic aneurysm and raises the question on the validity and efficacy of treatment in this patient cohort.

Endoleaks and Migration

Reporting methods and sources have been variable among studies, accounting for some of the large differences noted in endoleaks and migration rates. The TAG study relied on investigators reporting, whereas the other two trials relied mostly on a core laboratory. Persistent endoleaks at 1 year were noted in 12% of patients in the VALOR trial with 6.5% of patients requiring a secondary endovascular procedure and only 3.9% of patients in the STARZ trial. During long-term follow-up of the TAG study, approximately 4% of patients continued to have an endoleak at each yearly follow-up up to 5 years.[4-6] The incidence of endoleaks is decreasing with second-generation devices with design improvements and better conformability.[30] The distribution of endoleak type is also variable with the TAG reporting a majority of type I and III endoleaks whereas the other two studies show primarily type II endoleaks. Endoleaks in general occur less frequently after TEVAR than with EVAR and account for most of the reinterventions.

Device migration occurs rather infrequently with current devices with reported incidence ranging from 0.7% to 3.9%. Graft migration of more than 10 mm occurred in 2.8% (3/107) of patients at 12 months with TX2, although none resulted in endoleak or reintervention. All were noted to have had implantation of the barbed segment either in an acutely angled segment or within thrombus. With the Talent device, the incidence was 3.9%, resulting in one reintervention.

Sac Behavior and Ruptures

Aneurysm sac enlargement has been reported to occur in 7.1% to 14.5% of patients after TEVAR at 1 year.[17,31] The incidence appears similar among all three graft types.. In the only 5-year follow-up report, aneurysm sac decrease of $\geq$5 mm was observed in 50% of patients whereas it remained stable in 27% of patients in the TAG pivotal trial.[4] Sac growth of $\geq$5 mm, on the other hand, was observed in 19% of patients. These results, however, are from normal-porosity ePTFE grafts and may not reflect long-term performance of currently available devices that use low-porosity material. After the normal-porosity ePTFE material was found to result in significant sac growth in the infrarenal grafts, the material was changed to a low-porosity fabric.[3] With this change, the percentage of patients who had sac enlargement decreased from 12.9% to 2.9% in the confirmatory TAG trial. A similar increase in sac shrinkage rate was noted with the infrarenal Excluder using the low-porosity material.[32] Results with other devices are to be determined. Only one rupture has been reported in all three U.S. trial patients; one rupture in the Talent device resulted from fabric erosion.

Reinterventions

Reinterventions during the first year have been noted in only 2.1% in the TAG study, in 4.4% in the STARZ trial, and in 10.7% of the VALOR trial. The incidence for the open control group was 5.7% in the STARZ trial at 1 year. At 5 years secondary procedures were performed in 15% of TAG patients and 32% of open surgical controls.

Stent Graft Collapse

One of the more difficult challenges associated with thoracic endografts involves obtaining a proper seal in the curved aortic arch. This has been reported with several types of endografts but most commonly with the TAG device when used for traumatic aortic transection. This occurs frequently in younger patients with small, more dynamic aortas for which the current generations of endografts are oversized.[33] The phenomenon of "bird-beaking" is not unusual (Figure 43-7), and the lack of apposition to the inner curve of the arch may be the initiating factor of collapse presenting a leading edge for the high thoracic aortic flow. This can result in devastating consequences such as reperfusion of the pseudoaneurysm sac or aortic obstruction.

Fortunately, many of these situations can be fixed with further endovascular means. Hinchliffe et al.[34] demonstrated that in six of seven patients endograft collapse was repaired with either a balloon-expandable stent or further stent graft. In the setting of thoracic grafts placed for dissection or rupture, smaller aortas were more likely to result in this phenomenon, emphasizing the importance of not oversizing the graft more than the manufacturer's recommendation.[35]

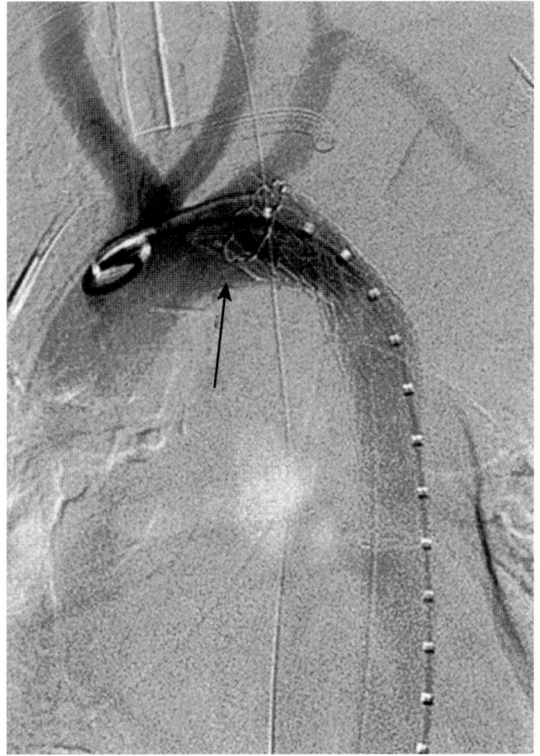

FIGURE 43-7 Angiogram demonstrating "bird-beaking" of graft as it rides off the lesser curvature of the aortic arch *(arrow)* with protrusion of the graft edge into the vessel lumen.

DISCUSSION

Relative to the fast progress in the development of and application of EVAR, the advances in the thoracic endografts have been slow because of a lower incidence of TAA, the need for larger device profile and delivery sheaths, the hostile hemodynamic forces in the thoracic aorta, and the proximity of the great vessels. Despite these hurdles, steady progress has been made to the point where, with three devices currently approved for commercial use by the U.S. FDA and another under a pivotal trial, TEVAR has secured its position as a safe and effective alternative, if not superior, to open surgical repair of TAA. High technical success rates with favorable mortality and paraparesis/paraplegia rates have been reported in all three FDA trials compared with open repairs of TAA. Device-specific adverse outcomes are rare but remain to be elucidated. Long-term results are not well understood.

Although these devices share similar traits, they also possess unique characteristics. Although the TAG device is very flexible, it also has the lowest radial force. This latter characteristic may predispose the device to infold and collapse when significant oversizing is used. Availability of smaller-diameter grafts with improved radial force is expected to help mitigate this problem. TX2 is unique in that it is the only device that uses an active fixation mechanism. This feature offers an advantage in a tortuous aorta and large aneurysm sacs helping to reduce both distal and proximal migration. This device, however, requires 3 cm of landing zones on both ends, which may limit the candidacy or increase the need for coverage of either the LSA and/or celiac axis. Both Talent and Relay devices are equipped with a longitudinal bar, which is designed to help orient and conform to the arch. Given its availability in short lengths only, the Talent endograft is not ideal for the treatment of long lesions because the use of multiple segments portends the risk of graft-related complications.

Obviously, none of these devices are perfect and suitable for all thoracic pathologies. Although current FDA approval is for TAA indication, there is widespread "off-label" use of these devices for other high-risk aortic pathologies. With continuing refinement of the stent grafts and development of pathology-specific devices, TEVAR is poised to expand its application to other complex aortic lesions beyond the atherosclerotic aneurysm.

References

1. Coselli JS, LeMaire SA, Conklin LD, et al: Left heart bypass during descending thoracic aortic aneurysm repair does not reduce the incidence of paraplegia, *Ann Thorac Surg* 77: 1298–1303, 2004.

2. Estrera AL, Miller CC III, Chen EP, et al: Descending thoracic aortic aneurysm repair: 12-year experience using distal aortic perfusion and cerebrospinal fluid drainage, *Ann Thorac Surg* 80:1290–1296, 2005.
3. Cho JS, Dillavou ED, Rhee RY, et al: Late abdominal aortic aneurysm enlargement after endovascular repair with the Excluder device, *J Vasc Surg* 39:1236–1241, 2004.
4. Makaroun MS, Dillavou ED, Wheatley GH, et al: Five-year results of endovascular treatment with the Gore TAG device compared with open repair of thoracic aortic aneurysms, *J Vasc Surg* 47:912–918, 2008.
5. Fairman RM, Criado F, Farber M, et al: Pivotal results of the Medtronic Vascular Talent Thoracic Stent Graft System: the VALOR Trial, *J Vasc Surg* 48:546–554, 2008.
6. Matsumura JS, Cambria RP, Dake MD, et al: International controlled clinical trial of thoracic endovascular aneurysm repair with the Zenith TX2 endovascular graft: 1-year results, *J Vasc Surg* 47:247–257, 2008.
7. Biglioli P, Roberto M, Cannata A, et al: Upper and lower spinal cord blood supply: the continuity of the anterior spinal artery and the relevance of the lumbar arteries, *J Thorac Cardiovasc Surg* 127:1188–1192, 2004.
8. Sunder-Plassmann L, Scharrer-Pamler R, Liewald F, et al: Endovascular exclusion of thoracic aortic aneurysms: mid-term results of elective treatment and in contained rupture, *J Card Surg* 18:367–374, 2003.
9. Rehders TC, Petzsch M, Ince H, et al: Intentional occlusion of the left subclavian artery during stent-graft implantation in the thoracic aorta: risk and relevance, *J Endovasc Ther* 11:659–666, 2004.
10. Riesenman PJ, Farber MA, Mendes RR, et al: Coverage of the left subclavian artery during thoracic endovascular aortic repair, *J Vasc Surg* 45:90–94, 2007.
11. Reece TB, Gazoni LM, Cherry KJ, et al: Reevaluating the need for left subclavian artery revascularization with thoracic endovascular aortic repair, *Ann Thorac Surg* 84:1201–1205, 2007.
12. Peterson BG, Eskandari MK, Gleason TG, et al: Utility of left subclavian artery revascularization in association with endoluminal repair of acute and chronic thoracic aortic pathology, *J Vasc Surg* 43:433–439, 2006.
13. Cina CS, Safar HA, Lagana A, et al: Subclavian carotid transposition and bypass grafting: consecutive cohort study and systematic review, *J Vasc Surg* 35:422–429, 2002.
14. Criado FJ, Abul-Khoudoud OR, Domer GS, et al: Endovascular repair of the thoracic aorta: lessons learned, *Ann Thorac Surg* 80:857–863, 2005.
15. Vaddineni SK, Taylor SM, Patterson MA, et al: Outcome after celiac artery coverage during endovascular thoracic aortic aneurysm repair: preliminary results, *J Vasc Surg* 45:467–471, 2007.
16. Fattori R, Nienaber CA, Rousseau H, et al: Results of endovascular repair of the thoracic aorta with the Talent thoracic stent graft: the Talent Thoracic Retrospective Registry, *J Thorac Cardiovasc Surg* 132:332–339, 2006.
17. Leurs LJ, Bell R, Degrieck Y, et al: Endovascular treatment of thoracic aortic diseases: combined experience from the EUROSTAR and United Kingdom Thoracic Endograft registries, *J Vasc Surg* 40:670–679, 2004.
18. Walsh SR, Tang TY, Sadat U, et al: Endovascular stenting versus open surgery for thoracic aortic disease: systematic review and meta-analysis of perioperative results, *J Vasc Surg* 47:1094–1098, 2008.
19. Cho JS, Haider SE, Makaroun MS: US multicenter trials of endoprostheses for the endovascular treatment of descending thoracic aneurysms, *J Vasc Surg* 43(Suppl A):12A–19A, 2006.
20. Buth J, Harris PL, Hobo R, et al: Neurologic complications associated with endovascular repair of thoracic aortic pathology: incidence and risk factors. a study from the European Collaborators on Stent/Graft Techniques for Aortic Aneurysm Repair (EUROSTAR) registry, *J Vasc Surg* 46:1103–1110, 2007.
21. Makaroun MS, Dillavou ED, Kee ST, et al: Endovascular treatment of thoracic aortic aneurysms: results of the phase II multicenter trial of the GORE TAG thoracic endoprosthesis, *J Vasc Surg* 41:1–9, 2005.
22. Stone DH, Brewster DC, Kwolek CJ, et al: Stent-graft versus open-surgical repair of the thoracic aorta: mid-term results, *J Vasc Surg* 44:1188–1197, 2006.
23. Cho JS, Rhee RY, Makaroun MS: Delayed paraplegia 10 months after endovascular repair of thoracic aortic aneurysm, *J Vasc Surg* 47:625–628, 2008.
24. Feezor RJ, Martin TD, Hess PJ, et al: Risk factors for perioperative stroke during thoracic endovascular aortic repairs (TEVAR), *J Endovasc Ther* 14:568–573, 2007.
25. Chiesa R, Melissano G, Marrocco-Trischitta MM, et al: Spinal cord ischemia after elective stent-graft repair of the thoracic aorta, *J Vasc Surg* 42:11–17, 2005.
26. Khoynezhad A, Donayre CE, Bui H, et al: Risk factors of neurologic deficit after thoracic aortic endografting, *Ann Thorac Surg* 83:S882–S889, 2007.
27. Gravereaux EC, Faries PL, Burks JA, et al: Risk of spinal cord ischemia after endograft repair of thoracic aortic aneurysms, *J Vasc Surg* 34:997–1003, 2001.
28. Neuhauser B, Perkmann R, Greiner A, et al: Mid-term results after endovascular repair of the atherosclerotic descending thoracic aortic aneurysm, *Eur J Vasc Endovasc Surg* 28:146–153, 2004.
29. Demers P, Miller DC, Mitchell RS, et al: Midterm results of endovascular repair of descending thoracic aortic aneurysms with first-generation stent grafts, *J Thorac Cardiovasc Surg* 127:664–673, 2004.
30. Appoo JJ, Moser WG, Fairman RM, et al: Thoracic aortic stent grafting: improving results with newer generation investigational devices, *J Thorac Cardiovasc Surg* 131:1087–1094, 2006.
31. Ellozy SH, Carroccio A, Minor M, et al: Challenges of endovascular tube graft repair of thoracic aortic aneurysm: midterm follow-up and lessons learned, *J Vasc Surg* 38:676–683, 2003.
32. Haider SE, Najjar SF, Cho JS, et al: Sac behavior after aneurysm treatment with the Gore Excluder low-permeability aortic endoprosthesis: 12-month comparison to the original Excluder device, *J Vasc Surg* 44:694–700, 2006.
33. Go MR, Barbato JE, Dillavou ED, et al: Thoracic endovascular aortic repair for traumatic aortic transection, *J Vasc Surg* 46:928–933, 2007.
34. Hinchliffe RJ, Krasznai A, Schultzekool L, et al: Observations on the failure of stent-grafts in the aortic arch, *Eur J Vasc Endovasc Surg* 34:451–456, 2007.
35. Muhs BE, Balm R, White GH, et al: Anatomic factors associated with acute endograft collapse after Gore TAG treatment of thoracic aortic dissection or traumatic rupture, *J Vasc Surg* 45:655–661, 2007.

CHAPTER

44

Endovascular Repair of Abdominal Aortic Aneurysm

Comparative Technique and Results of Currently Available Devices

Jon S. Matsumura, Colleen L. Jay

Abdominal aortic aneurysm (AAA) is a common and potentially life-threatening condition. It is the fifteenth leading cause of death in the United States in individuals aged 50 years or more, responsible for approximately 13,800 deaths in 2005.[1] According to Nationwide Inpatient Sample data, there are more than 58,000 AAA repairs in the United States each year with an in-hospital mortality rate of 5.3%.[2] As many as 2.7 million Americans are estimated to have AAAs, but only around half have been diagnosed. The overall mortality rate after rupture may exceed 90%.[3] In a review of a series of patients with ruptured AAAs at the University of California, Los Angeles (UCLA) Medical Center, 41% had known aneurysms and had decided not to have the aneurysm repaired previously because of fear of the operation or being advised not to because of the perceived high morbidity and mortality associated with conventional aneurysm repair.[4]

The introduction of endovascular techniques has provided the opportunity to repair aneurysms without performing a major intra-abdominal operation. With endovascular repair, patients may experience decreased hospital length of stay, less postoperative pain, and quicker recovery. In the Endovascular Aortic Repair (EVAR) trial 1, a randomized trial of 1082 patients with large aneurysms (mean diameter of 6.5 cm), in-hospital mortality was 2.1% with endovascular repair versus 6.2% with open.[5] This was the largest single randomized trial, enrolling patients over a 5-year period from 1999 to 2003. In a study by the Dutch Randomized Endovascular Aneurysm (DREAM) Management Trial Group, 351 patients were randomly assigned to endovascular versus open repair.[6] The rate of combined mortality and severe complications was 4.7% with endovascular repair compared with 9.8% with open repair. Furthermore, their results demonstrated equivalent 2-year cumulative survival rates. They also identified a trend toward lower short-term survival rates with endovascular repair, but these improvements in survival rates were not sustained after 1 year. The Open Versus Endovascular Repair (OVER) trial, which randomly assigned 881 Veterans Affairs patients, and the French Anevrysme Chirurgie de l'aorte contre Endoprothèse (ACE) trial are due to report 2-year results soon. In a propensity-score risk-adjusted analysis of the Nationwide Inpatient Sample, endovascular repair was associated with lower perioperative mortality compared with open repair (1.2% vs. 4.8%).[7] Late survival was similar for the two techniques. In sum, the current literature demonstrates that endovascular repair is associated with lower perioperative hazard but equivalent longer-term all-cause mortality rates compared with open repair and should be considered in patients with anatomically suited large aneurysms. This chapter traces the development of the procedure, reviews the various commercially available endografts, and updates results of current clinical trials.

BACKGROUND

The first percutaneous attempt to place a prosthesis within an arterial lumen was reported by Dotter in 1969.[8] This original report described the placement of a coiled spring in the popliteal artery of a dog. He demonstrated angiographically that the technique was feasible and that patency could be maintained. In 1983, Cragg et al.[9] described their experience with "nonsurgical" placement of an arterial endoprosthesis made from nitinol wire into canine aortas. In 1984, Lemole et al.[10] reported a nonsutured technique of inserting a prosthetic graft into the aorta. This was done through an open approach. The device was originally intended to treat thoracic aortic dissections and consisted of a prosthetic graft with rigid attachments at each end. After opening the thoracic aorta, the device was inserted and then rapidly attached at the proximal and distal ends. This endoprosthesis was subsequently reported to be effective in the treatment of infrarenal AAAs provided there was a satisfactory proximal and distal neck. However, their technique still required a thoracotomy or a laparotomy.

The current modern concept of repairing an AAA through remote deployment of an endograft may be credited to two investigators, Parodi of Buenos Aires and Lazarus of Salt Lake City. These investigators, unknown to each other, began to develop prototypes for tube graft repair in the late 1970s. Parodi was the first to insert an endograft for definitive treatment of AAA, which he reported in 1991.[11] His prosthesis used commercially available, off-label components including a lightweight fabric graft to which a balloon-expandable stent was sewn at the proximal end. The device was inserted through a sheath, and the proximal attachment system was placed just below the renal arteries and fixed in place by balloon expansion of the stent. Initially, the distal portion of the graft was not stented. Subsequently, a balloon-expandable stent was incorporated into the distal portion of the graft as well. Lazarus received a patent for his intraluminal device in 1988.[12] His prototype included transfemoral delivery of a lightweight woven polyester graft with a self-expanding stent and circumferential hooks on each end that were driven into the aortic wall with balloon expansion. After Food and Drug Administration (FDA) approval, the first successful clinical implant of this device took place at UCLA on February 10, 1993.[13]

Also in 1991, Volodos et al.[14] from the Soviet Union described a clinical experience with the use of a self-fixing synthetic prosthesis for repair of both thoracic and abdominal aneurysms. Since then, groups in Rochester, Malmo, Sydney, New York City, and elsewhere all contributed to the rapid advancement of the field.[15] At present, endovascular repair of AAAs is being performed worldwide with use of a variety of endograft designs.

ENDOGRAFT CONCEPTS

There are currently six commercially available endografts approved by the FDA in the United States. There are many similar and some varying design features across the available graft designs. Currently, most available devices employ a fully supported body and limbs to reduce risk of kinking and thrombosis. Some devices are of unibody construction and others of modular design. Current devices use a self-expanding stent design, in contrast to the original device described by Parodi, which had a balloon-expandable stent. There is also variation in the current attachment systems with some including anchors, hooks, or barbs at the attachment sites to retard migration. Other devices depend on friction and column strength generated from stent contact with the arterial wall. Finally, some devices include uncovered struts extending above the renal arteries for additional fixation. Table 44-1 summarizes the features of the currently available devices.

PATIENT SELECTION

Current indications for AAA repair include diameter greater than 5.5 cm, increase in size greater than 0.5 cm in 6 months, or symptoms attributable to the aneurysm.[16]

TABLE 44-1 Features of Currently Approved Endografts

Feature	AneuRx	Zenith Flex	Excluder	Ancure	Talent	Powerlink
Full support along graft	X	X*	X		X*	X
Self-expanding	X	X	X	X	X	X
Unibody				X		X†
Modular	X	X	X		X	
Hook/anchor/barb fixation		X	X	X		
Suprarenal attachment		X			X	X‡

**Some spacing between stent elements.*
†Aortic or iliac cuffs frequently required.
‡Suprarenal component on aortic cuff.

Many physicians consider a lower size threshold of 5 cm when evaluating female patients. These indications are based on annual risks of rupture with a 0.6% risk for AAAs less than 5.5 cm, 5% to 10% risk for aneurysms greater than 5.5 cm, and 20% risk for those greater than 7 cm. Size criteria are unchanged when considering endovascular repair.

As discussed above, large randomized controlled trials have been conducted comparing endovascular and open repair showing no difference in midterm cumulative survival between the two groups. There was noted to be a decrease in aneurysm-related deaths in the endovascular group accounted for by differences occurring in the perioperative period. In one study, health-related quality of life was also examined and demonstrated that there was little difference between the two groups at 12 months of follow-up.[6,17] Endovascular repair is typically more expensive because of the need for ongoing surveillance and a greater number of late complications and reinterventions.[17] Trials with longer follow-up and more modern devices may be informative.

Anatomic Considerations

When evaluating a patient for endovascular repair, an imaging study is obtained to assess aneurysm length, diameter, characteristics of proximal and distal necks, and characteristics of the access vessels including the amount of tortuosity and calcification. An abdominal and pelvic computed tomography (CT) scan with thin cuts and intravenous contrast provides the necessary detailed anatomic information. Using postprocessing reconstruction of CT data, the necessary preoperative measurements can typically be obtained (Figure 44-1). CT imaging also allows assessment of the major branch vessels of the aorta, as well as any aberrant vessels. Certain situations involving severe arterial tortuosity and kinking or questions regarding arterial response to stiff wires and devices may require an invasive arteriogram with a measurement catheter (Figure 44-2). Occasionally, device treatment lengths may be refined where device positioning is difficult to predict on CT data alone because of tortuous arterial anatomy or in large aneurysm sacs.[18]

For endovascular repair, certain anatomic criteria must be met with slight variations based on the particular type of endograft. The most important anatomic limitations involve the length, diameter, and angulation of the segment of the aorta ("neck") between the renal arteries and the aneurysm. A cylindrical neck, with a minimum length of 15 mm distal to the renal arteries and a diameter of 26 mm or less, is preferred. The neck should be relatively free of thrombus and heavy

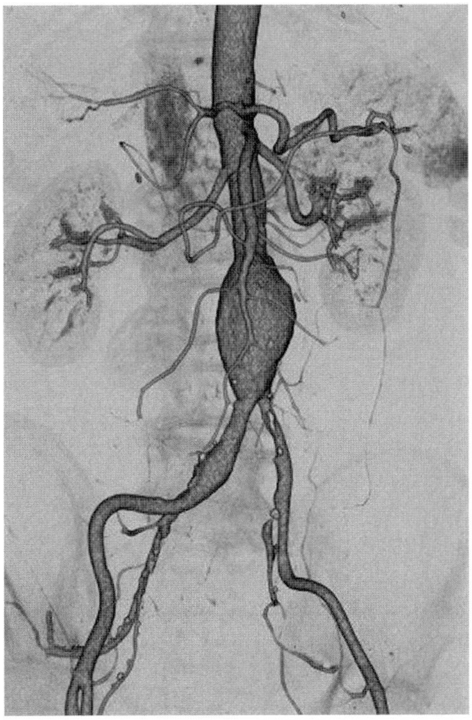

FIGURE 44-1 CT angiography has become the standard method of evaluating aneurysms for endovascular repair.

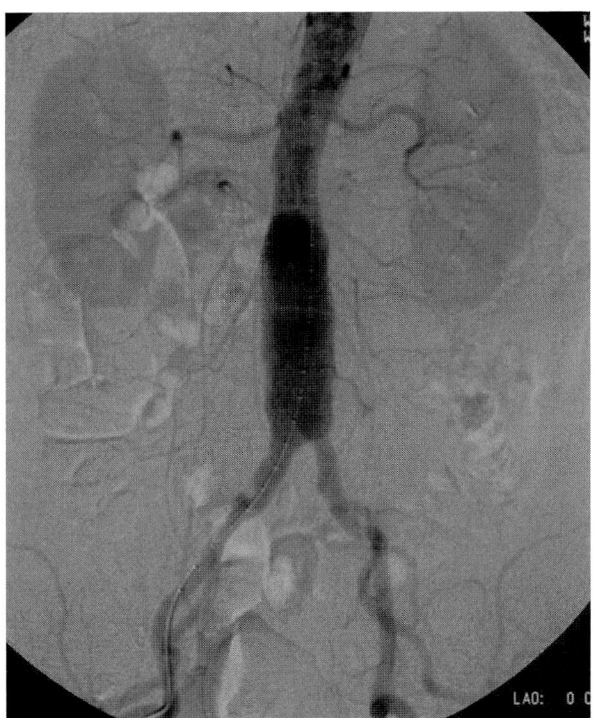

FIGURE 44-2 Aortogram performed with a measurement catheter. The aortogram delineates the anatomy from the renal arteries to the aortic bifurcation and the proximal iliac arteries and can be helpful in large tortuous aneurysms.

calcification. Conical necks flaring more than 3 to 4 mm in diameter from proximal to distal end are less suitable for device placement. Ideally, the angle between the proximal neck and suprarenal aorta should be less than 45 degrees for endovascular repair.[19-21] A few devices are approved for use in necks that are shorter (10 mm), have larger diameter (30 mm), or are more angulated (60 degrees). It may be prudent to consider alternative options in these patients with more challenging neck anatomy. Patency of the inferior mesenteric artery (IMA), as well as the status of the celiac and superior mesenteric arteries, should be evaluated. The origin of accessory renal arteries and the presence of iliac occlusive or aneurysmal disease must be considered in the management plan. The diameter of the external iliac and femoral arteries may be critical because small, calcified arteries may limit accessibility. Each of these anatomic constraints deserves detailed attention.

The target distal landing zone within the iliac arteries is of critical importance when deciding on device choice and size.[22,23] Severe circumferential calcification of the iliac arteries, greater than 90-degree angles, or a maximal distal seal-zone diameter less than 2 mm of the largest limb graft size available may be associated with suboptimal sealing results. If the common iliac artery is short and/or the external iliac artery must be used as the landing vessel, the internal iliac artery may require embolization either before or during the procedure to prevent a large back-bleeding endoleak.[22,24] In the presence of iliac artery ectasia without frank aneurysm, aortic or flared cuffs can be used to allow part of the enlarged iliac artery to function as a seal zone for the endograft; this has been referred to as the "bell-bottom."[25] Tortuous or heavily calcified vessels can cause graft kinking and prevent apposition.[26,27] Graft kinking can be particularly troublesome if the hypogastric artery has been occluded because severe limb ischemia may develop rapidly. Awareness of these iliac pitfalls can often allow the physician to overcome anatomic challenges with adjunctive procedures.

In considering the quality of the access vessels, the femoral and iliac vessel lumen diameter must be sufficient to allow access of the introducer sheath or bare device. Otherwise, a surgical conduit or endoconduit may be necessary.[28-30] The outer diameter, hydrophilicity, and trackability of the delivery sheaths vary depending on the device. The degree of vessel tortuosity should be carefully evaluated. However, tortuosity can often be straightened by using stiff guidewires and an introducer system or a brachial-femoral wire.[31] Most difficulties arise in situations of combined vessel tortuosity with small diameter, calcification, or focal stenoses. In some situations, vessel recoil may occur as the vessel tries to resume its original shape causing kinking, malpositioning, or limb dislocation. Partially supported or unsupported stent grafts may require adjunctive procedures.

Finally, if the IMA is patent, it is necessary to ensure that the superior mesenteric artery will provide adequate collateral circulation once the IMA is occluded. Occasionally, patients with large inferior pole renal arteries, aberrant large lumbar arteries, or widely patent IMAs undergo preemptive coil embolization. However, there are scant data on whether this strategy is effective in reducing type II endoleaks, and it does have additional costs and risks.

GRAFT PLACEMENT

Access to the common femoral arteries is obtained either through a surgical cutdown or percutaneously in combination with a large vessel closure device. Angiography is performed identifying the levels of the renal arteries, aortic bifurcation, and iliac bifurcations. Multiple magnified views with careful selection of imaging angles enable optimal placement of the endograft. The main body of the graft is inserted and positioned so the graft material is just inferior to the lowest renal artery. When positioning a modular graft, it is important to orient it such that the contralateral limb gate can be easily accessed. A repeated angiogram may be necessary to confirm the position of the lowest renal artery during and after retraction of stiff outer jackets that may shift anatomy. Deployment of the main body occurs next with some systems allowing for minor placement alterations at points of partial deployment.

With modular systems, a directional catheter and guidewire are advanced through the contralateral femoral artery, and the contralateral gate is selectively catheterized. This maneuver can be facilitated with a long sheath that overcomes iliac tortuosity and by frequently changing the gantry position to obtain different views of the relative positions of the target gate and selective catheter. Multiple oblique fluoroscopic views or free rotation of a curved catheter in the proximal neck can assist in verification of device cannulation. Once short limb cannulation is assured, an angiogram is performed through the side port of the sheath to ascertain the position of the hypogastric artery. The contralateral limb size is selected to extend down to the planned distal landing zone and overlap the contralateral gate. With unibody devices, the contralateral limb is snared and pulled into position. When necessary, balloons can be used to mold the graft at the proximal and distal fixation sites. A completion arteriogram is performed to check side branch patency, assess limbs for kinking, evaluate for endoleak, and monitor for access-related arterial injury. Each graft varies slightly regarding its introduction and deployment. The specifics for each graft are detailed in individual training courses and product manuals.

CURRENTLY APPROVED ENDOGRAFTS

Comparison of endograft systems is hampered by the multiple device iterations of each system, multiple cohorts within a trial including lead-in and high-risk subsets, a lack of uniform outcomes definitions, and a lack of consistent follow-up in regulatory trials. For example, most trials did not follow control patients longer than 1 year. Some trials discharged endovascular patients soon after conversion or open explantation of the endograft, and a few trials used control groups from other trials or controls with significantly larger aneurysms. Even definitions of aneurysm-related mortality have subtle differences between studies. Nevertheless, some patterns of outcomes can be recognized with each system, and it is important for physicians to be familiar with the mechanisms of failure for their preferred endograft system. Fortunately, randomized trials in which the device was selected before randomization will be forthcoming. Table 44-1 compares some basic features of each system.

Ancure System

The Ancure (Boston Scientific, Natick, MA) is a unibody bifurcated endograft that is supported at only the aortic and iliac attachment sites (Figure 44-3). The proximal attachment features fixation hooks and polyester fuzz to encourage sealing and ingrowth. This results in a durable attachment system. Because of the unsupported limbs, off-label adjunctive stenting has been frequently performed. The device is complicated to deploy and requires the largest ipsilateral sheath, approximately 27F after expansion, and a 12F contralateral sheath. The device is not currently manufactured. Aneurysm-related mortality at 5-year follow-up was 2.7% for the endograft cohort and 2.7% for the open repair controls.[32]

AneuRx System

The AneuRx (Medtronic, Santa Rosa, CA) graft is a bifurcated, modular graft made from woven polyester supported by a nitinol exoskeleton (Figure 44-4). Aortic diameters of 20 to 28 mm and iliac diameters of 12 to 24 mm are available. The ipsilateral sheath is 21F with contralateral sheaths available in 16F to 19F sizes. Often the device can be inserted bare with a tapered tip and hydrophilic system. The slow deployment and buttressing techniques allow very precise deployment of the

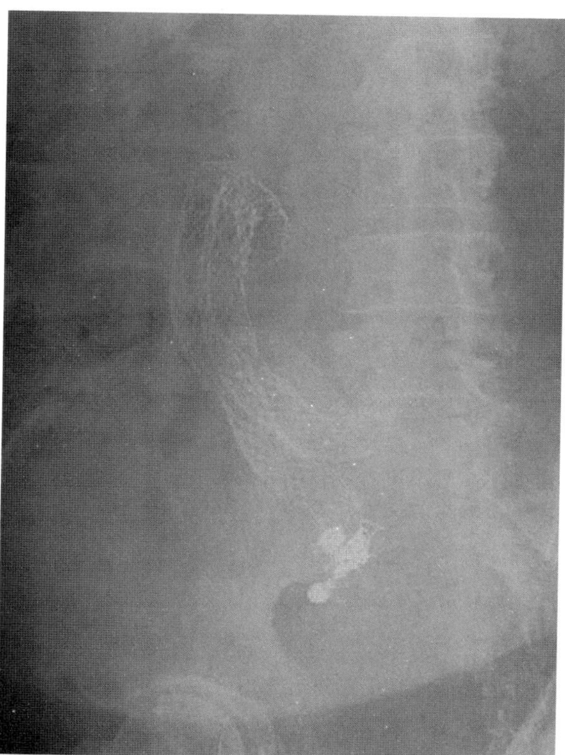

FIGURE 44-3 Radiograph showing device has migrated completely out of proximal neck.

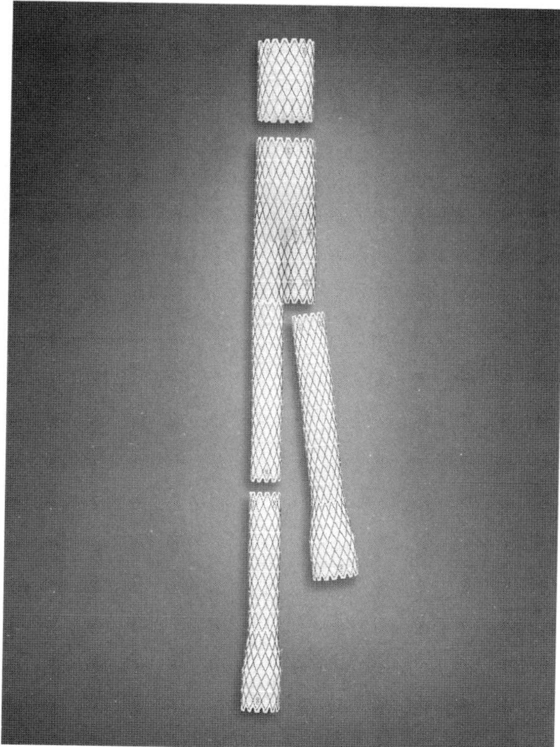

FIGURE 44-4 AneuRx system. *(Courtesy Medtronic Cardiovascular, Santa Rosa, CA.)*

proximal end of this device. This system has been in clinical use since 1996 with several device improvements, including a graft material change in 2004.

In a third FDA Public Health Notification in 2008, concern was raised about late mortality that was increasing and higher than previously reported. Specifically, late aneurysm-related mortality was less than 0.4% per year in the first 3 years, 1.3% in year 4, and 1.5% in year 5. This compares with an average late aneurysm-related mortality rate of 0.18% per year with open repair.[33] Five years after endovascular repair, cumulative aneurysm-related mortality was 3.9% per the 2005 clinical update but 5.3% per the 2008 FDA Public Health Notification. Increased late mortality after endovascular repair may be related to poor device fixation. There have been several published reports regarding migration rates with the AneuRx stent graft. Some studies used Society for Vascular Surgery reporting standards of device movement greater than 10 mm or movement of greater than 10 mm or less requiring a secondary intervention or producing symptoms. These studies found migration rates of 4% to 15%.[34-37] The device main trunk was modified for a longer main body component, and revised instructions for use were issued that may reduce the risk of late migration.

Excluder System

The Excluder (W. L. Gore & Associates, Flagstaff, AZ) is a modular system made from expanded polytetrafluoroethylene (PTFE) graft with nitinol exoskeleton (Figure 44-5). The device includes proximal covered flares, fixation anchors, and a sealing cuff. It comes in aortic diameters of 23 to 31 mm and iliac diameters of 10 to 20 mm. The ipsilateral sheath is 18F to 20F with a contralateral sheath of 12F to 18F. The contralateral gate includes a gold ring to increase radiopacity. The original device was deployed rapidly with a pull on a deployment cord. This device was first approved for commercial use in 2002. In 2004, the device was modified with a low permeability film because of a very high rate of aneurysm sac enlargement without endoleak.

Aneurysm-related mortality for this device was 2% with endovascular repair in the combined cohort and 2% with open controls at 5 years.[38]

Zenith System

The Zenith Flex (Cook Medical, Bloomington, IN) graft is a modular, bifurcated three-component system made from woven polyester sutured to stainless steel Z-stents including a bare suprarenal stent component for additional fixation at the proximal aortic attachment site (Figure 44-6). The device comes in a wide variety of aortic diameters of 22 to 36 mm and iliac diameters of 8 to 24 mm. The ipsilateral sheath comes in 18F to 20F sizes and the contralateral sheath 14F to 16F. The main body is long to facilitate gate cannulation and proximal sealing. The staged deployment system allows very precise deployment and permits off-label device

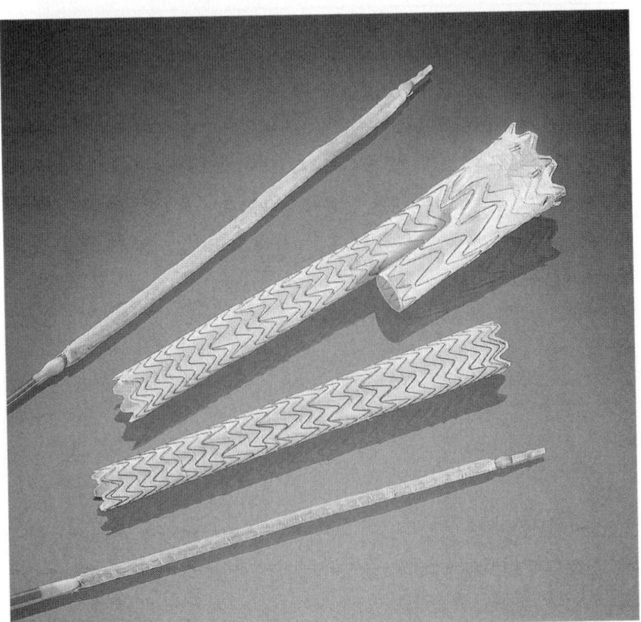

FIGURE 44-5 Excluder system. *(Courtesy Gore Medical, Newark, DE.)*

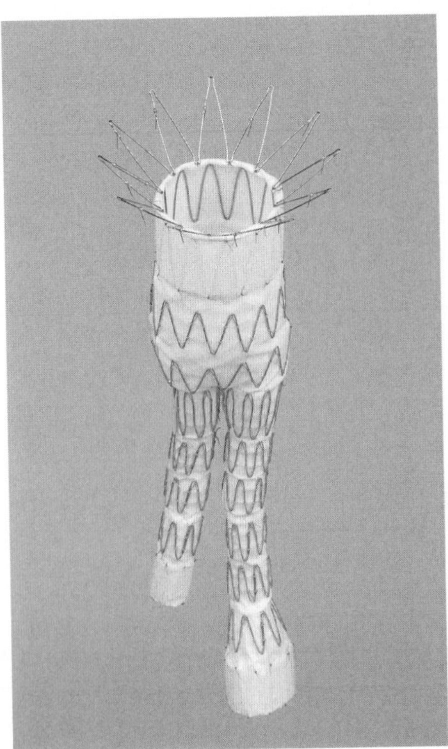

FIGURE 44-6 Zenith system. *(Courtesy Cook Medical Inc., Bloomington, IN.)*

modification with fenestrations. Aneurysm-related mortality at 5 years was 1.1% in "standard-risk" patients and 6.2% in the "high-risk" cohort.[39]

Powerlink System

The Powerlink (Endologix, Irvine, CA) endograft is a unibody design made with a long main body of a cobalt chromium alloy stent enveloped in PTFE (Figure 44-7). The device comes in aortic diameters of 25 to 28 mm and iliac diameters of 16 to 25 mm. Larger aortic extensions with suprarenal fixation are also available. The ipsilateral sheath is 21F and the contralateral sheath 12.5F to 19F. The device can be inserted bare. This device has been in commercial use since 2004. Aneurysm-related mortality was 2.1% at 5 years in the pivotal trial of 192 patients with a mean aneurysm diameter of 5.1 cm.[40,41]

Talent System

The Talent (Medtronic, Santa Rosa, CA) graft is made of woven polyester graft sutured to a nitinol lattice (Figure 44-8). Available diameters span a broad range from 22 to 36 mm, and the graft has flared, tapered iliac limbs ranging from 8 to 24 mm in diameter. The ipsilateral sheath is 22F to 24F. The contralateral sheath is 18F to 20F. The system includes suprarenal fixation and an additional sinusoidal proximal stent for improved conformability and sealing. This device was approved in the United States in 2008. Aneurysm-related mortality was 2.1% at 1-year follow-up.

COMPLICATIONS OF ENDOGRAFT REPAIR

Perioperative Complications

The most common complications in the immediate perioperative period are groin and wound complications, including bleeding, hematoma, and pseudoaneurysm formation. Liberal use of femoral completion arteriography and patch closure may minimize thromboembolic complications.

Injuries to the access vessels, particularly diseased or tortuous vessels, can occur when passing the large-bore catheters and sheaths. In situations of difficult access anatomy, access via the brachial artery with passage of a wire through the thoracic aorta and subsequent capturing of that wire with a snare catheter allows tension to be applied at both the femoral and brachial ends resulting in straightening of the iliac artery ("body-floss technique").[31] Alternatively, the use of iliac conduits through a limited retroperitoneal approach allows the operator to bypass unsuitable iliac anatomy.[28] In many situations, predilation with a dilator or balloon will allow the device to pass. The most catastrophic problem is iliac artery avulsion, which can result in cardiovascular collapse. If less-severe perforation or arterial dissection occurs, then stent grafts or stents may be used to repair the artery and avoid conversion to open repair.

Coverage of the internal iliac artery is frequently required. Studies have shown that the main trunk of the internal iliac artery can be occluded with minimal adverse consequences.[24] However, caution should be exercised when bilateral iliac artery occlusion is necessary, yet these patients often have the most extensive

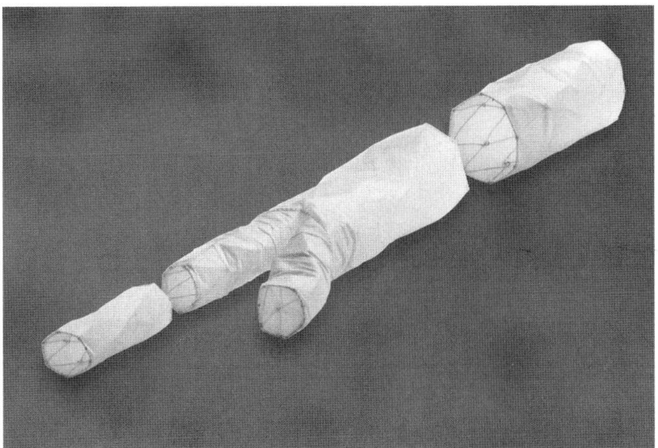

FIGURE 44-7 Powerlink system. *(Courtesy Endologix, Irvine, CA.)*

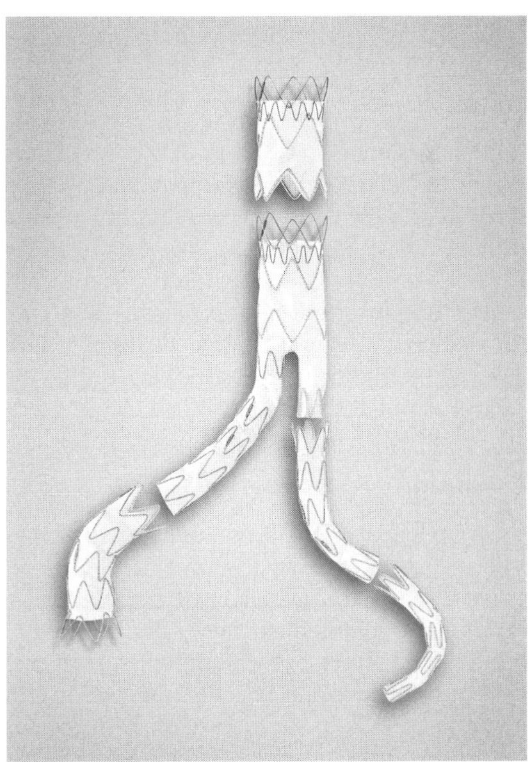

FIGURE 44-8 Talent system. *(Courtesy Medtronic Cardiovascular, Santa Rosa, CA.)*

iliac aneurysm disease and are at high risk with open repair as well. Occasionally, there is suitable anatomy for a creative solution in which one of the internal iliac arteries may be revascularized.[22]

Distal embolization to the lower extremities can occur because of manipulation of the endovascular devices within either the aneurysm sac or the access vessels.[42] Occasionally, microembolization can reflux into the kidneys. Care should be taken to reduce manipulations in the aneurysm and adjacent arteries, particularly if there is mural thrombus identified on CT scan. If distal embolization occurs, the same principles hold for endovascular repair as in open repair. Embolectomy catheters can be used to remove large pieces of distal debris. Bypass may be necessary to restore blood flow to the extremity.

Finally, postimplant syndrome may occur. This syndrome is characterized by fever, malaise, and back pain.[43] Cultures are usually negative, but these symptoms can last up to 10 days after implant. The etiology may be related to cytokine release related to thrombosis within the aneurysm sac. This is considered a benign, self-limited event.

Later Complications

Aneurysm rupture may occur after endovascular repair and may be related to device migration, graft material failure, neck dilation, metallic fatigue fracture, and endoleak. Surveillance and reintervention may reduce the risk of aneurysm rupture in many cases.

Migration

Migration is defined as 10-mm or more movement of a device or any endograft displacement associated with new symptoms, new endoleak, or requiring a secondary procedure[27,42] (see Figure 44-3). Migration can lead to types I or III endoleaks and is often a significant risk factor for late rupture. Migration seems less common with devices with strong positive fixation. It is rarely associated with dilation of the aortic neck or iliac arteries that enlarge above the nominal size of the device.[20]

Sac Expansion

Aneurysm sac size has been considered a proxy for procedural success and sac growth a cause for concern. This is particularly true when associated with an endoleak. Rates of sac enlargement vary with the type of graft, and some devices have been modified as graft material issues have been identified.[44-46] Ultrafiltration through graft material results in sac enlargement in the absence of an endoleak. It is characterized by a gray, gelatinous, nonbloody fluid found in the aneurysm sac.[47]

Limb Occlusion

Limb occlusion typically presents with acute onset of claudication, but if the ipsilateral hypogastric artery is occluded it may present with a threatened or even nonsalvageable extremity.[48,49] Most limb occlusions occur early and are more common with unsupported devices. Native vessel disease distal to the endograft or arterial injury caused by large sheaths can also cause limb occlusion. Finally, morphologic changes resulting from a shrinking aneurysm sac can lead to kinking of limbs with subsequent lower-extremity ischemia.[26]

Neck Dilation

A small fraction of patients have clinically important dilation in the first 3 years after endovascular repair.[50] The causes of late neck dilation include continuation of the original aneurysmal process and device oversizing. Neck enlargement with subsequent late endoleak can happen many years after repair, just as subsequent aneurysms are known to form decades after an open repair.

Graft Material Failure

Endovascular devices may frequently develop fabric defects related to weave deformation from sutures or abrasion with metallic components or calcified plaque. Rarely, large fabric tears may lead to clinically important aneurysm enlargement or even rupture more than 5 years after endovascular repair (Figures 44-9 and 44-10) There is no long-term experience with newer, modified graft materials that were introduced after observed failures with initial materials.

Fracture

Fatigue fractures are a risk with many medical devices, including stent grafts. Poor design predictions, welds, compression forces on the inner curve, distraction forces on the outer curve, lack of adequate surface polishing, off-label manipulation of devices, and placement in adverse anatomy are all potential contributing factors to device failure. When the metal elements are compromised, fixation, sealing, and luminal patency are all threatened.[51] Regulatory trials of stent grafts are poorly powered to detect low rates of fracture, and postmarketing surveillance is important to identify these late events.[52]

ENDOLEAK

Endoleak is the failure to exclude the aneurysm sac fully from arterial blood flow. Its presence raises the possibility of continuing aneurysm sac pressurization, enlargement, and subsequent rupture. White and colleagues[53,54] developed a classification that has been widely used. They divided endoleak into four categories depending on the source and mechanism.[53,54]

Type I Endoleak

A type I leak occurs when there is an incomplete seal of either a proximal or distal attachment system in the aorta or iliac arteries. There is ongoing blood flow between the prosthesis and the arterial wall maintaining blood flow into the aneurysm sac. Early type I endoleaks often seal, but persistent or late-appearing type I endoleaks seem to lead to sac enlargement and possibly rupture. As such, intervention is indicated to treat persistent or new type I endoleaks as long as there is a reasonably safe treatment available. Sometimes, treatment is not anatomically possible or the patient is too ill to undergo secondary intervention, and the patient is observed. Aneurysm rupture may not occur imminently, just as untreated aneurysms do not predictably rupture.

Type II Endoleak

This occurs when there is backflow from a patent lumbar artery, middle sacral artery, or IMA. The majority of these leaks are self-sealing, and as such observation is initially pursued. If the aneurysm sac is stable or shrinking on follow-up imaging, most physicians will elect to continue observing. If the sac enlarges, then embolization of the source can be attempted through a superselective approach or a translumbar direct puncture. Some clinicians will observe all type II endoleaks.

Type III Endoleak

A type III leak occurs when there is a component disconnection or a fabric tear or erosion. These usually are managed similarly to type I endoleaks (see Figures 44-9 and 44-10).

Type IV Endoleak

A type IV endoleak occurs when blood flows through a recently placed graft material. This happens when the graft material is highly porous allowing, transmural flow. Over time, the pores become sealed by fibrin deposition. These leaks are self-limited during the first 30 days by definition and are commonly observed.

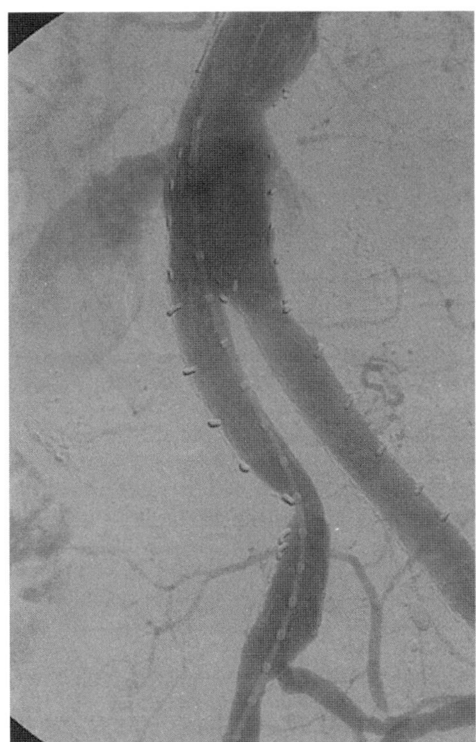

FIGURE 44-9 Type IIIb endoleak developed after many years following implantation with off-label iliac stents that eventually wore through graft material. *(Courtesy M. Eskandari.)*

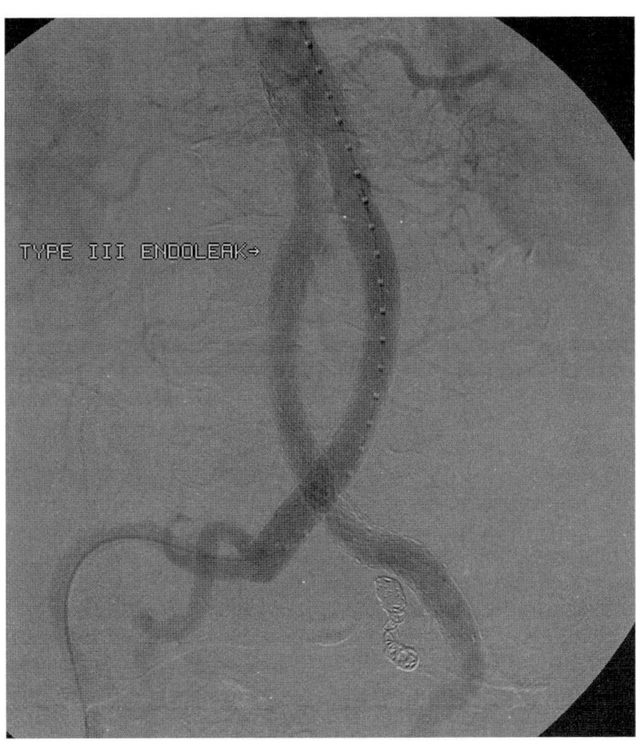

FIGURE 44-10 Type IIIb endoleak from fabric hole that led to aneurysm rupture 6 years after initial treatment.

CONCLUSION

Endovascular aneurysm repair has matured significantly since its introduction more than 2 decades ago. Clearly, specific device failure modes have been recognized, and engineering solutions have emerged. Device innovation and process of care improvements continue to address shortcomings that are identified through careful clinical research. Randomized trial data with newer devices and longer follow-up will clarify the precise benefits and costs of endovascular aneurysm repair.

References

1. Kung HC, Hoyert DL, Xu JW, et al. *National vital statistics report*, Rockville, MD, 2008, Healthcare Cost and Utilization Project.
2. HCUP reports: Healthcare Cost and Utilization Project (HCUP), *Agency for Healthcare Research and Quality*, October 2008.
3. Ernst CB: Abdominal aortic aneurysm [see comment], *N Engl J Med* 328(16):1167–1172, 1993.
4. Hiatt JC, Barker WF, Machleder HI, et al: Determinants of failure in the treatment of ruptured abdominal aortic aneurysm, *Arch Surg* 119(11):1264–1268, 1984.
5. Greenhalgh RM, Brown LC, Kwong GP, et al: Comparison of endovascular aneurysm repair with open repair in patients with abdominal aortic aneurysm (EVAR trial 1), 30-day operative mortality results: randomised controlled trial [see comment], *Lancet* 364(9437):843–848, 2004.
6. Blankensteijn JD, de Jong SE, Prinssen M, et al: Two-year outcomes after conventional or endovascular repair of abdominal aortic aneurysms [see comment], *N Engl J Med* 352(23): 2398–2405, 2005.
7. Schermerhorn ML, O'Malley AJ, Jhaveri A, et al: Endovascular vs. open repair of abdominal aortic aneurysms in the Medicare population [see comment], *N Engl J Med* 358(5):464–474, 2008.
8. Dotter CT: Transluminally-placed coilspring endarterial tube grafts: long-term patency in canine popliteal artery, *Invest Radiol* 4(5):329–332, 1969.
9. Cragg A, Lund G, Rysavy J, et al: Nonsurgical placement of arterial endoprostheses: a new technique using nitinol wire, *Radiology* 147(1):261–263, 1983.
10. Lemole GM, Spagna PM, Strong MD, Karmilowicz NP: Rigid intraluminal prosthesis for replacement of thoracic and abdominal aorta, *J Vasc Surg* 1(1):22–26, 1984.
11. Parodi JC, Palmaz JC, Barone HD: Transfemoral intraluminal graft implantation for abdominal aortic aneurysms, *Ann Vasc Surg* 5(6):491–499, 1991.
12. Lazarus H. Intraluminal graft device, system and method. US Patent No. 4787899, November 11, 1998.
13. Moore WS, Vescera CL: Repair of abdominal aortic aneurysm by transfemoral endovascular graft placement, *Ann Surg* 220 (3):331–339, 1994, discussion 339–341.
14. Volodos NL, Karpovich IP, Troyan VI, et al: Clinical experience of the use of self-fixing synthetic prostheses for remote endoprosthetics of the thoracic and the abdominal aorta and iliac arteries through the femoral artery and as intraoperative endoprosthesis for aorta reconstruction, *Vasa* [suppl] 33:93–95, 1991.
15. Chuter TA, Green RM, Ouriel K, et al: Transfemoral endovascular aortic graft placement [see comment], *J Vasc Surg* 18(2):185–195, 1993, discussion 195–197.
16. Lederle FA, Wilson SE, Johnson GR, et al: Immediate repair compared with surveillance of small abdominal aortic aneurysms [see comment], *N Engl J Med* 346(19):1437–1444, 2002.
17. EVAR trial participants: Endovascular aneurysm repair versus open repair in patients with abdominal aortic aneurysm (EVAR trial 1): randomised controlled trial.[see comment], *Lancet* 365 (9478):2179–2186, 2005.
18. Broeders IA, Blankensteijn JD, Olree M, et al: Preoperative sizing of grafts for transfemoral endovascular aneurysm management: a prospective comparative study of spiral CT angiography, arteriography, and conventional CT imaging, *J Endovasc Surg* 4 (3):252–261, 1997.
19. Albertini J, Kalliafas S, Travis S, et al: Anatomical risk factors for proximal perigraft endoleak and graft migration following endovascular repair of abdominal aortic aneurysms, *Eur J Vasc Endovasc Surg* 19(3):308–312, 2000.
20. Stanley BM, Semmens JB, Mai Q, et al: Evaluation of patient selection guidelines for endoluminal AAA repair with the Zenith Stent-Graft: the Australasian experience, *J Endovasc Ther* 8 (5):457–464, 2001.
21. Sternbergh WC 3rd, Carter G, York JW, et al: Aortic neck angulation predicts adverse outcome with endovascular abdominal aortic aneurysm repair, *J Vasc Surg* 35(3):482–486, 2002.
22. Rhee RY, Muluk SC, Tzeng E, et al: Can the internal iliac artery be safely covered during endovascular repair of abdominal aortic and iliac artery aneurysms? *Ann Vasc Surg* 16(1):29–36, 2002.
23. Schumacher H, Eckstein HH, Kallinowski F, Allenberg JR: Morphometry and classification in abdominal aortic aneurysms: patient selection for endovascular and open surgery [see comment], *J Endovasc Surg* 4(1):39–44, 1997.
24. Schoder M, Zaunbauer L, Holzenbein T, et al: Internal iliac artery embolization before endovascular repair of abdominal aortic aneurysms: frequency, efficacy, and clinical results, *AJR Am J Roentgenol* 177(3):599–605, 2001.
25. Kritpracha B, Pigott JP, Russell TE, et al: Bell-bottom aortoiliac endografts: an alternative that preserves pelvic blood flow, *J Vasc Surg* 35(5):874–881, 2002.
26. Carroccio A, Faries PL, Morrissey NJ, et al: Predicting iliac limb occlusions after bifurcated aortic stent grafting: anatomic and device-related causes, *J Vasc Surg* 36(4):679–684, 2002.
27. Dawson DL, Hellinger JC, Terramani TT, et al: Iliac artery kinking with endovascular therapies: technical considerations, *J Vasc Interv Radiol* 13(7):729–733, 2002.
28. Abu-Ghaida AM, Clair DG, Greenberg RK, et al: Broadening the applicability of endovascular aneurysm repair: the use of iliac conduits, *J Vasc Surg* 36(1):111–117, 2002.
29. Petersen BG, Matsumura JS: Creative options for large sheath access during aortic endografting, *J Vasc Interv Radiol* 19(suppl 6):522–526, 2008.
30. Peterson BG, Matsumura JS, Peterson BG, Matsumura JS: Internal endoconduit: an innovative technique to address unfavorable iliac artery anatomy encountered during thoracic endovascular aortic repair. [see comment], *J Vasc Surg* 47(2):441–445, 2008.
31. Criado FJ, Wilson EP, Abul-Khoudoud O, et al: Brachial artery catheterization to facilitate endovascular grafting of abdominal aortic aneurysm: safety and rationale, *J Vasc Surg* 32 (6):1137–1141, 2000.
32. *Annual clinical update for the Ancure System*, Santa Rosa, CA, 2008, Medtronic Cardiovasoular.
33. Food and Drug Administration, *Center for Devices and Radiological Health, FDA Public health notification: updated data on mortality associated with the Medtronic AneuRx Stent Graft System*, Silver Spring, MD, 2008, FDA.

34. Azizzadeh A, Sanchez LA, Rubin BG, et al: Aortic neck attachment failure and the AneuRx graft: incidence, treatment options, and early results, *Ann Vasc Surg* 19(4):516–521, 2005.
35. Cao P, Verzini F, Zannetti S, et al: Device migration after endoluminal abdominal aortic aneurysm repair: analysis of 113 cases with a minimum follow-up period of 2 years, *J Vasc Surg* 35 (2):229–235, 2002.
36. Fulton JJ, Farber MA, Sanchez LA, et al: Effect of challenging neck anatomy on mid-term migration rates in AneuRx endografts, *J Vasc Surg* 44(5):932–937, 2006, discussion 937.
37. Heikkinen MA, Alsac JM, Arko FR, et al: The importance of iliac fixation in prevention of stent graft migration, *J Vasc Surg* 43 (6):1130–1137, 2006, discussion 1137.
38. Gore. Gore Excluder AAA Endoprosthesis: Annual clinical update 2008, Flagstaff, AZ, 2008.
39. WL Gore Associates: Zenith® AAA Endovascular Graft five-year user report. 2007.
40. Wang GJ, Carpenter JP, Endologix I, et al: The Powerlink system for endovascular abdominal aortic aneurysm repair: six-year results, *J Vasc Surg* 48(3):535–545, 2008.
41. Endologix: Endologix Powerlink System: annual clinical update December 2007, Irvine, CA, 2007, Endolink Powerlink.
42. Hovsepian DM, Hein AN, Pilgram TK, et al: Endovascular abdominal aortic aneurysm repair in 144 patients: correlation of aneurysm size, proximal aortic neck length, and procedure-related complications, *J Vasc Interv Radiol* 12(12):1373–1382, 2001.
43. Blum U, Voshage G, Lammer J, et al: Endoluminal stent-grafts for infrarenal abdominal aortic aneurysms [see comment], *N Engl J Med* 336(1):13–20, 1997.
44. Ebaugh JL, Eskandari MK, Finkelstein A, et al: Caudal migration of endoprostheses after treatment of abdominal aortic aneurysms, *J Surg Res* 107(1):14–17, 2002.
45. Sternbergh WC 3rd, Money SR, Greenberg RK, et al: Influence of endograft oversizing on device migration, endoleak, aneurysm shrinkage, and aortic neck dilation: results from the Zenith Multicenter Trial, *J Vasc Surg* 39(1):20–26, 2004.
46. Zarins CK, Bloch DA, Crabtree T, et al: Stent graft migration after endovascular aneurysm repair: importance of proximal fixation, *J Vasc Surg* 38(6):1264–1272, 2003, discussion 1272.
47. Cho JS, Dillavou ED, Rhee RY, et al: Late abdominal aortic aneurysm enlargement after endovascular repair with the Excluder device, *J Vasc Surg* 39(6):1236–1241, 2004, discussion 2141–2142.
48. Carpenter JP, Endologix I, Carpenter JP: Midterm results of the multicenter trial of the powerlink bifurcated system for endovascular aortic aneurysm repair, *J Vasc Surg* 40(5):849–859, 2004.
49. Conner MS 3rd, Sternbergh WC 3rd, Carter G, et al: Secondary procedures after endovascular aortic aneurysm repair, *J Vasc Surg* 36(5):992–996, 2002.
50. Matsumura JS, Chaikof EL: Continued expansion of aortic necks after endovascular repair of abdominal aortic aneurysms. EVT Investigators. EndoVascular Technologies, Inc, *J Vasc Surg* 28 (3):422–430, 1998, discussion 430–431.
51. Coppi G, Silingardi R, Saitta G, et al: Single-center experience with the Talent LPS endograft in patients with at least 5 years of follow-up, *J Endovasc Ther* 15(1):23–32, 2008.
52. Rutherford RB, Krupski WC, Rutherford RB, Krupski WC: Current status of open versus endovascular stent-graft repair of abdominal aortic aneurysm, *J Vasc Surg* 39(5):1129–1139, 2004.
53. White GH, May J, Waugh RC, et al: Type III and type IV endoleak: toward a complete definition of blood flow in the sac after endoluminal AAA repair, *J Endovasc Surg* 5(4):305–309, 1998.
54. White GH, Yu W, May J, et al: Endoleak as a complication of endoluminal grafting of abdominal aortic aneurysms: classification, incidence, diagnosis, and management, *J Endovasc Surg* 4(2):152–168, 1997.

CHAPTER

45

Endovascular Repair of Ruptured Abdominal Aortic Aneurysms

Frank J. Veith, Nicholas J. Gargiulo III, Neal S. Cayne

When abdominal aortic aneurysms (AAAs) rupture and are not treated, they invariably lead to the patient's death. In addition, ruptured abdominal aortic aneurysms (RAAAs) have high mortality (35%-70%) and morbidity rates when treated by standard open surgical methods.[1-5] These high perioperative mortality and morbidity rates have not been substantially reduced despite the introduction of many improvements in open operative technique or perioperative care.[1-6] The introduction of endovascular approaches to treat AAAs in the early 1990s seemed like an opportunity to alter substantially the treatment outcomes when rupture occurred.[7,8] This chapter details how these endovascular approaches, which include endovascular stented grafts, can be applied to the treatment of RAAAs, and what advantages these new catheter-based approaches to treatment offer.

OBSTACLES TO USE OF ENDOVASCULAR GRAFTS IN THE RUPTURED ANEURYSM SETTING

The less-invasive nature of endovascular treatment of RAAAs offers many potential advantages. However, one obstacle in the early days of endovascular AAA treatment was the selection of the appropriate graft for each patient, which required complex measurements of aneurysmal and adjacent arterial lengths and diameters. These measurements are usually based on high-quality contrast computed tomographic (CT) scans or arteriography, which take time to perform and which may not be available in the RAAA setting. Moreover, it may not be possible to have available a stock of grafts suitable for most patients. A second obstacle to the use of endovascular grafts was that standard surgical practice mandated early proximal aortic control, and it was thought that this could be achieved most rapidly and most effectively by laparotomy with placement of a supraceliac or infrarenal aortic clamp.[9]

SUITABLE ENDOGRAFTS FOR ENDOVASCULAR REPAIR IN THE RUPTURED ABDOMINAL AORTIC ANEURYSM SETTING

To overcome the first obstacle, we have had available since 1993 a derivative of the original Parodi endograft[10] to treat aortic and aortoiliac aneurysms. This Vascular Innovation (VI) graft,* which is used in an aortofemoral configuration, is composed of a large proximal Palmaz balloon-expandable stent affixed to a long tulip-shaped polytetrafluoroethylene graft (Figure 45-1).[11] This graft is a "one size fits most" because the proximal diameter can vary between 20 and 27 mm depending on the inflation pressure applied to the deployment balloon, and the excess graft length can be cut off and tailored appropriately before the distal graft is sutured to the graft introduction site within the common femoral artery (Figure 45-2).

Having this graft sterilized and available has had the potential for eliminating the need for preoperative measurement and fabricating or procuring a suitable graft for use in the urgent RAAA setting. Moreover, as the commercially made modular endografts became

Supported in part by grants from the William J. von Liebig Foundation.

*This graft was originally made by us from available materials but is now to be commercialized as the Vascular Innovation (VI) Graft, Vascular Innovation, Inc., Perrysburg, OH.

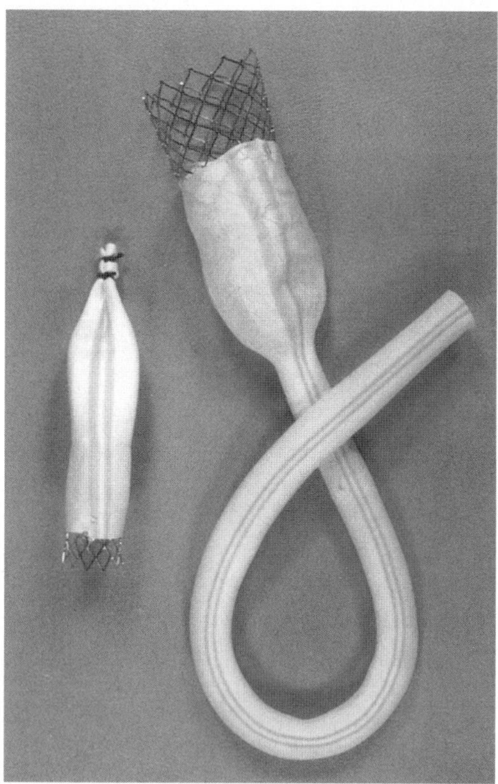

FIGURE 45-1 Vascular Innovation (VI) graft. A large Palmaz stent is attached to the polytetrafluoroethylene graft. A surgeon-made occluder device is shown on the left. However, there are many other commercially made occluders available, and any of these can be used to block the opposite common iliac artery.

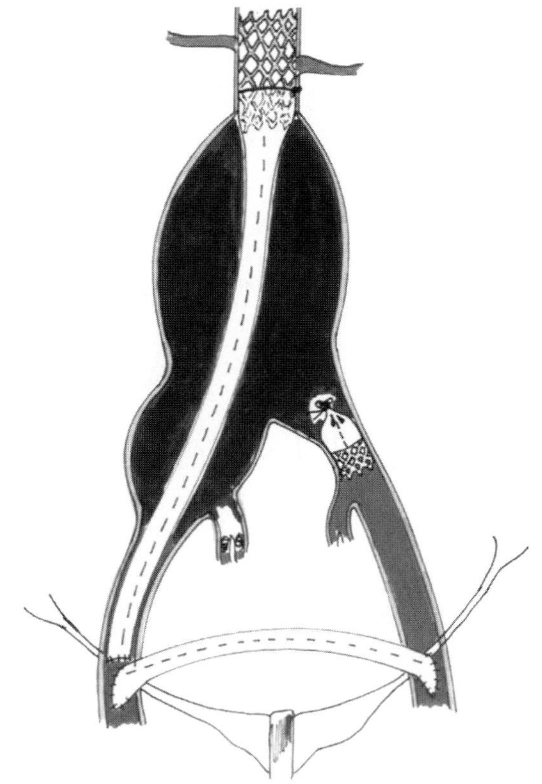

FIGURE 45-2 Schematic drawing illustrating how the VI graft is used This graft is fixed within the proximal neck with a large Palmaz stent. The cranial end of the graft is denoted by a metallic marker attached to the graft. The bare portion of the stent is deployed across the orifice of the renal arteries so that the graft is implanted immediately below the renal arteries. An endoluminal anastomosis is performed at the distal end of the endograft. The occluder device is deployed in the contralateral common iliac artery to preserve at least one internal iliac artery.

available, components of these grafts could be stocked in the operating room and could be used to treat RAAAs.

EARLY EXPERIENCE WITH ENDOVASCULAR TREATMENT OF RUPTURED ABDOMINAL AORTIC ANEURYSMS

Because we had available a surgeon-made VI graft, on April 21, 1994, we had a patient with a ruptured abdominal aorta and all the clinical sequelae thereof, that is, severe abdominal pain, hypotension, and a large pulsatile abdominal mass. Because the patient had had a total cystectomy and ileal bladder, and because he had severe symptomatic coronary artery disease with an ejection fraction of 20%, he was deemed unsuitable for an open repair of his ruptured aortic aneurysm. We were able to perform an endovascular graft repair of his RAAA along with placement of a right common iliac artery occluder and a femorofemoral bypass (Figure 45-3).[7] The patient did well after this procedure until he died of cardiac disease 3 years later. To our knowledge this was the first endovascular graft repair of a ruptured aortic aneurysm, although another early case was reported by Yusuf et al.[8]

After our experience with our first successful case we performed similar operations in another 11 patients with ruptured aortoiliac aneurysms.[11] All these patients had major contraindications to open operation with serious medical comorbidities (e.g., coincident major myocardial infarction, chronic obstructive pulmonary disease requiring home oxygen therapy) or surgical problems producing a hostile abdomen (e.g., abdominal infection or massive recurrent incisional hernias). All 12 of these first patients had been stable enough to undergo preoperative CT scanning to confirm the aneurysmal rupture. In all 12 of these original patients, the ruptured aneurysm was successfully excluded by the endovascular graft. Moreover, only 2 of the patients died within 2 months of the procedure, a 17% operative mortality.

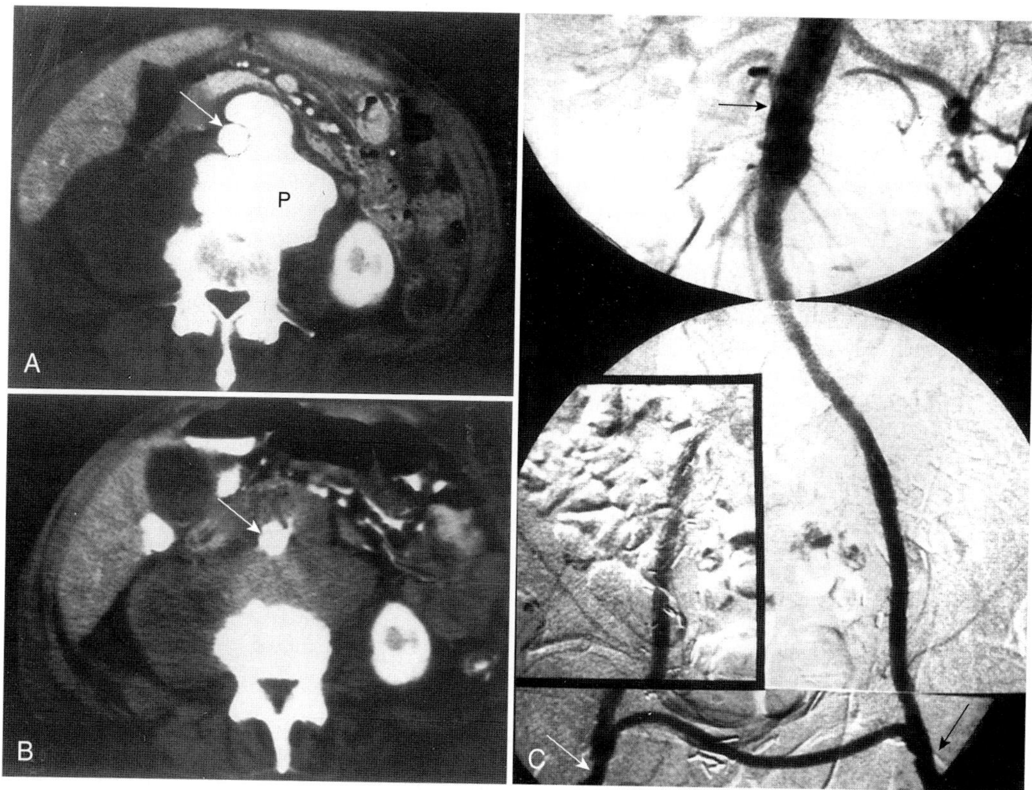

FIGURE 45-3 **A,** Transfemoral repair of a rupture of a distal aortic aneurysm. A spiral CT scan demonstrates extravasation of contrast material from the aorta *(arrow)* into a large, partially clot-filled pseudoaneurysm *(P)*. **B,** A spiral CT scan performed after transfemoral insertion of an endovascular graft demonstrates that the pseudoaneurysm is excluded and vascular continuity within the lumen of the aorta *(arrow)* is preserved. **C,** A postoperative transfemoral arteriogram at 1 week demonstrates vascular continuity between the aorta *(arrow)* and the common femoral arteries *(arrows)*. *Inset,* Flow up the external iliac artery to the right hypogastric artery. An occluder has been placed in the right common iliac artery. *(Reproduced with permission from Marin ML, Veith FJ, Cynamon J, et al: Initial experience with transluminally placed endovascular grafts for the treatment of complex vascular lesions,* Ann Surg *222:1-17, 1995.)*

HYPOTHESIS REGARDING ENDOVASCULAR TREATMENT OF RUPTURED ABDOMINAL AORTIC ANEURYSMS AND CURRENT MANAGEMENT PLAN

This low operative mortality prompted us to speculate that all RAAAs should be treated endovascularly. Such an approach might lead to better outcomes than were currently being achieved with open repair. In 1995, we therefore adopted the following treatment plan.[12] All patients with a *presumed diagnosis* of a RAAA were taken immediately to the operating room. A diagnosis of RAAA was presumed if two or more elements of the diagnostic triad were present, namely syncope, abdominal or back pain, and a known or palpable AAA.[9] In the operating room, with preparation for fluoroscopy of the patient from the neck to the knees, via a femoral or brachial puncture under local anesthesia a wire was placed in the supraceliac aorta. With use of this guidewire a catheter was placed to visualize the abdominal aorta and iliac arteries angiographically. This angiogram, which was best performed with a power injector, allowed a determination of whether or not an endovascular graft repair of the RAAA was possible on the basis of aortic neck and iliac artery anatomy. If not, a standard repair was carried out.

CONTROL OF BLEEDING AND BLOOD PRESSURE: RESTRICTED RESUSCITATION, HYPOTENSIVE HEMOSTASIS, AND PROXIMAL BALLOON CONTROL

As already noted, it is widely believed that with RAAAs it is necessary to perform immediate laparotomy to permit clamp control of the aorta proximal to the aneurysm. With major arterial bleeding in other circumstances, however, restricted fluid resuscitation and withholding blood transfusions have been shown to decrease blood loss and improve outcomes.[13-16] One editorial in 1991 also advocated restriction of fluid resuscitation in the preoperative management of

RAAAs.[17] We also believe that restriction of fluid resuscitation and blood transfusion in the RAAA setting is not only desirable but mandatory. If the blood pressure is in the 50– to 70–mm Hg range, it should be left there. If the patient is moving and talking, no fluids should be given. This should continue when the patient is first in the operating room being prepared for treatment and having a guidewire and catheter placed in the suprarenal aorta under local anesthesia via either a femoral or brachial puncture.

Patients with RAAAs frequently deteriorate with induction of anesthesia. If that occurs and the blood pressure falls below 50 mm Hg or is unobtainable, administration of fluid and blood becomes necessary. We believe such deterioration warrants proximal balloon control and have used this technique selectively in our current management plan for ruptured aneurysms.

PROXIMAL BALLOON CONTROL

If and when a patient's condition deteriorates before, during, or after induction of anesthesia, a larger size (14F-16F) hemostatic sheath is inserted over the previously placed guidewire via either the femoral or brachial artery. With the wire in place a 27-, 33-, or 40-mm compliant (latex) balloon is inserted through the sheath and inflated with dilute contrast under fluoroscopic control (Figure 45-4) in either the supraceliac or pararenal aorta (depending on the length of the infrarenal neck). If the femoral route is chosen for the balloon placement, the sheath must be kept in place in the aorta to support the balloon and to facilitate its removal after graft placement. With the balloon inflated, the remainder of the procedure is conducted as rapidly as possible to minimize the duration of visceral and renal ischemia. If the infrarenal neck is too short, too flared, or too angulated for an endovascular repair, open aortic control, preferably below the renal arteries, is obtained and a standard AAA repair performed. If a bifurcated endograft is inserted, an infrarenal balloon should be placed within the graft to replace the more proximal balloon as soon as possible. Then the endograft procedure is completed in a deliberate fashion. Details of the techniques for balloon control and endograft insertion without losing aortic control have been well described by Malina et al.[18]

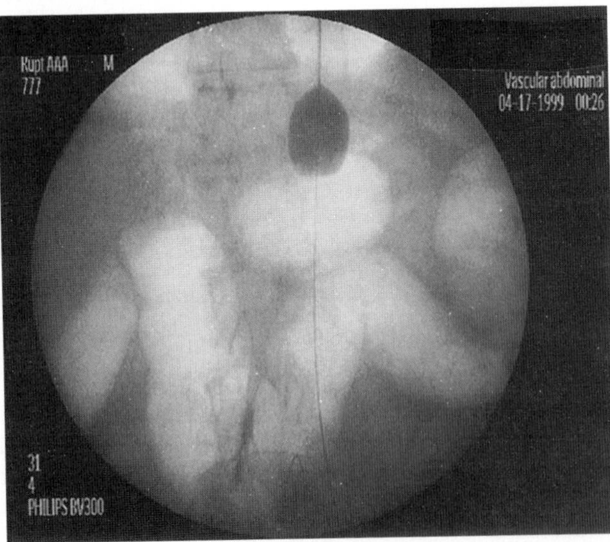

FIGURE 45-4 Fluoroscopic view of a proximal occlusion balloon introduced through the brachial artery.

EXPERIENCE WITH ENDOVASCULAR TREATMENT OF RUPTURED ABDOMINAL AORTIC ANEURYSMS

To date, we have treated 49 patients with ruptured aortoiliac aneurysms using endovascular techniques. Included are the 12 original patients already described and another 37 patients treated according to our current management plan. Of these 49 patients, 8 were deemed unsuitable for endovascular treatment because of their aortic neck or iliac anatomy. These 8 (16%) underwent open repair; only 3 required inflation of the proximal balloon. All survived for more than 2 months after operation.

Of the remaining 41 patients who received an endovascular graft, 32 had the graft inserted without the need for proximal balloon control. Only 9 of the 41 (or 12 of the total 49 patients [24%]) required balloon control. Twenty-five of the patients receiving an endograft were treated with a VI graft, and 16 received an industry-made graft (AneuRx Medtronic, Minneapolis, MN; Zenith, Cook Medical, Indianapolis, IN; Excluder, W. L. Gore & Associates, Flagstaff, AZ). In all 41 endograft-treated patients, the graft was deployed successfully and completely excluded the ruptured aneurysm. There were no significant endoleaks, and all surviving patients became and remained asymptomatic. Five of the 41 endograft-treated patients died during the 30 days after their procedure, but all had serious medical comorbidities (coincident major myocardial infarctions and/or oxygen-dependent chronic obstructive pulmonary disease). Thus, and in this entire series of 49 ruptured AAAs, there was a procedural mortality of only 10%.

Three patients receiving endovascular grafts required evacuation of a large retroperitoneal hematoma for abdominal compartment syndrome. In two of these patients the decompression was required immediately after graft placement; in the other it was required 7 days later. Details of optimal methods for diagnosing and treating abdominal compartment syndromes in the ruptured AAA setting have been described by

Lachat et al.[19] Two groin wound infections required drainage but healed without graft involvement.

COLLECTED WORLD EXPERIENCE WITH ENDOVASCULAR GRAFT TREATMENT OF RUPTURED ABDOMINAL AORTIC ANEURYSMS

Over the last 4 years, a collaborative group, the EVAR for Ruptured Aneurysm Investigators, have been pooling their results with the use of endovascular graft repair of RAAAs. The data collection is still in progress. However, to date many centers have submitted their results, which will be published as a multiauthored report. Of 583 patients with RAAA collected to date and treated with endografts, 470 have survived more than 30 days, giving an encouragingly low procedural mortality rate of 19%. Although patients were selected for endovascular treatment by a variety of criteria, some of the patients had free intraperitoneal rupture, and many had severe hypotension. In addition, many were at prohibitive risk for a standard open repair (Figure 45-5). The low mortality for endograft repair coupled with the inclusion of many high-risk patients with RAAA strongly suggests that endovascular graft repair, when feasible, will improve treatment outcomes for RAAAs.

ADVANTAGES OF ENDOVASCULAR TREATMENT OF RUPTURED ABDOMINAL AORTIC ANEURYSMS

Among the advantages of endovascular repair of ruptured aneurysms are the ability to obtain proximal control without general anesthesia, the ability to deploy the graft from a remote access site, reduced blood loss, and minimizing hypothermia by eliminating laparotomy.

Proximal Control Without General Anesthesia

Patients with ruptured AAAs may have severe hypotension. However, many patients may have their blood pressure stabilized at a nonlethal level. This is due to sympathetically mediated vasoconstriction in response to hypotension. It is not uncommon for this vasoconstriction to be released during the induction of general anesthesia, which results in a sudden drop in blood pressure. Therefore a relatively stable patient may become severely hypotensive, mandating urgent application of a proximal aortic clamp. However, a guidewire can be inserted in the upper abdominal or lower thoracic aorta through a percutaneous puncture under local anesthesia, while maintaining the vasoconstriction. Once the guidewire is inserted in the aorta, the patient can then safely undergo induction of general anesthesia because proximal control can be rapidly and relatively safely obtained by an occlusion balloon placed over the previously inserted guidewire.

Deployment of Graft From a Remote Access Site

Endovascular grafts can be inserted and deployed through a remote access site, thereby obviating the need for laparotomy and, more important, eliminating the technical difficulties that are encountered when performing a standard repair in the rupture setting. With the associated bleeding, the anatomy of the retroperitoneal structures is often distorted and obscured by a large hematoma, which may lead to technical difficulties, as well as inadvertent injury of the inferior vena cava, the left renal vein or its genital branches, the duodenum, or other surrounding structures. These iatrogenic injuries have been the cause of significant operative morbidity and mortality after standard surgery for RAAAs. In contrast, endograft repair is performed within the arterial tree, which is unaffected by extravasated blood or previous operative scarring. Thus the technical difficulty encountered when treating a RAAA with an endograft is similar to that for elective cases. Moreover, this approach completely eliminates the risk of inadvertent injury to surrounding structures.

Reduced Blood Loss

In our experience, endovascular repair for RAAAs was accomplished with a relatively small amount of additional blood loss (800 mL) compared with that which occurs during open RAAA repair. This advantage is more important in patients with RAAAs because these patients have already lost a significant amount of blood after rupture, and coagulopathy or disseminated intravascular coagulation resulting from further blood loss can be serious and often lethal complications. There are several reasons why blood loss was limited, including the maintenance of the tamponade effect within the retroperitoneum. In addition, back-bleeding from the iliac and lumbar arteries and bleeding from the anastomotic suture lines and from iatrogenic venous injuries are eliminated.

Minimizing Hypothermia

Hypothermia caused by poor perfusion and laparotomy can exacerbate coagulopathy, which is one of the causes of mortality after open surgical repair. Endovascular graft repair can minimize the extent of hypothermia by avoiding laparotomy.

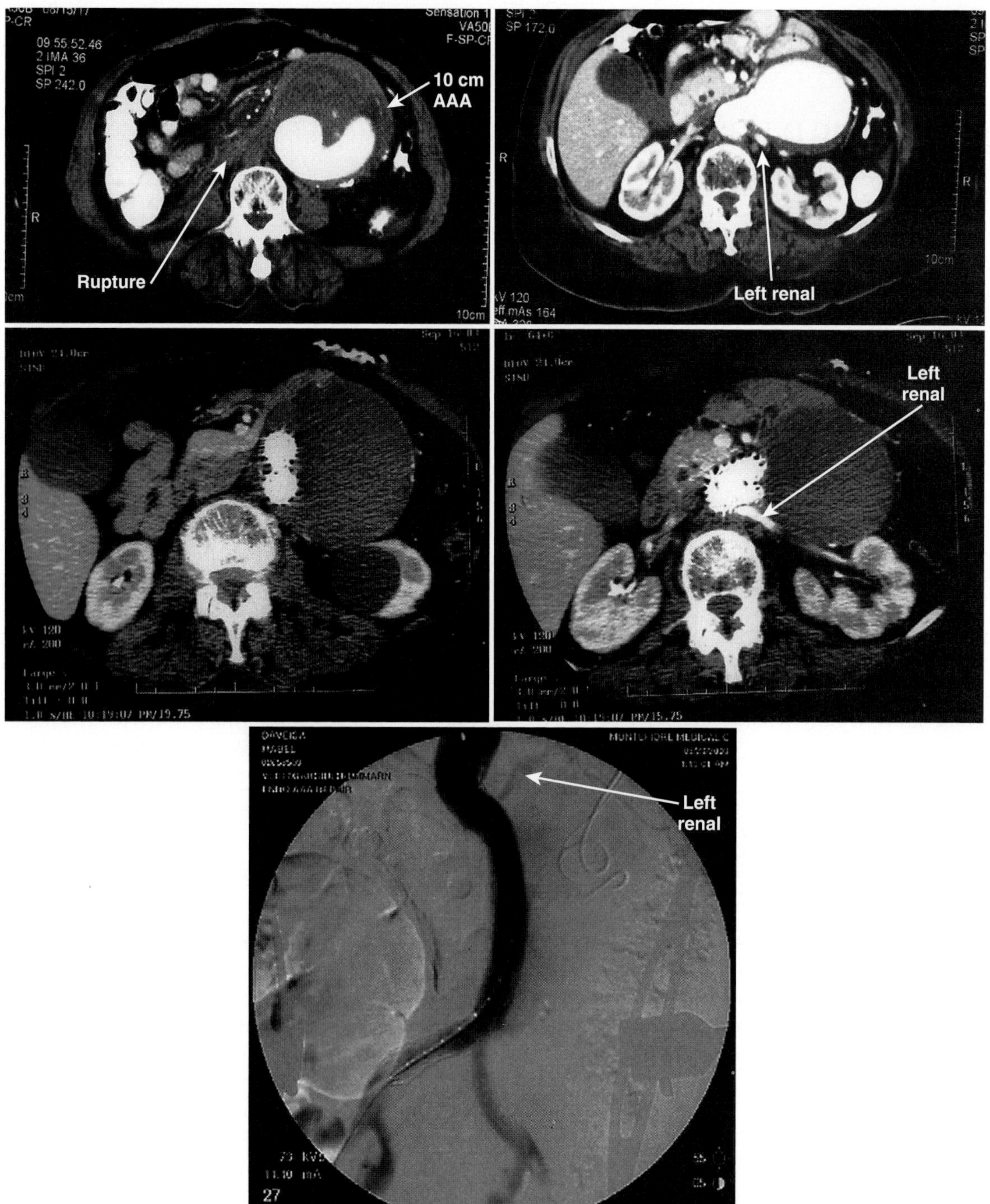

FIGURE 45-5 An 86-year-old patient with a 10-cm RAAA. **A,** Contrast CT showing RAAA. **B,** Contrast CT showing an unfavorable short angulated neck. Open repair was advised, but patient refused blood transfusion for religious reasons. The hematocrit fell to 17% and the systolic arterial blood pressure to 60 mm Hg. Open repair was thought to carry a prohibitive risk. **C,** Endovascular repair was performed despite the angulated short neck. Note left renal artery appearing to arise from the aneurysm. The endograft is in place but not yet deployed. **D,** Contrast CT scan 6 weeks after the procedure. The aneurysm sac is excluded from the circulation. **E,** Contrast CT scan 6 weeks after the procedure. The aneurysm is excluded. The left renal artery is perfused. The patient remains well more than 2 years later.

DISCUSSION

The relatively low mortality rates in patients with RAAA treated endovascularly are encouraging, particularly because many were high-risk patients who were poor surgical candidates.[12,20-24] These results show that endograft repair of RAAAs is feasible and effective in selected cases. However, before the universal use of these techniques is adopted, many questions must be answered. Should endovascular repair be attempted in all patients with RAAA or just those whose condition is relatively stable? In what proportion of patients with RAAA should an endograft repair be used? Should a CT scan be obtained before patients with RAAA are taken to the operating room or endovascular suite? In which patients should a proximal balloon be placed? How should this be done? Is a randomized prospective comparison with open repair necessary or justified? Should an aortounilateral graft be used or a modular bifurcated graft? What kind of anesthesia should be employed? What resources are required for an institution to undertake endograft repairs of RAAAs? Until these questions are answered, we will not know the optimal approach to endovascular repair of RAAAs. Nevertheless, we believe that endovascular grafts represent a potentially better way to treat this entity because previous open surgical methods have had such a persistently high morbidity and mortality. We currently believe that these endovascular grafts can and should be used in more than 50% to 60% of patients who present with a RAAA. Indeed some of the sickest, most urgent hypotensive patients may benefit the most from endograft treatment rather than subjecting them to an emergent open repair under suboptimal conditions. Moreover, we believe that the use of fluoroscopic techniques to facilitate the placement of proximal occlusion balloons, an old idea,[25-28] will make this endovascular adjunct a practical and valuable one, even if an endovascular graft procedure is not possible and an open repair is required. And finally, we believe that hypotensive hemostasis or restricted fluid resuscitation will prove valuable in the RAAA setting and will become the standard of care for this entity leading to improved treatment outcomes for this lethal condition.

References

1. Johansen K, Kohler TR, Nicholls SC, et al: Ruptured abdominal aortic aneurysm: the Harborview experience, *J Vasc Surg* 13:240–247, 1991.
2. Gloviczki P, Pairolero PC, Mucha P: Ruptured abdominal aortic aneurysms: repair should not be denied, *J Vasc Surg* 15:851–859, 1992.
3. Marty-Ane CH, Alric P, Picot MC, et al: Ruptured abdominal aortic aneurysm: influence of intraoperative management on surgical outcome, *J Vasc Surg* 22:780–786, 1995.
4. Darling RC, Cordero JA, Chang BB: Advances in the surgical repair of ruptured abdominal aortic aneurysms, *Cardiovasc Surg* 4:720–723, 1996.
5. Dardik A, Burleyson GP, Bowman H, et al: Surgical repair of ruptured abdominal aortic aneurysms in the state of Maryland: factors influencing outcome among 527 recent cases, *J Vasc Surg* 28:413–423, 1998.
6. Noel AA, Gloviczki P, Cherry KJ Jr, et al: Ruptured abdominal aortic aneurysms: the excessive mortality rate of conventional repair, *J Vasc Surg* 34:41–46, 2001.
7. Marin ML, Veith FJ, Cynamon J, et al: Initial experience with transluminally placed endovascular grafts for the treatment of complex vascular lesions, *Ann Surg* 222:1–17, 1995.
8. Yusuf SW, Whitaker SC, Chuter TA, Wenham PW, Hopkinson BR: Emergency endovascular repair of leaking aortic aneurysms, *Lancet* 344:1645, 1994.
9. Veith FJ: Emergency abdominal aortic aneurysm surgery, *Compr Ther* 18:25–29, 1992.
10. Parodi JC, Palmaz JC, Barone HD: Transfemoral intraluminal graft implantation for abdominal aortic aneurysms, *Ann Vasc Surg* 5:491–499, 1991.
11. Ohki T, Veith FJ, Sanchez LA, et al: Endovascular graft repair of ruptured aorto-iliac aneurysms, *J Am Coll Surg* 189:102–123, 1999.
12. Veith FJ, Ohki T: Endovascular approaches to ruptured infrarenal aorto-iliac aneurysms, *J Cardiovasc Surg* 43:369–378, 2002.
13. Andresen AFR: Results of treatment of massive gastric hemorrhage, *Am J Digest Dis* 6:641–650, 1939.
14. Andresen AFR: Management of gastric hemorrhage, *NY State J Med* 48:603–611, 1948.
15. Shaftan GW, Chiu CJ, Dennis C, Harris B: Fundamentals of physiologic control of arterial hemorrhage, *Surgery* 58:851–856, 1968.
16. Bickell WH, Wall MJ Jr, Pepe PE, et al: Immediate versus delayed fluid resuscitation for hypotensive patients with penetrating torso injuries, *N Engl J Med* 331:1105–1109, 1994.
17. Crawford ES: Ruptured abdominal aortic aneurysm: an editorial, *J Vasc Surg* 13:348–350, 1991.
18. Malina M, Veith FJ, Ivancev K, Jonesson F: Balloon occlusion of the aorta during endovascular repair of ruptured abdominal aortic aneurysm, *J Endovasc Ther* 12:556–559, 2005.
19. Lachat M, Mayer D, Labler L, et al: Abdominal compartment syndrome following ruptured AAA. In: Becquemin JP, Alimi YS, editors: *Controversies and updates in vascular surgery*, Turin, 2006, Minerva Medica, pp 103–107.
20. Yusuf SW, Whitaker SC, Chuter TAM, et al: Early results of endovascular aortic aneurysm surgery with aortouniiliac graft, contralateral iliac occlusion, and femorofemoral bypass, *J Vasc Surg* 25:165–172, 1997.
21. Yusuf SW, Hopkinson BR: Is it feasible to treat contained aortic aneurysm rupture by stent-graft combination? In: Greenhalgh RM, editor: *Indications in vascular and endovascular surgery*, London, 1998, Saunders, pp 153–165.
22. Greenberg RK, Srivastava SD, Ouriel K, et al: An endoluminal method of hemorrhage control and repair of ruptured abdominal aortic aneurysms, *J Endovasc Ther* 7:1–7, 2000.
23. Lachat ML, Pfammatter T, Witzke HJ, et al: Endovascular repair with bifurcated stent-grafts under local anaesthesia to improve outcome of ruptured aortoiliac aneurysms, *Eur J Vasc Endovasc Surg* 23:528–536, 2002.
24. Hechelhammer L, Lachat ML, Wildermuth S, et al: Midterm outcomes of endovascular repair of ruptured abdominal aortic aneurysms, *J Vasc Surg* 205; 41:752–757.

25. Hughes LCCW: Use of an intra-aortic balloon catheter tamponade for controlling intraabdominal hemorrhage in man, *Surgery* 36:65–68, 1954.
26. Hesse FG, Kletschka HD: Rupture of abdominal aortic aneurysm: control of hemorrhage by intraluminal balloon tamponade, *Ann Surg* 155:320–322, 1962.
27. Anastacio CN, Ochsner EC: Use of Fogarty catheter tamponade for ruptured abdominal aortic aneurysms, *Am J Roentgenol* 128:31–33, 1977.
28. Hyde GL, Sullivan DM: Fogarty catheter tamponade of ruptured abdominal aortic aneurysms, *Surg Gynecol Obstet* 154:197–199, 1982.

CHAPTER

46

Iliac Artery Aneurysms

Michael Wilderman, Luis Sanchez

An iliac artery aneurysm is any permanent, localized dilation of the iliac artery larger than 1.5 cm in maximal diameter as defined by the Subcommittee on Reporting Standards for Arterial Aneurysms of the Society for Vascular Surgery.[1] Many authors additionally consider an aneurysm to be a "localized" abnormal widening or ballooning of a portion of any artery, iliac included, greater than 50% of the normal caliber of the artery. Multiple reports suggest that most iliac artery aneurysms are associated with abdominal aortic aneurysms (AAAs), and they account for between 2% and 7% of atherosclerotic aneurysms of the aortoiliac segment.[2-7] Isolated aneurysms of the iliac artery are less common, having a prevalence of approximately 0.4 to 1.9% of all aneurysmal disease.[8] Brunkwall et al.[2] reported that in a population-based study their estimated prevalence is an even lower 0.03% based on autopsy findings. The vast majority of isolated iliac artery aneurysms (>70%) involve the common iliac artery (CIA), while about 20% arise from the internal iliac artery, and very few arise from the external iliac artery (EIA).[9] Iliac artery aneurysms may occur in multiple iliac segments and can also be bilateral. One report by Richards et al.[6] found that approximately two thirds of iliac artery aneurysms involved two or more iliac segments and one third were bilateral.

Similar to AAAs, isolated iliac artery aneurysms are more common in males than females. Depending on the series, there are reports of male-to-female ratios between 5:1 and 16:1, and most patients are older, presenting between 65 and 75 years of age.[4,6,10] A study by Lawrence and colleagues[11] found that the incidence of isolated iliac artery aneurysms in men 65 to 75 years of age is 70 per 100,000 person-years and only 2 per 100,000 in women of the same age. Pseudoaneurysms of iliac artery suture lines are also relatively rare, with incidences reported between 0.2% and 15% depending on the series.[10,12-16]

ETIOLOGY

The pathogenesis of iliac artery aneurysms is multifactorial and similar to that of AAAs. Etiologies that have been reported to contribute to iliac aneurysmal dilatation include atherosclerotic changes, inflammation, wall stress and wall tension, proteolytic degradation of arterial wall tissue, and molecular genetics.[17] Histologically, an iliac aneurysm, similar to an AAA, is characterized by macrophage degradation of the medial elastin lamellar architecture by metalloproteinases.[18-21] Other less-common causes include infection, trauma, arteritis, collagen vascular disease, and pregnancy.[22-26] Iliac artery pseudoaneurysms are caused by previous surgery, trauma, infection, or other intravascular interventions.

PRESENTATION AND EVALUATION

One of the clinical challenges for isolated iliac aneurysms is detection, given their location deep within the pelvis. Most patients with iliac artery aneurysms have no symptoms, although some may be seen with abdominal pain. Although rarely, others may present with compression of local structures: a ureter leading to hydronephrosis, pyelonephritis, or recurrent urinary tract infections; bowel compression leading to obstruction; nerve root pressure leading to a neurologic deficit or neurogenic pain; or iliac vein compression leading to swelling, deep venous thrombosis, or even a pulmonary embolism. Iliac artery aneurysms are rarely detected on physical examination unless they are larger than 4 cm and in patients with a favorable body habitus. With the increasing frequency of abdominal imaging being performed to aid in the diagnoses of various other entities, these aneurysms are being discovered more frequently than before, and at smaller sizes. Before this, most isolated iliac artery aneurysms presented ruptured and patients had a high mortality rate. Depending on the series, the mortality rate from a ruptured iliac artery aneurysm has been reported to be between 25% and 57%, whereas the mortality for elective repair is less than 5%.[4,6,10] Patients with untreated pseudoaneurysms are susceptible to the same outcomes as or worse outcomes than those with true aneurysms. Intraoperative and perioperative mortality rates can be higher, especially with emergent interventions that are usually reoperations.[12,15]

As with AAA, ultrasound is a simple and reliable study to diagnose iliac artery aneurysms. Given the availability of ultrasound and its relatively low cost compared with cross-sectional imaging studies such as computed tomography (CT) or magnetic resonance (MR), it is the diagnostic screening study of choice. CT scanning provides greater diagnostic imaging to allow for accurate measurements and exact location of an aneurysm to aid in operative planning (Figure 46-1). MR angiography is also an effective diagnostic tool (Figure 46-2), although given its higher cost and availability compared with CT, it is typically reserved for patients with contrast allergies or those at risk for dye-induced nephrotoxicity.[5,10,27] Its application in the latter group of patients has diminished with the increased reports of nephrogenic systemic fibrosis/nephrogenic fibrosing dermopathy associated with the use of gadolinium in patients with severe renal insufficiency or renal failure.[28,29]

As opposed to the well-documented progression and subsequent enlargement of AAAs,[30,31] there are no large prospective studies looking at the progression of iliac artery aneurysms. Santilli et al.[32] reported on 189 patients with 323 iliac artery aneurysms. They found that, for aneurysms smaller than 30 mm, the growth rate was 1.1 mm/yr; aneurysms between 30 and 50 mm had a growth rate of 2.6 mm/yr. The study also concluded that iliac artery aneurysms smaller than 3 cm could be followed with annual duplex ultrasonography, those between 3 and 3.5 cm could be followed every 6 months or considered for elective treatment in selected cases such as those with continued documented aneurysm growth, and those aneurysms larger than 3.5 cm should be repaired electively.[32] As with AAA, size is the most important factor in rate of rupture, with the average size of a ruptured iliac artery aneurysm being 5.6 cm.[4,6]

TREATMENT

The principal aim of surgical intervention is to eliminate aneurysmal flow and wall tension, thus preventing future dilatation and rupture.[33] As in patients with AAAs, a critical assessment of the patient's operative risk must be ascertained before any intervention. In addition, critical evaluation of the patient's arterial anatomy and, specifically, the location, size, and relationship of the iliac artery aneurysm to branch vessels and adjacent structures must be performed before planning any surgical procedure. In patients being considered for an elective repair, the surgeon should determine the best approach based on the patient's general state of health, longevity, aneurysm location, branch involvement and the repercussions of branch occlusion, bilaterality of the aneurysms, whether or not the aorta is involved, devices available for endovascular repair of the specific anatomy, along with the risks and benefits of both open and endovascular repair for the specific patient.[34]

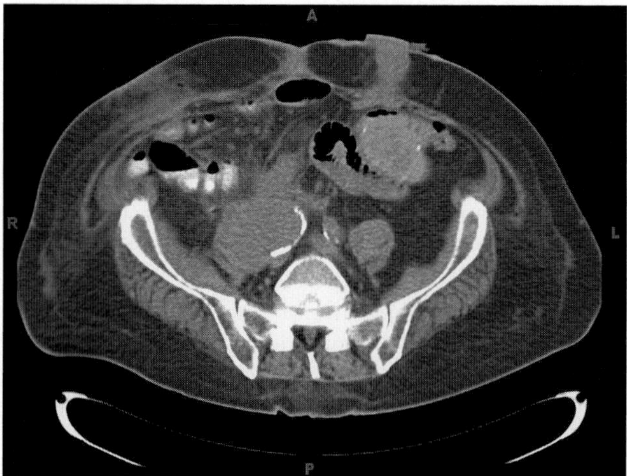

FIGURE 46-1 An example of an iliac artery aneurysm diagnosed by CT angiography.

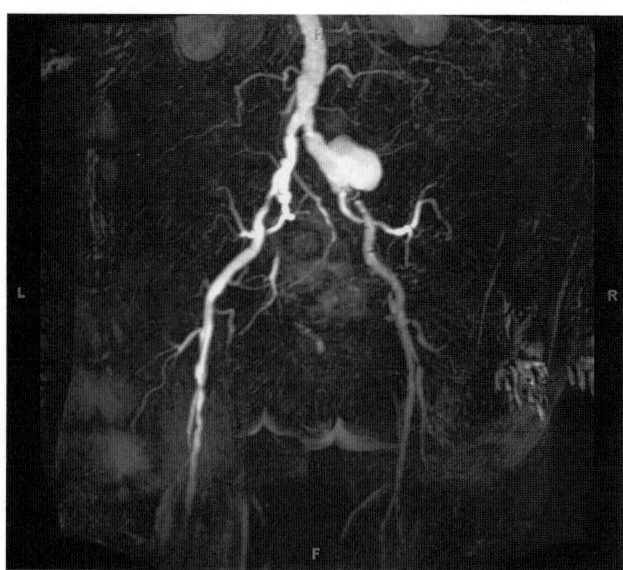

FIGURE 46-2 An example of an iliac artery aneurysm diagnosed by MR angiography.

An open surgical repair through either a midline incision or retroperitoneal approach, depending on the location of the aneurysm, with insertion of an interposition graft has been the standard of care for a long time (Figures 46-3 and 46-4). In one of the first reports, Krupski and colleagues[10] reported no deaths and a major complication rate of only 5%. The results of open repairs have continued to improve over the years. In one series of 320 operations between 1985 and 2001, the mortality for elective repair was 5% and 28% for an emergent repair.[9] A contemporary large series reported an elective mortality rate of 1%, but major complications were seen in 23% of the patients.[35]

More recently, the endovascular treatment of iliac artery aneurysms or pseudoaneurysms has been increasingly used. Endoluminal methods allow the surgeon to access the arterial system from the femoral arteries, rather than requiring a deep and extensive pelvic dissection, with its associated potential complications. This approach is even more useful in patients who are at high operative risk because of significant medical comorbidities, prior abdominal or pelvic surgery, abdominal or pelvic radiation, lower abdominal stomas, or morbid obesity.[36] Other advantages of the endoluminal approach are decreased blood loss, minimal trauma to the patient, faster recovery, and decreased length of hospital stay.[10] Sandhu and Pipinos[9] describe five broad categories of iliac artery aneurysms. Patients with aneurysms that are confined to the CIA, have a proximal and distal neck longer than 1 cm, and have minimal mural thrombus or calcification are in category A. These patients are suitable for either open aneurysmorrhaphy and interposition graft or an endoluminal repair with fixation entirely in the CIA. Patients whose aneurysms fall into category B are those whose proximal CIA neck is adequate, but whose aneurysm extends to the iliac artery bifurcation. These patients can undergo an open repair with the distal anastomosis secured to the iliac bifurcation. These aneurysms can also be repaired endoluminally. The graft would lie between the CIA and EIA with exclusion of the internal iliac artery. The internal iliac is often embolized proximally to prevent retrograde perfusion of the CIA aneurysm. Class C aneurysms extend from the common iliac into both the internal iliac artery and EIA. These can be repaired in an open or endovascular fashion similar to those in category B. The internal iliac is often embolized at its branches to prevent retrograde perfusion of the hypogastric aneurysm. Sandu and Pipinos[9] classify an aneurysm as a type D if it solely involves the internal iliac artery. Both endoluminal and open operations are possible for the treatment of this type of aneurysm, but open repair is technically challenging because of the deep pelvic location of internal iliac artery aneurysms. The most commonly used endoluminal method requires embolization of the distal branches of the internal iliac artery followed by exclusion of the internal iliac artery aneurysm by an endovascular graft deployed from the CIA to the EIA, similar to those patients in category C. Patients who have bilateral CIA aneurysms, those that involve both the abdominal aorta and the iliac artery, or those CIA aneurysms without a proximal neck are classified as type E. These patients can have a standard open aortic operation with a bifurcated graft or an endoluminal repair with a bifurcated endovascular system or an aortouni-iliac system, an iliac occlusion device and femoral-to-femoral bypass.[9]

The endovascular treatment of arterial aneurysms has flourished since Parodi et al.[37] published their groundbreaking experience with AAAs. Initially, physicians

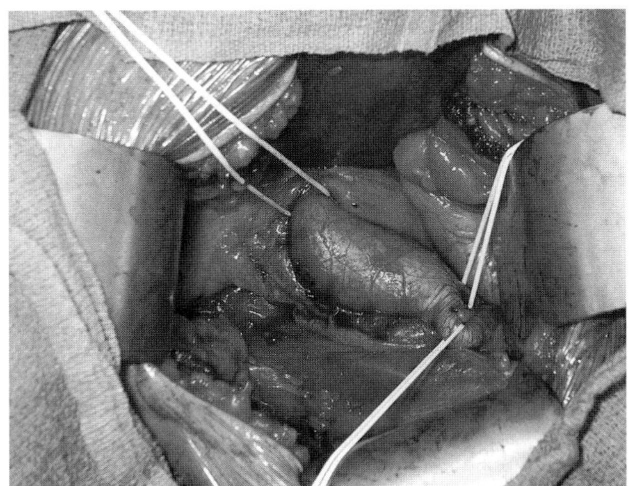

FIGURE 46-3 An example of an intraoperative exposure of an iliac artery aneurysm being repaired in an open fashion.

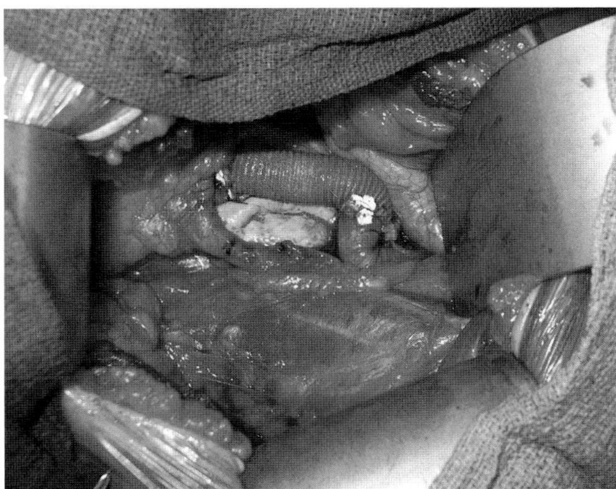

FIGURE 46-4 An example of a completed open repair of an iliac artery aneurysm.

began by using homemade devices composed of balloon-expandable stents and prosthetic grafts. Now physicians use commercially available covered stents, iliac limbs of aortic stent graft systems, or even full aortic endovascular grafts to repair these aneurysms with excellent results.

The basic technical procedure involves placing an endovascular graft across the iliac artery aneurysm to exclude it from arterial blood flow and systemic arterial pressure. This type of repair requires at least a 1-cm landing or attachment zone of normal CIA proximal and distal to the aneurysm. This situation is relatively uncommon in clinical practice. If there is not an adequate distal landing zone in the CIA, the stent graft can be brought lower to terminate in the EIA. Using this strategy requires the embolization of the internal iliac artery with either coils or an excluding plug (i.e., Amplatzer plug [AGA Medical Corp, Plymouth, MN] or others) to prevent retrograde perfusion and a potential type 2 endoleak (Figure 46-5). A frequently used option is to exclude the entire infrarenal aorta and bilateral iliac arteries with a bifurcated aortic graft. Iliac artery aneurysms rarely have a suitable proximal neck and require a bifurcated aortic graft.

One of the earliest series was reported out of New York by Sanchez et al.[38] They reported on a 5-year series of 40 patients with isolated iliac artery aneurysms and pseudoaneurysms treated with endovascular grafts. The majority (n = 37) of the patients were treated with endovascular grafts composed of 6-mm polytetrafluoroethylene grafts sutured onto a Palmaz balloon-expandable stent. There was a 100% technical success rate, and the 4-year primary patency rate was 94.5%. The perioperative complications were few and included one episode of colonic ischemia, one episode of distal embolization, five instances of graft kinking or compression, and one instance of graft thrombosis. There was only one perioperative death in a patient whose

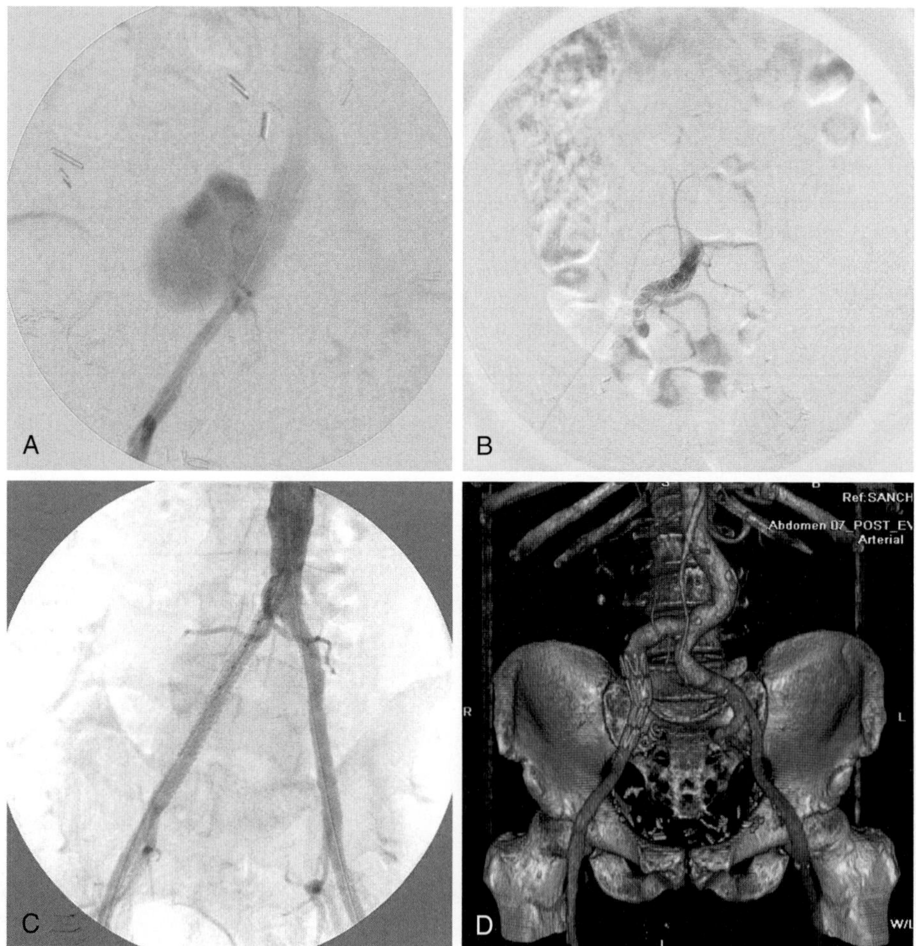

FIGURE 46-5 **A,** An example of an intraoperative angiograph performed to help localize an iliac artery aneurysm. **B,** An example of coils being placed in a hypogastric artery before placing a covered stent graft across the iliac bifurcation. **C,** An example of a completion arteriogram demonstrating the exclusion of an iliac artery aneurysm by a stent graft. **D,** An example of a postoperative CT angiogram demonstrating the successful exclusion of an iliac artery aneurysm via coil embolization of the hypogastric artery and placement of a covered stent graft.

aneurysm had ruptured before he entered the operating room. Longer term, there were two patients with endoleaks, and one required open repair. They concluded that this was certainly a safe and effective technique with outstanding midterm results despite the homemade devices used.[38] Parsons and colleagues[39] also reported similar results in their contemporaneous series of iliac artery aneurysms treated with endoluminal grafts.

Multiple small series have been published with the use of a variety of commercial endovascular devices over the past 15 years. Early reports were published about use of the Corvita endoluminal device (Corvita, Miami, FL),[40] the Endopro Stent Graft System (Boston Scientific, Natick, MA),[41,42] the Passenger Stent Graft (Boston Scientific), and Gore Hemobahn (W. L. Gore & Associates, Flagstaff, AZ).[43] All reports had excellent early success rates approaching 100% and consistent long-term results, even with these early generation devices as suggested by Stroumpouli et al.[38,40-45] At a mean follow-up of 51 months, Stroumpouli et al. reported stent graft patency was 100%. Reinterventions were performed in four patients: three with type 2 endoleaks and one with a type 1 endoleak.[43]

TREATMENT COMPLICATIONS

To date there have been numerous reports in the literature of patients treated with endovascular stent grafts for iliac artery aneurysms, and all have had very good outcomes (Table 46-1[46-53]). Despite their excellent results, endovascular repairs of iliac artery aneurysms have some unique complications compared with open surgery. The most common complication is that of an endoleak, with a rate of 0% to 36% in various series (see Table 46-1). Most of these are type 2 endoleaks that rarely require intervention, especially if the aneurysm is shrinking in size. In fact, early results are similar to those found with endovascular AAA repairs. If the aneurysm sac is still pressurized, the aneurysm is at risk for expansion and rupture. Sahgal et al.[54] reported that the enlargement of an iliac artery aneurysm, even without the presence of an endoleak, appears to be an ominous sign suggestive of impending rupture, and patients with this situation should be considered for open surgical repair. On the basis of their findings, at least a full evaluation of the endovascular graft is necessary because pressurization of the aneurysm sac through thrombus at poor attachment sites or caused by material failure can occur, and an endovascular procedure may be a reasonable alternative treatment.

Internal iliac artery exclusion or occlusion is often necessary to use endovascular techniques for the treatment of iliac artery aneurysms. Distal internal iliac artery occlusion at its branches has been associated with a significant risk of buttock claudication (10%-50%) as the most common complication, but others include bowel ischemia and impotence.[55-59] Most, if not all, authors have stated in their published series that buttock claudication improves over time. Proximal internal iliac artery embolization with preservation of the distal branches can significantly decrease the risk of buttock claudication and other associated complications by preserving cross-pelvic collaterals.[55-59] Lin et al.[52] reported that hypogastric artery exclusion with or without embolization is clearly associated with diminished pelvic blood flow as noted by penile brachial indices and manifested by buttock claudication or erectile dysfunction. They found that symptoms were more likely to occur after bilateral hypogastric artery embolization, and this technique should be avoided if possible. They also noted that patients with diseased profunda femoris arteries were at higher risk for ischemic complications. They suggested concomitant profundaplasty at the time of endografting to limit the risk of pelvic ischemia in selected patients who required hypogastric artery occlusion.[60] One study by Rayt et al.[61] reported that 178 of 634 (28%) patients

TABLE 46-1 Endovascular Treatment of Iliac Artery Aneurysms

Author	No.	Mean f/u (months)	Patency (%)	Complication rate (%)	Endoleak rate (%)	30 day mortality
Fahrni et al 2003[50]	19	21	100	21	21	0
Casana et al 2003[48]	16	18	100	0	6.2	0
Tielliu et al 2006[53]	40	31	97.5	8	5	0
Stroumpouli et al 2006[52]	31	51.2	100	19	19	0
Caronno et al 2006[47]	33	32	85	24	14	0
Boules et al 2006[46]	61	22	95	45	36	0
Pitoulias et al 2007[51]	32	35.2	97	3.1	0	0
Chaer et al 2008[49]	52	17	96	9.6	5.7	2%

who underwent unilateral or bilateral internal iliac artery embolization as a part of an endoluminal iliac or aortoiliac aneurysm repair had buttock claudication. Mehta et al.[58] looked at a large series of patients who underwent either unilateral or bilateral hypogastric artery embolization and found that although hypogastric artery flow should be preserved, selective interruption of one or both can be performed safely in selected patients. They thought that other comorbid factors, such as distal embolization, systemic hypotension, or failure to preserve collateral branches of the external or common femoral arteries, also contributed to pelvic ischemia.[58] Mehta's group also found that, within the first month of surgery, 40% of patients with bilateral embolization had buttock claudication and 36% with unilateral embolization did also. By 1 year, only 11% and 12% of patients still had lingering symptoms, respectively. Other series have reported similarly high early rates of buttock claudication that improved over time.[59,62-64] Mehta et al.[65] described a technique to accomplish bilateral hypogastric artery embolization with limited morbidity. They recommend interruption at the origin of the hypogastric artery to preserve pelvic collaterals, staging bilateral hypogastric embolizations, and preserving collateral branches of the EIA and common femoral artery, along with providing adequate heparinization during the procedure.[65] Most authors have suggested that preservation of pelvic circulation using a hypogastric artery bypass, open revascularization, or reimplantation to the EIA should be performed to one hypogastric artery if feasible and safe when bilateral hypogastric embolizations are necessary.[37,59,60,66-69]

Wyers et al.[70] reported on a series of patients who had endoluminal repairs of aortoiliac aneurysms that required coverage of the internal iliac artery. Their decision to cover the internal iliac artery without concomitant coil embolization was based on the presence or absence of adequate graft oversizing (>10%-15%) in the distal 5 mm of CIA and proximal 15 mm of EIA. Those that did not have the appropriate anatomy had their internal iliac artery coil embolized. They found that coverage without embolization in these selected patients had less severe and shorter-term pelvic ischemia.[70] Others have found similar results, suggesting that covering the internal iliac artery without embolization is safe and may even be safer than embolization, especially in the proper patient population.[71,72] All of the authors thought that, even if iliac artery embolization is required, distal internal iliac branches should be preserved to maintain cross-pelvic collaterals if possible.[59,62-64,70-72]

Another complication of decreased blood flow to the pelvis, especially after iliac artery embolization, is visceral ischemia. Although this complication can be catastrophic, it is much less common than buttock claudication. Many series report zero incidence of colonic ischemia.[65,70,72] Geraghty et al.[73] reported on a large series of patients treated with bifurcated endovascular grafts. Of those, 19% underwent perioperative hypogastric artery embolization. They found that four patients (1.7%) had signs or symptoms of ischemic colitis and three required a colectomy. All three patients who underwent a colectomy were found to have ischemia caused by atheroemboli and all had bilateral patent hypogastric arteries. They therefore concluded that, although elective embolization of one or both hypogastric arteries may contribute to pelvic ischemia and ischemic colitis, atheromatous debris rather than proximal hypogastric artery occlusion is the primary cause of ischemic colitis.[73] Another series, by Mehta et al.,[58] found the incidence of ischemic colitis from endovascular repair to be less than its incidence from an open repair (2%) and also suggested that embolization was the most common cause of ischemic colitis.

Other complications include lower-extremity ischemia caused by technical failure, graft thrombosis, or distal arterial embolization. These are rare and occur in fewer than 3% of patients. One final type of complication that is not present in open repairs is an access site complication such as a significant hematoma, arterial pseudoaneurysm, arterial dissection, or arteriovenous fistula. These occurred in 9% to 20% of early endovascular repairs of aortoiliac aneurysms performed in trials that led to device approval in the United States. These complications continue to decrease in frequency because of better surgical techniques and improved endovascular introducer systems.[38,40,74-78]

The percutaneous technique using "Perclose" devices was initially described by Haas et al.[79] in 1999.[80] Razavi et al.[80] described their percutaneous approach for endoluminal stenting of iliac aneurysms in eight patients. They reported successful deployment of stent grafts and aneurysm thrombosis in all patients. Patients with endoleaks underwent coil embolization of the branch vessels feeding the sac or further stent placement.[80] Krajcer et al.,[81] Lee et al.,[82,83] and Starnes et al.[84] along with other authors have promoted the use of these percutaneous techniques for the endovascular treatment of aortoiliac aneurysms. Depending on the graft selected, companies recommend introducer systems ranging in size from 7F (2.3 mm) to 24F (8.6 mm). Many reports in the literature, with use of a variety of commercially available closure devices, describe totally percutaneous aortoiliac aneurysm repair as technically feasible and safe with minimal effects on luminal diameter of the femoral artery. They report higher success rates with smaller sheaths (12F-16F) (94%-99%) than larger sheaths (18F-24F) (>92%). Most report higher complications in patients who are morbidly obese and those devices requiring larger sheaths. One study demonstrated a 75% complication rate with 24F sheaths.[79,81-84] As the profiles of the delivery systems improve and get smaller, a higher percentage of endovascular procedures will be safely performed entirely via percutaneous approaches.

FUTURE DEVICES

Another area for future development is branched devices that would decrease the need for hypogastric artery exclusion. The early generation of the Fortron endovascular device (Cordis Corp./Johnson & Johnson Inc, Miami Lakes, FL) included an iliac branch component, but the device never completed phase II trials in the United States. Ancillary branched iliac components for the Zenith Endovascular Graft (Cook, Inc., Bloomington, IN) have been developed and are used worldwide. Greenberg et al.[85] reported on 21 patients treated with a branched iliac artery device. They had technical success in 86% and after surgery found 15% acute and 11% late branch vessel thrombosis.[85] Ziegler et al.[86] reported on 6-year experience with branched iliac artery devices. They have found that, as the devices have improved, their technical success has also improved. In addition, their group has found favorable long-term outcomes.[86] Two different configurations, one straight and one spiral, are likely to be evaluated in prospective trials. Branched endografts are still early in development, and better devices and long-term clinical trials are still needed before significant conclusions can be drawn and widespread use can occur.

CONCLUSION

The endovascular repair of iliac artery aneurysms and pseudoaneurysms is a safe and effective technique with low periprocedural morbidity and mortality and good short-term and midterm results, especially in appropriately chosen patients. Given its shorter operative time, decreased blood loss, and shorter recovery, it is extremely beneficial for older, frail patients who have greater preoperative comorbidities. New, more versatile and durable commercially available devices are likely to further improve short-term, midterm, and long-term outcomes. In addition, with smaller access sheaths and more flexible devices, more patients may have suitable anatomy for an endovascular approach. However, longer-term data still need to be acquired to better answer the question of long-term durability and safety of this method of repair when compared with open surgical repair.

References

1. Johnston KW, Rutherford RB, Tilson MD, et al: Suggested standards for reporting on arterial aneurysms. Subcommittee on Reporting Standards for Arterial Aneurysms, Ad Hoc Committee on Reporting Standards, Society for Vascular Surgery and North American Chapter, International Society for Cardiovascular Surgery, *J Vasc Surg* 13(3):452–458, 1991.
2. Brunkwall J, Ahuksson H, Bengsston H, et al: Solitary aneurysms of the iliac arterial system: an estimate of their frequency of occurrence, *J Vasc Surg* 10(4):381–384, 1989.
3. Lowry SF, Kraft RO, Paizolero PC, Gilmore JC: Isolated aneurysms of the iliac artery, *Arch Surg* 113(11):1289–1293, 1978.
4. McCready RA, Paizolero PC, Gilmore JC, et al: Isolated iliac artery aneurysms, *Surgery* 93(5):688–693, 1983.
5. Nachbur BH, Inderbitzi RG, Bar W: Isolated iliac aneurysms, *Eur J Vasc Surg* 5(4):375–381, 1991.
6. Richardson JW, Greenfield LJ: Natural history and management of iliac aneurysms, *J Vasc Surg* 8(2):165–171, 1988.
7. Sacks NP, Huddy SP, Wegner T, et al: Management of solitary iliac aneurysms, *J Cardiovasc Surg (Torino)* 33(6):679–683, 1992.
8. Levi N, Schroeder TV: Isolated iliac artery aneurysms, *Eur J Vasc Endovasc Surg* 16(4):342–344, 1998.
9. Sandhu RS, Pipinos II: Isolated iliac artery aneurysms, *Semin Vasc Surg* 18(4):209–215, 2005.
10. Krupski WC, Selzman CH, Floridia R, et al: Contemporary management of isolated iliac aneurysms, *J Vasc Surg* 28(1):1–11. discussion 11-3, 1998.
11. Lawrence PF, Lorenzo-Rivero S, Lyon JL: The incidence of iliac, femoral, and popliteal artery aneurysms in hospitalized patients, *J Vasc Surg* 22(4):409–415, discussion 415-416, 1995.
12. Edwards JM, Teefey SA, Zierler RE, et al: Intraabdominal paraanastomotic aneurysms after aortic bypass grafting, *J Vasc Surg* 15(2):344–350. discussion 351-3, 1992.
13. Mikati A, Marache P, Watel A, et al: End-to-side aortoprosthetic anastomoses: long-term computed tomography assessment, *Ann Vasc Surg* 4(6):584–591, 1990.
14. Szilagyi DE, Smith RF, Elliott JP, et al: Anastomotic aneurysms after vascular reconstruction: problems of incidence, etiology, and treatment, *Surgery* 78(6):800–816, 1975.
15. Treiman GS, Weaver FA, Cossman DV, et al: Anastomotic false aneurysms of the abdominal aorta and the iliac arteries, *J Vasc Surg* 8(3):268–273, 1988.
16. van den Akker PJ, Brand R, van Schilfgaarde R, et al: False aneurysms after prosthetic reconstructions for aortoiliac obstructive disease, *Ann Surg* 210(5):658–666, 1989.
17. Ailawadi G, Eliason JL, Upchurch GR Jr: Current concepts in the pathogenesis of abdominal aortic aneurysm, *J Vasc Surg* 38(3): 584–588, 2003.
18. Curci JA, Liao S, Huffman MD, et al: Expression and localization of macrophage elastase (matrix metalloproteinase-12) in abdominal aortic aneurysms, *J Clin Invest* 102(11):1900–1910, 1998.
19. Thompson RW: Basic science of abdominal aortic aneurysms: emerging therapeutic strategies for an unresolved clinical problem, *Curr Opin Cardiol* 11(5):504–518, 1996.
20. Mertens RA, Holmes DR, Thompson RW, et al: Production and localization of 92-kilodalton gelatinase in abdominal aortic aneurysms: an elastolytic metalloproteinase expressed by aneurysm-infiltrating macrophages, *J Clin Invest* 96(1):318–326, 1995.
21. Thompson RW, Parks WC: Role of matrix metalloproteinases in abdominal aortic aneurysms, *Ann N Y Acad Sci* 800:157–174, 1996.
22. Brown T, Soule S: Aneurysms of the internal iliac artery complicating pregnancy, *Am J Obstet Gynecol* 27:766–767, 1934.

23. Feinsod FM, Norfleet RG, Hoehn JL: Mycotic aneurysm of the external iliac artery: a triad of clinical signs facilitating early diagnosis, *JAMA* 238(3):245–246, 1977.
24. Hennessy OF, Timmis JB, Allison DJ: Vascular complications following hip replacement, *Br J Radiol* 56(664):275–277, 1983.
25. Priddle HD: Rupture of an aneurysm of the left external iliac artery during pregnancy, *Am J Obstet Gynecol* 63(2):461–463, 1952.
26. Tsunezuka Y, et al: A solitary iliac artery aneurysm caused by *Candida* infection: report of a case, *J Cardiovasc Surg (Torino)* 39(4):437–439, 1998.
27. Jezic DV, Stonesifer GL Jr: Computed tomography for noninvasive imaging of the iliac arteries, *South Med J* 75(11):1385–1388, 1982.
28. Solomon GJ, Rosen PP, Wu E: The role of gadolinium in triggering nephrogenic systemic fibrosis/nephrogenic fibrosing dermopathy, *Arch Pathol Lab Med* 131(10):1515–1516, 2007.
29. Stratta P, Canavese C, Aime S: Gadolinium-enhanced magnetic resonance imaging, renal failure and nephrogenic systemic fibrosis/nephrogenic fibrosing dermopathy, *Curr Med Chem* 15 (12):1229–1235, 2008.
30. Cronenwett JL, Johnston KW: The United Kingdom Small Aneurysm Trial: implications for surgical treatment of abdominal aortic aneurysms, *J Vasc Surg* 29(1):191–194, 1999.
31. Limet R, et al: Pathogenesis of abdominal aortic aneurysm (AAA) formation, *Acta Chir Belg* 98(5):195–198, 1998.
32. Santilli SM, Wernsing SE, Lee ES: Expansion rates and outcomes for iliac artery aneurysms, *J Vasc Surg* 31(1 Pt 1):114–121, 2000.
33. Desiron Q, Detry O, Sakalihasan N, et al: Isolated atherosclerotic aneurysms of the iliac arteries, *Ann Vasc Surg* 9(Suppl):S62–S66, 1995.
34. Matsumoto K, et al: Surgical and endovascular procedures for treating isolated iliac artery aneurysms: ten-year experience, *World J Surg* 28(8):797–800, 2004.
35. Huang Y, Gloviczki P, Duncan AA, et al: Common iliac artery aneurysm: expansion rate and results of open surgical and endovascular repair, *J Vasc Surg* 47(6):1203–1210. discussion 1210-1211, 2008.
36. Sanchez LA, Marin ML, Veith FJ, et al: Placement of endovascular stented grafts via remote access sites: a new approach to the treatment of failed aortoiliofemoral reconstructions, *Ann Vasc Surg* 9(1):1–8, 1995.
37. Parodi JC, Palmaz JC, Barone HD: Transfemoral intraluminal graft implantation for abdominal aortic aneurysms, *Ann Vasc Surg* 5(6):491–499, 1991.
38. Sanchez LA, Patel AV, Ohki T, et al: Midterm experience with the endovascular treatment of isolated iliac aneurysms, *J Vasc Surg* 30 (5):907–913, 1999.
39. Parsons RE, Marin ML, Veith FJ, et al: Midterm results of endovascular stented grafts for the treatment of isolated iliac artery aneurysms, *J Vasc Surg* 30(5):915–921, 1999.
40. Sanchez LA, Veith FJ, Ohki T, et al: Early experience with the Corvita endoluminal graft for treatment of arterial injuries, *Ann Vasc Surg* 13(2):
151–157, 1999.
41. Cardon JM, Cardon A, Joueux A, et al: Endovascular repair of iliac artery aneurysm with Endoprosystem I: a multicentric French study, *J Cardiovasc Surg (Torino)* 37(3 Suppl. 1):45–50, 1996.
42. Gasparini D, et al: Percutaneous treatment of iliac aneurysms and pseudoaneurysms with Cragg Endopro System 1 stent-grafts, *Cardiovasc Intervent Radiol* 20(5):348–352, 1997.
43. Stroumpouli E, et al: The endovascular management of iliac artery aneurysms, *Cardiovasc Intervent Radiol* 30(6):1099–1104, 2007.
44. Buckley CJ, Buckley SD: Technical tips for endovascular repair of common iliac artery aneurysms, *Semin Vasc Surg* 21(1):31–34, 2008.
45 Henry M, Amor M, Henry I, et al: Endovascular treatment of internal iliac artery aneurysms, *J Endovasc Surg* 5(4):345–348, 1998.
46. Boules TN, Selzer F, Stanziali SF, et al: Endovascular management of isolated iliac artery aneurysms, *J Vasc Surg* 44(1):29–37, 2006.
47. Caronno R, Piffaretti G, Tozzi M, et al: Endovascular treatment of isolated iliac artery aneurysms, *Ann Vasc Surg* 20(4):496–501, 2006.
48. Casana R, Nano G, Dalainas I, et al: Midterm experience with the endovascular treatment of isolated iliac artery aneurysms, *Int Angiol* 22(1):32–35, 2003.
49. Chaer RA, Barbato JE, Lin SC, et al: Isolated iliac artery aneurysms: a contemporary comparison of endovascular and open repair, *J Vasc Surg* 47(4):708–713, 2008.
50. Fahrni M, Lachat MM, Wildermuth S, et al: Endovascular therapeutic options for isolated iliac aneurysms with a working classification, *Cardiovasc intervent Radiol* 26(5):443–447, 2003.
51. Pitoulias GA, Donas KP, Schulte S, et al: Isolated iliac artery aneurysms: endovascular versus open elective repair, *J Vasc Surg* 46(4):648–654, 2007.
52. Stroumpouli E, Nassef A, Loosemore T, et al: The IEndovascular management of iliac artery aneurysms, *Cardiovasc Intervent Radiol* 30(6):1099–1104, 2007.
53. Tielliu IF, Verhoeven EL, Zeebregts CJ, et al: Endovascular treatment of iliac artery aneurysms with a tubular stent-graft: mid-term results, *J Vasc Surg* 43(3):440–445, 2006.
54. Sahgal A, Veith FJ, Lipsitz E, et al: Diameter changes in isolated iliac artery aneurysms 1 to 6 years after endovascular graft repair, *J Vasc Surg* 33(2): 289–284; discussion 294-295, 2001.
55. Cynamon J, Lerer D, Veith FJ, et al: Hypogastric artery coil embolization prior to endoluminal repair of aneurysms and fistulas: buttock claudication, a recognized but possibly preventable complication, *J Vasc Interv Radiol* 11(5):573–577, 2000.
56. Cynamon J, Prabhaker P, Twersky T: Techniques for hypogastric artery embolization, *Tech Vasc Interv Radiol* 4(4):236–242, 2001.
57. Kickuth R, Dick F, Triller J, et al: Internal iliac artery embolization before endovascular repair of aortoiliac aneurysms with a nitinol vascular occlusion plug, *J Vasc Interv Radiol* 18(9):1081–1087, 2007.
58. Mehta M, Veith FJ, Ohki T, et al: Unilateral and bilateral hypogastric artery interruption during aortoiliac aneurysm repair in 154 patients: a relatively innocuous procedure, *J Vasc Surg* 33(2 Suppl):S27–S32, 2001.
59. Wolpert LM, Dittrich KP, Hallisey MJ, et al: Hypogastric artery embolization in endovascular abdominal aortic aneurysm repair, *J Vasc Surg* 33(6):1193–1198, 2001.
60. Lin PH, Bush RL, Chaikof EL, et al: A prospective evaluation of hypogastric artery embolization in endovascular aortoiliac aneurysm repair, *J Vasc Surg* 36(3):500–506, 2002.
61. Rayt HS, Bown MJ, Lambert KV, et al: Buttock claudication and erectile dysfunction after internal iliac artery embolization in patients prior to endovascular aortic aneurysm repair, *Cardiovasc Intervent Radiol* 2008.
62. Criado FJ, et al: Safety of coil embolization of the internal iliac artery in endovascular grafting of abdominal aortic aneurysms, *J Vasc Surg* 32(4):684–688, 2000.
63. Karch LA, Hodgson KJ, Mattos MA, et al: Adverse consequences of internal iliac artery occlusion during endovascular repair of abdominal aortic aneurysms, *J Vasc Surg* 32(4):676–683, 2000.

64. Yano OJ, Morrissey N, Eisen L, et al: Intentional internal iliac artery occlusion to facilitate endovascular repair of aortoiliac aneurysms, *J Vasc Surg* 34(2):204–211, 2001.
65. Mehta M, Ohki T, Veith FJ, et al: Effects of bilateral hypogastric artery interruption during endovascular and open aortoiliac aneurysm repair, *J Vasc Surg* 40(4):698–702, 2004.
66. Unno N, Inuzuka K, Yamamoto N, et al: Preservation of pelvic circulation with hypogastric artery bypass in endovascular repair of abdominal aortic aneurysm with bilateral iliac artery aneurysms, *J Vasc Surg* 44(6):1170–1175, 2006.
67. Arko FR, Lee WA, Hill BB, et al: Hypogastric artery bypass to preserve pelvic circulation: improved outcome after endovascular abdominal aortic aneurysm repair, *J Vasc Surg* 39(2):404–408, 2004.
68. Delle M, Lönn L, Wingren U, et al: Preserved pelvic circulation after stent-graft treatment of complex aortoiliac artery aneurysms: a new approach, *J Endovasc Ther* 12(2):189–195, 2005.
69. Lee WA, Berceli SA, Huber TS, et al: A technique for combined hypogastric artery bypass and endovascular repair of complex aortoiliac aneurysms, *J Vasc Surg* 35(6):1289–1291, 2002.
70. Wyers MC, Schermerhorn ML, Fillinger MF, et al: Internal iliac occlusion without coil embolization during endovascular abdominal aortic aneurysm repair, *J Vasc Surg* 36(6):1138–1145, 2002.
71. Lee CW, Kaufman JA, Fan CM, et al: Clinical outcome of internal iliac artery occlusions during endovascular treatment of aortoiliac aneurysmal diseases, *J Vasc Interv Radiol* 11(5):567–571, 2000.
72. Rhee RY, Eskandari M, Zajko A, et al: Can the internal iliac artery be safely covered during endovascular repair of abdominal aortic and iliac artery aneurysms?, *Ann Vasc Surg* 16(1):29–36, 2002.
73. Geraghty PJ, Sanchez LA, Rubin BG, et al: Overt ischemic colitis after endovascular repair of aortoiliac aneurysms, *J Vasc Surg* 40(3):413–418, 2004.
74. Adriaensen ME, Bosch JL, Halpern EL, et al: Elective endovascular versus open surgical repair of abdominal aortic aneurysms: systematic review of short-term results, *Radiology* 224(3):739–747, 2002.
75. Boules TN, Selzer F, Stanziale SF, et al: Endovascular management of isolated iliac artery aneurysms, *J Vasc Surg* 44(1):29–37, 2006.
76. Maher MM, McNamara AM, MacEneaney PM, et al: Abdominal aortic aneurysms: elective endovascular repair versus conventional surgery: evaluation with evidence-based medicine techniques, *Radiology* 228(3):647–658, 2003.
77. Saratzis N, Melas N, Saratzis LA, et al: EndoFit stent-graft repair of isolated common iliac artery aneurysms with short necks, *J Endovasc Ther* 13(5):667–671, 2006.
78. Fahrni M, Lachat MM, Wildermuth S, et al: Endovascular therapeutic options for isolated iliac aneurysms with a working classification, *Cardiovasc Intervent Radiol* 26(5):443–447, 2003.
79. Haas PC, Krajcer Z, Diethrich EB: Closure of large percutaneous access sites using the Prostar XL Percutaneous Vascular Surgery device, *J Endovasc Surg* 6(2):168–170, 1999.
80. Razavi MK, Dake MD, Semba CP, et al: Percutaneous endoluminal placement of stent-grafts for the treatment of isolated iliac artery aneurysms, *Radiology* 197(3):801–804, 1995.
81. Krajcer Z, Howell M: A novel technique using the percutaneous vascular surgery device to close the 22 French femoral artery entry site used for percutaneous abdominal aortic aneurysm exclusion, *Catheter Cardiovasc Interv* 50(3):356–360, 2000.
82. Lee WA, Brown MP, Nelson PR, et al: Total percutaneous access for endovascular aortic aneurysm repair ("Preclose" technique), *J Vasc Surg* 45(6):1095–1101, 2007.
83. Lee WA, Brown MP, Nelson PR, et al: Midterm outcomes of femoral arteries after percutaneous endovascular aortic repair using the Preclose technique, *J Vasc Surg* 47(5):919–923, 2008.
84. Starnes BW, Andersen CA, Ronsivalle JA, et al: Totally percutaneous aortic aneurysm repair: experience and prudence, *J Vasc Surg* 43(2):270–276, 2006.
85. Greenberg RK, West K, Pfaff K, et al: Beyond the aortic bifurcation: branched endovascular grafts for thoracoabdominal and aortoiliac aneurysms, *J Vasc Surg* 43(5):879–886, discussion 886-887, 2006.
86. Ziegler P, Avgerinos ED, Umscheid T, et al: Branched iliac bifurcation: 6 years experience with endovascular preservation of internal iliac artery flow, *J Vasc Surg* 46(2):204–210, 2007.

CHAPTER

47

Endovascular Management of Anastomotic Aneurysms

Karthikeshwar Kasirajan

Anastomotic aneurysms can occur because of a variety of etiologies ranging from true para-anastomotic aneurysm to pseudoaneurysms. Reoperative aortic surgery is associated with a high morbidity and mortality because of the often present comorbid conditions. A variety of endovascular techniques offer a less-invasive option for the management of these complex problems.

INCIDENCE

The reported prevalence of all true para-anastomotic aneurysms ranges from 2% to 29%.[1,2] Edwards et al.[3] reported a 5% prevalence at 8-year follow-up and 30% at 15 years. Para-anastomotic aneurysms are caused by true aneurysmal degeneration of the aorta proximal or distal to the prior open surgical repair. These may be differentiated from pseudoaneurysms by the presence of all three layers of the aortic wall. False or pseudoaneurysms result from late anastomotic dehiscence usually caused by low-grade infection or faulty technique or historically caused by use of silk sutures. False aneurysms are believed to be two to three times more common than true aneurysms. The average time interval between the original procedure and the development of the aneurysm is about 6.2 years.

NATURAL HISTORY

The natural history of para-anastomotic aneurysms can be complicated by rupture, thrombosis, embolism, and pressure on or erosion into adjacent structures.[4-6] Accurate estimation of the risk of rupture relative to the size of the aneurysm is not available, but it is generally accepted that this occurs less frequently when the diameter is not greater than 2 cm.[7]

ETIOLOGY

The causes of anastomotic aneurysm formation are various. Technical faults and surgical wound complications are responsible for the early development of false aneurysms or pseudoaneurysms.[8-10] Late predisposing factors resulting in juxta-anastomotic aneurysms include fatigue of the prosthesis or the suture material and most commonly degeneration of the host artery caused by atherosclerosis, excessive endarterectomy, inflammatory disease (Behçet's disease, Takayasu's arteritis), and other connective tissue disorders.

TRADITIONAL OPERATIVE MANAGEMENT

Elective open repair of anastomotic aneurysms is challenging for a variety of reasons. Patients are several years older than at the time of primary reconstruction, and dissection through previous scarred operative sites is required. Additionally, dissection is tedious because of the limited working length available, for example, the distance between the renal arteries and the prior infrarenal graft. This often requires a supraceliac clamp or a thoracoabdominal repair in patients with multiple comorbid conditions. In one large series reporting on open repair of proximal anastomotic aneurysms after open infrarenal abdominal aortic aneurysm (AAA) repair, renal artery reimplantation or bypass was required in 45% with significant surgical morbidity in 27%. In another series of patients with para-anastomotic aneurysms, emergency repair resulted in a 24% mortality, repair after rupture in 67% mortality, and elective repair in 11% mortality.[4,8,11] Hence mortality rates for elective open repair of para-anastomotic aneurysms are relatively high, ranging from 3% to 17%, with only two reports having a mortality rate <8% in patients with no symptoms.[3,4,8,11]

ENDOVASCULAR TREATMENT

Endovascular repair has been proposed as an alternative in properly selected patients as a less-invasive option to reduce the relatively poor results after open repair. In one series endovascular treatment reduced mortality to 3.6% and significant morbidity to 14.2%.[12] The largest series was reported by Faries et al.[13] Their experiences in endovascular repair of failed prior endovascular (n = 14) or conventional (n = 33) AAA repair is described with several different commercially available and physician-made devices. In this series, morbidity and mortality were low, but techniques and results were not differentiated between patients treated for complications after open or endovascular AAA repair.

TECHNICAL CHALLENGES TO ENDOVASCULAR TECHNIQUES

The major challenge to standard endograft placement is the limited landing zone for these stent grafts. Additionally, the often present short bifurcation and long limb lengths of traditional open grafts make it nearly impossible to use standard bifurcated endografts. If an adequate landing zone is present without compromising critical branch vessels standard endograft cuffs have been used in the infrarenal location. The techniques and devices have to be modified depending on the location of the anastomotic aneurysms.

Thoracic Anastomotic Aneurysms

Depending on the location, standard endografts are often adequate to treat these aneurysms. If located close to the cervical branch vessels a variety of arch debranching procedures can be used to improve the proximal landing zone. These range from total arch debranching procedures to carotid-to-carotid and carotid-to-subclavian bypass procedures. These are often quite well tolerated and we often combine them with the stent graft procedure.

Arch Debranching

Total Arch Debranching

The technique of total arch debranching involves the proximal relocation of all vessels from the aortic arch with the exception of the left subclavian artery (LSA) (the LSA in most patients is occluded proximally with coils or occlusion devices). Total arch debranching converts the distal ascending aorta and the arch as a proximal landing zone for the thoracic stent graft. The technique involves a median sternotomy and exposure of the proximal ascending aorta or prior ascending aortic graft followed by exposure of the innominate artery and the left common carotid artery. The brachiocephalic vein may be ligated for ease of exposure. We have not experienced significant postoperative arm swelling when this vein was sacrificed. Usually a 12-mm Dacron graft is anastomosed to the right lateral wall of the proximal ascending aorta. We have been able to perform this in all patients with a side-biting clamp to the ascending aorta. The graft is typically jumped off the lateral wall to avoid compression during closure of the median sternotomy. The distal end is then anastomosed to the innominate artery in an end-to-end fashion. Usually an 8-mm side limb is sewn to the 12-mm Dacron before the innominate bypass. This 8-mm limb is then anastomosed to the left common carotid in an end-to-end fashion (Figure 47-1). The proximal stump of the innominate and the left common carotid is then ligated. The LSA is not easily approached via the median sternotomy. We have either coil embolized this or placed vascular occlusion plugs (Figure 47-2) at the time of stent graft repair. If a left carotid–to–subclavian bypass is required, the subclavian is ligated at the time of the procedure proximal to the vertebral artery. The entire arch and the distal ascending aorta are then used as the proximal landing zone (Figure 47-3, *A*). Sternal wires may be placed around the proximal graft to mark the proximal landing site (see Figure 47-3, *B*).

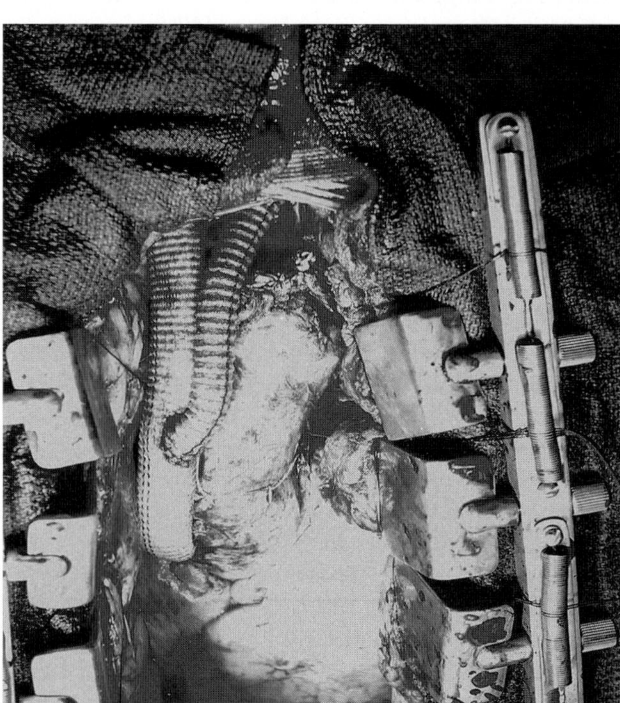

FIGURE 47-1 Inverted "Y" graft to relocate arch vessels to a more proximal location.

Carotid-to-Carotid Bypass and Carotid-to-Subclavian Bypass

Carotid-to-carotid bypass and carotid-to-subclavian bypass allow for the proximal end of the stent graft to land just distal to the origin of the innominate artery. Indications for revascularization of the LSA are given in Box 47-1. The ability to avoid an intracavitary procedure allows for a quicker recovery with minimal morbidity. The technique of a carotid-to-carotid bypass is quite similar to the exposure for a carotid-subclavian bypass. The common carotid artery is located on both sides of the neck, taking care to remain close to the artery to avoid any cranial nerve injury. I have preferred to tunnel subcutaneously with an 8-mm ringed expanded polytetrafluoroethylene graft, unless the patient is very thin. In this case I have used a retropharyngeal location for the tunnel, taking care to stay just anterior to the prevertebral fascia. If a simultaneous carotid subclavian bypass was required, my preferred technique is a right common carotid–to–left subclavian bypass with reimplant of the left common carotid into the graft (Figure 47-4). The left common carotid and the subclavian artery are then ligated in a proximal location.

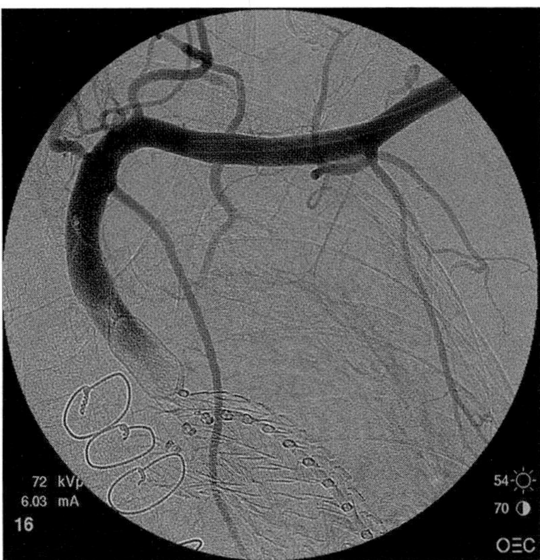

FIGURE 47-2 Amplatzer vascular plug seen occluding the proximal LSA.

Abdominal and Thoracoabdominal Anastomotic Aneurysms

The abdominal and thoracoabdominal anastomotic pseudoaneurysms are often located in close proximity to critical branch vessels preventing a straightforward endograft technique. A variety of debranching procedures can provide new landing zones for these complex aneurysms. Although this involved an operative procedure, extensive dissection through scar tissue can often be avoided, and the added stress of major ischemia and reperfusion can also be eliminated by these hybrid techniques.

Total Abdominal Debranching

Total abdominal debranching involves retrograde bypass to the hepatic artery, superior mesenteric artery (SMA), and both renal arteries. Typically, the abdomen is entered in the midline and the common hepatic artery is identified along the lesser curvature of the stomach. Next the duodenum and the ascending colon are mobilized and the right renal vein is identified; this is then retracted to expose the renal artery. The right common and external iliac artery can also be identified via the same exposure. The second stage of the procedure involves identification of the SMA and the left renal artery. Both of these vessels are identified in the midline, similar to a standard open AAA repair after ligation of the left renal vein. The left common iliac artery is also identified via the same exposure. A 14/7 bifurcated

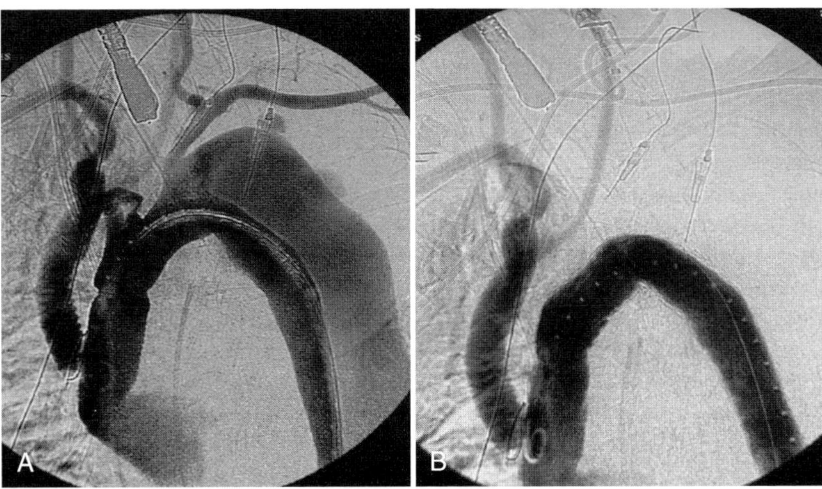

FIGURE 47-3 **A,** Patient with prior ascending aortic replacement for a type A dissection with subsequent visceral relocation to ascending aortic graft. **B,** After thoracic stent graft placement the entire arch and descending thoracic aorta are excluded.

BOX 47-1

INDICATIONS FOR CAROTID-TO-SUBCLAVIAN BYPASS

- Left internal mammary artery → coronary bypass
- Dominant left vertebral
- Right subclavian or innominate stenosis
- Aberrant origin of left vertebral (arch)
- Left brachial occlusion (? prior brachial access)
- Aberrant right subclavian origin
- Total arch and abdominal debranching

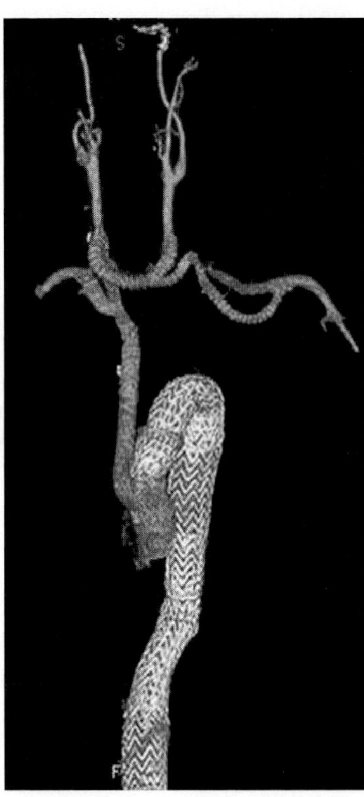

FIGURE 47-4 Carotid-to-carotid and carotid-to-subclavian bypass from a prior arch debranching.

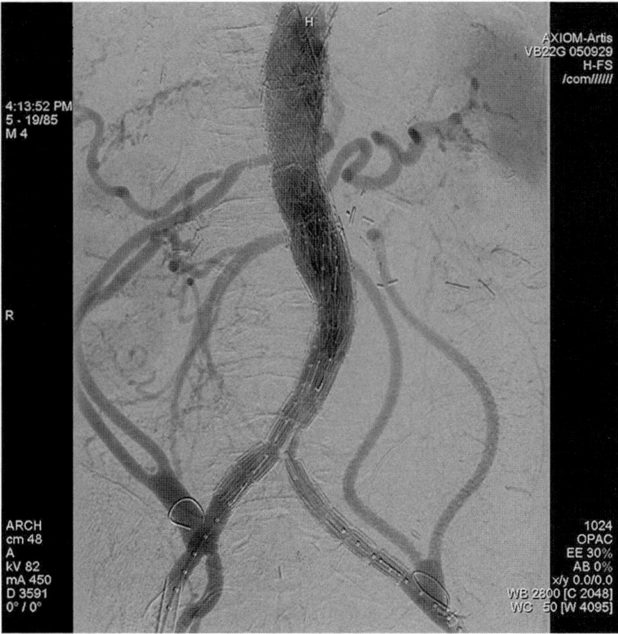

FIGURE 47-5 Total abdominal debranching; note sternal wires used to mark proximal anastomosis.

expanded polytetrafluoroethylene graft is most commonly used. Proximal anastomosis is performed in an end-to-side fashion at the common iliac artery bifurcation, and this location is marked with sternal wires (Figure 47-5). All distal anastomoses are end-to-end bypass except to the hepatic artery. The celiac artery is easily coiled by a transfemoral approach through the hepatic bypass at the time of the stent graft placement (Figure 47-6). This essentially converts the hepatic artery bypass to a functional end-to-end bypass. A variety of different bypasses can be done to exclude one or more visceral vessels that are modifications of the above procedure (Figures 47-7, 47-8, and 47-9). These are given in Box 47-2. The proximal location for the debranching can also be from the prior infrarenal graft.

Branched Stent Grafts

Although these are not commercially available in the United States a variety of branched and fenestrated grafts are in clinical trials and if and when available may offer a less-invasive alternative in patients requiring complex debranching procedures. Initial experience for thoracoabdominal aneurysm suggests that early results are comparable with those of open surgical techniques because of the complexity of these endovascular graft techniques.[14]

Management of Focal Anastomotic Pseudoaneurysms

Focal defects with a narrow neck lend themselves to coil embolization or use of the Amplatzer Plug (AGA Medical Corp., Plymouth, MN). Figures 47-10,

BOX 47-2

TYPES OF VISCERAL RELOCATION IN THE ABDOMEN

Partial

- Splenorenal
- Hepatorenal
- Iliorenal
- Axillary-celiac/SMA

Total

- Iliac-renal/SMA/celiac

SMA, Superior mesenteric artery.

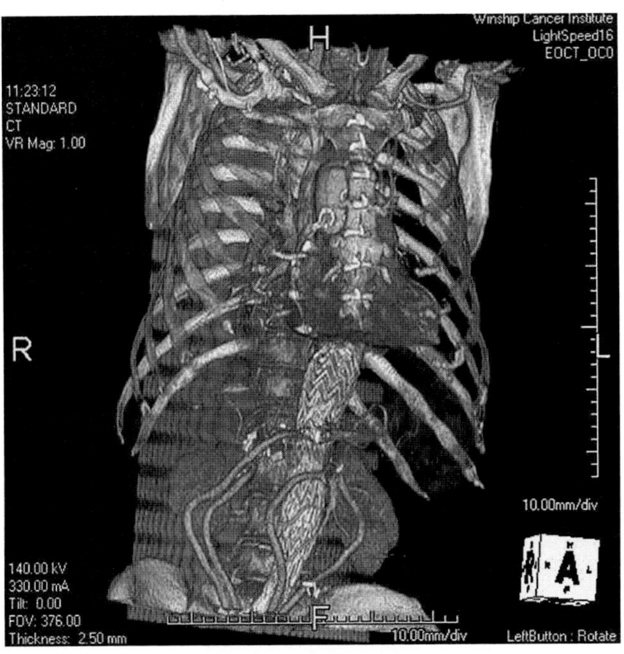

FIGURE 47-6 Coil embolization of celiac axis via the iliohepatic bypass.

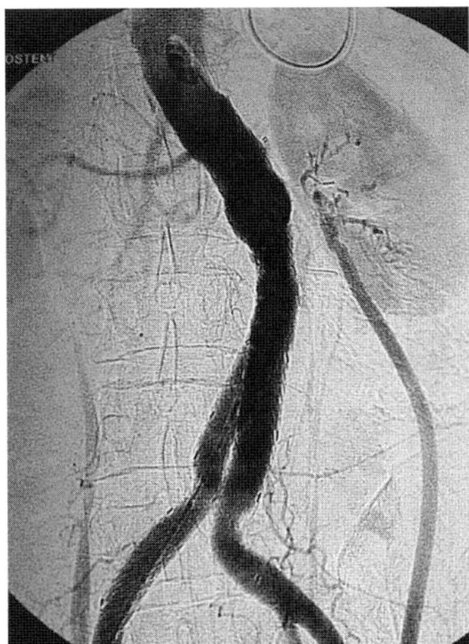

FIGURE 47-7 Iliorenal bypass.

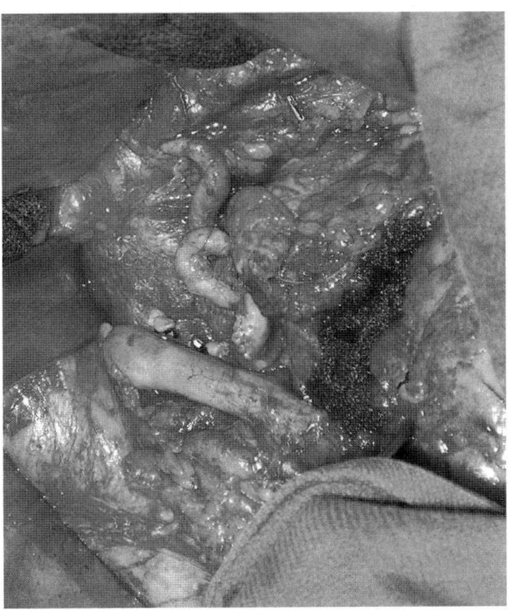

FIGURE 47-8 Splenorenal bypass.

47-11, 47-12, and 47-13 are of a patient who had a gunshot wound to the aorta between the celiac artery and the SMA. This was repaired by a standard open technique with debridement and reapproximation of the aortic wall. The patient was subsequently seen with a large pseudoaneurysm at the site of the open repair (see Figure 47-10). This was confirmed on a diagnostic angiogram (see Figure 47-11). An Amplatzer Plug was subsequently used to close the focal defect leading to the pseudoaneurysm. The celiac artery and SMA were at a safe distance from the plug as confirmed by an intraoperative intravascular ultrasound scan (see Figure 47-12). Computed tomography in 1 year confirmed total aneurysm exclusion (see Figure 47-13).

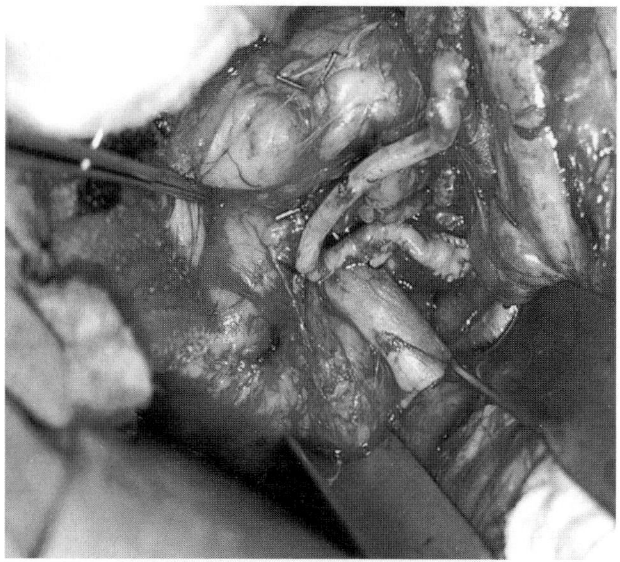

FIGURE 47-9 Hepatorenal bypass.

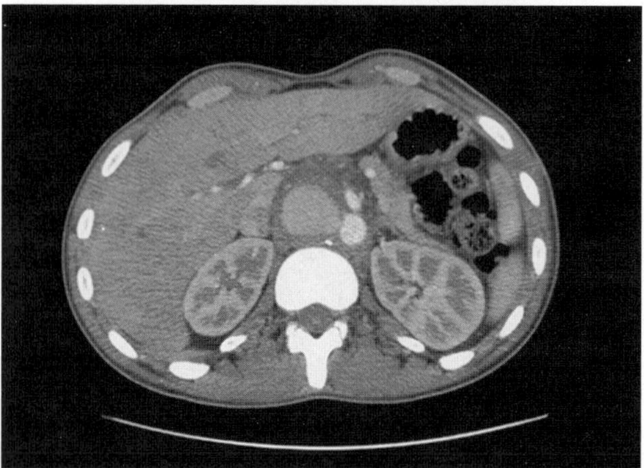

FIGURE 47-10 Computed tomogram of a pseudoaneurysm arising at the site of a prior gunshot wound to the visceral segment of the aorta.

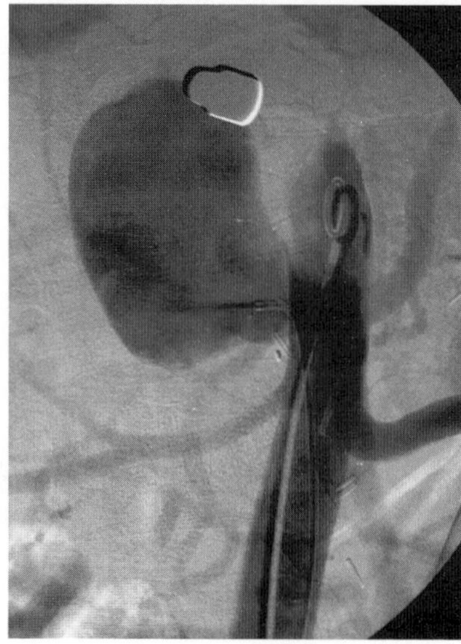

FIGURE 47-11 Diagnostic angiogram of patient in Figure 47-10.

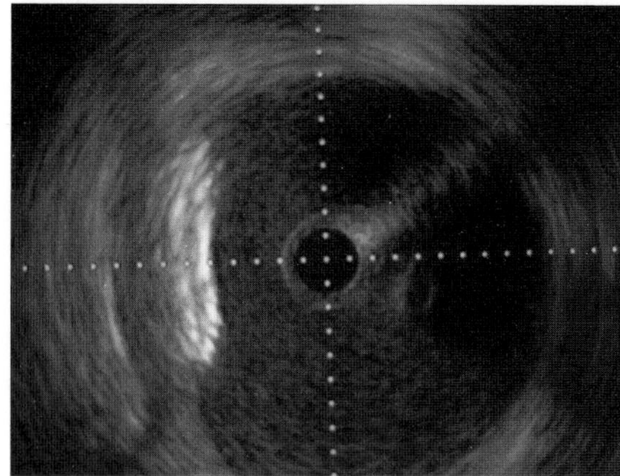

FIGURE 47-12 Intravascular ultrasound scan demonstrates the Amplatzer Plug used to exclude the focal defect in the aorta.

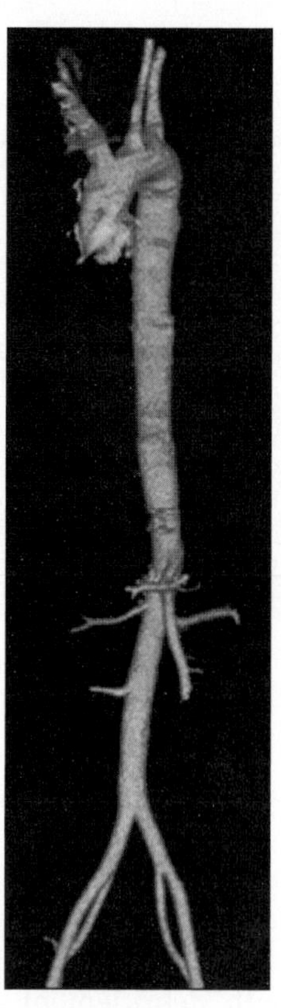

FIGURE 47-13 Computed tomograpy demonstrates the Amplatzer Plug with aneurysm exclusion at 1 year.

ENDOGRAFTS FOR FEMORAL ANASTOMOTIC ANEURYSMS

The majority of femoral anastomotic aneurysms have an infective etiology, hence not ideal for endograft exclusion because of the risk of graft infection. In most patients these are best treated by open surgical

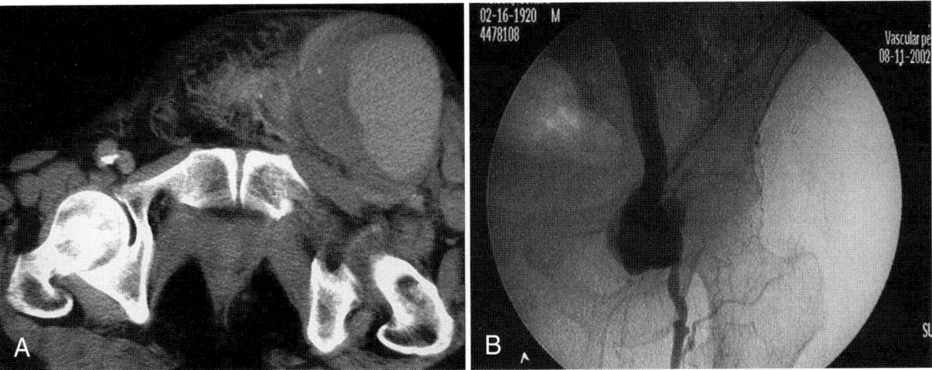

FIGURE 47-14 **A,** Ruptured femoral artery pseudoaneurysm in a patient with a remote aortobifemoral bypass as seen on a computed tomogram. **B,** Angiogram of patient with the ruptured femoral pseudoaneurysm.

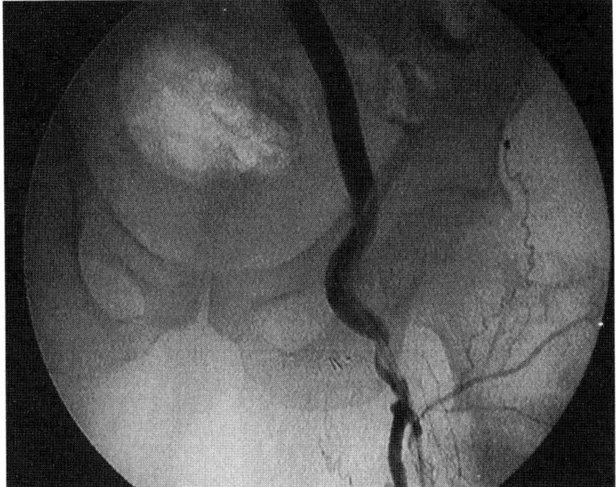

FIGURE 47-15 Viabahn used to exclude the ruptured femoral artery pseudoaneurysm of patient in Figure 47-14.

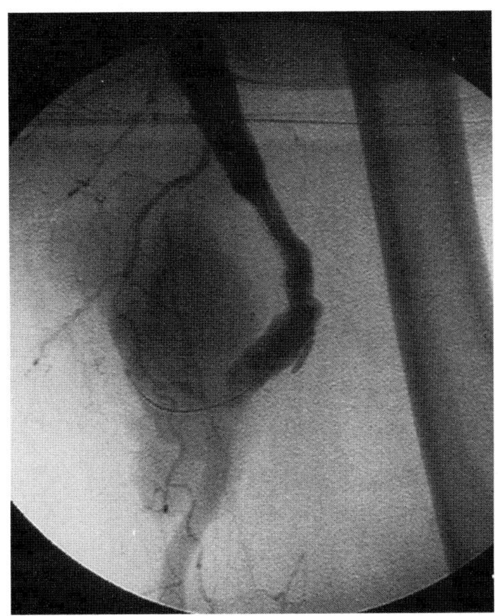

FIGURE 47-16 Ruptured pseudoaneurysm at the site of the distal anastomosis of a recent femoral–to–above-knee popliteal bypass.

techniques of an extra-anatomic bypass and aneurysm excision, or in situ replacement with a vein graft and a muscle flap. However, endografts may be used as a temporary means of aneurysm exclusion in patients in extremis to control hemorrhage. Patients can then be adequately resuscitated and optimally prepared for a semiemergent operation. Examples are provided below in two patients. The first was a patient with a ruptured femoral artery anastomotic aneurysm resulting from an aortobifemoral bypass done 11 years before this event (Figure 47-14, *A* and *B*). The patient's condition was too unstable for an axillopopliteal bypass and aneurysm excision. A Viabahn (W. L. Gore & Associates, Flagstaff, AZ) was rapidly inserted via a percutaneous profunda femoris approach (Figure 47-15). The patient was then adequately resuscitated and brought back 3 days later for an extra-anatomic bypass and aneurysm/graft excision.

The second example is a patient with infected femoral–to–above-knee popliteal bypass with warfarin anticoagulation performed 11 days before presentation to the emergency department. The patient was seen with extreme hypotension resulting from a distal anastomotic dehiscence (Figure 47-16) in the presence of a supratherapeutic international normalized ratio. The hemorrhage was rapidly controlled by placing a Viabahn across the dehiscence (Figure 47-17). The international normalized ratio was subsequently corrected, and the patient was brought back to the operating room the next day for an in situ replacement with the superficial femoral vein.

CONCLUSION

Endovascular options for these complex problems in often sick patients are an attractive option. In the

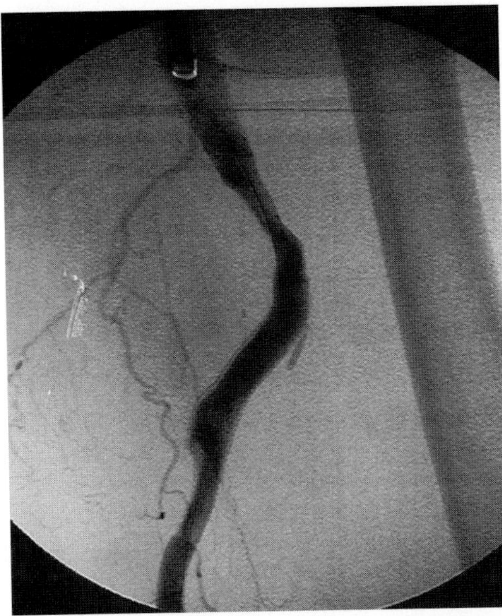

FIGURE 47-17 Viabahn used to exclude the ruptured pseudoaneurysm in patient in Figure 47-16.

absence of an obvious infective etiology endograft techniques appear to provide a stable repair. In patients with infective etiology endografts may help convert a major emergency procedure to a semielective procedure in a patient who has been optimally prepared.

References

1. van den Akker PJ, Brand R, van Schilfgaarde R, et al: Aortoiliac and aortofemoral reconstruction of obstructive disease, *Am J Surg* 167:379–385, 1994.
2. Kraus TW, Paetz B, Hupp T, et al: Revision of the proximal aortic anastomosis after aortic bifurcation surgery, *Eur J Vasc Surg* 8:735–740, 1994.
3. Edwards JM, Teefey SA, Zierler RE, et al: Intraabdominal paraanastomotic aneurysms after aortic bypass grafting, *J Vasc Surg* 15:344–350, 1992.
4. Allen RC, Schneider J, Longenecker L, et al: Paraanastomotic aneurysms of the abdominal aorta, *J Vasc Surg* 18:424–431, 1993.
5. Curl GR, Faggioli GL, Stella A, et al: Aneurysmal change at or above the proximal anastomosis after infrarenal aortic grafting, *J Vasc Surg* 16:855–859, 1992.
6. Treiman GS, Weaver FA, Cossman DV, et al: Anastomotic false aneurysms of the abdominal aorta and the iliac arteries, *J Vasc Surg* 8:268–273, 1988.
7. Levi N, Schroeder TV: True anastomotic femoral artery aneurysms: is the risk of rupture and thrombosis related to the size of the aneurysm? *Eur J Vasc Endovasc Surg* 18:111–113, 1999.
8. Mulder EJ, Van Bockel JH, et al: Morbidity and mortality of reconstructive surgery of noninfected false aneurysms detected long after aortic prosthetic reconstruction, *Arch Surg* 133:45–49, 1998.
9. Stern MS: Arteriosclerosis: considerations as to etiology, *South Med J* 32:370, 1939.
10. Orii M, Shirashugi N, Yamazaki M, et al: Pseudoaneurysm caused by disruption of an externally supported knitted Dacron graft for femoropopliteal by-pass, *J Exp Clin Med* 20:241–244, 1995.
11. Locati P, Socrate AM, Costantini E: Paraanastomotic aneurysms of the abdominal aorta: a 15-year experience review, *Cardiovasc Surg* 8:274–279, 2000.
12. Yuan JG, Marin ML, Veith FJ, et al: Endovascular grafts for noninfected aortoiliac anastomotic aneurysms, *J Vasc Surg* 26:210–212, 1997.
13. Faries PL, Won J, Morrissey NJ, et al: Endovascular treatment of failed prior abdominal aortic aneurysm repair, *Ann Vasc Surg* 17:43–48, 2003.
14. Greenberg RK, Lytle B: Endovascular repair of thoracoabdominal aneurysms, *Circulation* 117(17):2288–2296, 2008.

CHAPTER

48

Endovascular Treatment of Vascular Injuries

Jagajan Karmacharya, Sheela T. Patel, Omaida Velazquez, Juan C. Parodi

Management of vascular disease has significantly changed since the introduction of catheter-based interventions by Dotter and Judkins,[1,2] Volodos et al.,[3,4] Palmaz et al.,[5] and Parodi et al.[6] Over the past few decades, these same endovascular techniques have been used with increasing frequency for the management of trauma. The use of diagnostic angiography coupled with the ability for therapeutic intervention makes endovascular approaches appealing especially to stabilize patient in extremis or to serve as a bridge to future elective procedures. Historically, Gary Becker, when he was in the Miami Vascular Institute, described a temporary placement of a stent coated with silicone as a temporary bailout for acute bleeding, until a definitive open procedure could be carried out.[7] This same concept in selected pediatric patients may be also considered as a temporary bridge to a more definitive operative repair at a later stage as we have carried out in our center. In pediatric patients with life-threatening aortic disruption who have other concomitant injuries, it may be appropriate to perform endovascular repair to exclude the aortic injury until the patients fully recover from other injuries and can undergo an elective definitive open repair with proved long-term durability.

The benefits of minimally invasive endovascular techniques in vascular trauma are remote arterial access from site of injury, controlling bleeding, avoiding general anesthesia, minimizing hospital stay, and decreased blood loss.[8-10] Techniques such as coil embolization are well established in achieving hemostasis in uncontrollable pelvic hemorrhage where traditional access is fraught with difficulty. Balloon control of the hypogastric artery to temporize bleeding in pelvic fractures and recently remote temporary balloon control in traumatic and atherosclerotic rupture aneurysm have been well documented.[11-13] The acceptance and increased utilization of endovascular techniques in both civilian and military environments have brought the vascular surgeons newer challenges and tools in dealing with difficult vascular injuries.[14,15] Vascular surgeons have a wide range of tools from coils, glue, detachable balloons, and covered and uncovered stents to stop hemorrhage. Vascular injuries comprise approximately 3% of all civilian trauma. Trauma surgeons are increasingly asking vascular surgeons to bring endovascular skills in the management of vascular trauma that has been traditionally in the realm of open surgery.[12] The analysis by Reuben et al.[7] of the National Trauma Data Bank demonstrated the rapid use of endovascular therapy for arterial injuries in this decade. However, not all injuries are amenable to endotherapy, particularly in the presence of hard signs of active bleeding, or expanding hematoma (Box 48-1).

Endovascular treatment is not only helpful in the acute setting but has expanded indications to treat arteriovenous fistulas (AVFs) and pseudoaneurysms that result soon after the injury or has a history of trauma in the remote past. Parodi et al. in 1992 were the first in placing a permanent custom-made endograft in a police officer who had congestive heart failure and high-output subclavian AVF.[16] The initial insult was a gunshot wound to his subclavian artery. The treatment was performed via the right brachial artery access with the patient under local anesthesia and placement of a custom-made covered Palmaz stent (Figure 48-1). Subsequently, a 17-year-old Buenos Aires female patient with an iliac AVF was treated from the groin with a covered stent. In Montefiore, these same concepts were applied, and Marin et al. published their series in 1995.[5,17] Since then, endovascular techniques are increasingly being used as a multidisciplinary approach in the management of complex vascular injuries. This chapter is a review of the current techniques and guidelines in the endovascular management of blunt and penetrating vascular injury.

The basic principle of vascular trauma as dictated by advanced trauma life support should be followed. Attempting heroic endovascular procedures that are

BOX 48-1

HARD AND SOFT SIGNS OF TRAUMATIC ARTERIAL INJURY

Hard Signs

- Massive bleeding
- Pulsatile hematoma
- Severe ischemia
- Shock
- Thrill/bruit

Soft Signs

- Moderate hematoma
- Decreased ankle-brachial index
- Vessel close to the injury
- Dislocation of the knee
- Nerve injury

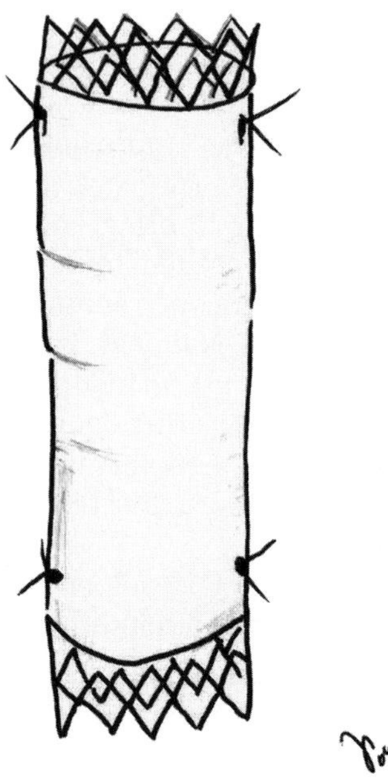

FIGURE 48-1 Drawing of custom-made endografts. The covered stents consisting of polytetrafluoroethylene, Dacron, or vein in some instances were fixed to metallic stent with sutures at about 180 degrees.

complex may be unwarranted in many situations. Patients should be carefully selected on the basis of history, physical examination, and review of imaging. Planning the approach and availability of appropriate tools must be accessed before any intervention. Before the surgeon's arrival the need for fluoroscopy and the assortment of wires, balloons, catheters, and stents should be thought through. Fluoroscopy must be available with all the necessary equipment in the room. Hemodynamically unstable patients may be unsuitable for transport to the operating room for intervention, ideally to an endovascular suite. Adequate resuscitation is a prerequisite. Vascular injuries as result of blunt or penetrating injury can result in a wide variety of presentations, ranging from intimal flaps, occlusions, dissections, pseudoaneurysms, AVFs, and transections. Success in treatment is a result of accurate assessment and the appropriate use of endovascular tools that should be readily available.

CAROTID ARTERY INJURIES

Carotid injuries are not common. The estimated incidence of blunt carotid injuries is around 0.08% to 0.33%. The cervical blood vessels are the most commonly injured structures.[18] Direct and indirect carotid artery injury may manifest in hemorrhage, formation of AVF, pseudoaneurysm, carotid-cavernous fistula, partial or complete transections, thrombosis, and dissections. Clinical findings other than the soft tissue injury in the neck include Horner's syndrome, carotid bruit, neck pain, tinnitus, and the presence of lateralizing focal neurologic symptoms and signs.[19] One must suspect blunt carotid injury if there is history of possible neck injury especially with history of high-velocity deceleration and soft-tissue signs indicative of neck injury. Direct or indirect violent forces to the head and face are responsible for most blunt carotid artery injuries; however, direct trauma to the artery (seat belt injury) may cause disruption of the vessel wall leading to thrombosis, dissection, or pseudoaneurysm formation. The mechanism of injury is related to the force of extension and contralateral rotation.[20] Hyperextension and rotation of the head stretch the tethered carotid artery over the transverse process of the second cervical vertebra, producing an intimal injury or a mural contusion most often in the distal carotid artery. The majority of patients with blunt carotid injury do not display immediate neurologic sequelae. More often, neurologic symptoms are delayed. One of the hallmarks of blunt carotid injury is presence of neurologic deficits out of proportion to the computed tomographic (CT) findings of the brain.

BOX 48-2

INDICATIONS FOR CAROTID STENT IN TRAUMA

- Progression of neurologic symptoms despite anticoagulation
- Persistent emboli
- Stenosis
- Arteriovenous fistula
- Pseudoaneurysm
- Contraindication for anticoagulation

Blunt carotid dissection is a rare injury and occurs in fewer than 1 in 1000 victims of blunt injuries.[21] The standard treatment of carotid dissections is nonoperative.[22] Conservative management with anticoagulation is well established in spontaneous carotid artery dissections.[23] This experience has been translated to acute traumatic carotid dissections. Most surgeons treat asymptomatic, non–flow-limiting traumatic carotid dissections with anticoagulation for 3 to 6 months and antiplatelet therapy (low-dose aspirin).[18] Level 1 evidence for duration of treatment and dosage of antiplatelet therapy does not exist. A prospective study using angiography as a screening tool for carotid artery injury recommends anticoagulation when there are no contraindications to antiplatelet therapy to prevent adverse neurologic sequelae.[24] The rationale for anticoagulation is to minimize the clot formation and propagation and prevent embolization.[25] Trials in patients with asymptomatic carotid artery stenosis caused by atherosclerosis recommend lifelong therapy with aspirin 81 to 325 mg.[26] Extrapolating these data to trauma patients may not be entirely correct. Most patients with traumatic dissections are younger and have healthier vessels. However, anecdotal evidence indicates that most surgeons would treat traumatic carotid dissections with dual antiplatelet therapy (aspirin 81-325 mg and clopidogrel 75 mg) for at least 6 weeks.[27] The long-term benefits and the prevention of stenosis are not known. Retrospective studies indicate that antiplatelet therapy does not reduce the incidence of recurrent stenosis.[28]

Carotid artery stents have been proposed for progression of neurologic symptoms, such as recurrence from emboli (despite anticoagulation),[19] stenosis, AVF, or pseudoaneurysm or in the setting of patients with solid-organ injuries or closed-head injuries when anticoagulation is contraindicated (Box 48-2). Persistent neurologic symptoms such as transient hemiparesis, amaurosis fugax, Horner's syndrome, unspecific headache, and aphasia are other indications for the use of carotid artery stents.[29] The goal of stenting is to cover the entry point of the dissection and restore flow in the true lumen of the internal carotid artery (ICA). The initial devices were custom-made or designed on the table. Fashioning Palmaz stent grafts (Cordis Endovascular, Warren, NJ) on autogenous veins or Wallgrafts (Boston Scientific, Natick, MA) were used to treat AVF and pseudoaneurysms in the carotid artery not approachable by traditional techniques.[8] Parodi et al.[8] reported eight traumatic internal or common carotid artery AVFs and pseudoaneurysms using these devices with good initial results (Figure 48-2). However, in one patient the Palmaz stent was too close to the base, resulting in external compression. Long-term studies in a controlled manner in larger series have not been reported. An Austrian group reported its successful long-term results in six patients without any adverse neurologic events.[30] Five patients had history of trauma. Stenosis greater than 80% was seen by magnetic resonance angiography and duplex ultrasound in four patients, and two patients had ICA aneurysms. Embolic protection devices were not used. After preoperative angiograms were performed, the common carotid artery was approached through a direct cutdown. The group's rationale for open hybrid approach was to allow for the

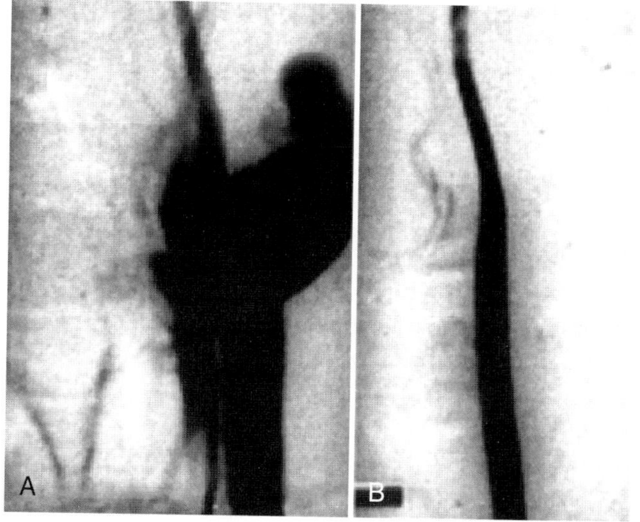

FIGURE 48-2 High-flow carotid-jugular AVF. **A,** Preoperative. **B,** Postoperative angiogram at 48 hours. *(From Parodi JC, et al. Endovascular stent-graft treatment of traumatic arterial lesions,* Ann Vasc Surg *13[2]:121-129, 1999.)*

implant with retrograde flow of the ICA to prevent embolization because the Parodi flow-reversal device was not available at time of its study; in addition, the Hemobahn (W. L. Gore & Associates, Flagstaff, AZ) is not of adequate length to reach the carotids from the groin. Bejjani et al.[31] treated four symptomatic carotid dissections with stents. All four patients had improvement in their neurologic deficits, and there were no complications.[31] Thrombosis of stents and clinical embolic events remain a concern after endovascular management of carotid trauma, but this is rarely documented. Broad application of routine carotid stenting is cautioned. A large retrospective analysis in a level I trauma center comparing carotid artery stenting with conservative management demonstrated a higher incidence of cerebrovascular accidents with the use of open cell carotid stents.[32]

Whereas the natural history of nonocclusive dissections appears to be resolution in about two thirds of patients with early anticoagulation, pseudoaneurysm develops in approximately one third of patients with initial dissections. Pseudoaneurysms of the ICA do not resolve with anticoagulation, and they are frequently the source of embolization or thrombosis. Therefore repair of carotid pseudoaneurysm is recommended in nearly all cases regardless of the patient's neurologic status. Many of these lesions are amenable to endovascular treatment. Parodi et al.,[8] when in Buenos Aires, described three patients with traumatic carotid artery pseudoaneurysm using Palmaz stents with autogenous vein. The first patient was a 20-year-old man who had a false aneurysm at the base of the common carotid artery. The ostia was occluded with a custom-made autologous vein stent. The rationale of using vein was to reduce the thrombogenic tendency and potential infection in a grossly contaminated wound. Recent advances in stent technology have led to commercially available smaller-diameter self-expanding covered stents for the treatment of pseudoaneurysms.[33]

External carotid artery pseudoaneurysms, on the other hand, can be managed by coil embolization. Recent wartime data in the battlefields of Iraq and Afghanistan were analyzed by Cox et al.[34] Of 124 significant penetrating injuries, 13 pseudoaneurysms of the head and neck were found. Most of the patients were treated by coil embolization with two patients requiring open repair. Two patients were treated with a stent and one stent occluded without any evidence of stroke.[34]

Bleeding carotid and vertebral artery injuries as a result of blunt or penetrating injury often are difficult vessels to approach and expose adequately, particularly injuries near the skull base. Anatomic division of the neck into zones allows a selective approach and planning the endovascular management. Zone I injury lies below the cricoid cartilage, zone II is between the clavicle and the angle of the mandible, and, last, zone III is higher than the angle of the mandible.[35] Penetrating zone I and III injuries that require immediate operative intervention are not candidates for endovascular treatment. The incidence of cranial nerve injury (58%) is higher when attempting open repair of these injuries.[36] Endovascular techniques may be used as an adjunct to support the standard open repair of these injuries. Endovascular approach to zone I injuries are useful in emergent situations when the balloon can be used to gain control of the more proximal vessel to allow for repair to be done in an controlled manner.[27] Alternatively, if the proximal vessel can be visualized from a cervical approach but not secured with a vascular clamp, a balloon catheter can be passed retrograde for temporary proximal control. With an occlusion balloon in place, an arteriogram can locate the injury and allow for operative planning. Zone II injuries are typically managed by direct approach through a cervical incision and repairing the vessel. However, blunt injuries to this region may be missed and may present later. Active bleeding in zone III is difficult to approach by endovascular means; however, successful management by endovascular techniques has been described in the literature.[37] Thus an endovascular approach avoids the morbidity of median sternotomy, a high thoracic incision, or difficult dissection at the base of the skull. In addition, endovascular treatment can be performed with the patient under local anesthesia, allowing the provider direct assessment of neurologic status.

Vertebral injuries can be difficult to expose and control.[38] Although the first portion of the vertebral artery is fairly accessible, the second portion (within the bony foramen of the cervical canal) and the third portion (as the vessel exits the bony foramen and enters the base of the skull) can be extremely difficult to control. Trauma to the vertebral artery can result in dissection of the vessel or thrombotic occlusion or result in the formation of a pseudoaneurysm and, in other cases, an AVF. These injuries can be traumatic or spontaneous.[39,40] Most traumatic fistulas are associated with penetrating neck injuries. The majority are asymptomatic. Auscultation may demonstrate a bruit. Other symptoms are neck pain, cervical radiculopathy, subarachnoid hemorrhage, stiff neck, tinnitus, spinal cord symptoms, vascular dementia syndrome, vertigo, and diplopia. Injuries commonly occur between C2 and C5 vertebrae. This correlates with the fact that the most frequent site of penetrating injuries is zone II.[41] Transcatheter embolization or detachable balloons are useful to control bleeding. These same maneuvers can used for vertebral artery transections, pseudoaneurysms, and AVFs.[41-50] Recent series of 18 traumatic injuries over an 8-year period demonstrated that an incidence of 89% injuries were AVFs and only 11% were pseudoaneurysms, and all were treated by an endovascular approach.[41] General anesthesia can be avoided in all these patients. It is often necessary to evaluate the collaterals' circulation. This should be done by injecting the contralateral vertebral artery and both carotid arteries during the balloon occlusion, before proceeding with coil embolization or the use of liquid *n*-butyl cyanoacrylate. If the collaterals' circulation is adequate after 20 minutes of balloon occlusion (with no neurologic signs), then one can proceed with coil embolization or detachment of the detachable balloons. If it is not, then the use of stents is necessary for revascularization.

THORACIC AORTIC INJURIES

Acute blunt rupture of the thoracic aorta is highly lethal. Blunt aortic injury ranks second to head injury as the most common cause of trauma-related deaths. The majority of patients (80%-85%) die at the scene of injury. Of those presenting to a trauma center, half die within 24 hours of injury and 90% die within the first month if the injury is not repaired. Most patients who survive a traumatic thoracic aortic disruption long enough to make it to a trauma center have a contained pseudoaneurysm and represent a precarious yet stable clinical condition. Furthermore, the magnitude of force necessary to cause blunt thoracic aortic injury results in a high proportion of concomitant injuries.[51] In patients whose condition is stable or unstable because of a clear source of hemorrhage other than the thoracic aorta, it is appropriate to delay treatment of the aortic disruption until other life-threatening injuries are stabilized. Contained injuries should be treated with antihypertensive to reduce the aortic wall stress.[52]

Acute ruptures of the thoracic aorta occur as a result of severe deceleration injury. The shearing forces result in aortic tears of varying degrees at the aortic isthmus, distal to the origin of the left subclavian artery (LSA) (Figure 48-3). The transition is at the ligamentum arteriosum (between the mobile distal aortic arch and the fixed descending thoracic aorta). The nature of the high forces involved in causing such aortic injuries resulting in other concomitant injuries often makes these patients poorly suitable to undergo cardiopulmonary bypass and its sequelae. Conventional treatment through a left posterolateral thoracotomy and cardiopulmonary bypass are associated with mortality rates ranging from 15% to 54% and paraplegia rates as high as 36%.[53-55] A meta-analysis of 1742 cases demonstrated that the overall mortality of patients who reached the hospital alive was 32%, with one third of these patients dying before definitive treatment. Postoperative paraplegia occurred in 9.9% of those surviving the repair.[56] Fabian et al.[54] published a landmark prospective study of blunt aortic injury inclusive of 50 trauma centers across North America. There were 274 cases of blunt aortic injury over a 2.5-year period with average time from injury to repair of 16.5 hours. Overall mortality was 31% with 63% of deaths attributable to aortic rupture. Postoperative paraplegia occurred in 8.7% of patients. The proximal descending aorta in the region of the aortic isthmus was the site of almost all aortic tears.[54] In stark contrast the current trend of thoracic aortic stenting results demonstrates a reduction in procedure time, blood loss, length of stay, and decreased morbidity and mortality.[57,58] This trend has steadily increased since Dake et al.[59] in 1998 first published their case series of thoracic stent grafts to treat blunt thoracic aortic injury. In a review of all existing published literature on the use of thoracic endovascular repair of blunt aortic injury excluding single case reports, a total of 235 patients underwent repair from 1997 to 2006. Overall mortality was 6.8% over a mean follow-up period of 21.7 months. There is no reported incidence of postoperative paraplegia.[27] Hoffer et al.[60] performed a meta-analysis of 19 publications that compared the outcomes of 262 stent graft repairs and 376 open repairs. The pooled 30-day mortality rates were 8.4% in the endovascular group and 20.2% in the open repair group. Pooled incidences of paraplegia were 0.83% for the stent graft group and 5.7% for the open repair group. Some authors have compared single-institution experience between open and endovascular repair. Rousseau et al.[61] reported mortality and paraplegia rates of 21% and 7%,

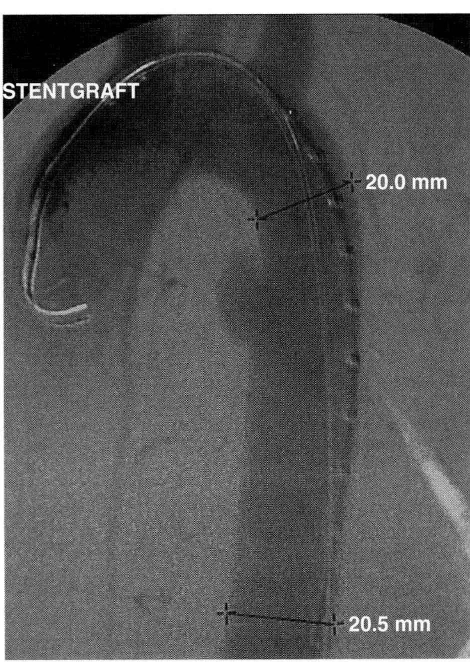

FIGURE 48-3 Contained thoracic aortic tear distal to the origin of the subclavian artery. The tears usually occur between the mobile distal aortic arch and the fixed descending portion of the aorta.

TABLE 48-1 Single-center Series of Thoracic Endografts Published Excluding Centers With Fewer Than 10 Cases

Year	Author	No.	Age (yr)	Follow-up	Mortality	Paraplegia	Stroke	Endoleak	Access	Total Complications
2002	Fattori	19	39.4	20	0	0	0	1		1
2002	Orend	11	46.7	14	1	0	0	2	1	4
2003	Karmy-Jones	11	33	—	3	0	0	1		2
2004	Bartone	14	30.8	14	0	0	0	0		0
2004	Dunham	16	33.7	10.7	1	0	1	0		0
2004	McInitchouk	15	44.9	34.1	1	0	0	1		2
2004	Scheinert	10	38.6	15	0	0	0	0		1
2005	Pacini	15	—	—	0	0	0	0		0
2006	Agostinelli	15	42.3	29	2	0	0	0		0
2006	Andrassy	15	39.1	15.1	2	0	0	1		6
2006	Broux	13	46	31	2	0	0	0		0
2006	Hoornweg	28	40.9	26.5	4	0	0	0		2
2006	Marchiex	33	38.2	32.4	0	0	0	3	3	9
2006	Pratesi	11	48	18.2	1	0	0	0		0
2006	Reed	13	54.8	12	3	0	0	1	1	3
2006	Steingruber	22	39.1	31.7	0	0	0	3		4
2006	Tehrani	30	43	11.6	2	0	1	0	1	2
Total		291			22	0	2	13		36
Average			41.27333333	21.09285714	2.588235294	0	0.117647059	0.764705882		2.1875
Percentage					7.5	0	0.7	4.5		12

Note: The mean age is 41 years. Follow-up ranges from not being reported to 34 months. The total accumulative complications are 12%. Most deaths were related to the nature of injury. Only a small percentage of open conversions were reported. The rate of neurologic complications is 0.1% in these series; this may be due to the young age of this patient population. Access-related complications in these reports were mostly in the brachial artery.

respectively, for 28 patients undergoing open repair versus 0% and 0%, respectively, for of 29 patients undergoing endovascular repair of blunt aortic injury. Despite the lack of prospective randomized studies, these compelling findings have elicited a dramatic shift in the primary management of blunt aortic injury. Most series are single institutional experiences that demonstrate favorable short-term outcomes (Table 48-1). Inherent in all stent graft repairs is that the technique avoids most physiologic insults of open repair: pulmonary impairment after thoracotomy, dissection through hematoma, blood pressure variations, coagulopathy of cardiopulmonary bypass or aortic cross-clamping, and single-lung ventilation. Heparinization is minimized, and general anesthesia can be avoided. In addition stent graft repair avoids distal ischemia from occlusion of the aorta, does not increase intracranial pressure, avoids aortic wall trauma produced by a cross-clamp, and does not require patients with spine injuries to be repositioned, thus minimizing potential factors leading to postoperative paresis.

The majority of aortic transections occur 2 to 3 cm distal to the origin of the LSA. In some patients, the LSA has to be intentionally covered to provide a sufficient proximal landing zone of at least 20 mm (Figure 48-4). The first case report describing intentional coverage of the LSA during endovascular repair was by Mattison et al. in 2001.[62] Coverage of the LSA origin is usually well tolerated as a result of the collateral flow via the vertebral artery. Some authors recommend coverage of the LSA because of energy forces directed on the graft, unless the patient has documented stenosis or occlusion of the right vertebral artery or prior use of left internal mammary artery bypass for coronary bypass grafting. In a review of 23 patients (11 blunt aortic injury) undergoing intentional coverage of the LSA during endovascular repair of thoracic aortic pathology, no patient had vertebrobasilar insufficiency–type symptoms or was symptomatic.[63] Woo et al.[64] reviewed the results of left subclavian coverage during thoracic endovascular aortic repair of 308 patients of whom 70 patients had

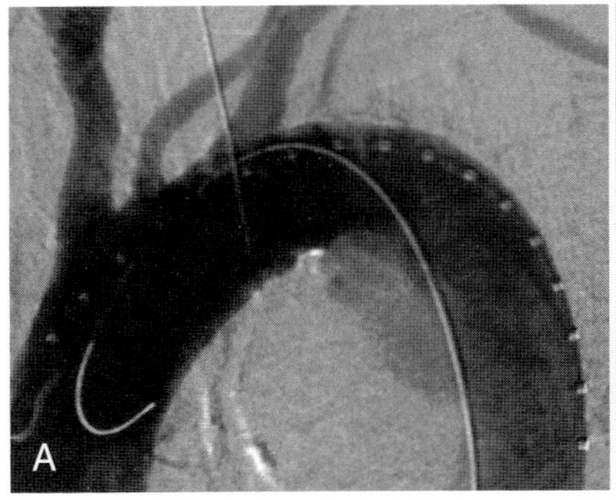

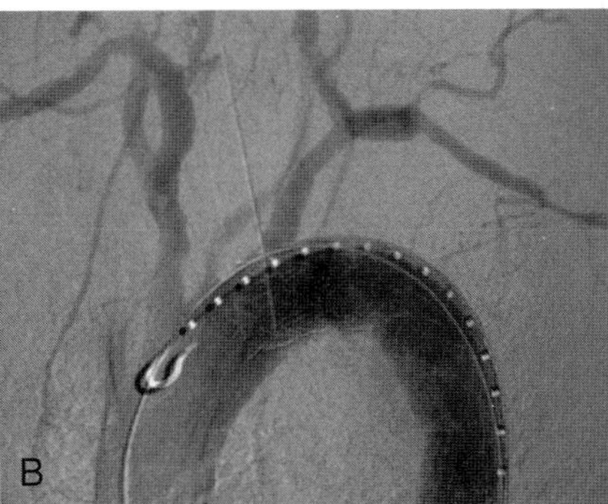

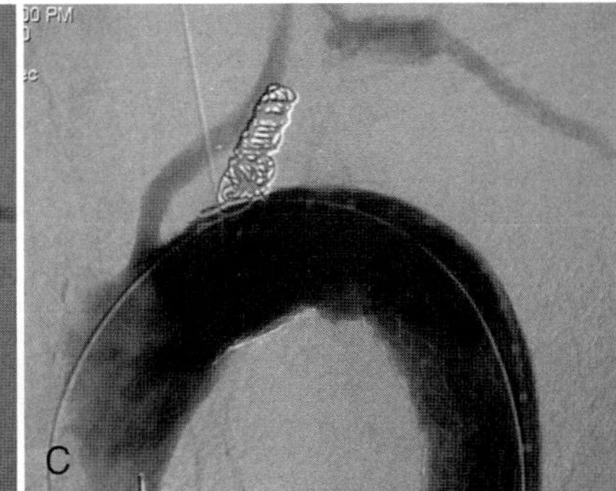

FIGURE 48-4 **A,** Contained pseudoaneurysm treated electively. **B,** Intentional coverage of the subclavian artery after carotid subclavian bypass to gain additional proximal landing zone. **C,** Coil embolization to prevent endoleaks from proximal landing zone.

BOX 48-3

ANATOMIC CRITERIA FOR THORACIC ENDOVASCULAR REPAIR

- Proximal neck at least 15 to 30 mm
- Distal neck at least 15 to 25 mm proximal to the origin of the celiac artery
- Adequate vascular access; small, noncompliant vessels, less than 7 mm may not be suitable especially if there is severe tortuosity, calcification, or atherosclerotic disease involving iliac vessels
- Transverse diameter of proximal and distal neck within the range of available devices

intentional coverage of the subclavian artery. Symptoms such as acute hand ischemia, discoloration of fingers, and severe claudication developed in 5 patients. Extra-anatomic bypass or transposition was not always necessary. Left carotid subclavian bypass should be reserved for patients in whom symptoms develop that necessitate intervention and in patients with left internal mammary artery–left anterior descending bypass.[64,65]

A majority of patients with blunt aortic injury are young and hence have small aortic anatomy measuring from 16 to 24 mm in diameter. Most commercially available grafts are designed for the treatment of aneurysmal disease and not meant for young aortas with smaller diameters and smaller arch radius of curvature (Box 48-3). The smallest commercially available grafts specifically designed for the thoracic aorta are 22 mm (Talent, Medtronic, Santa Rosa, CA) and 26 mm (TAG; W. L. Gore & Associates). At the time of this writing, the Gore TAG device and the Cook TX2 are the only Food and Drug Administration–approved devices in the United States. Most experts would recommend oversizing of 10% to 15% based on the aortic diameters of the landing zones. Therefore the 26-mm graft should be placed in a 22- to 24-mm aorta. The mean aortic diameter for patients who have blunt aortic injury is 19.3 mm.[66] Aggressive oversizing in similar vessels will lead to stent graft failures and "infolding" of the grafts resulting in annoying endoleaks and eventual collapse or demise of the patient.[67] Lack of apposition of the graft to the inner curve of the arch can result in stent collapsing. The graft tends to be pushed away from the inner curvature of the aortic arch as a result of the tendency of most stent grafts to recoil to their straight form. When encountering small aortas some authors have used a variety of infrarenal cuffs and limb extensions of abdominal aortic stents.[58,68] However, these cuffs may have shorter delivery devices that may require an iliac access to reach the arch. Not only should one know the current limitations of stent graft sizes but one should also be prepared to deal with the challenges of access. In patients with hemorrhagic shock, the transfemoral standard access might be challenging because of heavy arterial vasospasm or naturally small vessels in young people and in female patients, resulting in significant diameter mismatch with the delivery system of the stent graft. The outer size of the introducer sheath for the thoracic endograft (20F to 25F) requires a vessel lumen of more than 8 mm. To avoid iatrogenic dissection, rupture, or occlusion of the access vessels, it may be necessary to choose a retroperitoneal approach. A 10-mm Dacron graft is anastomosed end-to-side to the common iliac artery, providing excellent transprosthetic access through this conduit.[69] Planning is the key factor in avoiding complications. Most trauma patients in our center have high-resolution CT angiograms soon after blunt aortic injury is suspected. Postprocessing using 3D-rendering technology with either TerraRecon or M2S is invaluable in planning the approach. If the aorta is amenable to repair, depending on the available commercial device, it is important to plan the access. The size of the iliac artery will determine whether it is necessary to cut down and create a conduit. We frequently get brachial artery access of the left arm and place a 5F sheath. This can be used for coil embolization if it is necessary for subclavian coverage. Only occasionally have we had to start with a subclavian-carotid bypass. The use of intravascular ultrasound if available is helpful in measuring the necessary device length particularly if the preoperative CT angiography has not been adequate. It also provides a means to visualize the tear and adjust the determination of the landing zone. An adjunct such as transesophageal echocardiography is also helpful. Transesophageal echocardiography not only provides information on cardiac function but is a useful tool in guiding the placement of the graft and accessing whether the tears have been adequately sealed.

However, stent graft application requires appropriate anatomy and primary reliance on evolving technology and has device- and access-related complications. Device-related complications occur in an estimated 3% of patients undergoing endovascular repair of acute traumatic aortic disruption.[70] Women and those with small external iliacs are at increased risk for vascular injury during thoracic stent grafting.[71] The lack of proved long-term stent graft durability remains a concern, particularly for young patients because their aortas may become much larger over time, which may ultimately result in loss of fixation. In addition, material fatigue, such as stent fractures and fabric fatigue, worsen over time. Thus it is absolutely imperative that patients treated with stent grafts be followed with long-term surveillance and treated with a high index of suspicion for stent graft collapse, migration, or endoleak. Newer technical innovations such as smaller-diameter, shorter-length thoracic endografts with increased radial force, yet pliable; better attachment systems; and increased flexibility to better oppose the inner wall of the aortic arch will expand the current constraints for the treatment of thoracic aortic transection.

ABDOMINAL AND PELVIS INJURIES

Abdominal traumas both penetrating and blunt carry a high mortality. Mattox et al.[72] described abdominal vascular injuries accounting for 33.7% of all vascular injuries. Abdominal vascular injuries are the most common cause of death after penetrating abdominal trauma. Blunt abdominal injuries are frequently associated with other visceral injuries because the direct and indirect deceleration may result in tears of the solid and hollow organs. Contamination from hollow viscus injuries combined with the need for arterial repair in the same setting makes endovascular therapy appealing.[73] In patients in stable condition with hostile or grossly contaminated damage-controlled abdomen there is no doubt a role for endovascular approach. The role could be as a temporary method until definitive therapy can be planned or as a definitive procedure. Traumatic pseudoaneurysms of the visceral blood vessels can also be managed by endovascular repair.[74] Traditional approaches have been toward resuscitation, damage control, and trips to the angiographic suites for coil embolization of visceral and pelvic injuries. Current indications other than embolization are aortic dissections, aortocaval fistulas, iliac artery injuries, pseudoaneurysms, and AVFs. Most blunt and penetrating injuries to the abdomen with active hemorrhage are managed by open surgery. However, in a hostile abdomen an endovascular approach for temporary or definitive control can be achieved by balloon control or by placement of a stent.[75] These endovascular approaches to the treatment of vascular injuries to the abdomen have been fueled primarily from the success of endovascular treatment of infrarenal aortic aneurysm repair (EVAR) first described in 1991.[16,73,76] Scharrer-Palmer et al.[77] reported the first successful endovascular repair of an actively hemorrhaging infrarenal aortic rupture 6 days after blunt trauma. Yeh et al.[75] reported on the acute management of an actively hemorrhaging gunshot injury to the abdominal aorta. The patient was 2 weeks out from his initial penetrating injuries that included multiple bowel enterotomies and an aortic injury that was repaired primarily. Two weeks later, the patient was actively hemorrhaging from a ruptured mycotic pseudoaneurysm. A stent graft was placed to arrest the bleeding in the setting of a hostile abdomen with potential septic contamination.[76,78]

Blunt injuries of the abdomen can present from intimal flap injuries to aortic dissection with visceral malperfusion, lower-limb ischemia, and transection leading to frank exsanguination.[73] The mechanism of injury in a high-speed motor vehicle crash has been postulated as deceleration injury or a result of direct blunt trauma as the aorta is crushed against the spine.[79-82] A common terminology for the most common blunt aortic injury seen after motor vehicle accidents is the seat belt aorta. The seat belt aorta is defined as injury to the aorta after direct compression against the spine. The most common site of this injury is directly below the inferior mesenteric artery. Traumatic infrarenal aortic dissections can happen in the young, but it is far more common in older patients with preexisting atherosclerotic disease. However, aortic dissections of the

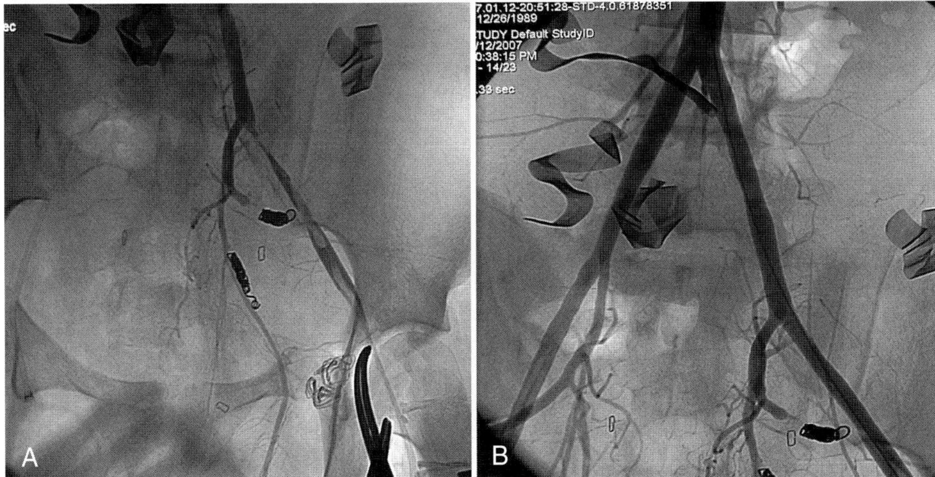

FIGURE 48-5 **A,** Degloving injury of iliac vessels treated with coil embolization and percutaneous transluminal angioplasty. The coils have been placed in the anterior hypogastric branches. The external iliac artery has a focal intimal injury mostly likely caused by the shearing force of the crush injury. **B,** This was treated by retrograde percutaneous approach with balloon angioplasty allowing restoration of flow.

infrarenal aorta are not so common. Traumatic dissections to the infrarenal portion of the aorta account for about 17% of all abdominal aortic dissections.[83] The most common mechanism of injury is motor vehicle crashes. The vectors of force working at the plaque intima interface may not necessarily be so high to start the dissection plane.[84,85]

Careful physical evaluation, CT, and angiography will reveal most abnormalities to plan the endovascular procedure.[86] CT angiogram with slices at 2 to 3 mm should include the thorax, abdomen, and pelvis for thorough evaluation. CT findings include double lumen, differential inflow patterns to aortic branches (evident by abnormal contrast opacifications of the aorta), and intraluminal flaps. Thrombosis, transections, and pseudoaneurysms may be evident in the scans.[86] Diagnostic angiography combined with intravascular ultrasound is our preferred technique in identifying the entry and exit tears. Intravascular ultrasound may not be available in all centers but in recent times is playing an increasing role in the management of aortic aneurysm and aortic dissections.[87,88] The aortic tear can often lead to visceral malperfusion combined with limb ischemia. Techniques such as fenestration may be necessary to establish flow at other times with use of Palmaz Wallstents, or aortic extension stents are usually enough.[89] Because of lack of randomized studies, most techniques are extrapolated from endovascular thoracic dissections and the treatment of degenerative and occlusive disease. The long-term effect of self-expanding stents in the distal aorta and iliac arteries still remains to be seen. What effect it will have as the patients age, whether the stents will lead to stenosis, erode, or lead to aortic dilation in the long term, is still not known. Endovascular treatment for celiac and superior mesenteric artery injuries is rare in literature. One case report describes a spontaneous dissection of the celiac artery and the other an iatrogenic dissection of the celiac artery that was treated by fenestration of the intima.[90,91]

Iliac injuries are difficult to approach and manage. Direct repair is possible in an acute setting, but in blunt injuries with associated pelvic fractures this may result in massive hemorrhage. The mechanism of injury may be due to blunt or penetrating injury or at times iatrogenic. Most injuries present several days or months and years after the injury. Parodi treated a 17-year-old girl in whom an iliac AVF fistula developed after a laparoscopic gynecologic operation; she was treated from the groin with a covered Palmaz stent successfully.[92] However, most pelvic blood vessel injuries are due to penetrating injuries. Pelvic blood vessel injuries resulting from blunt injuries occur in about 12% of all abdominal trauma.[93] Acute limb ischemia is an unusual presentation. In a series of eight patients, five were recognized within 6 hours and were treated by open techniques.[94] Degloving injuries resulting in limb ischemia in the face of pelvic fractures with associated colonic injuries place traditional use of interposition grafts as a potential threat to infection. We have treated these injuries percutaneously. A young female presented with lower-limb ischemia after being run over by a school bus. Bleeding of the pelvic blood vessels were coil embolized, the bowel injuries were stapled, and damage controlled. The degloving injury resulted in an intact adventitia of the external iliac artery. However, she had left lower limb ischemia because of intimal flaps and mural thrombi. We were able to treat this by crossing the lesion and simple angioplasty and flushed the thrombi out via an open cutdown of the groin, thus avoiding the need for placing a Dacron graft

(Figure 48-5). On other occasions it may be necessary to restore flow by placing covered stents across the iliac injury. At other times, when the injury is due to a dissection flap, placing a self-expanding stent may be all that is necessary. Access to both iliac vessels may be necessary in our opinion. The contralateral side can provide access for balloon control in case access cannot be gained or in face of frank extravasation for control.

The utility of angiographic embolization of bleeding pelvic vessels in association with severe blunt pelvic trauma is well documented in the literature since the late 1970s for life-threatening bleeding. Slurry of gel foam or coils can be used to embolize the internal iliac artery with high efficacy. The effects of embolization in a recent retrospective review of 100 trauma patients indicate no significant differences in regard to skin necrosis, sloughing, pelvic perineal infection, or nerve injury between embolized and nonembolized patients.[95] Similarly, claudication, skin ulceration, and regional pain at mean follow-up of 18 months were not statistically significant. However, there are numerous single case series and case reports of impotence, bowel infarction, rhabdomyolysis, bladder necrosis, and sciatic or sacral palsies.[96-99]

Blunt trauma is the most common cause of renal artery injury. There are few reports in the literature describing renal artery stenting for traumatic injury. Renal injury occurs in approximately 1% to 2% in the United States. The involvement of renal vessels occurs in only about 2.5% to 4%.[100,101] Treatment remains controversial when the end organ is not threatened. Most recommend treatment within 6 to 12 hours as the most critical factor in preserving renal function. Most patients with multiple injuries with major renal pedicle involvement and whose condition is unstable are treated with open surgery with nephrectomy as part of the damage-control concept.[102,103] Endovascular treatments of AVF caused by penetrating injuries to the renovascular pedicle with covered stents have been reported.[104,105] The role of endovascular surgery is limited to embolization only in approximately 3% to 4% of the patients in both segmental and main renal artery injuries.[106]

UPPER-EXTREMITY INJURIES

Civilian injuries are as a result of penetrating or blunt injuries caused by motor vehicle accidents, gunshot wounds, stab wounds, and sport-related injuries. The incidence of civilian vascular injuries is about 3%.[107] Presentation can be dramatic with obvious signs of injury and hemodynamic instability to delayed presentation with AVFs, pseudoaneurysms, limb ischemia from thrombosis, emboli, and intimal flaps. Most obvious penetrating peripheral upper-limb injuries are easy to control with direct pressure. Conventional open approach dictates proximal and distal control combined with wound exploration and direct repair depending on mechanism of injury with or without bypass. The use of endovascular techniques and their application in the injuries of the upper extremity are limited to diagnosis and getting proximal control of the subclavian and axillary vessels in penetrating and blunt injuries (Box 48-4). These vessels in the thoracic outlet are often difficult to approach in an acute setting. Traditional methods with right-sided lesions often require a median sternotomy, and the left-sided lesions require a high thoracotomy with extension of the incision with the excision of the clavicular head. Difficulty in anatomic localization in presence of hematoma and

BOX 48-4

INDICATIONS FOR INTERVENTION IN SUBCLAVIAN INJURIES

Indications

- Axillosubclavian pseudoaneurysms
- Arteriovenous fistulas
- First-order branch vessel injuries
- Intimal flaps
- Focal lacerations
- Upper-extremity compartment syndrome with neurovascular compression

Relative Contraindications

- Injury to the axillary artery's third portion
- Venous transection
- Refractory hypotension

Contraindications

- Long segmental injuries
- Injuries without sufficient proximal or distal vascular fixation points
- Subtotal/total arterial transection

Modified from Danetz et al.[117]

friable and "caput medusa–like" vessels may lead to further bleeding in both acute and delayed traumatic conditions. A placement of a remote balloon rather than direct exploration for proximal control can be life saving and allow exploration of the injury in a controlled setting.[108] Becker et al.[15] demonstrated initially that substantial hemorrhage could be controlled by remote access in preparation for more definitive repair. The first permanent treatment for a vascular trauma case was reported by us some years afterwards (1995). Trauma occurred in a police officer who had a gunshot wound in his right subclavian artery without immediate severe consequences until months later he had congestive heart failure because of the high-output subclavian AVF. Treatment was performed from the right brachial artery with the patient under local anesthesia, and a covered Palmaz stent (Dacron) was used. This resulted in closure of the false communication, reversing his congestive heart failure and cardiomegaly within a short period. Some years later we published the use of stents for traumatic arterial injuries in 29 patients.[8] Eleven patients had subclavian or axillary injuries resulting in AVFs or pseudoaneurysms as a result of gunshot or iatrogenic injuries. The initial stents that were used were Palmaz stents mounted in angioplasty balloon catheters secured by "U" stitches placed at the ends of the graft compressed into 11F or 12F introducer sheaths (see Figure 48-1).

Technical advancement of endovascular surgery has led to an explosion of case reports and anecdotal tips for the management of traumatic subclavian and axillary injuries. The use of covered stents in life-threatening subclavian and axillary injuries has been accepted despite lack of long-term and prospective data (Figure 48-6). Most studies continue to be small because of these injuries being rare in both civilian and military environments.[109-114] In a recent retrospective review of 27 patients with injury to subclavian or axillary injuries, 12 patients had lesions amenable to endovascular repair.[115] The 1-year axillosubclavian patency was similar when the patients treated by endoprosthesis were compared with patients treated by open means. However, to date, randomized data do not exist in providing guidelines for endovascular therapy for upper-limb vascular injuries. The only study that is prospective to demonstrate long-term data is a multicenter nonrandomized registry trial looking at the safety and efficacy of endovascular treatment of arterial trauma using the Wallgraft endoprosthesis.[116] They treated 18 patients with subclavian injuries over a 6-year period and demonstrated a patency rate of 85.6% in 1 year. Danetz et al.[117] in a retrospective analysis of penetrating upper limb injuries demonstrated that only 50% were potentially treatable by endovascular means. They cautioned the routine use of endovascular therapy because the approach may have limitations such as associated injuries, involvement of critical branch vessels, and the involvement of distal axillary vessels (Figure 48-7).

Injuries to the brachial artery can result from shoulder and elbow dislocations and fractures of the humerus. Lonn et al[118] reported the first use of angioplasty in brachial artery after blunt trauma. They describe intimal injury resulting in thrombosis that they were successfully able to recanalize by passing a hydrophilic wire past the lesion and using angioplasty to "glue the intima."[118] There is no doubt that further reports will be seen in the near future of more case series in the use of endovascular methods for more peripheral injuries not amenable to open repair; however, these peripheral injuries are best approached using open techniques. The role of

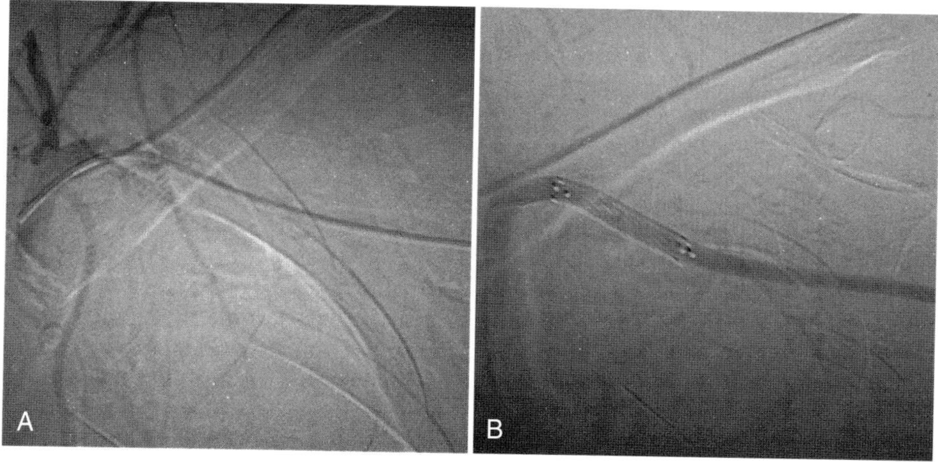

FIGURE 48-6 **A,** Subclavian injury behind the clavicle. **B,** Successful subclavian artery stent for injury distal to the vertebral artery in young female after a motor vehicle crash.

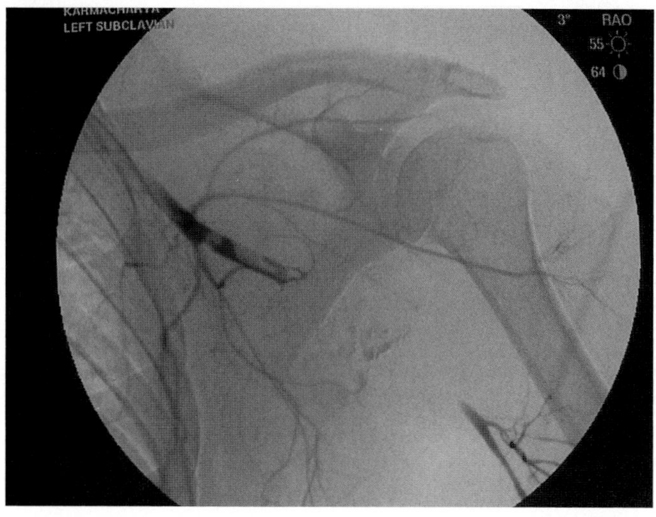

FIGURE 48-7 Acute transection of axillary artery injury from a degloving injury not amenable for endovascular repair. The length of the transection and the mobility of this region are the key reasons for not approaching this by endovascular techniques.

endovascular therapy to radial and ulnar arteries is limited because most can be treated by simple ligation or coil embolization.[108] Hand ischemia often requires urgent revascularization and fasciotomy. The treating surgeon must balance the clinical picture and the location of vessel injury in determining the endovascular approach.[117] The indications for an endovascular approach are outlined in Box 48-4.

Use of endovascular techniques in wartime is emerging as more qualified endovascular surgeons are deployed to war zones. In the most recent evaluation of wartime-related limb injuries, most injuries had been treated by open techniques.[119] In an evaluation of contemporary patterns of upper-extremity injury and effectiveness of management in Iraq, 2473 combat-related injuries in a tertiary surgical facility demonstrated 43 (1.7%) upper-extremity and 83 (3.3%) lower-extremity vascular injuries. Most of these injuries were treated in the forward locations, and six patients were brought to the tertiary center after insertion of temporary shunts. The techniques employed were interposition grafts, direct repair, or ligations with 9.3% of the patients requiring early amputation.[119] However, Rasmussen et al.[120] recently published the military experience of using endovascular techniques over a 3-period in the same war. The majority of endovascular techniques were in the deployment of inferior vena cava filters, angiography, and a handful of therapeutic procedures including the use of covered stents. The study does illustrate that endovascular approaches have increased the armamentarium of the military surgeon in the fronts of battle. Clearly, the visionary military surgeons have applied the civilian data of remote control in wartime to treat physiologically depleted soldiers and civilians with minimally invasive methods.[121,122]

LOWER-EXTREMITY INJURIES

Traumatic injuries of the lower extremity have been treated by endovascular techniques in the past decade by Marin and others.[8,17,123,124] These injuries were gunshot wounds or iatrogenic injuries that presented acutely or delayed, with AVFs or pseudoaneurysms of the common or superficial femoral artery. The majority of peripheral lower-limb injuries are easily approached by traditional open surgery. In a select few traumatic injuries that have AVF or pseudoaneurysms that are difficult to approach via traditional means, we have approached by endovascular repair. However, careful evaluation and the position of the injury in relation to the profunda are necessary before deployment of any covered stents to exclude the injury. Loss of the profunda circulation to the injured leg may result in loss of limb. The majority of peripheral injuries can be treated within 4 to 6 hours of presentation allowing for radiographic evaluation of associated injuries and angiographic evaluation.[108,125] Short stents measuring 6 to 8 mm are useful in the common femoral artery and in the superficial femoral artery. Uncovered stents are helpful if there is no extravasation of contrast and the injury is due to intimal tears or demonstration of residual flap. Covered stents (Viabahn, W. L. Gore & Associates) have been used to treat superficial femoral artery lesions and to cross the knee joint. We like most surgeons avoid using stents across the hip and knee joint for fear of stent occlusion caused by the restricted ability of a rigid stent to accommodate flexion around the joint. There is a paucity of randomized and long-term data in the use of stents for lower-extremity trauma. A prospective review by White and colleagues[116] described treatment of 11 femoral lesions with primary patency rates of 85.7%. Proponents of using endovascular therapy tout the decreased hospital stay, earlier recovery, decreased blood loss, and use of local anesthesia despite lack of long-term data regarding its use in acute trauma. Analysis of the National Trauma Data Bank indicates increasing use of endovascular therapy.[7] Numerous reports exist on the use of covered stents for the iatrogenic injury to the femoral artery after cardiac and neurovascular interventions,[126,127] particularly when ultrasound guide compressions and thrombin injections have failed.[128] Injuries to the tibial and peroneal vessels can be embolized when associated with active bleeding, pseudoaneurysm, or AVF formation.

CONCLUSION

In summary, there has been a vast improvement in technology to accommodate the needs of endovascular repair. The stents and the delivery systems have much improved since the initial reports of handmade devices. As the popularity of endovascular surgery has increased so has the number of vascular specialists with facility in dealing with complex vascular injuries. The management of traumatic injuries will continue to become more minimally invasive as time evolves. Hypogastric artery embolization, AVF management, and remote control of bleeding are well-established techniques of endotherapy. Thoracic stent grafts for aortic transection have gained widespread popularity both in the United States and abroad. Most thoracic aortic injuries in our center are treated with endovascular repair. As data continue to evolve and as our field continues to evolve there is an increasing need to maintain sensibility when approaching complex vascular injuries as endotherapy is rapidly being incorporated. The fate of graft erosion, fracture, development of endoleaks, migration, stenosis, and long-term outcome is not known in the mostly young patient population. The assumptions have been extrapolated from encouraging results of industry-sponsored trials and our atherosclerotic aging population.

Acknowledgment

We thank M. Guiseppe for his dedication to our endovascular program.

References

1. Dotter CT, Judkins MP: Transluminal treatment of arteriosclerotic obstruction: description of a new technic and a preliminary report of its application. 1964, *Radiology* 172(3 Pt 2):904–920, 1989.
2. Dotter CT, Judkins MP: Transluminal treatment of arteriosclerotic obstruction: description of a new technic and a preliminary report of its application, *Circulation* 30:654–670, 1964.
3. Volodos NL, et al: [A self-fixing synthetic blood vessel endoprosthesis], *Vestn Khir Im I I Grek* 137(11):123–125, 1986.
4. Volodos NL, et al: Clinical experience of the use of self-fixing synthetic prostheses for remote endoprosthetics of the thoracic and the abdominal aorta and iliac arteries through the femoral artery and as intraoperative endoprosthesis for aorta reconstruction, *Vasa Suppl* 33:93–95, 1991.
5. Palmaz JC, et al: Expandable intraluminal graft: a preliminary study: work in progress, *Radiology* 156(1):73–77, 1985.
6. Parodi JC, Palmaz JC, Barone HD: Transfemoral intraluminal graft implantation for abdominal aortic aneurysms, *Ann Vasc Surg* 5(6):491–499, 1991.
7. Reuben BC, et al: Increasing use of endovascular therapy in acute arterial injuries: analysis of the National Trauma Data Bank, *J Vasc Surg* 46(6):1222–1226, 2007.
8. Parodi JC, et al: Endovascular stent-graft treatment of traumatic arterial lesions, *Ann Vasc Surg* 13(2):121–129, 1999.
9. McArthur CS, Marin ML: Endovascular therapy for the treatment of arterial trauma, *Mt Sinai J Med* 71(1):4–11, 2004.
10. Arthurs ZM, Sohn VY, Starnes BW: Ruptured abdominal aortic aneurysms: remote aortic occlusion for the general surgeon, *Surg Clin North Am* 87(5):1035–1045, 2007, viii.
11. Sheldon GF, Winestock DP: Hemorrhage from open pelvic fracture controlled intraoperatively with balloon catheter, *J Trauma* 18(1):68–70, 1978.
12. Veith FJ, et al: Treatment of ruptured abdominal aneurysms with stent grafts: a new gold standard? *Semin Vasc Surg* 16 (2):171–175, 2003.
13. Veith FJ, Gargiulo NJ: Endovascular aortic repair should be the gold standard for ruptured AAAs, and all vascular surgeons should be prepared to perform them, *Perspect Vasc Surg Endovasc Ther* 19(3):275–282, 2007.
14. Rudstrom H, et al: Iatrogenic vascular injuries in Sweden: a nationwide study 1987-2005, *Eur J Vasc Endovasc Surg* 35(2): 131–138, 2008.
15. Becker GJ, Benenati JF, Zemel G, et al: Percutaneous placement of a balloon-expandable intraluminal graft for life-threatening subclavian arterial hemorrhage, *J Vasc Interv Radiol* 2:225–229, 1991.
16. Parodi JC: Endovascular repair of aortic aneurysms, arteriovenous fistulas, and false aneurysms, *World J Surg* 20(6):655–663, 1996.
17. Marin ML, et al: Initial experience with transluminally placed endovascular grafts for the treatment of complex vascular lesions, *Ann Surg* 222(4):449–465, 1995, discussion 465–469.
18. Fabian TC, Croce MA, et al: Blunt carotid injury. Importance of early diagnosis and anticoagulant therapy, *Ann Surg* 223: 513–525, 1996.
19. Duke BJ, Ryu RK, Coldwell DM, et al: Treatment of blunt injury to the carotid artery by using endovascular stents: an early experience, *J Neurosurg* 87:825–829, 1997.
20. Perry MO, Thal ER: Carotid artery injuries caused by blunt trauma, *Ann Surg* 192:74–77, 1980.
21. Davis JW, et al: Blunt carotid artery dissection: incidence, associated injuries, screening, and treatment, *J Trauma* 30(12): 1514–1517, 1990.
22. Schievink WI: The treatment of spontaneous carotid and vertebral artery dissections, *Curr Opin Cardiol* 15(5):316–321, 2000.
23. Chandra A, Suliman A, Angle N: Spontaneous dissection of the carotid and vertebral arteries: the 10-year UCSD experience, *Ann Vasc Surg* 21(2):178–185, 2007.

24. Cothren CC, et al: Anticoagulation is the gold standard therapy for blunt carotid injuries to reduce stroke rate, *Arch Surg* 139 (5):540–545, 2004, discussion 545–554.
25. Watridge CB, Muhlbauer MS, Lowery RD: Traumatic carotid artery dissection: diagnosis and treatment, *J Neurosurg* 71 (6):854–857, 1989.
26. Sobel M, Verhaeghe R: Antithrombotic therapy for peripheral artery occlusive disease: American College of Chest Physicians evidence-based clinical practice guidelines (ed 8), *Chest* 133 (suppl 6):815S–843S, 2008.
27. Starnes BW, Arthurs ZM: Endovascular management of vascular trauma, *Perspect Vasc Surg Endovasc Ther* 18(2):114–129, 2006.
28. Clagett GP, et al: Etiologic factors for recurrent carotid artery stenosis, *Surgery* 93(2):313–318, 1983.
29. Nakagawa N, et al: Endovascular stent placement of cervical internal carotid artery dissection related to a seat-belt injury: a case report, *Minim Invasive Neurosurg* 50(2):115–119, 2007.
30. Assadian A, et al: Long-term results of covered stent repair of internal carotid artery dissections, *J Vasc Surg* 40(3):484–487, 2004.
31. Bejjani GK, et al: Treatment of symptomatic cervical carotid dissections with endovascular stents, *Neurosurgery* 44(4): 755–760, 1999, discussion 760-1.
32. Cothren CC, et al: Carotid artery stents for blunt cerebrovascular injury: risks exceed benefits, *Arch Surg* 140(5):480–485, 2005, discussion 485-6.
33. Ahn JY, et al: Stent-graft placement in a traumatic internal carotid-internal jugular fistula and pseudoaneurysm, *J Clin Neurosci* 11(6):636–639, 2004.
34. Cox MW, et al: Traumatic pseudoaneurysms of the head and neck: early endovascular intervention, *J Vasc Surg* 46(6): 1227–1233, 2007.
35. Monson DO, Saletta JD, Freeark RJ: Carotid vertebral trauma, *J Trauma* 9(12):987–999, 1969.
36. Müller BT, Hort W, Neumann-Haefelin T, Aulich A, Sandmann W: Surgical treatment of 50 carotid dissections: indications and results, *J Vasc Surg* 2000(5):980–988, 2000.
37. Ditmars ML, Klein SR, Bongard FS: Diagnosis and management of zone III carotid injuries, *Injury* 28(8):515–520, 1997.
38. Debrun G, et al: Endovascular occlusion of vertebral fistulae by detachable balloons with conservation of the vertebral blood flow, *Radiology* 130(1):141–147, 1979.
39. Nagashima C, et al: Traumatic arteriovenous fistula of the vertebral artery with spinal cord symptoms: case report, *J Neurosurg* 46(5):681–687, 1977.
40. Hieshima GB, et al: Spontaneous arteriovenous fistulas of cerebral vessels in association with fibromuscular dysplasia, *Neurosurgery* 18(4):454–458, 1986.
41. Herrera DA, Vargas SA, Dublin AB: Endovascular treatment of traumatic injuries of the vertebral artery, *AJNR Am J Neuroradiol* 29(8):1585–1589, 2008.
42. Yi AC, et al: Endovascular treatment of carotid and vertebral pseudoaneurysms with covered stents, *AJNR Am J Neuroradiol* 29(5):983–987, 2008.
43. Miller RE, et al: Acute traumatic vertebral arteriovenous fistula: balloon occlusion with the use of a contralateral approach, *Neurosurgery* 14(2):225–229, 1984.
44. Ammirati M, Mirzai S, Samii M: Vertebral arteriovenous fistulae: report of two cases and review of the literature, *Acta Neurochir (Wien)* 99(3-4):122–126, 1989.
45. Higashida RT, et al: Interventional neurovascular treatment of traumatic carotid and vertebral artery lesions: results in 234 cases, *AJR Am J Roentgenol* 153(3):577–582, 1989.
46. Olteanu-Nerbe V, et al: Endovascular treatment of traumatic arterio-venous fistulas of the vertebral artery, *Neurosurg Rev* 16 (4):267–273, 1993.
47. Vinchon M, et al: Vertebral arteriovenous fistulas: a study of 49 cases and review of the literature, *Cardiovasc Surg* 2(3):359–369, 1994.
48. Gallo P, et al: Giant pseudoaneurysm of the extracranial vertebral artery: case report, *Arq Neuropsiquiatr* 54(2):297–303, 1996.
49. Higashida RT, et al: Endovascular surgical approach to intracranial vascular diseases, *J Endovasc Surg* 3(2):146–157, 1996.
50. Santos-Franco JA, Zenteno M, Lee A: Dissecting aneurysms of the vertebrobasilar system: a comprehensive review on natural history and treatment options, *Neurosurg Rev* 31(2):131–140, 2008, discussion 140.
51. Cook J, et al: The effect of changing presentation and management on the outcome of blunt rupture of the thoracic aorta, *J Thorac Cardiovasc Surg* 131(3):594–600, 2006.
52. Fabian TC, et al: Prospective study of blunt aortic injury: helical CT is diagnostic and antihypertensive therapy reduces rupture, *Ann Surg* 227(5):666–676, 1998, discussion 676-7.
53. von Oppell UO, et al: Acute traumatic rupture of the thoracic aorta. A comparison of techniques, *S Afr J Surg* 34(1):19–24, 1996.
54. Fabian TC, et al: Prospective study of blunt aortic injury: Multicenter Trial of the American Association for the Surgery of Trauma, *J Trauma* 42(3):374–380, 1997, discussion 380-3.
55. Smith RS, Chang FC: Traumatic rupture of the aorta: still a lethal injury, *Am J Surg* 152(6):660–663, 1986.
56. von Oppell UO, et al: Traumatic aortic rupture: twenty-year metaanalysis of mortality and risk of paraplegia, *Ann Thorac Surg* 58(2):585–593, 1994.
57. Moainie SL, et al: Endovascular stenting for traumatic aortic injury: an emerging new standard of care, *Ann Thorac Surg* 85 (5):1625–1629, 2008, discussion 1629-1630.
58. Karmacharya JJ, Woo EY, Fairman RM: Endovascular repair of a ruptured thoracic aortic aneurysm with the use of aortic extension cuffs, *J Vasc Surg* 39(5):1128, 2004.
59. Dake MD, et al: The "first generation" of endovascular stent-grafts for patients with aneurysms of the descending thoracic aorta, *J Thorac Cardiovasc Surg* 116(5):689–703, 1998, discussion 703-4.
60. Hoffer EK, et al: Endovascular stent-graft or open surgical repair for blunt thoracic aortic trauma: systematic review, *J Vasc Interv Radiol* 19(8):1153–1164, 2008.
61. Rousseau H, et al: Acute traumatic aortic rupture: a comparison of surgical and stent-graft repair, *J Thorac Cardiovasc Surg* 129 (5):1050–1055, 2005.
62. Mattison R, et al: Stent-graft repair of acute traumatic thoracic aortic transection with intentional occlusion of the left subclavian artery: case report, *J Trauma* 51(2):326–328, 2001.
63. Gorich J, et al: Initial experience with intentional stent-graft coverage of the subclavian artery during endovascular thoracic aortic repairs, *J Endovasc Ther* 9(suppl 2):II39–II43, 2002.
64. Woo EY, et al: Left subclavian artery coverage during thoracic endovascular aortic repair: a single-center experience, *J Vasc Surg* 48(3):555–560, 2008.
65. Peterson BG, et al: Utility of left subclavian artery revascularization in association with endoluminal repair of acute and chronic thoracic aortic pathology, *J Vasc Surg* 43(3):433–439, 2006.
66. Borsa JJ, et al: Angiographic description of blunt traumatic injuries to the thoracic aorta with specific relevance to endograft repair, *J Endovasc Ther* 9(suppl 2):II84–II91, 2002.

67. Steinbauer MG, et al: Endovascular repair of proximal endograft collapse after treatment for thoracic aortic disease, *J Vasc Surg* 43(3):609–612, 2006.
68. Thompson JK, Reed AB, Giglia JS: Novel endovascular treatment of blunt thoracic aortic trauma with a self-expanding stent lined with aortic extender cuffs, *Ann Vasc Surg* 20(2):271–273, 2006.
69. Parmer SS, Carpenter JP: Techniques for large sheath insertion during endovascular thoracic aortic aneurysm repair, *J Vasc Surg* 43(suppl A):62A–68A, 2006.
70. Lin PH, et al: Endovascular treatment of traumatic thoracic aortic injury–should this be the new standard of treatment? *J Vasc Surg* 43(suppl A):22A–29A, 2006.
71. Jackson BM: *Vascular access for thoracic stent grafting: approaches & complications, in Society of Vascular Surgery,* San Diego, 2008, Vascular Annual Meeting 2008, p. 312
72. Mattox KL, et al: Management of upper abdominal vascular trauma, *Am J Surg* 128(6):823–828, 1974.
73. Michaels AJ, et al: Blunt force injury of the abdominal aorta, *J Trauma* 41(1):105–109, 1996.
74. Miller MT, et al: Endoluminal embolization and revascularization for complicated mesenteric pseudoaneurysms: a report of two cases and a literature review, *J Vasc Surg* 45(2):381–386, 2007.
75. Yeh MW, et al: Endovascular repair of an actively hemorrhaging gunshot injury to the abdominal aorta, *J Vasc Surg* 42(5): 1007–1009, 2005.
76. Vernhet H, et al: Dissection of the abdominal aorta in blunt trauma: management by percutaneous stent placement, *Cardiovasc Intervent Radiol* 20(6):473–476, 1997.
77. Scharrer-Pamler R, et al: Emergent endoluminal repair of delayed abdominal aortic rupture after blunt trauma, *J Endovasc Surg* 5(2):134–137, 1998.
78. Hussain Q, et al: Endovascular repair of an actively hemorrhaging stab wound injury to the abdominal aorta, *Cardiovasc Intervent Radiol* 31(5):1023–1025, 2008.
79. Campbell DK, Austin RF: Seat-belt injury: injury of the abdominal aorta, *Radiology* 92(1):123–124, 1969.
80. Garrett JW, Braunstein PW: The seat belt syndrome, *J Trauma* 2:220–238, 1962.
81. Nunn DB: Abdominal aortic dissection following nonpenetrating abdominal trauma, *Am Surg* 39(3):177–179, 1973.
82. Dajee H, Richardson IW, Iype MO: Seat belt aorta: acute dissection and thrombosis of the abdominal aorta, *Surgery* 85 (3):263–267, 1979.
83. Fann JI, Miller DC: Aortic dissection, *Ann Vasc Surg* 9 (3):311–323, 1995.
84. Borja AR, Lansing AM: Thrombosis of the abdominal aorta caused by blunt trauma, *J Trauma* 10(6):499–501, 1970.
85. Brunsting LA, Ouriel K: Traumatic fracture of the abdominal aorta: rupture of a calcified abdominal aorta with minimal trauma, *J Vasc Surg* 8(2):184–186, 1988.
86. Berthet JP, et al: Dissection of the abdominal aorta in blunt trauma: endovascular or conventional surgical management? *J Vasc Surg* 38(5):997–1003, 2003, discussion 1004.
87. Nyman R, Eriksson MO: The future of imaging in the management of abdominal aortic aneurysm, *Scand J Surg* 97 (2):110–115, 2008.
88. Lai KM, Coleman P: Endovascular repair of abdominal aortic aneurysm with chronic dissection using an intravascular ultrasound-guided reentry catheter, *Vasc Endovascular Surg* 42(5): 462–465, 2008.
89. Peterson AH, et al: Percutaneous treatment of a traumatic aortic dissection by balloon fenestration and stent placement, *AJR Am J Roentgenol* 164(5):1274–1276, 1995.
90. Chaillou P, et al: Spontaneous dissection of the celiac artery, *Ann Vasc Surg* 11(4):413–415, 1997.
91. So YH, Chung JW, Park JH: Balloon fenestration of iatrogenic celiac artery dissection, *J Vasc Interv Radiol* 14(4):493–496, 2003.
92. Parodi JC, Marin ML, Veith FJ: Transfemoral, endovascular stented graft repair of an abdominal aortic aneurysm, *Arch Surg* 130(5):549–552, 1995.
93. Tyburski JG, et al: Factors affecting mortality rates in patients with abdominal vascular injuries, *J Trauma* 50(6):1020–1026, 2001.
94. Sternbergh WC 3rd, et al: Acute bilateral iliac artery occlusion secondary to blunt trauma: successful endovascular treatment, *J Vasc Surg* 38(3):589–592, 2003.
95. Travis T, et al: Evaluation of short-term and long-term complications after emergent internal iliac artery embolization in patients with pelvic trauma, *J Vasc Interv Radiol* 19(6):840–847, 2008.
96. Perez JV, Hughes TM, Bowers K: Angiographic embolisation in pelvic fracture, *Injury* 29(3):187–191, 1998.
97. Suzuki T, et al: Clinical characteristics of pelvic fracture patients with gluteal necrosis resulting from transcatheter arterial embolization, *Arch Orthop Trauma Surg* 125(7):448–452, 2005.
98. Sieber PR: Bladder necrosis secondary to pelvic artery embolization: case report and literature review, *J Urol* 151(2): 422, 1994.
99. Piotin M, et al: Percutaneous transcatheter embolization in multiply injured patients with pelvic ring disruption associated with severe haemorrhage and coagulopathy, *Injury* 26(10): 677–680, 1995.
100. Carroll PR, et al: Renovascular trauma: risk assessment, surgical management, and outcome, *J Trauma* 30(5):547–552, 1990, discussion 553–554.
101. Cass AS, et al: Renal pedicle injury in the multiple injured patient, *J Urol* 122(6):728–730, 1979.
102. Ivatury RR, Zubowski R, Stahl WM: Penetrating renovascular trauma, *J Trauma* 29(12):1620–1623, 1989.
103. Nash PA, Bruce JE, McAninch JW: Nephrectomy for traumatic renal injuries, *J Urol* 153(3 Pt 1):609–611, 1995.
104. Areste N, et al: [Endovascular treatment with "covered stent" of arteriovenous fistula secondary to percutaneous renal biopsy], *Nefrologia* 25(4):449–450, 2005.
105. Sprouse LR 2nd, Hamilton IN Jr: The endovascular treatment of a renal arteriovenous fistula: placement of a covered stent, *J Vasc Surg* 36(5):1066–1068, 2002.
106. Elliott SP, Olweny EO, McAninch JW: Renal arterial injuries: a single center analysis of management strategies and outcomes, *J Urol* 178(6):2451–2455, 2007.
107. Austin OM, et al: Vascular trauma: a review, *J Am Coll Surg* 181 (1):91–108, 1995.
108. Arthurs ZM, Sohn VY, Starnes BW: Vascular trauma: endovascular management and techniques, *Surg Clin North Am* 87 (5):1179–1192, 2007.
109. Criado E, et al: Endovascular repair of peripheral aneurysms, pseudoaneurysms, and arteriovenous fistulas, *Ann Vasc Surg* 11 (3):256–263, 1997.
110. Dinkel HP, et al: Emergent axillary artery stent-graft placement for massive hemorrhage from an avulsed subscapular artery, *J Endovasc Ther* 9(1):129–133, 2002.
111. Fass G, et al: Endovascular treatment of axillary artery dissection following anterior shoulder dislocation, *Acta Chir Belg* 108 (1):119–121, 2008.
112. Herbreteau D, et al: Endovascular treatment of arteriovenous fistulas arising from branches of the subclavian artery, *J Vasc Interv Radiol* 4(2):237–240, 1993.

113. Piffaretti G, et al: Endovascular treatment for traumatic injuries of the peripheral arteries following blunt trauma, *Injury* 38 (9):1091–1097, 2007.
114. Valentin MD, Tulsyan N, James K: Endovascular management of traumatic axillary artery dissection: a case report and review of the literature, *Vasc Endovascular Surg* 38(5):473–475, 2004.
115. Xenos ES, et al: Covered stents for injuries of subclavian and axillary arteries, *J Vasc Surg* 38(3):451–454, 2003.
116. White R, et al: Results of a multicenter trial for the treatment of traumatic vascular injury with a covered stent, *J Trauma* 60 (6):1189–1195, 2006; discussion 1195–1196.
117. Danetz JS, et al: Feasibility of endovascular repair in penetrating axillosubclavian injuries: a retrospective review, *J Vasc Surg* 41 (2):246–254, 2005.
118. Lonn L, et al: Should blunt arterial trauma to the extremities be treated with endovascular techniques? *J Trauma* 59(5): 1224–1227, 2005.
119. Clouse WD, et al: Upper extremity vascular injury: a current in-theater wartime report from Operation Iraqi Freedom, *Ann Vasc Surg* 20(4):429–434, 2006.
120. Rasmussen TE, et al: Development and implementation of endovascular capabilities in wartime, *J Trauma* 64(5):1169–1176, 2008; discussion 1176.
121. Fox CJ, et al: Contemporary management of wartime vascular trauma, *J Vasc Surg* 41(4):638–644, 2005.
122. Rosa P, et al: Endovascular management of a peroneal artery injury due to a military fragment wound, *Ann Vasc Surg* 17 (6):678–681, 2003.
123. Durai R, Kyriakides C: Stenting as an alternative to open repair in traumatic superficial femoral artery injuries, *South Med J* 101 (9):963–966, 2008.
124. Risberg B, Lonn L: Management of vascular injuries using endovascular techniques, *Eur J Surg* 166(3):196–201, 2000.
125. Wolma FJ, Larrieu AJ, Alsop GC: Arterial injuries of the legs associated with fractures and dislocations, *Am J Surg* 140 (6):806–809, 1980.
126. Arat A, et al: Emergent treatment of an iatrogenic arterial injury at femoral puncture site with Symbiot self-expanding PTFE-covered coronary stent-graft, *Australas Radiol* 51(suppl): B331–B333, 2007.
127. Waigand J, et al: Percutaneous treatment of pseudoaneurysms and arteriovenous fistulas after invasive vascular procedures, *Catheter Cardiovasc Interv* 47(2):157–164, 1999.
128. Lonn L, et al: Prospective randomized study comparing ultrasound-guided thrombin injection to compression in the treatment of femoral pseudoaneurysms, *J Endovasc Ther* 11 (5):570–576, 2004.

CHAPTER

49

Endovascular Treatment of Visceral Artery Aneurysms

Todd D. Reil, Alexander Gevorgyan, Juan Carlos Jimenez, Samuel S. Ahn

Visceral artery aneurysms (VAAs) are being diagnosed with increasing frequency in asymptomatic patients because of enhanced noninvasive imaging techniques.[1,2] The majority of the surgical literature related to endovascular treatment of VAAs is limited to retrospective single-center case series with limited numbers and case reports. Associated risk factors include atherosclerosis, hypertension, systemic inflammation, trauma, collagen vascular disease, infection, fibromuscular dysplasia, and cirrhosis.[3,4]

Although their estimated incidence is only 0.1% to 2%, VAAs present with rupture in 30% to 40% of patients, with mortality rates of 25% to 70%.[4-6] Pregnant patients are especially at risk with mortality reaching up to 75%, and pregnancy is associated with 20% to 50% of all ruptures.[7,8] The clinical symptoms and natural history of VAAs vary depending on the location of the aneurysm. The most common locations for VAAs are splenic (60%), hepatic (20%), superior mesenteric (5%), and celiac (4%) arteries. Less likely affected are the gastroduodenal, renal, pancreatic-duodenal, jejunal, ileocolic, and inferior mesenteric arteries.[9,10]

Rupture occurs more frequently when the maximum diameter exceeds 2 cm, which is the currently accepted threshold for treatment of asymptomatic lesions.[11,12] We generally recommend treating asymptomatic VAAs greater than 2 cm and symptomatic ones regardless of size. The most common open surgical options include aneurysm ligation, resection with or without revascularization, and/or end-organ resection.

With ongoing advances in endovascular therapy, increasing options are available for minimally invasive treatment of VAAs with low morbidity and excellent outcomes reported in selected patients.[11,13] Various techniques including aneurysm sac embolization and stent graft exclusion have been described. Documented early and late failures of endovascular aneurysm therapy have been documented, including ruptures, and can range as high as 20% to 40% in some series.[14,15] Therefore close follow-up with serial imaging is required in these patients.

SPLENIC ARTERY ANEURYSM

Splenic artery aneurysms (SAAs) represent approximately 60% of all VAAs.[1] The majority are asymptomatic, and they are often discovered incidentally by abdominal imaging for unrelated symptoms. Although the overall rupture risk is actually quite low, rupture is associated with high mortality. Associated risk factors for rupture include pregnancy, portal hypertension, and liver transplantation.[2] Acute rupture may occur into the lesser sac or freely into the peritoneum leading to a severe hypovolemia and exsanguination. Treatment is warranted in patients with associated risk factors, as well as patients with symptomatic, expanding, or large (>2 cm) aneurysms.[16,17] Smaller aneurysms require close outpatient observation with serial imaging to monitor aneurysm growth.

Traditionally SAAs have been treated with open aneurysmorrhaphy, ligation, and/or splenectomy. Resection and patch angioplasty may also be used for saccular SAAs. Recent advances in minimally invasive techniques have led to more frequent use of endovascular treatment for these patients. Endovascular approaches to managing VAAs and visceral artery pseudoaneurysms offer an alternative to conventional open surgery with the benefit of low procedural morbidity and mortality.[6] Patients with cardiac and pulmonary comorbidities or prior abdominal surgery who are poor candidates for open visceral aneurysm repair may benefit from these less-invasive options. Transcatheter embolization or stent graft placement may be preferred in patients with portal hypertension caused by extensive arterial collaterals and high bleeding risk.[18-20]

Coil embolization is the most frequently described endovascular technique for SAAs (Figure 49-1, *A* and *B*). The arterial supply of the spleen contains rich collateral beds that may allow for splenic viability despite thrombosis of the main splenic artery. The placement of coils into the aneurysm sac promotes thrombosis of the SAA and diminishes inline flow through the aneurysm sac.

If an SAA has a defined neck, simple packing of the aneurysm sac with coils allows exclusion and thrombosis of the aneurysm while preserving splenic perfusion. Various coil sizes and configurations are available and may be used. We prefer the use of 0.0889-cm/0.035-inch fibered coils. Microcoils delivered through smaller-profile catheters can also be used for smaller aneurysms.[21]

We have used an alternative approach that can be used to help preserve splenic artery perfusion. A bare metal stent is deployed in the splenic artery across the involved aneurysmal segment. This is followed by cannulation of the aneurysm sac through the interstices of the stent with an appropriate-sized catheter to allow coil placement. Placing coils through the stent interstices into the aneurysm prevents embolization of coils downstream while preserving splenic flow. Glue or thrombin can also be injected into the coil-filled sac to aid in thrombosis.[21]

Another method for SAA exclusion is coil placement in the splenic artery proximal and distal to the aneurysm, the so-called sandwich technique. This eliminates prograde and retrograde flow into the aneurysm.[21] It is also important in this setting to coil any communicating side branches to completely exclude the SAA. In the majority of patients, perfusion of the spleen is maintained through collateral circulation via the short gastric arteries.

Technical success of percutaneous transcatheter coil embolization has been acceptable in most series with reported primary success rates ranging from 66.7% to 92%.[3,13,22,23] Other complications include migration of coils (leading to organ infarction), abscess formation, and, rarely, aneurysm rupture.[24] Recanalization after successful embolization is rare but has been reported.[13]

Coil embolization of the splenic artery can lead to splenic infarction. This is noted primarily after distal or hilar branch embolization and has a reported incidence of approximately 25% in our experience. Symptoms range from abdominal pain and/or low-grade fevers to sepsis, pancreatitis, and infection or abscess of the splenic parenchyma.[2] A high index of suspicion for splenic infarction must be maintained during the perioperative period. Clinical signs of worsening abdominal pain, leukocytosis, and fever may indicate the need for laparoscopic versus open splenectomy. Follow-up after coil embolization may be difficult because of scatter and artifact caused by coils on imaging studies, and magnetic resonance angiography may be preferred to computed tomography (CT) for postprocedural imaging.

Therapeutic chemoembolization has traditionally been reserved for poor surgical candidates, but recent advances have made this a primary option for treatment. The use of agents, such as gel foam, fibrin and thrombin glue, inert particles, and detachable balloons, has been described.[2,15,25,26] Kemmeter et al.[27] reported successful percutaneous thrombin injection in two patients with ruptured splanchnic artery aneurysms. Successful treatment of hepatic artery aneurysms (HAAs) with percutaneous thrombin injection has

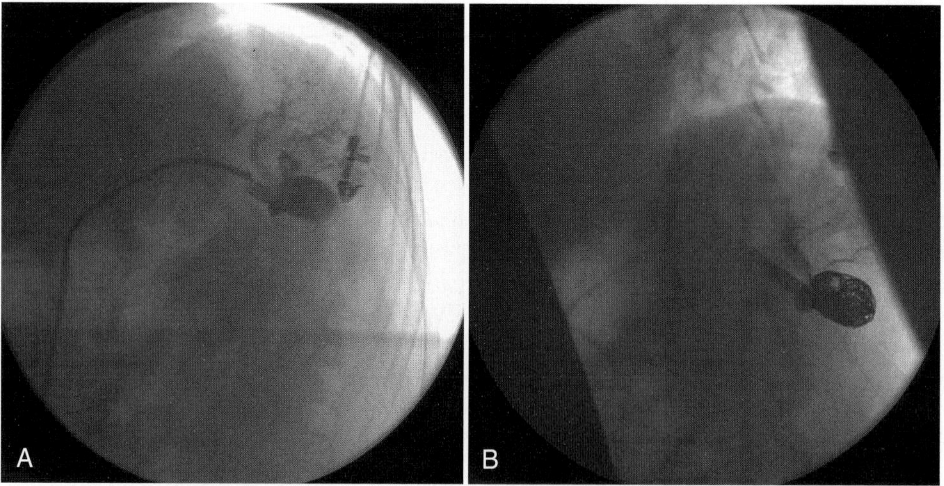

FIGURE 49-1 **A,** Angiogram demonstrating the presence of a large SAA before treatment. **B,** Completion angiogram after coil embolization of SAA.

also been reported.[28] Embolization using *N*-butyl-2-cyanoacrylate has also been described. A potential serious complication to this method is pancreatitis.[29] This occurs as a result of obliteration of small arterioles to the pancreas that come off the splenic artery.

Success rates in literature have varied from 75% to 100% with morbidity rates ranging from 14% to 25%.[22,23] Most of the complications reported in literature include pain, fever, transitory increased pancreatic or hepatic enzymes, migration of embolizing materials or stent graft, and access site complications.[30]

Lower stent profiles and improved delivery systems have allowed greater opportunities with endovascular aneurysm exclusion using covered stent grafts.[31-34]

An advantage of this method includes preservation of direct arterial splenic perfusion. The use of stent grafts, however, is frequently limited by tortuous splenic artery anatomy and device-specific considerations including size and delivery. The careful use of stiff wires may facilitate advancement of covered stents through the splenic artery. With the introduction of more flexible stent grafts and smaller delivery systems, it may be possible to offer this therapy to a wider population.

HEPATIC ARTERY ANEURYSM

HAAs are the second most common VAA. Most occur in males, are solitary, and are extrahepatic.[35] Almost 50% of HAAs are pseudoaneurysms. This reflects the increased use of interventional procedures of the biliary tract and CT after blunt abdominal trauma.[36] True aneurysms occur four times more frequently in the extrahepatic arteries, usually involve the common hepatic artery, and are associated mainly with arteriolosclerosis and acquired medical degeneration.[35,37,38] Mycotic aneurysms are rare (<5% of HAAs). Other causes include polyarteritis nodosa, pancreatitis, liver transplantation, neurofibromatosis, Wegener's granulomatosis, and tuberculosis.[35,38]

The majority of HAAs are asymptomatic. Symptomatic patients may present with hemobilia, jaundice, and pain. Mortality rates of greater than 50% have been reported after acute rupture.[39] Twenty percent to 30% of HAAs may rupture into the peritoneal cavity and manifest symptoms of abdominal pain with hypovolemic shock.[35,36] Risk factors for rupture of true aneurysms include multiple HAAs and a nonatherosclerotic etiology of the aneurysm.[36]

The location of the HAA, as well as the collateral blood supply to the liver, is critical to choosing endovascular versus surgical treatment. Traditional surgical treatment involves open aneurysm ligation or resection with bypass to preserve inline arterial flow (Figure 49-2, *A* and *B*). The blood supply to the liver is provided by both the hepatic artery and portal vein. The main arterial collateral supply comes from the gastroduodenal artery (GDA). This is important in determining which treatment method to offer the patient. If there is good collateralization from the GDA to the distal hepatic artery, the common hepatic artery can be embolized without significant clinical sequelae. Tulsyan et al.[6] reported their experience at the Cleveland Clinic with coil embolization of HAAs and pseudoaneurysms. Twelve total aneurysms were treated with a technical success rate of 100%. There were no perioperative (30 day) deaths, and no patients had signs of end-organ ischemia.[6]

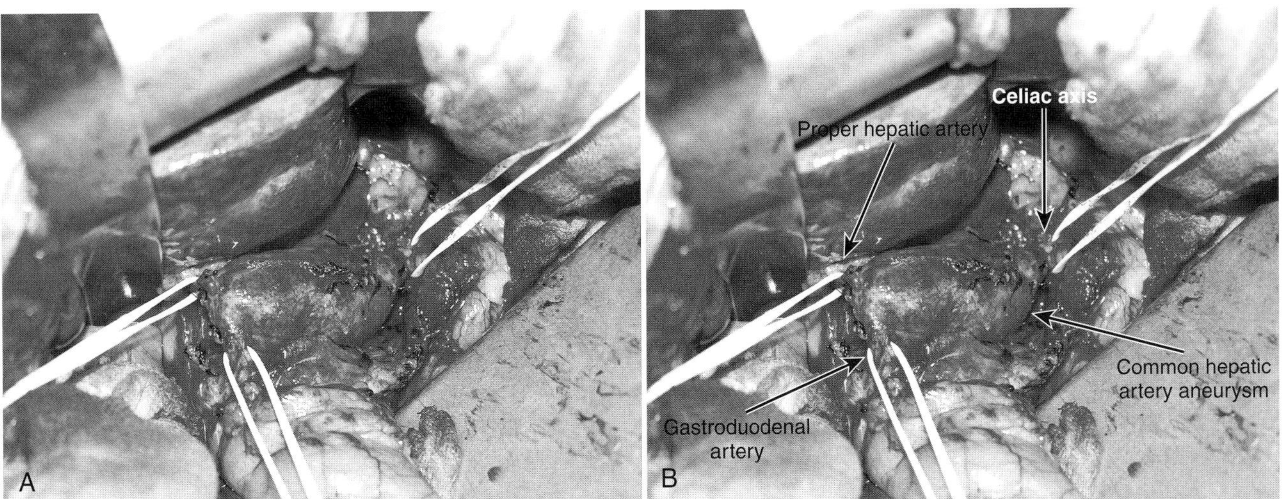

FIGURE 49-2 **A,** Traditional surgical management of HAAs traditionally involves surgical exposure through laparotomy. **B,** Resection of large common HAA and reconstruction with interposition Dacron graft.

However, if the aneurysm is distal to the GDA, surgical repair may be preferable. If adequate proximal and distal landing zones are present (≥2 cm), covered stent treatment is an alternative to surgical ligation and bypass and has been described in multiple case reports for both ruptured and nonruptured HAAs.[40-42]

Intrahepatic aneurysms are best treated with endovascular techniques because open surgical repair often necessitates liver resection. Most intrahepatic aneurysms can be treated with coil occlusion or embolization. Extensive collateral circulation and contribution of portal flow to the oxygen supply of the liver limits significant ischemia in this situation. In the absence of collateral hepatic perfusion, covered stent placement has also been described, preserving direct blood-flow to the liver bed.[31,34] Currently, there are no studies comparing the efficacy of coil embolization versus stent graft treatment for HAA.

CELIAC ARTERY ANEURYSM

Celiac artery aneurysms (CAAs) occur in approximately 0.2% of the overall population and constitute approximately 4% of all VAAs.[43,44] Their risk of rupture is estimated at 10% to 15% and is associated with high mortality.[41] Shanley et al.[36] reported mortality rates of approximately 20% for HAAs to 100% for more proximal aneurysms of the celiac artery in their experience. The most common etiology appears to be atherosclerosis and medial degeneration. Other etiologies include infection, trauma, connective tissue disorders, or vasculitis (Takayasu arteritis, polyarteritis nodosa, fibromuscular dysplasia, Behçet's disease).[45-47] Syphilitic aneurysms are now uncommon. CAAs can present with epigastric pain or upper gastrointestinal hemorrhage. Worsening abdominal pain usually indicates a rapidly expanding aneurysm or rupture. Dysphagia may occur from esophageal compression.[48]

Traditional surgical management of CAAs frequently requires supraceliac aortic clamping, and mortality exceeds 5%.[49] CAAs can be treated surgically with celiac ligation, followed by aortohepatic bypass or direct aortic reimplantation. In patients undergoing revascularization both prosthetic and saphenous vein grafts may be used for arterial reconstruction. If the aneurysm ruptures, intervention may include ligation or percutaneous transcatheter embolization.

More recently, percutaneous and endovascular techniques have offered patients other alternatives for treatment of CAAs and pseudoaneurysms. Reports of endotherapy of CAAs is limited to case reports. Carrafiello et al.[50] described a successful combined endovascular repair of a celiac trunk aneurysm using a celiac-splenic stent graft and hepatic artery embolization. Postoperative CT confirmed preservation of flow to the hepatic and splenic arteries with successful exclusion of the CAA.[50] Basile et al.[51] reported successful treatment of a CAA using a combined hepatic artery stent graft and splenic artery embolization. Although partial splenic infarction was noted during the perioperative period, the patient did not require splenectomy and recovered fully. Postoperative CT confirmed a patent hepatic artery without evidence of liver ischemia.[51]

SUPERIOR MESENTERIC ARTERY ANEURYSM

Superior mesenteric artery (SMA) aneurysms represent approximately 5% of all VAAs.[2] The most common etiology is infectious or mycotic. Other causes include trauma, dissection, atherosclerosis, polyarteritis nodosa, pancreatitis, and neurofibromatosis. Patients with symptomatic SMA aneurysms are seen with intermittent upper abdominal pain. Symptoms may be caused by both thrombosis and distal embolization. Open surgical intervention has been the mainstay of therapy for this type of aneurysm because of multiple side branches frequently encountered on the main SMA trunk. Traditional surgical options include resection with bypass versus ligation alone, if adequate collateralization is present.

Endovascular options include stent graft placement or stenting with coil embolization. Transcatheter embolization of SMA aneurysms has been reported in several case reports in selected patients.[52,53] However, this is generally limited to a few, select patients because there frequently is no good landing zone to achieve seal and multiple branch points involved. We reported a successful endovascular exclusion of a superior mesenteric pseudoaneurysm in a patient with multiple prior abdominal operations including open gastric bypass and partial nephrectomy for renal cell cancer.[54] We deployed a Gore Viabahn covered stent (W. L. Gore & Associates, Flagstaff, AZ) across the length of the SMA pseudoaneurysm, which resulted in complete exclusion with preservation of distal mesenteric perfusion without endoleak. The patient has remained asymptomatic 4 years after her procedure (Figure 49-3).

GASTRODUODENAL/ PANCREATICODUODENAL ARTERY ANEURYSMS

True aneurysms of the GDA and pancreaticoduodenal artery (PDA) are often degenerative whereas pseudoaneurysms are often complications from acute and chronic pancreatitis. Many present with significant symptoms including intraperitoneal or retroperitoneal

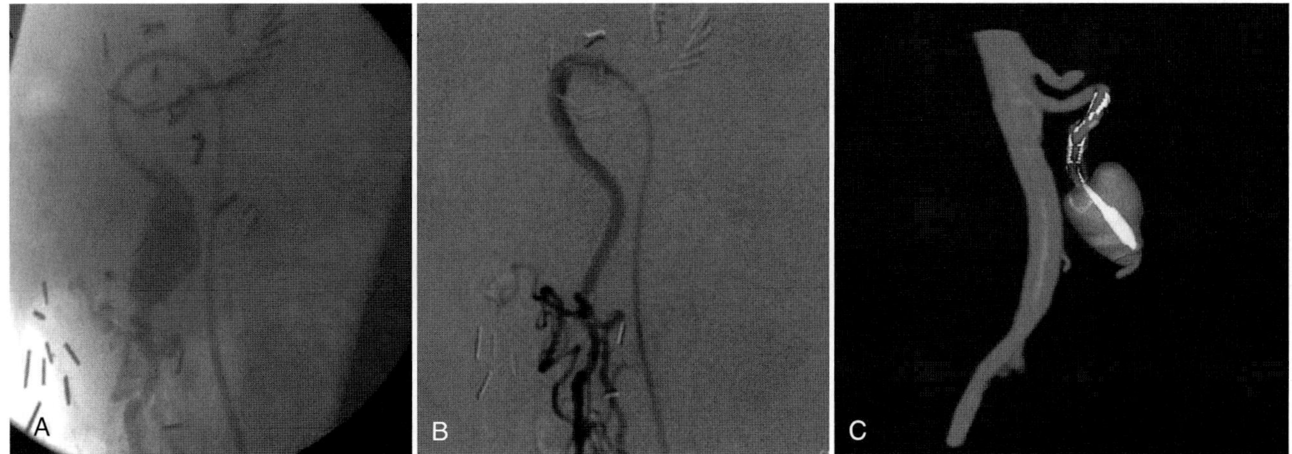

FIGURE 49-3 **A,** Angiogram demonstrating a large pseudoaneurysm of the SMA. Note the presence of surgical clips from multiple prior laparotomies. **B,** Completion angiogram after complete exclusion of SMA aneurysm with covered stent graft. **C,** Three-dimensional reconstruction demonstrates direct flow through the covered stent with excluded SMA aneurysm sac.

bleeding. Coil embolization is the endovascular treatment of choice for these aneurysms because of the presence of extensive end-organ collaterals.[21]

When treating aneurysms in the pancreaticoduodenal distribution, a thorough search for collateral supply to these aneurysms is essential. Endovascular approaches to aneurysms of the GDA and/or PDA should be considered first-line treatment whenever possible because surgical exposure can prove difficult in this anatomic region. Descriptions in the surgical literature are limited to case reports. Kueper et al.[55] reported excellent results after coil embolization of a ruptured GDA aneurysm. Endovascular coiling of both the GDA and PDA were performed, and active bleeding was stopped. The patient was remained asymptomatic in the postoperative period and was released 18 days later.

RENAL ARTERY ANEURYSMS

Renal artery aneurysms (RAAs) are the third most common visceral aneurysm with a reported incidence from 0.6% to 1% in angiography studies.[56,57] Most are asymptomatic. The most common cause is typically fibromuscular dysplasia. Other etiologies include degenerative disorders, trauma, and vasculitis. Treatment is generally recommended for any RAA greater than 2 cm. However, other patient and anatomic factors should also be considered including age of the patient, comorbidities, gender, and combined renal-vascular hypertension. Females tend to have a higher rupture risk, especially if pregnant. The mortality for rupture in pregnancy is reported to be 60% to 80%.[58-60]

Treatment is traditionally open surgery with aneurysm resection, ligation, and surgical bypass. Resection with patch angioplasty may be used in the presence of saccular aneurysms of the renal artery.[61] If branches are involved, explantation with repair and subsequent reimplantation is sometimes necessary.[62] Occasionally, nephrectomy may even be required.[54]

Endovascular approaches have been reported; however, they are limited by the renal artery anatomy and end-organ limitations of renal perfusion. Patients with main RAAs can potentially be treated with covered stent graft placement if an adequate landing zone to allow seal is present.[63-66] This method provides exclusion of the aneurysm while maintaining renal perfusion. As stent graft size, flexibility, and design methods improve, this treatment modality may increase in frequency.

If the aneurysm is saccular and has a narrow neck, packing the aneurysm sac with coils to cause thrombosis of the sac but maintain patency of the renal artery is another treatment option. Superselective embolization is possible with new advances in microcatheter technology and embolization methods. The use of platinum detachable coils, glue, and innovative techniques, such as balloon remodeling to prevent the migration of coils, has also been proposed.[67] Injection of other materials to induce aneurysm thrombosis including aneurysm sac injection of thrombin and ethylene-vinyl alcohol has been described.[68,69]

INFERIOR MESENTERIC ARTERY ANEURYSM

Aneurysms of the inferior mesenteric artery (IMA) are very rare, representing about 0.5% of all VAAs. Etiologies include mycotic, Takayasu's disease, iatrogenic pseudoaneurysm, and polyarteritis nodosa.[70] Case reviews have reported the presence of IMA aneurysms associated with occlusion of both the celiac artery and

SMA.[71,72] This particular etiology is believed to be caused by increased flow through the IMA in the presence of mesenteric occlusive disease. Surgical treatment of IMA aneurysm includes resection, ligation with exclusion, resection and reimplantation into the aorta, hypogastric artery, or prosthesis, and resection with bypass reconstruction. Endovascular coiling and laparoscopic and robotic clipping of the IMA have all been described, particularly for treatment of endoleak after endovascular aortic aneurysm repair.[73-75] However, endovascular therapy for treatment of an IMA aneurysm has not been described.

CONCLUSION

Although VAAs are relatively rare, they can be rapidly fatal if acute rupture occurs. The mainstay of treatment has been open laparotomy before the advent of endovascular techniques. Endovascular treatment of VAAs can be performed with a variety of techniques with excellent outcomes and minimal patient morbidity. There are limited prospective data, and most of the current treatment recommendations are based on case reports and data from small single-center series. Rapidly improving endovascular technology will continue to facilitate the efficacy and outcomes of these minimally invasive techniques.

References

1. Stanley JC, Thompson NW, Fry WJ: Splanchnic artery aneurysms, *Arch Surg* 101(6):689–697, 1970.
2. Berceli SA: Hepatic and splenic artery aneurysms, *Semin Vasc Surg* 18(4):196–201, 2005.
3. Salam TA, Lumsden AB, Martin LG, et al: Nonoperative management of visceral aneurysms and pseudoaneurysms, *Am J Surg* 164:215–219, 1992.
4. Wagner WH, Allins AD, Treiman RL, et al: Ruptured visceral artery aneurysms, *Ann. Vasc. Surg* 11:342–347, 1997.
5. Hossain A, et al: Visceral artery aneurysms: experience in a tertiary-care center, *Am Surg* 67(5):432–437, 2001.
6. Tulsyan N, et al: The endovascular management of visceral artery aneurysms and pseudoaneurysms, *J Vasc Surg* 45(2):276–283, discussion 283, 2007.
7. Stanley JC, Fry WJ: Pathogenesis and clinical significance of splenic artery aneurysms, *Surgery* 76:898–909, 1974.
8. Trastek VF, Pairolero PC, Joyce JW, et al: Splenic artery aneurysms, *Surgery* 76:898–909, 1974.
9. Lagana Domenico, Gianpaolo, et al: Multimodal approach to endovascular treatment of visceral artery aneurysms and Pseudoaneurysms, *Eur J Radiol* 59:104–111, 2006.
10. Sessa C, Tinella G, Porcu P, et al: Treatment of visceral artery aneurysm: description of a retrospective series of 42 aneurysm in 34 patients, *Ann Vasc Surg* 18:695–703, 2004.
11. Carr SC, Mahvri DM, Hoch JR, et al: Visceral artery aneurysm rupture, *J Vasc Surg* 33:806–811, 2001.
12. Eskandari MK, Resnick SA: Aneurysms of the renal artery, *Semin Vasc Surg* 18:202–208, 2005.
13. Carr SC, Pearce WH, Vogelzang RL, et al: Current management of visceral artery aneurysms, *Surgery* 120:627–633, 1996.
14. Parildar M, Oran I, Memis A: Embolization of visceral pseudoaneurysms with platinum coils and N-butyl cyanoacrylate, *Abdom Imaging* 28(1):36–40, 2003.
15. Guillon R, et al: Management of splenic artery aneurysms and false aneurysms with endovascular treatment in 12 patients, *Cardiovasc Intervent Radiol* 26(3):256–260, 2003.
16. Roland J, Brody F, Venbrux A: Endovascular management of a splenic artery aneurysm, *Surg Laparosc Endosc Percutan Tech* 17(5):459–461, 2007.
17. Trastek VF, et al: Splenic artery aneurysms, *Surgery* 91(6): 694–699, 1982.
18. Pasha SF, Gloviczki P, Stanson AW, et al: Splanchnic Artery Aneurysms, *Mayo Clin Proc* 82(4):472–479, April 2007.
19. McDermott VG, Shlansky-Goldberg R, Cope C: Endovascular management of splenic artery aneurysm and pseudoaneurysms, *Cardiovasc Intervent Radiol* 17:179–184, 1994.
20. Arepally A, Dagli M, Hofmann LV, et al: Treatment of splenic artery aneurysm with use of a stent-graft, *J Vasc Interv Radiol* 13:631–633, 2002.
21. Nosher JL, et al: Visceral and renal artery aneurysms: a pictorial essay on endovascular therapy, *Radiographics* 26(6):1687–1704, 2006.
22. Kasirajan K, Greenberg RK, Clair D, et al: Endovascular management of visceral artery aneurysms, *J Endovasc Ther* 8: 150–155, 2001.
23. Gabelmann A, Gorich J, Merkle EM: Endovascular treatment of visceral artery aneurysms, *J Endovasc Ther* 9:38–47, 2002.
24. Reidy JF, Rowe PH, Ellis FG: Splenic artery aneurysm embolisation: the preferred technique to surgery, *Clin Radiol* 41:281–282, 1990.
25. Carr JA, Cho JS, Shepard AD, et al: Visceral pseudoaneurysms due to pancreatic pseudocysts: rare but lethal complications of pancreatitis, *J Vasc Surg* 32:722–730, 2000.
26. Mandel SR, Jaues PF, Sanofsky S, et al: Nonoperative management of peripancreatic arterial aneurysms: a 10-year experience, *Ann Surg* 205:126–128, 1987.
27. Kemmeter P, Bonnell B, VanderKolk W, et al: Percutaneous thrombin injection of splanchnic artery aneurysms: two case reports, *J Vasc Interv Radiol* 11:469–472, 2000.
28. Puri S, Nicholson AA, Breen DJ: Percutaneous thrombin injection for the treatment of a post-pancreatitis pseudoaneurysm, *Eur Radiol* 13:79–82, 2003.
29. Parildar M, Oran I, Memis A: Embolization of visceral pseudoaneurysms with platinum coils and N-butyl cyanoacrylate, *Abdom Imaging* 28(1):36–40, 2003.
30. Brountzon EN, Vagenas K, Apostolopoulou SC, et al: Pancreatitis-associated splenic artery pseudoaneurysm: endovascular treatment with self-expandable stent-graft, *Cardiovasc Intervent Radiol* 26:88–91, 2003.
31. Rossi M, et al: Endovascular exclusion of visceral artery aneurysms with stent-grafts: technique and long-term follow-up, *Cardiovasc Intervent Radiol* 31(1):36–42, 2008.
32. Guller J, et al: Repair of a splenic artery aneurysm using a novel balloon-expandable covered stent, *Vasc Med* 11(2):111–113, 2006.
33. Karaman K, et al: Endovascular stent graft treatment in a patient with splenic artery aneurysm, *Diagn Interv Radiol* 11(2):119–121, 2005.
34. Larson RA, Solomon J, Carpenter JP: Stent graft repair of visceral artery aneurysms, *J Vasc Surg* 36(6):1260–1263, 2002.
35. Abbas MA, Fowl RJ, Stone WM, et al: Hepatic artery aneurysm: factors that predict complications, *J Vasc Surg* 38:41–45, 2003.
36. Shanley CJ, Shah NL, Messin LM: Common splanchnic artery aneurysms: splenic, hepatic, and celiac, *Ann Vasc Surg* 10:315–322, 1996.

37. Kibbler CC, Cohen DL, Cruicshank JK, et al: Use of CAT scanning in the diagnosis and management of hepatic artery aneurysm, *Gut* 26:752–756, 1985.
38. O'Driscoll D, Olliff SP, Oliff JF: Hepatic artery aneurysm, *Br J Radiol* 72:1018–1025, 1999.
39. Carroccio A, et al: Endovascular treatment of visceral artery aneurysms, *Vasc Endovascular Surg* 41(5):373–382, 2007.
40. Ginat DT, Saad WE, Waldman DL, et al: Stent-graft placement for management of iatrogenic hepatic artery branch pseudoaneurysm after liver transplantation, *Vasc Endovasc Surg* 43:513–517, 2009.
41. Won YD, Ku YM, Kim KH, et al: Successful management of a ruptured hepatic artery pseudoaneurysm with a stent-graft, *Emerg Radiol* 16:247–249, 2009.
42. Narumi S, Hakamda K, Toyoki Y, Noda H, et al: Endovascular treatment of a life-threatening pseudoaneurysm of the hepatic artery after pancreaticoduodenectomy, *Hepatogastroenterology* 54:2152–2154, 2007.
43. Veraldi GF, Dorrucci V, de Manzoni G, et al: Aneurysm of the celiac trunk: diagnosis with US-color-Doppler: presentation of a new case and review of the literature, *Hepatogastroenterology* 46:781–783, 1999.
44. Vohra R, Carr HMH, Welch M, et al: Management of celiac artery aneurysms, *Br J Surg* 78:1373, 1991.
45. Lukes P, Wihed A, et al: Angiography of visceral aneurysms, *Eur Radiol* 4:75–79, 1994.
46. Basaranoglu G, Basaranglu M: Behçet's disease complicated with celiac trunk aneurysm, *J Clin Gastroenterol* 3:174–175, 2001.
47. Parfitt J, Chalmers RTA, Wolfe JHN: Visceral aneurysms in Ehlers-Danlos syndrome: case report and review of literature, *J Vasc Surg* 31:1248–1251, 2000.
48. Saliou C, Kassab M, Duteille F: Aneurysm of the celiac artery, *Cardiovasc Surg* 4:552–555, 1996.
49. Messina LM, Shanley CJ: Visceral artery aneurysms, *Surg Clin North Am* 77:425–441, 1997.
50. Carrafiello G, Rivolta N, Fontana F, et al: Combined endovascular repair of a celiac trunk aneurysm using celiac-splenic stent graft and hepatic artery embolization, *Cardiovasc Intervent Radiol* 33(2): 352–354, 2010.
51. Basile A, Lupattelli T, Magnano M, et al: Treatment of a celiac trunk aneurysm close to the hepato-splenic bifurcation by using hepatic stent-graft implantation and splenic artery embolization, *Cardiovasc Intervent Radiol* 30:126–128, 2007.
52. Stone WM, Abbas M, Chry KJ, et al. Superior mesenteric artery aneurysms: is presence an indication for intervention? *J Vasc Surg* 19, Number 2, 234–237, 2002.
53. Stambo GW, Hallise MJ, Gallagher JJ: Arteriographic embolization of visceral artery pseudoaneurysms, *Ann Vasc Surg* 10:476–480, 1996.
54. Jimenez JC, Lawrence PF, Reil TD: Endovascular exclusion of superior mesenteric pseudoaneurysms: an alternative to laparotomy in high risk patients, *Vasc Endovasc Surg* 42:184–186, 2008.
55. Kueper MA, Ludescher B, Koenigsrainer I, et al: Successful coil embolization of a ruptured gastroduodenal artery aneurysm, *Vasc Endovasc Surg* 41:568–571, 2008.
56. Tham G, et al: Renal artery aneurysms. Natural history and prognosis, *Ann Surg* 197(3):348–352, 1983.
57. Stanley JC, et al: Renal artery aneurysms: significance of macroaneurysms exclusive of dissections and fibrodysplastic mural dilations, *Arch Surg* 110(11):1327–1333, 1975.
58. Yang JC, Hye RJ: Ruptured renal artery aneurysm during pregnancy, *Ann Vasc Surg* 10(4):370–372, 1996.
59. Rijbroek A, van Dijk HA, Roex AJ: Rupture of renal artery aneurysm during pregnancy, *Eur J Vasc Surg* 8(3):375–376, 1994.
60. Cohen JR, Shamash FS: Ruptured renal artery aneurysms during pregnancy, *J Vasc Surg* 6(1):51–59, 1987.
61. Chandra A, O'Connell JB, Quinones-Baldrich WJ, et al: Aneurysmectomy with arterial reconstruction of renal artery aneurysms in the endovascular era: a safe, effective treatement for both aneurysm and associated hypertension, *Ann Vasc Surg* May 24(4):503–510, 2010.
62. Pfeiffer T, et al: Reconstruction for renal artery aneurysm: operative techniques and long-term results, *J Vasc Surg* 37(2):293–300, 2003.
63. Sahin S, et al: Wide-necked renal artery aneurysm: endovascular treatment with stent-graft, *Diagn Interv Radiol* 13(1):42–45, 2007.
64. Malacrida G, et al: Endovascular treatment of a renal artery branch aneurysm, *Cardiovasc Intervent Radiol* 30(1):118–120, 2007.
65. Klonaris C, et al: Renal artery aneurysm endovascular repair, *Int Angiol* 26(2):189–192, 2007.
66. Gutta R, et al: Endovascular embolization of a giant renal artery aneurysm with preservation of renal parenchyma, *Angiology* 59 (2):240–243, 2008.
67. Mounayer C, et al: Balloon-assisted coil embolization for large-necked renal artery aneurysms, *Cardiovasc Intervent Radiol* 23 (3):228–230, 2000.
68. Corso R, et al: Pseudoaneurysm after spontaneous rupture of renal angiomyolipoma in tuberous sclerosis: successful treatment with percutaneous thrombin injection, *Cardiovasc Intervent Radiol* 28(2):262–264, 2005.
69. Bratby MJ, et al: Endovascular embolization of visceral artery aneurysms with ethylene-vinyl alcohol (Onyx): a case series, *Cardiovasc Intervent Radiol* 29(6):1125–1128, 2006.
70. Huang YK, Hsieh HC, Tsai FC, et al: Visceral artery aneurysm: risk factor analysis and therapeutic opinion, *Eur J Vasc Endovasc Surg* 33:293–301, 2007.
71. Mandeville KL, Bicknell C, Narula S, et al: Inferior mesenteric artery aneurysm with occlusion of the superior mesenteric artery, celiac trunk and right renal artery, *Eur J Vasc Endovasc Surg* 35:312–313, 2008.
72. Le Bas P, Batt M, Gagliardi JM, et al: Aneurysm of the inferior mesenteric artery associated with occlusion of the celiac axis and superior mesenteric artery, *Ann Vasc Surg* 1:254–257, 1986.
73. Lin JC, Eun D, Shrivastava A, et al: Total robotic ligation of inferior mesenteric artery for type II endoleak after endovascular aneurysm repair, *Ann Vasc Surg* 23(255e):19–21, 2009.
74. Conrad MF, Adams AB, Guest JM, et al: Secondary intervention after endovascular abdominal aortic aneurysm repair, *Ann Surg* 250(3):383–389, 2009.
75. Zhou W, Lumsden AB, Li J: IMA clipping for a type II endoleak: combined laparoscopic and endovascular approach, *Surg Laparosc Endosc Percutan Tech* 16:272–275, 2006.

CHAPTER

50

Endovascular Management of Popliteal Aneurysms

Timothy K. Liem, Gregory J. Landry

Popliteal artery aneurysms are typically defined as a diameter increase of greater than 50%, compared with the adjacent normal artery. Although popliteal aneurysms comprise about 80% of all peripheral aneurysms, their prevalence is fairly low, occurring in only 0.01% of all hospitalized patients.[1] However, they are associated with a significant incidence of ischemic complications caused by aneurysm thrombosis, distal thromboembolism, and, less commonly, aneurysm rupture.

Open surgical repair has been the mainstay of treatment for popliteal aneurysms, using either a medial or posterior approach. However, experience with endovascular stent graft repair is expanding. This chapter will review the anatomy and natural history of popliteal aneurysms, as well as indications for repair. The results of open surgery will be covered, because this is the benchmark by which endovascular therapy must be compared. Endovascular techniques, including catheter-directed thrombolysis and endovascular popliteal aneurysm repair, early results, and potential complications will be addressed.

ANATOMY, EPIDEMIOLOGY, AND NATURAL HISTORY

The normal popliteal artery originates at the adductor hiatus and typically ends at the inferior margin of the popliteus muscle, where it branches into the anterior tibial artery and tibioperoneal trunk. Smaller branches also arise from the popliteal artery, including the sural artery, and superior, middle, and inferior geniculate arteries. The diameter of the normal popliteal artery is not uniform throughout its length. The proximal and mid popliteal segments are typically larger than the distal popliteal artery, and these are the same segments that are more prone to aneurysmal degeneration.[2]

Popliteal artery aneurysms have a prevalence of about 1% in men between 65 and 80 years of age.[3] Men are far more commonly affected (95% to 99%), and the median age is 60 to 69 years. They occur much less commonly than aortic aneurysms, and patients with abdominal aortic aneurysms have a 1% to 2% prevalence of concomitant popliteal artery aneurysms. Conversely, patients with popliteal artery aneurysms have a greater than 40% chance of having an abdominal aortic aneurysm. Popliteal aneurysms are bilateral in more than 50% of cases.[4]

Patients may present with acute ischemia (approximately 20%), chronic ischemia (up to 40%), or symptoms caused by compression on adjacent structures (neurologic or venous, 4% to 10%), or they may have no symptoms (40% to 55%).[1,4-6] Aneurysm size and the presence of distortion and angulation correlate with the development of symptoms. Galland and Magee[7] found that the mean diameter of asymptomatic aneurysms was 2.0 cm, whereas the popliteal artery diameters in patients with acute ischemia and compression were 3.0 cm and 3.45 cm, respectively. Larger-diameter popliteal aneurysms also are more likely to contain intraluminal thrombus.[8]

In patients without symptoms, multiple case series document the natural history of conservatively treated popliteal aneurysms. Smaller aneurysms may develop ischemic complications in up to 8% of cases.[9] Dawson and colleagues[10] described the natural history of larger asymptomatic aneurysms (mean diameter 3.1 cm) that were followed for a mean of 6.2 years. The cumulative risk for development of ischemic complications was 24% at 1 year and 68% at 5 years. Using a Markov decision analysis, Michaels and Galland[11] had similar findings, estimating that asymptomatic popliteal aneurysms develop complications at a rate of 14% per year.

OPEN SURGICAL THERAPY: INDICATIONS AND RESULTS

Open surgical repair may be accomplished via a medial approach, performing a bypass with autogenous vein or prosthetic graft material. The popliteal aneurysm usually is ligated at both ends, excluding the aneurysm and preventing distal thromboembolism. Aneurysms localized within the popliteal fossa may be treated via a posterior approach with endoaneurysmorrhaphy and placement of a venous or prosthetic interposition graft.

Surgical repair of popliteal aneurysms should be performed in patients with ischemic or compressive symptoms. Regarding nonsymptomatic aneurysms, many surgeons recommend repair when the diameter reaches 2 cm or when intraluminal thrombus is present. Support for this comes from an earlier report that an aneurysm diameter of 2 cm, the presence of intraluminal thrombus, and poor runoff were risk factors for the development of complications in 67 popliteal aneurysms that were treated conservatively.[12] In addition, Galland and Magee[7] reported that larger aneurysm diameter correlated with the presence of ischemic or compressive symptoms. Otherwise, there are few other clinical data to support use of this particular threshold for repair.

Several large case series have shown that emergent popliteal aneurysm repair is an independent predictor of complications or the need for amputation.[4,13,14] Repair of nonsymptomatic popliteal aneurysms is associated with consistently higher rates of graft patency and limb salvage, when compared with symptomatic aneurysms, including those causing acute limb ischemia. Mahmood et al.[15] reported a 12-year experience, with an overall 5-year primary patency of 69%, secondary patency of 87%, and limb salvage rate of 87%. However, patients with no symptoms had a significantly higher secondary patency (100%) when compared with patients with symptoms (84%).[15] Shortell et al.[16] reported a 5-year patency and limb salvage of 92% and 100%, respectively, for asymptomatic aneurysms, compared with 39% and 84% for aneurysms causing limb-threatening ischemia. More recently, the Mayo Clinic reported similar findings with an overall 5-year primary and secondary patency of 76% and 87%, respectively, and a limb salvage rate of 97%. Again, the limb salvage rate was significantly higher in patients without symptoms (100%), when compared with patients with acute ischemia (85%).[4] These higher rates of patent grafts and limb salvage in patients without symptoms appear to support early surgical intervention, before the development of symptoms or acute ischemia.

Graft patency also may be influenced by other factors, including the choice of conduit, the quality of runoff, and the location of the distal target artery.[4,13] On average, venous conduit fares better than prosthetic graft material when repairing a popliteal aneurysm. However, this may only hold true for repairs performed via a medial approach. In a review of their experience with the posterior approach using prosthetic graft material, Beseth and Moore[17] reported a 96% secondary graft patency at 2 years and 100% limb salvage. The large experience reported by the Swedish Vascular Registry demonstrated that use of a venous conduit was associated with a significantly higher primary patency when a medial approach was performed. With the posterior approach, however, there was no significant advantage to venous conduit.[13]

The medial surgical approach, with bypass grafting and aneurysm ligation, may be complicated by continued aneurysm growth in up to 33% of patients.[13] Surgical repair of the expanding aneurysm was required only in about 2% to 5% of patients.[4,13] Reintervention commonly consists of endoaneurysmorrhaphy via a posterior approach.

CATHETER-DIRECTED THROMBOLYSIS

Catheter-directed thrombolysis is an important adjunctive therapy for patients with acute ischemia caused by popliteal aneurysm thrombosis or thromboembolism. It was in use at least a decade before the first popliteal artery stent grafts were described.[18] The primary indication for preoperative lysis is to recanalize a distal popliteal or tibial artery, in patients with acute limb ischemia and no visible target vessels. Preoperative thrombolysis may be performed via retrograde access of the contralateral common femoral, or antegrade access of the ipsilateral common femoral artery. Typically, a 5F multi—side-hole infusion catheter (with various infusion lengths) is advanced over a guidewire into the popliteal and/or tibial arteries. Tissue plasminogen activator is the most commonly used thrombolytic agent.

A recent report from the Swedish National Registry described 229 patients with popliteal aneurysms and acute limb ischemia.[19] Forty-two percent underwent preoperative thrombolysis with delayed surgery, and 58% underwent immediate surgery. In patients receiving thrombolysis, the median infusion time was 23.7 hours (range 0.5-75 hours). Lysis improved the runoff target vessel in 87%, and it was associated with decreased rates of amputation and fasciotomy. However, patients were selected for various treatments in a complex manner, and it is possible that patients who underwent immediate surgery had a more profound degree of ischemia. However, other large studies also report that preoperative thrombolysis is associated with improved patency rates and limb salvage, when compared with patients who undergo immediate surgery.[4,20]

Given the potentially large thrombus burden within the popliteal aneurysm and/or tibial runoff vessels, thrombolysis may be associated with worsening ischemia in a minority of patients. Galland et al.[21] reported that 13% of patients who underwent lysis of a popliteal aneurysm had deterioration, compared with 2% who had lysis of a nonaneurysmal artery or bypass graft. These authors prefer intraoperative thrombolysis, while other portions of the popliteal aneurysm repair are being performed. Although an appealing concept, the shorter infusion times may limit the degree of thrombus clearance.

ENDOVASCULAR REPAIR OF POPLITEAL ANEURYSMS

Stent graft insertion for the repair of a popliteal aneurysm was described in 1994, with use of a 6-mm polytetrafluoroethylene graft and two balloon-expandable stents.[22] Since then, numerous case reports, case series, and one small prospective randomized trial using commercially available stent grafts have been published.[23-30] Older series used a variety of stent graft designs including Wallstents (Boston Scientific, Natick, MA), Cragg EndoPro grafts (Mintec, Freeport, Bahamas), Corvita grafts (Schneider, Bülach, Switzerland), Passager grafts (Boston Scientific), and Hemobahn grafts (W. L. Gore & Associates, Inc., Scottsdale, Flagstaff, AZ). The Viabahn endoprosthesis (W. L. Gore & Associates, Inc.) is perhaps the most commonly used stent graft for endoluminal repair of popliteal aneurysms (Figures 50-1 and 50-2). However, none of these grafts has received Food and Drug Administration approval for the repair of peripheral aneurysms.

The Viabahn endoprosthesis currently is approved for patients with symptomatic peripheral arterial disease, in superficial femoral artery lesions. It uses expanded polytetrafluoroethylene with an external self-expanding nitinol support. Lengths range from 2.5 to 15 cm, with diameters of 5 to 8 mm, and a 0.035-inch guidewire platform. Larger-diameter stent grafts ranging from 9 to 13 mm (indicated for tracheobronchial strictures) also are available with a 0.025-inch guidewire platform. The delivery systems range from 7F to 12F, depending on the stent graft diameter, with catheter lengths ranging from 75 to 120 cm.

Anatomic inclusion criteria for the placement of a popliteal stent graft have not been strictly established. Criteria and contraindications for endovascular repair have been suggested by Siauw et al.[31] These are listed in Box 50-1. The insertion site may include retrograde access of the contralateral common femoral artery with a crossover cannulation technique, or antegrade access of the ipsilateral common femoral or superficial femoral artery. The choice of access would depend, in part, on the length of the delivery catheter and the angulation of the aortic bifurcation. Mini cutdown incisions often are used for larger catheter and sheath sizes. Although some authors use a 20% to 25% oversizing compared with the native popliteal artery,[27] we and others prefer a more modest 10% to 15% oversizing to avoid longitudinal graft infolding.[23] Some centers use proximal and distal landing zones ranging from 1 to 1.5 cm in length, whereas other large centers use a 2- to 3-cm landing zone.[23,24,27] When possible, a single stent graft should be used to cross the entire aneurysm. If multiple stent grafts are required, however, a minimum of 2- to 3-cm overlap is critical to avoid dislodging the grafts in an area that is subject to significant repetitive stress-strain cycles.

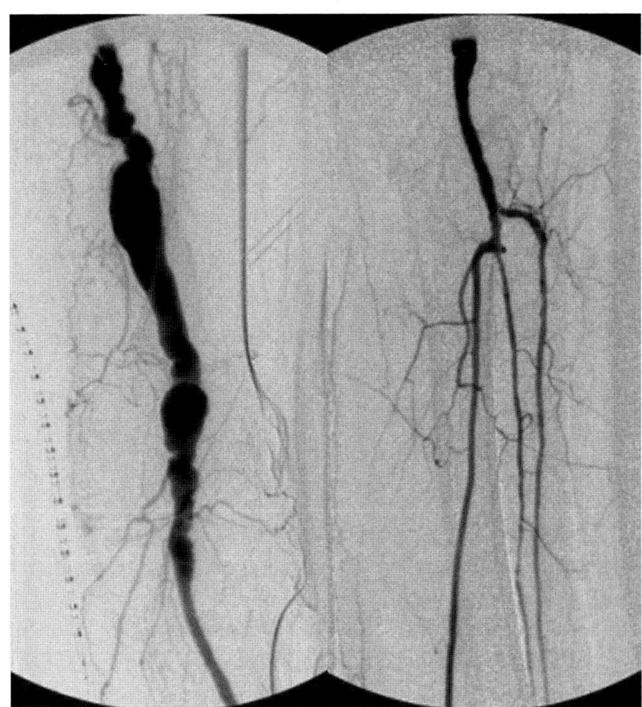

FIGURE 50-1 Popliteal aneurysm before stent graft deployment. This patient had concomitant bilateral common femoral aneurysms (>6 cm) and a large aortoiliac aneurysm.

The results of endovascular popliteal aneurysm repair have varied widely, with 12-month primary patency rates ranging from 47% to 93%, and reintervention rates as high as 26%. In part, this may be due to differences in stent graft design and advances in technique and postprocedure management. Earlier reports were smaller and described the use of multiple stent

BOX 50-1

CURRENT CRITERIA AND CONTRAINDICATIONS FOR ENDOVASCULAR POPLITEAL ANEURYSM REPAIR

Current Criteria for Endovascular Popliteal Aneurysm Repair

1. Popliteal aneurysm that is symptomatic or 2 cm diameter or contains intraluminal thrombus
2. Suitable proximal and distal landing zones
3. At least two-vessel calf runoff

Contraindications to Endovascular Popliteal Aneurysm Repair

1. Extensive aneurysmal dilatation of the distal superficial femoral artery or aneurysmal disease distal to the origin of the anterior tibial artery
2. Excessive popliteal artery tortuosity
3. Large symptomatic aneurysms where simple exclusion may not immediately resolve vascular or nerve compression

Modified from Siauw R, Koh EH, Walker SR. Endovascular repair of popliteal artery aneurysms: techniques, current evidence and recent experience, ANZ J Surg *2006, 76:505–511, 2006.*

TABLE 50-1 Case Series and One Prospective Randomized Trial Describing Endovascular Stent Graft Repair of Popliteal Aneurysms

Author, year	Stent graft	No. of limbs treated	Primary patency (%)
Curi et al., 2007[23]	Viabahn	56	83 at 24 mo
Rajasinghe et al., 2007[24]	Viabahn	23	93 at 12 mo
Tielliu et al., 2007[33]	Hemobahn	73	77 at 36 mo
Mohan et al., 2006[26]	Hemobahn Viabahn Passager AneuRx Homemade device	35	74.5 at 36 mo
Antonello et al., 2005[27]	Hemobahn	15	86.7 at 12 mo
Gerasimidis et al., 2003[28]	Hemobahn Wallgraft Passager	9 total	47 at 12 mo
Howell et al., 2002[29]	Wallgraft	13	69 at 12 mo
Henry et al., 2000[30]	Cragg/Passager Corvita Expander Wallstent	14 total	74 at 12 mo

graft designs. Later studies tended to be larger and report the use of single devices (Table 50-1). Stent graft–related complications also were more common during the early experience at some institutions.[25]

Lovegrove et al.[32] performed a recent meta-analysis that compared endovascular and open management for nonthrombosed popliteal aneurysms. Only three studies, comprising 141 patients (37 endovascular, 104 open surgery), met the inclusion criteria. Endovascular repair was associated with an unexpectedly longer operative time, a shorter length of stay (−3.9 days), and a higher 30-day reintervention rate. However, the

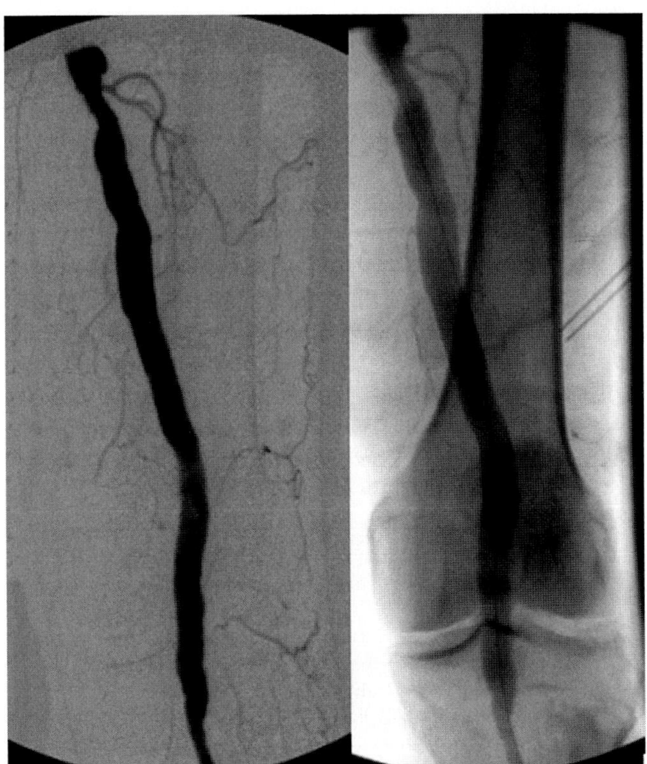

FIGURE 50-2 Popliteal aneurysm, status post placement of Gore Viabahn stent graft. This was performed simultaneous to open repair of the large common femoral aneurysms and endovascular repair of an aortoiliac aneurysm.

long-term graft patency was not significantly different between the two groups.

At present, the indications for endovascular management of a popliteal aneurysm include the primary or secondary prevention of limb ischemia caused by arterial thromboembolism or popliteal artery thrombosis. Until further data demonstrate otherwise, a threshold diameter of 2 cm, the presence of intraluminal thrombus, or a history of ischemic symptoms is a reasonable indication for endovascular treatment. Endovascular management is not likely to be effective in patients who present with a large aneurysm causing compressive symptoms. In this latter setting, placement of an endoprosthesis will not reliably decrease the size of the aneurysm or alleviate compression of an adjacent nerve or vein. Endoaneurysmorrhaphy is likely to be more effective.

POSTPROCEDURE MANAGEMENT

The postprocedure management of patients with popliteal artery stent grafts should include surveillance duplex scans to monitor stent graft patency and popliteal aneurysm diameter. Just as open surgical bypass grafting via a medial approach may be complicated by continued expansion of the ligated aneurysm sac, endovascular repair also is vulnerable to the development of type II endoleaks. The clinical significance of this finding has yet to be determined. It will likely have more significance in patients with larger preoperative aneurysm diameters. In addition, many authors use clopidogrel as an adjunctive antiplatelet agent during the postoperative period. One large study identified that postoperative clopidogrel (75 mg/day for 6 weeks) was the only significant predictor for graft patency.[33]

Other complications of endovascular popliteal aneurysm repair include stent graft occlusion, fracture, migration, kinking, and distal thromboembolism. Tielliu et al.[33] reported on 57 Hemobahn/Viabahn stent graft placements, 12 (21%) of which developed thrombosis at a mean of 8 months (range 1-28 months) after the procedure. Catheter-directed thrombolysis was able to recanalize five of seven stent grafts, but a slight majority went on to reocclude.[33] Fortunately, stent graft thrombosis was not associated with critical limb ischemia or lower-extremity amputation in any of the patients.

CONCLUSION

In summary, popliteal artery aneurysms are associated with a significant incidence of complications, including the development of acute or chronic limb ischemia. These aneurysms should be repaired if they are symptomatic. Reasonable indications for repair of nonsymptomatic aneurysms are diameter greater than 2 cm and the presence of intraluminal thrombus. Preoperative catheter-directed thrombolysis is effective at recanalizing the native popliteal or tibial arteries, and it may decrease the magnitude of subsequent surgical or endovascular procedures. Patients with acute ischemia and no visible distal popliteal or tibial arteries likely will derive the most benefit from preoperative lysis, assuming the ischemia is not too profound.

In carefully selected patients, endovascular popliteal aneurysm repair is a valid alternative to open surgery, especially in patients with significant comorbidities. Intermediate-term patency rates for endovascular popliteal aneurysm repair are approaching those for open surgical repair. However, the reintervention rates do seem to be higher. Patients should be monitored for stent graft thrombosis and continued expansion of the popliteal aneurysm.

References

1. Hamish M, Lockwood A, Cosgrove C, et al: Management of popliteal artery aneurysms, *ANZ J Surg* 76:912–915, 2006.

2. Wolf YG, Kobzantsev Z, Zelmanovich L: Size of normal and aneurysmal popliteal arteries: a duplex ultrasound study, *J Vasc Surg* 43:488–492, 2007.
3. Trickett JP, Scott RA, Tilney HS: Screening and management of asymptomatic popliteal aneurysms, *J Med Screen* 9:92–93, 2002.
4. Huang Y, Gloviczki P, Noel AA, et al: Early complications and long-term outcome after open surgical treatment of popliteal artery aneurysms: is exclusion with saphenous vein bypass still the gold standard? *J Vasc Surg* 45:706–715, 2007.
5. Gifford RW Jr, Hines EA Jr, Janes JM: An analysis and follow-up study of one hundred popliteal aneurysms, *Surgery* 33:284–293, 1953.
6. Whitehouse WM Jr, Wakefield TW, Graham LM, et al: Limb-threatening potential of arteriosclerotic popliteal artery aneurysms, *Surgery* 93:694–699, 1983.
7. Galland RB, Magee TR: Popliteal aneurysms: distortion and size related to symptoms, *Eur J Vasc Endovasc Surg* 30:534–538, 2005.
8. Varga ZA, Lock-Edmonds JC, Baird RN: A multicenter study of popliteal aneurysms: joint Vascular Research Group, *J Vasc Surg* 20:171–177, 1994.
9. Schellack J, Smith B III, Perdue GD: Nonoperative management of selected popliteal aneurysms, *Arch Surg* 122:372–375, 1987.
10. Dawson I, Sie R, van Baalen JM, et al: Asymptomatic popliteal aneurysm: elective operation versus conservative follow-up, *Br J Surg* 81:1504–1507, 1994.
11. Michaels JA, Galland RB: Management of asymptomatic popliteal aneurysms: the use of a Markov decision tree to determine the criteria for a conservative approach, *Eur J Vasc Surg* 7:136–143, 1993.
12. Lowell RC, Gloviczki P, Hallet JW, et al: Popliteal artery aneurysms: the risk of nonoperative management, *Ann Vasc Surg* 8:14–23, 1994.
13. Ravn H, Wanhainen A, Björck M, et al: Surgical technique and long-term results after popliteal artery aneurysm repair: results from 717 legs, *J Vasc Surg* 46:236–243, 2007.
14. Johnson ON III, Slidell MB, Macsata RA, et al: Outcomes of surgical management for popliteal artery aneurysms: an analysis of 583 cases, *J Vasc Surg* 48:845–851, 2008.
15. Mahmood A, Salaman R, Sintler M, et al: Surgery of popliteal artery aneurysms: a 12-year experience, *J Vasc Surg* 37:586–593, 2003.
16. Shortell CK, DeWeese JA, Ouriel K, et al: Popliteal artery aneurysms: a 25-year experience, *J Vasc Surg* 14:771–776, 1991.
17. Beseth BD, Moore WS: The posterior approach for repair of popliteal artery aneurysms, *J Vasc Surg* 43:940–944, 2006.
18. Taylor LM, Porter JM, Baur GM, et al: Intraarterial streptokinase infusion for acute popliteal and tibial artery occlusion, *Am J Surg* 147:583–588, 1984.
19. Ravn H, Björck M: Popliteal artery aneurysm with acute ischemia in 229 patients: outcome after thrombolytic and surgical therapy, *Eur J Vasc Endovasc Surg* 33:690–695, 2007.
20. Dorigo W, Pulli R, Turini F, et al: Acute leg ischaemia from thrombosed popliteal artery aneurysms: role of preoperative thrombolysis, *Eur J Vasc Endovasc Surg* 23:251–254, 2002.
21. Galland RB, Earnshaw JJ, Baird RN, et al: Acute limb deterioration during intra-arterial thrombolysis, *Br J Surg* 80:1118–1120, 1993.
22. Marin ML, Veith FJ, Panetta TF, et al: Transfemoral endoluminal stented graft repair of a popliteal artery aneurysm, *J Vasc Surg* 19:754–757, 1994.
23. Curi MA, Geraghty PJ, Merino OA, et al: Mid-term outcomes of endovascular popliteal artery aneurysm repair, *J Vasc Surg* 45:505–510, 2007.
24. Rajasinghe HA, Tzilinis A, Keller T, et al: Endovascular exclusion of popliteal artery aneurysms with expanded polytetrafluoroethylene stent-grafts: early results, *Vasc Endovasc Surg* 40:460–466, 2007.
25. Tielliu IF, Verhoeven EL, Zeebregts CJ, et al: Endovascular treatment of popliteal artery aneurysms: is the technique a valid alternative to open surgery? *J Cardiovasc Surg (Torino)* 48:275–279, 2007.
26. Mohan IV, Bray PJ, Harris JP, et al: Endovascular popliteal aneurysm repair: are the results comparable to open surgery? *Eur J Vasc Endovasc Surg* 32:149–154, 2006.
27. Antonello M, Frigatti P, Battocchio P, et al: Open repair versus endovascular treatment for asymptomatic popliteal artery aneurysm: results of a prospective randomized study, *J Vasc Surg* 42:185–193, 2005.
28. Gerasimidis T, Sfyroeras G, Papazoglou K, et al: Endovascular treatment of popliteal artery aneurysms, *Eur J Vasc Endovasc Surg* 26:506–511, 2003.
29. Howell M, Krajcer Z, Diethrich EB, et al: Wallgraft endoprosthesis for the percutaneous treatment of femoral and popliteal artery aneurysms, *J Endovasc Ther* 9:76–81, 2002.
30. Henry M, Amor M, Henry I, et al: Percutaneous endovascular treatment of peripheral aneurysms, *J Cardiovasc Surg (Torino)* 41:871–883, 2000.
31. Siauw R, Koh EH, Walker SR: Endovascular repair of popliteal artery aneurysms: techniques, current evidence and recent experience, *ANZ J Surg* 76:505–511, 2006.
32. Lovegrove RE, Javid M, Magoo TR, et al: Endovascular and open approaches to non-thrombosed popliteal aneurysm repair: a meta-analysis, *Eur J Vasc Endovasc Surg* 36:96–100, 2008.
33. Tielliu IFJ, Verhoeven ELG, Zeebregts CJ, et al: Endovascular treatment of popliteal artery aneurysms: results of a prospective cohort study, *J Vasc Surg* 41:561–566, 2005.

CHAPTER

51

Combined Endovascular and Surgical Approach to Thoracoabdominal Aortic Pathology

William J. Quinones-Baldrich

Surgical repair of thoracoabdominal aortic aneurysm (TAAA) is perhaps one of the most complex procedures performed by vascular surgeons. The results of surgical repair have improved over the years since the original description of the inclusion technique by Crawford et al.[1] The risk for paraplegia and other major complications has been reduced with the use of adjunctive techniques including spinal catheter drainage, left-sided heart bypass, and individual visceral catheter perfusion.[2-5] Additional techniques intended to reduce complications have been described including multigraft repair,[6] which avoids global visceral ischemia, and avoidance of division of the diaphragm.[7] However, patients presenting with thoracoabdominal aortic pathology requiring intervention frequently have significant comorbidities, which increase operative risk and contraindicate repair.

Endovascular repair of thoracoabdominal aortic pathology has emerged as an alternative to open surgical repair. The results to date have documented a low acceptable risk of paraplegia, with significant decrease in morbidity. The initial concern that extensive coverage of the descending thoracic and visceral aorta would lead to an increased risk for spinal cord injury has not materialized.[8] This has led to the recognition that spinal cord injury during TAAA repair is a multifactorial process. Global visceral ischemia, intraoperative hypotension, in addition to decreasing spinal cord perfusion by exclusion of important intercostal vessels, all play a role in this complication. Unfortunately, patients with thoracoabdominal aneurysms frequently do not have the appropriate anatomy for a purely endovascular approach. It is in these instances that a combined endovascular and surgical approach to TAAAs has emerged as an alternative for high-risk patients.

A combined endovascular and surgical approach to thoracoabdominal aortic pathology has potential benefits. It avoids a thoracotomy and supravisceral aortic cross-clamping and limits the ischemia time to the viscera to one organ at a time. Intraoperative hypotension is rare, thus further contributing to a decreased risk for spinal cord complications. Importantly, in specific situations, it allows for staging of the procedure, which may also decrease morbidity.

This chapter presents the evolution of a combined endovascular and surgical approach (hybrid) to thoracoabdominal aortic pathology including the aortic arch, descending thoracic aorta, and visceral aorta. An emphasis is placed on patient selection, technical considerations, preoperative planning, staging, and other important aspects particular to this combined approach. Results, as published in the literature to date, are presented.

HISTORY

The evolution of endovascular technology has given vascular surgeons new tools that reduce the magnitude of procedures and often allow intervention in higher-risk patients. An example has been the introduction of endovascular grafts for repair of infrarenal abdominal aortic aneurysms (AAAs). Similarly, endovascular thoracic grafts have decreased the morbidity associated with surgical repair of descending thoracic aneurysms, with similar or perhaps reduced risk of paraplegia. Combining surgical procedures using extra-anatomic reconstructions to create a landing zone for endovascular grafts has reduced the limitations presented by unfavorable anatomy for endovascular repair.

In 1998, we evaluated a patient who presented with a type IV thoracoabdominal aneurysm, bilateral renal artery aneurysms, celiac and superior mesenteric artery (SMA) aneurysms, and two prior infrarenal aortic repairs after aneurysm rupture (Figure 51-1). The first aneurysm rupture had occurred 1 year prior and was repaired by

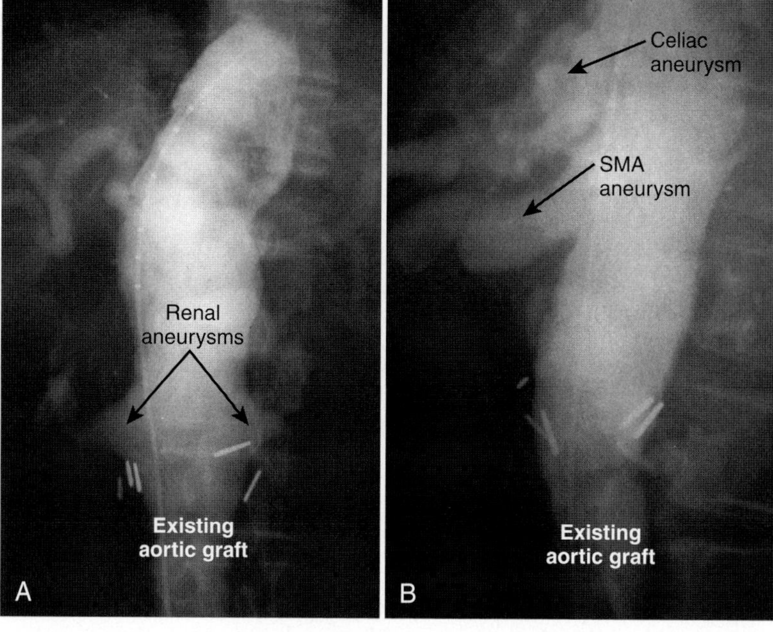

FIGURE 51-1 Anteroposterior **(A)** and lateral **(B)** aortogram in a patient presenting with a type IV thoracoabdominal aneurysm with bilateral renal artery aneurysms, SMA aneurysm, and celiac aneurysm. The patient had two prior infrarenal aortic replacements for aneurysm rupture.

using a transperitoneal approach and tube graft aortic replacement. The second rupture occurred several months later, distal to the prior tube graft, and was repaired by using a retroperitoneal approach with a bifurcated graft to both iliac arteries. Surgical repair of his type IV thoracoabdominal process would have required a redo retroperitoneal exposure and individual grafts to each one of the visceral vessels distal to their origin aneurysms. As an alternative, the patient was offered a combined endovascular and surgical approach, which would avoid some of the difficulties with the standard surgical procedure. After obtaining regulatory approval at our institution, this type IV thoracoabdominal aneurysm was repaired by using retrograde bypasses based on the right limb of the prior bifurcated graft to each one of the visceral vessels distal to their aneurysm with ligation proximal to the anastomosis. A Corvita endovascular graft (Corvita Corp, Miami, FL) was selected, because this was the only endovascular graft available of the size needed to exclude the aneurysmal portion of the distal descending and visceral aorta. Because this device was only available in a trial, special permission was obtained from the company. Dr. Thomas Panetta, the principal investigator in the Corvita trial, provided the endovascular grafts and assisted in the procedure. Access for placement of the endovascular graft was obtained through the right axillary artery and a conduit surgically placed at the right limb of the aortofemoral graft, distal to the takeoff of the retrograde bypasses. A Lunderquist guidewire (Cook Medical, Bloomington, IN) was passed through the right axillary artery and out the conduit. After deploying two endovascular grafts, completion angiography showed complete exclusion of the aneurysm and patency of the retrograde bypasses (Figure 51-2). The patient has done well clinically, and a computed tomographic (CT) scan 9 years later continued to show complete exclusion of the aneurysm and patency of his bypasses (Figure 51-3).

Since the original report of this case in 1999,[9] several reports of a combined endovascular and surgical repair of thoracoabdominal aortic pathology have been published. In an extensive review of the literature on the results of hybrid procedures for TAAA published in 2007, Donas et al.[10] found an overall early and long-term mortality for completed procedures of 15.5%. Reintervention rate for occluded graft occurred in 1 of 58 patients (1.6%). No paraplegia had been reported at the time of the review. The overall incidence of endoleak was 20.6% with 13.7% of patients requiring reintervention. They concluded that a hybrid approach for TAAAs showed promising midterm outcomes for high-risk patients.[10] They could not, however, conclude whether the technique was better than, worse than, or equivalent to open repair or medical treatment alone.

Patients chosen for the hybrid procedure tend to be at higher risk, with significant comorbidities. Patient selection bias will not allow direct comparisons with published reports on surgical repair of similar pathologies. In addition, follow-up is limited. Therefore no definitive conclusions can be made as to the role of the hybrid repair to thoracoabdominal aortic pathology. Experience to date suggests that a combined endovascular and surgical approach can be applied successfully in high-risk patients and that the risk of paraplegia may be lower.

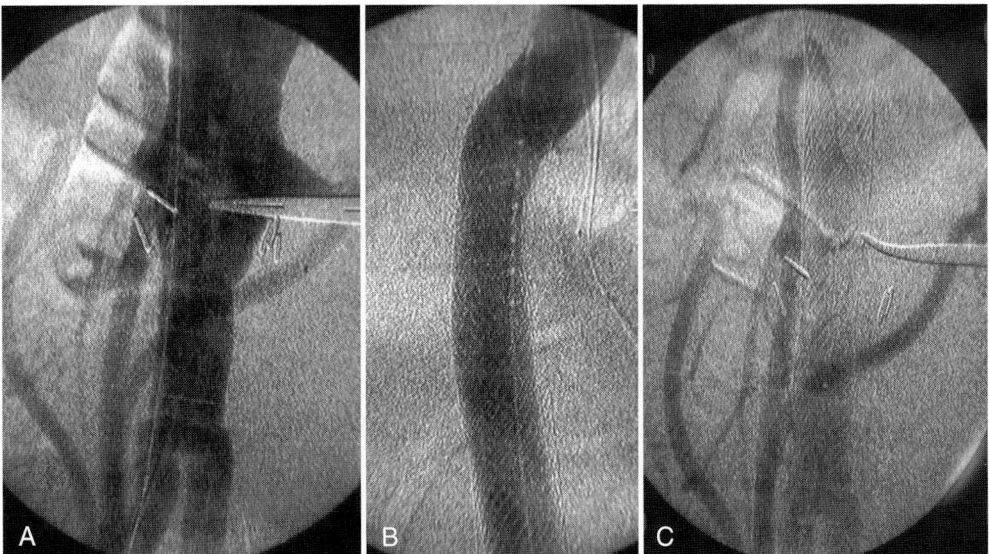

FIGURE 51-2 **A,** Intraoperative arteriogram after completion of retrograde bypasses to renal arteries, SMA, and celiac artery in the patient presented in Figure 51-1. **B,** Intraoperative aortogram after deployment of thoracic endograft to exclude type IV thoracoabdominal aneurysm. **C,** Intraoperative arteriogram showing patency of retrograde bypasses to visceral vessels.

Until the durability of this approach is better established, wider application cannot be recommended.

PATIENT SELECTION

Traditional indications for intervention in patients with thoracoabdominal aneurysms include size greater than 6 cm, growth of more than 0.5 cm/yr, aneurysm-related pain, and symptoms related to decreased perfusion of the viscera such as postprandial pain (chronic mesenteric ischemia), or renovascular hypertension. In patients with aortic dissection, these latter symptoms may be caused by malperfusion. Malperfusion may be related to a static obstruction of a visceral vessel or dynamic obstruction created by the dissection flap.

Patients in unstable condition with contained rupture or patients with free rupture are not candidates for a hybrid approach and are best treated with prompt surgical repair. Patients who present with aneurysm-related pain often have hypertension. Control of hypertension may relieve the pain, in which case, in the absence of other indications, continued observation is an option. If the hypertension is difficult to control, a renovascular process should be suspected. Management of this particular presentation will largely depend on whether a less-invasive alternative to improve control of the hypertension is possible without the need to completely repair the aneurysm. On the other hand, caution should be exercised with renal angioplasty in the presence of aneurysmal dilation of the visceral aorta, which can increase the risk of arterial tear or rupture.

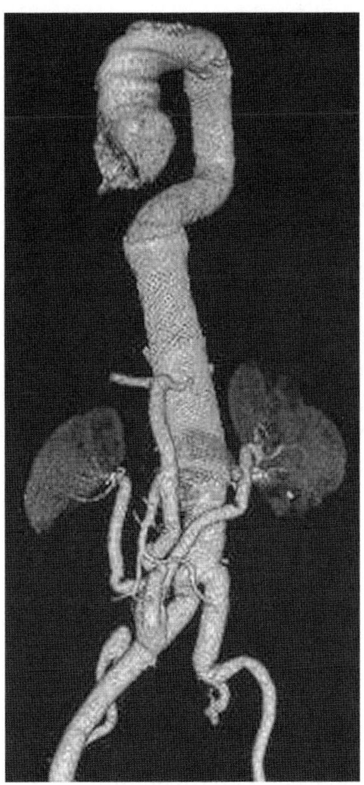

FIGURE 51-3 Three-dimensional reconstruction of CT scan 9 years after a combined endovascular and surgical repair of a type IV thoracoabdominal aneurysm in the patient presented in Figures 51-1 and 51-2.

The decision to proceed with a combined endovascular and surgical approach is largely based on patients' comorbidities, overall surgical risk, anatomy of the process, and prior surgical intervention. Patients with history of a left thoracotomy, particularly if they had left-sided heart bypass for prior surgical repair, are particularly challenging for any type of redo surgical intervention. Similarly, patients with prior TAAA repair who present with a patch aneurysm should be considered for a hybrid approach. Patients with prior infrarenal AAA repair may be considered candidates for a hybrid procedure mostly based on their comorbidities. Prior infrarenal AAA repair in a good-risk patient does not necessarily increase the risk of surgical intervention because the prior graft can be used for the distal anastomosis. On the other hand, the existing infrarenal graft is also an excellent source of inflow for retrograde bypasses and offers a landing zone for the thoracoabdominal endovascular graft. Clearly, an appropriate proximal landing zone must be present or created in the distal aortic arch.

Patients presenting with TAAA frequently have significant chronic obstructive pulmonary disease. This is a major risk factor for surgical intervention often requiring prolonged respiratory support. Avoidance of a thoracotomy in the hybrid approach may offer a reasonable alternative to surgical repair in these patients. Decreased cardiac function and/or aortic insufficiency significantly increases the risk in surgical repair with the need for high aortic cross-clamping. In these patients, a hybrid approach may be better tolerated. Patients with significant renal insufficiency may be better approached with a hybrid procedure because ischemia to the renal parenchyma is reduced compared with standard surgical intervention. These remain potential advantages, because the experience to date is limited.

One of the more difficult decisions in recommending intervention for TAAAs, whether surgical or hybrid approach, revolves around life expectancy. The presence of a malignancy, significant cardiac dysfunction, and preoperative level of activity should all be considered. Recent analysis on outcomes has shown a significant 1-year mortality for patients having repair of thoracoabdominal aneurysm.[11] Therefore the clinician must consider these factors on an individual basis.

PREOPERATIVE EVALUATION AND PREPARATION

One of the key elements in planning a combined endovascular and surgical approach to thoracoabdominal aortic pathology is appropriate imaging. Proximal and distal landing zones for the endovascular graft must be either present or created during the procedure. CT angiography with thin cuts and three-dimensional reconstruction is the study of choice. This should provide accurate information regarding the proximal landing zone, the length of the endovascular reconstruction, and patency of the visceral vessels. It will also assist in determining the best inflow source for the retrograde bypasses.

If the proximal landing zone requires coverage of the left subclavian artery (LSA), assessment of the vertebral circulation is critical. We will routinely obtain a duplex scan with particular attention to the vertebral circulation to determine whether the patient requires revascularization of the LSA as part of the procedure. If both vertebral arteries are of adequate size, coverage of the LSA without revascularization is preferred. Alternatively, if the left vertebral artery is dominant, a preparatory left carotid subclavian bypass should be performed. On occasion, the patient may have symptoms after coverage of the LSA. This can be treated on a semielective basis with either a left carotid–to-subclavian bypass or transposition. In these cases, ligation of the subclavian artery proximal to the vertebral artery takeoff is recommended.

Given the extensive coverage that is often required, and/or the presence of previous aortic surgery, spinal catheter drainage during the endovascular portion of the procedure is recommended. We routinely use spinal catheter drainage and prefer to place the catheter the night before the intervention. This will avoid having to postpone the surgery if bloody drainage is initially obtained. If this were to occur the night before surgery, allowing the catheter to drain overnight might permit proceeding with the intervention if the drainage clears.

In the presence of aortic dissection, the proximal landing zone for the endovascular graft must be in the true lumen. This will ensure adequate inflow and closure of the fenestrations by the endovascular graft. Intravascular ultrasound can provide the necessary information to ensure placement of the endovascular graft in the true lumen. We prefer transesophageal echocardiography, because it will allow real-time visualization of the true and false lumen without the need for catheter exchanges (Figure 51-4). An experienced anesthesiologist in transesophageal echocardiography can be extremely helpful in the performance and interpretation of the study. In some cases, when patients have had an interposition graft as the initial treatment for their dissection in the proximal descending thoracic aorta, and the distal end of the endovascular graft will be in either a normal nondissected segment of the aorta or a surgically placed infrarenal graft, the false lumen can be used for placement of the endovascular graft because it is often the larger of the two lumens and thus will allow complete expansion of the endovascular graft (Figure 51-5).

Mechanical bowel preparation is performed routinely. The presence of stool in the colon cannot only interfere with fluoroscopic visualization particularly in obese patients but will also increase the risk of bacterial translocation during ischemia of the bowel. The patient should receive a clear liquid diet 24 hours before the

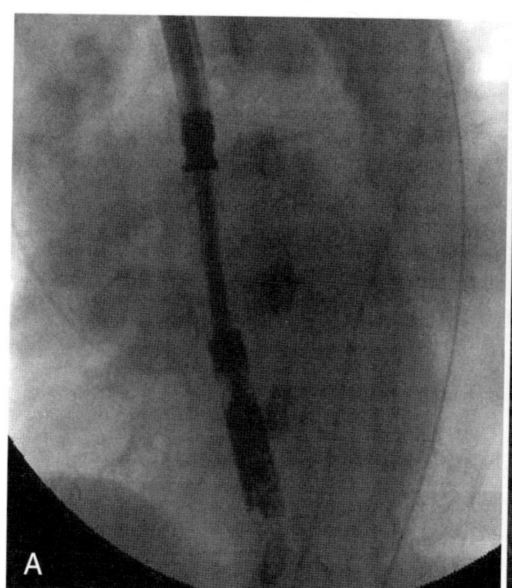

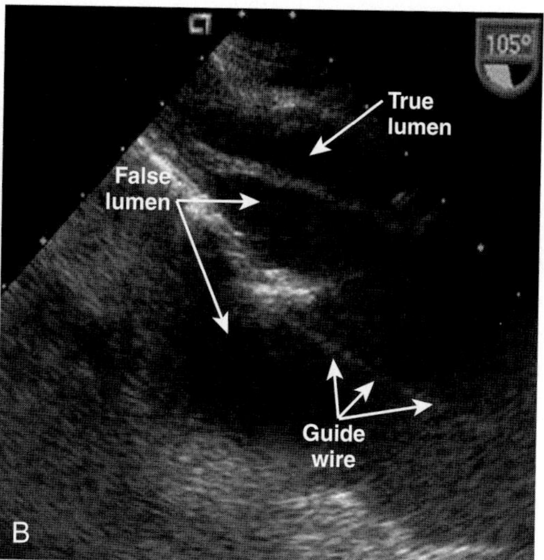

FIGURE 51-4 Intraoperative transesophageal echocardiography used during deployment of endovascular graft in a patient with TAAA with dissection. Identification of the guidewire in the true or false lumen can be determined so that deployment of the endovascular graft can be performed safely.

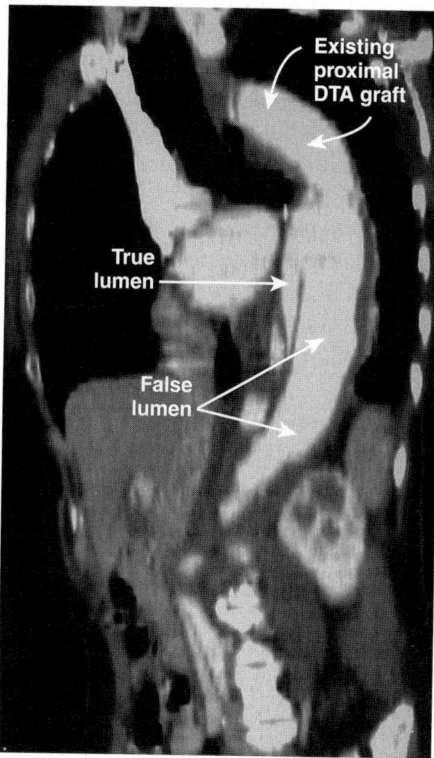

FIGURE 51-5 Preoperative CT scan reconstruction of a patient with aortic dissection who had undergone a previous interposition graft replacement in the proximal descending thoracic aorta *(DTA)*. The endovascular graft was purposely deployed from the interposition graft through the false lumen down to an infrarenal aortic graft to allow complete expansion of the endovascular graft.

procedure and a mechanical bowel cleansing, which can be done with either GoLYTELY (Braintree Laboratories, Braintree, MA) in the hospital or laxatives and an enema as an outpatient. Oral antibiotics are not recommended, whereas prophylactic intravenous antibiotics administered 1 hour before the procedure are routine.

SINGLE- VERSUS TWO-STAGE PROCEDURE

One major controversy related to hybrid procedures for thoracoabdominal aortic pathology remains the single- versus the two-stage approach. In the single-stage approach, both the surgical portion and the endovascular procedure are completed as a single intervention. This has the advantage of a single anesthetic for the patient and reduction or elimination of the potential for rupture of the aneurysm and thus would be clearly the preferred method in patients with symptoms. On the other hand, these are long operative interventions usually taking 6 to 9 hours and often require extensive coverage of the thoracoabdominal aorta. The arguments for staging the procedure include allowing the patient to recover from the more prolonged intervention (surgical portion) and thus performing the endovascular portion with less risk of hypotension (from the prolonged surgical procedure) and allowing the circulatory system to stabilize to the new flow pattern.

Another argument expressed for the single-stage approach relates to access for introduction of the endovascular graft. Clearly, at the time of the surgical procedure, access can be accomplished with placement of a conduit. In patients with small iliac arteries in whom access through the femoral artery is not advisable, placement of a subcutaneous conduit to be used at the second stage resolves this issue. We now routinely place a conduit in the subcutaneous tissue to be accessed at the second stage in all patients in whom a two-stage approach is chosen (see the following).

Our experience to date suggests that in patients who require extensive coverage of the thoracoabdominal aorta, particularly if the infrarenal aorta is to be excluded either surgically or by the endovascular graft, a two-stage approach is preferred. Our only case of paraplegia was in a patient who had complete coverage from the subclavian artery down to the iliac arteries. In retrospect, this procedure could have been staged after placement of the infrarenal bifurcated graft and the first distal thoracic endograft (Figure 51-6). We believe that each case should be individualized. Patients with symptoms presenting with pain or patients in stable condition with a contained rupture clearly should be approached in a single stage. When the procedure is limited to the descending thoracic and visceral aorta, a single stage is also appropriate. In patients who require more extensive coverage or whose condition is unstable during the surgical portion, a two-stage approach should be strongly considered. In either case, maintenance of the mean blood pressure above 80 mm Hg offers protection to spinal cord perfusion.

DEBRANCHING: EXTRA-ANATOMIC BYPASSES

Visceral Aorta

The surgical approach to perform the extra-anatomic bypasses will be either a transperitoneal approach if all four visceral vessels require revascularization or a retroperitoneal approach if the right renal artery does not require a bypass. The latter is the case if the right kidney is atrophic, if the patient is in renal failure already, or if the revascularization is limited to the suprarenal visceral aorta. Although access to the right renal artery can be done from a left retroperitoneal approach, it is often difficult in the presence of aneurysmal dilation of the perirenal segment of the aorta. In a recent case, even though we were able to expose the origin of the right renal artery, a very proximal bifurcation of this vessel prevented us from ligating the artery and having enough length to perform the distal anastomosis. Therefore an early bifurcation of the right renal artery should also be considered in determining a transperitoneal or a retroperitoneal approach. The approach should also take into account the potential sources of inflow for the retrograde revascularization. This is most often the distal infrarenal aorta close to the bifurcation, or one of the two common iliac arteries. When the latter is chosen, adequate size of the iliac artery must be ensured, because this will be perfusing not only the lower extremity but also most or all visceral vessels. Atherosclerotic disease in the proximal common iliac artery (CIA) should indicate an alternative source of inflow or correction at the time of the procedure. This can be done by extending the arteriotomy to the distal infrarenal aorta just proximal to the bifurcation originating the graft from both the distal aorta and the proximal CIA. The external iliac artery can be used as inflow source provided it is of adequate size and in the absence of occlusive disease. In these cases, an alternative route for introduction of the endovascular graft should be used to avoid visceral ischemia and/or embolization during the endovascular component of the procedure (see the following).

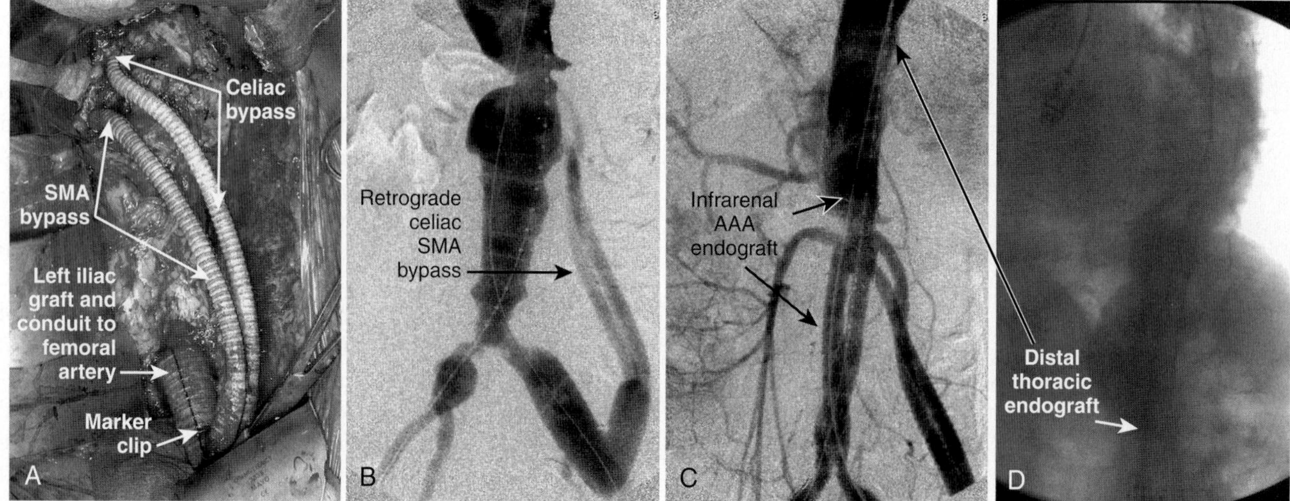

FIGURE 51-6 Combined endovascular and surgical repair of a type II thoracoabdominal aneurysm with iliac aneurysms performed in a single stage with use of both an endovascular AAA endograft and three thoracic endografts. **A,** Retroperitoneal approach for retrograde bypasses to celiac and SMA. The patient was in chronic renal failure, and therefore renal revascularization was not necessary. **B,** Anteroposterior arteriogram before deployment of endovascular grafts. **C,** Completion anteroposterior intraoperative angiogram of the hybrid procedure carried in a single stage. Unfortunately, the patient had spinal cord injury likely resulting from the extensive aortic coverage. **D,** Alternatively, the procedure could have been carried out in two stages after deployment of the infrarenal aortic endograft and the first distal thoracic endograft.

The surgical approach will also be influenced by any prior abdominal or retroperitoneal surgery. However, this becomes a secondary issue particularly if all visceral vessels require revascularization. The retroperitoneal approach is preferred when only the SMA and the celiac axis require revascularization. Patients tend to recover quicker with lower pulmonary morbidity from a retroperitoneal exposure. A retroperitoneal approach is preferred, when possible, particularly in patients with prior infrarenal aortic surgery.

One of the potential issues on the durability of combined endovascular and surgical approach relates to the use of retrograde bypass for visceral revascularization. In a comparison of antegrade and retrograde mesenteric bypass, Kansal et al.[12] concluded that the long-term durability of retrograde and antegrade mesenteric bypass was similar with a lower mortality for the retrograde approach. Avoidance of supraceliac aortic cross-clamping likely contributed to a lower mortality for retrograde bypasses. Familiarity with the construction of retrograde revascularization to visceral vessels is a key component to the success of the hybrid approach.

The source of inflow for revascularization of the visceral vessels will frequently be the distal infrarenal aorta and/or one of the iliac arteries. Proximal iliac occlusive disease should be addressed by either local endarterectomy or extension of the arteriotomy above the aortic bifurcation. We prefer to use a bifurcated or trifurcated graft making the body of the graft long enough to accept the conduit in the hood of the anastomoses, which avoids interference with flow during endograft placement (Figure 51-7). Alternatively, the conduit can be placed in the contralateral iliac artery avoiding this problem altogether. Dacron grafts are easier to route with less tendency to kink. New grafts are being developed for this purpose, which may help in the construction of these retrograde bypasses.

For renal revascularization, the right limb of the bifurcated retrograde graft is tunneled either posteromedial to the vena cava for proximal right renal revascularization or anterior to the vena cava for more distal access to the right renal artery. Exposure of the distal right renal artery is obtained by medial mobilization of the right colon, takedown of the hepatorenal ligament, and kocherization of the duodenum. The left renal artery can be approached either medial to the mesocolon for proximal revascularization or posterior to the mesocolon for access to the distal left renal artery. Medial approach to the left renal artery is best accomplished by ligation of the inferior mesenteric vein and gonadal vein with complete mobilization of the left renal vein. Lateral exposure of the distal left renal artery is done by medial rotation of the descending colon and careful division of the lienocolic ligament. Care must be taken that a proximal bifurcation or multiple renal arteries are properly addressed. The renal arteries should be ligated proximal to the distal anastomosis to avoid a type II endoleak. We prefer an end-to-end anastomosis with ligation of the proximal renal artery close to its origin.

Exposure of the SMA must be done proximal to the takeoff of the middle colic artery. This can be accomplished in two ways. The SMA can be approached by elevation of the mesocolon and following the course of the middle colic artery, which will lead to the SMA at the base of the mesentery. This is the typical approach for a SMA embolectomy. The middle colic artery, the SMA proximal to this vessel, and jejunal and distal SMA branches are carefully controlled. The anastomosis is performed in an end-to-side manner just distal to the middle colic artery with ligation of the SMA proximal to the latter (Figures 51-8 and 51-9). Alternatively, the SMA can be approached near its aortic origin. After ligation of the inferior mesenteric vein, gonadal vein, and adrenal vein, the left renal vein is fully mobilized. The third and fourth portion of the duodenum are mobilized to the right side identifying the SMA origin posterior to the pancreas and superior to the left renal artery. This is the preferred approach when the retrograde bypass originates from the left aortoiliac segment (Figure 51-10). It is easier to perform the anastomosis in an end-to-side manner with ligation of the SMA proximal to the anastomosis. An end-to-end anastomosis can also be performed.

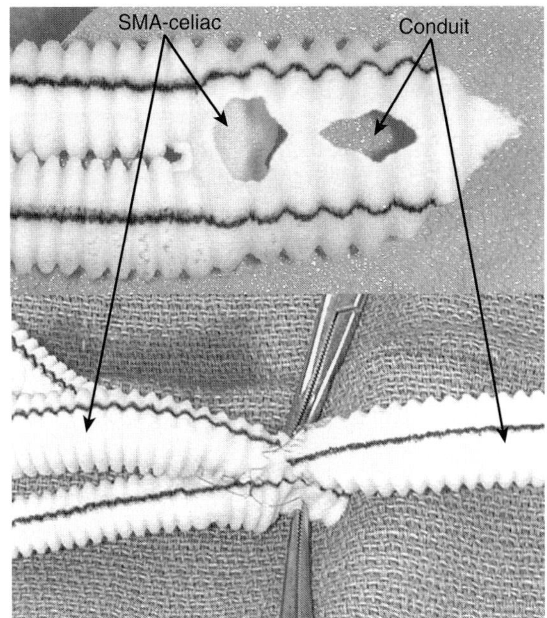

FIGURE 51-7 Construction of typical retrograde bypasses for distal revascularization. Note that the graftotomy for the conduit is placed in the hood of the bifurcated graft to prevent flow restriction during placement of the sheath for the endovascular procedure and allow natural passage of the guidewire into the native system.

Exposure of the celiac artery and its branches is best accomplished by entering the lesser sac through the gastrohepatic ligament. Placement of a nasogastric tube will keep the stomach decompressed and at the same time make identification of the esophagogastric junction easier. The very dense celiac plexus needs to be divided. The coronary vein (left gastric pain) is ligated. Frequently the left gastric artery is also ligated. By following either the hepatic or the splenic artery, the bifurcation of the celiac artery is exposed encircling the celiac artery proximal to the bifurcation. This will allow ligation of the artery once revascularization is completed to avoid a type II endoleak. The anastomosis is carried out in an end-to-side manner to either the hepatic or splenic artery (see Figure 51-9, C). Although the anastomosis can be performed at the bifurcation, this often proves to be more difficult and requires additional mobilization of the proximal celiac artery.

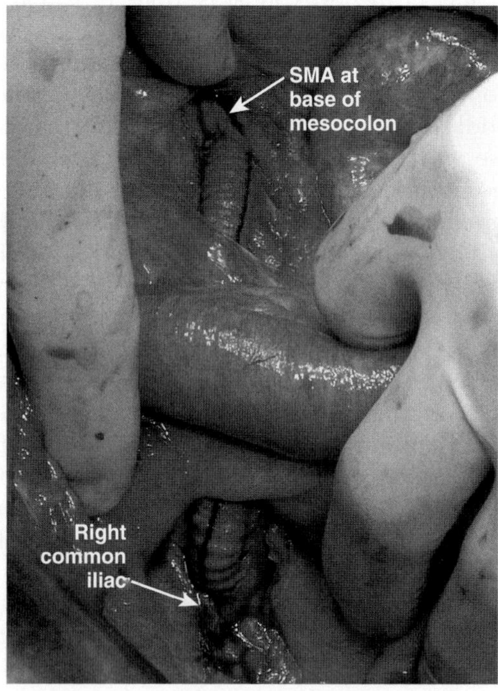

FIGURE 51-8 Right CIA–to–SMA bypass for SMA retrograde revascularization. The SMA is exposed at the base of the mesocolon, and the graft is tunneled between the anterior and posterior leaves of the mesentery.

Routing of the retrograde bypasses for visceral revascularization is also critical. When the retrograde bypass to the SMA originates in the right common iliac system, we prefer to tunnel this graft between the leaves of the base of the mesentery toward the retrocolic portion of the SMA (see Figure 51-8). A second graft is then anastomosed end to side to this graft and tunneled anterior to the pancreas for celiac revascularization (see Figure 51-9). When the SMA bypass originates from the left CIA, this graft is routed toward the origin of the SMA exposed behind the pancreas with complete mobilization of the third and fourth portion of the duodenum. A second graft is then anastomosed end to side and tunneled behind the pancreas for celiac revascularization (Figures 51-10 and 51-11). Alternatively, a C-loop configuration has been used successfully. In our experience, however, this is not necessary and makes it more difficult to isolate this graft from the intestines. In all

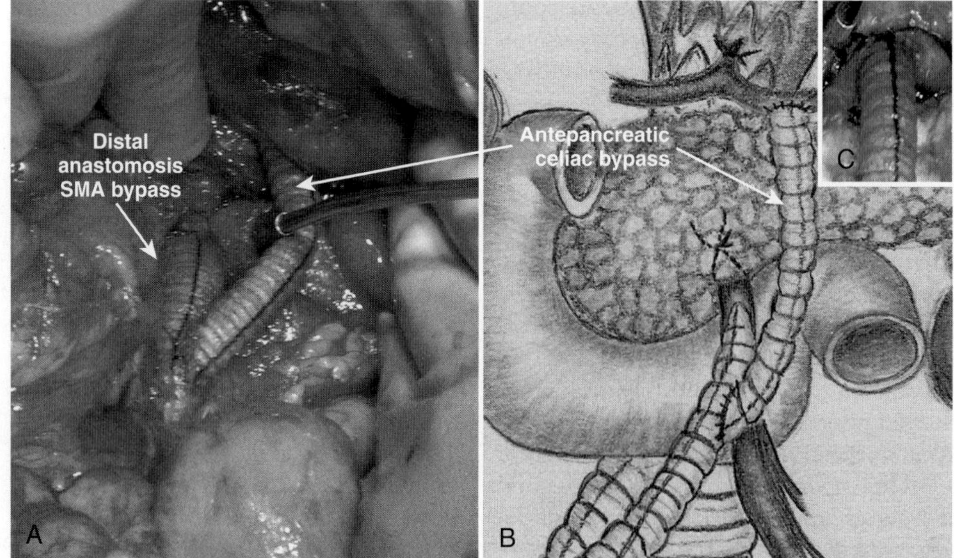

FIGURE 51-9 **A,** Retrograde bypass for celiac revascularization originating proximal to the distal anastomosis to the SMA. **B,** In this configuration, the celiac bypass is tunneled anterior to the pancreas. **C** *(inset),* Distal anastomosis of retrograde celiac bypass performed in an end-to-side manner to the splenic artery. Note that the celiac artery is ligated proximal to this anastomosis.

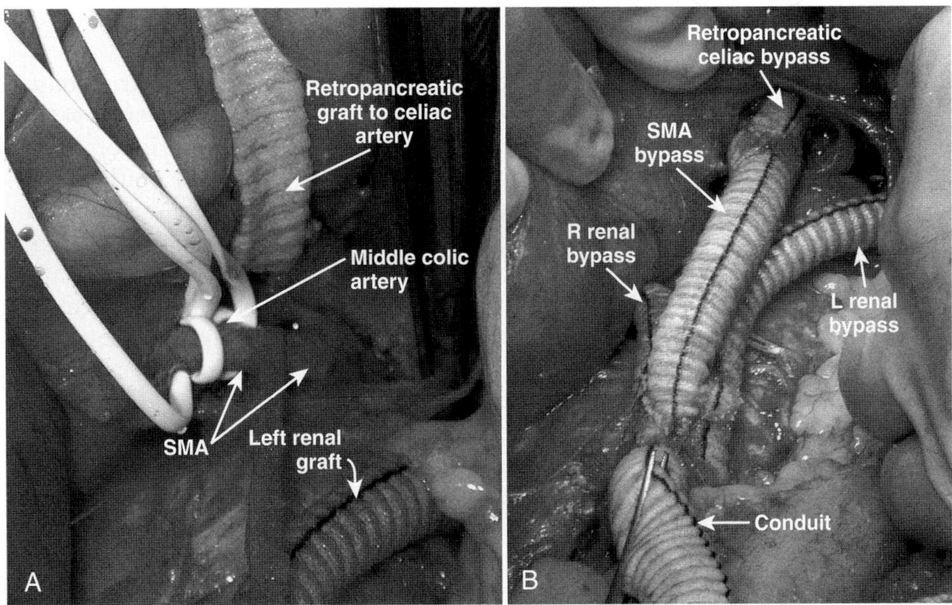

FIGURE 51-10 **A,** Exposure of the SMA near its origin in preparation for retrograde SMA and celiac revascularization originating in the left aortoiliac segment. The third and fourth portion of the duodenum had been mobilized to the right. **B,** Completion of the retrograde bypasses for visceral revascularization. Note that the celiac artery bypass has been tunneled posterior to the pancreas, which is best in this configuration. The conduit will be used in this case for a single-stage approach. On completion, it will be ligated.

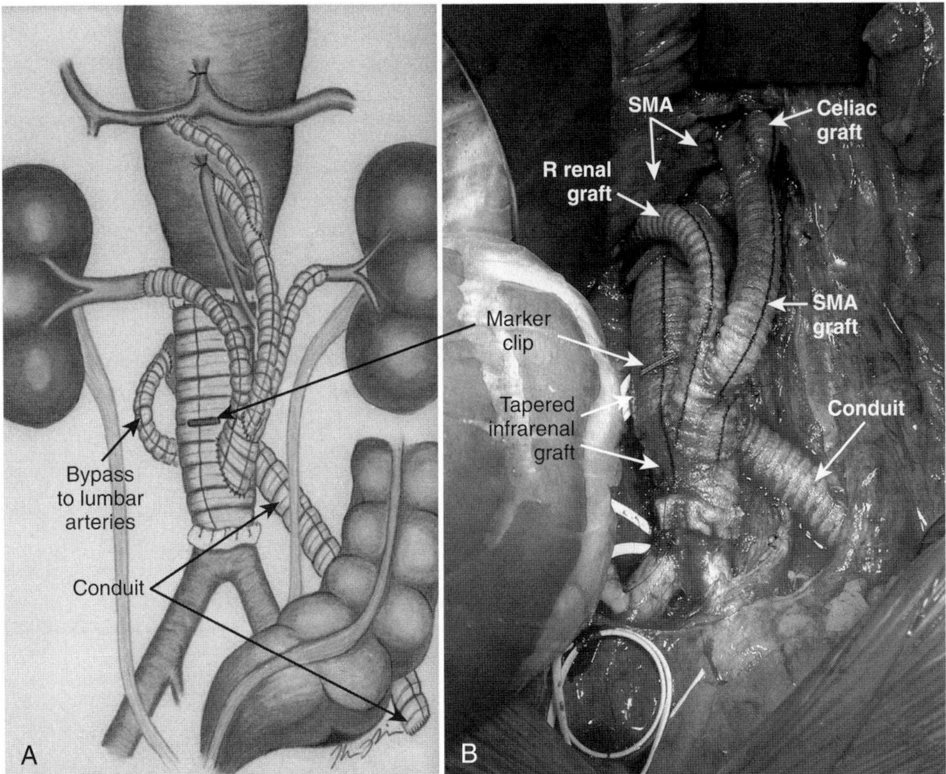

FIGURE 51-11 Intraoperative appearance of the infrarenal and retrograde reconstruction during stage 1 of the patient presented in Figure 51-5. A short bypass was performed to an island of two lumbar arteries just below the proximal anastomosis of the infrarenal graft. Note the marker clips, which will aid in the performance of the endovascular portion in stage 2. The conduit was placed posterior to the ureter and sigmoid colon and left in the subcutaneous tissue in the left lower quadrant.

instances, the artery is ligated proximal to the distal anastomosis of each inflow graft.

Inspection of the grafts should be performed once the viscera are returned to their anatomic position to ensure that no kinking or flow restriction occurs. If this is noted, reimplantation of the proximal end of the graft to a more suitable site within the reconstruction can solve this problem. Inspection of the viscera on completion of the procedure should be routine.

Surgical clips can be placed proximal to the takeoff of the retrograde bypasses to identify fluoroscopically the most distal landing site of the endovascular graft (Figures 51-11, 51-12, and 51-13). This helps limit the amount of contrast needed to identify the distal portion of the endovascular reconstruction. Similarly, if a subcutaneous conduit is created, a surgical clip placed at the distal end will help to identify its location with use of fluoroscopy at the second stage of the procedure.

Protection of the extra-anatomic intracavitary grafts in the abdomen is important to avoid the potential for long-term complication of graft enteric erosion and/or fistula. In most instances, the surrounding tissue can be used for this purpose. If more extensive coverage is needed, an omental flap can be developed and passed in a retrocolic fashion to the retroperitoneal area (see Figure 51-12). All grafts should be inspected and contact with the bowel avoided.

Aortic Arch

For complete arch reconstructions, a median sternotomy is the surgical approach of choice. This allows revascularization of the innominate and left carotid artery with a bifurcated graft. The hood of this graft, with placement of a conduit, will serve as access for the endovascular portion of the procedure. A left carotid subclavian bypass is often recommended as part of revascularization of all four extracranial vessels and provides inflow to the LSA through the left common carotid revascularization. This is best done before the median sternotomy either during the same intervention or as a preparatory procedure. Antegrade placement of the endovascular graft is usually best unless the landing zone is distal to the innominate artery. For antegrade deployment, a bifurcated graft is constructed with a conduit on the hood of the anastomosis to the ascending thoracic aorta. The aortic anastomosis should be placed as proximal as possible to provide an adequate landing zone for the endovascular graft. The right limb of the bifurcated graft is then anastomosed end to end to the innominate artery and the left limb to the left carotid artery (see Figure 51-13). The mediastinal grafts are best routed anterior to the innominate vein to avoid compression of this vein between the grafts and the sternum. In all instances, the arteries should be ligated proximal to the distal anastomosis and, in the case of

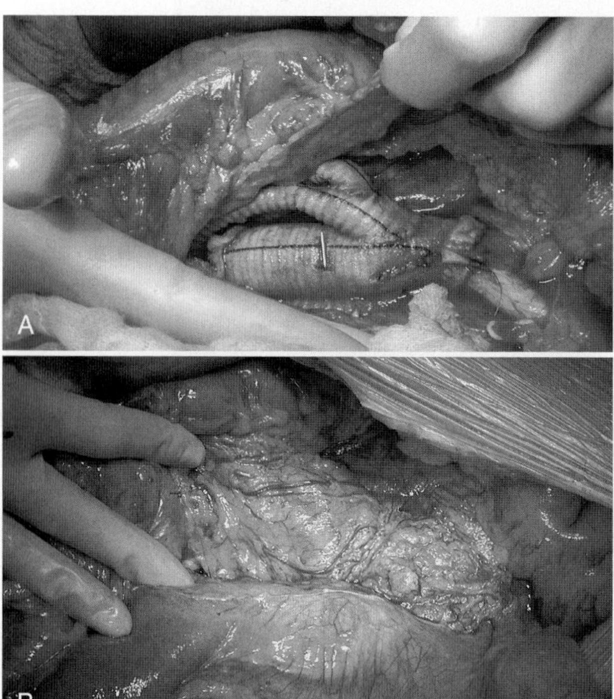

FIGURE 51-12 **A,** Development of omental flap passed in a retrocolic fashion to protect the retrograde grafts. **B,** Complete graft coverage with omental flap will prevent adherence of the intestines to the retrograde bypasses.

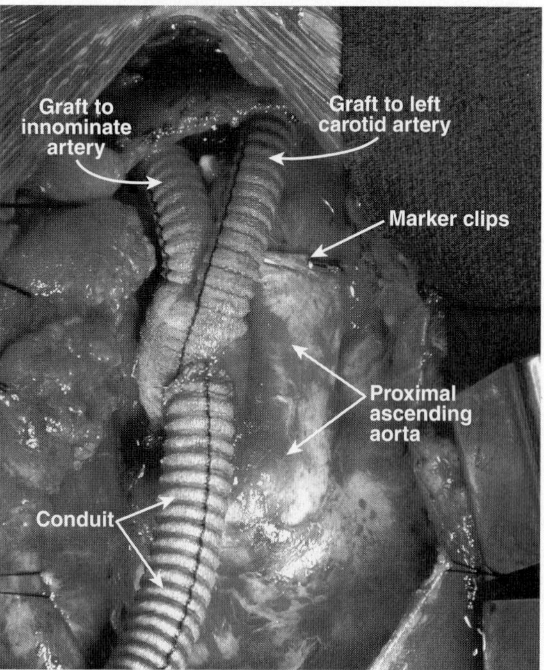

FIGURE 51-13 Complete arch reconstruction for treatment of large arch aneurysm just distal to the innominate artery. Note the marker clip on the ascending thoracic aorta, which will aid in accurate placement of the endovascular graft.

the LSA, proximal to the left vertebral artery. If the LSA is covered without preparatory revascularization, a type 2 endoleak can occur. This can be corrected with endovascular closure through a left brachial approach with use of coils or an Amplatzer occlusion device (AGA Medical Corp, Plymouth, MN) proximal to the vertebral artery origin.

Depending on the proximal landing site for the endovascular graft, complete debranching of the arch may not be necessary. In these instances, a carotid-carotid bypass for revascularization of the left common carotid artery, with or without a left carotid—to—subclavian bypass, can be used to land the endovascular graft proximal to the left common carotid artery. Therefore a median sternotomy is avoided. The carotid-carotid bypass can be performed either retrosternal or retropharyngeal. The latter is preferred, because it will allow unimpeded median sternotomy if necessary. Berguer et al.[13] have described the technique for retropharyngeal carotid-carotid bypass, and the reader is referred to this description for details on the technique. When the reconstruction is distal to the innominate artery, a femoral approach for introduction of the endovascular graft is preferred, which potentially reduces the risk for embolization present in the antegrade approach and avoids a median sternotomy. If a median sternotomy is performed, access for delivery of the endovascular graft can be antegrade through a conduit in the ascending aorta. The curvature, configuration, and specific anatomy in each case should be taken into consideration when deciding the access for delivery of the endovascular graft (see the following).

In cases of arch reconstructions that terminate in the mid descending thoracic aorta or higher, spinal catheter drainage is not indicated. In patients with prior infrarenal aortic replacement, particularly when revascularization of the LSA is not performed, spinal catheter drainage should be considered. If the endovascular graft is to cover the distal descending thoracic aorta, spinal catheter drainage is also recommended. In all instances, mean blood pressure should be maintained at 80 mm Hg or higher.

Endovascular Component

One of the main elements of the endovascular component of the approach will be access for deployment of the endovascular graft. Assessment of the size of the femoral and external iliac arteries on CT scan will determine whether this will be an adequate route for the deployment of the grafts. The planning should take into consideration whether, during deployment of the endovascular devices, compromise to the inflow of the retrograde graft will occur. This is to be avoided. One alternative is to use the iliofemoral system contralateral to the takeoff of the retrograde bypasses. When the retrograde inflow is from the infrarenal aorta, the larger of the two iliofemoral systems should be chosen.

In the single-stage approach, a conduit placed on the hood of the retrograde bifurcated graft allows retrograde flow during deployment. The location of this conduit to graft anastomosis should be such that it will naturally allow preferential entry into the native system (see Figure 51-7). With the current available endovascular deployment catheters, a 10-mm graft will permit both the main delivery sheath and a 5F sheath in parallel to use for control angiography. The conduit can be brought up to the surface of the lower abdominal wall, temporarily covering the viscera with a moist towel and a plastic drape. This will prevent the possibility of contamination from the fluoroscopy equipment (Figure 51-14). On completion of the deployment, the conduit can be ligated flush with its proximal anastomosis.

In a two-stage approach, if the iliofemoral system contralateral to the takeoff of the retrograde bypasses is of adequate size, this should be chosen preferentially. If the retrograde grafts originate from the infrarenal aorta, the larger iliofemoral segment should be chosen for the main delivery system. The contralateral side is then used percutaneously for control angiography. We have found that the placement of a subcutaneous conduit at the first stage either at the femoral level below the inguinal ligament, or in the flank, provides easy access for both the main delivery system and control angiography (Figures 51-11 and 51-15). The procedure in this case is initiated by thrombectomy of the graft conduit with retrograde angiography to document the absence of any luminal defects (see Figure 51-15, *B*).

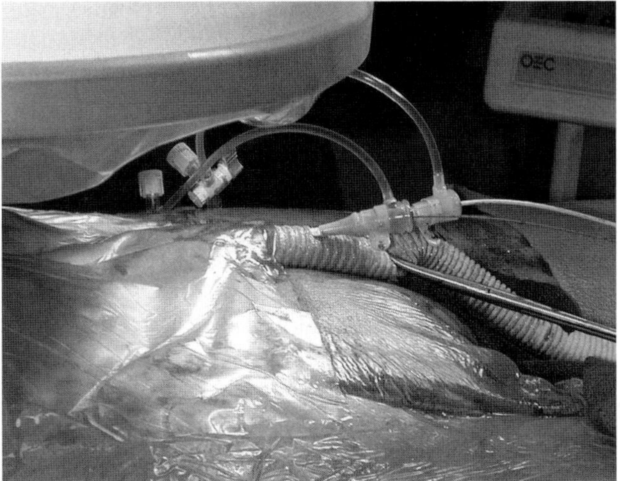

FIGURE 51-14 Ten-millimeter Dacron graft being used as a conduit for both the delivery sheath and a smaller sheath for control angiography in a single-stage combined endovascular and surgical repair. Placement of a protective drape over the wound will help stabilize the conduit and prevent contamination.

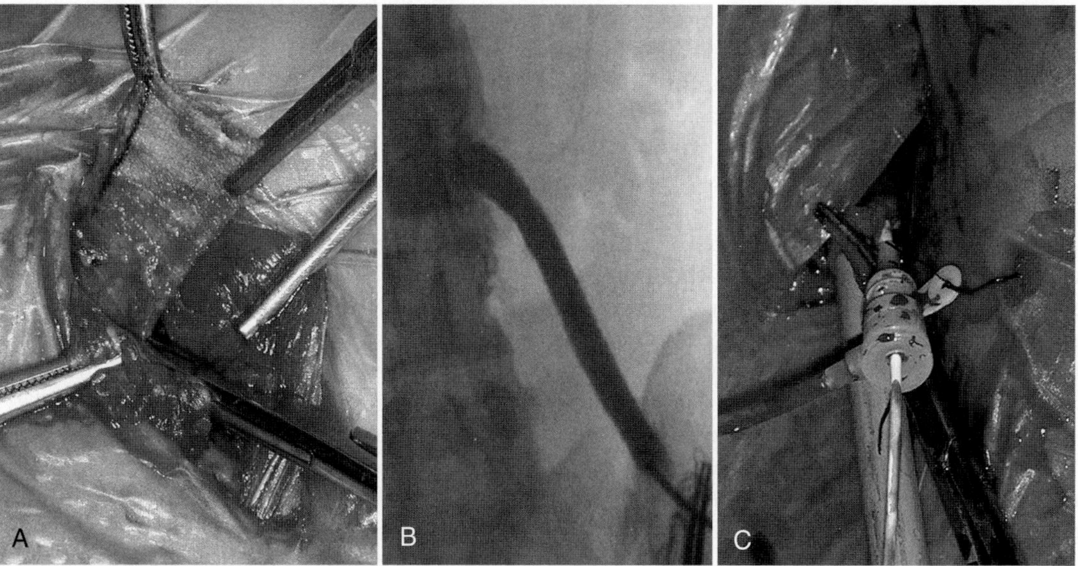

FIGURE 51-15 **A,** Exposure of distal end of subcutaneous conduit through a small cutdown in the left lower quadrant during stage 2 of a combined endovascular and surgical approach to repair a dissecting thoracoabdominal aneurysm depicted in Figures 51-5 and 51-11. **B,** Completion arteriogram after thrombectomy of subcutaneous conduit. **C,** Conduit being used for access for the main sheath and a smaller sheath for control angiography.

A 10-mm subcutaneous conduit will allow access for both the delivery system and control angiography. Once the delivery is completed, the conduit is ligated as proximal as possible and left in place. One concern of this approach is the potential for infection of the conduit left behind. If this were to occur, and the conduit originates from the retrograde bypass origin, it would have major consequences. It is therefore critical that at the second stage the patient receive prophylactic antibiotics, and there should be strict observance of sterile technique. Once ligated, the conduit should be separated from the skin by at least a two-layer closure. Alternatively, the subcutaneous conduit placed at the first stage can originate from the contralateral iliac system, away from the main retrograde bypasses.

As mentioned earlier, access for reconstructions of the aortic arch can be either from a femoral approach if the grafts are distal to the innominate artery or from a conduit placed through the original median sternotomy at the hood of the extra-anatomic bypasses. We have found the latter to be preferable in a single-stage approach because it provides excellent control for deployment of the endovascular graft particularly in instances where the curvature of the aortic arch may be difficult to negotiate through a femoral approach.

The order of deployment of multiple thoracic endografts will be dictated by the anatomy. This is no different than for endovascular repair of a descending thoracic aneurysm. Care should be taken, however, after deployment of distal grafts when the more proximal endovascular deployment is being performed. Because the proximal end of the distal graft is usually in an aneurysmal portion of the aorta, migration can occur with passage of the deployment system of the more proximal graft. On occasion, we have used a trilobed balloon catheter to fix the more distal portion of the initial endovascular component while passing the delivery system for the more proximal endograft. In any case, when the order of deployment is from distal to proximal, balloon inflation of the distal seal zone before passage of the delivery system for the more proximal graft is recommended.

COMPLICATIONS

One of the more feared complications of TAAA repair is paraplegia. We recommend routine use of spinal catheter drainage in all patients undergoing hybrid procedures for TAAA repair. In addition, maintaining the mean blood pressure of 80 mm Hg or higher during the intraoperative and postoperative periods reduces the risk of this complication. Spinal catheter pressure is maintained at 10 cm H_2O with use of a Becker drain system, which is leveled with the spinal column. Spinal catheter drainage is maintained for 72 hours after surgery. If there is no evidence of spinal cord injury, the spinal drainage pressure is raised to 20 cm H_2O for 6 hours, and, if no neurologic deficit is seen, the spinal drain is removed. Patients should be maintained relatively flat in bed to avoid spinal headache. If a spinal cord injury deficit is seen in the postoperative period, a magnetic resonance (MR) image of the lumbosacral spine should be obtained if the patient's condition is otherwise stable. This will exclude the possibility of compression of the cord by a hematoma as a complication of the spinal catheter drain. The blood pressure should be raised with pressors to improve spinal cord perfusion. If spinal catheter drainage was not used, or the drain has been removed, prompt insertion with reinstitution of spinal catheter drainage has been associated with resolution of the deficit in some cases.

One of the potential complications for combined endovascular and surgical repair is occlusion of the extra-anatomic or retrograde bypasses. In aortic arch reconstructions, this can be asymptomatic or manifested with a transient or permanent neurologic deficit. Management of this particular complication will be dictated by the patient's overall condition. If the stroke is severe particularly with loss of consciousness, revascularization can be associated with a significant risk for mortality. If the neurologic deficit is transient or minor, thrombectomy and/or revision of the involved bypass should be considered. On occasion, the proximal end of the thoracic endograft may be partially occluding the artery supplying the affected territory. In these cases, antegrade or retrograde placement of a stent can correct the problem.

In reconstructions involving the visceral aorta, occlusion of a retrograde bypass can be asymptomatic particularly to either the celiac or renal arteries. If occlusion of the bypass to the celiac artery occurs without evidence of liver dysfunction, conservative management is appropriate. Similarly, thrombosis of a renal artery bypass without significant deterioration of renal function can be managed conservatively. If significant organ dysfunction results from occlusion of one of these bypasses, more aggressive management is indicated including reoperation and revision. Occlusion of a retrograde bypass to the SMA should be suspected in patients with persistent acidosis, severe abdominal pain, or poor clinical progress. Prompt intervention is indicated. Evaluation of patency of these retrograde bypasses can be done with a variety of imaging techniques. Abdominal duplex scan will frequently document patency of these reconstructions. Evaluation of renal perfusion can also be obtained with use of MAG3 nuclear renal scan. CT angiography or MR angiography can also be very helpful, particularly in patients whose condition is otherwise stable. Fortunately, experience to date suggests that occlusion of these retrograde bypasses is a rare event.

Embolic stroke is a potential complication of any type of endovascular reconstruction in the area of the aortic arch. This is usually the result of embolization during placement of the thoracic endograft. Guidewire manipulation should be minimized, and accurate deployment of the endograft without the need for additional extensions or revisions will reduce the risk of this complication. Management of patients with embolic stroke after thoracic endograft placement is beyond the scope of this chapter. Careful evaluation with imaging of the reconstruction will exclude correctable technical issues as described earlier.

Respiratory complications can occur in patients with significant chronic obstructive pulmonary disease. One of the potential advantages of the combined endovascular and surgical approach is reduction in pulmonary morbidity. Occasionally, however, significant deterioration in pulmonary function can occur, because these patients tend to be in the high-risk category. Preoperative optimization is important in reducing the risk of this complication. The usual precautions to prevent aspiration in the postoperative period with early removal of the nasogastric tube in patients undergoing laparotomy and early mobilization will all help maintain adequate pulmonary function. We prefer retroperitoneal approach when possible, because this is also associated with a reduced risk of pulmonary complications.

In our experience, we have seen one patient in our series with chylous ascites after retrograde revascularization. This was successfully managed conservatively maintaining the patient to receive nothing by mouth with intravenous hyperalimentation. The source of the chylous leak was unclear, but we suspect that it may have been related to the SMA exposure at its origin.

LONG-TERM MANAGEMENT

An important component of the management of patients undergoing a hybrid procedure is careful follow-up of the endovascular component of the approach. In a review of the available literature on combined endovascular and surgical repair of thoracoabdominal aneurysms, the overall long-term endoleak rate was 20.6% and the reintervention rate was 13.7%.[10] Patients should have routine imaging, because it is standard for follow-up of endovascular repair of thoracic aneurysms. We recommend a CT scan with intravenous contrast within the first few weeks after discharge, at 6 months, and yearly thereafter. In patients with elevated creatinine level, an MR angiogram can be done if the creatinine is less than 2.0 mg/dL. In patients with creatinine greater than 2.0, a CT scan without contrast can be used to monitor the size of the aneurysm. If there is no evidence of aneurysm growth, or there is aneurysm shrinkage around the endovascular graft, one can be reassured that no significant endoleak is present. Type I endoleaks should be corrected as soon as identified. Type II endoleak has occurred once in our series related to incomplete ligation of the visceral artery proximal to the bypass. We recommend correction of type II endoleaks when they arise from one of the major aortic branches. For example, a type II endoleak from the covered but not ligated LSA should be corrected. In our case, back-bleeding into the aneurysm from the partially ligated celiac artery was corrected by placement of a covered endograft through the retrograde bypass into the hepatic artery, excluding flow to the splenic artery. Type II endoleaks arising from intercostal vessels can be managed conservatively as long as there is no aneurysm growth.

Long-term complications can be related either to the extra-anatomic or retrograde bypass or to the endovascular component of the repair. Aortoenteric erosion or fistula is a potential complication of retrograde revascularization of the visceral vessels. It is imperative that these grafts be covered and separated from the intestines. This complication has not been reported to date. With increased use of the hybrid technique for repair of thoracoabdominal aortic pathology, it is likely that this complication will occur. Graft occlusion over the long term has been reported to occur infrequently. In a review of the literature, with a mean follow-up of 14.5 months, a 97.8% retrograde graft patency was documented.[10] Management will be dictated by the clinical consequence of such occurrence. Patients without symptoms, who have adequate collateral circulation, can be managed conservatively. Graft revision and/or replacement are indicated in patients with symptoms.

Aneurysm rupture in patients who undergo a two-stage procedure has occurred once in our series and underscores the importance of patient selection for a single- or two-stage approach. Patients undergoing a two-stage approach should be monitored carefully and educated in terms of potential symptoms that would warrant proceeding with the endovascular repair as early as possible.

RESULTS

Results of the reported series with more than 10 patients are summarized in Table 51-1. Lee et al.[14] reported in 2005 a retrospective review of 17 patients who had renal and visceral revascularization as a first stage of a hybrid procedure for repair of TAAA. The first stage of the procedure was associated with a mortality of 24% and a morbidity of 25%. The second stage of the procedure was completed in 11 patients noting no additional deaths or postoperative complications. There was no paraplegia. At a mean follow-up of 8 months in the 11 patients completing both stages there were no deaths, and the primary patency for the renal and visceral grafts was 96%. The authors concluded that this was a difficult operation for both the patient and the surgeon. They also stated that a hybrid approach was not likely to be the final word in the treatment of patients with TAAA.

In 2006, Resch et al.[15] reported on 13 patients who underwent visceral bypass followed by endovascular thoracoabdominal aneurysm repair. There were three patients with symptoms, and two patients presented with rupture. All patients were thought to be unfit for conventional thoracoabdominal repair because of comorbid conditions. Six patients required either a proximal or distal direct aortic repair, and three patients also had a left carotid subclavian bypass. There were two patients with paraplegia, one of them with a ruptured aneurysm, and two patients with transient paraparesis. There were two patients in whom transient renal failure developed. Mortality was 23%, and there were two late aneurysm-related deaths. They concluded that staged

TABLE 51-1 Reported Series of a Combined Endovascular and Surgical Approach to Thoracoabdominal Aortic Pathology (10 or More Patients)

Author (reference)	Year	No. of patients	TAAA/arch (n)	Mortality 30 days (%)	Permanent paraplegia (%)	Overall morbidity (%)	Median follow-up (mo)	Survival (%)
Lee et al.[14]	2005	17*	17/0	24	0	25	8	100
Resch et al.[15]	2006	13	13/0	23	30	46	NA	NA
Black et al.[16]	2006	22	22/0	13	0	54	8	NA
Zhou et al.[17]	2006	31	16/15	3.2	0	9.6	16	90
Chiesa et al.[18]	2007	13†	13/0	23	0	31	14.9	76.9
Bockler et al.[19]	2008	28	28/0	14.3	11	59	22	70
Quinones et al.[20]	2008	17	15/2	0	5.8	12	17	81‡

* *All staged procedures.*
† *Seven patients with aortic dissection.*
‡ *Cumulative survival.*
NA, Not available; *TAAA*, thoracoabdominal aortic aneurysm.

endovascular and open procedures are feasible for treatment of thoracoabdominal aneurysm in patients with prohibitive risk for open surgery. They noted that this approach still carries a significant risk of perioperative morbidity and mortality.

In 2006 Black et al.[16] published a series of 29 consecutive patients where a hybrid procedure was used to treat complex TAAAs. Twenty-two patients electively had retrograde visceral revascularization with endovascular exclusion. Four patients were treated either urgently or emergently because of symptomatic aneurysms or true rupture respectively. Forty-five percent of the patients had previous aortic surgery, and severe preoperative comorbidity was present in 80%. In three patients, the procedure was not completed because of myocardial instability and/or poor inflow in a patient with a type B aortic dissection. Elective mortality was 13% whereas all three patients who presented with a ruptured aneurysm died. The three deaths in elective procedures were a result of pulmonary embolism, myocardial infarction, and trash embolization, respectively. There was no incidence of paraplegia. The authors compared these results with their own series of open thoracoabdominal aneurysm repair and concluded that the hybrid approach, in their hands, improved outcomes.

Zhou and colleagues[17] reported their experience in 2006 with a hybrid approach to complex thoracic aortic aneurysm in high-risk patients. Thirty-one patients underwent combined open and endovascular approach for complex aneurysms. Sixteen patients had ascending and arch aneurysm and 15 patients aneurysms involving the visceral vessels. There was one death for a mortality of 3.2%. Procedure-related complications included renal bypass thrombosis in two patients and a retroperitoneal hematoma managed conservatively. There was no paraplegia or stroke. There were two early type II endoleaks, one that resolved spontaneously. During a mean follow-up of 16 months, two patients died of unrelated causes, but the others had no aneurysm enlargement and remained without symptoms.

In 2007, Chiesa et al.[18] reported their experience with a combined endovascular and surgical approach to thoracoabdominal aneurysms in patients with prior aortic surgery. Thirteen patients underwent a one-stage hybrid repair of their TAAA. All patients were American Society of Anesthesiologists (ASA) class 3 or 4. The results were compared with a similar group of 29 patients from within their series of 246 patients who had surgical repair of TAAA. There were no intraoperative deaths in either group. Perioperative mortality was 23% in the hybrid group and 17.2% in the surgical group. Morbidity was slightly higher in the surgical group (44.8%) versus the hybrid group (30.8%). In the hybrid group there was one delayed transient paraplegia whereas in the surgical group three patients had this complication. At a median follow-up of 14.9 months in the hybrid group, all grafts were patent and there was no aneurysm-related death, endoleak, stent graft migration, or morbidity related to visceral revascularization. In the surgical group, at a median follow-up of 5.4 years there were no significant complications related to the aortic repair except for three patients with dilation of the visceral aortic patch. The authors concluded that the hybrid repair did not lead to significant improvement in outcome and that further follow-up and larger series were necessary to evaluate this approach. The lower incidence of paraplegia in the hybrid group, however, should not be ignored.

Bockler et al.[19] reported in 2008 on 28 patients treated with a hybrid approach for TAAA. Seven patients had concomitant aortic dissection. Elective mortality was 14.3%, and 11% of patients had paraplegia. Overall morbidity was 59%. At a median follow-up of 13 months, graft patency was 86%. They found no significant difference between single-stage and two-stage procedures in regard to paraplegia and complications. A significant difference in mortality was noted between emergency and elective cases (28% vs. 12%). Overall survival at 3 years was 70%. They concluded that the early results of the hybrid repair for high-risk patients with complex thoracoabdominal aneurysms were encouraging.

Our experience at the University of California, Los Angeles, Medical Center to date consists of 17 high-risk patients approached with either a single- or two-stage procedure.[20] Six patients had prior aortic surgery adjacent to the presenting thoracoabdominal aneurysm. One patient had a functional renal transplant, and all patients were considered high risk on the basis of preoperative comorbidities. Spinal catheter drainage was used routinely. A single-stage procedure was performed in 10 patients, and in 6 patients the procedure was completed in two stages with use of a subcutaneous conduit constructed at the first stage. One patient had a fatal myocardial infarction before completing the second stage. There were no perioperative deaths. One patient with complete aortic coverage from left subclavian to bilateral iliac bifurcation in the single-stage group had the only case of paraplegia. In this patient in retrospect the procedure could have been performed in two stages. Two type II endoleaks without aneurysm growth are under observation, and two patients had successful reintervention for a type I and II endoleak respectively. There has been no graft thrombosis or aneurysm growth or rupture during a mean follow-up of 16.5 months (2-120 months) in 16 patients with a completed procedure. Cumulative survival at 2 years is 81%. Continued surveillance is critical after a completed repair and to date, in our experience, the combined approach has been effective in management of the high-risk patient with thoracoabdominal aortic pathology (Figure 51-16).

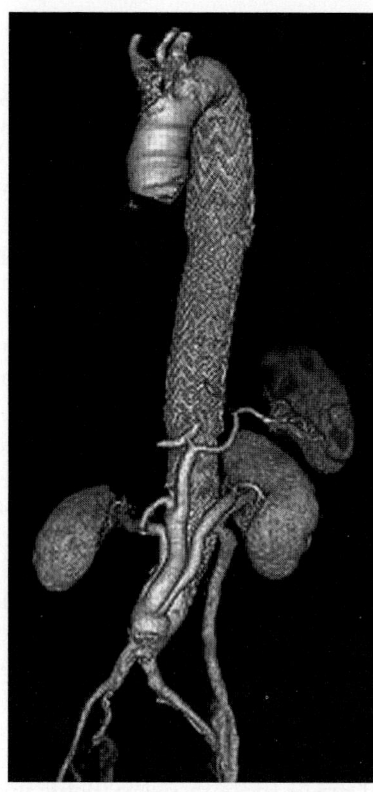

FIGURE 51-16 Three-dimensional reconstruction 4 years after combined endovascular and surgical repair of a type II thoracoabdominal aneurysm.

Overall, encouraging midterm results continue to support using a hybrid approach to TAAA in selected patients. However, the mixed results reported to date underscore that the role of the hybrid approach for thoracoabdominal aortic pathology remains ill-defined. The longest follow-up available is from our original patient whose case was reported in 1999. This patient is now 9 years after a combined endovascular and surgical approach to his thoracoabdominal aneurysm and is doing well (see Figure 51-3). His course suggests that a hybrid approach for thoracoabdominal aortic pathology can be durable. Additional long-term follow-up certainly will be needed to refine patient selection criteria for a hybrid approach to thoracoabdominal aortic pathology. Development of branched endografts will likely add to the alternatives available for management of these cases.[21,22] Younger patients and good-surgical-risk patients should be offered standard surgical repair. High-risk patients with significant comorbidities should be considered for a combined approach.

CONCLUSION

A combined surgical and endovascular approach to thoracoabdominal aortic pathology can be performed with acceptable results in high-risk patients. The durability of retrograde or extra-anatomic bypasses and the long-term complications of endovascular repair are potential drawbacks to this approach. Experience to date, however, suggests that these concerns have not significantly affected the midterm results of these reconstructions. Additional experience will help in selecting patients, refining surgical technique, staging the procedures, and managing complications. Longer follow-up is needed to better define the role of a combined endovascular and surgical approach in the management of thoracoabdominal aortic pathology at a time of rapid evolution and improvements in endovascular technologies.

Acknowledgment

Special thanks to Kristy Biggs, MD, for providing the illustrations.

References

1. Crawford ES, Snyder DM, Cho GC, et al: Progress in treatment of thoracoabdominal and abdominal aortic aneurysms involving celiac, superior mesenteric, and renal arteries, *Ann Surg* 188:404–410, 1978.
2. Safi HJ, Miller CC III, Huynh TT, et al: Distal aortic perfusion and cerebrospinal fluid drainage for thoracoabdominal and descending thoracic aortic repair: Ten years of organ protection, *Ann Surg* 238:372–380, 2003.
3. Coselli JS, Conklin LD, LeMaire SA: Thoracoabdominal aortic aneurysm repair: review and update of current strategies, *Ann Thorac Surg* 74:S1881–S1884, 2002.
4. Quinones-Baldrich WJ: Descending thoracic and thoracoabdominal aortic aneurysm repair: 15-year results using a uniform approach, *Ann Vasc Surg* 18:335–342, 2004.
5. Coselli JS: The use of left heart bypass in the repair of thoracoabdominal aortic aneurysms: current techniques and results, *Semin Thorac Cardiovasc Surg* 15:326–332, 2003.
6. Ballard JL, Abou Zamzam AM Jr, Teruya TH: Type III and IV thoracoabdominal aortic aneurysm repair: results of a trifurcated/two-graft technique, *J Vasc Surg* 36(2):211–216, 2002, discussion 216.
7. Engle J, Safi HJ, Miller CC III, et al: The impact of diaphragm management on prolonged ventilator support after thoracoabdominal aortic repair, *J Vasc Surg* 29(1):150–156, 1999.
8. Walsh SR, Tang TY, Sadat U, et al: Endovascular stenting versus open surgery for thoracic aortic disease: systematic review and meta-analysis of perioperative results, *J Vasc Surg* 47(5):1094–1098, 2008.
9. Quinones-Baldrich WJ, Panetta TF, Vescera CL, et al: Repair of type IV thoracoabdominal aneurysm with a combined endovascular and surgical approach, *J Vasc Surg* 30:555–560, 1999.
10. Donas KP, Czerny M, Guber I, et al: Hybrid open endovascular repair for thoracoabdominal aortic aneurysms: current status and level of evidence, *Eur J Vasc Endovasc Surg* 34:528–533, 2007.
11. Rigberg D, McGory ML, Zingmond DS, et al: Thirty-day mortality statistics underestimate the risk of repair of thoracoabdominal aortic aneurysms: a statewide experience, *J Vasc Surg* 43(2):217–222, discussion 223, 2006.
12. Kansal N, LoGerfo FW, Belfield AK, et al: A comparison of antegrade and retrograde mesenteric bypass, *Ann Vasc Surg* 16:591–596, 2002.

13. Berguer R: Revascularization across the neck using a retropharyngeal route. In Veith FJ, editor: *Current clinical problems in vascular surgery,* St. Louis, 1996, Quality Medical Publishing.
14. Lee WA, Brown MP, Martin TD, et al: Early results after staged hybrid repair of thoracoabdominal aortic aneurysms, *J Am Coll Surg 2007*:420–431, 2005.
15. Resch TA, Greenburg RK, Lyden SP, et al: Combined staged procedures for the treatment of thoracoabdominal aneurysms, *J Endovasc Ther* 13(4):481–489, 2006.
16. Black SA, Wolfe JH, Clark M, et al: Complex thoracoabdominal aortic aneurysms: endovascular exclusion with visceral revascularization, *J Vasc Surg* 43:1081–1089, 2006.
17. Zhou W, Reardon M, Peden EK, et al: Hybrid approach to complex thoracic aortic aneurysms in high-risk patients: surgical challenges and clinical outcomes, *J Vasc Surg* 44:688–693, 2006.
18. Chiesa R, Melissano G, Civilini E, et al: Two-stage combined endovascular and surgical approach for recurrent thoracoabdominal aortic aneurysm, *J Endovasc Ther* 11:330–333, 2004.
19. Bockler D, Kotelis D, Geisbusch P, et al: Hybrid procedures for thoracoabdominal aortic aneurysms and chronic aortic dissections: a single center experience in 28 patients, *J Vasc Surg* 724–732, 2008.
20. Quinones-Baldrich W, Jimenez JC, Moore WS: Combined endovascular and surgical (hybrid) approach to thoracoabdominal aortic pathology: a ten year experience, *J Vasc Surg* 49:1125–1134, 2009.
21. Anderson JL, Adam DJ, Berce M: Repair of thoracoabdominal aortic aneurysms with fenestrated and branched endovascular stent grafts, *J Vasc Surg* 600–607, 2005.
22. Chuter TA: Branched and fenestrated stent grafts for endovascular repair of thoracic aortic aneurysms, *J Vasc Surg* 43(suppl A): A111–A115, 2006.

CHAPTER

52

Endovascular Repair of Abdominal Aortic Aneurysm Using Fenestrated Grafts

Tara M. Mastracci, Roy K. Greenberg

The evolution of endograft technology has largely involved the migration of covered stents into more complex and proximal portions of the aorta. Simple infrarenal devices informed the innovation of thoracic devices, and lessons learned in these territories are being used to develop fenestrated and branched technology. Fenestrated endografts were first developed to accommodate complex infrarenal neck anatomy and were tested in a canine model in 1999.[1] Extending the sealing zone of infrarenal devices into the visceral segment of aorta expands the number of people eligible for aortic repair. Published series show encouraging results for both perioperative and long-term outcomes. In this chapter we review the history and rationale for development of fenestrated devices, outline the basic procedure for planning and performing cases, and review the outcomes reported by centers with expertise.

EVOLUTION AND DESIGN

Endovascular repair of infrarenal abdominal aortic aneurysms was first described in humans in 1991 with use of a tubular stent graft deployed into normal-caliber segments of aorta.[2] Subsequent iterations of endografts have evolved into the modern-day modular systems that include iliac arteries in a bifurcated configuration. The change in endograft design has evolved with the increasing understanding of the dynamic displacement forces that act on an endograft over time and through the cardiac cycle. As a result, methods for sealing and fixation have become more sophisticated and now are often independent mechanisms. Fixation is the process of holding a stent graft in the position in which it is deployed and may be active or passive. Passive fixation uses radial force to secure the stent graft in place, where active fixation uses barbs, screws, or suprarenal uncovered stents to resist displacement forces. Both the fixation system in the proximal and distal areas of the stent and the structure of stent itself combine to overcome the dynamic forces that threaten the integrity of the repair over time. Planning of a stent graft must be done with the anticipation that the device will have to adapt to changes in the morphology of the aneurysm over time.

Sealing is the process of excluding the aneurysm from circulatory flow and requires sufficient graft material to wall apposition that no flow channels will develop around the stent graft. With a sturdy fixation system and a landing zone in nondilating aorta, the sealing present on deployment of the device should be maintained throughout the lifespan of the device. The failure of current commercial infrarenal endovascular devices occurs when there is insufficient wall apposition in the infrarenal neck because of an intrinsic short or large-diameter neck or angulation of the infrarenal region. It is accepted that all the commercially available infrarenal stent grafts require the presence of at least 10 mm of normal-caliber aorta in the infrarenal segment, in the absence of significant angulation, to ensure sealing. For patients in whom these criteria cannot be met, alternative methods for sealing and fixation are needed.

Fenestrated endografts were developed to address the need for a device to accommodate patients with complex infrarenal neck anatomy either who were found to be ineligible for standard endovascular aneurysm repair (EVAR) for anatomic reasons or in whom a standard EVAR procedure had failed for reasons related to the neck. It is estimated that the rate of ineligibility for infrarenal endovascular repair using standard devices is 25% to 40% among patients with aneurysms whose maximum diameter has met operative threshold.[3,4] In patients found ineligible, the cause is proximal neck anatomy in 74% of patients,[3] and this can be due to length, diameter, or angulation.[3,5] Failed endovascular repair can also be a surrogate indicator of unrecognized complex aortic neck anatomy or the evolution of disease into proximal segments of aorta. In the Eurostar Registry, 17.8% of patients who required placement of proximal aortic cuffs had type I endoleaks.[6]

Proximal fenestrations were first described in 1996[7] but were further tested and refined in a canine model in 1999,[1] where it was found that stents could be mated to the main body of the device without jeopardizing the integrity of the repair. Since that time, fenestrated designs have been used in patients with short-neck infrarenal aneurysms. In effect, this extends the sealing zone for aneurysm repair into healthy, normal-caliber aorta, leading to a more durable design (Figure 52-1).

PLANNING AND SIZING

The era of fenestrated endografting has solidified the importance of three-dimensional imaging in the armamentarium of the vascular surgeon. High-quality, contrast-enhanced computed tomography (CT) should be performed in patients to determine candidacy for fenestrated devices. Postprocessing software, with the capability of multiplanar reconstruction and center lumen of flow analysis, is essential to device design, because generation of a stretched view (Figure 52-2) allows for relational analysis of branched vessels. Determining a healthy segment of aorta, in both diameter and length, should be the first goal of image analysis. Presently, the only manufactured and available fenestrated graft is the Zenith platform (Cook Medical, Bloomington, IN). Proper sizing for a Zenith fenestrated device requires assessing a length of aorta of normal caliber (<30 mm) approximately 25 mm long, which marks the position of the first sealing stent and forms the basis of the remainder of the graft design. Fenestrations are then planned, on the basis of relative distance from the proximal edge of the graft and clock position, to accommodate all branch vessels incorporated in the repair. A bifurcated component is then designed to mate with the fenestrated tube component and sit on the aortic bifurcation. Overlap between these components should be maximized to avoid late component separation as the graft moves to accommodate the anterior wall of the aneurysm sac.[8] Finally, limb extensions are planned to extend the graft distally into normal-caliber iliac arteries. Care is taken to ensure sound proximal and distal fixation and sealing, as well as a bifurcation well placed on the aortic bifurcation, to maintain the stability of the repair.

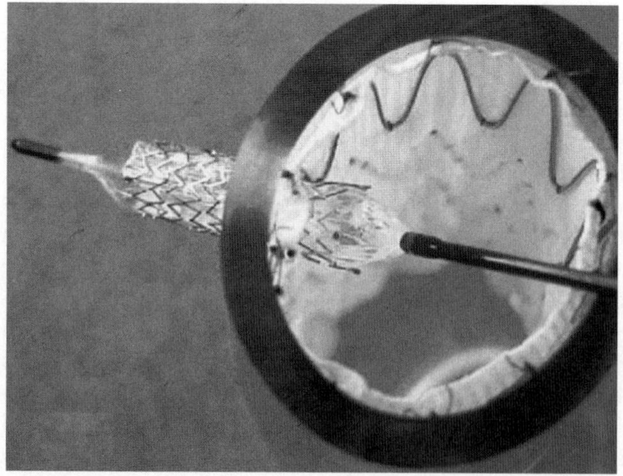

FIGURE 52-1 Ex vivo Zenith fenestrated graft (Cook, Inc). Uncovered, balloon-expandable stent is placed in a reinforced fenestration. (From Greenberg et al. *J Vasc Surg* 43:879–86, 2006.)

PERIOPERATIVE DETAIL

Because the conduct of a fenestrated repair is planned entirely in advance, careful attention to detail when designing the graft is paramount. Specifically, the conduct of the operation is determined by the need for improved access, and placement of an iliofemoral conduit is usually done in a staged procedure well before the implantation of the device, if possible.[9] Preoperative evaluation consists of cardiac, pulmonary, and renal workup to risk stratify before the procedure. In our current population, patients are candidates for fenestrated repair if they are high risk for conventional open surgery and have anatomic contraindications to a commercially available infrarenal graft. For this reason, optimizing pulmonary function before surgery and investigating coronary artery disease with stress echocardiography are our standard protocol. Renal function is assessed with serum creatinine and glomerular filtration rate (GFR) measurement, and patients found to have renal insufficiency are usually hydrated with a sodium bicarbonate infusion before the procedure. For patients with a more significant degree of kidney disease, *N*-acetylcysteine is commonly administered orally in the 24-hour preoperative period. Evaluation by the anesthesia team is also a preoperative requisite, and patients are given the option of regional or general anesthesia.

Once in the operating room, bilateral groin exposures are performed through transverse incisions, and the common femoral arteries are isolated. After systemic heparin administration (100 units/kg, intravenous), wire access is gained through the right common femoral artery, and a stiff wire is carefully advanced into the ascending aorta. A 20F or 22F sheath is advanced into the aorta at the level of the iliac bifurcation, and this Check-Flo sheath (Cook Medical) is punctured multiple times for placement of short 5F sheaths. An aortogram is performed to confirm location of the branch vessels, and commonly two branches are accessed to provide positioning landmarks for the graft. The contralateral femoral artery is then accessed, and a second stiff wire is advanced into the ascending aorta. The fenestrated component of the device is oriented extracorporeally and then introduced into the aorta. The gold markers on the device that correspond to branch vessels are positioned appropriately, and the graft is unsheathed. All fenestrations and corresponding branch vessels are then accessed with stiff wires and 7F or 8F sheaths. Covered balloon-expandable stents are then positioned in the branch vessels. Before deployment of the branch stents, the diameter-reducing ties are removed, and the top cap is released. Once the branch stents are deployed and flared, angiograms are performed selectively in all the branch vessels to ensure no kinking or dissection. The remainder of the case proceeds much like an infrarenal graft, with the bifurcated component introduced from the contralateral side, the short limb cannulated, and the final limb extensions put into place. Completion angiography is done to confirm stent patency and identify endoleaks.

In the postoperative period, the patient is monitored in an intensive care unit. Renal function is monitored, and hydration provided if necessary. When confirmed stable, the patient undergoes a repeated CT scan. Follow-up is scheduled for 1 month, with CT, x-ray examination of the kidneys, ureter, and bladder, and ultrasonography of mesenteric vessels, and then annually thereafter.

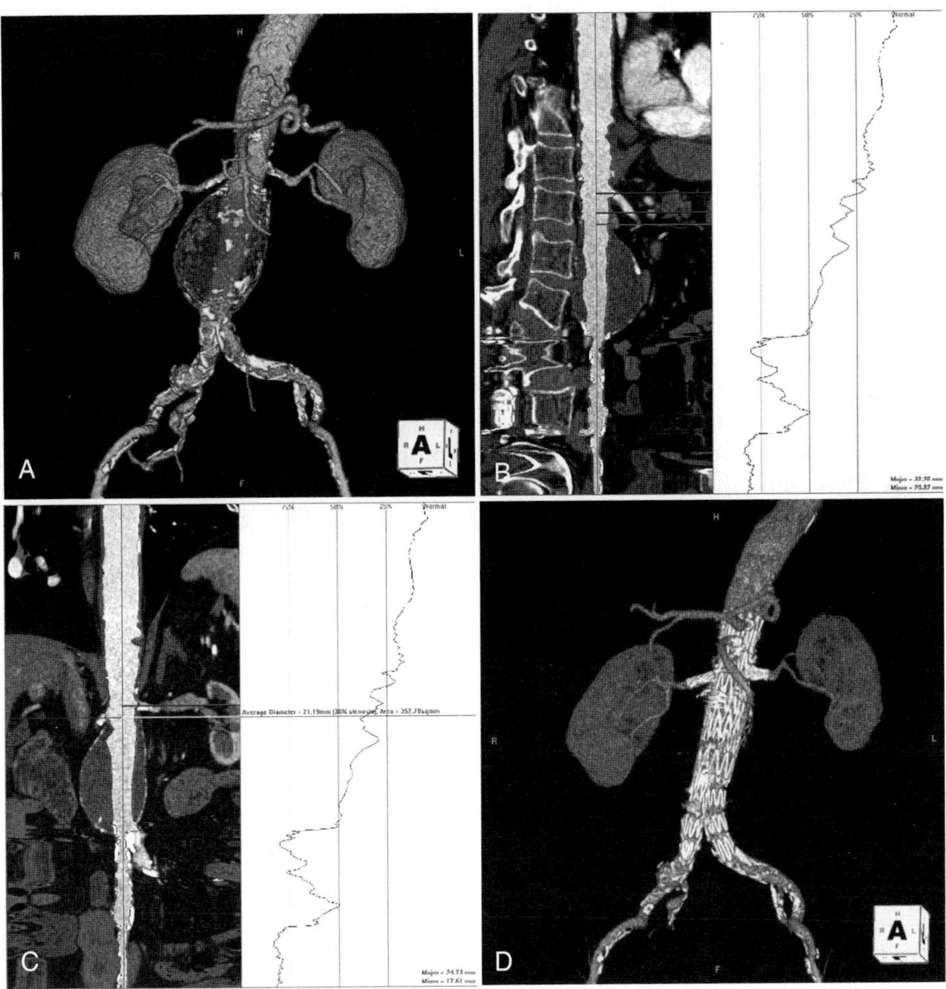

FIGURE 52-2 Preoperative imaging and planning. Postprocessing software (TeraRecon Inc., San Mateo, CA) is used to generate three-dimensional images. **A,** A three-dimensional representation of the aneurysm and its proximity to the renal arteries. A center lumen of flow is then calculated, and a stretched view is generated, from which relational anatomy of the branches is determined. **B,** Relation of the renal arteries to the superior mesenteric artery. **C,** The aneurysm in relation to the superior mesenteric artery. **D,** After stent graft implantation, the same software allows for postoperative surveillance.

TABLE 52-1 Perioperative and Long-term Mortality for Reported Series of Fenestrated Endograft Repair

Author (reference)	30-day mortality, n (%)	Median follow-up, mo (range)	Late mortality, n (%)
Semmens et al., 2006[17]	2/58 (3.4)	16.8 (3-30)	6/58 (10.3)
O'Neill et al., 2006[18]	1/119 (0.8)	19 (0-42)	15/119 (12.6)
Muhs et al., 2006[19]	1/30 (3.3)	25.8 (13-39)	—
Halak et al., 2006[20]	0/15 (0)	20.5 (4-40)	1/15 (6.7)
Ziegler et al., 2007[21]	0/59 (0)	23 (5-41)	14/63 (22)
Scurr et al., 2008[22]	1/45 (2.2)	24 (1-48)	4/45 (8.8)

EVIDENCE AND EXPERIENCE

A thorough review of the literature reveals that only a few centers have published experience with fenestrated grafts, although there have been more than 2000 implanted to date (Cook Medical, personal communication). This reflects the substantial training and unique skill set required to perform these procedures, with limited formal training programs available globally, as well as the inaccessibility of most centers in the United States to use these devices because they are not commercially available. Although some clinicians have developed experience with "back-table" fenestrations or in vivo fenestrated devices,[10,11] these topics are beyond the scope of this review. Thus the centers with the greatest expertise are likely those reporting higher volumes, which means that the current literature likely reflects the efficacy, rather than the effectiveness, of this procedure using a manufactured device and does not predict outcomes for other off-label or homemade devices. However, even with these limitations, the results to date are promising.

The perioperative and late mortality for fenestrated repair is presented in Table 52-1. Determining the appropriate group of patients who have undergone conventional, open repair to provide context or comparison for these results is challenging, because patients who require fenestrated grafts may include those who fit the traditional definition of "juxtarenal" but also may be pure infrarenal repairs. If the juxtarenal cohort is considered, published outcomes from high-volume centers of expertise are presented in Table 52-2. Although statistical comparison is not appropriate, it does appear that published mortality rates for these groups are similar, which is compelling given that fenestrated endovascular interventions are commonly performed in a more high-risk cohort of patients.

Because the instrumentation of renal arteries and use of potentially nephrotoxic contrast are both required for fenestrated repair, it is necessary to also consider renal dysfunction as an important outcome. In the published series, the definitions of renal insufficiency or impairment vary, but the reported outcomes are presented in Table 52-3. A detailed report of renal outcomes for fenestrated devices was published for the first 72 patients treated at the Cleveland Clinic, where it was found that most renal events occurred within the first month after surgery.[12] Deterioration in renal function (GFR <30% of baseline) is more common in patients with baseline renal insufficiency (GFR $\leq$60 mL/min/1.73 m^3) compared with those who have normal preoperative renal function, 39% versus 16.3%, p=.04. Only four patients in this group required any dialysis, all of whom had baseline renal dysfunction. If these results are once again compared with the reported outcomes for juxtarenal aneurysms, there is a striking difference. Qvarfordt et al.[13] reported a rate of 23% renal insufficiency in the perioperative period (defined as serum creatinine >1.2 mg/dL) of which 44% were transient and 89% mild (serum creatinine level rose <1.0 mg/dL), and similarly Sarac et al.[14] reported a rate of renal insufficiency of 27.5% overall, which was higher in patients who had a supravisceral clamp. In the report by Pearce et al.,[15] 14% of patients had acute tubular necrosis, with a 9% in-hospital dialysis rate. The apparent preservation of renal function, despite the use of potentially nephrotoxic contrast and renal artery instrumentation, is encouraging.

TABLE 52-2 Published Reports of Juxtarenal Aneurysms

Author (reference)	30-day mortality	%
Qvarfordt et al., 1986[13]	1/77	1.30
Sarac et al., 2002[14]	7/138	5.07
Pearce et al., 2007[15]	4/134	2.99
Chiesa et al., 2005[23]	4/85	4.71

Beyond the immediate perioperative risk of renal dysfunction, the consequences of long-term renal stenting on renal function have also been studied. Experience at the Cleveland Clinic investigating renal impairment

TABLE 52-3 Renal Impairment

Author (reference)	Transient renal impairment, n (%)	Permanent renal impairment, n (%)	Dialysis, n (%)	Definition
Semmens et al., 2006[17]	N/R	4/58 (6.9)	N/R	Serum creatinine >2 mg/dL
O'Neill et al., 2006[18]	30(25)	2(2)	2(2)	Increase in serum creatinine >30%
Muhs et al., 2006[19*]	N/R	2/38	0/38 (0)	Increase in serum creatinine >50%
Halak et al., 2006[20]	N/R	N/R	1/17 (5.8)	N/R
Ziegler et al., 2007[21*]	8/63 (12.7)	6/63 (9.5)		Serum creatinine >2 mg/dL or >30% compared with baseline
Scurr et al., 2008[22]	N/R	N/R	N/R	

N/R, Not reported.
*Results include patients with thoracoabdominal and thoracic aneurysms because data could not be extracted separately.

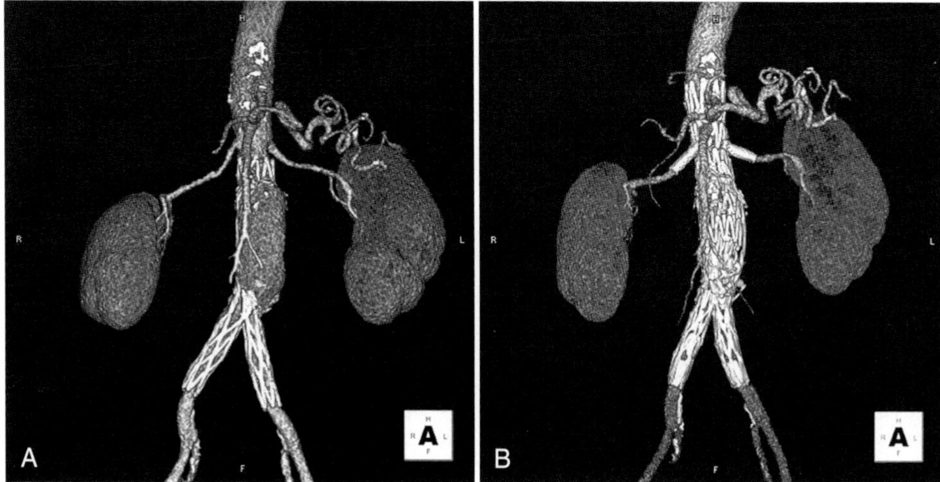

FIGURE 52-3 Preoperative **(A)** and postoperative **(B)** images of migrated infrarenal EVAR graft requiring a fenestrated graft for conversion because of proximal endoleak. Note the sealing zone extension afforded by the fenestrated component.

in fenestrated endografting specifically has found that the rate of renal events decreases with use of covered stents in fenestrations in both fenestrated and branched graft population.[16] With a mean follow-up of 26 months, 518 renal arteries were treated with renal stents or stent grafts (287 patients), and the estimated freedom from stenosis at 12, 24, and 36 months was 95%, 92%, and 89%, respectively, for uncovered stents and 98, 97, and 95, respectively, for covered stents (log rank $p = .04$). Overall, 13 of 287 (4.5%) uncovered stents and 5 of 231 (2.2%) covered stents occluded on follow-up imaging. There were 11 patients whose stent was found occluded at the first postoperative visit, and, when etiology was determined, it was a procedural dissection in 4 arteries, smaller distal renal artery in 3 arteries, and narrowing across the fenestration in 3 arteries. Renal stent occlusions developed in the remaining 7 patients between the 1- and 6-month visit.

Target vessel loss is a commonly reported outcome in endovascular series of fenestrated grafts. Patency of branches is greater than 91% in all series, over variable periods of follow-up.[17-22] Branch occlusion seems more likely to occur in the first year. Multiple causes could contribute to this number, including, in the short term, vessel dissection, inadequate caliber and flow, or graft migration and ostial occlusion. Lack of adequate flow, fracture or in-stent stenosis, and graft migration may be causes. The most important of these factors is migration. Although migration standards in infrarenal grafts are measured significant when greater than 10 mm, movement of the main body more than 1 or 2 mm could compromise a branch stent and cause occlusion. This brings to bear the importance of a stable proximal fixation system, which should be considered and designed in the planning and sizing stages of the preoperative period.

Recently, fenestrated endografts have also been used to repair failed infrarenal EVAR. In these patients, a proximal type 1 endoleak leads to continued aneurysm growth and an aneurysm that is not excluded from circulatory flow. This occurs because of either migration or unfavorable anatomy. Because repair requires extending the sealing zone into the branched segment of the abdominal aorta, a fenestrated "cuff" is used (Figure 52-3). The challenges of this repair are imposed by the configuration of the previously implanted graft. Grafts with intrinsically short bodies leave limited body length for sealing and thus may require conversion to a uni-iliac repair with femoral-femoral bypass by necessity. The role of fenestrated grafts in this scenario will likely expand as early generation grafts mature.

FUTURE DIRECTIONS

There are endovascular options available for abdominal aneurysms with short infrarenal necks or for infrarenal repairs that have failed with conventional devices. Outcomes are promising and rival those of conventional open repair. The next steps will be the conduct of a trial to further refine the indications for this technology in the aneurysm population.

References

1. Browne TF, Hartley D, Purchas S, et al: A fenestrated covered suprarenal aortic stent, *Eur J Vasc Endovasc Surg* 18:445–449, 1999.
2. Parodi JC, Palmaz JC, Barone HD: Transfemoral intraluminal graft implantation for abdominal aortic aneurysms, *Ann Vasc Surg* 5:491–499, 1991.
3. Arko FR, Filis KA, Seidel SA, et al: How many patients with infrarenal aneurysms are candidates for endovascular repair? The Northern California experience, *J Endovasc Ther* 11:33–40, 2004.
4. Cotroneo AR, Iezzi R, Giancristofaro D, et al: Endovascular abdominal aortic aneurysm repair: how many patients are eligible for endovascular repair? *Radiol Med (Torino)* 111(4): 597–606, 2006.
5. Hobo R, Kievit J, Leurs LJ, et al: Influence of severe infrarenal aortic neck angulation on complications at the proximal neck following endovascular AAA repair: a EUROSTAR study, *J Endovasc Ther* 14:1–11, 2007.
6. Hobo R, Laheij RJ, Buth J: The influence of aortic cuffs and iliac limb extensions on the outcome of endovascular abdominal aortic aneurysm repair, *J Vasc Surg* 45:79–85, 2007.
7. Park JH, Chung JW, Choo IW, et al: Fenestrated stent-grafts for preserving visceral arterial branches in the treatment of abdominal aortic aneurysms: preliminary experience, *J Vasc Interv Radiol* 7:819–823, 1996.
8. Dowdall JF, Greenberg RK, West K, et al: Separation of components in fenestrated and branched endovascular grafting: branch protection or a potentially new mode of failure? *Eur J Vasc Endovasc Surg* 36(1):1–9, 2008.
9. Abu-Ghaida AM, Clair DG, Greenberg RK, et al: Broadening the applicability of endovascular aneurysm repair: the use of iliac conduits, *J Vasc Surg* 36:111–117, 2002.
10. Ricotta JJ, Oderich GS: Fenestrated and branched stent grafts, *Perspect Vasc Surg Endovasc.Ther* 20:174–187, 2008.
11. Uflacker R, Robison JD, Schonholz C, et al: Clinical experience with a customized fenestrated endograft for juxtarenal abdominal aortic aneurysm repair, *J Vasc Interv Radiol* 17:1935–1942, 2006.
12. Haddad F, Greenberg RK, Walker E, et al: Fenestrated endovascular grafting: the renal side of the story, *J Vasc Surg* 41:181–190, 2005.
13. Qvarfordt PG, Stoney RJ, Reilly LM, et al: Management of pararenal aneurysms of the abdominal aorta, *J Vasc Surg* 3:84–93, 1986.
14. Sarac TP, Clair DG, Hertzer NR, et al: Contemporary results of juxtarenal aneurysm repair, *J Vasc Surg* 36:1104–1111, 2002.
15. Pearce JD, Edwards MS, Stafford JM, et al: Open repair of aortic aneurysms involving the renal vessels, *Ann Vasc Surg* 21:676–686, 2007.
16. Mohabbat W, Greenberg RK, Mastracci TM, et al: Revised duplex criteria and outcomes for renal stents and stentgrafts following endovascular repair of juxtarenal and thoracoabdominal aneurysms, *J Vasc Surg* 49(4):827–837, 2009.
17. Semmens JB, Lawrence-Brown MM, Hartley DE, et al: Outcomes of fenestrated endografts in the treatment of abdominal aortic aneurysm in Western Australia (1997-2004), *J Endovasc Ther* (13):320–329, 2006.
18. O'Neill S, Greenberg RK, Haddad F, et al: A prospective analysis of fenestrated endovascular grafting: intermediate-term outcomes, *Eur J Vasc Endovasc Surg* 32:115–123, 2006.
19. Muhs BE, Verhoeven EL, Zeebregts CJ, et al: Mid-term results of endovascular aneurysm repair with branched and fenestrated endografts, *J Vasc Surg* 44:9–15, 2006.
20. Halak M, Goodman MA, Baker SR: The fate of target visceral vessels after fenestrated endovascular aortic repair: general considerations and mid-term results, *Eur J Vasc Endovasc Surg* 32:124–128, 2006.
21. Ziegler P, Avgerinos ED, Umscheid T, et al: Branched iliac bifurcation: 6 years experience with endovascular preservation of internal iliac artery flow, *J Vasc Surg* 46:204–210, 2007.
22. Scurr JR, Brennan JA, Gilling-Smith GL, et al: Fenestrated endovascular repair for juxtarenal aortic aneurysm, *Br J Surg* 95:326–332, 2008.
23. Chiesa R, Marone EM, Brioschi C, et al: Open repair of pararenal aortic aneurysms: operative management, early results, and risk factor analysis, *Ann Vasc Surg* 20:739–746, 2006.

CHAPTER

53

Repair of Thoracoabdominal Aortic Aneurysms Using Branched Endografts

Timothy A.M. Chuter, Linda M. Reilly

The thoracoabdominal aorta occupies an inaccessible location high in the abdomen behind the liver, stomach, and pancreas, and its branches supply organs that have a limited tolerance for ischemia. Open surgical repair of a thoracoabdominal aneurysm (TAAA) involves a large incision, extensive dissection, aortic cross-clamp, visceral ischemia, spinal ischemia, and reperfusion injury, all of which contribute to high rates of mortality, morbidity, and disability.[1-6] Although many high-volume surgeons and centers report acceptable results,[4-6] statewide audits show that most patients have a far worse outcome.[1,2]

Endovascular techniques have the potential to avoid many of the more destabilizing aspects of aortic aneurysm repair. A transarterial route of access eliminates the need for a large incision and extensive dissection, and an intact aneurysm and rapid, stent-mediated methods of graft attachment eliminate the need for flow interruption. Endovascular repair would long ago have assumed a prominent role in the management of TAAA, were it not for the presence of indispensable branches to the abdominal organs. One cannot exclude flow to a TAAA without doing something to maintain visceral and renal perfusion.

One approach, described in Chapter 51, employs surgical bypass from a remote location to "debranch" the visceral segment, which then becomes amenable to endovascular repair using simple aortoaortic, or aortoiliac, stent grafts.[7-9] The alternative is to provide the stent graft with branches of its own, which carry blood to corresponding branches of the thoracoabdominal aorta while isolating the aneurysm from the circulation.

Branched stent grafts vary according to the type of attachment between the trunk of the graft and the branches. Unibody stent grafts are inserted whole with the branches already sewn in place.[10] Modular stent grafts[11-17] are assembled in situ from separately inserted components. The main advantage of a unibody stent graft is freedom from risk of component separation. The main disadvantage is the complexity of stent graft construction and insertion, which increases exponentially with each additional branch. Modular stent grafts tend to be simpler, easier to insert, and easier to modify during insertion. These characteristics assume an overriding importance in the endovascular repair of TAAA, with use of a multibranched stent graft.

There are two main types of modular multibranched stent graft: cuffed and fenestrated. A cuffed stent graft has short, axially oriented branches (cuffs) to enhance attachment between its trunk and the self-expanding covered stents that form its branches. Fenestrated stent grafts have no cuffs, only holes (fenestrations) where balloon-expanded covered stents exit the stent graft.

Dr. Chuter receives the following support from Cook, Inc., the manufacturer of the Zenith stent graft: royalties from licensed patents, travel expenses, research funding.

FENESTRATED BRANCHED STENT GRAFTS

The key innovation in stent graft fenestration, the use of a bridging catheter to ensure precise apposition between each fenestration and the orifice of the corresponding renal artery, was first used clinically in 1998 and first reported in 2001.[17] Since then, fenestrated stent grafts have been used to treat juxtarenal aneurysms of the abdominal aorta in thousands of patients. The substitution of a covered stent for the uncovered bridging stent of the standard technique converts the fenestration into a branch. As long as the ring of contact between the fenestration and the stent remains both hemostatic and secure, each branch conveys blood from the primary stent graft to the target artery, while isolating the intervening aneurysm from flow and pressure.

The technique of fenestrated stent graft insertion for juxtarenal abdominal aortic aneurysms is described in Chapter 52. Endovascular repair of TAAA follows essentially the same steps with three notable exceptions: the number of fenestrations is usually higher, covered stents take the place of uncovered stents, and an aneurysm sac lies between the fenestrations and the target artery orifices. These apparently simple differences impart a far higher degree of procedural complexity.

A stent graft with one fenestration is easy to plan and easy to insert; there is only one target. The addition of a second fenestration restricts the options for intraoperative adjustment of position and orientation, and, if the relative positions of the fenestrations fail to match the relative positions of the renal arteries, one may have to choose which of the two will be deployed accurately. This is a problem when angulation of the aorta in the coronal plane introduces uncertainty regarding the final lie of the stent graft. Two more fenestrations, one for the superior mesenteric artery and one for the celiac artery, add even more complexity to device planning and insertion and even more dimensions to the matrix of possible errors.

Covered stents are larger and stiffer than uncovered stents. They often require more support from sheaths and guidewires before they will traverse the path from the lumen of the stent graft to the lumen of the target artery, especially when the target artery in question is short, caudally oriented, or far from the wall of the stent graft.

Covered stents flare less easily than uncovered stents. In TAAA repair the covered stent has to flare both inside and outside the fenestration to help maintain a secure hemostatic intercomponent connection. Ideally, the covered stent should occupy the same transaxial orientation during balloon-driven flange creation as it will when all the wires and balloons have been removed. This can be a difficult goal; angioplasty balloons tend to stand up straight in the aorta on balloon inflation, and the longer they are the more they assume the axial orientation of the aorta, not the transaxial orientation of the branch. The remedy is to use a short balloon and push up on the back end of the balloon (using the sheath) during inflation.

CUFFED BRANCHED STENT GRAFTS

Cuffed stent grafts have been used in TAAA repair almost as long as fenestrated stent grafts have been used to treat juxtarenal aneurysms.[11] Indeed, both techniques were first reported in the same 2001 issue of the *Journal of Endovascular Surgery*. The fundamental aspects of cuffed TAAA repair have changed very little in the past 10 years. The main features of the original physician-made device, namely stainless steel Z-stents, polyester fabric, barb-mediated attachment, caudally oriented cuffs, a tapered trunk, and polytetrafluoroethylene-covered, self-expanding branches, are all present on the current industry-made device. Nevertheless, refinements in stent graft design and insertion technique have changed the operation from an unpredictable 9-hour ordeal into a highly choreographed 4- or 5-hour intervention. Although new applications, such as aortic dissection, continue to provide new challenges, the multibranched endovascular repair of a typical TAAA has been standardized to the point where most repairs can be accomplished with use of off-the-shelf inventory.

Most aspects of the current design of a cuffed stent graft design reflect the characteristics of the Zenith platform, with one exception: there is no uncovered stent. The Z-stent exoskeleton extends throughout the length of the stent graft, except for the ends where the stents are on the inside to enhance apposition between the graft and the implantation site. The proximal ends carry caudally oriented barbs.

Cuff Shape and Orientation

The cuffs are intended to provide a zone of overlap between the trunk of the stent graft and its separately inserted branches. In theory, they can be outside or inside, short or long, straight or helical, and oriented up, down, or out. In practice, most are straight, roughly 2 cm long, and tilted slightly outward relative to the long axis of the trunk with their proximal orifices on the inside and their distal orifices on the outside.

Helical cuffs wrap around the trunk of the stent graft.[13] They are longer than the usual straight cuffs, the idea being that their additional length provides a more stable connection and their changing orientation provides a smoother, more kink-resistant path to the target artery. However, there is no evidence that these putative advantages have any effect on stent graft stability. Moreover, the additional length and bulk of the helical cuff increase the overall delivery system profile and limit the number of helical cuffs to two per device, so helical cuffs to the celiac and superior mesenteric artery are usually used in combination with fenestrations for branches to the renal arteries.

The orientation of the cuff dictates the orientation of the covered stent. When that orientation approximates the longitudinal orientation of the aorta, variation in the relative positions of the cuff and the target artery up and down the aorta affect the length of the covered stent, and variations in the relative positions of the cuff and the target artery around the circumference of the aorta affect the curvature of the covered stent. Both allow intraoperative adjustments in the length, overlap, position, and curvature of the branches to accommodate for preoperative errors in graft design and intraoperative errors in graft deployment. Our 100% success rate in branch insertion (>150 branches) reflects the forgiving nature of the axially oriented cuffs used in the majority of our cases as much as it does the accuracy of stent graft sizing and deployment. Some alarming errors in stent graft design and position early in our experience had surprisingly little effect on the outcome of the procedure.

The vast majority of superior mesenteric and celiac arteries take origin from the aorta in a caudal direction. This is also true of most renal arteries, but not all. Some, most often the left, run in a cranial direction before turning posteriorly to enter the kidney. These cranially oriented renal arteries are most easily catheterized through cranially oriented cuffs. However, we have largely abandoned this approach for three reasons. First, experience has cast doubt over the long-term patency of the cranially oriented branch. Second, with the proper wire and sheath guidance, a covered stent has little difficulty navigating the curved path from a caudally oriented cuff into a cranially oriented renal artery. Third, with the proper stent lining, the covered stent never kinks, however acute the angle between the cuff and the renal artery. The majority of our TAAA repairs are now performed with use of only caudally oriented cuffs. We use very few cranially oriented cuffs and almost no fenestrations (Figure 53-1).

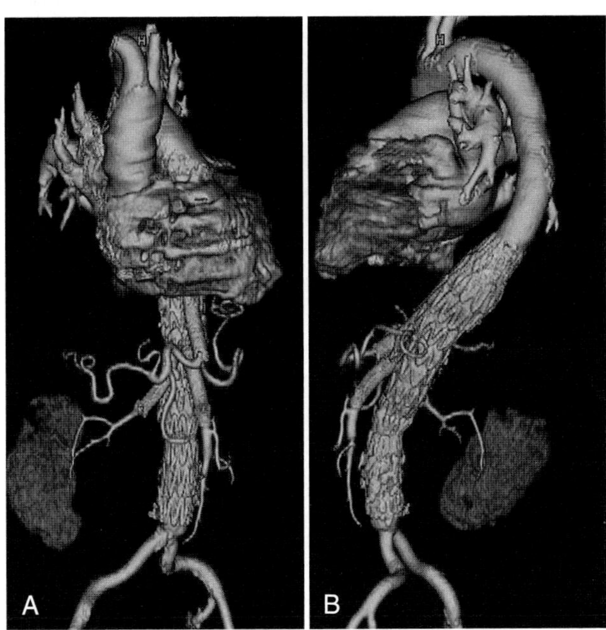

FIGURE 53-1 **A,** AP view of a contrast-enhanced CT scan after endovascular repair of a TAAA using a stent graft with three branches, one to the superior mesenteric artery, one to the celiac artery, and one to the sole renal artery. **B,** Lateral view of the same CT scan as in **A**.

Tapering of the Stent Graft

Because the branches of a cuffed stent graft parallel the trunk before turning outward and exiting the aorta, the trunk and branches compete for space. This is not an issue when the entire visceral segment is both dilated and devoid of mural thrombus, but in many cases the residual lumen may be quite small, especially when the primary pathology was aortic dissection. Our preferred design has a narrow (18 mm wide) distal segment where the branches originate and a wider proximal segment where the stent graft attaches to the native aorta or the distal end of a supraceliac stent graft (Figure 53-2). We used to worry that such a dramatic reduction in the diameter of the trunk of the stent graft would generate a hemodynamic load on the stent graft and cause migration. Although we may be right about the forces on the stent graft, long-term results show that these forces have little effect on the position of the stent graft. With a total experience of 50 cases and follow-up of as much as 4 years, we have never seen any evidence of instability. The stent grafts have neither moved nor changed shape. This stability may be attributable in part to barb-mediated proximal attachment and in part to the bracing provided by four short, stiff caudally oriented branches. Unless these branches buckle or break, which seems unlikely given their structure, the stent graft simply cannot migrate, at least not in a caudal direction.

Proximal and Distal Extensions

Patients with TAAA have widely varying aortic anatomy. However, most of this heterogeneity is the result of variation in the extent of the aneurysm or the extent of prior reconstructive surgery. The relative positions of the visceral arteries are surprisingly consistent, and most of that variability can be accommodated by intraoperative adjustments in the length and orientation of the stent graft branches, as described earlier.

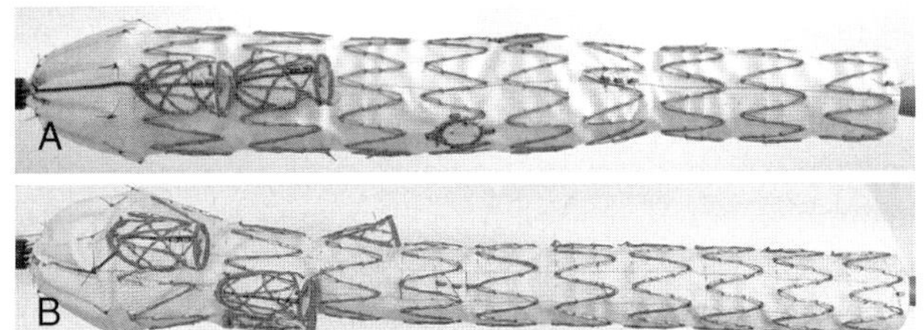

FIGURE 53-2 **A,** A photograph of the primary aortic stent graft for use in a case of TAAA, showing two cuffs and a fenestration. Note the uniform diameter of the trunk necessitated by the presence of a fenestrated branch. **B,** A photograph of the primary aortic stent graft for use in another case of TAAA, showing four cuffs. Note the tapered shape of the trunk, which is typical of a stent graft with multiple cuffed branches.

Consequently, the majority of patients can be treated with use of the same off-the-shelf cuffed stent grafts in combination with a small range of proximal and distal extensions. Our off-the-shelf inventory currently comprises the following: two tapered thoracic aortic stent grafts of different lengths, one cuffed stent graft with four caudally oriented cuffs, one bifurcated distal extension for bi-iliac implantation, and one flared distal extension for aortic implantation. To these we add various commercially available Zenith ZTEG (thoracic) and TFLE (iliac) components.

STAGED REPAIR

In the presence of complicating factors such as branch artery stenosis or iliac artery disease, we try to stage the repair in the belief that high-risk patients tolerate two small operations better than one large one. We have found that the total blood loss, for example, is greatly reduced by allowing coagulation to return to normal after iliac bypass operation. Proceeding directly from retroperitoneal surgery to stent graft implantation requires continued anticoagulation, which perpetuates oozing within the surgical field for the duration of the endovascular procedure. In general we perform the first operation a week or more before stent graft insertion to allow time for recovery, but the interval may be even longer when the findings of the first operation influence the design of the stent graft.

Iliac Bypass

If the external iliac artery is tortuous or narrow, we create an ilioiliac bypass between an end-to-end anastomosis with the proximal common iliac or proximal external iliac artery, and an end-to-side anastomosis with the distal external iliac artery. The intra-abdominal termination of an ilioiliac bypass avoids the increased risk of infection that would otherwise result from serial surgical exposure of an iliofemoral bypass. If both common iliac arteries are aneurysmal, we combine iliofemoral bypass with a rerouting of flow to the ipsilateral internal iliac artery.

If the renal or mesenteric arterial orifices are stenotic, we perform balloon angioplasty and stent placement through a brachial sheath, taking care to ensure that very little, if any, of the stent protrudes into the aortic lumen. Balloon-expanded stents are used in the renal arteries and self-expanding stents in the celiac and superior mesenteric arteries. Sometimes we cannot tell from the computed tomographic angiography (CTA) whether the celiac artery is occluded or severely stenotic. The proximal orifice may be occluded while the trunk remains patent because of retrograde perfusion through the left gastric artery. In addition, the celiac artery often runs parallel to the aorta for 10 to 20 mm where it is compressed by the diaphragm. Lateral views, high frame rates, and selective superior mesenteric injections all help make the diagnosis.

If there are two renal arteries on one side, we perform angiography to decide whether one, both, or none are suitable recipient sites for a branch of the stent graft. Arteries wider than 4 mm or more are preserved, arteries narrower than 2 mm are ignored, and arteries of 2 to 4 mm are embolized to prevent type II endoleak.

If the left brachial artery pressure is less than the right, we perform carotid-subclavian bypass in the belief that the left subclavian artery is a potential source of collateral perfusion to the spine. This operation is often indicated when the distal aortic arch has already undergone endovascular repair of a type B dissection or descending thoracic aortic aneurysm because the subclavian artery has a rich collateral supply and direct subclavian inflow has long been considered dispensable.

If the underlying pathology is aortic dissection, there may be multiple anatomic obstacles to endovascular repair to be overcome at a preliminary operation. For example, true lumen compression may require the insertion of conventional single-lumen stent graft into the proximal descending thoracic aorta to seal the primary tear, induce false lumen thrombosis, and promote true lumen expansion. In addition, we sometimes have to fenestrate the interluminal septum to gain access to all four arterial orifices, or insert kissing stents to connect the true lumens of the aorta and the iliac arteries.

Stent Graft Insertion

The basic steps in cuffed branched stent graft insertion have changed very little since 2000 when the operation was first performed.[11] We still insert the aortic components through surgically exposed femoral arteries, starting with the most proximal, and the branched stents through surgically exposed brachial arteries, starting with the most distal. Each branch consists of a self-expanding covered stent and a self-expanding uncovered stent. A long sheath from the brachial artery to the inside of the stent graft protects the aortic arch from the embolic risks for repeated instrumentation. A catheter is directed through one of the cuffs into the perigraft aorta and then into the target artery. After angiographic identification of the orifice and branches of the target artery, the catheter is exchanged over a stiff wire for the covered stent delivery system. The covered stent is deployed with at least 10 mm of overlap into the target artery, then lined with an uncovered stent, which projects approximately 5 mm from both ends of the covered stent. This sequence is repeated until all the branches are in place.

Although the principles remain the same, the details of stent graft insertion have gradually evolved over the years. Our current approach includes the following technical refinements.

Selective Visceral Angiography

We seldom inject contrast into the main lumen of the aorta. Direct selective injection of 3 to 5 mL of half-strength contrast through a catheter with its tip in the target artery generally provides the superior localizing information. Once in place, the radiopaque catheter serves as a marker for the visceral orifice even as the field of view changes to track the movement of the stent graft delivery system. Using this approach we have been able to implant multi-branched thoracoabdominal stent grafts using as little as 28 mL of contrast and never more than 100 mL.

Sheath Support

The path from the left brachial artery to the visceral aorta is both long and tortuous. When the brachial sheaths, or their contents, encounter resistance to insertion they tend to coil at points of angulation such as the aortic arch, whereupon their tips "push back" out of target arteries. Stiff guidewires and additional sheath provide some support, but the best prophylaxis against coiling is provided by a brachiofemoral guidewire.

Once we have deployed the cuffed stent graft we withdraw the visceral selective catheter into the aorta and redirect it through one of the cuffs into the lumen of the stent graft. Then we pass it proximally over a guidewire to the distal aortic arch. We exchange the catheter for a 6F sheath and triple-loop snare, with which we retrieve a floppy transbrachial guidewire. Tension on the ends of this 0.035-inch guidewire provides the support needed to insert a 10F sheath through the left brachial artery, around the distal aortic arch, and down the descending thoracic aorta. Once the sheath is in place within the cuffed stent graft, we exchange the 0.035-inch wire for a 0.014-inch coronary wire, which remains in place for the rest of the operation. This wire actually bridges a relatively short distance between two sheaths, one in the left femoral artery and one in the brachial artery. These sheaths protect the iliac arteries and subclavian orifice from cheese-wire injury when tension is applied to the brachiofemoral wire. We perform all subsequent transbrachial instrumentation through a separate puncture in the margin of the valve of the 10F brachial sheath. The alternative is to link two Tuohy-Borst ports to create a dual access sheath. The diaphragms of the Tuohy-Borst assembly provide better hemostasis than the double-punctured valve, but the additional length may limit catheter choice.

Atraumatic Visceral Artery Instrumentation

The delivery system used for the usual 7- and 9-mm covered stents (Fluency, C.R. Bard, Inc, Murry Hill, NJ) is relatively large (9F outer diameter) and blunt-ended. Attempts to introduce this device through areas of angulation or luminal irregularity sometimes destabilize the position of guidewires, catheters, and sheaths. Unless one is very careful, the resulting paradoxical movements can injure the target artery, causing extravasation or dissection. Renal artery injury used to be our commonest serious complication, but not anymore. A few simple changes in insertion technique have simplified covered stent insertion and eliminated this source of perioperative morbidity and mortality.

The brachiofemoral coronary wire stabilizes sheath and guidewire position, even when the tip of the Fluency delivery system encounters resistance and the curled tip of the Rosen guidewire (Cook Medical, Bloomington, IN) extends only a short way into the trunk of the left renal artery.

In those rare instances when the target artery will not admit the uncovered tip of the covered stent delivery system it will admit the smaller, more flexible delivery system of an uncovered stent, such as a Wallstent (Boston Scientific, Natick, MA), with or without the aid of a Shuttle Select (Cook Medical) sheath. The Wallstent then smoothes and straightens the pathway enough for the Flexor to pass.

Covered Stent Support

Having never inserted the covered Fluency stent without the additional luminal support of a vascular Wallstent, we cannot really say whether the Wallstent made any difference to the stability or patency of the stent graft but are reluctant to change such a successful approach. This practice was originally based on the observation that, in the absence of additional stent support, the Fluency covered stent tends to kink, whereas the supported Fluency tolerates bends of 90 degrees, or more, without any evidence of luminal compromise. The Wallstent may also contribute to stent graft stability by sticking out of the ends of the Fluency. The distal end of the Wallstent keeps the artery from folding over the distal end of the Fluency. It may also become incorporated into the surrounding artery, thereby holding both the Wallstent and the Fluency in position. The proximal end of the Wallstent may have a similar stabilizing effect. Outside the confines of the Fluency it expands into a short cone that is too wide to pull out through the cuff of the stent graft.

MEASURES TO PREVENT PARAPLEGIA

A rich network of collateral arteries feeds the intercostal and lumbar branches of the thoracoabdominal aorta, all of which remain patent after endovascular TAAA repair.[18] Inflow to this collateral network is through the left subclavian and internal iliac arteries, and loss of either one has been shown to increase the rate of lower-extremity weakness. Spinal perfusion also depends heavily on systemic blood pressure. In our experience, lower-extremity weakness only ever occurs when the systolic pressure falls below 90 mm Hg, and the prompt elevation of blood pressure, with or without a reduction in cerebrospinal fluid (CSF) pressure, produces a prompt resolution of symptoms.[18] In our experience, permanent weakness occurred only when hypotension persisted.

We have never had a patient wake from anesthesia with lower-extremity weakness. Nevertheless, on insertion of the last branch of the stent graft we take the precaution of raising systolic pressure to at least 130 mm Hg and draining 20 mL of CSF per hour through a previously placed spinal catheter. We continue spinal drainage at the rate of 10 mL/hr to keep the catheter patent for at least 24 hours after the operation, because experience has shown that prompt spinal drainage is an effective adjunct to blood pressure elevation in cases of lower-extremity weakness. Blood pressure is monitored closely and maintained pharmacologically during the first postoperative night. Most patients are then allowed to become moderately hypertensive after the perioperative withdrawal, or reduction, of antihypertensive medications.

Although these measures appear to have been effective, we are starting to reevaluate the role of the spinal catheter. It has been more than a year since we had a case of lower-extremity weakness and more than 2 years since we had a case of permanent lower-extremity weakness, during which time the only neurologic complication was caused by hydrocephalus from catheter-related bleeding into the subarachnoid space. In the meantime, cases have been canceled when blood-tinged CSF precluded the administration of heparin.

PATIENT SELECTION

The proper management of a TAAA depends on the relative risks of five alternatives: no treatment, conventional surgical repair, visceral bypass combined with endovascular repair, endovascular repair using a fenestrated multibranched stent graft, and endovascular repair using a cuffed multibranched stent graft. These decisions depend to some extent on patient-specific characteristics such as the extent of the aneurysm, the general health of the patient, the presence of concomitant arterial disease, and prior surgical repair and to some extent on technique-specific constraints such as regulatory barriers to device availability, delays in manufacture, and local experience with multibranched stent graft implantation.

When we first started to used branched stent grafts we decided to use this investigational technology only in patients whose large aneurysms and poor health precluded all the other management options. Our current results, with perioperative mortality and paraplegia rates less than 5%, probably warrant a reassessment of these selection criteria. These results compare favorably with the published results of both open repair and hybrid repair, especially when undertaken for extensive aneurysms (types 2 and 3). Although the extent of the TAAA is a major determinant of outcome after open surgical repair, we have not found the same to be true of endovascular repair. One would not expect it to be; the length of a multibranched stent graft has little bearing on the complexity of the operation, the size of the incision, the extent of the dissection, the amount of blood loss, or the duration of visceral ischemia. In our experience, the extent of the repair did not even seem have any effect on the rate of lower-extremity weakness.

However good the short-term results of endovascular TAAA repair may be, we still lack the long-term results to advocate this form of repair for patients whose general health is either very good or very poor. Those in very poor health do not live long enough to reap the benefits of freedom from risk of rupture, whereas those in very good health may live long enough to see the device fail, not that we have seen any long-term changes in the position, structure, or function of any multibranched stent graft. The only late problems have been stent graft erosion in one unusual case and branch artery stenosis or occlusion in fewer than 5%. All presented within 6 months of stent graft implantation, and, in all but one, the distal end of the covered stent abutted an area of angulation or branching in the renal artery. We have modified implantation technique accordingly and added antiplatelet agents to the postoperative regimen.

Very few patients lack the anatomic substrate for endovascular aneurysm repair using a branched stent graft. The procedure may be easier in the absence of aortic tortuosity, aortic dissection, iliac stenosis, iliac aneurysm, and visceral artery stenosis, but far from impossible, if one is prepared to apply some of the adjunctive maneuvers described above. A particular pattern of anatomic distortion sometimes calls for a particular form of branched repair. However, we have found a branching pattern based on caudally directed cuffs to be the safest, most predictable, and most effective solution in the majority of cases. Moreover, the adaptability of the cuffed approach permits the use of standard off-the-shelf components, which have the potential to eliminate the manufacturing delays that would otherwise prevent the inclusion of patients with symptoms. We seldom use fenestrated branches, except in cases of pararenal aneurysm where a balloon-expanded covered stent bridges a very short gap with little potential for intercomponent movement, separation, or fracture. But we would not use fenestrated branches to treat more extensive aneurysms, which require more than two branches, and we have used cuffed branches in areas where the lumen, or true lumen, of the aorta measures only 12 mm in transverse diameter.

CONCLUSION

For all its advantages, endovascular TAAA repair has yet to achieve widespread application. The situation is changing as centers in Europe, Canada, Australia, and South America acquire the necessary skills and facilities, but nothing of the sort can occur in the United States where regulatory barriers to device availability will remain in place until some manufacturer sees a potential market large enough to justify the cost of an Investigational Device Exemption study. However safe, effective, and durable multibranched repair proves to be, it suffers from one major limitation that may keep it forever out of the hands of U.S. surgeons, and that is the combination of multiple components from multiple manufacturers.

References

1. Rigberg DA, McGory ML, Zingmond DS, et al: Thirty day mortality statistics underestimate the risk of repair of thoracoabdominal aortic aneurysms: a statewide experience, *J Vasc Surg* 43:217–223, 2006.
2. Cowan JA Jr, Dimick JB, Henke PK, et al: Surgical treatment of intact thoracoabdominal aortic aneurysms in the United States: hospital and surgeon volume-related outcomes, *J Vasc Surg* 37:1169–1174, 2003.
3. Gloviczki P: Surgical repair of thoracoabdominal aneurysms: patient selection, techniques and results, *Cardiovascular Surg* 10:434–441, 2002.
4. Coselli JS, LeMaire SA, Miller CC 3rd, et al: Mortality and paraplegia after thoracoabdominal aortic aneurysm repair: a risk factor analysis, *Ann Thorac Surg* 69:409–414, 2000.
5. Safi HJ, Miller CC 3rd, Carr C, et al: Importance of intercostal artery reattachment during thoracoabdominal aortic aneurysm repair, *J Vasc Surg* 27:58–66, 1998.
6. Jacobs MJ, Mommertz G, Koeppel TA, et al: Surgical repair of thoracoabdominal aortic aneurysms, *J Cardiovasc Surg* 48:49–58, 2007.
7. van de Mortel RHW, Wahl AC, Balm R, et al: Collective experience with hybrid procedures for suprarenal and thoracoabdominal aortic aneurysms, *Vascular* 16:140–146, 2008.
8. Black SA, Wolfe JHN, Clark M, et al: Complex thoracoabdominal aortic aneurysms: endovascular exclusion with visceral revascularization, *J Vasc Surg* 43:1081–1089, 2006.
9. Resch TA, Greenberg RK, Lyden SP, et al: Combined staged procedures for the treatment of thoracoabdominal aneurysms, *J Endovasc Ther* 13:491–499, 2006.
10. Inoue K, Iwase T, Sato M, et al: Transluminal endovascular branched graft placement for a pseudoaneurysm: reconstruction of the descending thoracic aorta including the celiac axis, *J Thorac Cardiovasc Surg* 114:859–861, 1997.
11. Chuter TA, Gordon L, Reilly LM, et al: Multi-branched stent-graft for type III thoracoabdominal aortic aneurysm, *J Vasc Interv Radiol* 12:391–392, 2001.
12. Chuter TA, Rapp JH, Hiramoto JS, et al: Endovascular treatment of thoracoabdominal aortic aneurysms, *J Vasc Surg* 47(1):6–16, 2008.
13. Greenberg RK, West K, Pfaff K, et al: Beyond the aortic bifurcation: branched endovascular grafts for thoracoabdominal and aortoiliac aneurysms, *J Vasc Surg* 43:879–886, 2006.
14. Verhoeven EL, Tielliu IF, Muhs BE, et al: Fenestrated and branched stent-grafting: a 5-years experience, *Acta Chir Belg* 317–322, 2006.
15. Anderson JL, Adam DJ, Berce M, et al: Repair of thoracoabdominal aortic aneurysms with fenestrated and branched endovascular stent-grafts, *J Vasc Surg* 42:600–607, 2005.
16. Chuter TA, Hiramoto JS, Chang C, et al: Branched stent-grafts: will these become the new standard? *J Vasc Interv Radiol* 19:S57–S62, 2008.
17. Stanley BM, Semmens JB, Lawrence-Brown MM, et al: Fenestration in endovascular grafts for aortic aneurysm repair: new horizons for preserving blood flow in branch vessels, *J Endovasc Ther* 8:16–24, 2001.
18. Chang CK, Chuter TA, Reilly LM, et al: Spinal arterial anatomy and risk factors for lower extremity weakness following endovascular thoracoabdominal aortic aneurysm repair with branched stent-grafts, *J Endovasc Ther* 15(3):356–362, 2008.

CHAPTER

54

Endovascular Repair of Acute and Chronic Thoracic Aortic Dissections

Karthikeshwar Kasirajan

The most revolutionary management option for descending aortic dissections was first introduced by Wheat et al.[1] in 1965, when they described medical therapy directed toward lowering blood pressure and the aortic pulsation. Various other investigators have made significant advances in the detection, characterization, and treatment of aortic dissection; however, the morbidity and mortality remain relatively high, with an overall in-hospital mortality of 27.4% reported by the International Registry of Aortic Dissection.[2] The latest additions to the armamentarium to treat dissection have been based on thoracic stent graft techniques aimed at covering the primary entry point. The less-invasive nature of this technique makes it an attractive alternative to open surgical intervention with continued improvement in techniques and dissection-specific devices.

CLASSIFICATION

The most frequently used anatomic classifications of aortic dissection are the DeBakey and Stanford classifications. In the DeBakey system, type I dissection begins in the proximal aorta and involves both the ascending and descending thoracic aorta, type II dissection is confined to the ascending aorta, and type III is confined to the descending aorta. In the Stanford system, type A dissection involves the ascending aorta, whereas type B dissection does not. The convenience and clinical value of the Stanford system have resulted in its being most commonly used. Both these classifications do not typically address the location of the primary entry point. The location of the entry point is the focus of treatment in the use of currently available endografts. For example, in a typical type A dissection, the primary tear is located in the ascending aorta, making this a non-endograft zone. However, in a retrograde type A dissection, the entry tear maybe located in the descending aorta, hence presenting the potential for stent graft treatment. Thus the location of the entry point has a profound influence on the current feasibility of stent graft management. A new proposed entry point–based classification of dissections is provided in Table 54-1.

A time-from-event–based nonanatomic classification is also frequently used. This classifies a dissection as acute when identified ≤2 weeks from the onset of symptoms and chronic when identified more than 2 weeks from the onset of symptoms. This classification was proposed on the basis of the fact that the highest morbidity and mortality occur during the first 2 weeks. Some investigators further classify the acute phase as early (<24 hours) and late (≥24 hours to 2 weeks) from the onset of symptoms. If stent grafts are used to cover the entry point, the false-lumen elimination is based on the mobility of the septum. The mobility and pliability of the septum in turn depend on the time for the initial event (Figure 54-1). In the early phase the septum is thin and very mobile, allowing for complete aortic remodeling after endograft treatment (Figure 54-2, *A* and *B*). However, in the chronic phase despite false-lumen thrombosis the thickened septum is quite immobile preventing total resolution of the false channel. On the basis of the author's experience, the septum continues to remodel and reposition up to 3 months, potentially classifying the initial 3 months as the "dynamic" or "acute" phase of the dissections. Additionally, up to another 12 months stent grafts have been noted to produce total aortic remodeling; hence we classify these as the "subacute phase" or the "compliant" phase of dissections. The real "chronic" or the "noncompliant" phase is probably best represented by patients beyond the 12-month period. Thoracic stent grafts have the least complications and best anatomic result when used in the subacute and chronic phase of dissections.

TABLE 54-1 Dissection Classification Based on the Primary Entry Point

Dissection	Location of entry point
Zone I	Ascending aorta to left common carotid
Zone II	Distal to left common carotid artery
IIa	Distal extension only
IIb	Associated with retrograde extension

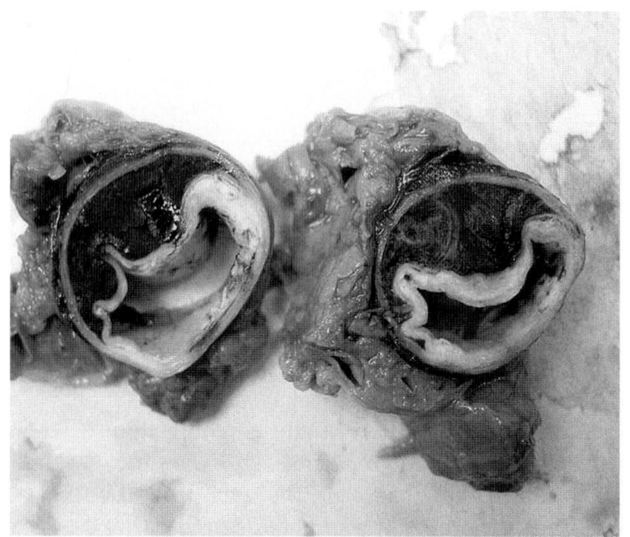

FIGURE 54-1 Difference in thickness of septum between acute *(left)* and chronic *(right)* dissection.

NATURAL HISTORY AND CONVENTIONAL MANAGEMENT

The mortality associated with acute uncomplicated distal aortic dissection managed medically is quite low (≤10%). If complications arise that require surgical intervention, this figure increases to 30% or more. Hence, because of the small risk of aortic rupture and sudden death and the high morbidity and mortality associated with surgical repair of the descending aorta in the acute phase, medical treatment alone has historically been advocated for uncomplicated type B dissection. Because medical therapy alone does not stop flow within the false lumen, in 20% to 50% of patients who survive the acute phase, aneurysmal dilatation of the false lumen develops within 1 to 5 years after onset. Dialetto et al.[3] reported that 28.5% of uncomplicated type B dissections managed medically progressed to aneurysmal dilatation at a mean of 18.1 ± 16.9 months. Risk factors for progressive aneurysmal degeneration were patency of the false lumen or patients in whom the distal aortic diameter was ≥40 to 45 mm. Adequate management of hypertension does not appear to have a protective effect. The majority of late deaths that occur in patients with type B dissection initially managed by medical therapy are due to rupture, extension of dissection, and perioperative mortality of the subsequent surgery. In fact, the long-term survival after the acute phase of patients with type B dissection remains worse than that of patients with type A dissection, because the majority of type A dissections are repaired in the acute phase.

A report from the International Registry of Aortic Dissection database analyzing outcomes of acute type

FIGURE 54-2 **A,** Preprocedural image of patient with acute dissection. **B,** Postprocedure image demonstrating complete aortic remodeling.

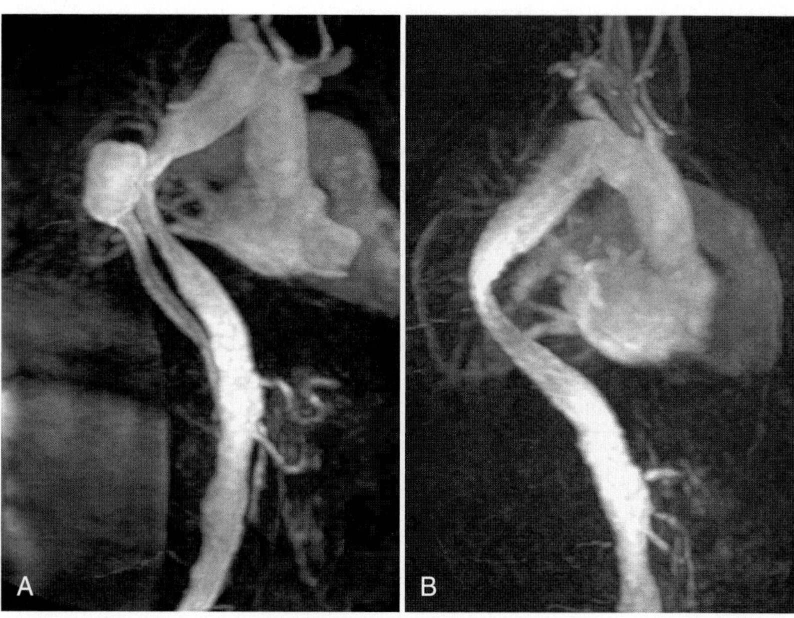

B dissection in 242 patients who survived initial hospitalization showed 3-year survival for medical therapy to be 77.6% ± 6.6%, surgical repair 82.8% ± 18.9%, and endovascular therapy 76.2% ± 25.2%, respectively.[2]

CURRENT INDICATIONS FOR INVASIVE MANAGEMENT OF DESCENDING AORTIC DISSECTIONS

Uncomplicated Acute and Subacute Descending Aortic Dissections

The majority of patients presenting with an acute descending (zone II) dissection can be managed medically. There is no role for routine open surgical management in this patient population. The routine use of thoracic stent grafts in all patients at the initial presentation has the theoretic advantage of preventing delayed false lumen enlargement and the potential for complete aortic remodeling. However, complications associated with the use of the current generation of stent grafts do not warrant their routine use in uncomplicated zone II dissections. The INSTEAD trial (INvestigation of STEnt grafts in patients with type B Aortic Dissection) is a prospective trial designed to compare outcomes of patients randomly assigned to either stent graft or best medical management.[21] Inclusion criteria include age greater than 18 years, uncomplicated type B dissection, and lack of spontaneous thrombosis in the false lumen 14 days after the index event. Although the INSTEAD data have not yet been published, the initial report has demonstrated superiority in the medically treated group primarily because of device-specific complications.

Complicated Acute and Subacute Descending Thoracic Dissections

A variety of complications can happen in the acute phase as given in Box 54-1. In patients with complicated dissection, the mortality was significantly greater (18%) compared with uncomplicated dissection (1.2%). Certain indications require emergent treatment for survival, such as rupture and mesenteric ischemia. Certain other indications for stent graft therapy can be quite "soft." These include refractory hypertension, persistent back pain, and even acute paraplegia. Indeed, hypertension that is difficult to control or refractory to medical management can be present in nearly two thirds of patients in some reports. Estrera et al.[4] followed 159 consecutive patients, admitted between January 2001 and April 2006, who had acute type B dissection, all initially managed medically. In their report the median time to obtain a systolic blood pressure less than 140 mm Hg and to control primary pain was 48 hours. Presentation with paralysis is reported to occur in 2% to 8% of patients who had distal dissection. Similar to our experience they observed that limb, spinal, and visceral malperfusion could in a significant number of cases spontaneously resolve. Overall, in two thirds of patients presenting with paraplegia the condition resolved spontaneously. An overtly aggressive approach to blood pressure control may also exacerbate the renal and visceral ischemia. Hence, deciding when to intervene in any given patient may not be straightforward and may require multiple imaging studies and the operator's experience. A complication-specific treatment plan is recommended, with rupture being addressed with stent grafting and malperfusion issues addressed predominantly by endovascular stent grafting with or without branch artery stenting.

Chronic Dissections

The primary indication for treatment in this phase is dilatation of the false lumen. Once aneurysmal degeneration has set in during the chronic phase, it generally recommended that patients with an aortic diameter greater than 50 mm (or 55 mm) or growth of greater than 5 mm over a 6-month period seek treatment. This recommendation is extrapolated from the encouraging data in the population with atherosclerotic aneurysm,

BOX 54-1

COMPLICATIONS IN THE ACUTE PHASE THAT WOULD PROMPT INVASIVE TREATMENT

- Rupture
- Refractory hypertension
- Persistent back pain
- Acute false-lumen enlargement
- Mesenteric ischemia
- Limb ischemia
- Acute renal failure
- Retrograde dissection
- Paraplegia

BOX 54-2

ENDOGRAFT PRINCIPLES FOR DISSECTIONS

1. Size endograft to normal proximal aorta between the left common carotid and subclavian artery.
2. Use minimal stent-graft over sizing (5%-10%).
3. Limit coverage to 20 cm or less.
4. Do not balloon dilate the stent graft after deployment.
5. Routinely deploy device just distal to the left common carotid artery (cover subclavian).
6. Strict postoperative blood pressure control in the intensive care unit.

particularly with the reduced incidence of spinal cord injury, although how well this translates to the population with chronic dissection is currently unknown. With use of traditional open surgery the indications for repair have been 6.5 cm, given the high incidence of postoperative complications. We currently offer endovascular treatment for patients with total aortic diameter of ≥5.5 cm or patients with rapid expansion or new onset back pain. The majority of our chronic patients (74%) had chronic back pain at time of treatment, and interestingly after treatment 12 (34%) had resolution in back pain.

Several studies have demonstrated higher in-hospital mortality rates and major complication rates for patients treated with stent graft placement for descending aortic dissection in the acute phase compared with the chronic phase. Specifically, these include device collapse and retrograde dissection into the ascending aorta. Kato et al.[5] speculated that worse outcomes in the acute phase after endograft treatment may reflect sequelae caused by unfavorable morphologic alterations of a fragile dissection membrane compared with manipulation of a more fibrotic and stable flap in the subacute. This has led us to delay stent graft treatment if possible to the subacute or chronic phase.

PRINCIPLES OF ENDOGRAFT TREATMENT

The goal of endograft treatment is to cover the entry point.[6] This is most commonly located just distal to the left subclavian artery (LSA). In the acute phase of dissection the entire descending thoracic aorta is very fragile and the intima can quite easily be perforated. The most stable portion of the thoracic aorta is the arch proximal to the LSA. Hence, I routinely extend the proximal portion of the stent graft to cover the LSA and land it just distal to the left common carotid artery (CCA). Postdeployment balloon dilatation of the stent graft should be avoided. Sizing is based on the normal aorta located between the left CCA and the LSA. Minimal oversizing at 5% to 10% is recommended. Strict control of the blood pressure to avoid hypertension in the postoperative period is also vital in avoiding stent graft–induced complications. These four principles (Box 54-2) have helped minimize complications such as stent collapse and proximal extension of the dissection. Type A conversion is also more likely in devices with proximal bare springs (Figure 54-3). In the future, dissection-specific endografts will eliminate proximal bare springs, optimize radial force, and better approximate to the inner curve of the aorta. Single side-branch devices may also help to maintain flow through the LSA. With a few exceptions (Box 54-3) the LSA can be covered. It is important to image the termination of the left vertebral artery that is most often not properly evaluated. In about 15% of patients the left vertebral can end in the posterior inferior cerebellar artery and not in the basilar artery. Covering the left vertebral artery that terminates in the posterior inferior cerebellar artery can result in a vertebrobasilar stroke. We either get a preoperative computed tomographic (CT) angiogram or magnetic resonance (MR) angiogram of both vertebral arteries

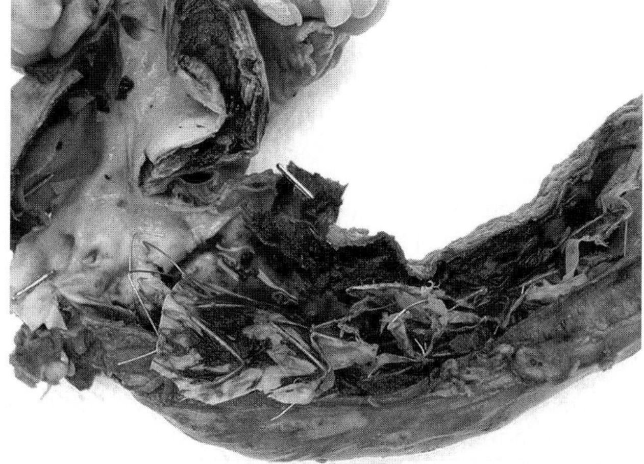

FIGURE 54-3 Retrograde extension of the dissection in a proximal bare spring device (Talent, Cordis, Warren, NJ).

BOX 54-3

INDICATIONS FOR LEFT CAROTID–SUBCLAVIAN BYPASS OR TRANSPOSITION

1. Left internal mammary artery bypass
2. Left vertebral terminating in the posterior inferior cerebellar artery
3. Dominant left vertebral artery
4. Innominate or right subclavian stenosis/occlusion
5. Dialysis graft or fistula in left arm
6. Left brachial occlusion (beware of prior brachial catheterization)
7. Anomalous origin of left vertebral from the aortic arch
8. Dysphagia lusoria
9. Prior left axillofemoral bypass graft

or perform a selective left vertebral angiogram at the time of the procedure.

TECHNICAL ASPECTS

A preoperative CT scan is evaluated in detail to access the access vessels, branch vessel involvement, extent of dissection, and diameter of the normal proximal aorta for stent graft selection.[7] Most often the dissection extends to both iliac arteries. The site for insertion of the endograft is based on adequate external iliac diameter and the limb best supplied by the true lumen. Once this has been determined the common femoral artery on the selected side is exposed. In our experience a conduit is rarely required in patients with dissections. An 8F sheath is then introduced in the exposed common femoral artery and an intravascular ultrasound examination (IVUS) is used to follow to the glidewire to confirm true lumen location at all points. If the glidewire is seen exiting the true lumen to the false lumen (Figure 54-4, *A* and *B*), we then can use fluoroscopic guided manipulation with an angled catheter at this point to get back in the true lumen. A transbrachial wire placement does not guarantee true lumen location at all times (Figure 54-5, *A* and *B*). This always needs to be confirmed with the help of an IVUS catheter. Once we confirm guidewire location in the true lumen from femoral to the ascending aorta, the IVUS is used to confirm the aortic diameter for stent graft selection. A contralateral 5F sheath is used for the diagnostic pigtail catheter placement. This can be manipulated on the basis of the location of the prior guidewire but may occasionally require the use of an IVUS or a transbrachial pigtail placement for the diagnostic angiogram.

The endograft is oversized 5% to 10% on the basis of the normal proximal aorta. We use the longest graft available for that given diameter (usually a 15-cm or 20-cm device). The graft is then deployed on the basis of the angiographic location of the left CCA. The

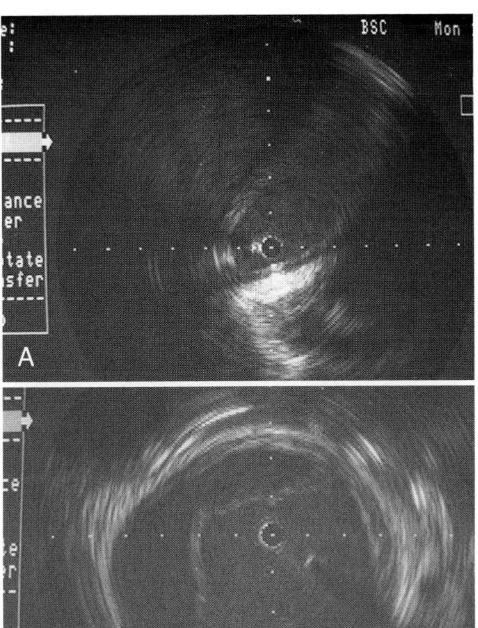

FIGURE 54-4 **A,** Intravascular ultrasound of catheter located in the true lumen, **B,** Same patient in **A** with catheter now in the false lumen.

proximal end of the graft is deployed immediately distal to the left CCA. We avoid post–stent graft balloon angioplasty, especially in the acute phase, to avoid the possibility of a acute retrograde dissection. A completion angiogram at this point should confirm elimination of the entry point into the false lumen. A small blush of contrast if seen will usually disappear with continued graft expansion. The distal end of the graft may appear compressed, and this often fully expands in less than 24 hours. A very significant proximal or distal compression may require relining the graft (this doubles the radial force) or a gentle balloon dilatation. I have never had

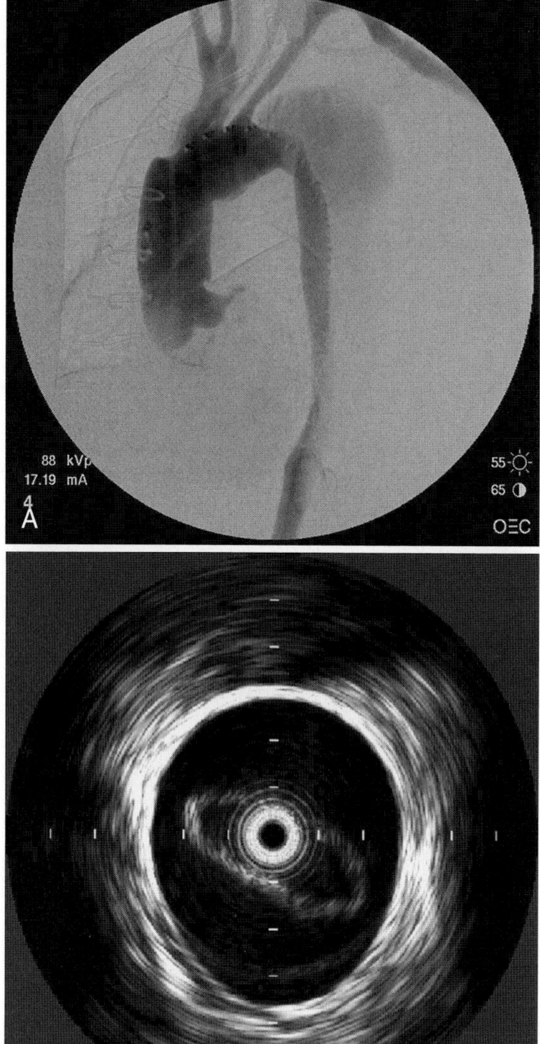

FIGURE 54-5 **A,** Two-dimensional image created by conventional angiogram. **B,** IVUS of patient in **A** demonstrates the complex three-dimensional nature of dissections.

to do this at the primary procedure in acute dissections. A completion angiogram is then performed of the thoracic aorta distal to the stent graft in addition to an abdominal aortogram. I do not primarily treat reentry points with the exception of ruptures. The false lumen in patients with acute dissection will gradually remodel to a predissection state. In patients with chronic dissection the false lumen distal to the stented segment is almost always patent. This has not been a problem in our chronic dissection subset because the aneurysmal portion of the false lumen across the stented segment thrombosis often shrinks or stabilizes (Figure 54-6, *A* and *B*).

Routinely extending the stent graft in all patients to the level of the celiac axis is not required with the exception of patients presenting with a rupture. The incidence of paraplegia in patients with dissections is clearly related to the length of coverage. This is unlike true aneurysms of the thoracic aorta that often have a layer of thrombus that has allowed for a gradual intercostal occlusion and compensation. In contrast, patients with dissections have open intercostals that are acutely lost with stent graft coverage. Routine cerebrospinal fluid (CSF) drains are not used, paraplegia/paraparesis when observed is often delayed, and most of the time patients recover with a CSF drain instituted at that point. Similarly, routine carotid-to-subclavian bypass cannot currently be recommended with an intent to prevent paraplegia on the basis of current literature.

Occasionally, the LSA is in direct communication with the false lumen resulting in a retrograde type II endoleak. This is managed by transbrachial placed coils or an Amplatzer plug (AGA Medical, Plymouth, MN) (Figure 54-7). If this is quite obvious before surgery, the Amplatzer plug can be placed before the stent graft procedure via the femoral route. Because of the size of the sheath required for the Amplatzer plugs, an axillary cutdown may often be required if the upper arm is the selected route for delivery.

Leurs et al.[8] presented a combined report from the EUROSTAR and United Kingdom Thoracic Endograft registries. One hundred thirty-one patients underwent endografting, 57% for complications of dissection and the remainder being without symptoms. Primary success rate was 89%, 30-day mortality overall was 6.5% (12% if emergent), and paraplegia occurred in 0.8%. Overall 1-year survival of the 67 who had follow-up was 90%. Xu et al.[9] reviewed 63 patients who presented with acute type B dissection and were managed with endovascular stents, 59 after 2 weeks of medical therapy. The primary entry site was completely sealed at the initial procedure in 95% of cases, 30-day mortality was 3.2%, retrograde dissection occurred in 3.2%, and the false lumen was completely thrombosed in the thoracic aorta at 1 year in 98%. Follow-up averaged 11.7 ± 10.6 months, during which time 3 (4.8%) died.

Techniques to Increase Proximal Landing Zone

Ideally a 1.5- to 2-cm proximal normal aorta is recommended for a durable and adequate seal. This may be less than ideal in some patients because of the proximity of the entry tear to the LSA and subsequently the proximity of the LSA to the left CCA. Landing zones can be increased via a variety of debranching procedures such as a carotid-to-carotid bypass or even ascending aorta–to–arch vessel bypass procedures.[10] These have been described previously and will not be further discussed in this chapter.

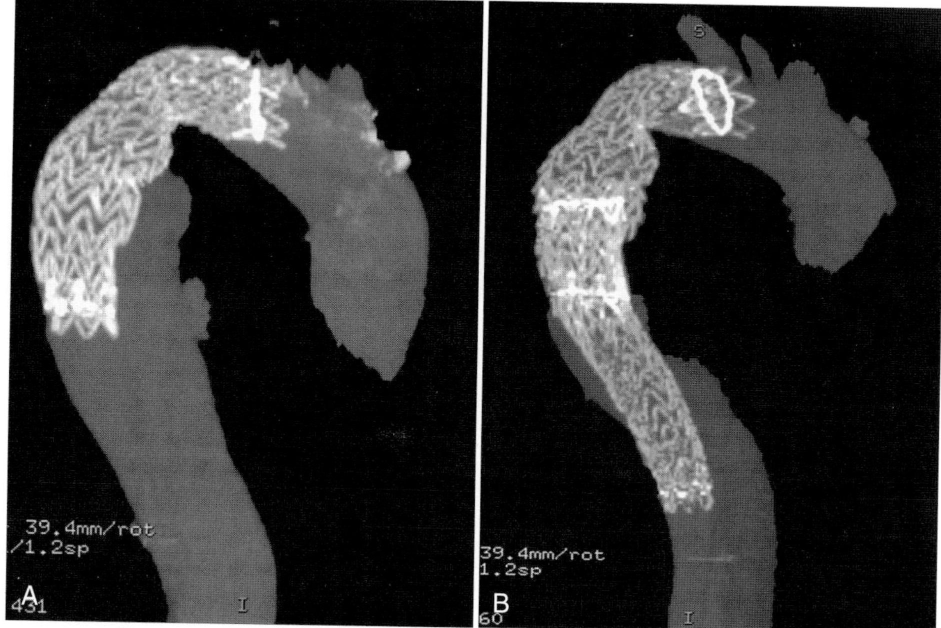

FIGURE 54-6 **A,** Chronic dissection with false-lumen thrombosis across stented segment. **B,** Same patient in **A** with distal stent graft extension and thrombosis now extends lower down, but only across stented segment.

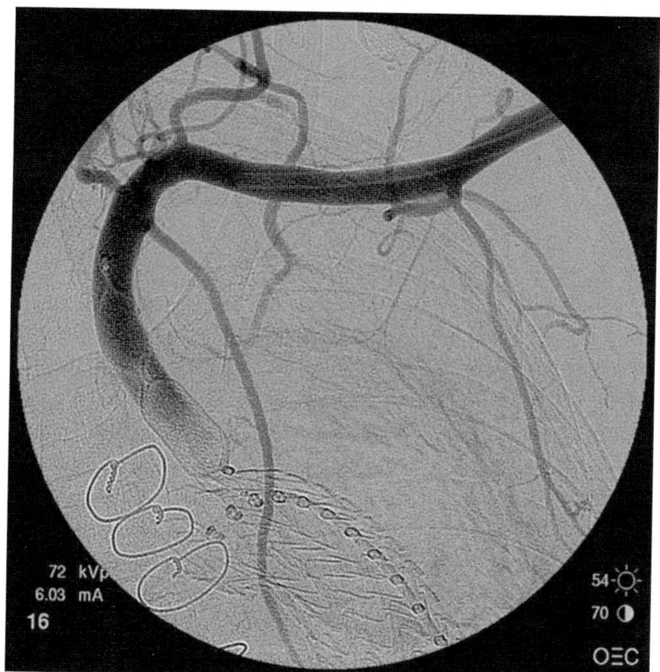

FIGURE 54-7 Amplatzer plug used to occlude proximal portion of the LSA.

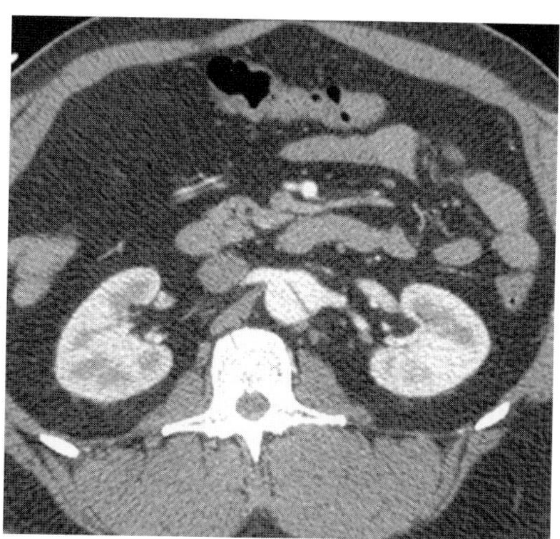

FIGURE 54-8 CT demonstrates the right renal artery compromise with the dissection flap.

Branch Vessel Stenting

The preoperative CT scan and intraoperative IVUS can help establish true lumen compromise in any of the branch vessels (Figure 54-8). The major vessels that can be compromised by the dissection are the celiac, superior mesenteric artery (SMA), renal arteries, and the iliac arteries. These are not treated unless patients have symptoms. In the acute phase, proximal stent graft exclusion of the entry point is often sufficient to relieve true-lumen compromise of the branch vessels. Hence, we often treat the primary entry point and reimage the patient with IVUS and abdominal aortograms. If progressive expansion of the true lumen is noted these are not acutely treated.

In patients with abdominal pain, unexplained lactic acidosis, and unexplained hypotension mesenteric ischemia should be suspected. This involved an

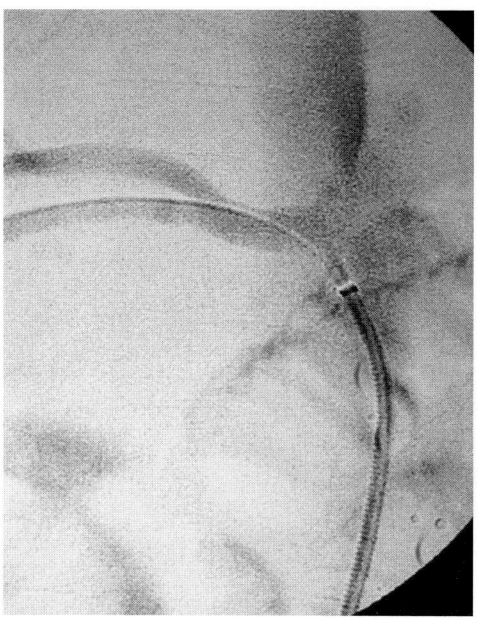

FIGURE 54-9 Angiogram with right renal artery seen extending across the false lumen.

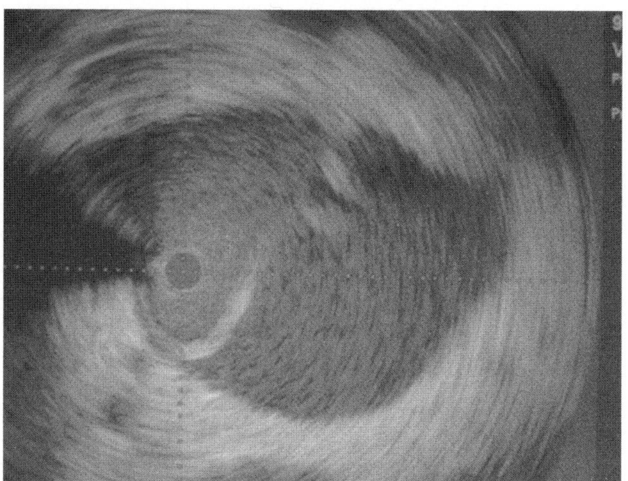

FIGURE 54-10 Pretreatment IVUS of the renal artery.

exploratory laparotomy with possible mesenteric artery stenting. Similarly, patients with dissection flaps that extend into the renal arteries with true lumen compromise need to be addressed for symptoms/signs of uncontrolled hypertension or acute/progressive renal failure. Acute limb ischemia often resolves with proximal stent graft placement; if this does not help iliac stents may be required with occasional thrombectomy.

Technique of Branch Vessel Stenting

A femoral approach is most often used with placement of an 8F sheath to confirm true lumen location with the help of an IVUS. I then place a 6F hockey-stick Pinnacle Destination sheath via the 8F sheath in the groin and then selectively cannulate the target branch vessel. An SOS (Cook Medical, Bloomington, IN) or a JR4 is the most frequently used preshaped catheter that helps with the selective cannulation. True-lumen location in the branch vessels can also be confirmed at this point via an angiogram through the Pinnacle sheath (Terumo, Somerset, NJ) (Figure 54-9) or a 0.018-inch or 0.014-inch IVUS catheter (Figure 54-10). A self-expanding (nitinol)–based stent is then deployed extending from the branch vessel across the false lumen into the true lumen (Figure 54-11). Renals most frequently require an 8- × 2- or 8- × 3-mm nitinol stent and the SMA may require a 10- or 12- × 30-mm stent. Usually the radial force of the stents is adequate at this point to displace the intimal flap, causing the dynamic obstruction to be held open (Figure 54-12). Balloon dilatation is rarely required. It is not recommended to use balloon-mounted stents,

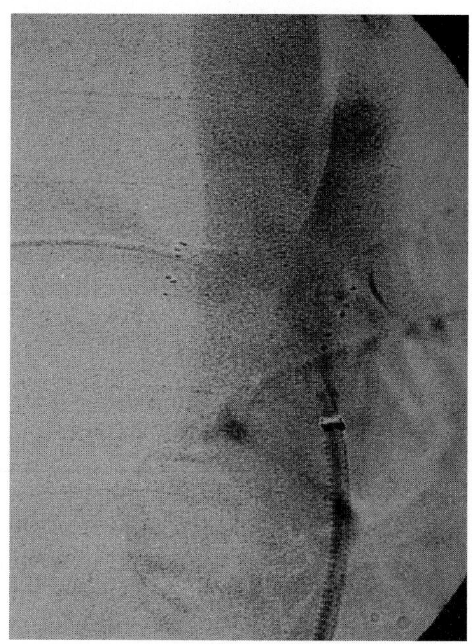

FIGURE 54-11 Self-expanding renal stent to avoid dynamic obstruction.

because of the risk of crush injury to the stent. We have also not had the need for covered stents in this location.

Fenestration

Endovascular fenestrations were done in the past to treat acute true lumen compromise. Rather than treating the entry tear, which increases the resistance to false-lumen inflow, fenestration is aimed at artificially creating a distal reentry channel, which decreases the resistance to false-lumen outflow. Technique involves cannulation of the true lumen from one femoral and cannulation of the false lumen from the other femoral. The wires are

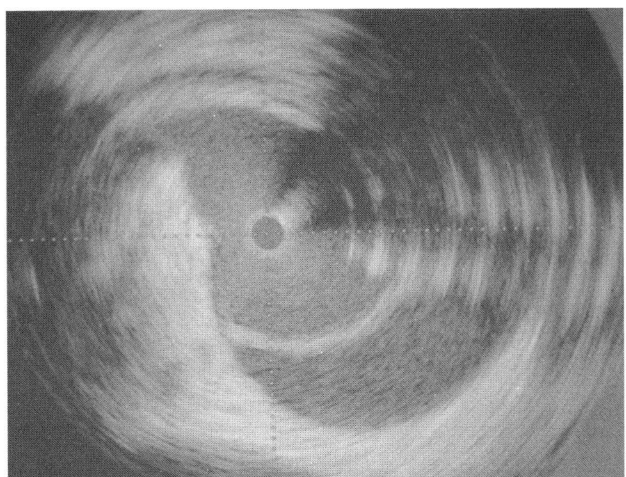

FIGURE 54-12 IVUS after renal stent demonstrates open renal artery.

then snared across the septum and a single wire is then held entering one common femoral into the true lumen across the septum into the false lumen and out via the contralateral femoral artery. A downward pulling motion and gently sawing back and forth causes a sizable rent in the septum, equalizing pressure in both true and false lumen and thereby reperfusing organs supplied from branches coming off the true lumen. We have not had to perform these fenestrations with the availability of stent grafts. Additionally, once a fenestration has been performed follow-up images have always demonstrated rapid increase in size of the false lumen requiring complex open thoracoabdominal reconstructions. Hence, fenestration is mentioned only to be abandoned.

COMPLICATIONS

Access Related

Because of the large sheath diameter (>9 mm for some devices) required for the thoracic stent grafts a careful preoperative evaluation of the external iliac artery (EIA) needs to done. Not just the diameter but calcification and tortuosity also play a major role in the ability of the sheath to track through the EIA. The combination of calcification with tortuosity in a patient with a borderline vessel diameter can be a far greater problem than in a noncalcified vessel. Fortunately, dissection is often seen in younger patients with minimal calcification. When in doubt it is always better to have a conduit for access. It is also easier to get sheaths to advance than it is to withdraw them in tight EIAs. In the event of a possible iliac rupture, it always advisable to leave the guidewire in place and have ready access to aortic occlusion balloons and covered stents.

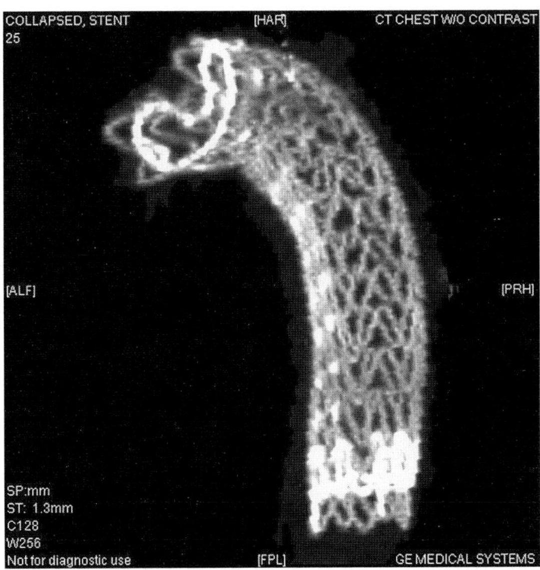

FIGURE 54-13 TAG device collapse in patient with acute type B dissection.

Stent Graft Procedure Related

Two complications that are unique to dissection-related stent grafts are type A conversion and device compression.[11]

Device compression tends to happen on the outer aspect of the stent graft as opposed to the compression/collapse seen in trauma or coarctation (Figure 54-13). This points to a variety of factors that include false-lumen pressure on the outer curvature of the graft, true-lumen compression distally, and inadequate radial force of the graft. This appears to be a unique phenomenon related to the TAG (W. L. Gore & Associates, Inc., Flagstaff, AZ) graft that may be a function of its radial force. This can best be avoided by preventing aggressive oversizing, preventing the proximal end of the graft from being deployed in the junction between the arch and the descending thoracic aorta, and adequate postprocedural blood pressure control. When noticed, it can be managed by relining the graft with a second device of same length and diameter. This doubles the radial force and adequately addresses the problem. Relining with a Palmaz stent or grafts with greater radial force have also been used.

Type A conversion is one of the most dreaded complications of stent graft treatment of dissections. This is often related to the use of devices with proximal bare springs and tends to be fatal if not recognized immediately. In patients with acute dissection, the tear can be immediately fatal with proximal extension into the aortic valve, coronary arteries, and/or the pericardium. Proper graft positioning with good blood pressure control can minimize this complication. New-onset stroke or back pain in the postprocedure period should

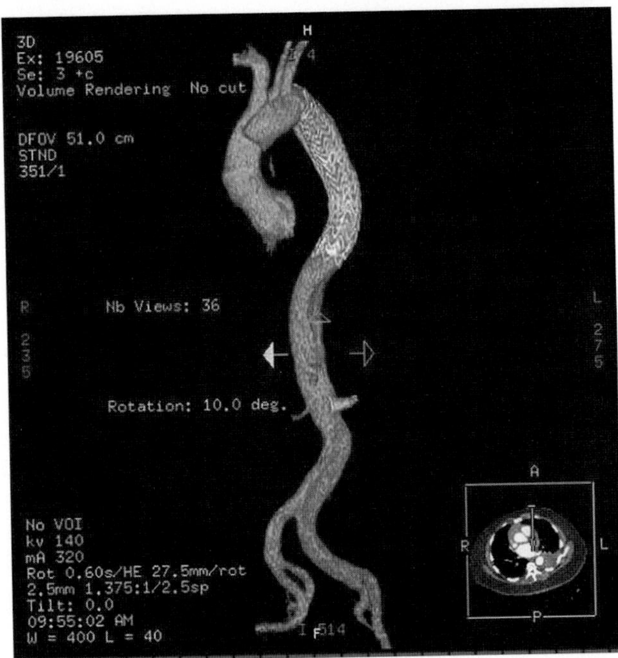

FIGURE 54-14 Proximal extension of dissection seen after stent graft placement for dissection.

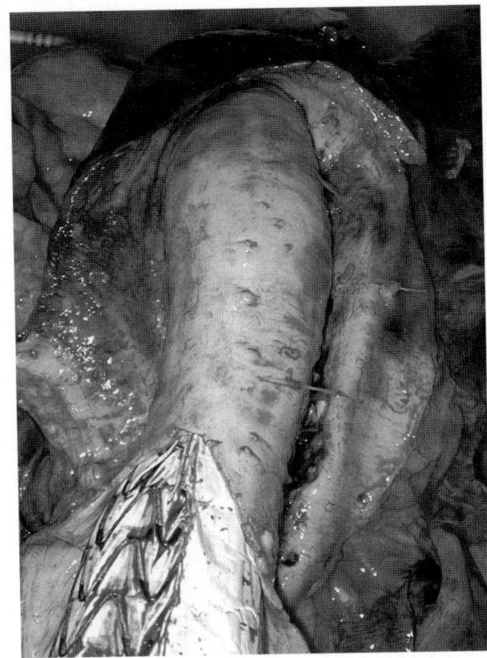

FIGURE 54-15 Distal flare perforation in patient with acute dissection and rupture.

always prompt a repeated CT to evaluate for a proximal extension (Figure 54-14). This is an open surgical emergency and often needs a prompt trip to the operating room. The reported incidence, in larger series of dissection cases, is roughly 0.5% to 3% but has been reported in as many as 10%.

Distal Flare Perforation

Distal flare perforation can also be seen, especially in patients with poor blood pressure control (Figure 54-15). This can present as new-onset acute limb, renal, or mesenteric ischemia. A distal extension of the stent graft often resolves this complication.

Other complications such as stent graft migration, type III endoleaks, and retrograde type II endoleaks via the subclavian artery have been reported with equal incidence as degenerative aneurysms. Treatment is similar to routine thoracic stent graft procedures such as proximal extension, bridging grafts (for type III), and occlusion of the proximal subclavian artery for type II endoleaks. Overall endoleaks are less common in patients treated for dissection than aneurysmal disease, being reported at 6% or less. True type I endoleak (proximal) is uncommon in dissection patients treated with stent grafts. In up to one third of cases, small, late-appearing proximal endoleaks have sealed at follow-up studies. Other reported complications include aortoesophageal fistula and mobile thrombus within the stent graft lumen. These complications, in addition to retrograde dissection, stent graft collapse, endoleak, and late rupture underscore the importance of close and lifelong imaging follow-up of these patients. We routinely obtain a CT angiogram or MR angiogram at 1 month and every 6 months thereafter for the life of the patient.

Dissection Related

Other complications such as stroke, paraplegia, mesenteric ischemia, renal failure, and limb ischemia can be related to the acute dissection or noted in the perioperative period. In patients with dissection (acute and chronic) the reported incidence of spinal cord injury is approximately 0% to 6%. Risk factors have included prior abdominal aortic aneurysm repair; hypogastric disease; coverage of more than 20 cm of thoracic aorta; or complete coverage, including the LSA or coverage below T8. The use of lumbar drains in these higher-risk cases (keep the CSF pressure ≤10-14 mm Hg) does seem to provide additional protection.

AUTHOR'S PERSPECTIVE: DISSECTIONS ARE NOT ANEURYSMS

Results with increased operator experience have been demonstrated to get better, with consistently less morbidity and mortality in patients in the chronic phase compared with the acute phase. However, in patients in the chronic phase false-lumen thrombosis is consistently

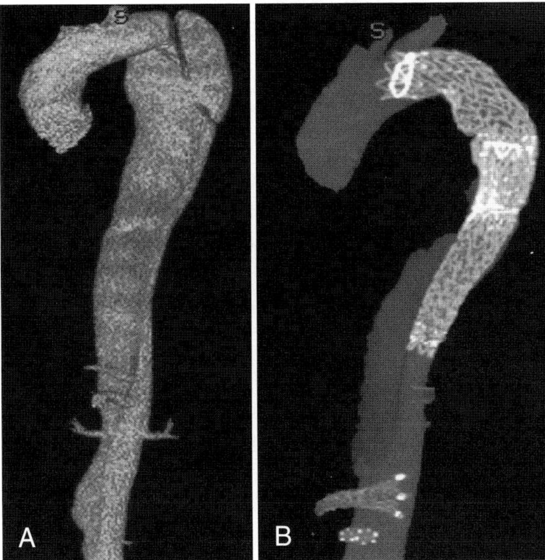

FIGURE 54-16 **A,** Preprocedural CT of patient with chronic descending thoracic dissection. **B,** Post–stent graft treatment with branch vessel stenting (SMA and renal artery).

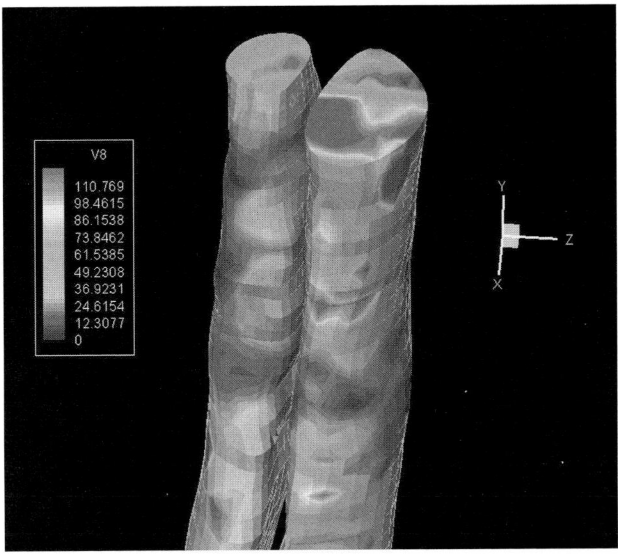

FIGURE 54-17 Calculation of peak systolic velocity with flow studies (*red* represents areas of maximum velocity).

seen across the level of the implanted stent graft, but thrombosis distal to the implant is less common. This is often related to persistent flow through distal flap fenestrations. The author treated a total of 34 patients with chronic dissections (20 males; mean age 56 ± 3 years) over a 4-year period with custom (2) or the TAG endografts for proximal thoracic false-lumen enlargement. The majority of patients were treated with a single component (n = 28 [82%]). The mean maximal thoracic aneurysm diameter was 6.9 ± 1 cm. The majority (n = 25 [74%]) of patients had symptoms of chronic back pain. The mean time from the initial acute dissection was 4.3 ± 0.8 years. Two patients had Marfan's syndrome. All but one patient had successful exclusion of the proximal entry point on completion angiogram (97% primary success). The majority (n = 31 [91%]) of patients had routine coverage of the LSA. Bypass adjuncts to improve proximal landing zone included three ascending aorta–to–innominate and CCA bypasses, two carotid-to-carotid and carotid-to-subclavian bypasses, one bilateral carotid-to-subclavian bypass, and one total thoracic and abdominal visceral vessel debranching. None of the patients with isolated LSA occlusion required an adjunctive procedure. Perioperative complications included two deaths, one transient paraparesis, and one paraplegia. One patient with a persistent proximal flow on completion angiogram had a successful open surgical conversion. Secondary endovascular interventions were required for two patients with type II endoleaks, one with a type III endoleak, and one distal flare perforation. An asymptomatic proximal extension of the aortic dissection was noted in one patient 6 months after initial treatment. At a mean follow-up of 14 ± 8 months, all but one patient had complete false-lumen thrombosis across the stented segment. Among patients with false-lumen thrombosis (n = 30), 24 (80%) patients had no growth in the size of the aneurysm and 6 (20%) patients had a mean 3.3 ± 1 mm decrease in the size of the maximal thoracic aortic diameter. Two patients required distal stent graft extension after 12 months because of false-lumen enlargement distal to the stented segment. Interestingly, even in these two patients the proximal false lumen (across the prior stented segment) was stable and thrombosed (Figure 54-16, *A* and *B*). This underscores the importance of treatment being directed to exclusion of the primary entry point and time of initial treatment. Close follow-up can detect and treat delayed distal problems if and when this happens. Avoiding extensive coverage at the primary operation may help decrease the most dreaded complication of paraplegia.

To evaluate the etiology for delayed false-lumen enlargement, eight patients presenting with acute type B dissection were followed with serial pressure measurements in the true and false lumen and phase-contrast MR angiograms and CT angiograms every 6 months. Flow information was fused with anatomic data obtained via CT/MR angiography. The composite data sets were used to evaluate a number of fluid dynamic parameters including wall shear stress, peak flow velocities, and flow volumes in both true and false channels. Idealized models were also analyzed with computational fluid dynamics for comparison (Figure 54-17). Wall shear stresses were significantly higher in patients with early false-lumen enlargement, with a stress ratio of 1.37 ± 0.06 (Figure 54-18). In

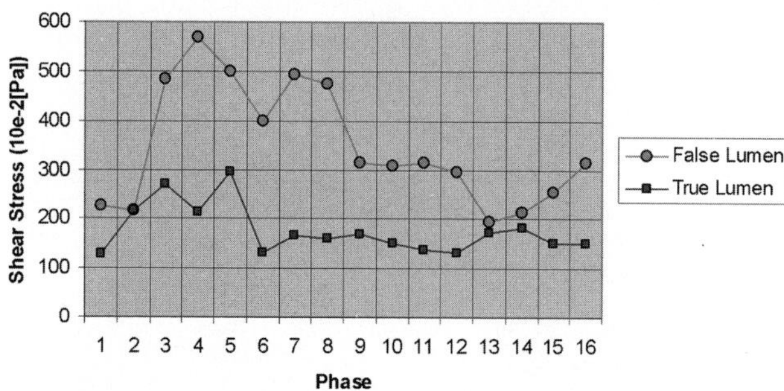

FIGURE 54-18 Graphic representation of difference in the shear stress between true and false lumens.

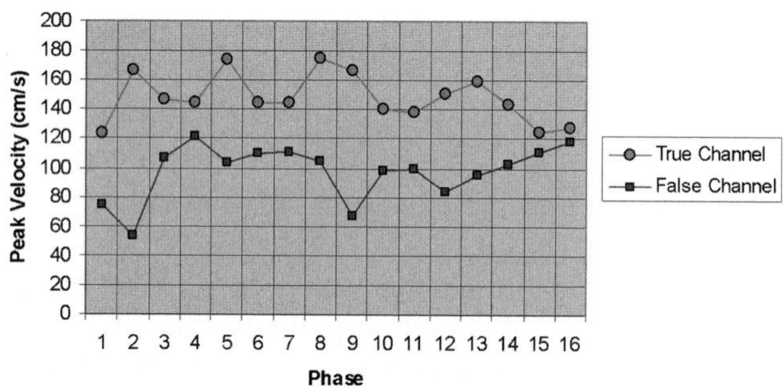

FIGURE 54-19 Graphic representation of difference in peak velocity between true and false lumens.

addition, we observed that peak velocities (Figure 54-19) were consistently higher in the false lumen as compared with the true lumen in patients with progressive false-lumen enlargement (158.8 ± 8.8 vs. 108.3 ± 14.5 cm/s; $p < .05$). Strong agreement was observed between clinical and computational fluid dynamics data sets. There was no difference in the pressure measurements between the true and the false lumen, and additionally this did not correlate with delayed false-lumen enlargement. These data suggest that wall shear stress at the entry point and increased peak flow velocities in the false lumen may be the primary driving forces for progressive late false-lumen expansion. The concept of sac pressurization, borrowed from the treatment of degenerative aneurysms, may have little role to play in the evaluation and treatment of patients with dissections.

CONCLUSION

Data continue to accumulate on the etiology and management of dissections with interest in the development of dissection-specific devices. Currently, acute uncomplicated dissections are best managed medically with delayed stent graft treatment if false-lumen enlargement is noted. Complications during the acute phase are best managed with thoracic stent graft exclusion of the entry point and possible branch vessel stenting. Thoracic stent grafts for chronic dissections have demonstrated promising midterm results. Longer follow-up and prospective studies will throw more light on the best approach for these complex aortic pathologies.

References

1. Wheat MW Jr, Palmer RF, Bartley TD, Seelman RC: Treatment of dissecting aneurysms of the aorta without surgery, *J Thorac Cardiovasc Surg* 50:364–373, 1965.
2. Hagan PG, Nienaber CA, Isselbacher EM, Bruckman D, Karavite DJ, Russman, et al: The International Registry of Acute Aortic Dissection (IRAD): new insights into an old disease, *JAMA* 283:897–903, 2000.
3. Dialetto G, Covino FE, Scognamiglio G, et al: Treatment of type B aortic dissection: endoluminal repair or conventional medical therapy? *Eur J Cardiothorac Surg* 27:826–830, 2005.
4. Estera AL, Miller CC, Goodrick J: Update on outcomes of acute type B dissection, *Am Thorac Surg* 83(2):5842–5845, 2007.
5. Kato N, Shimono T, Hirono T, et al: Mid-term results of stent graft repair of acute and chronic aortic dissection with descending tears: the complication-specific approach, *J Thorac Cardiovasc Surg* 124:306–312, 2002.
6. Song TK, Donayre CE, Walot I, Kopchok GE, Litwinski RA, Lippmann M, et al: Endograft exclusion of acute and chronic descending thoracic aortic dissections, *J Vasc Surg* 43:247–258, 2006.
7. Kasirajan K: Thoracic endografts: procedural steps, technical pitfalls and how to avoid them, *Semin Vasc Surg* 19(1):3–10, 2006.
8. Leurs LJ, Bell R, Degrieck Y, et al: Endovascular treatment of thoracic aortic diseases: combined experience from the EUROSTAR and United Kingdom Thoracic Endograft registries, *J Vasc Surg* 40:670–679, 2004, [discussion: 679–80].
9. Xu SD, Huang FJ, Yang JF, et al: Endovascular repair of acute type B aortic dissection: early and mid-term results, *J Vasc Surg* 43:1090–1095, 2006.
10. Dietl CA, Kasirajan K, Pett SB, Wernly JA: Off-pump management of aortic arch aneurysm by using an endovascular thoracic stent graft, *J Thorac Cardiovasc Surg* 126(4):1181–1183, 2003.
11. Kasirajan K, Milner R, Chaikof EL: Late complications of thoracic endografts, *J Vasc Surg* 43(Suppl A):94A–99A, 2006.

CHAPTER

55

Endovascular Repair of Aortic Arch Aneurysm Using Supra-Aortic Trunk Debranching

Edward B. Diethrich, Julio A. Rodriguez-Lopez, Dawn Olsen, Venkatesh J. Ramiah, Grayson H. Wheatley, Khalid Irshad, Donald B. Reid

There can be few procedures more challenging in vascular surgery than the treatment of aneurysms in the aortic arch. Open surgery in this territory for arteriosclerotic or dissecting aneurysms has always carried a high morbidity and mortality for a variety of reasons: the patients are usually old with comorbid disease, the surgery is difficult and very invasive, access requires a sternotomy, and the blood supply to the brain and upper limbs must be maintained.[1,2] Although open surgery has been the mainstay of treatment for many years, the development of endovascular surgery and particularly endoluminal grafting of the descending thoracic aorta has pushed the boundaries proximally into the arch.[3] Initially this began by endovascular surgeons occasionally covering the left subclavian artery (LSA). Then, as experience and endograft technology improved, so did the ability of endovascular surgeons to treat what has become the final frontier of endovascular intervention: aneurysms in the aortic arch.

Debranching is the term used when an endoluminal graft covers the origin of one or more of the supra-aortic vessels. Although the LSA may compensate through its extensive collateral blood supply, debranching of the left carotid or innominate arteries requires revascularization. This extra-anatomic surgical revascularization is generally described as either partial or total, depending on how many of the supra-aortic vessels are involved.[4]

This chapter describes the endovascular management of aneurysms in the aortic arch and the surgical techniques required to debranch the supra-aortic vessels and yet maintain their blood supply. It also compares the results of endovascular debranching using a variety of different endoluminal grafts with open surgery and reports the authors' own experience with this technique.

OPEN SURGERY

Currently, treatment of aneurysms in the aortic arch is recommended when their maximum diameter exceeds 5 to 5.5 cm, or when the annular dilation creates marked aortic insufficiency.[5] There are a variety of different, purely open surgical procedures performed, and these tend to depend on the extent of the aneurysm and the degree of involvement of the different supra-aortic vessels.[6] The surgery involves replacing the arch with a prosthetic Dacron graft, and either the supra-aortic vessels can be revascularized with Dacron branched grafts or a cuff of aorta containing the origins of the supra-aortic vessels is sutured onto the side of an aortic tube graft (the island technique).[7]

Replacement of the aortic arch may also be part of the management of a thoracoabdominal aneurysm.[8] In this situation, a staged repair using the "elephant trunk" technique has been developed: in stage 1, the ascending aorta and arch are repaired through a sternotomy and a long cuff or "trunk" of Dacron is left hanging inside the descending aorta; in stage 2, the descending aortic aneurysm is repaired making use of the trunk of Dacron through a lateral thoracotomy.[9,10] This elephant trunk technique helps the surgeon to avoid the potentially dangerous and difficult dissection of the proximal descending aorta and also avoids the patient having a much larger operation.

Arch replacement surgery involves the most demanding challenges for the patient and surgeon, using hypothermic cardiopulmonary bypass and antegrade (or retrograde) cerebral perfusion methods for the prevention of cerebral ischemia.[11] All open surgery in the thoracic aorta carries a high mortality and morbidity, whether involving just the arch or the whole thoracic aorta. The 30-day

TABLE 55-1 Mortality and Stroke Rates in Recent Published Series of Open Surgery in the Aortic Arch for Aneurysms and Dissection

Author	Year	N	Mortality (%)	Stroke (%)
Tabayashi et al.[12]	1993	20	15	0
Okita et al.[13]	1999	39	11	18
Jacobs et al.[14]	2001	50	6	6
Kikuchi et al.[15]	2002	60	3.3	1.6
Matsuda et al.[16]	2002	101	6.9	1
Nakai et al.[17]	2002	109	14.7	17.4
Matalanis et al.[18]	2003	62	8	6.4
Niinami et al.[19]	2003	43	11.6	11.6

perioperative mortality and stroke rates for open surgery are shown in Table 55-1, based on the eight largest recently published series.[12-19]

DEVELOPMENT OF ENDOGRAFTS FOR THE THORACIC AORTA

In 1988, Volodos et al.[20] reported from the Ukraine on their clinical use of an endoluminal graft to treat a thoracic aneurysm. Subsequently, Dake et al.[3] at Stanford University began an investigational program of thoracic endografting in 1992. Their use of a custom-made device using a stainless steel Z-stent covered with polyester was an important contribution because the configuration of the stents allowed the endoluminal graft to conform with the curvature of the thoracic aorta. In the late 1990s, experience in thoracic endografting rapidly increased in Europe, the Far East, and also North America. Although most of this experience was in the descending aorta, investigators reported the first debranching cases in 1999 and described covering the LSA and also the complications that arose.[21,22]

Endoluminal grafting in the aortic arch has special challenges for any device. The arch is a substantial distance away from the femoral artery access site, and therefore control, torque, and accurate placement are much more difficult. The delivery sheath is greater than 20F diameter, and the device must traverse through the fragile bends of the iliac arteries and any concurrent arterial disease. The potential for cerebral embolization resulting from manipulation within the diseased arch is substantial. Accurate device placement is also made more difficult because of the curvature of the arch, and careful fluoroscopy alignment is essential. Despite these problems, several commercially available devices have been introduced in recent years with favorable midterm results.[23]

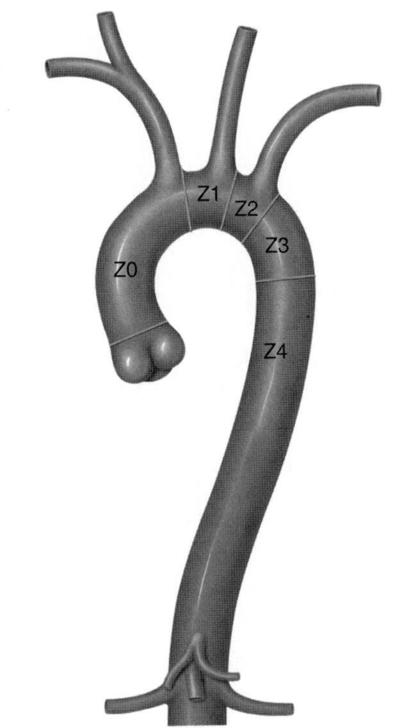

FIGURE 55-1 Anatomic landing zone map.

ANATOMIC LANDING ZONES

For any endoluminal graft to successfully exclude an aneurysm, it must seal between the proximal fabric of the device and the aortic wall. This "neck" or landing zone has been classified in the aortic arch depending on its anatomic relationship to the supra-aortic vessels. Two classifications have been described. Although Bergeron et al.[4] have recently described the "retrograde landing zone classification," the First International Summit on Thoracic Aortic Endografting produced its own classification, which has become more universally applied (Figure 55-1) and is used in this chapter.[24]

HYBRID SURGICAL TECHNIQUES

Any endovascular treatment in this territory requires an experienced and highly skilled team in a dedicated endovascular suite. The very best preoperative imaging and careful clinical judgment are required. In cases of thoracic aneurysm requiring debranching, the preliminary bypass surgery to maintain cerebral and upper limb perfusion depends on the site of the landing zone. Placing an endograft in zone Z2 (see Figure 55-1) may require partial revascularization with a left carotid subclavian bypass.[25] Deploying an endograft at zone Z1 will require a carotid-carotid bypass to maintain blood

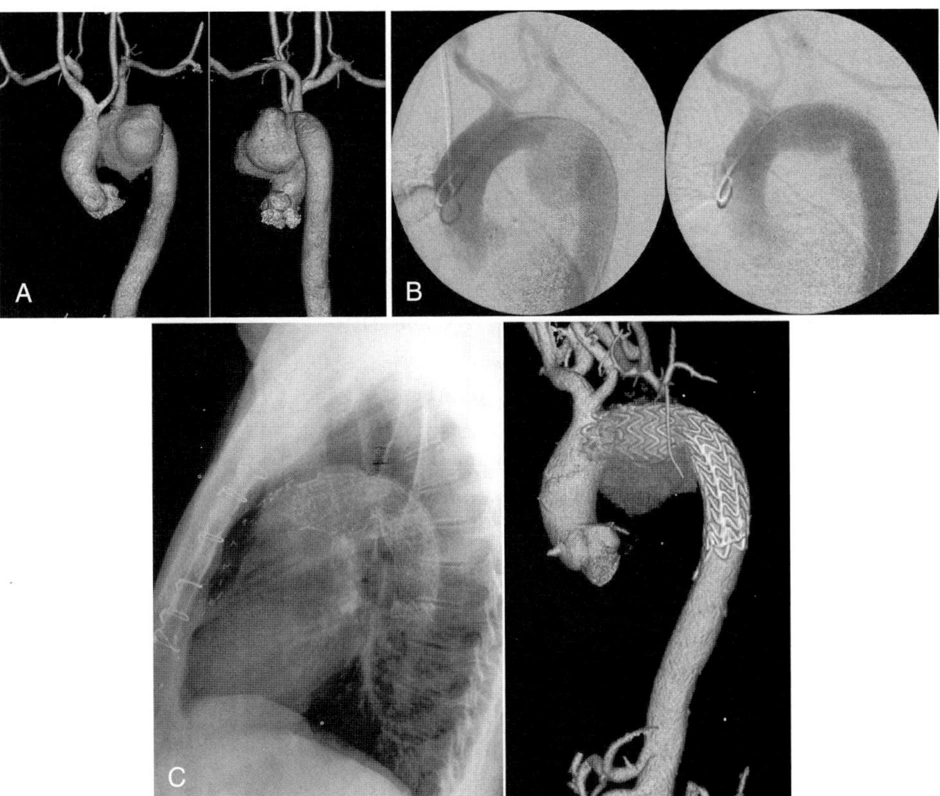

FIGURE 55-2 **A,** Sixty-four–slice CT angiography demonstrates a large aneurysm arising from the anterior wall of the aortic arch. The left common carotid artery takes its origin from the innominate (bovine arch). **B,** Digital subtraction aortograms before and after deployment of an endoluminal graft. Note the slight kink where the endograft stents do not entirely conform to the curvature of the aortic arch. **C,** Plain x-ray and three-dimensional reconstruction of CT angiography after successful exclusion of the aneurysm.

supply to the left cerebral hemisphere (unless there is bovine anatomy; Figure 55-2). Placing an endograft in zone Z0 will require total revascularization. This is usually performed with a bifurcated "Y" graft taken from the ascending aorta to the innominate artery and the left carotid artery. It has become our preference to perform carotid subclavian and carotid-carotid artery bypasses using an end-to-side interposition prosthetic graft. We have found that transposing the patient's native artery can be difficult, because the origin of the LSA or left carotid artery is often involved with the inflammation that is associated with a thoracic aneurysm. Although transposition of these vessels is an alternative used by other investigators, it can lead to kinking that, in the case of the LSA, can pinch the origin of the vertebral artery.[4] In carotid-carotid artery bypass, we prefer to place the 7-mm Dacron graft such that it lies in a tunnel anterior to the trachea. These revascularization operations are generally performed a day or so before endoluminal grafting to allow the new circulation to establish itself.

Total revascularization is performed through a medium sternotomy, and a side-biting vascular clamp is used to isolate a portion of the anterior wall of the ascending aorta, to maintain aortic blood flow. The body of the bifurcated Dacron graft is anastomosed to the ascending aorta in an end-to-side configuration; then the limbs are anastomosed end-to-end to the innominate and left common carotid arteries.

Multislice computed tomographic (CT) scanning has greatly assisted the operator in knowing where to land the endograft. It has also proved invaluable for measuring the device size. Three-dimensional reconstruction has also allowed a much greater understanding of the extent of the aneurysm and its relation to the anatomy, the supra-aortic vessels, and the shape of the curve of the arch and aortic knuckle. We also use the CT angiogram to decide whether we will pass the endoluminal graft through the left or right iliac systems. With the patient under general anesthesia, a small incision is made over the appropriate femoral artery to gain vascular control. Initially, a soft Glidewire (Meditech/Boston Scientific, Natick, MA) is passed up into the arch, and a pigtail catheter is passed over it. With a road mapping arch aortogram being followed and an oblique view and digital subtraction used, the endoluminal graft is deployed over a very stiff guidewire. Just before the graft is deployed, the anesthesiologist brings down the systolic blood pressure in an effort to prevent distal migration while the graft is being deployed in the strong aortic circulation. We have found that intravascular ultrasound (IVUS) and transesophageal echocardiography are outstandingly helpful in accurately placing these endografts.[26,27]

CASE ILLUSTRATIONS

Case Illustration 1

A 53-year-old man was referred from Pakistan to the Arizona Heart Hospital with an expanding 6-cm aneurysm in his aortic arch (see Figure 55-2). He had been known to have hypertension for 10 years and had undergone coronary artery bypass grafting 4 years previously. He had a 6-month history of hoarseness and breathlessness. Laryngoscopy confirmed a left vocal cord paralysis. We used 64-slice CT scanning to identify the extent of the aneurysm along the aortic arch and to find a suitable landing zone. A left carotid subclavian bypass was performed with a 7-mm Dacron tube graft. IVUS was performed to assist with device sizing and to identify a suitable landing zone. The following day, a TAG (W. L. Gore & Associates, Flagstaff, AZ) thoracic endograft was deployed in zone Z1 (because the left common carotid artery came off the innominate artery, that is, bovine arch) without any complication. Access for this was gained through a retrograde femoral artery approach. Complete seal and exclusion of this expanding aneurysm was confirmed by aortography and subsequent CT scanning. This patient has no leak more than a year after surgery, despite the very short arterial "neck" left to use in repair.

Case Illustration 2

A 70-year-old man presented with an extensive aneurysm of the aortic arch. Preoperative 64-slice CT scanning confirmed that it would be necessary to deploy an endograft in zone Z0 (Figure 55-3). A median sternotomy was performed. An aortic side clamp was placed over a portion of the ascending aorta, and a Dacron graft was sutured to an arteriotomy in the ascending aorta. This Dacron graft had been custom-made in the operating room immediately before surgery and incorporated three limbs. One limb was used for wire access, and the two main limbs were anastomosed end-to-end to the divided innominate and left carotid arteries. This third limb allowed control of the stiff guidewire and prevented the wire from entering the heart. It was also used for selective arteriography to demonstrate the patency of the grafts to the innominate and carotid

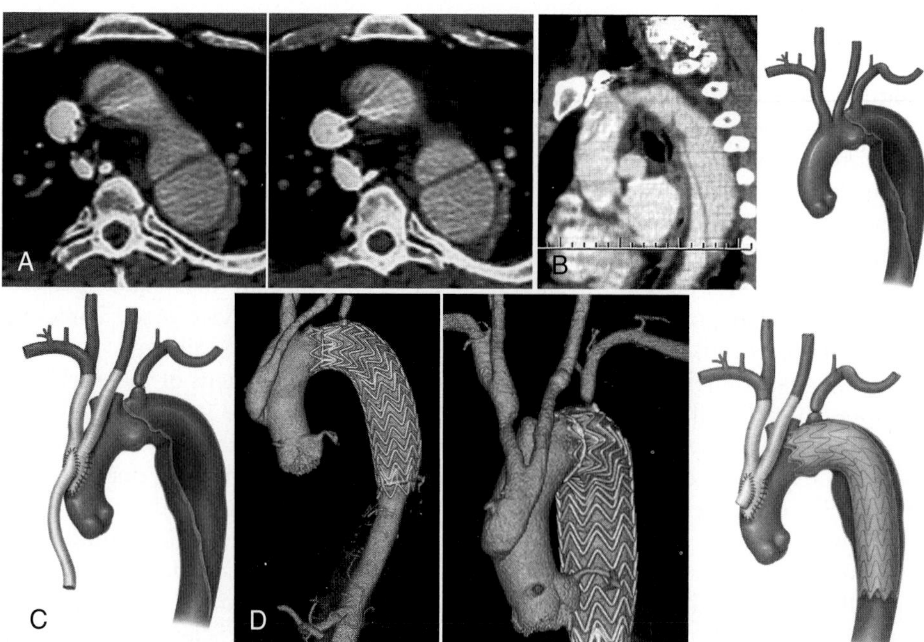

FIGURE 55-3 **A,** CT angiography of a dissecting aneurysm of the aortic arch. **B,** CT angiography and artist's impression of the dissecting aneurysm. **C,** Total revascularization is performed before debranching in this patient with a dissecting aneurysm. A Dacron graft with three branches is taken from the ascending aorta to the innominate and left carotid arteries. The third branch was used temporarily for wire access to deploy an endoluminal graft from a retrograde femoral artery approach. **D,** Postoperative CT scanning confirms successful deployment of the thoracic endograft with correction of the dissection, and debranching and total revascularization.

arteries. In the same procedure, a TAG (W. L. Gore & Associates) thoracic endograft was then deployed into zone Z0 from a retrograde femoral artery approach. After successful deployment and exclusion of this aneurysm, the third Dacron limb, which had been used for wire access, was divided near its origin and closed with sutures. This patient recovered without any complication. Follow-up shows no endoleak.

INSTITUTIONAL EXPERIENCE WITH THORACIC DEBRANCHING

Between October 2001 and May 2008, we treated 22 cases of thoracic aortic endografting using debranching in an overall experience of more than 500 cases during this period of time. Of the 22 patients, 12 were men and 10 women. The average age was 78 years (range 42-90 years). There were 17 patients who had total revascularizations, 5 patients who had carotid-carotid bypass, and 1 patient who had a carotid-subclavian bypass. Four of the patients were operated on emergently.

The 30-day perioperative mortality was 6 of 22 (27%). One patient died of a cerebrovascular accident with an intracranial hemorrhage, and another patient had a fatal stroke when the endograft migrated covering the extra-anatomic bypass. One patient died of hemorrhage with a suspected injury to the pulmonary artery, and another patient died of a suspected pulmonary embolism. One patient died of sepsis with mediastinitis and a suspected infected graft, and another patient died of multisystem organ failure and sepsis. Morbidity was also significant: one patient had a myocardial infarction, another patient had a degree of paraplegia, and three patients had ruptured iliac arteries (two out of the six who died). Six patients had acute respiratory failure. In follow-up, one further patient died 6 months after his procedure when another distal thoracic aneurysm ruptured.

DISCUSSION

Repair of a thoracic aneurysm situated in the aortic arch is an extremely complex and difficult problem that has challenged cardiovascular surgeons for many years. The open surgery is so invasive and carries such high risks that the concept of being able to use a less-invasive endovascular method has stimulated many centers around the world to investigate and apply this new technique.

The two illustrative cases and our institution's experience demonstrate the very high-risk nature of treating patients with aneurysms and dissecting aneurysms in the aortic arch. The results of other investigators who have used debranching endovascular techniques for aneurysm and dissection are shown in Table 55-2, although it should be noted that these published series are mostly cases of debranching of the LSA.[4,28-33] Some variation in the results of these series probably reflects caseload mix and the proportion of emergent cases performed.

Debranching of the supra-aortic vessels clearly carries the risk of major stroke. However, not all of the supra-aortic vessels require revascularization. The LSA has excellent collateral branches that can compensate and provide a viable blood supply to the left arm when it is occluded. It has three major branches that are relevant to endovascular repair in the thoracic aorta. The internal mammary artery is often used as a bypass graft for coronary reperfusion. The vertebral artery provides spinal branches before it links with the contralateral vertebral artery to become the basilar artery, which is the main blood supply to the hindbrain. The costocervical trunk leads into intercostal arteries, which also contribute to spinal cord perfusion.

We practice selective revascularization of the LSA and only perform carotid subclavian bypass when we believe that there is either a threat to an internal mammary artery coronary graft or a risk of cerebral or spinal ischemia. A careful assessment of the

TABLE 55-2 Mortality and Stroke Rates in Recent Published Series of Endografts in the Aortic Arch for Aneurysms and Dissection

Author	Year	N	Z0	Z1	Z2	Z3	Mortality (%)	Stroke (%)
Bergeron et al.[4]	2006	25	15	—	—	—	8	8
Kwok et al.[28]	2006	15	1	1	1	12	13	13
Peterson et al.[29]	2006	30	0	0	30	0	3.3	16.7
Reece et al.[30]	2007	27	0	0	27	0	0	11
Melissano et al.[31]	2007	64	14	12	38	0	6.3	3.1
Czerny et al.[32]	2007	27	—	—	—	—	7.4	0
Riesenman et al.[33]	2007	28	1	3	24	0	11	10.1

NOTE: Where available details of the landing zones (Z0, Z1, Z2, Z3) are included.

contralateral vertebral artery is therefore important; however, spinal ischemia is more difficult to predict because there are other factors in its etiology during thoracic endografting. Preliminary transient balloon occlusion of the LSA can be used to test for ischemic consequences of debranching.[34]

Accurate placement of a thoracic endograft encounters different problems in different landing zones. Whatever the location, it is essential to have modern high-definition fluoroscopy in the operating room with digital subtraction for road mapping. Although we like to lower the systolic blood pressure at the moment of deployment, other investigators have used different techniques for precise deployment, which include sodium nitroprusside titration, venacaval occlusion, intra-atrial balloon, adenosine-induced transient cardiac arrest, and rapid right ventricular pacing.[35] Rapid pacing appears to be a safe maneuver that has been shown to provide an accurate deployment.[36]

IVUS also assists accurate placement, despite some limitations in imaging the curvature of the arch.[37] We use an 8.4F IVUS catheter (Volcano Therapeutics, Rancho Cordova, CA), which is advanced into the arch after aortography over a 0.35-inch guidewire, and a manual pullback is performed. This provides diameter measurements and an indication of required length, which can be compared with the CT scan. The location of the landing site can also be positioned precisely by using the IVUS and the road map. In this setting, IVUS provides the operator with a much better spatial understanding of the three-dimensional shape of the arch and its branches.

Transesophageal echocardiography and IVUS are also useful in thoracic dissecting aneurysms to show the operator the true lumen and the extent of dissection. Although transesophageal echocardiography can help visualize the actual deployment of the endograft, it cannot show the whole of the thoracic aorta because of its location inside the esophagus. Another simple but effective method to identify anatomic landmarks in debranching the arch is the placement of either a guidewire or a pigtail catheter in the innominate artery from a retrograde brachial approach.[4]

Although accurate deployment of an endoluminal graft helps to obtain seal, endoleak and migration are potential complications given the curvature of the arch and the limitations of the current devices.[23] It is difficult to completely appose an endograft to the curve when the contact with the vessel wall is determined by the length of each stent unit. One recent report suggested customized in situ bending of the stent graft for each individual case.[38,39] It has also been reported that the more proximal the endograft is implanted in the aortic arch, the higher the incidence of stroke and endoleak.[31] Such complications also highlight the requirement for a thorough program of long-term follow-up.

Different commercially available endografts have been developed, modified, and manufactured over the last few years, each with their own special features. Although there are approximately a dozen endografts available in Europe, the United States currently only has three with Food and Drug Administration (FDA) approval.

W. L. Gore & Associates were the first to gain FDA approval. Their TAG (formerly called the Excluder) device is made of polytetrafluoroethylene (PTFE) and has a very rapid deployment that uses a mechanism to expand the middle of the graft first, thus avoiding the "wind sock" phenomenon. The self-expanding stents are placed along the entire graft surface outside the PTFE. A circumferential PTFE sealing cuff is located on the external surface of the endograft at the base of each flared scalloped end.

The Zenith TX2 endograft (Cook Medical, Bloomington, IN) received FDA approval in May 2008. Stainless steel Z-stents are sewn to Dacron fabric. It comes in two variants: the TX1 is one piece, and the TX2 is modular with two pieces. The proximal portion is covered, and caudally oriented hooks prevent distal migration.

The Talent device (formerly World Medical Corporation, now Medtronic, Santa Rosa, CA) received FDA approval in June 2008. It is available with a range of diameters up to 46 mm in size with bare stents proximal to the covered material. Medtronic also manufactures the Valiant thoracic endograft, a third-generation device with a self-expanding nitinol wire scaffold sewn to a low-profile polyester graft.

The Relay device (Bolton Medical, Sunrise, FL) is in FDA-approved trials. Sinusoidal-shaped, self-expanding nitinol stents are sutured to a polyester fabric. A longitudinal wire is sutured to the outer curve to provide longitudinal support. It comes in straight and tapered forms with diameters up to 46 mm and a length of up to 25 cm.

The Endofit device (LeMaitre Vascular, Burlington, MA) uses laminate PTFE and a nitinol stent, which makes it a very flexible graft for the aortic arch. It has the advantage of coming in more than 250 custom-made sizes with straight and tapered varieties.

FUTURE DEVELOPMENTS IN AORTIC ARCH ENDOGRAFTING

Given the fact that debranching the supra-aortic vessels requires extra-anatomic bypass, some investigators are developing branched and fenestrated endografts that directly maintain blood flow into the origins of the supra-aortic vessels.[40-43] Inoue et al.[44] have reported single-branched and multibranched stent grafts for aneurysms involving the supra-aortic vessels. They have reported short- to medium-term results in 17 patients using a branched endograft for the LSA: 3 of 17 patients had type I endoleaks with a mean follow-up of just over 2 years. One patient had paraparesis.[45]

Chuter et al.[46] have designed a bifurcated stent graft that is deployed in the ascending aorta. This technique of repair involves total revascularization but without a sternotomy.[46] Extra-anatomic revascularization is combined with supraclavicular access to deploy the bifurcated endograft from the right carotid or innominate artery. A modular portion is connected from a retrograde femoral approach, entirely covering the arch. Although the technical successes of placing any branched endografts in the aortic arch may well be an indication of the future, the early results indicate just how challenging and unforgiving this territory is.

CONCLUSION

Endovascular repair with supra-aortic debranching has developed as a less-invasive alternative to open surgery in the treatment of aneurysms involving the aortic arch. Preoperative assessment with detailed multislice CT angiography is crucial in planning a suitable landing zone, and this then indicates the type of revascularization required to maintain cerebral and upper limb perfusion. At present, a sternotomy is required to provide total revascularization for zone Z0 cases; however, lesions that are more distal in the arch can be corrected without a thoracotomy. Any surgeon who performs this kind of work is rapidly aware of the hazards and complicated issues that are ever present in treating this difficult condition. Yet the hybrid combination of extra-anatomic surgical revascularization and endoluminal grafting from a retrograde femoral artery approach greatly reduces the morbidity, making it much lighter on the patient. With advances in graft technology and increasing clinical experience, the management of aneurysms in the aortic arch is more than likely to improve.

References

1. Cooley DA, Mahaffey DE, DeBakey ME: Total excision of the aortic arch for aneurysm, *Surg Gynecol Obstet* 42(1):101–120, 1957.
2. Griepp RB, Stinson EB, Hollingsworth JF, Buehler D: Prosthetic replacement of the aortic arch, *J Thorac Cardiovasc Surg* 70:1051–1063, 1975.
3. Dake MD, Miller DC, Semba CP, et al: Transluminal placement of endovascular stent/grafts for the treatment of descending thoracic aortic aneurysms, *N Engl J Med* 331:1729–1734, 1994.
4. Bergeron P, Mangialardi N, Costa P, et al: Great vessel management for endovascular exclusion of aortic arch aneurysms and dissections, *Eur J Vasc Endovasc Surg* 32:38–45, 2006.
5. Coady MA, Rizzo JA, Hammond GL, et al: Surgical intervention criteria for thoracic aortic aneurysms: a study of growth rates and complications, *Ann Thorac Surg* 67:1922–1926, 1999.
6. Kazui T, Washiyama N, Muhammed BAH, et al: Total arch replacement using aortic arch branched grafts with the aid of antegrade selective cerebral perfusion, *Ann Thorac Surg* 70:3–9, 2000.
7. Kazui T, Washiyama N, Muhammed BAH, et al: Improved results of atherosclerotic arch aneurysm operations with a refined technique, *J Thorac Cardiovasc Surg* 121:491–499, 2001.
8. Safi HJ, Miller CC, Estrera AL, et al: Optimization of aortic arch replacement: two-stage approach, *Ann Thorac Surg* 83:S815–S818, 2007.
9. Borst HG, Walterbusch G, Schaps D: Extensive aortic replacement using "elephant trunk" prosthesis, *Thorac Cardiovasc Surg* 31:37–40, 1983.
10. Karck M, Shaven A, Khaladj N, et al: The frozen elephant trunk technique for the treatment of extensive thoracic aortic aneurysms: operative results and follow up, *Eur J Cardiothorac Surg* 28:286–290, 2005.
11. Safi HJ, Brien HW, Winter JN, et al: Brain protection via cerebral retrograde perfusion during aortic arch aneurysm repair, *Ann Thoracic Surg* 56:270–276, 1993.
12. Tabayashi K, Ohmi M, Togo T, et al: Replacement of the transverse aortic arch for type A acute aortic dissection, *Ann Thorac Surg* 55(4):864–867, 1993.
13. Okita Y, Ando M, Minatoya K: Predictive factors for mortality and cerebral complications in arteriosclerotic aneurysm of the aortic arch, *Ann Thorac Surg* 67(1):72–78, 1999.
14. Jacobs MJ, De Mol BA, Veldman DJ: Aortic arch and proximal supra-aortic arterial repair under continuous antegrade cerebral perfusion and moderate hypothermia, *Cardiovasc Surg* 9(4): 396–402, 2001.
15. Kikuchi Y, Sakurada T, Hirano T, et al: Long-term results of the operation for the aortic arch aneurysm, *Kyobu Geka* 55 (4):309–313, 2002.
16. Matsuda H, Hino Y, Matsukawa R, et al: Mid-term results of the surgery for aortic arch aneurysm, *Kyobu Geka* 55(4):340–346, 2002.
17. Nakai M, Shimamoto M, Yamazaki F, et al: Long-term results after surgery for aortic arch nondissection aneurysm, *Kyobu Geka* 55(4):280–284, 2002.
18. Matalanis G, Hata M, Buxton BF: A retrospective comparative study of deep hypothermic circulatory arrest, retrograde, and antegrade cerebral perfusion in aortic arch surgery, *Ann Thorac Cardiovasc Surg* 9(3):174–179, 2003.
19. Niinami H, Aomi S, Chikazawa G, et al: Progress in the treatment of aneurysms of the distal aortic arch: approach through median sternotomy, *J Cardiovasc Surg (Torino)* 44(2):243–248, 2003.
20. Volodos NL, Karpovich IP, Shekhanin VE, et al: A case of distant transfemoral endoprosthesis of the thoracic artery using a self-fixing synthetic prosthesis in traumatic aneurysm (in Russian), *Grudn Khir* 6:84–86, 1988.
21. Mitchell RS, Miller DC, Dake MD, et al: Thoracic aortic aneurysm repair with an endovascular stent graft: the "first generation," *Ann Thorac Surg* 67:1971–1974, 1999.
22. Greenberg RK, Resch T, Nyman U, et al: Endovascular repair of descending thoracic aortic aneurysms: an early experience with intermediate-term follow up, *J Vasc Surg* 31:147–156, 2000.
23. Ishimaru S: Endografting of the aortic arch, *J Endovasc Ther* 11 (Suppl II): II-62-II-71, 2004.

24. Mitchell RS, Ishimaru S, Ehrlich MP, et al: First International Summit on Thoracic Aortic Endografting: roundtable on thoracic aortic dissection as an indication for endografting, *J Endovasc Ther* 9(suppl II): 11-98-II105, 2002.
25. Diethrich EB, Garrett HE, Ameriso J, et al: Occlusive disease of the common carotid and subclavian arteries treated by carotid subclavian bypass: analysis of 125 cases, *Ann J Surg* 114(5): 800–808, 1967.
26. Irshad K, Rahman N, Bain D, et al: The role of intravascular ultrasound and peripheral endovascular interventions. In Heuser RR, Henry M, editors: *Textbook of peripheral vascular interventions*, London, 2004, Martin Dunitz, pp 25–34.
27. Bergeron P, De Chaumaray T, Gay J, et al: Endovascular treatment of thoracic aortic aneurysms, *J Cardiovasc Surg (Torino)* 44 (3):349–361, 2003.
28. Kwok PC, Ho KK, Ma CC, et al: The short-to-midterm results of endovascular stent grafting for acute thoracic aortic diseases in Chinese patients, *Hong Kong Med J* 12:355–360, 2006.
29. Peterson BG, Eskandari MK, Gleason TG, et al: Utility of left subclavian artery revascularization in association with endoluminal repair of acute and chronic thoracic aortic pathology, *J Vasc Surg* 43:433–439, 2006.
30. Reece TB, Gazoni LM, Cherry KJ, et al: Re-evaluating the need for left subclavian artery revascularization with thoracic endovascular aortic repair, *Ann Thorac Surg* 84:1201–1205, 2007.
31. Melissano G, Civilini E, Bertoglio L, et al: Results of endografting of the aortic arch in different landing zones, *Eur J Vasc Endovasc Surg* 33:561–566, 2007.
32. Czerny M, Gottardi R, Zimpfer D, et al: Mid-term results of supraaortic transpositions for extended endovascular repair of aortic arch pathologies, *Eur J Cardiothorac Surg* 31:623–627, 2007.
33. Riesenman PJ, Farber MA, Mendes RR, et al: Coverage of the left subclavian artery during thoracic endovascular aortic repair, *J Vasc Surg* 45:90–94, 2007.
34. Noor N, Sadat U, Hayes PD, et al: Management of the left subclavian artery during endovascular repair of the thoracic aorta, *J Endovasc Ther* 15:168–176, 2008.
35. Diethrich EB: A safe, simple alternative for pressure reduction during aortic endograft deployment (commentary), *J Endovasc Surg* 3:275, 1996.
36. Nienaber CA, Kische S, Rehders TC, et al: Rapid pacing for better placing: comparison of techniques for precise deployment of endografts in the thoracic aorta, *J Endovasc Ther* 14:506–512, 2007.
37. Fernandez JD, Donovan S, Garrett HE, et al: Endovascular thoracic aortic aneurysm repair: evaluating the utility of intravascular ultrasound measurements, *J Endovasc Ther* 15:68–72, 2008.
38. Colbel T, Lee T, Ivancev K, et al: In situ bending of a thoracic stent-graft: a proposed novel technique to improve thoracic endograft seal, *J Endovasc Ther* 15:62–66, 2008.
39. Criado FJ: Following the curve in TEVAR: adapting stent-grafts to the aortic arch, *J Endovasc Ther* 15:67, 2008.
40. Inoue K, Sato M, Iwasc T, et al: Clinical endovascular placement of branched graft for type B aortic dissection, *J Thorac Cardiovasc Surg* 112:1111–1113, 1996.
41. Chuter TAM, Schneider DB, Reilly LM, et al: Modular branched stent graft for endovascular repair of aortic arch aneurysm and dissection, *J Vasc Surg* 38:859–863, 2003.
42. Chuter TAM: Fenestrated and branched stent grafts for thoraco abdominal, pararenal and juxtarenal aortic aneurysm repair, *Semin Vasc Surg* 20:90–96, 2007.
43. Baldwin ZK, Chuter TAM, Hiramoto JS, et al: Double-barrel technique for endovascular exclusion of an aortic arch aneurysm without sternotomy, *J Endovasc Ther* 15:161–165, 2008.
44. Inoue K, Hosokawa H, Iwasc T, et al: Aortic arch reconstruction by transluminally placed endovascular branched stent graft, *Circulation* 100:316–321, 1999.
45. Saito N, Kimura T, Odashiro K, et al: Feasibility of the Inoue single-branched stent-graft implantation for thoracic aortic aneurysm or dissection involving the left subclavian artery: short-to medium-term results in 17 patients, *J Vasc Surg* 41:206 – 212, 2005.
46. Chuter TAM, Schneider DB: Endovascular repair of the aortic arch, *Perspect Vasc Surg Endovasc Ther* 19:188–192, 2007.

CHAPTER

56

Management of Complications After Endovascular Abdominal Aortic Aneurysm Repair

Sharif Ellozy, Daniel Silverberg

Endovascular stent graft repair for abdominal aortic aneurysms has gained wide acceptance since it was first reported in 1991.[1] Randomized controlled trials have shown decreased short-term morbidity and mortality when compared with open controls.[2,3] Refinements in device design and improvements in preoperative imaging have led to improved outcomes and widespread adoption of this technique as the first-line therapy for suitable abdominal aortic aneurysms. However, as with any therapy, the potential for complications exists. This chapter reviews the common short- and long-term complications of endovascular aneurysm repair, as well as their prevention and management options.

ENDOVASCULAR ANEURYSM REPAIR COMPLICATIONS

It is useful to classify complications of stent grafting according to their temporal occurrence. Early complications may be related to passage of the device, failure at a seal zone, or accidental coverage of a side branch such as the renal artery. Late complications are most often related to endoleaks but can include other entities such as limb occlusion, degeneration of the proximal neck, device fatigue, graft infection, and rupture.

Early Complications

Access Vessels

Appropriate iliac access is the cornerstone of successful endovascular aneurysm repair. Although long-term durability is most dependent on the anatomy of the seal zones, challenges related to the access vessels can result in significant perioperative morbidity and potentially mortality.[4,5] Iliac artery rupture during passage of the device can lead to significant blood loss and, if it is not controlled expeditiously, can be potentially lethal. Fortunately, with the quality of current computed tomographic (CT) imaging, it is possible to anticipate the majority of access problems. Most commercially available endografts require a delivery system with an outer diameter of anywhere from 20F to 25F. Therefore, depending on the device, the iliac arteries should have a minimal luminal diameter of anywhere from 7 to 9 mm. Apart from diameter, other anatomic factors need to be considered, such as the extent of calcification and tortuosity (Figure 56-1). In general, if only one of these factors is marginal, transfemoral delivery can be attempted. However, if more than one factor is marginal, an alternative access such as an iliac conduit should be considered.

Two classes of conduits have been described: open and endovascular. Open conduits are typically performed through a retroperitoneal incision. It is the authors' preference to construct this conduit with the patient under combined spinal-epidural anesthesia. A 10-mm crimped Dacron graft is sewn in an end-to-side fashion to the distal common iliac artery (CIA), and the graft is clamped distally. The graft can then be punctured and used analogously to a native vessel to allow for delivery of the device. After delivery of the device, the graft can simply be ligated, or it can be tunneled down to the groin and anastomosed to the femoral artery to treat any significant iliac occlusive disease. An open conduit also maintains perfusion to the ipsilateral internal iliac artery (Figure 56-2).

Endoluminal conduits consist of a balloon-expandable stent sewn to a thin-walled, 8-mm polytetrafluoroethylene

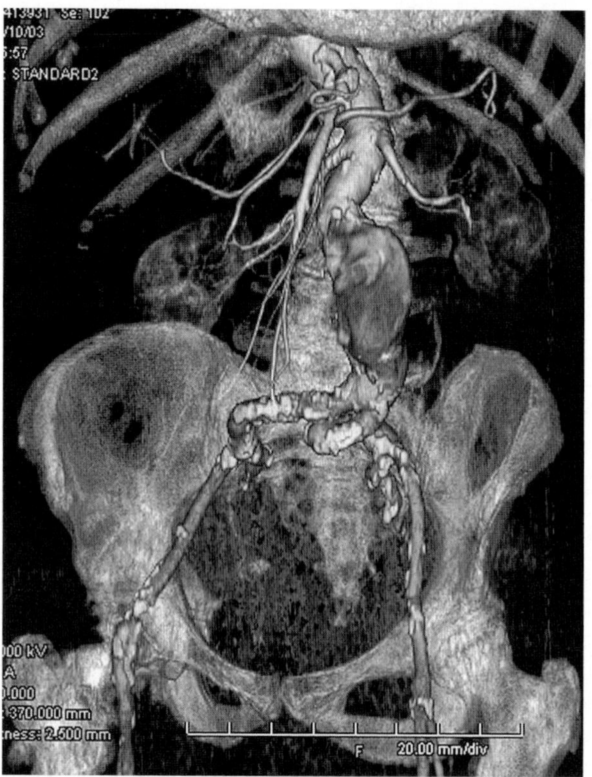

FIGURE 56-1 Challenging iliac access vessels. Note the calcification and severe tortuosity.

(PTFE) graft. The PTFE is predilated at the tip to an appropriate diameter (the diameter of the CIA at the seal zone), sewn to an appropriately sized balloon-expandable metal stent, and then crimped onto a balloon sized for the iliac seal zone (Figure 56-3, *A* and *B*). The balloon, stent, and PTFE graft are then back-loaded into a sheath (typically 16F to 18F), and an angioplasty balloon (typically 6 mm by 2 cm) is used to form a tapered tip for the delivery system. This conduit can be placed with use of only local anesthesia if necessary. The endoluminal conduit is delivered transfemorally after judicious predilatation of the iliacs. Once the stent is in the CIA, the sheath is withdrawn, the stent is expanded, and the PTFE is then dilated to at least 10 mm throughout its entire length down to the groin. At this point, the endoluminal conduit can be accessed in a similar fashion to a native vessel to allow for delivery of the device (see Figure 56-3, *B* and *C*). On completion of the procedure, the PTFE is anastomosed to the femoral artery. The benefit of an endoluminal conduit is that it obviates a retroperitoneal incision in a patient with a hostile abdomen. Additionally, in patients with circumferential iliac calcification, the conduit does not need to be sutured to the artery. Disadvantages include the fact that the ipsilateral internal iliac artery needs to be covered. Variations of the endoluminal conduit have been described, such as placement of a commercially available self-expanding stent graft in the iliac artery before delivery of the stent graft.[6]

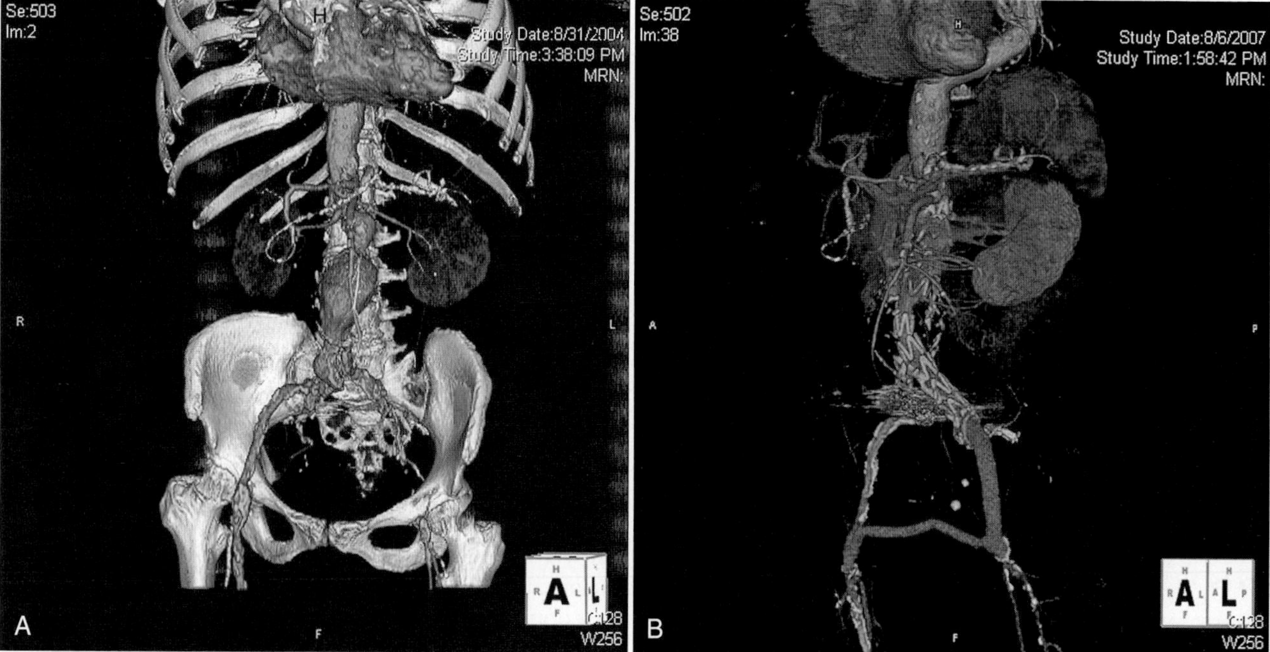

FIGURE 56-2 Open iliac conduit. **A,** Preoperative CT angiogram demonstrating occlusion of the left external iliac artery, with tortuosity, stenosis, and calcification seen on the right. **B,** Follow-up CT angiogram after repair with an aortouniiliac device delivered via a left common iliac conduit. The conduit was then anastomosed to the left common femoral artery, and a femorofemoral bypass was performed.

Despite adequate planning, access vessel rupture can occur (Figure 56-4). Two conditions are necessary to allow for a safe outcome. First, prompt recognition of the rupture is mandatory. Any unexplained hypotension during surgery should be investigated with a retrograde injection of contrast through the iliac artery. Second, it is absolutely essential to maintain wire access. This allows for placement of a compliant aortic occlusion balloon to control hemorrhage. Because the balloon is compliant, it can be inflated in the CIA just proximal to the site of rupture to allow for continued perfusion of the contralateral iliac artery. At this point, a decision can be made as to how to repair the iliac rupture. If the device has already been delivered, an extension limb or a commercially available stent graft can be deployed over the site of rupture. There are several types available (Viabahn, W.L. Gore & Associates, Flagstaff, AZ; Fluency, Bard Peripheral Vascular, Temple AZ; Atrium icast, Atrium Medical Corp., Hudson, NH), and the delivery systems range in size from 7F to 11F. If the rupture is not amenable to repair with a stent graft, then a retroperitoneal incision can be made in a controlled fashion, and either direct repair of the artery or placement of an open iliac conduit can be performed at this time.

A small-caliber, calcified distal aorta may present access problems as well, especially when a bifurcated device is planned. A narrow lumen in the distal aorta may not allow full deployment of the main device, making access of the contralateral gate difficult. If possible, partial deployment of the device with constraint of the iliac limb can be performed. Then, after cannulation of the contralateral gate, the device can be fully deployed. This will, it is hoped, prevent jailing out the contralateral gate. Once the aneurysm is excluded, judicious postdilatation of the iliac limbs should be performed to eliminate any stenoses. An alternative strategy is to employ an aortouniiliac device.

Acute Neck Complications

Although access vessel issues are responsible for the majority of acute complications, the long-term success of endovascular aneurysm repair (EVAR) is ultimately

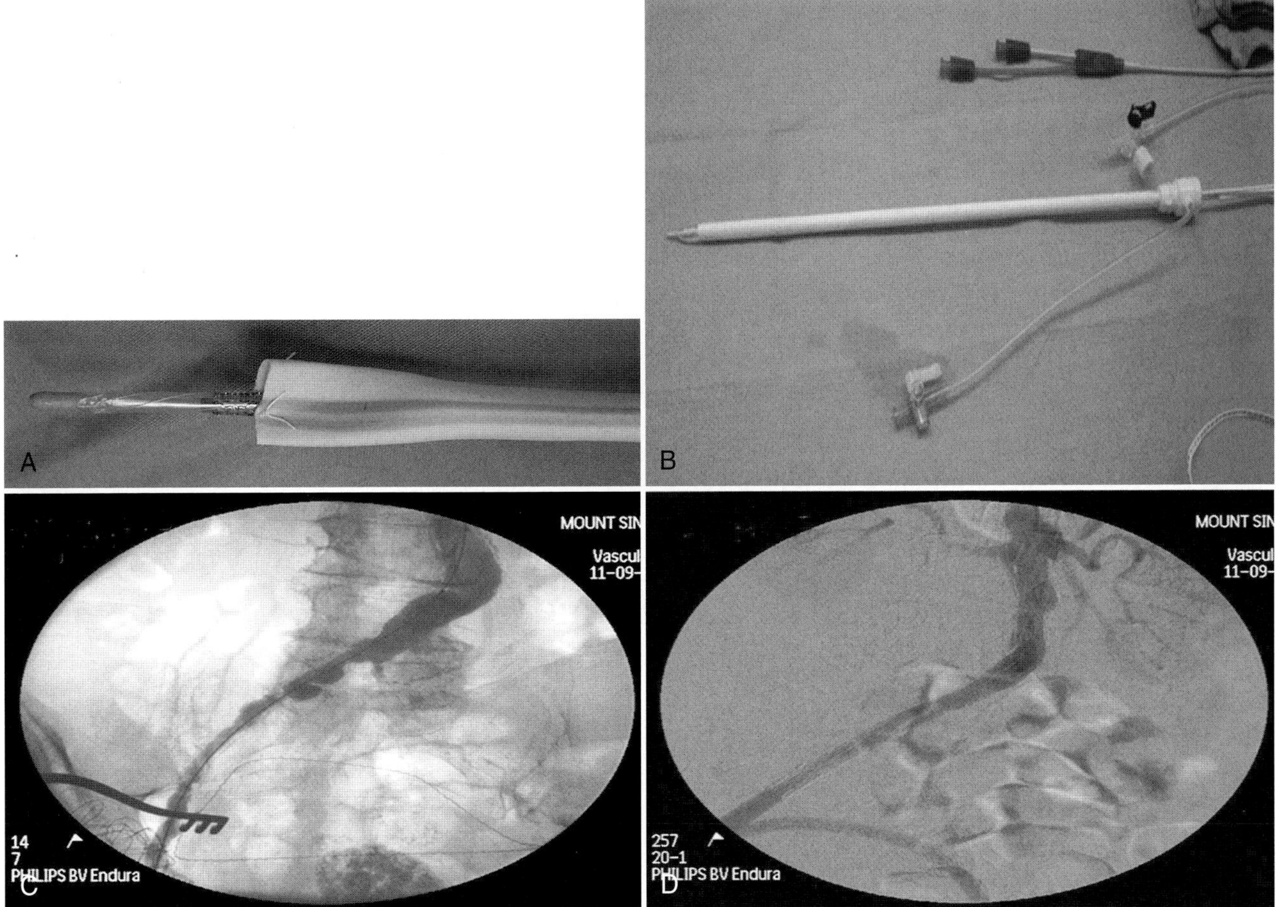

FIGURE 56-3 Endoluminal conduit. **A,** Balloon-expandable stent sewn to expanded PTFE graft. **B,** Endoluminal conduit in its delivery sheath. **C,** Predeployment angiogram demonstrating occlusion of the left common iliac and right internal iliac arteries, with a stenosed and calcified right iliac system. **D,** Completion angiogram after delivery of an aortouniiliac device through the endoluminal conduit.

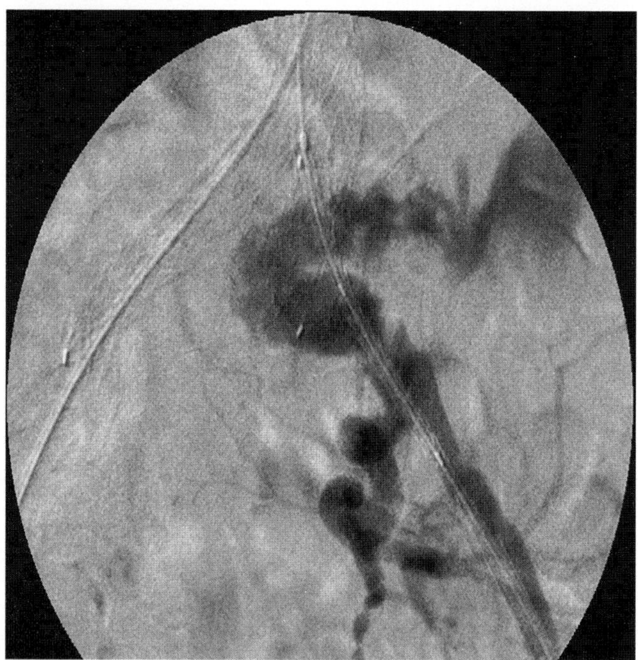

FIGURE 56-4 Retroperitoneal rupture after dilatation of left iliac limb.

dependent on the seal zone at the proximal neck. Four anatomic characteristics of the proximal neck determine suitability: angulation, length, shape, and the extent of mural thrombus. In general, long, straight necks with minimal thrombus are ideal. Preoperative assessment with three-dimensional CT angiography is essential in assessing these characteristics. Center-line reformatted images can provide an accurate assessment of neck length, shaded surface reconstructions can give an accurate view of the angulation and shape of the neck, and orthogonal reconstructions allow for accurate diameter measurements and assessment of the extent of mural thrombus (Figure 56-5). If one anatomic factor is unfavorable, one can consider attempting EVAR. However, if multiple factors are unfavorable, the likelihood of long-term failure increases significantly.[7]

The choice of device may contribute to the success or failure of the proximal seal zone. However, there are no definitive data proving superiority of any one graft over another.[8] The clinician should base his or her choice of device on several factors, such as diameter, conformability, trackability, and precision of deployment. Additionally, the importance of operator familiarity with the device cannot be overemphasized.

Accurate sizing and placement of the device are key. Angiography from multiple projections should be performed to identify the true origin of the lowest renal artery. The entire length of suitable neck should be used to allow for durable fixation of the stent graft. If a proximal type I endoleak is present after placement of the main device, several maneuvers may be helpful. It is the authors' practice to complete deployment of the contralateral limb before addressing the proximal leak. This provides additional column strength to the device before any salvage maneuvers are undertaken. At this point, the cause of the endoleak needs to be determined. If the device is too low, then placement of an extension cuff is generally the first step. Occasionally, the device abuts the lowest renal artery but does not cover the entire length of neck on the opposite wall because of neck angulation. In this case, a second cuff may be helpful, because it may position itself in a different fashion once the main body is in place (Figure 56-6).

If a proximal endoleak persists despite coverage of the entire available neck, then the mechanism of the endoleak needs to be determined. Occasionally, the device may be correctly sized and positioned, but it does not seal because of conformability issues. Should this be the case, a large balloon-expandable stent may help seal the endoleak. Care should be taken when inflating the stent so as not to overdilate the aortic neck (Figure 56-7). It should be noted that the durability of a balloon-expandable stent deployed inside a commercially approved device has not been rigorously studied.

Accidental coverage of a renal artery can be a challenging complication. Other authors have described pulling the devices downward using either an aortic occlusion balloon or a wire and a catheter pulled over the device bifurcation and grasped from both femoral arteries.[9] These maneuvers can be challenging to perform with any amount of control. Should there be any residual renal lumen, it is the preference of the authors to simply stent the renal arteries to maintain patency. As with most endovascular interventions, the key is to establish wire access. Brachial access can be particularly helpful, because the stent grafts cover the inferior aspect of the renal ostium. Low-profile systems are preferable (Figure 56-8). Long-term salvage of renal function after accidental renal artery coverage is possible.[10,11]

Late Complications

Endoleak

Endoleaks are defined as any persistent perfusion seen inside the aneurysm sac. They are classified by their point of origin (Table 56-1). The incidence of endoleak has been reported to be from 15% to 50%.[12-14] The majority of these endoleaks are type II, resulting from retrograde filling of the sac via patent side branches. In the absence of sac enlargement, most clinicians believe that these endoleaks are benign and do not warrant intervention. Type I or type III endoleaks, however, are thought to convey systemic pressure to

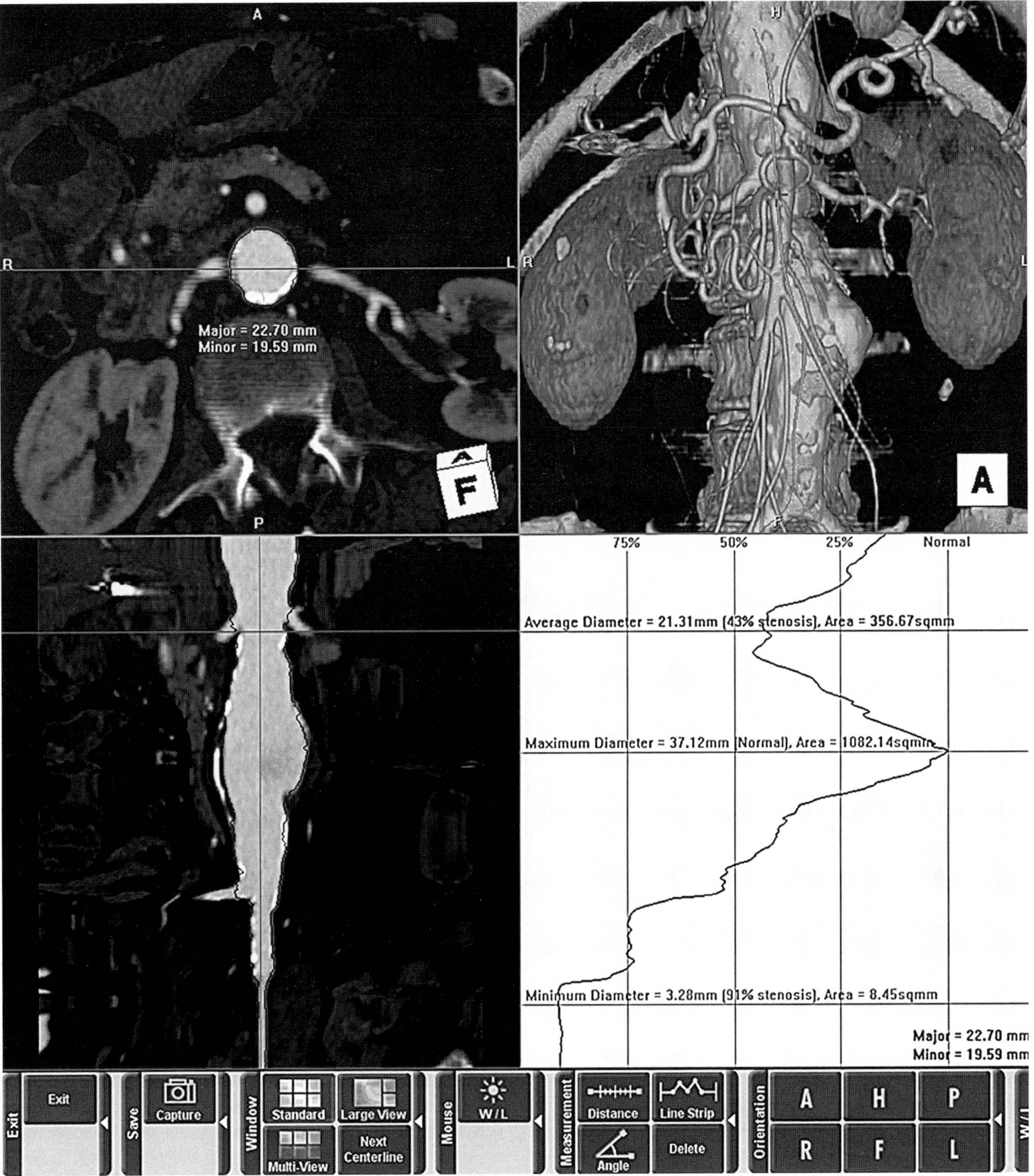

FIGURE 56-5 Three-dimensional CT reconstruction showing orthogonal, shaded surface, and stretched views of the abdominal aorta.

the aneurysm sac. Patients with type I or III endoleaks are thought to be at risk of rupture, and the presence of one of these endoleaks mandates correction. Any patient with an enlarging sac and a persistent type II endoleak should be investigated further, as there exists the possibility that this may represent an unappreciated type I endoleak.

Accurate characterization of an endoleak is the key to its management. CT angiography is the most common form of surveillance after EVAR, and it is highly

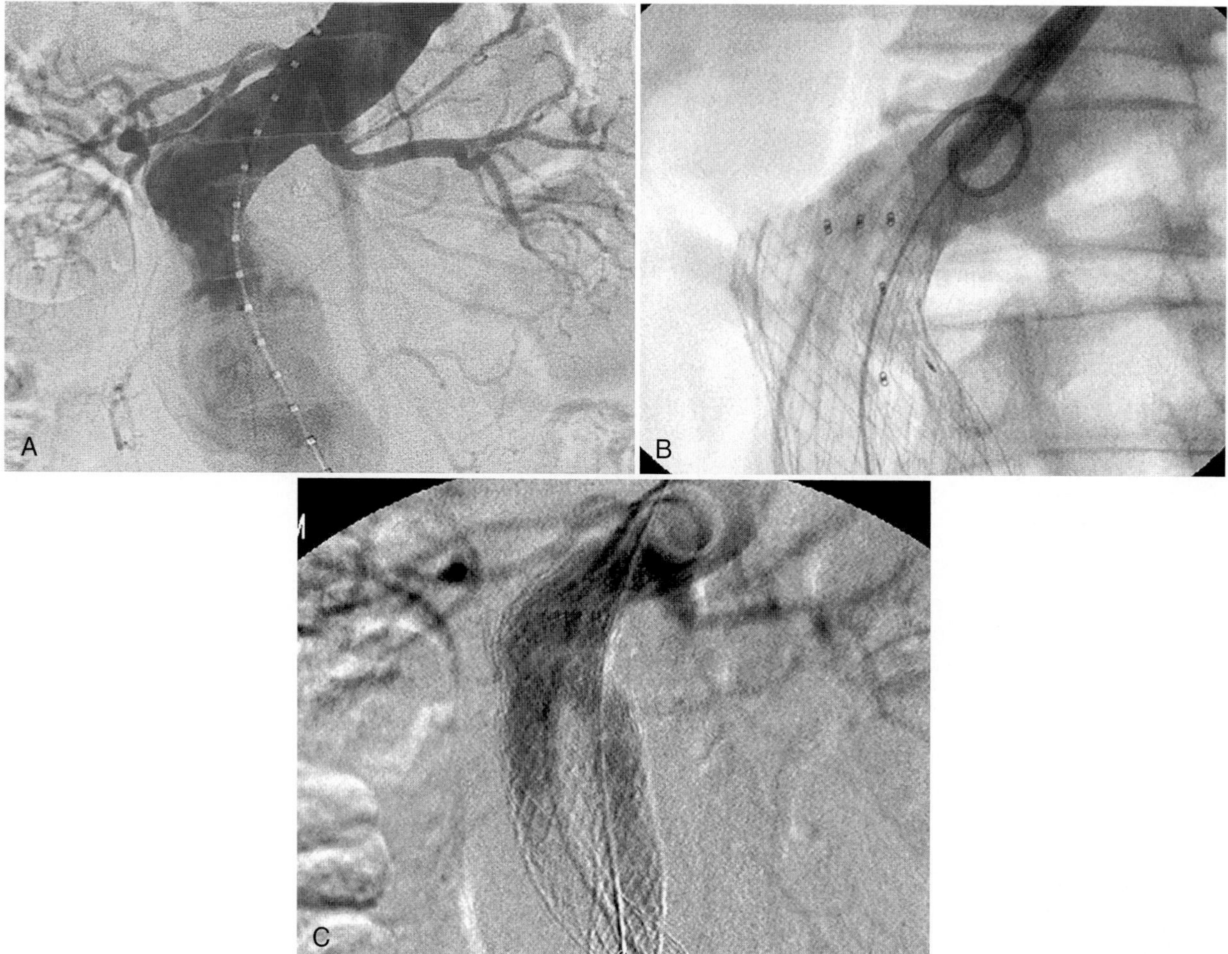

FIGURE 56-6 **A,** Angled neck. **B,** Deployment of the main body. The graft is low on the greater curve despite being just below the left renal artery on the lesser curve. This is primarily due to the stiffness of the device preventing it from conforming to the neck angulation. **C,** Deployment of a proximal cuff allows for better coverage on the greater curve.

sensitive for the presence of an endoleak. However, CT angiography is a static study and does not demonstrate direction of flow. This is of clinical significance, because type I endoleaks often show flow in patent aortic side branches. The flow is antegrade, in contrast to the retrograde flow seen in type II endoleaks. As such, CT angiography may not always differentiate between a type I and type II endoleak. A dynamic study, such as conventional angiography or time-resolved MR angiography, is needed to tell the direction of flow in the endoleak.

Conventional angiography can be both diagnostic and therapeutic in the management of endoleaks. Flush aortography, selective injection of the superior mesenteric and both internal iliac arteries, and interrogation of the seal zones may be needed to define the nature of the endoleak. The type of treatment depends entirely on the character of the endoleak. Should the sac enlargement be due to a type II endoleak, embolization at the time of angiography can be performed. Access to the sac can be gained typically in one of two ways: either via a microcatheter through the superior mesenteric artery and the marginal artery into the inferior mesenteric artery or through direct translumbar puncture. Both methods have their advantages, but it should be kept in mind that a translumbar puncture cannot definitively define the origin of an endoleak, because it will only demonstrate the outflow from the sac. Therefore a transfemoral angiogram needs to be performed first for diagnostic purposes. Once a catheter has been introduced into the aneurysm sac, a variety of embolic agents, such as coils or glue, can be used (Figure 56-9).

Delayed failure of the proximal seal zone is perhaps the most challenging complication of endovascular stent grafting. If the endoleak is demonstrated to be a proximal type I endoleak, then the determination needs to be made as to whether this can be salvaged with another endovascular device or whether the patient will require open conversion. The same anatomic criteria for endovascular suitability exist for a revision as they do for a primary repair: length, shape, angulation, and

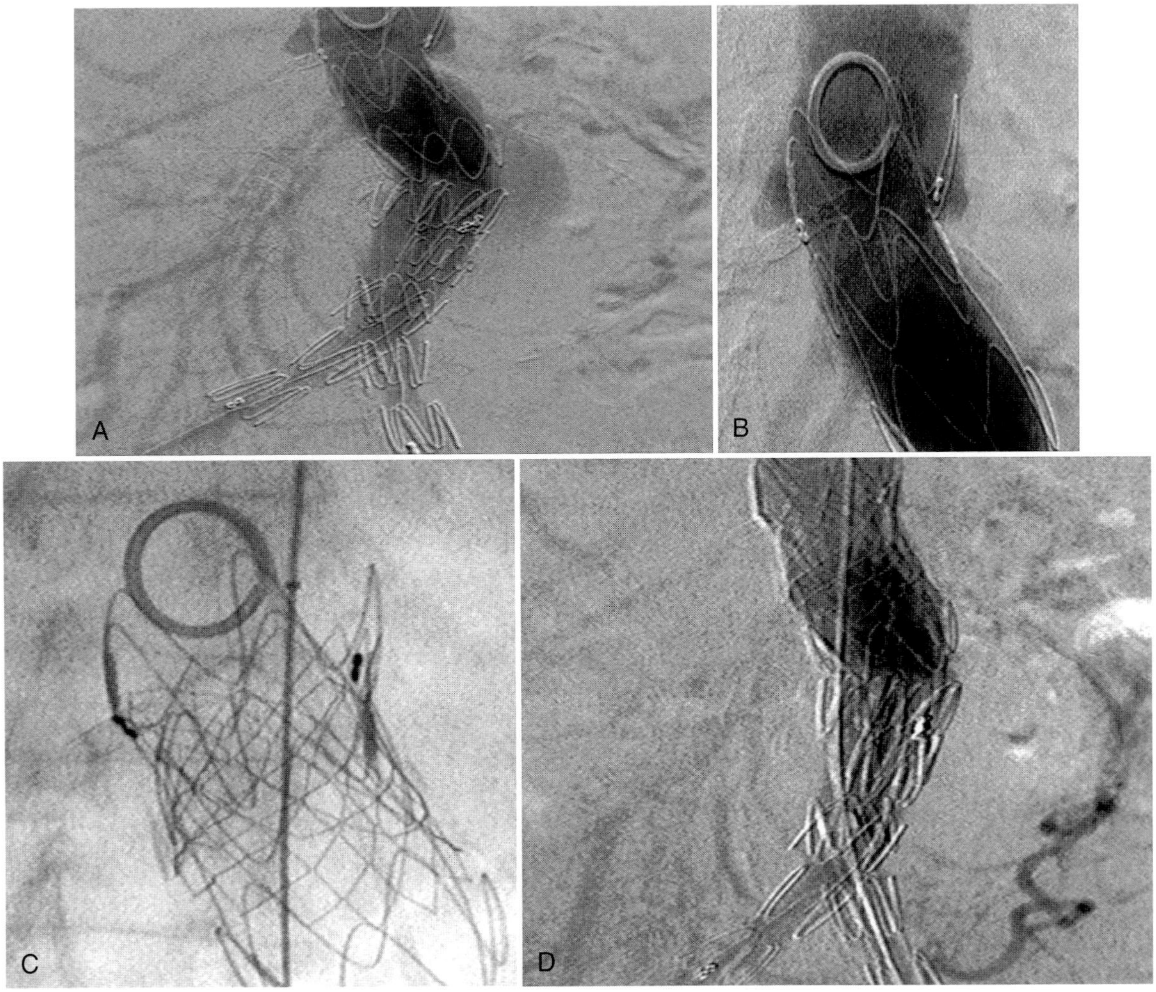

FIGURE 56-7 Neck irregularity treated with a large balloon-expandable stent. **A,** Proximal type I endoleak noted despite adequate position and sizing of the graft. **B,** Poor apposition of the graft against the aortic wall calcification (note the calcification in the wall). **C,** Improved device apposition against the wall after stent placement. **D,** Resolution of the proximal type I endoleak.

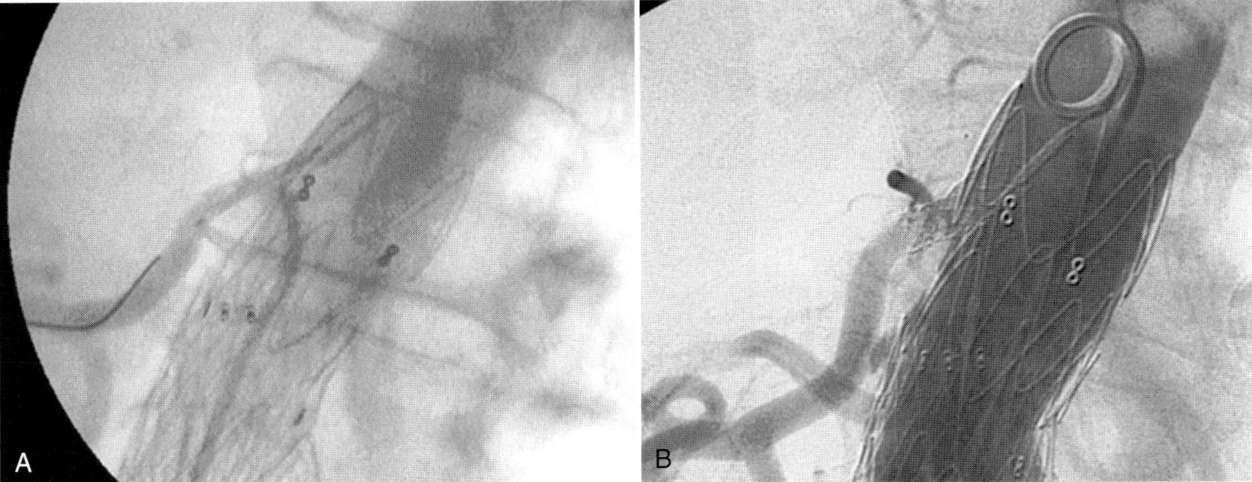

FIGURE 56-8 **A,** Significant impingement of a single renal artery orifice by stent graft fabric. Renal wire access has been obtained from a brachial approach. **B,** Completion angiography after stent deployment demonstrates a widely patent renal artery.

TABLE 56-1 Endoleak Classification

Endoleak type	Point of origin
Type I	Proximal or distal seal zone
Type II	Patent aortic side branch (inferior mesenteric artery or lumbar arteries)
Type III	Failure of device integrity (fabric tear or junctional leak)
Type IV	Endotension (enlarging sac with no demonstrable endoleak)

presence of thrombus in the neck. Review of the original, pretreatment images can be useful in determining further therapy. If the original device was undersized or misdeployed, then repeated endovascular repair may be feasible. However, if the original films demonstrate circumferential thrombus in the neck, or if the device failed despite adequate sizing and deployment, endovascular revision is likely to fail. Additionally, the presence of a device in the aneurysm may complicate access issues, because it can make passage of a secondary device more difficult. Two approaches have been typically used for endovascular salvage: placement of a proximal cuff or conversion to an aortouniiliac device with a femorofemoral bypass. Although the placement of a cuff is simpler, it relies on a seal between the old device and the new device for long-term fixation. This may be difficult to achieve if there is significant angulation in the neck. The aortouniiliac repair is more labor intensive, because the goal is to reline the entire aorta from the renal arteries to the iliac seal zone and it requires creation of a femorofemoral bypass (Figure 56-10). However, it does not depend on the integrity of the old device or on a seal between the old and the new device. In the authors' institutional experience, aortouniiliac repairs seemed to be more durable.[15] The use of a device with a suprarenal stent should be considered when revising proximal failures.

Distal type I endoleaks can easily be treated with internal iliac artery embolization and extension of the limb to the external iliac artery. This can be usually be performed percutaneously with the use of a closure device.

Type III endoleaks can often be salvaged endovascularly by relining the stent graft, because the seal zones are still intact. Although rare, fatigue and junctional failures can be seen with all devices[16] (Figure 56-11). It is essential to characterize the site of failure to correct it. If the endoleak is junctional, then simply placing a limb to bridge the leak typically solves the problem. If, however, the problem with device integrity is in the body of the graft, then the entire device needs to be excluded. This usually requires an aortouniiliac device with a femorofemoral bypass, because a second bifurcated device cannot be placed inside the first.

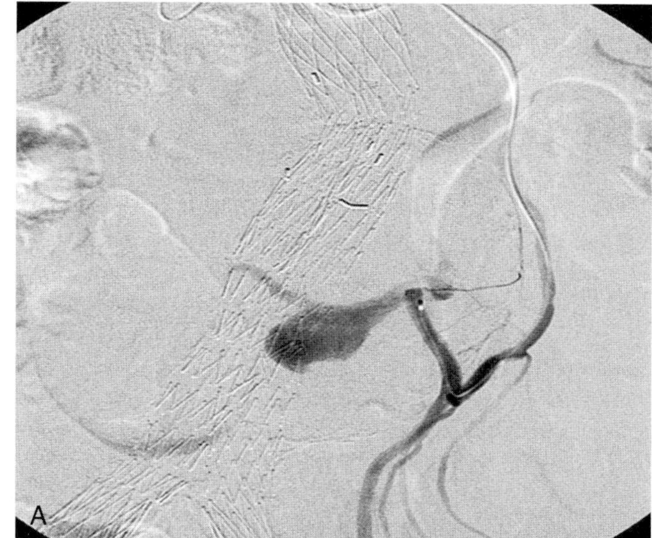

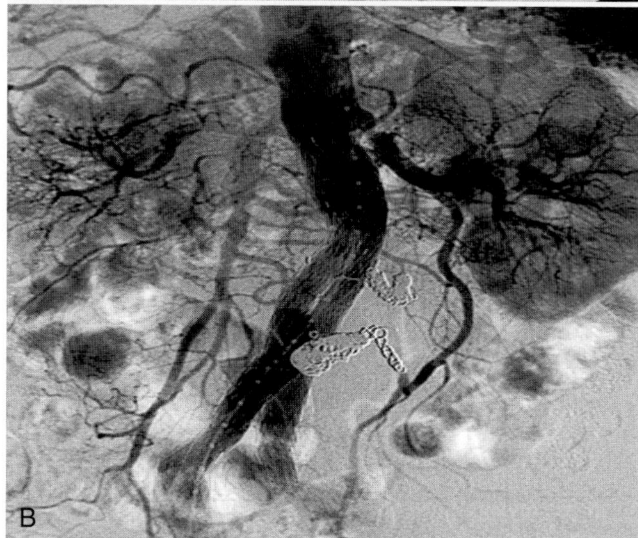

FIGURE 56-9 **A,** Type II endoleak through a patent inferior mesenteric artery. The microcatheter was advanced into the sac through the superior mesenteric artery via the arc of Riolan. **B,** Completion angiogram after embolization of the sac with microcoils demonstrates no further endoleak.

Limb Occlusion

Iliac limb occlusion after endovascular stent graft occurs with a reported incidence of 3% to 7% of patients. The risk factors for limb occlusion include extension of the limb to the external iliac, extensive calcification, the use of unsupported graft limbs, kinking of the graft limbs, and small-caliber vessels.[17-19] The clinical presentation can vary from an incidental finding on surveillance CT to an acutely ischemic, threatened limb, depending on the collateral circulation. Important collaterals around the area of occlusion include the internal iliac artery and the profunda femoris (Figure 56-12).

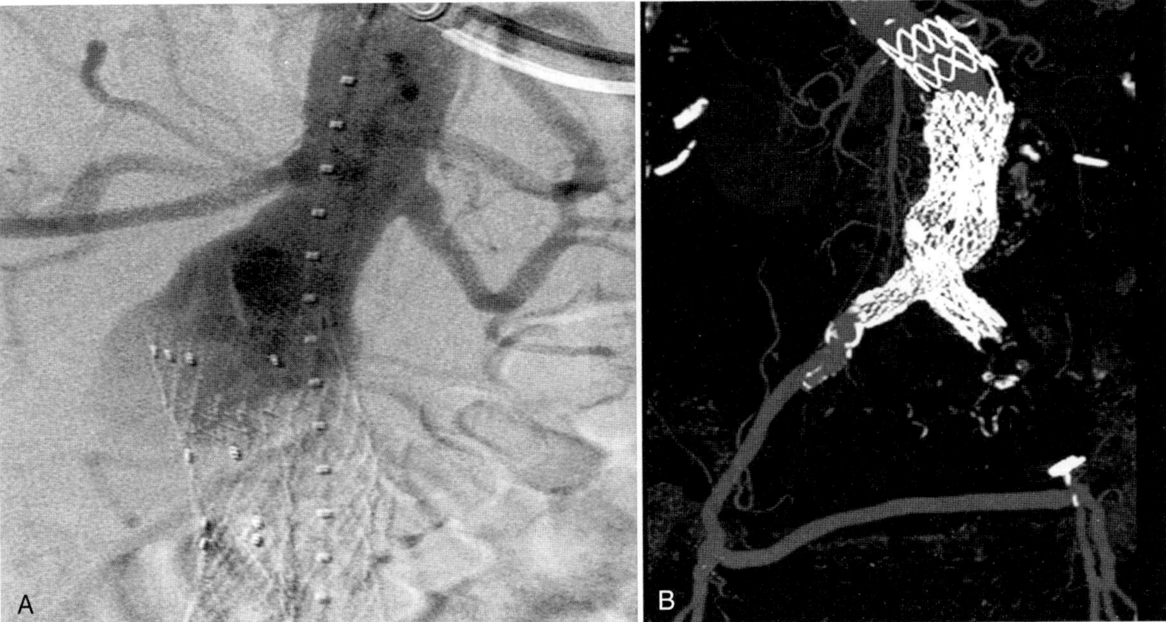

FIGURE 56-10 **A,** Delayed proximal type I endoleak. Note that the device is sitting in the aneurysm sac. **B,** CT reconstruction after conversion to an aortouniiliac device with a femorofemoral bypass.

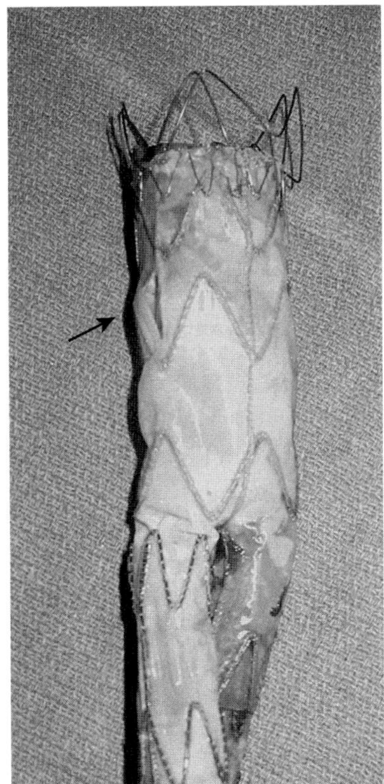

FIGURE 56-11 Fabric tear noted at explant.

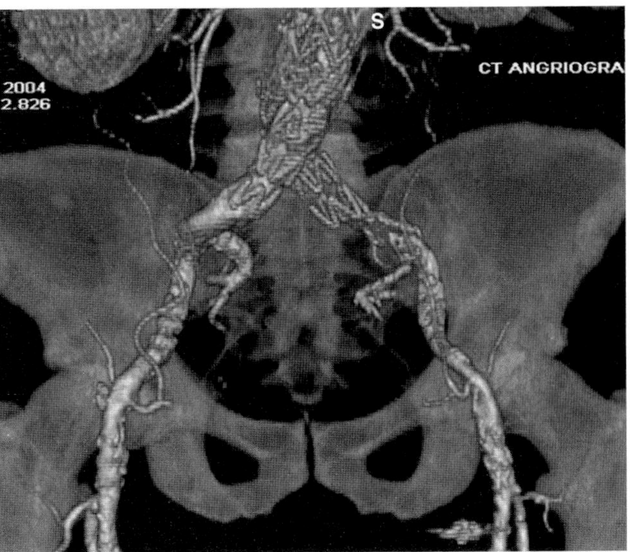

FIGURE 56-12 Occlusion of the left iliac limb with reconstitution at the level of the iliac bifurcation via pelvic collaterals.

The management of an iliac limb occlusion depends on the acuity of the ischemia and the underlying anatomic defect. Certain authors have described endovascular approaches to limb occlusion. Catheter-directed thrombolysis and thrombectomy will reveal any contributing stenosis. This may then be managed with angioplasty and stenting.[18] This strategy offers the potential benefit of a completely percutaneous approach. However, in the acutely ischemic patient, it may take several hours to restore perfusion. An additional concern is that it may be difficult to correct the anatomic cause of the occlusion. An alternative approach, generally favored by the authors, is to simply perform a femoral-femoral bypass. This avoids the risk for thrombolysis and allows for rapid restoration of perfusion. Long-term patency of the femoral-femoral bypass in this setting is very good.[20,21]

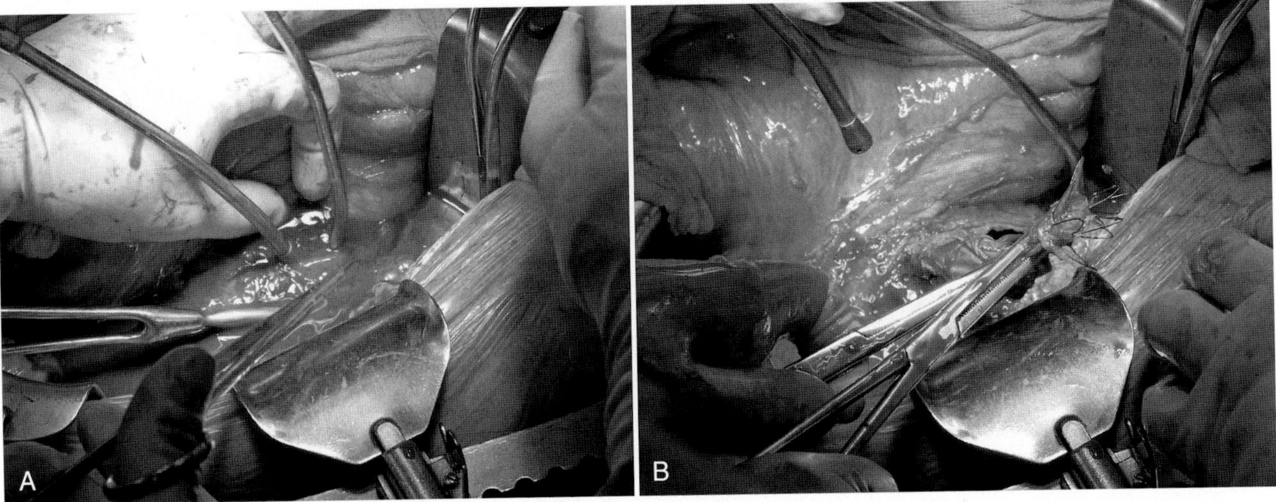

FIGURE 56-13 Stent graft infection. **A,** Grossly infected sac contents. **B,** Removal of the stent graft.

Graft Infection

Endovascular stent graft infection is a rare but potentially lethal complication. It can arise in the setting of an aortoenteric fistula or may come about because of contamination of the graft. Graft infection may be suspected if air is seen in the aneurysm sac on CT more than 1 month out from the initial implantation, or if the patient has inflammatory findings around the aneurysm with systemic signs of infection. When feasible, the treatment of choice is graft excision with extra-anatomic bypass and debridement of all infected tissue (Figure 56-13).

Open Conversion

Open conversion after failed endovascular repair can be facilitated with several techniques. Positioning of the proximal clamp is determined by the presence or absence of suprarenal stents. If there are bare stents across the renal arteries, an initial supraceliac clamp can be placed until the device is out, and then the clamp can be moved into the infrarenal position. Balloon occlusion catheters, deployed either transfemorally or transbrachially, can be helpful in patients with challenging anatomy. Some authors have even described deploying the catheters directly through the indwelling stent graft. Care should be taken in removing the device to prevent damage to the aorta at the pararenal segment. If the suprarenal stents are embedded in the wall of the aorta, a sterile wire cutter can be used to leave the wires in situ. Distally, the iliac arteries and the device limbs can be clamped directly. Vascular clamps with Fogarty inserts can facilitate occlusion of the stent graft limbs. If the distal seal is intact, the iliac limbs do not need to be removed. The limbs can be transected, and an end-to-end anastomosis can be fashioned to the limbs with use of the native iliac as an external pledget. Despite the increased complexity of repair in the setting of a failed stent graft, some authors have reported good long-term outcomes.[22]

CONCLUSION

The key to managing complications in endovascular aneurysm repair is anticipation and case selection. The most serious acute complications are related to access vessels, and these are typically predictable. The liberal use of conduits in challenging cases allows for safe endovascular repair. Close surveillance after repair, with the use of dynamic imaging in equivocal cases, allows for early identification and safe treatment of late complications. Precise imaging is key in determining whether endovascular revision of failed stent grafts is possible. Should the patient need open conversion, balloon occlusion catheters, Fogarty vascular clamps, and sterile wire cutters can significantly simplify the operation.

References

1. Parodi JC, Palmaz JC, Barone HD: Transfemoral intraluminal graft implantation for abdominal aortic aneurysms, *Ann Vasc Surg* 5(6):491–499, 1991.
2. Greenhalgh RM, Brown LC, Kwong GP: (EVAR Trial Participants) et al: Comparison of endovascular aneurysm repair with open repair in patients with abdominal aortic aneurysm (EVAR trial 1) 30-day operative mortality results: randomised controlled trial, *Lancet* 364(9437):843–848, 2004.
3. Prinssen M, Verhoeven EL, Buth J: (Dutch Randomized Endovascular Aneurysm Management (DREAM) Trial Group, et al: A randomized trial comparing conventional and endovascular repair of abdominal aortic aneurysms, *N Engl J Med* 351 (16):1607–1618, 2004.
4. Fairman RM, Velazquez O, Baum R: Endovascular repair of aortic aneurysms: critical events and adjunctive procedures, *J Vasc Surg* 33(6):1226–1232, 2001.

5. Henretta JP, Karch LA, Hodgson KJ, et al: Special iliac artery considerations during aneurysm endografting, *Am J Surg* 178(3):212–218, 1999.
6. Peterson B, Matsumura J: Internal endoconduit: an innovative technique to address unfavorable iliac artery anatomy encountered during thoracic endovascular aortic repair, *J Vasc Surg* 47(2):441–445, 2008.
7. Sampaio SM, Panneton JM, Mozes GI, et al: Proximal type I endoleak after endovascular abdominal aortic aneurysm repair: predictive factors, *Ann Vasc Surg* 18(6):621–628, 2004.
8. Abbruzzese TA, Kwolek CJ, Brewster DC, et al: Outcomes following endovascular abdominal aortic aneurysm repair (EVAR): an anatomic and device-specific analysis, *J Vasc Surg* 48(1):19–28, 2008.
9. Lin PH, Bush RL, Lumsden AB: Endovascular rescue of a maldeployed aortic stent-graft causing renal artery occlusion: technical considerations, *Vasc Endovascular Surg* 38(1):69–73, 2004.
10. Baril DT, Lookstein RA, Jacobs TS, et al: Durability of renal artery stents in patients with transrenal abdominal aortic endografts, *J Vasc Surg* 45(5):915–920. discussion 920–921, 2007.
11. Hedayati N, Lin PH, Lumsden AB, Zhou W: Prolonged renal artery occlusion after endovascular aneurysm repair: endovascular rescue and renal function salvage, *J Vasc Surg* 47(2): 446–449, 2008.
12. Silverberg D, Baril DT, Ellozy SH, et al: An 8-year experience with type II endoleaks: natural history suggests selective intervention is a safe approach, *J Vasc Surg* 44(3):453–459, 2006.
13. Sampram ES, Karafa MT, Mascha EJ, et al: Nature, frequency, and predictors of secondary procedures after endovascular repair of abdominal aortic aneurysm, *J Vasc Surg* 37(5):930–937, 2003.
14. van Marrewijk C, Buth J, Harris PL, et al: Significance of endoleaks after endovascular repair of abdominal aortic aneurysms: The EUROSTAR experience, *J Vasc Surg* 35(3):461–473, 2002.
15. Baril DT, Silverberg D, Ellozy SH, et al: Endovascular stent-graft repair of failed endovascular abdominal aortic aneurysm repair, *Ann Vasc Surg* 22(1):30–36, 2008.
16. Jacobs TS, Won J, Gravereaux EC, et al: Mechanical failure of prosthetic human implants: a 10-year experience with aortic stent graft devices, *J Vasc Surg* 37(1):16–26, 2003.
17. Carroccio A, Faries PL, Morrissey NJ, et al: Predicting iliac limb occlusions after bifurcated aortic stent grafting: anatomic and device-related causes, *J Vasc Surg* 36(4):679–684, 2002.
18. Erzurum VZ, Sampram ES, Sarac TP, et al: Initial management and outcome of aortic endograft limb occlusion, *J Vasc Surg* 40(3):419–423, 2004.
19. Cochennec F, Becquemin JP, Desgranges P, et al: Limb graft occlusion following EVAR: clinical pattern, outcomes and predictive factors of occurrence, *Eur J Vasc Endovasc Surg* 34(1):59–65, 2007.
20. Clouse WD, Brewster DC, Marone LK, et al: Evt/Guidant Investigators. Durability of aortouniiliac endografting with femorofemoral crossover: 4-year experience in the Evt/Guidant trials, *J Vasc Surg* 37(6):1142–1149, 2003.
21. Heredero AF, Stefanov S, Riera Del Moral L, et al: Long-term results of femoro-femoral crossover bypass after endovascular Aortouniiliac Repair of Abdominal Aortic and Aortoiliac aneurysms, *Vasc Endovascular Surg* 42(5):420–426, 2008.
22. Jimenez JC, Moore WS, Quinones-Baldrich WJ: Acute and chronic open conversion after endovascular aortic aneurysm repair: a 14-year review, *J Vasc Surg* 46(4):642–647, 2007.

SECTION IX

DIALYSIS ACCESS SALVAGE

CHAPTER

57

Duplex Ultrasound Surveillance of Dialysis Access Function

Joe P. Chauvapun, Martin R. Back, Dennis F. Bandyk

Maintenance of a functional dialysis access requires vigilance in caring for patients with end-stage renal disease. Both autogenous fistulas (AVFs) and prosthetic bridge grafts are associated with a spectrum of problems that threaten or terminate dialysis access site function. The failure rate, that is, primary patency rate based on "intention to treat" reporting standards, has been reported as high as 40% at 1 year for both autogenous and prosthetic dialysis accesses.[1,2] The most frequently occurring complications are those associated with thrombosis, infection, false aneurysm formation, venous hypertension producing limb edema, and arterial steal syndrome producing hand ischemia. In the majority of patients, salvage of dialysis access grafts is possible, but the subsequent failure rate is substantial with secondary patency rates at 1 year of 60% to 80% for AVFs and 50% to 70% for polytetrafluoroethylene (PTFE) bridge grafts.[1,2] The rationale for dialysis access surveillance is rooted in belief that surgical or endovascular intervention to maintain functional patency is more successful when performed on a patent but "failing" vascular access than on one that has thrombosed. The most common secondary procedure is repair of an access venous outflow stenosis that reduces flow to a level that hemodialysis is inadequate. Monitoring of dialysis access function is a recommended "quality assurance" guideline, but the efficacy of duplex ultrasound surveillance to improve patency is at present an unproved clinical application in part because a properly designed, randomized clinical trial has not been conducted.

Surveillance of dialysis access function requires use of accurate diagnostics and effective interventions to restore access anatomy and hemodynamics for access cannulation and hemodialysis. The goal is to maintain a high-flow, subcutaneous conduit that can be easily accessed to deliver blood to and from a dialysis machine. In general, three-times-weekly hemodialysis requires at least a 10-cm length of subcutaneous conduit for needle cannulation and volume flow rate of greater than 600 mL/min. The National Kidney Foundation (http://www.kidney.org) in its Dialysis Outcome Quality Initiative guidelines 9 through 11 recommends "prospective surveillance of dialysis access grafts for hemodynamically significant stenosis." Evidence-based data indicate that surveillance combined with lesion repair "improves patency and decreases the incidence of thrombosis." The surveillance protocol should include weekly physical examination in the dialysis unit and the use of anatomic and physiologic techniques to detect access stenosis or flow reduction. Diagnostic methods available to clinicians include access recirculation calculations, venous line pressures, ultrasonic dilution techniques, duplex ultrasound testing for stenosis detection and volume flow measurement, and contrast fistulography.[3] The best surveillance method is one that is accurate, inexpensive, safe, and, for practical considerations, reimbursed by the Centers for Medicare & Medicaid Services (CMS) or other health care providers. Although duplex ultrasound appears ideally suited for dialysis access surveillance, the current CMS payment guidelines for CPT 93900 (duplex scan of hemodialysis access) will not pay for routine surveillance. Payment is provided if any sign or symptom of access dysfunction exists including decreased thrill on physical examination, difficulty in needle cannulation, clot formation during hemodialysis, an elevated venous line dynamic pressure (>200 mm Hg) during dialysis at a flow of 200 mL/min, access recirculation of 12% or greater, or an otherwise unexplained urea reduction ratio of less than 60%. Also, CMS will not pay for a duplex scan and a fistulogram unless documentation of medical necessity for both diagnostic tests is provided.[4]

The development of a segmental stenosis in the venous outflow vessels is the most common mechanism for dialysis access failure, including failure to mature after access construction. Clinical features of the common types of upper-extremity dialysis access are detailed in Table 57-1, including expected maturation times. Stenotic lesions can also develop at the arterial anastomosis, within the prosthetic graft, and in the central veins of the thorax. Significant stenosis, that is, greater than 50% diameter reducing (DR), is found in 80% to 90%[5-7] of thrombosed access grafts. In the remaining failures, no causative anatomic lesion is identified, suggesting other etiologies such as transient hypotension, hypovolemia, hypercoagulability, excessive access compression, and improper access cannulation or puncture site compression. Duplex ultrasound is ideally suited to noninvasively image the dialysis conduit for stenotic lesions and quantify volume flow. Documentation of normal access anatomy and hemodynamics is useful for patient management, including the initial decision to begin using a newly constructed dialysis conduit. By using appropriate interpretation criteria, duplex testing enables the clinician to access the significance of stenotic segments on the basis of access volume flow changes to a level that would compromise hemodialysis. Other lesions may also interfere with access function or longevity, such as pseudoaneurysm formation, mural thrombus, cannulation site hematoma, and perigraft seroma, which are also readily detected by duplex testing.

Repair of duplex- or fistulogram-detected stenosis by open surgical revision or percutaneous transluminal balloon angioplasty can restore functional patency and extend access survival.[2,3,8-11] Prospective clinical studies comparing results of surgical versus endovascular intervention have reported equivalent success in the management of the "thrombosed" or "stenotic" access conduit. Intervention decisions are typically based on nature and site of the lesions, the age of dialysis access, conduit type, and experience of the operator. Because most lesion development occurs within the first year, access surveillance should be most rigorous during this time. Also, the efficacy of access surveillance may differ between prosthetic bridge grafts and autologous AVFs, and thus the optimal surveillance algorithm should be tailored to the various types of access conduits constructed. The goal of this chapter is to review dialysis access surveillance methods and detail a protocol using duplex ultrasound to evaluate access function after construction and during long-term hemodialysis usage.

ACCESS SURVEILLANCE METHODS

Historically, access surveillance relied on anatomic assessment using contrast digital subtraction arteriography to assess access dysfunction or failure. Current recommendations support the application of physiologic testing methods for surveillance including duplex ultrasound, venous line pressure measurements, and Doppler volume flow measurements. These techniques can identify the "low" volume flow or failing dialysis access—a hemodynamic characteristic predictive of thrombosis or difficult hemodialysis. The minimum volume flow threshold for satisfactory hemodialysis is approximately 500 mL/min. Volume flow rates of clinically functional upper-extremity dialysis accesses are much higher, in the range of 800 to 1200 mL/min depending on access type and its age. After dialysis access construction, volume flow increases during the first several weeks. Overall, autogenous forearm accesses have a lower flow rate than arm or prosthetic bridge grafts because of smaller outflow vein caliber and radial artery inflow hemodynamics. As the fistulas

TABLE 57-1 Features of Common Upper-Extremity Dialysis Access Procedures

Type of access	Inflow artery	Outflow vein	Anastomotic configuration	Time to maturation*
Arteriovenous fistula				
Brescia-Cimino	Radial	Cephalic	Side-to-side	8-12 wk
	Brachial	Cephalic	End-to-side	8-12 wk
Autologous vein				
Transposition	Radial/brachial	Basilic/cephalic	End-to-side	8-12 wk
Saphenous graft	Radial/brachial	Basilic/brachial		6-8 wk
Prosthetic bridge graft†				
PTFE 6 mm diameter or 4-7 mm taper	Radial/brachial	Basilic/cephalic/brachial	Side-to-side	2-4 wk

PTFE, Polytetrafluoroethylene.
*Maturation time dependent on initial vein diameter and development of sufficient volume flow for hemodialysis.
†Graft configuration may be a straight or loop connection between any suitable artery and vein.

"mature," vein and radial artery caliber increases as does volume flow. Thus volume flow is an important criterion of dialysis access maturation and should be measured before initial cannulation.

A stenosis that reduces lumen diameter greater than 50%, that is, 80% cross-sectional area reduction, is associated with a resting pressure gradient, and therefore basal volume flow is reduced. Documentation of a 50% to 60% DR venous stenosis by contrast fistulogram is anatomic evidence of access dysfunction but may be observed in patients with clinically functioning vascular accesses. The intent of surveillance is through sequential monitoring of access function to identify hemodynamic changes before access thrombosis, for example, volume flow reduction below a critical (<300-500 mL/min) level.

Contrast Fistulography

Angiography by direct injection of iodinated contrast agents is considered the "gold standard" for imaging of access conduits. Use of digital subtraction techniques, multiplane imaging, and proper catheter positioning facilitates full delineation of the arterial inflow, access conduit, venous outflow, and anastomotic regions. Stenosis grading by fistulogram requires accurate measurements of narrowed luminal dimensions and comparison with adjacent, minimally diseased vessel or conduit segments. Fistulography can also detect true and false aneurysms associated with arteriovenous hemodialysis conduits—lesions that increase thrombotic risk and require repair. Because testing is invasive and expensive and has associated risks, it should not be used as a primary method for screening dialysis access grafts for anatomic lesions but is rather reserved for evaluation of documented failing access. Iodinated contrast exposure in those patients not yet receiving hemodialysis with recently constructed, but dysfunctional access conduits should also be avoided to prevent acceleration of renal failure. In such cases, duplex ultrasonography alone may be used to identify stenoses for intervention. Fistulography is indicated without prior surveillance study when access dysfunction is severe enough to hinder adequate hemodialysis or there is marked change in the palpable thrill normally felt over an existing conduit. A fistulogram produces high-resolution anatomic imaging of the dialysis access found to be abnormal by noninvasive physiologic testing and can aid in selection of the most appropriate intervention when a lesion is identified. A catheter-directed venography is the preferred technique to evaluate the central (axillary, subclavian, brachiocephalic, superior vena cava) venous system for obstruction or stenotic lesions produced by prior venous catheters.

Access Recirculation

Recirculation within a hemodialysis access conduit is defined as dialyzed blood returning through the venous needle that reenters the extracorporeal circuit through the arterial needle. If measured accurately, access recirculation does not occur unless the blood flow rate through the access conduit is less than that prescribed through the dialyzer circuit.[12] Measurement of recirculation percentage of 12% or greater correlates with low volume flow and is an indicator of inefficient hemodialysis. Access recirculation is calculated by using the measured concentration of blood urea nitrogen (BUN) according to the formula:

$$U_s - U_a / U_s - U_v \times 100\%$$

where U_s is systemic [BUN], U_a is arterial blood line [BUN], and U_v is venous blood line [BUN]. Existing methods (three-needle, peripheral vein techniques) of measurement of systemic [BUN] are prone to error and overestimation of recirculation because of arteriovenous and venovenous disequilibrium. Alternatively, a two-needle, slow/stop flow method for urea recirculation may decrease these errors.[13] Techniques to directly measure access recirculation without urea measurement include newer saline or temperature dilution techniques. Recirculation measurements are made during hemodialysis and can be repeated serially over time.

Recirculation measurements have not generally been predictive of dialysis access thrombosis, and uniformly accepted threshold values for urea recirculation do not exist to prompt further evaluation of a suspected failing access. Urea recirculation values of greater than 15% at a dialyzer flow rate of 400 mL/min have had an acceptable accuracy for identifying access conduits with stenoses according to Windus et al.[14] and Daniels et al.[15] These results have not been reproduced in the prospective studies of others.[2,5,16,17] Measurement of access recirculation should not be considered a preferred method for identification of a failing access and is not suited for surveillance.

Venous Line Pressure

Elevation of pressure measured in the drip chamber of the venous cannula downstream of the dialysis pump and membrane unit can occur with significant obstructions at the venous anastomosis or venous outflow. Because venous outflow stenosis is a common cause of access failure, serial measurement of venous line pressures has been proposed as a surveillance method. The pressure measurement accuracy is highly dependent on proper matching of the dynamic response of the catheter-transducer system, transducer zeroing relative to height differences in the system, and elimination of air bubbles or blood clots. Although both static (measured under no dialyzer flow condition) and dynamic (with dialyzer flow) venous line pressures have been used, line pressure with the dialysis flow rate held constant at 200 to 250 mL/min for several minutes is the preferred technique. Testing is performed before proceeding with hemodialysis at a flow rate of 300 to 400 mL/min with a line pressure less than 150 mm Hg considered normal.

The diagnostic accuracy of venous line pressures in detection of greater than 50% DR access is sufficient for surveillance testing. A dynamic venous pressure greater than150 mm Hg during three consecutive dialysis sessions had a 86% sensitivity and 93% specificity for detection of greater than 50% venous outflow stenosis by fistulography.[9] Mean dynamic venous line pressure was significantly higher in patients with greater than 50% DR angiographic-confirmed stenosis (126 ± 35 mm Hg SD) than in accesses without stenosis (95 ± 22 mm Hg).[18] When used alone, venous line pressure measurements had not been predictive of access thrombosis in three prospective studies.[5,17,18] Testing is most sensitive to the development of anastomotic or venous outflow stenosis because lesions proximal to venous cannula will not be detected. Thus, serial venous line pressure measurements can recognize the "failing" access, and a threshold value in the 150 to 200 mm Hg range is an appropriate indication to proceed with additional diagnostic testing such as duplex ultrasound.

Measurement of Dialysis Access Volume Flow

Serial measurement of blood flow rates within functioning access grafts holds promise as the most accurate method for access surveillance. An association between low access volume flow rate and risk of thrombosis has been demonstrated, but the relationship between presence of stenosis and conduit flow rates has not yet been fully defined. In general, a high-grade stenosis (<2 mm residual lumen, end-diastolic velocity >250 cm/s) is associated with "low" or "reduced" dialysis access flow.

Doppler-derived volume flow calculations and newer ultrasonic dilution techniques have been used to estimate time-averaged blood flow rates. Because the diameter of the vessel and time-averaged velocity can be measured by ultrasound methods, volume flow can be calculated by using the formula:

$$Q = vA = v(\pi d^2)/4$$

where v is time- and spatially averaged velocity over the lumen cross-section, and d and A are the lumen diameter and cross-sectional area at the site of velocity measurement. Assumptions made in this calculation

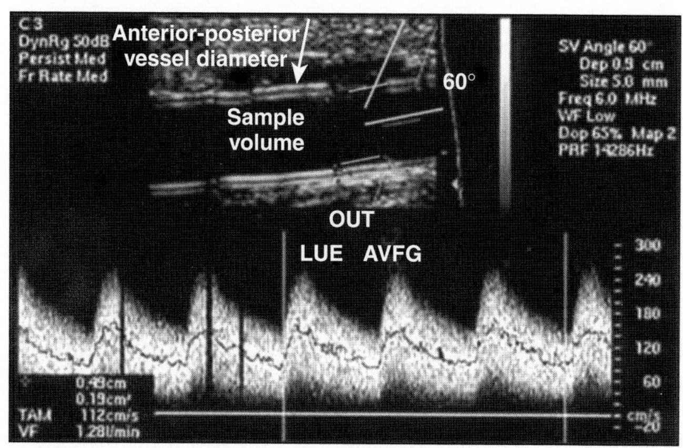

FIGURE 57-1 Duplex ultrasound image of a 6-mm–diameter dialysis bridge graft with a calculated volume flow of 1.28 L/min. NOTE: Velocity spectra were recorded at a 60-degree Doppler angle, the pulsed-Doppler sample volume encompasses the entire lumen, and time-averaged, mean velocity was measured over three pulse cycles.

are that blood flow is minimally disturbed and axial-symmetric at the recording site, and the lumen cross-section is circular. Testing should not be performed during or after dialysis, because reduction in blood pressure is a potential source of error. Dialysis access evaluation is best performed in a vascular laboratory on a nondialysis day by a certified technologist.

Volume flow calculations are possible with use of software packages available on essentially all high-resolution duplex ultrasound units. For upper-extremity autogenous accesses with variable vein diameter, volume flow measurement from the inflow artery is an appropriate option. Site of flow measurement should be carefully selected. No stenosis or lumen narrowing should be imaged, and pulsed Doppler velocity spectra should demonstrate mild-to-moderate spectral broadening (Figure 57-1). Vessel diameter (anterior-posterior dimension) is measured with transducer scan lines perpendicular to the long axis of the conduit. The pulsed Doppler sample volume is sized to encompass the entire lumen, and the velocity spectra recorded at a Doppler angle of 60 degrees. The time-averaged velocity is calculated over two or three pulse cycles. Measurements are obtained at two to three locations along the access graft, typically four vessel diameters downstream of the arterial anastomosis, at midgraft, and proximal to the venous anastomosis (Figure 57-2). Experimental validation of duplex-derived volume flow measurements have been performed in baboons with an average error of 13% and good correlation ($r = 0.9$) with timed blood collection at flow rates in the range of 300 mL/min.[19] Similar validation data does not exist for the high-volume and disturbed flow conditions present in arteriovenous access conduits, but it is estimated that the accuracy is ±20% to 25%.

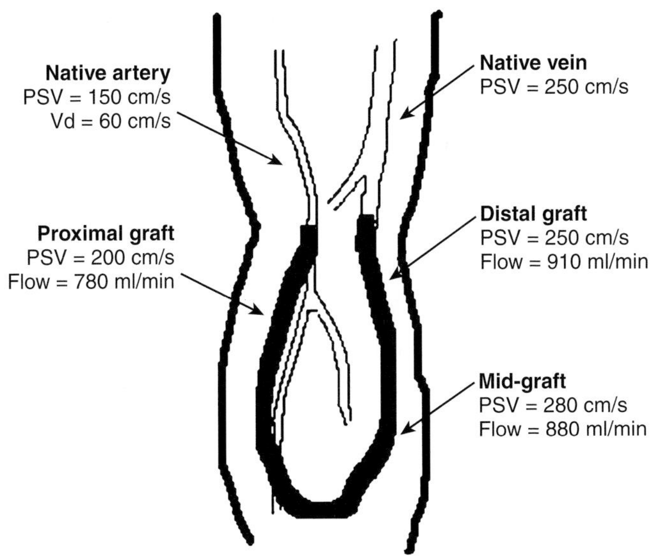

FIGURE 57-2 Schematic of forearm loop prosthetic bridge graft for dialysis showing typical duplex scan recording sites of PSV (centimeters per second) and volume flow (milliliters per minute) measurements. Mean graft flow calculated as the average of measurements recorded from three graft sites.

Access flow can be measured during hemodialysis sessions using the transit-time, ultrasonic dilution method. Separate ultrasound transducers are placed on the arterial and venous dialysis tubing and the lines are reversed so that the arterial line is downstream of the venous line within the access conduit. The dialysis circuit flow is fixed at 200 to 300 mL/min and ultrafiltration turned off. Rapid injection of 5 to 10 mL of normal saline solution at body temperature into the venous line dilutes the red cell mass in blood flowing through the access and results in alteration of the Doppler-derived velocity waveform recorded by the arterial line transducer. The measured areas under the perturbed velocity versus time curve at the venous (S_v) and arterial (S_a) lines and the known dialyzer flow rate (Q_b) allows calculation of the access flow rate by the relation:

$$Q = Q_b(S_v/S_a - 1)$$

Accuracy of the access flow calculation appears independent of dialyzer flow rates between 177 and 350 mL/min but requires careful positioning of the arterial needle within the center stream of the access flow.[20] Two or three access flow measurements should be made for reproducibility because the error between consecutive measurements averages 5%.[19] Clinical comparison of ultrasound dilution and Doppler-derived flow rate measurements have yielded acceptable agreement (correlation coefficients 0.79-0.83) over a wide range of access flows.[16,21,22] The ultrasound dilution technique did not have a tendency to overestimate or underestimate flow rates except in accesses with conduit stenosis where dilution measurements were lower than those obtained by duplex ultrasound.[21]

Low access flow rates are strongly predictive of limited conduit patency in PTFE bridge grafts (Table 57-2).[5,16-18,23-25] Thrombotic risk increases greatly with falling bridge graft flows whether measured by Doppler-derived or ultrasound dilution techniques. The association between flow rate and patency of AVFs is not as strong as for prosthetic bridge grafts because lower flow rates may support autologous conduits but not more thrombogenic PTFE grafts. Lower access flow rates are also predictive of patent conduits with stenoses in several studies.[5,18] Flow rates were significantly less in conduits with stenosis than in functioning conduits with a maintained stenosis-free patency. In fact, the flow rate values in stenotic conduits were similar to those measured in accesses with subsequent thrombotic events.[5] These observations suggest that access stenosis may compromise access flow rate and increase thrombotic risk. It should be noted that some access grafts can demonstrate reduced volume flow rates without anatomic evidence of arterial inflow, within conduit or venous outflow obstruction. Mechanisms of failure in low-flow grafts include development of heart failure, hypotension, hypercoagulability, or extrinsic pressure on the graft.

Controversy exists regarding the threshold access volume flow that should prompt intervention or additional imaging studies such as contrast fistulography. On the basis of current retrospective and uncontrolled prospective data, PTFE bridge grafts with access flow rates below 700 to 800 mL/min and reduced peak systolic velocities (PSVs) in the inflow brachial/radial artery less than 90 cm/s should be imaged with duplex scanning. Strauch et al.[7] have used a lower volume flow cutoff (357 cm/s) to identify grafts that will likely fail without intervention. Similarly, measured flow rates less then 400 mL/min in AVFs should prompt angiographic assessment. Back et al.[26] found that a threshold conduit flow rate of 800 mL/min was a better discriminant of failing and functional AVFs and bridge grafts (with accuracy of 77%) than a flow rate greater than or less than 500 mL/min (accuracy of 67%). Regardless of the threshold levels chosen, grafts demonstrated to have flow-reducing stenosis should be monitored for concomitant reduction in volume flow. Optimal intervals for surveillance measurement of access flow rates have not been specified and may differ with access type and graft diameters. Because access failure is most common during the first postoperative year, surveillance at 3-month intervals is recommended.

TABLE 57-2 Correlation of Hemodialysis Access Blood Flow Rate Measurements With Arteriography and Graft Failure

Author	Access type	Technique	Threshold value (mL/min)	Validation angio ?	Findings
Rittgers et al.[23]	PTFE	Doppler	<450	No	100% failure 2 wk
Shackleton et al.[24]	PTFE	Doppler	<450	No	83% sensitivity, 75% specificity failure 2-6 wk
Sands et al.[25]	PTFE	Doppler	<800	No	93% failure 6 mo*
Johnson et al.[34]	PTFE	Doppler	<400	No	64% failure 3 mo*
	AVF	Doppler	<320	No	Lower primary and secondary patency rates*
May et al.[16]	PTFE	Dilution	1150	No	Relative risk failure 3 mo = 1
			750		1.5*
			300		2.4*
Bay et al.[17]	PTFE	Doppler	700-1000	No	Relative risk intervention/failure 6 mo = 1
			300-500		1.4*
			<300		2.0*
Bosman et al.[18]	Graft	Dilution	1061	Yes	Nonstenotic
			664		> 50% stenosis*
Besarab et al.[5]	PTFE	Dilution	1121	Yes	No event
			605		Stenosis/intervention*
			540		Failure*
	AVF	Dilution	1057	Yes	No event
			313		Stenosis/intervention*
			475		Failure*

*$p<.05$, statistically different group.
Angio, Angiogram; *AVF,* autogenous fistula; *PTFE,* polytetrafluoroethylene.

Color Duplex Ultrasonography

Duplex ultrasound interrogation of dialysis accesses aims to directly identify stenotic or occluded segments within the arterial inflow, conduit, and venous outflow with precision similar to contrast fistulography. Color duplex ultrasound like Doppler-derived volume flow rate measurements can be done serially and is best performed in an accredited vascular laboratory. The subcutaneous location of arteriovenous access conduits allows the use of high-frequency (7.5-10 MHz) linear array transducers to obtain high-resolution vessel imaging. Both transverse and longitudinal B-mode and color Doppler imaging should be performed along the entire access length, anastomotic regions, arterial inflow, and venous outflow including central veins to the extent possible. The technique of duplex mapping is identical to peripheral artery scanning with color/power Doppler imaging for stenosis and pulsed-wave Doppler velocity spectra recording for stenosis classification in DR categories of less than 50% and greater than 50% based on PSV, end-diastolic velocity (EDV). The velocity spectra of dialysis access hemodynamics are those of high flow and low resistance with "normal" dialysis conduit PSV greater than 150 cm/s (see Figure 57-1). The resistive index should be 0.7 or less. Spectral broadening is typically present especially within the arterial anastomotic regions because of PSV greater than 200 cm/s and vessel tortuosity producing highly disturbed flow conditions. Proper selection of the color bar and velocity scale helps to minimize aliasing artifacts associated with color Doppler imaging.

Access graft stenosis is identified by color flow imaging of a narrowed lumen and at least doubling of PSVs compared with adjacent graft segments (Figures 57-3 and 57-4). A perivascular color artifact may be present and represents a graft bruit caused by turbulent flow and vessel wall/tissue vibration. A duplex classification criteria for interpretation of dialysis access stenosis is listed in Table 57-3. In the presence of a high-grade, flow-reducing stenosis of the access venous outflow, high resistance (resistive index >0.7) and lower PSV (<150 cm/s) will be recorded from the dialysis conduit and arterial inflow artery. When the access is thrombosed, the inflow artery will demonstrate

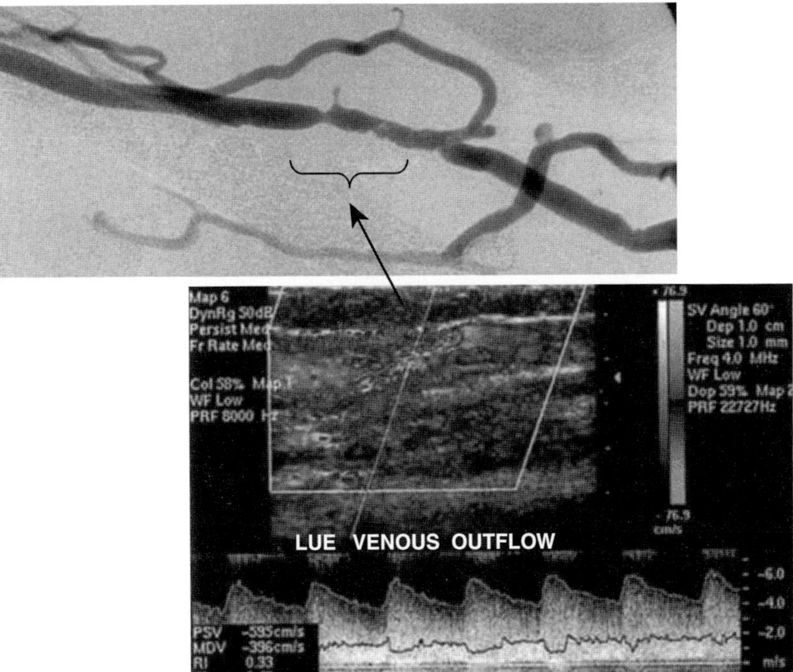

FIGURE 57-3 Contrast fistulogram and duplex scan of a >50% DR venous outflow stenosis. PSV of 600 cm/s and EDV of 400 cm/s predictive of >50% stenosis. Volume flow was measured at 0.7 L/m. The PSV ratio across the stenosis was 4.8. NOTE: Red color pixels outside the vessel in the duplex scan image are caused by a tissue bruit.

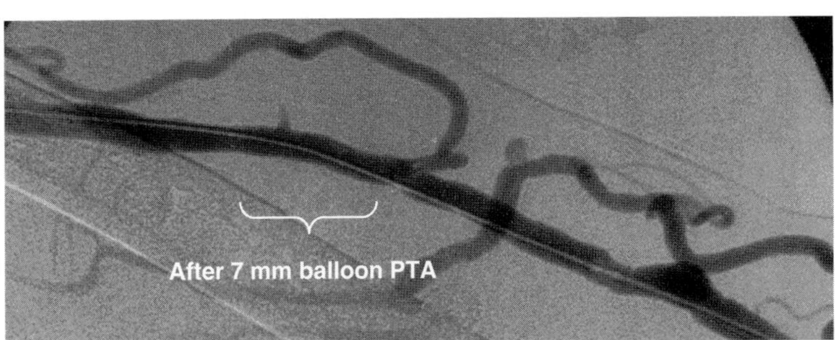

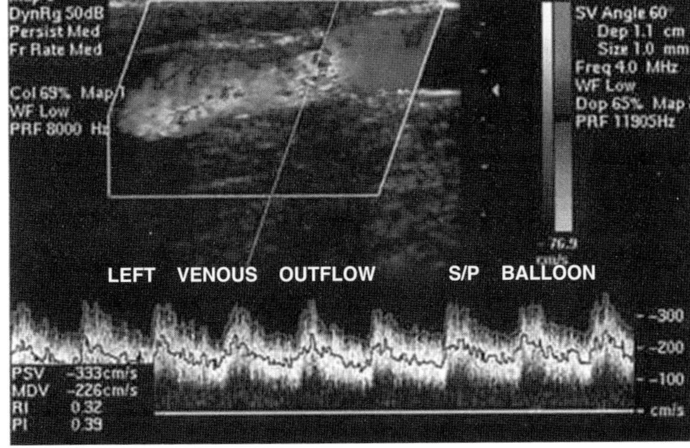

FIGURE 57-4 Contrast fistulogram and intraprocedural duplex scan of vein segment shown in Figure 57-2 after 7-mm–diameter balloon angioplasty. Volume flow has increased to 1.4 L/min with reduction in PSV (330 cm/s), EDV (226 cm/s), and PSV ratio (1.8) indicating a less than 50% DR residual stenosis, which corresponds to the fistulogram findings. *s/p*, Status post.

multiphasic, high-resistance velocity spectra and no Doppler signal will be recorded within the occluded access conduit. In general, a hemodynamically significant (>50% DR) stenosis that impairs volume flow and should be repaired has the duplex features of a PSV above 400 cm/s, EDV greater than 250 cm/s, and a residual power Doppler flow lumen ≤2 to 3 mm in diameter.

The diagnostic accuracy (sensitivity, specificity, positive predictive value) of duplex testing compared with contrast fistulogram for the detection of greater than 50% DR stenosis is approximately 80% (Table 57-4).[16,27-32]

TABLE 57-3 Duplex Classification of Dialysis Access Stenosis

Scan Interpretation	Recorded Velocity Spectra	Color Doppler Imaging
Normal	Arterial anastomosis >200 cm/s	No graft stenosis imaged; patent venous outflow
	Midgraft >150 cm/s	
<50% stenosis	PSV anastomosis 200-400 cm/s	Focal decrease in lumen diameter
	PSV conduit lesion <300 cm/s	PSV ratio across lesion <2
	Midgraft 100-150 cm/s	At stenosis
>50% stenosis	PSV anastomosis >400 cm/s	>50% DR lumen stenosis
	Midgraft velocity <100 cm/s	<2- to 3-mm residual lumen
	PSV conduit lesion >300 cm/s	PSV ratio across lesion >2
Occlusion	No Doppler signal	Intraluminal graft echoes; occluded vein may be imaged

DR, Diameter reducing; *PSV*, peak systolic velocity.

TABLE 57-4 Results of Duplex Surveillance of Dialysis Access Grafts

Author	Access type	Threshold value	Validation fistulogram	Diagnostic accuracy
Middleton et al.[27]	PTFE + AVF	>50% DR	Yes	87% sensitivity
Dousset et al.[28]	Graft	>50% DR	Yes	86% sensitivity, 60% specificity
MacDonald et al.[29]	PTFE	>50% DR	Yes	84% sensitivity
Lumsden et al.[30]	PTFE	>50% DR	Yes	76% sensitivity
Tordoir et al.[31]	Graft	>50% DR	Yes	
		PSV >300		92% sensitivity, 84% specificity
		PSV ratio >3.5		75% sensitivity, 96% specificity
	AVF	PSV >375	Yes	79% sensitivity, 84% specificity
	Venous outflow	PSV >250	Yes	95% sensitivity, 97% specificity
Older et al.[32]	PTFE + AVF	PSV >400	Yes	83% positive predictive value
		PSV ratio >3		

AVF, Autogenous fistula; *DR*, diameter reducing; *PSV*, peak systolic velocity (cm/s); *PSV ratio*, maximum PSV at stenosis divided by PSV in proximal vessel; *PTFE*, polytetrafluoroethylene.

Several reports used direct measurement of DR by B-mode and color flow imaging for identification of greater than 50% stenoses. Tordoir et al.[31] used duplex-measured velocity criteria for greater than 50% DR stenosis within bridge grafts, AVFs, and venous outflow. In a smaller clinical series, Older et al.[32] showed that 83% of duplex-detected lesions with greater than 50% DR stenosis confirmed by fistulography had a threshold PSV greater than 400 cm/s or PSV ratio greater than 3. Diagnostic errors are primarily due to the limited ability of duplex testing to identify central vein obstruction or stenosis.[29,30] Passman et al.[33] reported a diagnostic sensitivity of 81% for greater than 50% DR axillary, subclavian, or brachiocephalic venous stenosis or occlusion.

Routine surveillance of dialysis access has demonstrated the prevalence of greater than 50% DR stenosis (based on PSV and PSV ratio values, fistulogram) in the range of 30% to 48%.[17,29-31] Thus access stenosis is a common finding, especially for PTFE bridge grafts, despite sufficient functional patency that hemodialysis is not compromised. The mean number of stenoses identified in the conduit or outflow veins ranged from 1.4 to 1.8. Correlation studies of duplex-detected stenosis with subsequent access thrombosis have yielded mixed results. Although duplex-detected stenosis within a dialysis access has been associated with reduced primary patency compared with "normal" scans, prospective clinical trials and prophylactic endovascular treatment

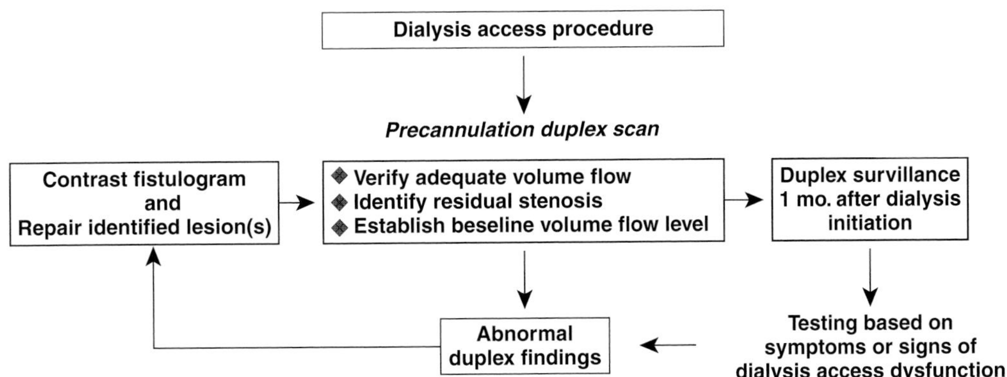

FIGURE 57-5 Duplex ultrasound surveillance algorithm.

of detected lesions did not demonstrate significant improvement in assisted primary patency.[16,17,30] These results suggest that the presence of an access stenosis alone should not be the sole criterion for intervention. Because dialysis access failure is related to volume flow, duplex surveillance should include both imaging for stenosis and measurement of volume flow.

Duplex testing can also detect other dialysis graft/fistula abnormalities that interfere with hemodialysis or threaten patency. Aneurysms or pseudoaneurysms are readily detected by color flow imaging and are easily distinguished from hematoma by the presence of flow. Small pseudoaneurysms (<5 mm diameter) caused by cannulation tend to remain stable whereas large pseudoaneurysms (>1 cm diameter) typically enlarge and should be repaired. Lumen thrombus can also be detected by duplex scanning and is a sign of access dysfunction and associated with eventual access thrombosis.

APPLICATION OF DUPLEX SURVEILLANCE

At present, duplex ultrasound is the preferred method for dialysis access surveillance. Whether testing is provided depends on the patient's nephrologist's willingness to participate in a surveillance program and the availability and expertise of the vascular laboratory in performing dialysis access studies. There must be a medical indication for testing for reimbursement. Because a minimum access volume flow rate is necessary for hemodialysis, testing before initial access usage to confirm "maturation" and subsequent testing to detect and manage "developing" stenotic segments based on both stenosis severity and level of access flow are recommended. Well-conducted clinical studies have showed volume flow rates in PTFE bridge grafts to be the only reliable predictor of access thrombosis.[16,17] Weekly measurement of dynamic venous line pressures has acceptable sensitivity for detection of venous outflow obstruction, and when a high (>200 mm Hg) dynamic pressure is recorded, ordering a duplex ultrasound evaluation that includes volume flow determination is appropriate.[5,14,15,18,21]

At the University of South Florida, our vascular group has used duplex surveillance routinely to evaluate dialysis access hemodynamics before approving cannulation and initial hemodialysis usage. If a newly constructed dialysis access is found to have a lower than expected volume flow, a detected stenosis or small-caliber vein segment is repaired to ensure that successful dialysis can be performed. Our surveillance algorithm (Figure 57-5) begins with a precannulation duplex scan followed by a second scan approximately 1 month after hemodialysis usage to verify "normal" functional patency and adequate volume flow. The second scan allows assessment of vein and valve site adaptation, that is, early myointimal hyperplasia development, to arterial pressure and elevated flow velocity. Thereafter, dialysis access surveillance is applied selectively on the basis of patient characteristics, prior access site intervention or failure, or medical indication for testing based on signs or symptoms of access dysfunction. When a "hemodynamically significant" access stenosis is identified and volume flow reduced to a lower than normal level, the lesion is repaired and duplex testing performed to confirm access hemodynamic improvement (see Figure 57-3). Testing is repeated within 1 to 2 months to detect restenosis.

Data regarding "expected" volume flow rate based on dialysis access type are limited. It is known that the initial volume flow of forearm AVFs is less than that of a prosthetic bridge graft constructed in either the forearm or arm. Basilic vein transpositions exhibit volume flow and other duplex ultrasound characteristics similar to 6- or 7-mm–diameter bridge grafts. Duplex surveillance of 125 consecutive dialysis access procedures (34 forearm fistulae, 53 arm fistulae, 38 prosthetic bridge grafts) performed in 108 patients

(82 men, 26 women; mean age of 58 years) demonstrated that initial volume flow rates differ on the basis of access configuration—radiocephalic 771 ± 435 mL/min; brachiocephalic, 1616 ± 790 mL/min; brachiobasilic transposition, 1185 ± 585 mL/min, and prosthetic bridge graft, 1270 ± 604 mL/min. PSV at the arterial anastomosis (approximately 400 cm/s) and midconduit recording site (approximately 250 cm/s) were similar in the various access types.[26]

On the basis of initial duplex testing performed within 4 to 6 weeks of the procedure, the access sites were deemed "adequate" for dialysis or "nonmaturing" by the presence of detected high-grade stenoses (PSV >400 cm/s, velocity ratio greater than 3, and minimal diameter less than 2 to 3 mm) and subjected to remedial interventions (endovascular or open). Remedial interventions were needed in 10 (26%) bridge grafts and 18 (21%) fistulae "nonmaturing" because of occlusive lesions. Conduit flow rates differentiated "nonmaturing" (606 ± 769 mL/min) from "maturing" (1140 ± 857) fistulae ($p = .01$). After remedial procedures to improve access function, the volume flow increased to 1159 ± 502 cm/s, a level similar to that of access conduits not requiring a remedial procedure (1374 ± 805 mL/min).

Analysis of subsequent patient outcomes over a 2- to 3-year period demonstrated that a threshold conduit flow rate of 800 mL/min was a better discriminator of "failing" versus functional fistulae and bridge grafts (accuracy 77%) than flow rate greater or less than 500 mL/min (accuracy 67%). Overall, remedial procedures were required in 42% of accesses with initial flow less than 800 mL/min compared with 12% of accesses with initial flow greater than 800 mL/min ($p < .05$). The average mean duration of primary (no intervention performed) patency was similar in access requiring (11.5 months) or not requiring a remedial (12.9 months) procedure.

Routine duplex surveillance after dialysis access does not yield similar assisted primary patency rates

BOX 57-1

GUIDELINES FOR DIALYSIS ACCESS TESTING USING COLOR DUPLEX ULTRASOUND

Access Site Imaging

- Scanning is performed in both longitudinal and transverse planes.
- Location and extent of perigraft fluid collections and masses are documented.
- Mapping sequence should proceed from artery inflow, through the arterial anastomosis, the entire length of the dialysis conduit, through the venous anastomosis if present, and into outflow veins.
- Native artery is imaged proximal to the arterial anastomosis and volume flow measured.
- Volume flow measurements are calculated at several locations along the access conduit at sites of normal lumen caliber and minimally disturbed flow conditions.
- Sites of lumen abnormality (stenosis, thrombus, aneurysm) are documented in a schematic of the dialysis access.
- Sites of lumen stenosis are classified on the basis of velocity spectra recorded proximal to stenosis, at the site of stenosis, and distal to stenosis.

Documentation

- PSV within native inflow artery (radial, brachial)
- PSV in dialysis graft or along autologous venous conduit
- PSV in arterial and venous anastomotic regions
- PSV and EDV at site of stenosis, including calculation of velocity ratio
- Volume flow calculations at sites measured—averaged to determine a mean volume flow rate for the access type
- Images of all pathology (thrombus, hematoma, seroma, abscess); measurement of aneurysm or pseudoaneurysm size and indication of presence of thrombus

Diagnostic Criteria

- Normal arterial velocities: PSV 100-400 cm/s, EDV 60-200 cm/s
- Normal venous velocities: PSV 50-200 cm/s
- Access stenosis: PSV >400 cm/s and velocity ratio >2
- High-resistance flow pattern suggests low volume flow and impending graft occlusion.
- Retrograde flow in the native inflow artery indicates arterial steal.
- Severe arterial steal is associated with digit pressure <60 mm Hg.
- Perigraft fluid collections indicate absence of graft healing and may be sign of infection when found along entire prosthetic graft length.

EDV, End-diastolic velocity; *PSV*, peak systolic velocity.

to those obtained after lower-extremity vein bypass grafting. Assisted patency rates are in the rage of 50% compared with 80% to 90%. Several prospective but uncontrolled studies documented a significant decrease in number of thrombotic events and increased conduit patency after elective surgical or endovascular intervention for duplex- or fistulogram-identified dialysis access stenosis.[3,8,9] Benefit is most likely to occur when the surveillance technique is conducted by experienced clinicians and the lesions treated are truly "hemodynamically" important based on both anatomic and physiologic criteria. Because access stenosis is a relatively common finding on imaging studies and not predictive of thrombotic failure, duplex testing with volume flow measurement has the potential to improve the efficacy of surveillance.

On the basis of the Dialysis Outcome Quality Initiative guidelines and available data, routine surveillance after dialysis access procedures is warranted. Refinements of the surveillance algorithm including testing intervals, test interpretation criteria, and subsequent access evaluation require further development. At present, a baseline duplex evaluation is recommended at the time of "anticipated" graft maturation followed by subsequent serial evaluations based on patient characteristics and signs of access dysfunction (Box 57-1). Access imaging combined with the calculation of volume flow by Doppler-derived techniques should be the primary surveillance methods for both autogenous and prosthetic dialysis accesses. The "low-flow" (<800 mL/min) conduits typically harbor a stenotic lesion and should be considered for remedial intervention to improve access hemodynamics and functional patency. When flow rates fall below 500 to 800 mL/min for either PTFE bridge grafts or AVFs, contrast fistulography should be considered unless duplex imaging clearly identifies a significant graft or anastomotic stenosis. Access flow in this range is associated with an increased thrombotic risk, and additional diagnostic testing is appropriate. If measurement of volume flow is not possible or deemed unreliable, intervention for a progressive duplex-identified stenosis with velocity spectra consistent with a critical stenosis (PSV >400 cm/s, EDV >250 cm/s, velocity ratio >3, midgraft velocity <150 cm/s, residual lumen <2 mm diameter) is recommended. Elective surgical or endovascular treatment of fistulogram-confirmed greater than 50% DR stenosis should be pursued. An important feature of a duplex surveillance program is confirmation of improved access flow rate and hemodynamic correction of access stenosis after intervention. Validation of the routine duplex surveillance would require a well-designed, prospective, randomized clinical trial, a difficult task given the patient population with end-stage renal disease and variable expertise in duplex ultrasound testing.

References

1. Hodges TC, Fillinger MF, Zwolak RM, et al: Longitudinal comparisons of dialysis access methods: risk factors for failure, *J Vasc Surg* 26:1009–1019, 1997.
2. Cinat ME, Hopkins J, Wilson SE: A prospective evaluation of PTFE graft patency and surveillance techniques in hemodialysis access, *Ann Vasc Surg* 13:191–198, 1999.
3. Beathard GA: Percutaneous transvenous angioplasty in the treatment of vascular access stenosis, *Kidney Int* 42:1390–1397, 1992.
4. Bowser A, Bandyk D: Surveillance program for hemodialysis access. In Yao JST, Pearce WH, editors: *Trends in vascular surgery,* Chicago, 2002, Appleton-Lange.
5. Besarab A, Lubkowski T , Frinak S, et al: Detecting vascular access dysfunction, *ASAIO Journal* 43:M539–M543, 1997.
6. Palder SB, Kirkman RL, Wittemore AD, et al: Vascular access for hemodialysis: patency rates and results of revision, *Ann Surg* 202:235–239, 1985.
7. Strauch BS, O'Connell RS, Geoly KL, et al: Forecasting thrombosis of vascular access with Doppler color flow imaging, *Am J Kidney Dis* 19:554–557, 1992.
8. Sands JJ, Miranda CL: Prolongation of hemodialysis access survival with elective revision, *Clin Nephrol* 44:329–333, 1995.
9. Schwab SJ, Raymond JR, Saeed M, et al: Prevention of hemodialysis fistula thrombosis: early detection of venous stenoses, *Kidney Int* 36:707–711, 1989.
10. Brooks JL, Sigley RD, May RJ Jr, et al: Transluminal angioplasty versus surgical repair for stenosis of hemodialysis grafts: a randomized study, *Am J Surg* 153:530–531, 1987.
11. Dapunt O, Feurstein M, Rendl KH, et al: Transluminal angioplasty versus conventional operation in the treatment of hemodialysis fistula stenosis: results from a 5 year study, *Br J Surg* 74:1004–1005, 1987.
12. Besarab A, Sherman R: The relationship of recirculation to access blood flow, *Am J Kidney Dis* 29:223–229, 1997.
13. National Kidney Foundation: Dialysis outcome quality initiative clinical practice guidelines for vascular access, *Am J Kidney Dis* 30(suppl 3):S150–S191, 1997.
14. Windus DW, Audrain J, Vanderson R, et al: Optimization of high-efficiency hemodialysis by detection and correction of fistula dysfunction, *Kidney Int* 38:337–341, 1990.
15. Daniels ID, Berlyne GM, Barth RH: Blood flow rates and accesses recirculation in hemodialysis, *Int J Artif Organs* 15:470–474, 1992.
16. May RE, Himmelfarb J, Yenicesu M, et al: Predictive measures of vascular access thrombosis: a prospective study, *Kidney Int* 52:1656–1662, 1997.
17. Bay WH, Henry ML, Lazarus JM, et al: Predicting hemodialysis access failures with color flow Doppler ultrasound, *Am J Nephrol* 18:296–304, 1998.
18. Bosman PJ, Boereboom FTJ, Smits HFM, et al: Pressure or flow recordings for the surveillance of hemodialysis grafts, *Kidney Int* 52:1084–1088, 1997.
19. Zierler BK, Kirkman TR, Kraiss LW, et al: Accuracy of duplex scanning for measurement of arterial volume flow, *J Vasc Surg* 16:520–526, 1992.
20. Depner TA, Krivitski NM: Clinical measurement of blood flow in hemodialysis access fistulae and graft by ultrasound dilution, *ASAIO J* 41:M745–M749, 1995.
21. Besarab A, Lubkowski T, Frinak S, et al: Detection of access strictures and outlet stenoses in vascular accesses: Which test is best? *ASAIO J* 43:M543–M547, 1997.
22. Sands J, Glidden D, Miranda C: Hemodialysis access flow measurement: comparison of ultrasound dilution and duplex ultrasonography, *ASAIO J* 42:M899–M901, 1996.

23. Rittgers SE, Garcia-Valdez C, McCormick JT, et al: Noninvasive blood flow measurement in expanded PTFE grafts for hemodialysis access, *J Vasc Surg* 3:635–642, 1986.
24. Shackleton CR, Taylor DC, Buckley AR, et al: Predicting failure in PTFE vascular access grafts for hemodialysis: a pilot study, *Can J Surg* 30:442–444, 1987.
25. Sands J, Young S, Miranda C: The effect of Doppler flow screening studies and elective revisions on dialysis access failure, *ASAIO J* 38:M524–M527, 1992.
26. Back MR, Maynard M, Winkler A, et al: Expected Flow Parameters Within Hemodialysis Access and Selection for Remedial Intervention of Nonmaturing Conduits, *Vasc Endovascular Surg* 42 (2):150–158, 2008.
27. Middleton WD, Picus DD, Marx MV, et al: Color Doppler sonography of hemodialysis vascular access: comparison with angiography, *AJR* 152:633–639, 1989.
28. Dousset V, Grenier N, Douws C, et al: Hemodialysis grafts: color Doppler flow imaging correlated with digital subtraction angiography and functional status, *Radiology* 181:89–94, 1991.
29. MacDonald MJ, Martin LG, Hughes JD, et al: Distribution and severity of stenoses in functioning arteriovenous grafts: a duplex and angiographic study, *J Vasc Technology* 20:131–136, 1996.
30. Lumsden AB, MacDonald MJ, Kikeri D, et al: Prophylactic balloon angioplasty fails to prolong the patency of PTFE arteriovenous grafts: results of a prospective randomized study, *J Vasc Surg* 24:382–392, 1997.
31. Tordoir JHM, deBruin HG, Hoeneveld H, et al: Duplex ultrasound scanning in the assessment of arteriovenous fistulas created for hemodialysis access: comparison with digital subtraction angiography, *J Vasc Surg* 10:122–128, 1989.
32. Older RA, Gizienski TA, Wilkowski MJ, et al: Hemodialysis access stenosis: early detection with color Doppler ultrasound, *Radiology* 207:161–164, 1998.
33. Passman MA, Criado E, Farber MA, et al: Efficiency of color flow duplex imaging for proximal upper extremity venous outflow obstruction in hemodialysis patients, *J Vasc Surg* 28:869–875, 1998.
34. Johnson CP, Zhu Y, Matt C, et al: Prognostic value of intraoperative blood flow measurements in vascular access surgery, *Surgery* 124:729–738, 1998.

CHAPTER

58

Percutaneous Thrombectomy Devices in Thrombosed Dialysis Access

Nicolas A. Nelken

Hemodialysis access is the most common service performed by most vascular surgeons, as well as one of the most problematic. Though selected articles demonstrate good overall patency, Medicare data nationwide tell a different story. Access is expensive, dangerous, painful, and temporary. The prevalence and incidence of renal failure itself are increasing as the population ages and as diabetes rates increase in parallel.[1]

Because the failure rate is high, there are an ever-growing number of techniques that have been developed to solve various aspects of access salvage. Unfortunately, in any situation in which many competing solutions exist, it is axiomatic that none of them works particularly well. Percutaneous thrombectomy devices (PTDs) currently offer 3-month patency of 37% to 70%, 6-month patency of 26% to 60%, and 1-year primary patency of 12% to 17%. Mean primary patency is only 14 weeks.[2-5]

Endoluminal solutions to vascular problems in general are enjoying a particularly fertile period of development, and dialysis access management is no exception. Different hospital services, and now free-standing dialysis access units,[6] are competing to treat clotted access, which brings other political biases to bear on an already complex situation. These outpatient vascular access centers decrease cost, hospital utilization, and missed dialysis. The question often asked in the literature is which technique is the best for patients, but, not surprisingly, the answer seems to be strongly influenced by whether the author primarily performs endoluminal or surgical treatment. Since the last publication of this chapter, however, an endoluminal-first policy appears to be considerably more popular than in 2003,[7] although subsequent surgical salvage of a failed endoluminal intervention has a dismal success rate of only about 8%.[8]

Purported advantages to PTDs in clotted hemodialysis access include (in decreasing order of likelihood)

1. Access to surgically inaccessible locations
2. Decreased discomfort
3. Vein preservation
4. Increased patient satisfaction
5. Almost certain improvement over surgery for native, autogenous fistulas[9]
6. Improved definition of anatomy both during the endoluminal procedure and in prior knowledge of the underlying anatomy from previous contrast studies when surgery becomes necessary
7. Ability to treat repetitively with percutaneous means without detriment to immediate outcome
8. Decreased success of repetitive surgical salvage
9. Improved patient "flow" through an overcrowded medical system (easier scheduling) leading to decreased use of percutaneous catheters as temporary access
10. Choice
11. Cost-effectiveness
12. Decreasing complication rate

Note that nowhere is it claimed that percutaneous management of thrombosed grafts (as opposed to autogenous fistulas) leads to increased primary patency even among its most ardent supporters, although there are some claims that secondary patency of the original anatomy may be increased with repeated reintervention.[10] Whether or not this is "cost-effective" is another issue entirely.

In fact, the 2002 meta-analysis by Green et al.[11] of all randomized controlled trials comparing endoluminal techniques with open surgery strongly suggested that open surgery significantly reduces the likelihood of subsequent thrombosis by a relative risk of about 1.3 for time points at 1, 2, 3, and 12 months. Technical failure rates were almost twice as likely in endoluminal procedures versus open surgery. It has further been noted that immediate success of percutaneous thrombectomy fares much better in retrospective trials (95%+) than in prospective randomized trials (70%-80%),[12-15] a fact that on its surface further supports the conclusions of Green et al. Why then should we even consider percutaneous methods for the thrombectomy of dialysis access?

Discomfort and patient preference notwithstanding, the tradeoff seems to be that surgical treatment lasts longer as long as some sort of stenosis management is employed[16] but uses up more vein than endoluminal procedures. "Primary patency after treatment after successful recanalization is relatively short, but long-term patency is improved substantially with retreatment of recurrent failure of the access with repeat thrombolysis and/or angioplasty."[15] The real value of any technique centers on the ultimate long-term patency rate of a dialysis access as opposed to the outcome after treatment of a single episode of access thrombosis,[17] and this has not been adequately studied with respect to the two techniques. Beathard,[10] however, has demonstrated a significant decrease in the percentage of patients with thrombosis who required graft replacement, after surgery was replaced by percutaneous therapy as the primary treatment method. Although unstratified randomized prospective trials are statistically more powerful because of larger numbers of patients, not all arteriovenous grafts present the same way. It is perhaps a weakness of the current literature that better stratified studies do not yet exist and may be a byproduct of the need for statistical power in the design of such studies. For practitioners who perform a large number of percutaneous thrombectomies, however, an initial success rate of 70% to 80% (as demonstrated in prospective trials[10,13-15]) would be considered a terrible outcome, a fact that implies selection bias in *retrospective* studies.

As surgeons are now more than ever before in a position to offer more than one solution, maybe it is better to examine the strengths and weaknesses of each technique and then apply each to the appropriate patient, in other words to intentionally apply selection bias to our own patients in practice. Arguing for one solution for all patients is becoming harder and harder to justify, even if patient preference were not part of the equation. In addition, because different providers have different skill sets, this too may have some bearing on what an individual practitioner should do. I will say at the outset that type I data supporting these conclusions do not yet exist and, given current trends, may never exist. "All dialysis grafts ultimately will fail again regardless of the treatment method. The ideal study would compare treatment algorithms, combinations of percutaneous and surgical treatments that depend on the lesion location or the graft type."[17]

Strengths of surgery include optimal outflow revision and definitive repair of focal problems. A new surgically created outflow is much less likely to suffer elastic recoil and rapid closure. However, surgery as practiced by most surgeons does not include a complete postprocedure angiogram, defined as inflow, access, and venous outflow to the right atrium.[18] At least 15% of access failures are caused by more central vein stenoses, and anywhere from 5% to 15% are caused by arterial inflow problems. With the consequent poor anatomic information, decisions are based more on probability than data, on feel and blind passage than image-directed access; lesions are missed, and revisions wasted. Furthermore, there is the danger that patch angioplasty may be performed in a venous outflow that does not need it, because this is usually performed presumptively with thrombectomy.

Conversely, endoluminal strengths include excellent anatomic data almost by definition, considerably decreased discomfort, and a trend toward decreased hospitalization (or no hospital utilization whatsoever using outpatient units) although this has become less marked in the last few years with increased outpatient surgery. Endoluminal thrombectomy has also been used to correct failed surgical thrombectomy[19] and also allows traversal of difficult lesions under fluoroscopy, which may not be amenable to traversal by blind Fogarty passage.[20]

Angioplasty, however, is just not as effective as surgery in modifying anatomy, which leaves the unstratified patient much more likely to have failure in the short term. Underscoring the fact that the technique of thrombectomy itself is not the problem, in patients whose outflow undergoes balloon angioplasty there is little difference whether the thrombectomy portion is performed endoluminally or open.[21] Additionally, although percutaneous chemical thrombolysis is not the subject of this chapter, studies have shown it to be equivalent in success rates with percutaneous thrombectomy.[22,23] Because tissue plasminogen activator is now available in considerably less-expensive 2-mg aliquots (Cathflo Alteplase, Genentech South San Francisco, CA), supplementation of mechanical thrombectomy with thrombolytic agents is common.

Surgeons have approached the solution to this problem in different ways. In an opinion paper, Gelbfish[20] suggests that thrombosed access be opened first with use of endoluminal techniques and, after these fail, then move on to surgery. The advantage to this approach is that surgeons would not be working blindly, having the endoluminal data at their disposal. Disease Outcomes Quality Initiative guidelines support this premise in suggesting that three percutaneous failures within a 3-month period define the need for a surgical solution.[1] Surgeon access to C-arm technology has greatly increased since 2003, so visualization of end points is no longer hard to obtain and visualization should be routine if there is any question of adequacy of venous outflow.

This approach may yet be too general. As grafts age, they suffer progressive breakdown, scarring, and disruption, which leads to increased anatomic irregularities within the same graft. As definitive anatomic changes are more likely to be provided by surgery than angioplasty, as grafts and fistulas age, surgery becomes a more attractive option. In addition, it has been noted that surgical revision of grafts previously treated by endoluminal means results in particularly poor outcomes,[24] and replacement of these grafts may be a better long-term option.

On the other hand, thrombosis of younger grafts is more likely to be the result of a single anatomic problem, or even hypercoagulability, which is just as likely to be solved percutaneously as open. It is important to note that grafts less than 1 month old present a different problem for percutaneous management because the potential space around the graft has not yet been obliterated by scar, and large postprocedure "sausage-like" hematomas can ruin a successful endoluminal thrombectomy.

SUGGESTIONS

Patent Graft

Repair should almost always be percutaneous at least for the first attempt unless there is evidence of a long stenosis greater than 4 cm or infection. Infection is an absolute contraindication to endoluminal management at any stage. Large pseudoaneurysms used to be a contraindication to endoluminal repair but are now often treated with stent grafts.[25]

Thrombosis Within the First Month

Repair should always be performed in the operating room itself. Percutaneous thrombectomy can be performed there carefully especially if a patient is known to be hypercoagulable. Perigraft hematoma is much more likely, and angioplasty of a fresh anastomosis can easily disrupt it, leading to emergency surgery. If the patient is in the angiography suite at the time of disruption, the only solution is inflation of a balloon to stop hemorrhage and emergency transfer to the operating room. Because rapid failures of recently placed grafts tend to be the result of surgical issues, performing thrombectomy outside of the operating room in these early patients makes little sense.

One Month to 1 Year

Lean toward endoluminal management, especially in a patient with known hypercoagulability, and those grafts that appear more normal morphologically. Physical examination can tell you a lot; unfortunately, few nephrologists or technicians either examine grafts or appear to be qualified to describe suspected anatomic problems with grafts, so this decision is hard to make over the phone. Very scarred irregular grafts and those with large pseudoaneurysms are poor candidates for endoluminal repair because the anatomic problems tend to be more numerous. Any graft that has failed three times in 3 months requires a surgical revision. Meta-analysis has demonstrated effectiveness of antiplatelet treatment in preventing thrombosis, but the complication rate of warfarin is too high for routine use in nonhypercoagulable patients.[26]

Greater Than 1 Year

Lean toward surgical repair, but there are many old grafts that are still morphologically mostly intact on physical examination and have limited anatomic problems. Do not waste time and resources percutaneously opening scarred, obviously damaged grafts and fistulas. Replace them immediately in the operating room if simple open Fogarty thrombectomy does not significantly change their appearance.

Old Thrombus (>7 Days)

Consider "lyse and wait technique"[27] followed by percutaneous thrombectomy if anatomy is favorable and the need arises. This is performed by injecting 4 mg tissue plasminogen activator (Cathflo, Alteplase, Genentech) through a small needle into the graft in the preoperative area to soften and partially dissolve clot during the normal preparation for the operating room or specials suite (about 45 minutes). Bleeding may be slightly more problematic and will likely require purse-string suture through puncture sites.[28]

It may make sense to perform *either* approach if scheduling opportunities for one allow you to avoid the need for percutaneous temporary access.

If you are in the position to choose the right venue:

Specials Suite

Better visualization and equipment (usually)
Scheduling often easier (depending on local patterns)
Faster turnover
However, sterile technique is often poor, and, if crossover is needed for surgery, the patient will need a separate procedure.

Operating Room

Any patient in regard to whom you feel ambivalent
Any patient with possible infected graft
Disease Outcomes Quality Initiative guidelines for intervention exceeded

Of course the last 5 years have seen the advent of fully equipped operating rooms with current-generation ceiling- or floor-mounted C-arms, which is the ideal solution but an expensive one.

Bottom Line

The mechanism of thrombectomy is not the problem—anatomy is, and examination of the graft or fistula before thrombectomy can give a good idea of how it will respond to endoluminal management. As the field matures, studies will more likely be tailored to addressing which patients are better candidates for endoluminal versus open surgical procedures, rather than trying to put all patients in the same basket.

Although it is not the subject of this chapter, always look to see whether a potential autogenous fistula may have been previously overlooked. Consider whether graft surveillance protocols are sufficient in each individual dialysis unit and whether anything could be done to improve detection of the failing graft so thrombectomy need not be done in the first place.

DEVICES

History

In the 1980s percutaneous balloon thrombectomy and saline-injection thrombectomy were used in some institutions. These techniques were simple and involved central embolization of the entire thrombus. The rationale for routine central embolization was based on studies pertaining to volume of pulmonary embolus necessary to produce definable physiologic changes in experimental animals.[29] Although serious consequences were rare, they were still occasionally seen,[30] though most studies did not have enough patients at that time to detect a meaningful sample of catastrophic outcomes. An editorial written by Dolmatch et al.[31] brought into question the validity of using healthy animals as a model for patients with multiple cardiopulmonary comorbidities. The possibility of not only acute but also chronic pulmonary circulatory changes was described and stimulated a more circumspect analysis of the problem. In the early 1990s there was an explosion of new devices and techniques to not only "move" thrombus but also entrain, dissolve, and often dispose of it.[32] It should be noted that, to date, none of the current devices is able to effectively remove the arterial-end "meniscus," the fibrin-rich plug at the arterial end of the thrombosed graft, the removal of which is the sine qua non of a successful thrombectomy.[33] With the use of all current devices, some of the meniscus is centrally embolized, although the total volume of embolus is probably less than a milliliter in spite of the fact that the meniscus is the least likely portion of the clot to be capable of endogenous thrombolysis. This may yet be problematic, although with the continued use of devices over a decade, there are few documented cases of pulmonary hypertension ascribed to such devices.[34]

Classification

There are many ways to classify PTDs, and, given the multitude of designs, all have merit.[23,27] For this chapter they will be divided into wall contact and non–wall contact (maceration vs. rheolytic) devices and a couple of unique outliers. Devices will be described according to classification, and applicability, strengths, and weaknesses discussed. The devices highlighted in this chapter have been chosen for their demonstration of principle. Actually, little has changed since 2003 other than the success and failure of different devices in the marketplace, as well as patent infringement suits that constantly change the specific devices available. After 16 years of devices, it is clear that the device itself is probably not really important as long as it is safe and removes thrombus.

Wall Contact Devices

Arrow-Trerotola Device (Arrow International, Reading, PA)

The first widely employed device (which was still available in 2008) used a wire basket rotating at about 3000 rpm. Thrombus is fragmented into small pieces but not microscopic particles (1-mm to 3-mm fragments). It has no built-in aspiration port, and removal of the slurry is performed by suction through the sheath after removal of the instrument. Because of significant wall contact it is not recommended for use in the native circulation, although case reports demonstrate its uses even in venous thrombectomy. Studies have shown higher rates of endothelial damage when used in native vessels.[35] It is Food and Drug Administration (FDA) approved for dialysis graft thrombectomy only. Two units are available, a 5F device that does not go over a wire and a 7F over-the-wire device.

Advantages: Inexpensive, disposable unit noted for ease of use. Over-the-wire model available. "Low tech," long history of use.
Disadvantages: Endothelial damage if carried into the native circulation, no aspiration port, fairly inflexible shaft. Large residual particles (1-3 mm).

Castañeda Over-the-Wire Brush (Micro Therapeutics, San Clemente, CA)

Wall contact soft brush spins within the lumen over a guidewire (related to the nonguidewire Cragg brush). Designed to be used in conjunction with thrombolytic agents. Technically the brush is used to mix the thrombolytic agent with the thrombus for later aspiration after lysis has had a chance to proceed. Studies have shown that there is less residual adherent mural thrombus with this device than any other tested.[36]

Advantages: Very complete thrombectomy, minimal residual mural thrombus. Disposable unit, over-the-wire construction.
Disadvantages: Added cost of thrombolytic agent by design (some have performed without lytic agent), wall contact endothelial damage if strays into the native circulation, no built-in aspiration port.

Percutaneous Aspiration Thrombectomy

This requires no "device" at all, just 7F to 8F sheaths.[37] Aspiration is performed through crossing sheaths, which are manipulated through the entire graft, and a large syringe supplies suction.

Advantages: Inexpensive, equipment readily available.
Disadvantages: Probably the most technically demanding procedure in which experience is most necessary. Although there are no data to support it, I would assume this would leave the most residual adherent mural thrombus in inexperienced hands.

Non–Wall Contact Devices

Maceration Systems

HELIX, CLOTBUSTER (EV3, NORTH PLYMOUTH, MN)

A gas-powered encapsulated impeller system spins at 125,000 rpm creating a vortex, which macerates and remacerates circulating thrombus. Particles are reduced to between 13 and 1000 μm.[38] Slurry is aspirated after removal of the catheter. Device has an inexpensive reusable pedal attachment for control. New design increases shear forces on the graft wall, decreasing residual mural thrombus, which was a problem in comparative studies using the older Amplatz Thrombectomy Device.[36] 7F.

Advantages: Fast maceration. Inexpensive reusable hardware. Small residual sized particles. Long history of use.
Disadvantages: Hemolysis (moderate and related to duration of use), does not go over a guidewire, which may make tracking difficult. Drive shaft periodically breaks, but company will replace broken devices. No built-in aspiration port. Some data to suggest detectable damage to endothelium when used in native vessels.

X-SIZER MECHANICAL THROMBECTOMY DEVICE (EV3, NORTH PLYMOUTH, MN)

Disposable unit uses an encapsulated screw-type impeller. Battery-powered, self-contained, handheld unit contains aspiration port and uses disposable vacuum bottles. Does go over a guidewire. 6F and 7F.

Advantages: Completely self-contained unit, guidewire traversal, flexible, simple system.
Disadvantages: Not as powerful as some other devices.

Rheolytic Systems (Flow Related, Bernoulli Principle)

These devices work by injecting jets of saline solution at high velocity to create vortices that not only entrain and macerate clot but also aspirate it.

POSSIS ANGIOJET (POSSIS MEDICAL, MINNEAPOLIS, MN)

Most powerful device of its class, the Angiojet currently comes in multiple sizes and models that change constantly. All thread over a guidewire and are used for vessels of different sizes. Jets of saline solution are pumped past open vents in a sheath at 350 mph, creating a vortex that fragments clot, and particles are evacuated by the Venturi effect. As of 2008, the AVX catheter is designed specifically for dialysis use (only 50 cm long with simpler catheter for cost containment) and goes over a 0.035-inch wire. Other models are FDA approved for coronary and peripheral arterial uses. New drive-pump design allows certain catheters to be used for "power-pulse" delivery (pulse-spray) of thrombolytic agent through the same catheter.

Advantages: By far the most versatile system with multiple uses and approvals. Very powerful system. Different catheters thread over different guidewire sizes with catheters ranging from 3F to 6F. A 2F system is being developed for potential neurovascular use, and studies are currently being performed to assess its effectiveness in acute myocardial infarction, as well as peripheral arterial thrombosis. Because it is a non–wall contact device it may be used in native fistulas, as well as dialysis grafts.
Disadvantages: Hemolysis. Very expensive drive pump. The company has creative financing schedules, but the bottom line is either pay for the unit or buy many catheters. Useful for the full-service endovascular center because it can be utilized for so many on- and off-label uses, as well as by cardiology. Too expensive for small centers with limited volume. Also the new drive pump, though substantially easier to set up compared with the old system 3000, has

internal programming that makes it impossible to use the new catheter for off-label "power-pulse" uses.

OASIS THROMBECTOMY SYSTEM (BOSTON SCIENTIFIC, MEDITECH, QUINCY, MA)

Similar in concept to the Angiojet, but powered by dye injector commonly found in endovascular suites, so expensive equipment purchase, or catheter "amortization" is avoided. The Venturi jet is not sheathed. 6F.

Advantages: Dye injectors usually already present in endovascular suites. Non–wall contact device. Threads over a guidewire (0.018 inch). Affordable. Requires no additional hardware if dye injector is present.
Disadvantages: Less powerful than the Angiojet; not FDA approved for nondialysis use. Company does not seem to be pushing its use very strongly.

HYDROLYSER (CORDIS, MIAMI, FL)

Very similar to the Oasis device; also uses dye injector. Older device with extensive European experience.[36] 6F to 7F systems. An over-the-wire and non–over-the-wire system exist.

Advantages: Same as Oasis. System is probably the best-studied device in this field.
Disadvantages: Aspiration port is on one side of the catheter that may require twisting the catheter for multiple passes. Some have complained that it is "stiff."

Other Systems

EXCIMER LASER THROMBECTOMY (SPECTRANETICS, COLORADO SPRINGS, CO)

The 308-nm laser works by three mechanisms: disruption of carbon-carbon bonds, agitation, and steam disruption. It breaks carbon-carbon bonds through resonant frequency. Each photon can break a single C-C bond with an efficiency of about 2%. This decreases heat transfer and allows laser to work not only against plaque but also against thrombus, the idea behind using it in clotted dialysis grafts. Although it is not FDA approved for this purpose, and currently too expensive to be practical, Dahm et al.[39] demonstrated effectiveness of excimer 308-nm laser in dialysis graft thrombectomy.

TECHNIQUE

Preparation: Obtain informed consent, and make the decision in which venue to perform the procedure depending on contingencies as outlined earlier. I give antibiotic prophylaxis if opening a nonautogenous graft. Obtain history of allergies to contrast, and obtain appropriate laboratory studies. Perform a full sterile preparation, and use local anesthesia. Sedation is not always necessary. In patients with moderately maintained urinary output, arrange for postprocedure dialysis to remove contrast to preserve any residual renal function.

Do not prepare the thrombectomy device yet. Perform antegrade puncture as near the arterial end as possible using as long a subcutaneous tunnel as practical. Puncture can be tricky in soft grafts because there is no flow within the graft, and it may be difficult to know whether you are actually in the lumen (ultrasound can help). Use a very light touch because the thrombosed graft can collapse after compression of the thrombus and will not refill because of absence of inflow. Advance a guidewire into the lumen gently. It is important to confirm the position of the guidewire fluoroscopically before continuing with the procedure. Manipulate a guidewire into the venous outflow and then place a catheter over the guidewire past the venous anastomosis (this can be tricky in patients with tight venous-end stenoses). Obtain a complete outflow venogram (all the way to the right atrium) (Figure 58-1). Assess whether thrombectomy is worthwhile given the anatomic data from the venogram. If not, abort here and save resources. Up to 30% of patients have been noted to have long venous-end stenoses, which argue for surgical repair, and 15% of patients demonstrate the need for central venous angioplasty proximal to the venous anastomosis.[12]

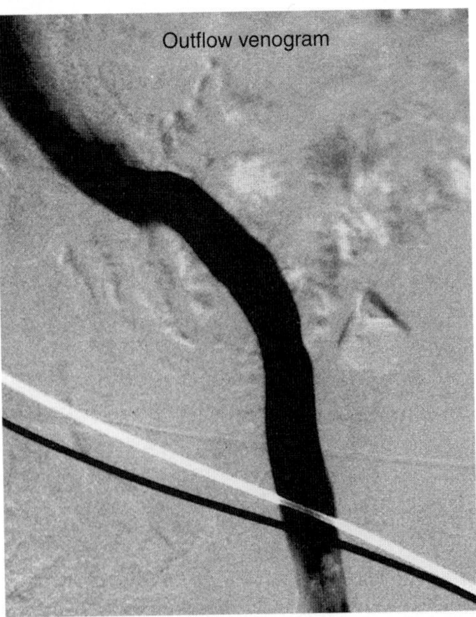

FIGURE 58-1 First in a series of illustrations showing percutaneous thrombectomy and angioplasty of a clotted thigh arteriovenous fistula. Access is obtained near the arterial end of the graft. A straight catheter is placed through the venous anastomosis into the outflow vein to determine whether thrombectomy is worthwhile. In this case, iliac venous outflow is normal.

If proceeding, heparinize the patient. Place the appropriate antegrade (radiopaque tipped) sheath for the device to be used. I place sterile needles in the skin at the location of presumed graft puncture so that this site is visible fluoroscopically. Perform mechanical thrombectomy of the body and venous end of the graft (Figure 58-2). If the device does not aspirate lysed thrombus, manually aspirate through the sheath before continuing. It is helpful to pass the effluent through a gauze sponge to check for embologenic material before continuing. If midprocedure fistulography demonstrates that residual thrombus is difficult to lyse (Figure 58-3), sometimes manual compression of the graft over the end of the thrombectomy device can help macerate thrombus and entrain it into the device. As one gains skill, less and less fluoroscopy is used during the thrombectomy portion of the procedure.

Thrombectomy will uncover any venous outflow stenosis. Balloon angioplasty (or very occasionally stent) the outflow if necessary (Figures 58-4 and 58-5). Because venous-end stenoses are neointimal tissue, they can be very hard to stretch. High-pressure balloons can be useful to overcome tight elastic scars, though they are not necessary if target diameter is reached with a conventional balloon, as it is the diameter, not the pressure, that determines outcome. New very-high-pressure balloons are now available up to 30 atm (Conquest PTA Balloon Dilation Catheter and Dorado Kevlar High Pressure Balloon, Bard Peripheral Vascular, Tempe, AZ).[41]

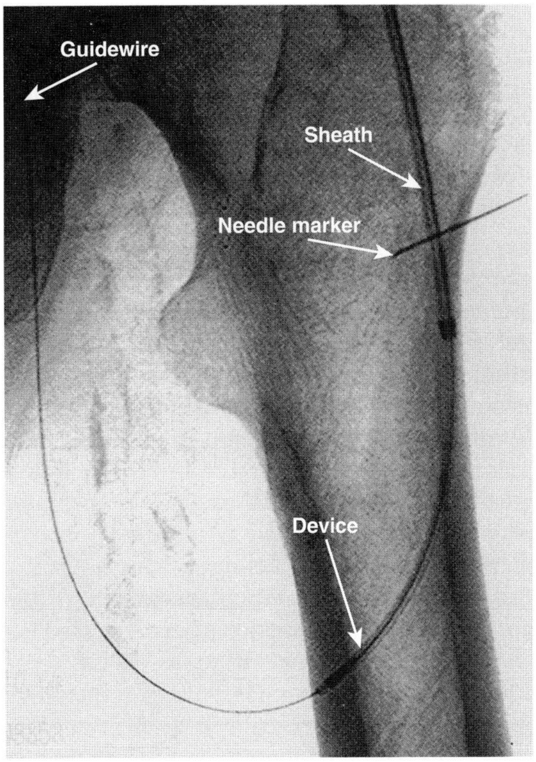

FIGURE 58-2 Unsubtracted view shows 6F sheath access near the arterial end of the graft. A needle marker is shown at the insertion site of the graft, which makes manipulation more secure under fluoroscopy and prevents unwanted removal of the sheath from the graft during position changes. Note the radiopaque tip, which is also helpful. The device is seen partially deployed near the apex of the graft (in this case, a Boston Scientific Oasis catheter).

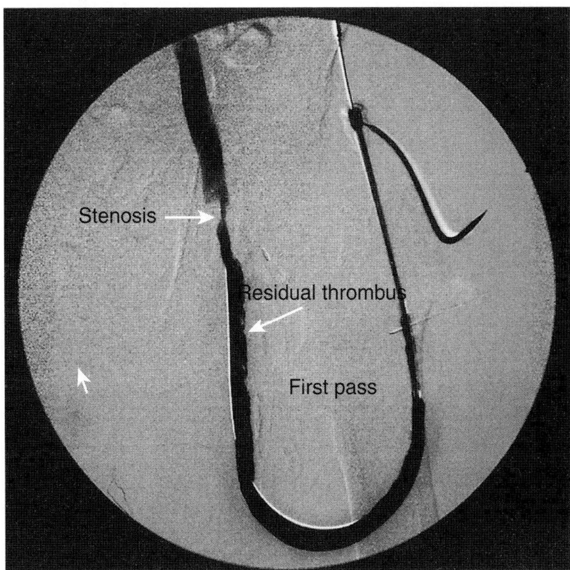

FIGURE 58-3 Fistulogram after first pass of the device. Note residual thrombus on the wall of the graft and venous-end stenosis.

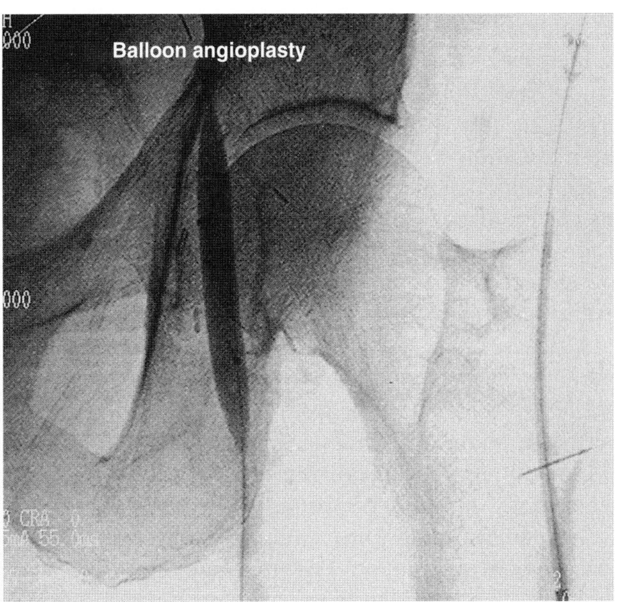

FIGURE 58-4 Balloon angioplasty. In this case, an 8-mm balloon was used. The graft was a 7-mm polytetrafluoroethylene graft. Slight oversizing is well tolerated with polytetrafluoroethylene, so long as dilation occurs in areas without much previous damage from dialysis needle insertions. Long inflation times can improve results.

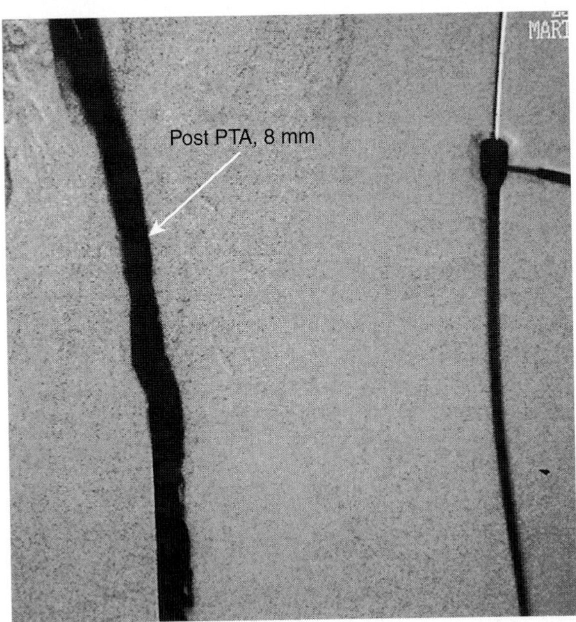

FIGURE 58-5 Post–percutaneous transluminal angioplasty *(PTA)* view showing good results. The venous end of the graft has undergone thrombectomy, but the arterial end is still thrombosed proximal to the sheath.

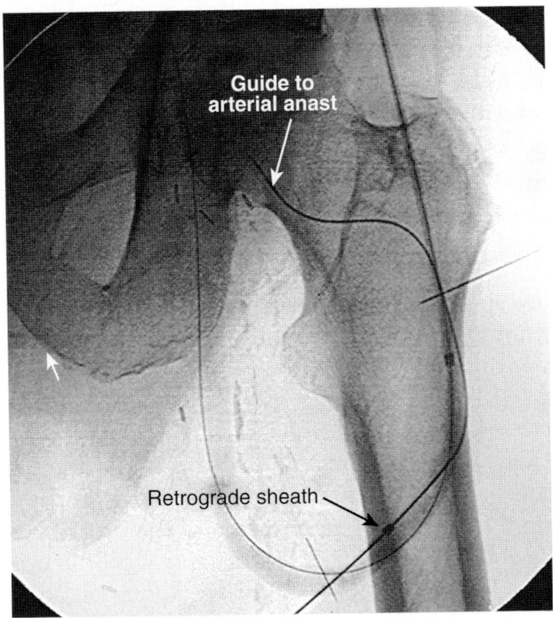

FIGURE 58-6 Access is now obtained in the opposite (crossed) direction, seen at the apex of the graft. Another marking needle is placed at the entry site. *Arrows* point to the radiopaque tip of the retrograde 5F sheath and the guidewire, which is advanced retrograde to the arterial anastomosis. A balloon embolectomy catheter is then placed through the retrograde sheath and is advanced through the arterial anastomosis. It is inflated, and the arterial-end thrombus and meniscus are pulled back to the tip of the antegrade sheath. The thrombectomy device is then passed through this thrombus to macerate it as much as possible before deflating the balloon and restoring flow. Aspiration of luminal contents can be performed through the antegrade sheath before balloon deflation to diminish the likelihood of central embolization.

I keep the balloons inflated for 5 minutes, although others claim this is not necessary.[18] I also repeat the angiogram just before the end of the procedure to make sure there is no elastic recoil. If the balloon cannot be fully inflated, do not use a stent, as it will not help with dilation. In spite of increased cost, we often use the cutting balloon for venous-end stenoses although the data are conflicting regarding efficacy.[42-44] It consists of a balloon in which three microtomes have been folded, which cuts the scar as the balloon is slowly inflated. Although first designed for calcific lesions, its most useful purpose may be in controlled cutting of scar. Balloon angioplasty of anastomoses within 1 to 2 months of surgery can be dangerous and must be performed with extreme caution.

After the antegrade work is finished, perform retrograde puncture at a convenient portion of the graft, preferably at least 10 cm from the original antegrade puncture, and cross guidewires (Figure 58-6). Place a 5F radiopaque-tipped sheath retrograde in the graft, and again mark its location with a needle. Place a standard 4F balloon thrombectomy catheter through the arterial anastomosis and inflate. Pull the meniscus only as far back as just beyond the marker of the original antegrade sheath, and leave the balloon inflated using a stopcock or flow switch. Reintroduce the thrombectomy device into the antegrade sheath, and macerate the meniscus as much as possible, aspirating as much of the residual as possible before deflating the thrombectomy balloon and sending whatever is left to the pulmonary circulation. Pass the thrombectomy catheter as often as necessary to clear the meniscus. A thrill should be noted at this stage.

Arterial-end angiography can be performed by occluding the lumen with the thrombectomy catheter just central to the antegrade sheath and injecting contrast slowly into the antegrade sheath (Figure 58-7). For the first view, I inject slowly to decrease the possibility of arterial embolization. The graft will slowly back-fill, and the arterial anastomosis can be studied. Arterial-end intervention, though less common, can be performed through the retrograde sheath if necessary.

Before completion of the procedure a repeated venous-end fistulogram is important to assess any possible remaining stenoses, or elastic restenosis of the previously angioplastied segments (Figure 58-8). Manual compression of the arterial end of the graft slows down the contrast bolus for better detail, but open-graft fistulograms demonstrate the presence of collateral filling that may be a clue to other missed hemodynamically significant stenoses. Palpation is important, and, if the graft is overly pulsatile or the thrill is weak, search for missed stenoses. Sometimes pullback pressures are necessary.

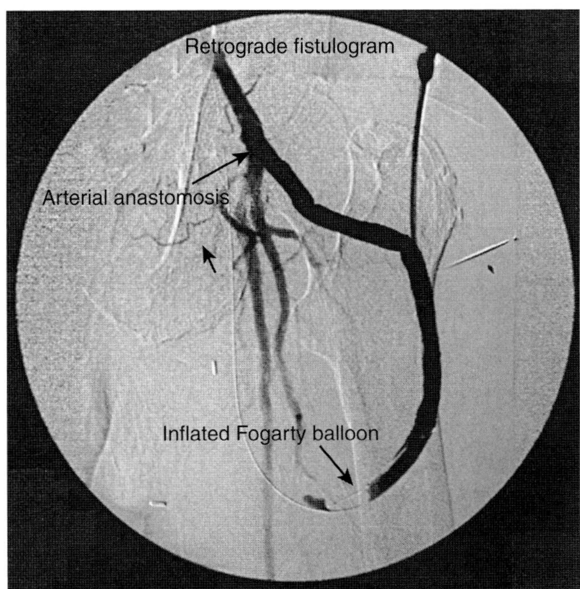

FIGURE 58-7 Retrograde fistulogram is performed by injecting contrast through the antegrade sheath with an inflated balloon distally. Excellent inflow is demonstrated, with minimal residual thrombus. Care should be exercised during contrast injection to avoid arterial embolism of residual thrombus.

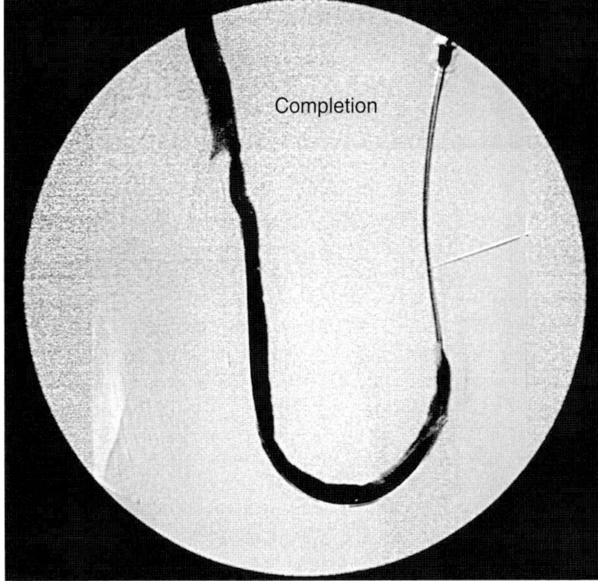

FIGURE 59-8 Completion view showing almost complete removal of thrombus and good result of angioplasty. Thrill is palpated at this time to confirm excellent flow. On occasion, elastic recoil of the segment undergoing angioplasty can be seen at this time, requiring further dilation or, rarely, stenting. Comparing this view with Figure 58-5 shows that a small amount or recoil has occurred in this case.

Central gradients of 5 to 10 mm Hg are considered significant, or more peripheral gradients of 20 mm Hg, and should be treated.

Pull the catheters and close the puncture sites with purse-string sutures in mature grafts. Perform finger-pressure hemostasis in immature grafts, because the graft tunnel has not yet scarred and hematoma might result. Pressure for hemostasis should not occlude the graft and can be performed with a surprisingly light touch at the end of a gloved finger. Patients may undergo dialysis immediately after the procedure.

COMPLICATIONS

Complications include bleeding, thrombosis, pulmonary embolus, arterial embolus, infection, dye-related complications, rupture, and death because of paradoxical embolus.[45] Trerotola has developed an ingenious technique for solving distal arterial embolus. If the arterial inflow *above the graft* is occluded by either balloon placement or percutaneous pressure, there is then a direct communication of the distal arterial tree where the embolus is lodged with the venous outflow through the graft. After occlusion of inflow the patient is instructed to make a fist repeatedly, and the embolus is often pushed retrograde out the arterial system into the fistula and out the central venous circulation, which tolerates small emboli considerably better than the hand does.

COMMENTS

Dialysis patients may live for many years and require functional access throughout. Conservation of sites should be the overriding goal in the management of vascular access whether by endoluminal, surgical, or a combination of means.

Clearly, technical excellence is important in the performance of open surgery, and, likewise, technical excellence is critical to percutaneous techniques. "Wide variations in the results suggest that the degree of commitment of physicians might be as important as the type of technique used."[45] Although clearly not a panacea, percutaneous thrombectomy of dialysis access provides a solution to many problems related to thrombosed dialysis access. Clinicians reading this chapter will have to contend with a spectrum of large versus small hospitals, easy versus difficult scheduling, radiologists limited to the angiography suite, surgeons limited to the operating room with potentially inferior equipment, and all combinations in between. The ultimate answer to the question of which technique to use in an individual patient is probably more regional than the answer to many other questions in surgery. Each clinician will have to weigh the potential benefits, costs, and risks with respect to his or her own environment. It is hoped that this chapter has outlined the technical issues to help make that individual decision.

References

1. NKF-DOQI clinical practice guidelines for vascular access. *Am J Kidney Dis* 30(4 suppl 3):S152–S189, 1997.
2. Beathard GA, Welch BR, Maidment HJ: Mechanical thrombolysis for the treatment of thrombosed hemodialysis access grafts, *Radiology* 200(3):711–716, 1996.
3. Trerotola SO, Vesely TM, Lund GB, et al: Treatment of thrombosed hemodialysis access grafts: Arrow Trerotola percutaneous thrombolytic device versus pulse-spray thrombolysis. Arrow-Trerotola percutaneous thrombolytic device clinical trial, *Radiology* 206(2):403–414, 1998.
4. Soulen MC, Zaetta JM, Amygdalos MA, et al: Mechanical declotting of thrombosed dialysis grafts: experience in 86 cases, *J Vasc Interv Radiol* 8(4):563–567, 1997.
5. Dougherty MJ, Calligaro KD, Schindler N, et al: Endovascular versus surgical treatment for thrombosed hemodialysis grafts: A prospective, randomized study, *J Vasc Surg* 30(6):1016–1023, 1999.
6. Singh MJ, Rhodes JM, Lee D, et al: Percutaneous therapy to maintain dialysis access successfully prolongs functional duration after primary failure, *Ann Vasc Surg* 21(4):474–480. Epub 2007 May 14, 2007.
7. Mishler R, Sands JJ, Ofsthun NJ, et al: Dedicated outpatient vascular access center decreases hospitalization and missed outpatient dialysis treatments, *Kidney Int* 69(2):393–398, 2006.
8. Maya ID, Smith T, Young CJ, et al: Is surgical salvage of arteriovenous grafts feasible after unsuccessful percutaneous mechanical thrombectomy? *Semin Dial* 21(2):174–177. Epub 2008 Jan 23, 2008.
9. Haage P, Vorwerk D, Wildberger JE, et al: Percutaneous treatment of thrombosed primary arteriovenous hemodialysis access fistulae, *Kidney Int* 57(3):1169–1175, 2000.
10. Beathard G: Percutaneous transvenous angioplasty in the treatment of vascular access stenosis, *Kidney Int* 42:1390–1397, 1992.
11. Green LD, Lee DS, Kucey DS: Metaanalysis comparing surgical thrombectomy, mechanical thrombectomy, and pharmacomechanical thrombolysis for thrombosed dialysis grafts, *J Vasc Surg* 36(5):939–945, 2002.
12. Marston WA, Craido E, Jaques PF, et al: Prospective randomized comparison of surgical versus endovascular management of thrombosed dialysis access grafts, *J Vasc Surg* 26:373–381, 1997.
13. Marston WQ, Mauro A, Keagy B, et al: Comparison of the AngioJet Rheolytic Catheter to surgical thrombectomy for the treatment of thrombosed hemodialysis grafts, *J Vasc Interv Radiol* 11:1095–1096, 2000.
14. Trerotola SO, Lund GB, Scheel PJ Jr, et al: Dialysis access grafts: percutaneous mechanical declotting without urokinase, *Radiology* 191(3):721–726, 1994.
15. Cohen MA, Kumpe DA, Durham JD, et al: Treatment of thrombosed hemodialysis access sites with thrombolysis and angioplasty, *Kidney Int* 46(5):1375–1380, 1994.
16. Liu YH, Hung YN, Hsieh HC, et al: Surgical thrombectomy for thrombosed dialysis grafts: comparison of adjunctive treatments. *World J Surg* 32(2):241–245. Erratum in: *World J Surg* 2008 32 (4):658, 2008.
17. Gray R: Regarding "Prospective randomized comparison of surgical versus endovascular management of thrombosed dialysis access grafts" (letter), *J Vasc Surg* 27(2):392–393, 1998.
18. Trerotola S: Interventional radiologic approach to hemodialysis access management. In: Savader S, Treotola S, editors: *Venous Interventional radiology with clinical perspectives*, New York, 1996, Thieme Medical Publishers, pp 178–211.
19. Berger MF, Aruny JE, Skibo LK: Thrombosis of polytetrafluoroethylene dialysis fistulas after recent surgical thrombectomy: salvage by means of thrombolysis and angioplasty, *J Vasc Interv Radiol* 5(5):725–730, 1994.
20. Gelbfish GA: Surgery versus percutaneous treatment of thrombosed dialysis access grafts: is there a best method? *J Vasc Interv Radiol* 9(6):875–877, 1998.
21. Anain P, Shenoy S, O'Brien-Irr M, et al: Balloon angioplasty for arteriovenous graft stenosis, *J Endovasc Ther* 8(2):167–172, 2001.
22. Barth KH, Gosnell MR, Palestrant AM, et al: Hydrodynamic thrombectomy system versus pulse-spray thrombolysis for thrombosed hemodialysis grafts: a multicenter prospective randomized comparison, *Radiology* 217(3):678–684, 2000.
23. Sofocleous CT, Cooper SG, Schur I, et al: Retrospective comparison of the Amplatz thrombectomy device with modified pulse-spray pharmacomechanical thrombolysis in the treatment of thrombosed hemodialysis access grafts, *Radiology* 213(2): 561–567, 1999.
24. Alexander J, Hood D, Rowe V, et al: Surgical intervention significantly prolong the patency of failed angioaccess grafts previously treated with percutaneous techniques? *Ann Vasc Surg* 16(2):197–200. Epub 2002 Feb 15, 2002.
25. Barshes NR, Annambhotla S, Bechara C, et al: Endovascular repair of hemodialysis graft-related pseudoaneurysm: an alternative treatment strategy in salvaging failing dialysis access, *Vasc Endovascular Surg* 42(3):228–234. Epub 2008 Mar 28, 2008.
26. Osborn G, Escofet X, Da Silva A: Medical adjuvant treatment to increase patency of arteriovenous fistulae and grafts, *Cochrane Database Syst Rev* (4):CD002786, 2008.
27. Cynamon J, Lakritz PS, Wahl SI, et al: Graft declotting: description of the "lyse and wait" technique, *J Vasc Interv Radiol* 8 (5):825–829, 1997.
28. Vogel PM, Bansal V, Marshall MW: Thrombosed hemodialysis grafts: lyse and wait with tissue plasminogen activator or urokinase compared to mechanical thrombolysis with the Arrow-Trerotola Percutaneous Thrombolytic Device, *J Vasc Interv Radiol* 12(10):1157–1165, 2001.
29. Marston WA, Criado E, Mauro MA, et al: Regarding "Prospective randomized comparison of surgical versus endovascular management of thrombosed dialysis access grafts": Reply, *J Vasc Surg* 27 (2):393, 1998.
30. Haskel Z: Mechanical thrombectomy devices for the treatment of peripheral arterial occlusions, *Rev Cardiovasc Med* 3(suppl 2): S45–S52, 2002.
31. Dolmatch BL, Gray RJ, Horton KM: Will iatrogenic pulmonary embolization be our pulmonary embarrassment? *Radiology* 191 (3):615–617; discussion 618, 1994.
32. Stainkin B: Mechanical thrombectomy: basic principles, current devices and future directions, *Tech Vasc Interv Radiol* 6(1):2–5, 2003.
33. Etheredge E, Haid S, Maeser M, et al: Salvage operations for malfunctioning polytetrafluoroethylene hemodialysis access grafts, *Surgery* 94:464–470, 1983.
34. Harp RJ, Stavropoulos SW, Wasserstein AG, et al: Pulmonary hypertension among end-stage renal failure patients following hemodialysis access thrombectomy, *Cardiovasc Intervent Radiol* 28 (1):17–22, 2005.
35. Trerotola SO, Davidson DD, Filo RS, et al: Preclinical in vivo testing of a rotational mechanical thrombolytic device, *J Vasc Interv Radiol* 7(5):717–723, 1996.
36. Muller-Hulsbeck S, Grimm J, Leidt J, et al: Comparison of in vitro effectiveness of mechanical thrombectomy devices, *J Vasc Interv Radiol* 12(10):1185–1191, 2001.
37. Sharafuddin MJ, Kadir S, Joshi SJ, et al: Balloon-assisted aspiration thrombectomy of clotted hemodialysis access grafts, *J Vasc Interv Radiol* 7(2):177–183, 1996.

38. Yasui k, Qian Z, Nararian G, et al: recirculation-type Amplatz clot macerator: determination of particle size and distribution, *J Vasc Interv Radiol* 4:275–278, 1993.
39. Dahm JB, Ruppert J, Doerr M, et al: Percutaneous laser-facilitated thro-mbectomy: an innovative, easily applied, and effective therapeutic option for recanalization of acute and subacute thrombotic hemodialysis shunt occlusions, *J Endovasc Ther* 13(5): 603–608, 2006.
41. Ross J: Ultrahigh-pressure PTA for hemodialysis, *Endovascular Today*, 23–28, 2003.
42. Bittl J, Feldman R: Cutting balloon angioplasty for undilatable venous stenoses causing dialysis graft failure, *Cathet Cardiovasc Intervent* 58:524–526, 2003.
43. Kariya S, Tanigawa N, Kojima H, et al: Primary patency with cutting and conventional balloon angioplasty for different types of hemodialysis access stenosis, *Radiology* 243(2):578–587. Epub 2007 Mar 30, 2007.
44. Vesely TM, Siegel JB: Use of the peripheral cutting balloon to treat hemodialysis-related stenoses, *J Vasc Interv Radiol* 16 (12):1593–1603, 2005.
45. Turmel-Rodrigues L, Pengloan J, Bourquelot P: Interventional radiology in hemodialysis fistulae and grafts: a multidisciplinary approach, *Cardiovasc Intervent Radiol* 25(1):3–16. Epub 2002 Jan 17. Review, 2002.

CHAPTER

59

Thrombolysis in Dialysis Access Salvage

Daniel I. Obrand, Reda Jamjoom

In patients with end-stage renal disease, autogenous fistulas are the preferred access modalities followed by prosthetic arteriovenous grafts (AVGs). Maintaining dialysis access patency is an expensive proposition. It is estimated that 50% of dialysis access sites will require revision within 2 years of creation, accounting for 16% of hospitalizations for patients undergoing dialysis.[1,2] Thrombotic occlusions account for the majority of these complications usually because of intimal hyperplasia at the venous anastomosis site. This is followed by the graft filling with thrombus and an arterial plug forming at the arterial anastomosis. As the life expectancy of patients receiving dialysis increases, salvage procedures for arteriovenous fistulas (AVFs) that can preserve venous locations for new shunts have become imperative. Debate exists over the optimal management of a thrombosed AVF: the surgical option of thrombectomy with or without revision (patch angioplasty, balloon angioplasty, or extension graft) versus percutaneous thrombectomy/thrombolysis versus thrombolytic therapy with or without revision. No universally accepted techniques for mechanical treatment exist, and consideration should be given to the costs of the various interventions, the time involvement, and the time until the fistula can be reaccessed. The goals of thrombolysis are the removal of the thrombus and restoration of flow in a short time frame allowing the return of function of the AVF.

CONTRAINDICATIONS

Absolute contraindications to thrombolytic therapy of clotted dialysis access grafts are the same as those for any thrombolysis treatment. As well, patients with a history of right-sided heart failure, pulmonary hypertension, cardiac dysrhythmias, or right-to-left cardiac shunts should not be considered for thrombolysis because of the risk of pulmonary emboli.[3] Relative contraindications include thrombosis of the fistula within 3 weeks of construction, ongoing graft infection, or allergy to iodine. AVGs composed of prosthetic material respond to thrombolysis and dilatation with better results than do native vessel fistulas.[4,5] In native vessel fistulas, the multiple venous side branches are often filled with thrombi of varying age. As well, multiple sites of venous stenosis may be present, requiring dilatation. Results of thrombolysis are not as good for this group as for grafts, and salvage may not be possible.

TECHNIQUE

Serum electrolytes should be checked, because markedly elevated potassium levels may require medical intervention or emergent dialysis with temporary catheter placement. The fistula should be examined to determine its location and configuration. The presence of a pseudoaneurysm may change the entry site. Large pseudoaneurysms may contain a large amount of thrombus and be more difficult to treat. The operative note should be reviewed with regard to the course and the type of AVF constructed. The patient can be premedicated with diphenhydramine (Benadryl), aspirin, or cimetidine to reduce the rigors associated with high-dose urokinase (UK) infusion. The four basic steps in performing an endovascular thrombectomy are the venogram to evaluate the central and peripheral veins, removal of the thrombus from the AVF, treatment of all underlying stenosis, and dislodgment of the arterial plug.

SYNTHETIC GRAFTS

Crossed Catheter Technique

The crossed catheter technique involves the placement of two catheters—one through the arterial anastomosis and one through the venous anastomosis.[3] The skin of the arm should be prepped and draped with use of sterile techniques. One percent lidocaine for local anesthesia is injected as a skin wheal at the entry sites. Straight grafts are entered at the center of the graft with approximately 5 to 8 cm separating the two catheters. Loop grafts are entered at each side of the apex of the graft. If the graft is longer (50 to 60 cm), the two entry sites should be made closer to the venous side separated by 8 to 10 cm. This makes it easier to manipulate the venous anastomosis or gain access to the axillary, the subclavian, or the jugular vein, if necessary. Once the skin has been anesthetized, the graft is entered with a 22-gauge needle at a 45-degree angle to the skin, aimed toward the venous anastomosis. A 0.018-inch guidewire is passed into the lumen of the graft; it should pass easily in a freshly thrombosed graft. With use of fluoroscopy, the guidewire is advanced. A 4F dilator is placed over the guidewire. The 0.018-inch guidewire is replaced with a 0.035-inch guidewire. The guidewire is passed through the venous anastomosis, where there is often stenosis. The 4F dilator is replaced with a 5F dilator over the guidewire. A 5F pulse-spray catheter is placed over the wire across the venous anastomosis into the native vein. The guidewire is removed, and contrast material is instilled to confirm intraluminal placement of the catheter. Formal venography of the venous outflow is performed to determine whether any mechanical obstruction in the native circulation is present. The pulse-spray catheter is positioned under fluoroscopic guidance (injecting contrast material as necessary) until its tip is just beyond the extent of the thrombus. (This may be at or beyond the venous anastomosis.)

A second catheter is now placed to access the arterial side of the graft. The skin entry site is proximal (toward the venous anastomosis) to the original catheter but is aimed toward the arterial anastomosis. The graft is entered with a 22-gauge needle at a 45-degree angle to the skin, aimed toward the arterial anastomosis. A 0.018-inch guidewire is passed into the lumen of the graft, over which a 4F dilator is placed. A 0.035-inch guidewire is then passed through the arterial anastomosis, and the 4F dilator is replaced with a 5F dilator, which is in turn replaced with a 5F pulse-spray catheter across the arterial anastomosis. Contrast material is instilled gently until a patent arterial segment is noted. Care must be taken when manipulating the arterial side not to dislodge thrombus into the arterial system. The patient is given 2500 units of heparin intravenously or through the venous side of the catheter system. Then 250,000 units of UK is reconstituted in 10 mL of sterile water to which 1250 units of heparin is added. Pulse-spray thrombolysis is instituted with infusion of 0.3 mL (7500 units) of UK pulsed through each catheter every 30 seconds. The entire graft is laced with 500,000 units of UK with use of this technique by manipulating the catheter. Repeated angiography is performed. Once antegrade flow of contrast material is seen in the graft, the thrombolytic therapy is terminated. If after instilling 500,000 units of UK no antegrade flow is seen, an additional 250,000 units of UK is pulsed through the catheter system (125,000 units through each catheter). This may be repeated if recanalization has not occurred. If a total of 1 million units of UK has been infused and no antegrade flow is seen within the graft, a drip infusion of 240,000 units of UK is given through the catheter placed at the arterial anastomosis. This infusion can be continued outside the angiography suite or the operating theater. When a return of Doppler flow within the graft is noted, repeated angiography is used to confirm antegrade flow. Any underlying stenosis can be treated with balloon angioplasty with use of the same access site.

Alternative Urokinase Infusion Protocols

Davis Protocol

In the Davis protocol, the crossed catheter technique (proximal and distal placement near the arterial and the venous anastomoses) is used.[6] The thrombus is laced with 50,000 to 75,000 units of UK per catheter (25,000 units/mL). UK is infused via each catheter at a rate of 2000 units/min. A bolus of 2000 to 3000 units of heparin is given, and then a continuous infusion of 1000 units/hr is given. Mean infusion time is 86 minutes.

Kumpe Protocol

In the Kumpe protocol, the crossed catheter technique (proximal and distal placement near the arterial and the venous anastomoses) is used.[1] The thrombus is laced with 150,000 to 500,000 units of UK and an infusion of 125,000 units/hr per catheter for 1 to 2 hours. An angiogram is repeated, and the infusion is continued at the same rate for 2 hours if necessary.

Brunner Ultrarapid Protocol

In the Brunner ultrarapid protocol, two multiple—side-hole catheters are placed with their tips at the arterial and the venous anastomoses.[7] UK is reconstituted to 50,000 units/mL in normal saline solution, and the patient is systemically heparinized with 5000 units of heparin. The UK is infused at 20,000 units/min for 50 minutes (1 million units). A repeated angiogram is performed. An additional 250,000 units of UK can be infused for residual thrombus.

Native Vessel Fistulas

The arm is prepped and draped, and local anesthesia is instilled at the entry point, which is chosen antegrade to the anastomosis. A retrograde entry toward the anastomosis may be required simultaneously if there is thrombus at the anastomosis. The fistula is entered with an 18- or 19-gauge angiocatheter sheath. Contrast material is injected, with identification of patent veins before thrombolysis. A small guidewire can be used to probe the thrombus and the small side branches gently to help the lytic agent reach these areas. A constant agent infusion of UK is given through the angiocatheter. Three vials of 250,000 units of UK are reconstituted with 5 mL of nonbacteriostatic water and are added to 235 mL of normal saline solution or 5% dextrose in water (final concentration 3000 units/mL). This is infused at 240,000 units/hr (80 mL/hr) for 2 hours, then 120,000 units/hr (40 mL/hr) for 2 hours; 80,000 units/hr (27 mL/hr) is infused overnight if necessary. Repeated angiography is performed in the morning or when a bruit is heard to assess the patency of the fistula and the side branches (compared with the original film). Stenoses are balloon dilated as needed.

POSTPROCEDURE MANAGEMENT

If the patient is to receive dialysis immediately after thrombolytic therapy, 7F high-flow catheters with internal stiffeners can be placed over the guidewires (which are then removed). The catheters are placed in the same crossed position, with indications for the hemodialysis staff. The catheters are flushed with heparinized saline solution and can be removed after dialysis when the activated coagulation time is less than 180 seconds. Patients can be discharged on the same day if no complications are noted. Routine repeated fistulograms are recommended in 1 month to assess the angioplasty sites.

COMPLICATIONS

Bleeding from the puncture site can be treated with application of direct pressure. Bleeding may also occur from previously made puncture sites and can be controlled with manual pressure. Rupture from guidewire manipulation or following angioplasty can be controlled with occluding balloon catheters deployed proximal and distal to the site until repair can be undertaken. A proximally occluding tourniquet can also temporize the situation. Distal embolization is unusual and has been reported to occur in fewer than 1% of procedures; it usually occurs distal (to the hand) from the arterial anastomosis.[8]

Fluid overload may be seen and should be treated with emergent dialysis. The risk of bleeding at distal sites is similar to the risks with other uses of systemic thrombolytic therapy.

RESULTS

Salvage of dialysis grafts is defined as patency after thrombolysis or angioplasty, or both, of greater than 1 month.

Synthetic Grafts

The usual time until successful lysis is 2 to 3 hours, with doses of UK ranging from 250,000 to 1 million units. Immediate technical success is reported to be greater than 90%. Long-term patency is less encouraging, with 30-day primary salvage rates of 70%. Six-month patencies are 40%, and the 1-year primary salvage rate is 20% to 30%. Secondary patency rates of 50% with repeated interventions have been reported.[8]

Native Vessels

The 1-month primary patency rate is 70% (89% for stenoses, 45% for occlusions).[9] Secondary patency rates are 93% at 6 months, 91% at 1 year, and 57% at 2 years for failing fistulas with stenoses. For patients with occlusions, the secondary patency rates at 6 months, 1 year, and 2 years are 80%, 50%, and 14%, respectively. Saeed and colleagues[4] reported 6-month patency after balloon angioplasty of anastomotic lesions to be 65%; there was 100% patency in nine patients with more proximal lesions.

References

1. Kumpe DA, Cohen MAH: Angioplasty/thrombolytic treatment of failing and failed hemodialysis access sites: comparison with surgical treatment, *Prog Cardiovasc Dis* 34:263–278, 1992.
2. Feldman HI, Held PH, Hutchinson JT, et al: Hemodialysis vascular access morbidity in the United States, *Kidney Int* 43:1091–1096, 1993.
3. Aruny JE: Dialysis access shunt and fistula recanalization. In: Kandarpa K, Aruny JE, editors: *Handbook of interventional radiologic procedures*, Boston, 1996, Little, Brown, pp 115–129.
4. Saeed M, Newman GE, McCann RL, et al: Stenoses in dialysis fistulas: treatment with percutaneous angioplasty, *Radiology* 164:693–697, 1987.
5. Glanz S, Gordon DH, Lipkowitz GS, et al: Axillary and subclavian vein stenosis: percutaneous angioplasty, *Radiology* 168:371–373, 1988.
6. Davis GB, Dowd CF, Bookstein JJ, et al: Thrombosed dialysis grafts: efficacy of intrathrombic deposition of concentrated urokinase, clot maceration, and angioplasty, *Am J Radiol* 149:177–181, 1987.
7. Brunner MC, Matalon TA, Patel SK, et al: Ultrarapid urokinase in hemodialysis access occlusion, *J Vasc Interv Radiol* 2:503–506, 1991.
8. Valji K, Bookstein JJ, Roberts AC, et al: Pharmacomechanical thrombolysis and angioplasty in the management of clotted hemodialysis grafts: early and late clinical results, *Radiology* 178:243–247, 1991.
9. Gmelin E, Winterhoff R, Rinast E: Insufficient hemodialysis access fistulas: late results of treatment with percutaneous balloon angioplasty, *Radiology* 171:657–660, 1989.

CHAPTER

60

Clinical Decision Making and Hemodialysis Graft Thrombosis

Hugh A. Gelabert

Hemodialysis access grafts and fistulas are essential life-preserving conduits. Their continuous function is imperative for patient survival. Loss of dialysis access, even for short periods of time, exposes patients to a series of metabolic processes that are inevitably fatal.

The object of this chapter is to provide a decision-making guide for approaching patients with access thrombosis. Implementing a successful endovascular intervention will require more than knowing the technical procedures; it also requires choosing the correct treatment in a given circumstance.

Endovascular therapy plays an important role in the management of the most common complications of hemodialysis: access insufficiency and thrombosis. Endovascular techniques offer the means of assessing the causes of graft failure. Endovascular interventions may correct the underlying causes of graft failure. By these means, endovascular therapy may extend the functional lifespan of an access site.

DIALYSIS ACCESS FAILURE

There are two basic ways in which an arteriovenous (AV) access may fail: (1) it may be unable to provide adequate efficient dialysis (because of restricted blood flow), or (2) it may be unable to provide any dialysis because of thrombotic occlusion (Box 60-1).

Recirculation of blood through the dialysis circuit is the primary cause of poor dialysis efficiency or clearance.[1,2] Recirculation results in inadequate flow and leads to poor dialysis and poor clearance of metabolic products. The amount of recirculation can be quantified and expressed as a percentage. Recirculation may be due to technical problems with access site location or poor inflow to the shunt. The principal cause of recirculation is outflow obstruction of the graft. As the obstruction increases, the recirculatory index rises. An increased recirculation fraction may be an indication of a failing graft and should prompt evaluation of the AV access for possible stenosis.

The most common causes of dialysis graft thrombosis are pseudoaneurysms, coagulation abnormalities, and stenosis (occlusive lesions).[3] *Pseudoaneurysms* develop in a graft because of overuse of a limited portion of the graft. Repeated graft punctures at a single site will result in disruption of graft integrity and development of a pseudoaneurysm. Once a pseudoaneurysm is sufficiently large, blood within it forms thrombus along the dilated graft wall. This clot can then act as a ball valve, obstructing blood flow through the graft and allowing the graft to thrombose.

Coagulation abnormalities may lead to graft thrombosis. Hypercoagulability disorders, such as protein S or C deficiencies or the presence of anticardiolipin antibodies, result in the formation of thrombus within the graft lumen. Common hypercoagulation disorders are listed in Box 60-2. If a graft or fistula thromboses and no hemodynamic or mechanical causes are discovered, a hypercoagulable condition may be present. Investigation of a coagulation abnormality should include screening for the most common known coagulation abnormalities. Empirical anticoagulation therapy with warfarin is frequently implemented and is often successful.[4]

Normal endothelial cells possess several antithrombotic properties. As a consequence, synthetic AV grafts (AVGs) are more prone to thrombosis than a native AV fistula. The grafts are less tolerant of impeded blood flow, less tolerant of blood stasis, and more vulnerable to the procoagulant effect of the hypercoagulation disorders. (Box 60-3 lists factors in the endothelial modulation of thrombosis.)

Occlusive lesions resulting in graft stenosis are the most common cause of thrombosis of an AVG. By far, the most common cause of graft stenosis is fibrointimal hyperplasia. Fibrointimal stenosis develops as a result of repeated and continued injury to both the vessels and the graft caused by flowing blood. The abrupt transition from normal vessel to prosthetic graft results in dramatic shear stress. This translates into mechanical damage to the cellular elements that line the anastomosis. One result of this damage is the fibrointimal hyperplastic lesion, a fibrous lesion with abnormal endothelial cell function.

The primary cell type encountered within grafts and at anastomotic sites is the myofibroblast. This cell is of uncertain origin but is thought to represent migrated subendothelial smooth muscle cells that have undergone a process of dedifferentiation as they replicate within the pseudointima at the juncture between graft and native vessel. The myofibroblasts replicate and secrete matrix. The result is a fibrous lesion that gradually increases in size as it grows into the lumen of the graft. Eventually, the mass of fibrointimal tissue will be sufficiently large to obstruct the flow of blood through the graft.

In addition to myofibroblasts, endothelial cells are present in varying numbers at the anastomotic regions. The endothelial cells that populate the vessel near the fibrointimal lesions are thought to be abnormal in regard to their functional characteristics. They are morphologically and synthetically impaired and are unable to provide the vessel lumen with the same antithrombotic and vasodilatory properties as a normal vessel. This altered ability is thought to contribute to the development of stenosis at the anastomotic junction.

The final element in the pathogenesis of the failing graft is abnormal endothelial function. Normal endothelial cells modulate the coagulation of blood in several ways: anticoagulation, vasodilation, modulation of platelet adhesion and activation, and modulation of fibrin

BOX 60-1

CAUSES OF ARTERIOVENOUS GRAFT FAILURE

- Aneurysm
- Hypercoagulability
- Stenosis
  - Intragraft
  - Anastomosis: artery/vein
  - Inflow/runoff vessels
  - Subclavian vein

BOX 60-2

COMMON HYPERCOAGULATION DISORDERS

- Antithrombin III deficiency
- Protein C deficiency
- Protein S deficiency
- Resistance to activated protein C
- Presence of antiphospholipid antibodies
- Presence of antibodies to platelets
- Presence of antibodies to heparin
- Presence of antibodies to thrombin
- Elevated factor VIII
- Elevated C-reactive protein

BOX 60-3

ENDOTHELIAL MODULATION OF THROMBOSIS

Anticoagulant Function (Normal Function)

- Tissue plasminogen activator synthesis
- Urokinase VIII synthesis
- Nitric oxide synthesis
- Prostaglandin I_2 (prostacyclin)
- Thrombomodulin synthesis
- Protein S synthesis
- Heparin sulfate synthesis

Procoagulant Function (Seen With Injury)

- Tissue factor expression
- Prostaglandin
- Plasminogen activator inhibitor synthesis
- Factor VIII: von Willebrand factor synthesis
- Factor V synthesis
- Prothrombinase complex receptor expression

polymerization and clot stabilization. In contrast, the damaged endothelial cell lacks anticoagulant abilities and expresses procoagulant elements. The procoagulant elements are also able to promote proliferation of cellular elements such as myofibroblasts and may enhance the development of hyperplastic lesions.

PRESENTATIONS AND CLINICAL CONSIDERATIONS

The most common presentation of a failed AVG is thrombosis. The graft clots, and the absence of blood flow is detected by cessation of the palpable thrill or the auscultated bruit. The event may be detected by the patient or by a dialysis unit worker. Assessing patient physiologic needs is important in deciding what intervention may be safely possible. Foremost is the consideration of time since the last hemodialysis session. Some patients with residual renal function may be able to survive several days without hemodialysis. However, for those without renal function (the vast majority) the time from last dialysis may be an important indicator as to whether a critical metabolic alteration may preclude intervention. At the very least it would indicate that an assessment of the metabolic state is warranted.

Residual Renal Function

If the patient has residual renal function, contrast administration may present a prohibitive risk, and surgical intervention would be preferred. The residual renal function provides the patient with significant benefit even if he or she is dialysis dependent. The residual renal function may make the patient less vulnerable to volume changes, may allow a less-restricted volume intake, and may allow a greater margin of safety in the event of access failure. Endovascular interventions based on contrast radiography should be avoided because the impaired kidney will be more sensitive to contrast agents, and the risk of inducing permanent complete renal failure in these patients is far greater than in a patient with normal or marginally impaired renal function. Instead mechanical thrombectomy and ultrasound guidance may be the safest approach.

Metabolic Anomalies

Significant hyperkalemia, congestive failure, and systemic acidosis are the common denominators of absent renal function and failed dialysis access. All patients will incur these anomalies and will be at risk for fatal myocardial arrhythmias and death. The patient's vital signs and weight, which are significant clues to the possibility of critical volume overload, should be registered. (Steps in the evaluation of patients are outlined in Box 60-4.) Endovascular intervention may offer the most rapid means of restoring dialysis and averting these problems. It is important to assess patients for these problems before beginning endovascular interventions such as thrombolysis and angioplasty. The risk in proceeding with endovascular treatment in the face of these metabolic anomalies is that the patient may die on the procedure table. If the patients demonstrate any of these anomalies then the appropriate intervention may be to provide temporary catheter access and return for more definitive treatment after hemodialysis is performed.

Anticoagulation

Patients with a history of repeated thrombotic events may be given anticoagulants. Because many of these patients are maintained with anticoagulants to improve the function and the patency of the dialysis graft, coagulation parameters must be checked before thrombolysis. Thus it is important to review the patient's medication list and to check coagulation tests before proceeding with any intervention. Those parameters that are grossly abnormal and that require correction should be addressed. Ideally, the patient's platelet count should be more than 60,000, and the international normalized ratio should be less than 2.0. Proceeding with thrombolysis in the face of anticoagulation may expose the patient to considerable risk. At the very least it is imperative to assess the coagulation status before proceeding with administration of lytic agents.

BOX 60-4

EVALUATION OF PATIENTS*

1. What is the patient's volume status?
2. Is the patient acidemic?
3. Is the patient hyperkalemic?
4. Is the patient anemic?
5. Is the patient euglycemic?
6. Are coagulation parameters acceptable?
7. Is the patient able to follow instructions and cooperate?

*To ensure the safety of endovascular intervention in patients undergoing hemodialysis, these seven questions must be addressed before the start of the procedure. The most frequent problems (volume overload, hyperkalemia, and acidosis) are common causes of cardiac arrest in this population. No absolute answers exist for any of these parameters, but careful clinical assessment and common sense should reduce the incidence of untoward events.

Timing of Thrombolysis

The time interval from thrombosis to the commencement of thrombolysis is a significant element in determining the likelihood of success of returning a clotted graft to good working order. Veins react to intraluminal thrombus by developing an intense inflammatory response. This response develops rapidly, so that within a few days of thrombosis the veins are seldom able to be salvaged. The inflammatory reaction results in loss of normal endothelial function. The endothelial cells are damaged or denuded, and the resultant vein is little more than a collagen and elastin tube. In such circumstances, the vein after removal of the thrombus is very thrombogenic.

Grafts, unlike veins, are largely unaffected by thrombus. Because the graft does not rely on endothelial function, clot within a graft does not have the pejorative effect on coagulation that occurs in veins. In addition, because the graft material is inert and nonreactive, the presence of clot within the graft does not have an adverse effect on the ability of thrombolysis to reestablish patency or return to function. Accordingly, thrombus within a graft may be successfully cleared up to several months after a graft clots.

GOALS OF ENDOVASCULAR THERAPY FOR OCCLUDED ARTERIOVENOUS ACCESS

Endovascular therapy for dialysis grafts has several goals that guide the exercise. The first is to clear the graft of clot and allow blood flow to resume. The second goal is to image the graft to evaluate the cause of graft failure. Imaging the graft will reveal stenosis within the graft or the graft anastomosis. The third goal is to treat the cause of graft failure. Should a stenotic lesion be identified then the goal would be endovascular repair of the stenosis. This may involve angioplasty, stenting, or atherectomy.

Goal 1: Clearing the Clot: Thrombolysis and Thrombectomy

The endovascular techniques for clearing thrombus from a graft include thrombolysis and thrombectomy. Thrombolysis refers to the dissolution of thrombus by degradation of the thrombus components. This is most commonly accomplished by enzymatic degradation of fibrin cross-links within the clot. It may also be achieved by mechanical disruption of the clot. A combination of mechanical and enzymatic thrombolysis occurs when the lytic agent is pressure sprayed into the clot, disrupting the thrombus mechanically as the infusion is delivered. This has been referred to as pharmacomechanical thrombolysis.

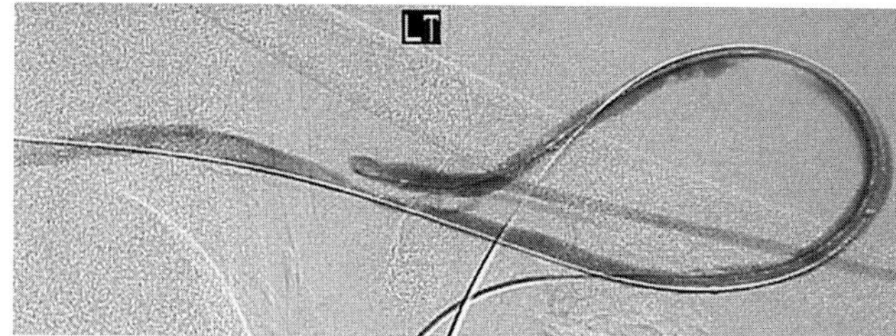

FIGURE 60-1 A thrombosed AVG partially cleared with AngioJet.

Thrombolysis

Enzymatic or pharmacologic thrombolysis has been implemented in a variety of manners, including pressure infusion, bolus administration, and clot lacing. It has been used in conjunction with mechanical clot disruption and clot removal. None of these variations in the technique of administration has had significant impact on the ultimate efficacy of thrombolysis. In most instances, the technical success rate (i.e., the ability to clear the clot from within the graft) is about 80% to 90%. In a prospective study comparing pulse-spray versus continuous urokinase infusions, Goodwin and associates[5] noted no significant difference in the time to thrombolysis, the total dose of urokinase required for thrombolysis, the success rate in clearing the grafts, or the 60-day patency rate (Figure 60-1).

Complications of Thrombolysis

By its very nature, endovascular therapy exposes patients to the risks of angiography: allergic reactions to contrast material, acute renal toxicity, and prothrombotic effects. Although most patients receiving hemodialysis are anephric, some may have mild residual renal function. Use of contrast agents in such patients presents a severe risk of complete renal failure. The incidence of acute renal insufficiency in large angiography series is generally between 1% and 10%. Of importance is that, in patients with preexisting renal insufficiency, the risk of contrast-related renal toxicity is much increased. In a study in 400 patients undergoing arteriographic procedures, the incidence of acute renal insufficiency (elevation of creatinine level) in patients with normal renal function was 8.2%.[6] In the same study, patients with elevated creatinine level who were undergoing angiography had a 41% incidence of deterioration in renal function. About 8% of those with renal insufficiency ultimately required permanent hemodialysis.[6] Therefore in patients with residual renal function, endovascular interventions will almost certainly result in complete renal failure. Although not unexpected, this is a significant issue for some patients.

Other potential complications of thrombolysis include pyrogenic reaction, pulmonary or arterial embolization, and hemorrhage. The pyrogenic reaction is a response to the lytic agents and the by-products of thrombolysis. It is usually self-limited and more of an inconvenience than a grave concern. The greater concerns associated with febrile responses during and after thrombolysis are the potential for allergic reactions to the lytic agents and the possibility of inoculating the graft with bacteria and causing a graft infection.

Embolization is a significant concern during thrombolysis. Pulmonary emboli are generally accepted to be commonplace, but most are subclinical, and patients tolerate these well. The specific means of clearing the graft will have dramatic bearing on the impact of the pulmonary emboli. Trerotola et al.[7] have reported segmental filling defects in as many as 90% of their experimental subjects undergoing pulse-spray thrombolysis. In contrast, they reported only a 10% incidence of similar emboli when using mechanical thrombolysis. The impact of pulmonary embolization is largely dependent on the amount and the nature of the embolic material. Most of the clot in an acutely thrombosed AVG is soft, fresh, semiliquid red clot. This clot dissolves rapidly with thrombolysis, and, when it embolizes, it appears to cause little problem. Some of the clot, however, is organized compacted white clot. This clot is typically found at the arterial anastomosis. Because it is well organized and firm, it is resistant to thrombolysis; when it embolizes, it is less likely to dissolve within the pulmonary capillary bed. Because of concerns about embolic potential, patients who are not able to tolerate pulmonary embolization (e.g., those with severe pulmonary hypertension) should not be considered candidates for percutaneous thrombolysis or thrombectomy. Similarly, patients with right-to-left intracardiac shunts would be considered at increased risk for stroke and should not undergo endovascular treatment of AVGs.[8]

Arterial embolization is a serious and fortunately less-common complication of endovascular therapy of AVGs. The event may occur as the wires and the catheters are passed through the graft or in the course of attempting to remove the compacted clot that invariably forms at the arterial anastomosis. Embolization into the arterial tree is significant because of the possibility of creating an ischemic lesion in the patient's hand. The incidence of these events is between 1.5% and 5%. Most are asymptomatic. Endovascular techniques such as catheter-directed thrombolysis, mechanical disruption, or retrieval with balloon catheters will succeed in treating most symptomatic lesions. Valji et al.[9] indicated that only one patient in a series of 272 cases required surgical thrombectomy.

Bleeding is a logically anticipated complication of thrombolytic therapy. Because the nature of the treatment is to dissolve clot, bleeding may ensue at any site where the vascular tree has been recently disrupted. Clinical practice guidelines have been drafted regarding the common circumstances that would impede thrombolysis. Reports of large series of thrombolysis for AVGs suggest that the incidence of major hemorrhagic complications (for which blood transfusion is required) is less than 1%. Experience and familiarity with thrombolytic agents, the duration of thrombolysis, the dose of agent used, and the use of adjunctive anticoagulants will all affect the probability of uncontrolled or prolonged bleeding.

Thrombectomy

Percutaneous thrombectomy includes the use of balloon catheters placed via percutaneous graft cannulas to dilate the graft and to push clot out of the graft into the venous circulation. In a report of 24 patients thus treated, Trerotola et al.[10] noted that the technique was successful in clearing clot in 94% of cases. The 24-hour success rate was 82%, but, at the end of 1 week, the clinical success rate had fallen to 59%. Of particular importance is the observation that no "symptomatic" pulmonary emboli were noted.

A more recent development in use of percutaneous thrombectomy is the addition of motor-driven mechanical clot disruption. The Cragg brush and the Trerotola fragmentation device are examples. The Cragg brush is a soft, low-speed brush that is introduced into the graft lumen via percutaneous puncture. Its mechanical action assists in the disruption of clot within the graft. It has been used effectively in conjunction with thrombolytic infusion. The addition of the soft brush results in a reduction of the dose of thrombolytic required. The complication rate associated with the use of the Cragg brush is not greater than for pulse-spray therapy alone.[11]

The Arrow-Trerotola Percutaneous Thrombolytic Device is a motor-driven fragmentation cage that is delivered on a 5F catheter (via a 6F sheath) into the graft lumen. The fragmentation cage self-expands as it rotates at 3000 to 4500 rpm. The mechanical disruption of the clot occurs as the fragmentation cage beats through the thrombus. It has the ability to dissolve fresh thrombus, as well as compacted white thrombus found at the arterial anastomosis.[12] In a randomized trial comparing the Trerotola cage with pulse-spray thrombolysis, results of the two techniques were comparable.[13] The immediate technical patency rates were equal (95%), the complication rates were equivalent (8% vs. 9%), and the 3-month patency rates were equivalent (39% vs. 40%). There was a minor difference in the procedure time (75 vs. 85 minutes).

Hydrodynamic thrombectomy is defined as disruption of thrombus using a pressurized stream of saline solution injected via a multilumen catheter. The secondary lumen is used as a means of egress of the injected fluid. The process creates Venturi-effect suction while the pressurized stream erodes the thrombus. The effect is to dissolve and to aspirate the thrombus simultaneously. Two such devices are currently in clinical use: the Hydrolyser (Cordis Endovascular Warren, NJ) and the AngioJet (Medrad, Warrensdale, PA). The principal differences between these two devices are the design of the catheter and how this affects the direction and the flow of the saline solution. The most recent modification of the Hydrolyser has added a third lumen to allow improved clot aspiration. Laboratory comparison of the catheters indicates that they both perform well and that both cause a moderate amount of hemolysis.[14-17]

The Hydrolyser catheter has been tested in a clinical multicenter study.[17] This demonstrated an initial success rate of 89% with early reocclusion in another 17%, yielding an early (1 week) success rate of 72%. The median duration of primary patency was 14 weeks. Complications occurred in 15%, including two arterial emboli, one pulmonary embolus, and one hematoma. The authors concluded that the effectiveness of the device is comparable with that of thrombolysis.

A similar device, the AngioJet, has been compared with surgical thrombectomy in a randomized trial.[18] A total of 153 patients were randomly assigned to the two treatment arms. Technical success was achieved in 73% of AngioJet and 78% of surgical cases. Patency at 3 months was 15% with AngioJet and 26% with surgery. The complication rates were identical, although the surgical complications were more serious. In all, the authors found both techniques comparable, although the 78% initial success rate is lower than expected for a surgical group.[18]

The mechanical methods of clearing grafts have several advantages that make them attractive alternatives to pharmacologic thrombolysis. Because they mechanically disrupt and liquefy the clot, they may reduce the potential for significant hemorrhagic or embolic events. Removal of the clot may reduce the incidence of pyrogenic reactions. Finally, these are generally rapid and effective methods, thus making them convenient and accessible. The speed of these devices in clearing clot is a significant advantage. The mechanical devices clear the clot in a graft within minutes.[8]

Goal 2: Endovascular Assessment of Cause of Clotting

If the initial goal of endovascular therapy is the removal of clot, the second goal is assessing the cause of the clot's formation. The most common mechanical cause of graft clotting is stenosis at the venous anastomosis of a dialysis graft. Thus it is imperative that the venous anastomosis be carefully examined with contrast agent injection and biplanar views once the clot has been removed. The second most common lesion is stenosis of the arterial anastomosis, followed by a lesion within the graft.

Other areas of concern are the runoff veins in the arm and in the chest. Subclavian or innominate vein stenosis is particularly common in the dialysis population. Use of temporary percutaneous subclavian catheters for urgent and intermittent hemodialysis results in the development of scar tissue within the subclavian and the innominate veins. This scar tissue, along with the increased flow generated by the AVG, results in the development of dense fibrointimal hyperplasia within the vein. Eventually, this hyperplastic tissue occludes the runoff veins and results in decreased flow in the graft and ultimately graft thrombosis.

Stenosis of the arterial inflow vessels is relatively uncommon but may be suspected on the basis of a weak arterial pulse in the limb. If this concern arises, noninvasive testing may suggest the presence of stenosis. If the latter is suspected during angiographic examination of a dialysis graft, retrograde arteriography may help establish the condition of the inflow vessels. For optimal viewing of the subclavian artery origin, however, femoral puncture and aortography are best. An additional benefit is that the femoral approach offers ready access for angioplasty and stenting of the subclavian artery if these are necessary. Sites of stenotic lesions in failed arteriovenous grafts are listed in Table 60-1.

If imaging of the graft reveals the absence of a mechanical cause of thrombosis, then the two most likely causes of graft thrombosis are either coagulation abnormality or hypotensive episode. In such cases, after thrombolysis the patient should be evaluated and managed medically. Anticoagulation with warfarin and correction of cardiac arrhythmias are the mainstay of medical management. Finally, if imaging of the graft reveals obstruction that cannot be repaired or stenosis that cannot be traversed with guidewires, the patient should be considered for a new access surgery.

TABLE 60-1 Sites of Stenotic Lesions in Failed Grafts

	Valji et al.[9]	Glanz et al.[3]	Kanterman et al.[36]
Patients (N)	272	63	215
Venous anastomosis (%)	79	59	58
Runoff vein (%)	20	10	35
Arterial anastomosis (%)	10	1	4
Intragraft lumen (%)	6	9	2
Arterial inflow (%)	3	0	0
Graft pseudoaneurysms (%)	1	23	0
No source identified (%)	3	6	11

Goal 3: Treatment of Stenosis

Endovascular therapy offers several methods (e.g., balloon angioplasty, intraluminal stenting, and atherectomy) of treating stenosis within the AVG and its related arteries and veins. It is important to be aware of the type graft used as this will present limits to the balloons that may be employed and the degree to which the graft may be angioplastied. Standard grafts include "straight" 6-mm polytetrafluoroethylene (PTFE) grafts and "step" 4- to 6-mm or 4- to 7-mm PTFE grafts. In the step graft, the graft is constructed so that one end has a smaller diameter (4 mm) and the other end is larger (6 or 7 mm). Usually, the smaller-diameter segment is anastomosed to the inflow artery, and the larger end is joined to the outflow vein. Thus it would be reasonable to use a 6- or 7-mm balloon in the venous limb of such a graft but not in the arterial limb (Figure 60-2).

Another consideration is the technique of graft construction. Different manufacturers employ differing techniques of graft construction. The net effect is that some grafts are incapable of stretching, and others will expand radially under pressure from an intraluminal balloon. Gore-Tex grafts (W. L. Gore & Associates, Flagstaff, AZ) are sheathed by a circular fiber in an outer layer, which makes them very difficult to stretch beyond their manufactured diameter. The IMPRA company's PTFE grafts (Bard/Impra, Temple, AZ) will stretch radially when a balloon is inflated within the graft. This has several consequences: A stricture involving the anastomosis of an IMPRA graft can be dilated more than a similar stricture involving a Gore-Tex graft. At the same time, the hypothetical risk of disruption of the graft, the anastomosis, or the attached vessel may be increased with the more expansible graft.

More recently, stents have been used as adjuncts to angioplasty. The rationale for the use of stents is to improve results in the face of dissection of the vessels and the lesions or to overcome the elastic recoil of dense fibrous lesions. When considering the use of stents in an AVG it is important to consider the possible future surgical revisions. Stenting may limit the ability to surgically revise a graft anastomosis. The presence of a stent across a graft anastomosis frequently results in loss of the site for further surgical repair. The metallic stent becomes imbedded in the vessel wall and prohibits surgical revision. Removal of the stent will damage the vessel to the point of destroying it. For this reason a stent placed across an anastomosis will result in abandonment of the site. When choosing to place a stent across an anastomosis of an AVG it should be done with certain knowledge that the site will be abandoned if the stented graft fails.

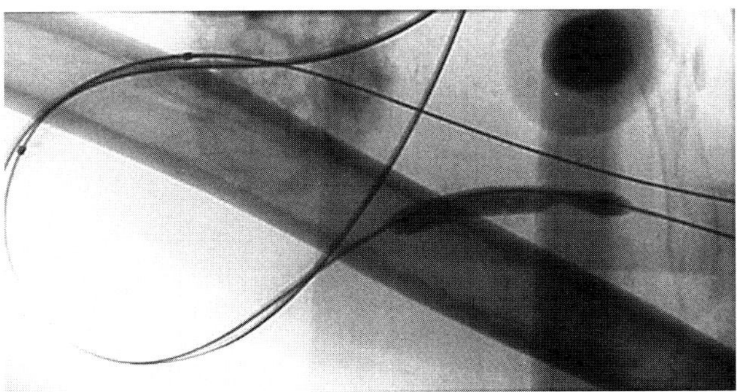

FIGURE 60-2 Balloon angioplasty of venous anastomosis.

Atherectomy, the mechanical removal of lesions within the graft or anastomosis by a mechanical device, is enjoying renewed interest. Several atherectomy devices have been developed and are in use for coronary and peripheral applications. Of these, the Rotablator and the Simpson (FoxHollow Technologies, Redwood City, CA) atherectomy devices have been most popular. All atherectomy devices remove small particles of the lesion, reducing its size and profile and thus improving flow through the graft. The devices are moderately effective, especially with atherosclerotic plaque. They remove some of the fibrointimal lesions but not as effectively. Because of the risk of disrupting a suture line they are not used across anastomosis. Accordingly they are best suited to eccentric lesions with high-profile intrusion into the lumen of the vessel or the graft.

CLINICAL OUTCOMES: ENDOVASCULAR DIALYSIS INTERVENTIONS

Surgery Versus Angioplasty and Stenting

The traditional surgical approach to graft thrombosis is balloon thrombectomy to clear the graft, patch angioplasty to repair stenosis, and bypass to overcome an occluded segment of vessel. Traditional surgical procedures are more painful and require anesthesia. The administration of anesthetics introduces yet another level of complications and concerns to the care of these ill patients. Finally, the availability of operating rooms and the need for preoperative fasting reduce the flexibility and the accessibility of surgical care when compared with endovascular care. Prospective randomized trials of these two treatments have demonstrated comparable results.

Quinn et al.[19] reported on a series of 87 patients who were randomly assigned to undergo percutaneous transluminal angioplasty (PTA) alone or primary stenting. They found no difference in the rate of success, primary patency, or secondary patency at 2, 6, and 12 months. At 12 months, the primary patency rate was 10% for PTA versus 11% for stenting, and the secondary patency rates were 71% and 64%, respectively. In a similar study, Hoffer et al.[20] reported the results of PTA and PTA with stenting in 37 grafts. They were initially successful in all patients (100% success rate for both groups). The primary and the secondary patency for both groups was essentially the same. The addition of stenting increased the cost of the procedure by 90%. They concluded that there was no advantage to primary use of stenting in stenosis that could be adequately dilated by means of angioplasty.

In a comparison of angioplasty and stenting with surgical thrombectomy and revision, Polak et al.[21] noted that surgical thrombectomy alone was the least successful intervention. They reported a series of 96 interventions in a population of 18 patients who presented with recurrent thrombosis of their dialysis grafts. Angioplasty and stenting were equivalent to surgical thrombectomy and revision in terms of durability of repair. They noted the relative risks of repeated occlusion after thrombolysis/angioplasty and thrombectomy/surgical revision. They thus concluded that thrombolysis with angioplasty was equivalent to thrombectomy with surgical revision.[21]

Angioplasty of Central Venous Stenosis

When the stenotic lesion is in the central veins (subclavian or innominate), angioplasty and stenting may be used in an attempt to prolong subclavian vein patency and graft function. The results of these attempts are less than encouraging and have not been tested in a prospective randomized trial. Lumsden et al.[22] have reported that the incidence of unsuspected central venous stenosis in patients with functioning grafts is 29%. Furthermore, the use of angioplasty and stenting results in a 1-year patency rate of only 17%. They conclude that, although these results are suboptimal, there are really no better alternatives available.

More recently Bakken et al.[23] at the University of Rochester have reported a series comparing results of angioplasty versus primary stenting for central venous stenosis in patients receiving dialysis. They followed 73 patients over a period of 8 years and noted that the primary patency, assisted primary patency, and ipsilateral dialysis access survival were equivalent between the two groups. They concluded that primary stenting does not improve access patency rates and does not increase access site survival when compared with angioplasty alone.[23]

Prospective Randomized Trials of Surgery Versus Endovascular Management

To date, there have been at least five prospective randomized trials comparing surgery with endovascular treatment of failing or thrombosed AVGs. The results have been remarkably consistent. The initial success rate in clearing the graft is 80% to 95% for the surgical approach versus 70% to 88% for the endovascular approach. The most common causes of early failure or inability to reestablish graft function are a lesion that cannot be traversed with guidewires, extensive venous occlusions, and degeneration of the grafts.

In the grafts that are amenable to repair, long-term patency is poor. The primary patency rate for the surgical approach at 12 months is 23% to 40%, versus 9% to 25% for the endovascular approach. Statistically, these are not significantly different. When long-term success is expressed as mean patency over a period of time, the result for surgery is 3.1 to 3.3 months; the mean duration of patency for endovascular treatment is 2.7 to 4.6 months.[18,24-28] Table 60-2 lists prospective randomized trials comparing surgical and endovascular therapy.

The cost of endovascular treatment has been compared with the cost of surgical treatment by several authors, with a wide variety of findings. Perhaps the most striking revelation is the cost of treating graft failure. Comparison of these studies is difficult because of dramatic changes in reimbursement for medical care

TABLE 60-2 Prospective Randomized Trials Comparing Surgical and Endovascular Therapy

			Initial success (%)		Long-term success	
Author	**Year**	**No.**	**Surgery**	**Endovascular therapy**	**Surgery**	**Endovascular therapy**
Dougherty et al.[24]	1999	80	93	72	23%	18% (12 mo)
Vesely et al.[18]	1999	153	78	73	26%	15% (3 mo)
Marston et al.[25]	1997	115	83	72	25%	9% (12 mo)
Vesely et al.[26]	1996	20	80	70	3.1 (mean, mo)	2.7 (mean, mo)
Schwartz et al.[27]	1995	61	87	88	3.3 (mean, mo)	4.6 (mean, mo)
Brooks et al.[28]	1987	43	95	79	40%	25% (12 mo)

NOTE: No significant differences were noted among groups.

in the short period of time during which the data became available. Thus what Summers et al. reported in 1993 bears little resemblance to the figures reported by Dougherty et al. in 1999.[24-26,29] Table 60-3 outlines studies comparing the cost of surgical versus endovascular management.

The absence of a standard for reporting has allowed a number of minor discrepancies to be incorporated into the literature in such a manner as to make comparison more difficult. Several aspects can vary: the difference between charges and collections, the inclusion or the exclusion of professional fees, and the accounting for unusual supplies and equipment. Finally, the methods used have a significant impact: an intention-to-treat analysis, in which failure of treatment in one arm leads to intervention in the other, results in a vastly different analysis from one that limits cost data collection to the moment of discharge. There is no agreement about how far to follow patients or how to account for the cost over the lifetime of the graft or the patient. There are no studies that count the cumulative cost of repeated failed interventions and compare this with the cost of new grafts. These same issues belie the decisions faced by clinicians in deciding on care for these patients. Despite this, many investigators note a similarity in the cost of both endovascular and surgical care. Thus ancillary considerations become very important in determining the choice of treatment: convenience, comfort, cosmesis, and access. Consumer issues become deciding elements in choice of care.

Endovascular care offers the advantages associated with less-invasive procedures: the incisions are smaller, and there is less pain during and after the procedure. There is less disability during recovery, which in turn means that patients are able to return to work sooner and that graft thrombosis is less of a disruption to their lives. Therefore patient acceptance of endovascular therapy is strongly favorable.

There are also technical advantages of endovascular therapy over conventional surgery. The use of contrast angiography to guide therapy results in superior imaging of the stenotic lesions and the graft lumen. Thus the endovascular approach offers better insight into the nature and the causes of graft failure. Traditional surgery may be supplemented with intraoperative angiography, but this is frequently not the case because most operating rooms are not configured as endovascular suites, and thus the time and the effort required to use these techniques is discouraging. For similar reasons, balloon angioplasty and stenting are not as frequently used in the traditional surgical approach. On the other hand, endovascular treatment, although effective, is limited in what can be offered. Should the lesion not be crossed by the guidewire, or should the graft deteriorate to the point where replacement is the best alternative, surgical care is needed. Ultimately, both open traditional surgery and endovascular approaches are complementary in the optimal management of dialysis graft failure.

Prophylactic Angioplasty

In an effort to improve the long-term patency of dialysis grafts, prophylactic angioplasty based on ultrasonic graft surveillance has been attempted. In prospective randomized trials, only those grafts with greater than 50% stenosis that had never undergone revision, thrombolysis, or angioplasty derived benefit from preemptive intervention (angioplasty).[30] This is in dramatic distinction to the unselected larger group of patients who underwent prophylactic angioplasty whenever stenosis greater than 50% was identified. When compared with a control group who were observed until the point of thrombosis, the group undergoing prophylactic angioplasty had identical patency at 6 months (69% for PTA vs. 70% in controls) and at 12 months (51% for PTA vs. 47% for controls).[31]

These results are echoed in a more recent publication by Shahin et al.[32] They compared the use of access monitoring and prophylactic intervention (prophylactic care) with intervention on the basis of clinical evidence of access failure (standard care) in a cohort of 22 patients. They noted that there was a sevenfold increase in the number of angioplasty procedures in the prophylactic

TABLE 60-3 Studies Comparing Cost of Surgical Versus Endovascular Management

			Initial success (%)		Cost ($)	
Author	**Year**	**No.**	**Surgery**	**Endovascular therapy**	**Surgery**	**Endovascular therapy**
Dougherty et al.[24]	1999	80	93	72	1,512	2,945*
Marston et al.[25]	1997	115	83	72	8,472	8,006
Vesely et al.[26]	1996	20	80	70	5,580	6,062†
Summers et al.[29]	1993	43	85	76	10,000	14,900

*Calculations did not include professional fees.
†Calculations include professional fees.

group. At the same time they noted no improvement in the thrombosis rate or cumulative fistula patency. On the basis of this they concluded that ultrasound monitoring and prophylactic angioplasty resulted in shorter primary patency but did not improve cumulative patency and did not reduce graft thrombosis rate.[32]

FUTURE DIRECTIONS

The future of endovascular therapy for dialysis access grafts rests with the development of adjunctive means of impeding fibrointimal hyperplasia. To this effect, investigators have used radiation therapy, photodynamic therapy, and gene therapy. Research in gene therapy is directed at identifying specific genes that are targeted for suppression or amplification. Current research focuses on the use of adenoviral vectors for delivery of a wide spectrum of genes to the endothelial cells that line the anastomotic sites. Genes such as those for nitric oxide, epidermal growth factor receptor, and thrombin receptor are currently being tested for potential application. In addition, more exotic means of modulating hyperplasia with photodynamic therapy and laser light are being researched.

External-beam radiation has been studied in a prospective randomized trial.[33] Cohen et al.[35] compared angioplasty with stenting and angioplasty with stenting plus external beam radiation at a dose of 7 Gy. They failed to find a significant difference in patency of the grafts between the groups.

ANGIOPLASTY AND COVERED STENT

Although the use of angioplasty alone for management of dialysis access stenosis has had moderate benefit, this are far form ideal. The use of stents or covered stents has been proposed as a means of improving the results of angioplasty. Recent publications have reported prospective randomized trials comparing angioplasty alone with angioplasty plus stent and angioplasty plus covered stent in management of AV access stenosis.

Shemesh et al.[33] reported use of covered stents as an adjunct to angioplasty when used in native arteriovenous fistulas. In a cohort of 25 patients randomized between angioplasty with bare stent and angioplasty plus covered stent, they noted a significant reduction in restenosis at 3 months: 70% in the bare stent group versus 18% in covered stent group. They concluded that the use of covered stents significantly improved short-term restenosis rates and long-term patency compared with the use of bare stents. Further because of the dramatic results, they were ethically forced to stop further recruitment to their study.[33]

In a publication released in February 2010, Haskal et al.[34] reported a prospective randomized trial comparing angioplasty alone with angioplasty plus covered stent in management of failing dialysis access grafts. They randomized 190 patients between two treatment arms. At the end of 6 months they noted a significant difference in graft patency in favor of stent grafts (51 vs. 23%). Similarly, they noted a significant improvement in the freedom from subsequent interventions and decrcase in incidence of severe restenosis (>50%). They conclude that use of stent grafts results in improved long-term patency and reduce need for subsequent interventions compared to balloon angioplasty alone.[34]

Taken together these two reports offer evidence of a significant benefit to be accrued by use of covered stents in management of dialysis access stenosis. Although further confirmation of these reports is expected, the use of covered stents in management of fistula and graft stenosis is anticipated to become a standard feature of the endovascular care of dialysis patients with graft thrombosis.

SUMMARY

Endovascular therapy is superior to traditional surgical approaches for those graft failures caused by hypercoagulable thrombosis and hypotensive episodes. The role of endovascular care in recurrent stenosis remains challenging: early success is still attended by relatively poor long-term results. Future innovations such as radiation treatment or photodynamic therapy may yield further improvements.[36]

Endovascular therapy remains an exciting and rapidly evolving method of treating hemodialysis graft failure. As the range of techniques and capabilities continues to expand, a major difficulty lies in choosing the techniques to apply and identifying the limits of endovascular care. The results of many endovascular interventions are comparable with those obtained with standard surgical techniques. A singular difference is patient acceptance of these procedures, which makes endovascular management a standard for patient care. It is less painful, more convenient, less invasive, and less disruptive.

References

1. Van Stone JC, Jones M, Van Stone J: Detection of hemodialysis access outlet stenosis by measuring outlet resistance, *Am J Kidney Dis* 23:562–568, 1994.
2. Lindsay RM, Rothera C, Blake PG: A comparison of methods for the measurement of hemodialysis access recirculation, *ASAIO J* 44:191–193, 1998.

3. Glanz S, Bashist B, Gordon AH, Adamson R: Angiography of upper extremity access fistulas for dialysis, *Radiology* 143:45–52, 1982.
4. O'Shea SI, Lawson JH, Reddan D, et al: Hypercoagulable states and antithrombotic strategies in recurrent vascular access site thrombosis, *J Vasc Surg* 38(3):541–548, 2003.
5. Goodwin SC, Arora LC, Razavi MK, et al: Dialysis access graft thrombolysis: randomized study of pulse-spray versus continuous urokinase infusion, *Cardiovasc Intervent Radiol* 21:135–137, 1998.
6. Martin-Paredero V, Dixon SM, Baker JD, et al: Risk of renal failure after major angiography, *Arch Surg* 118:1417–1420, 1983.
7. Trerotola SO, Johnson MS, Shah H, et al: Incidence and management of arterial emboli from hemodialysis graft surgical thrombectomy, *J Vasc Interv Radiol* 8:557–562, 1997.
8. Trerotola SO: Pulse-spray thrombolysis of hemodialysis grafts: not the final word, *AJR Am J Roentgenol* 164:1501–1503, 1995.
9. Valji K, Bookstein JJ, Roberts AC, et al: Pulse-spray pharmacomechanical thrombolysis of thrombosed hemodialysis access grafts: long-term experience and comparison of original and current techniques, *AJR Am J Roentgenol* 164:1495–1500, 1995.
10. Trerotola SO, Lund GB, Scheel PJ Jr, et al: Thrombosed dialysis access grafts: percutaneous mechanical declotting without urokinase, *Radiology* 191:721–726, 1994.
11. Dolmatch BL, Casteneda F, McNamara TO, et al: Synthetic dialysis shunts: thrombolysis with the Cragg thrombolytic brush catheter, *Radiology* 213:180–184, 1999.
12. Trerotola SO, Johnson MS, Schauwecker DS, et al: Pulmonary emboli from pulse-spray and mechanical thrombolysis: evaluation with an animal dialysis-graft model, *Radiology* 200:169–176, 1996.
13. Trerotola SO, Vesely TM, Lund GB, et al: Treatment of thrombosed hemodialysis access grafts: Arrow-Trerotola Percutaneous Thrombolytic Device versus pulse-spray thrombolysis. Arrow-Trerotola Percutaneous Thrombolytic Device Clinical Trial, *Radiology* 206:403–414, 1998.
14. Muller-Hulsbeck S, Bathe M, Grimm J, Heller M: Enhancement of in vitro effectiveness for hydrodynamic thrombectomy devices. Simultaneous high-pressure rt-PA application, *Invest Radiol* 34:536–542, 1999.
15. Muller-Hulsbeck S, Schwarzenberg H, Bathe M, et al: In vitro effectiveness study for hydrodynamic thrombectomy devices of the second generation, *Invest Radiol* 34:477–484, 1999.
16. Muller-Hulsbeck S, Bangard C, Schwarzenberg H, et al: In vitro effectiveness study of three hydrodynamic thrombectomy devices, *Radiology* 211:433–439, 1999.
17. Overbosch EH, Pattynama PM, Aarts HJ, et al: Occluded hemodialysis shunts: Dutch multicenter experience with the Hydrolyser catheter, *Radiology* 201:485–488, 1996.
18. Vesely TM, Williams D, Weiss M, et al: Comparison of the AngioJet Rheolytic catheter to surgical thrombectomy for the treatment of thrombosed hemodialysis grafts. Peripheral AngioJet Clinical Trial, *J Vasc Interv Radiol* 10:1195–1205, 1999.
19. Quinn SF, Schuman ES, Demlow TA, et al: Percutaneous transluminal angioplasty versus endovascular stent placement in the treatment of venous stenoses in patients undergoing hemodialysis: intermediate results, *J Vasc Interv Radiol* 6:851–855, 1995.
20. Hoffer EK, Sultan S, Herskowitz MM, et al: Prospective randomized trial of a metallic intravascular stent in hemodialysis graft maintenance, *J Vasc Interv Radiol* 8:965–973, 1997.
21. Polak JF, Berger MF, Pagan-Marin H, et al: Comparative efficacy of pulse-spray thrombolysis and angioplasty versus surgical salvage procedures for treatment of recurrent occlusion of PTFE dialysis access grafts, *Cardiovasc Intervent Radiol* 21(4):314–318, 1998.
22. Lumsden AB, MacDonald MJ, Isiklar H, et al: Central venous stenosis in the hemodialysis patient: incidence and efficacy of endovascular treatment, *Cardiovasc Surg* 5:504–509, 1997.
23. Bakken AM, Protack CD, Saad WE, et al: Long-term outcomes of primary angioplasty and primary stenting of central venous stenosis in hemodialysis patients, *J Vasc Surg* 45(4):776–783, 2007.
24. Dougherty MJ, Calligaro KD, Schindler N, et al: Endovascular versus surgical treatment for thrombosed hemodialysis grafts: a prospective, randomized study, *J Vasc Surg* 30:1016–1023, 1999.
25. Marston WA, Criado E, Jaques PF, et al: Prospective randomized comparison of surgical versus endovascular management of thrombosed dialysis access grafts, *J Vasc Surg* 26:373–381, 1997.
26. Vesely TM, Idso MC, Audrain J, et al: Thrombolysis versus surgical thrombectomy for the treatment of dialysis graft thrombosis: pilot study comparing costs, *J Vasc Interv Radiol* 7:507–512, 1996.
27. Schwartz CI, McBrayer CV, Sloan JH, et al: Thrombosed dialysis grafts: comparison of treatment with transluminal angioplasty and surgical revision, *Radiology* 194:337–341, 1995.
28. Brooks JL, Sigley RD, May KJ, Mack RM: Transluminal angioplasty versus surgical repair for stenosis of hemodialysis grafts, *Am J Surg* 153:530–531, 1987.
29. Summers S, Drazan KK, Gomes A, Freishclag J: Urokinase therapy for thrombosed hemodialysis access grafts, *Surg Gynecol Obstet* 176:534–538, 1993.
30. Martin LG, MacDonald MJ, Kikeri D, et al: Prophylactic angioplasty reduces thrombosis in virgin ePTFE arteriovenous dialysis grafts with greater than 50% stenosis: subset analysis of a prospectively randomized study, *J Vasc Interv Radiol* 10:389–396, 1999.
31. Lumsden AB, MacDonald MJ, Kikeri D, et al: Prophylactic balloon angioplasty fails to prolong the patency of expanded polytetrafluoroethylene arteriovenous grafts: results of a prospective randomized study, *J Vasc Surg* 26:382–392, 1997.
32. Shahin H, Reddy G, Sharafuddin M, et al: Monthly access flow monitoring with increased prophylactic angioplasty did not improve fistula patency, *Kidney Int* 68(5):2352–61.
33. Shemesh D, Goldin I, Zaghal I, et al: Angioplasty with stent graft versus bare stent for recurrent cephalic arch stenosis in autogenous arteriovenous access for hemodialysis: a prospective randomized clinical trial, *J Vasc Surg* 48:1524–1531, 2008.
34. Haskal ZJ, Trerotola S, Dolmatch B, et al: Stent graft versus balloon angioplasty for failing dialysis-access grafts, *N Engl J Med* 362:494–503, 2010.
35. Cohen GS, Freeman H, Ringold MA, et al: External beam irradiation as an adjunctive treatment in failing dialysis shunts, *J Vasc Interv Radiol* 11:321–326, 2000.
36. Kanterman RY, Vesely TM, Pilgram TK, et al: Dialysis access grafts: anatomic location of venous stenosis and results of angioplasty, *Radiology* 195:135–139, 1995.

CHAPTER

61

Central Venous Catheter Malfunction

Hugh A. Gelabert

Central venous catheters are used for the administration of medications, the sampling of blood, the provision of nutrition, and the removal and return of blood for plasmapheresis and hemodialysis. These are frequently critical and vital to the survival of the patient. The proper function of central catheters is important in providing for the patient's health.

Given the importance of central venous catheters in current care, there has been a dramatic proliferation of catheters. The names and device specifications vary significantly. For this reason it is difficult to address each specific catheter type. Fortunately a generic approach will allow understanding of the evaluation and correction of catheter malfunction.

MODALITIES OF FAILURE

Central catheter malfunction may present in a wide range of failure modalities. These include difficulty withdrawing blood, difficulty infusing, intermittent function, and insufficient flow volume. Box 61-1 presents a more complete listing of catheter failure modalities. The most common form of central venous catheter malfunction is inability to withdraw blood. Although this is an important function of the catheter, frequently blood drawing may be done peripherally, and if the catheter remains patent for infusion then it may still be of use. The second most common problem with central venous catheter function is difficulty infusing. This is a fundamental catheter function, and the inability to infuse will render a catheter useless and result in its removal. If a catheter is not able to infuse it becomes a liability to patient care.

Recirculation is a problem unique to dialysis and pheresis catheters. These catheters are intended to both withdraw and reinfuse blood. In this process some of the reinfused blood may be reaspirated and withdrawn before it has the opportunity to circulate through the patient's body. This phenomenon is termed recirculation. A small fraction of recirculation is common and in part determines the efficiency of a dialysis or pheresis technique. A high recirculation quotient is a problem that may negate the utility of these catheters.[1]

CAUSES OF CATHETER MALFUNCTION

The two fundamental reasons account for most catheter failure: (1) malpositioning of the catheter tip and (2) thrombosis associated with the catheter restricting the catheter's function. The position of the catheter tip is recognized to bear directly on catheter function and longevity. Correctly positioned catheters have a lower incidence of complications such as catheter obstruction, central venous stenosis, and venous thrombosis.[2-4] Properly positioning a catheter tip may be difficult because the position of the catheter is dynamic—the catheter moves within the patient as the patient moves. The position of the catheter at the time of implantation will be different from that when the patient is upright. An average migration of 3 cm is common. Large patients, obese patients, and patients with large chest wall mass or pendulous breasts will all magnify the change in catheter position with upright posture. The access point for the catheter (jugular versus subclavian vein) will impact this phenomenon.

Catheter obstruction is most often due to thrombus. Other causes may include kinking or compression. Most often, kinking results from technical error in tunneling the catheter on the chest wall. Frequently the catheter must make a sharp bend to enter the jugular or subclavian veins. If the angle is acute then the catheter may kink, and the result is a catheter obstruction. Extrinsic compression may occur for several reasons. The sutures required to hold the catheter in place may have been tightly applied to the catheter. The catheter may pass through a restricted anatomic location such as the costoclavicular space. The thrombus impeding the catheter lumen has several origins: it may result

BOX 61-1

MODALITIES OF FAILURE OF CENTRAL VENOUS CATHETERS

Amenable to Endovascular Treatment

- Failure to withdraw blood
- Failure to allow infusion
- Insufficient catheter flow volume
- Intermittent function (ball valve effect)
- Thrombosis of catheter
- Thrombosis of central venous structures
- Fracture of catheter
- Embolization of catheter fragments
- Perforation of vascular structures
- Withdrawal of catheter (pulled out)

Not Amenable to Endovascular Treatment

- Catheter infection
- Erosion through skin (reservoir port)
- Kinking in subcutaneous tunnel
- Fragmentation of catheter

BOX 61-2

CAUSES OF CENTRAL VENOUS CATHETER MALFUNCTION

- Malposition
- Catheter thrombosis
- Central venous thrombosis
- Central venous stenosis

from inadequate maintenance (poor flushing after use); it may arise around the catheter tip, enfolding the tip and obstructing it (such as a fibrin sheath or a thrombus over the catheter tip); or it may be part of a larger problem (e.g., central venous thrombosis). Central vein thrombosis may itself be the result of critical central venous stenosis, which in turn may be the consequence of incorrect catheter positioning.

These problems may be addressed with a variety of endovascular techniques, including catheter repositioning, stripping, or lysis; thrombolysis of central veins; and angioplasty of central venous strictures. Other causes of catheter malfunction, such as reservoir erosion or infection, do not lend themselves to endovascular treatment and are not included in this discussion (Box 61-2).

CATHETER POSITION

The location of the catheter tip is important in allowing correct catheter function. A catheter that is malpositioned will be prone to complications such as deep vein thrombosis and occlusive malfunction. The ideal location for a catheter tip is in the larger central veins: the superior vena cava (SVC), the inferior vena cava, the vena cava–atrial junction, or slightly inside the right atrium.[4] When thus positioned, the catheter tip is surrounded by vessels that are large enough to carry the volume of blood needed for the catheter to function optimally.

A malpositioned catheter will present as difficulty in aspirating blood. The reason for this is that the catheter tip comes to rest against the wall of the vein. When an attempt is made to aspirate the catheter, the vacuum forces the vein wall into the catheter opening, which blocks the further flow of blood. In effect, the vein wall acts as a ball valve to the catheter's tip.[3]

In smaller veins, such as the iliac or the subclavian or innominate vessels, a smaller volume of blood is carried as a result of the reduced diameter. Catheter function may be impaired because of close apposition of the catheter to the vein wall. The smaller veins allow less space for thrombus to develop before it engulfs and occludes the catheter. Deep vein thrombosis becomes much more common.

In the smaller vessels, infusion of potentially caustic material, such as total parenteral nutrition or chemotherapeutic agents, results in damage to the vein wall. This may result in the development of stricture or central venous thrombosis.[2]

When a catheter is located in a vein that is slowly developing stricture, the patient may remain without symptoms even after the vein has occluded. Should the process occur at an accelerated pace, the patient may then have symptoms. The most common symptoms of subclavian vein occlusion include arm swelling, aching, congestion, and blue discoloration. Jugular vein occlusion occasionally gives rise to fullness and venous prominence on the affected side. If the jugular occlusion is accompanied by more extensive occlusion of the central venous system, SVC syndrome may result, in which the patient has severe facial swelling, congestion, cyanosis, and dyspnea. Eastridge and Lefor[5] related catheter position to the probability of central venous thrombosis. They found that the probability of a catheter-related thrombosis occurring with a malpositioned catheter may be as much as 10 to 13 times more than the expected rate.

Ideal Catheter Position

The ideal catheter tip location is well into the SVC at the atrial-cava junction or slightly within the right atrium. Catheters deep within the right atrium may present problems with arrhythmias. Another problem with catheters far within the right atrium is that they may cross the tricuspid valve and result in valvular damage. For these reasons a measured approach to positioning the catheters is necessary. On the other hand, catheters that are barely into the SVC will invariably withdraw to more peripheral veins and in that location are at increased risk of complications. Position within the innominate, jugular, or subclavian veins is inadequate for these reasons.[2-4]

Assessment of Catheter Malfunction

The assessment of catheter malfunction should follow a routine approach: first an anteroposterior chest radiograph should be obtained. This should be inspected to determine the location of the catheter tip. It should be compared with the initial postplacement chest radiograph to assess migration of the catheter tip. By themselves these steps may identify the cause of catheter malfunction. If the catheter tip is evidently kinked, is abutting a vessel wall, or has redirected away from the central venous system then the diagnosis is established.

Ideally, the chest x-ray film should clearly show the catheter oriented along the vertical axis, with the tip well within the vena cava or the atrial–vena caval junction. The chest x-ray film should be compared, if possible, with the x-ray film obtained at the time of implantation. This comparison will help determine the mechanism by which the catheter came to be malpositioned: either it was malpositioned at the time of placement, or it migrated. The distinction is important and has bearing on the subsequent remedial actions. Malpositioning at the time of implantation may happen for two reasons: (1) an insufficient length of catheter was placed within the venous system, or (2) sufficient length was placed, but the catheter tip ended in the wrong place. If there is sufficient length, correction of the problem requires simply moving the catheter tip into the correct position. If there is not sufficient length of catheter, then either the catheter is advanced or it will not be able to be placed properly. Catheter tip migration may occur with smaller, more flexible catheters. Among the mechanisms that may account for catheter migration are the mechanical properties of the catheter itself. A more flexible catheter such as small-diameter (6F) silicone elastomer (Silastic) catheters are much more flexible than larger catheters. If such a catheter is forcefully flushed with saline solution or heparin, the jet effect may whip the catheter tip out of position.

Migration of Central Venous Catheters

Central venous catheters may be placed correctly but later migrate out of position. This is more common when the catheter length is marginally adequate and the catheter is of a smaller diameter. If the catheter length is only marginally adequate, the catheter tip is subject to migration by virtue of changes in the relative anatomy of the central venous structures and the chest wall that occur with patient movement. As the patient moves from the recumbent to the upright position, the catheter in effect migrates peripherally. The tip of the catheter is then farther away from the heart when the patient is upright than when the patient is supine. This occurs because the weight of the mediastinal structures and of the chest wall draws both chest and mediastinum toward the feet. The catheter, which straddles the clavicle or the first rib and is tethered to the chest wall by its cuff and sutures, is pulled along with the chest wall. The tip moves toward the thoracic inlet while the mediastinum moves away, toward the feet. This shifting of the catheter is accentuated in larger people, those with a long torso, and those with large chest walls. Women with pendulous breasts are also at risk. As the catheter tip pulls back, it may become lodged in the opening of the subclavian vein and become trapped there. In a report of 50 patients undergoing catheter placement, Kowalski et al.[6] noted that virtually all catheters demonstrate some degree of migration. Most catheters (49/50) migrated peripherally (they pulled out of the patient); very few (1/50) migrated centrally (they moved into the patient). The average migration distance was 3.2 cm. They advise placing the catheters about 3 to 4 cm more centrally than the desired final position.[6]

In the event of a catheter appearing to be in a correct position yet not working properly then a "catheter gram" should be obtained. This requires infusing radiopaque contrast under fluoroscopic imaging to determine the pattern of flow at the catheter tip. In those instances where the catheter tip is enveloped with a sheath of fibrin or thrombus the flow will be distorted and may appear to return in a backward direction along the catheter before entering the venous stream. In the case where a thrombus has formed over the catheter tip, then a globular mass is seen attached to the catheter tip.

Management

Repositioning of a misplaced catheter may be accomplished by means of endovascular technique with guidewires and snares. If the malposition is the result of catheter tip migration, the catheter may be salvaged with a repositioning procedure. A flexible Glidewire (Terumo Medical, Somerset, NJ) is passed through the catheter under fluoroscopic imaging. Occasionally, manipulation of the Glidewire will lead it into the vena cava. Further manipulation of the wire may then lead the catheter back to the correct position. If this is not successful then a second wire of catheter is placed via the femoral vein and may be used to trap and pull the catheter tip. A pigtail catheter may be used to try to hook the wire exiting the tip of the malpositioned central line. Another technique replaced the pigtail catheter with a looped snare wire. The goal of this approach is to snare the catheter tip or snare a Glidewire passed through the malpositioned catheter. The snare is then used to pull the catheter tip into place.

If the malposition is the result of too short a catheter, then repositioning will not result in a durable solution. In these instances the most effective correction is to replace the catheter. In certain instances in which a tunneled cuffed catheter is found to be short of its ideal position, it may be advanced into a correct position by snaring the catheter tip and pulling it forward. This is done by approaching the catheter from a femoral puncture with a snare wire, capturing the catheter tip with the snare wire, and pulling the catheter forward into the central venous system. This technique depends on the catheter being mobile, the catheter length being sufficient, and the attached catheter cuff not being firmly held by scar tissue. Attempts at "pulling" a catheter forward will more likely succeed in the early postoperative period before the attached cuff has had time to develop a thick fibrous encasement. If the catheter is attached to a nonmobile element such as a subcutaneous port, then it is also unlikely that pulling the catheter tip into position will be successful.

CATHETER THROMBOSIS

Thrombosis of a catheter occurs when blood coagulates within the catheter itself. Thrombosis within the catheter occurs when blood is allowed to rest stagnant within the catheter lumen. This occurs most commonly when catheters are used for blood aspiration and are not completely cleared with flushing solutions. The normal capillary effect draws blood into the open end of the catheter. When the catheter is not well primed with heparin, this blood may thrombose and occlude the catheter.

A second mechanism of thrombotic occlusion of a catheter is entrapment and surrounding of the catheter tip by a thrombus. Most catheters stimulate the development of a fibrin sheath, which surrounds the catheter's intravascular length. On occasion, this fibrin sheath progresses to become a thrombus within the vein. If this thrombus grows to the point of surrounding the catheter tip, it will initially act as a ball valve and will prevent aspiration of blood from the catheter. Should the thrombus consolidate and adhere tightly to the catheter and the vein wall, it could encase the catheter and obstruct the infusion of medication. Accordingly, catheter thrombosis may present as the inability to draw blood from the catheter or, more commonly, as the inability to infuse through the catheter. Dialysis catheters that become entrapped in this manner demonstrate a decrease in their maximum flow rate. The reduction of the maximum flow to less than 200 mL/min is generally considered a sign of a failing catheter.[7]

Management

Thrombosis of a catheter is initially managed by flushing the catheter with normal saline solution in an attempt to dislodge any thrombus within the catheter lumen. Care should be taken in forcing fluids into the obstructed catheter as too much pressure may fracture the catheter. Should this fail, the second step is instillation of a thrombolytic agent such as urokinase or tissue plasminogen activator into the obstructed catheter. The thrombolytic agent is then allowed to dwell within the catheter for a period of time, and a subsequent attempt is made to flush the line. Administration of the lytic agent may be repeated two or three times.[8,9]

Should instillation of thrombolytic agents fail, the catheter may be reamed with a guidewire. A flexible but moderately rigid hydrophilic wire, such as the Glidewire, may be passed into the obstructed catheter to clear a passage mechanically through the thrombus. The principal risk of this procedure is inadvertent perforation of a central vein with the wire. To reduce this risk, it is prudent to pass the wire under fluoroscopy so that the position of the wire in the catheter may be observed at all times. Once the catheter has been cleared with the guidewire, thrombolytic agents may be used to clear residual fibrin that remains within the catheter.[8,9]

Catheter entrapment should be suspected if passage of a Glidewire does not result in free flow through the catheter. In this instance, the possibility of extrinsic entrapment of the catheter tip by a thrombus should be considered. Angiography should be performed with the injection of contrast dye to demonstrate the presence of the intravenous thrombus, thrombus around the catheter tip, or a fibrin sheath entrapping the distal catheter.

This situation may be managed in one of two ways: (1) treat the thrombus with infusion of lytic agents, or (2) attempt to mechanically dislodge the thrombus from the catheter tip. The decision is based on one's impression of the extent of the thrombus in the central veins. Thrombus obstructing a catheter may be treated with an infusion of thrombolytic agent through the catheter itself. The thrombolytic infusion is administered over a several-hour time period. The catheter is manually aspirated to test for resolution of the occlusion. Repeated venography should be performed if there are concerns regarding compete resolution of the thrombus. In a prospective report, Savader and associates[10] noted 100% immediate technical success with infusion of 2.5 mg of recombinant tissue plasminogen activator infused over a 3-hour period. The mean duration of catheter function after infusion was 41 days. They comment that these results were comparable with other published results of thrombolysis with urokinase, catheter exchange, and sheath stripping.[10]

Mechanical disruption of the fibrin sheath surrounding the catheter may be achieved in two ways: balloon disruption of the fibrin sheath and catheter striping. To disrupt the fibrin tract with a balloon, the catheter must be withdrawn over a wire; then a balloon is advanced over the wire and inflated within the fibrin sheath and thus disrupts the sheath. The catheter is then replaced over the wire.

Catheter stripping is accomplished by passage of a snare wire into the central venous system in proximity to the entrapped catheter tip. A second wire is passed through the lumen of the obstructed central catheter and into the central venous system. This second wire is captured by the snare wire (Figure 61-1). Both wires are then pulled back to remove the catheter tip from the vein wall. Once the catheter tip is free of the vein wall, the snare wire is relaxed, allowing the snare loop to open. The snare is advanced over the catheter tip and then slightly tightened. Ideally the snare wire will be close to the catheter but not tightly applied. The intention is to allow the snare wire to strip the fibrin off of the catheter.[7,11] At this point, a repeated contrast study should be performed to evaluate the result of the procedure. The overall efficacy of this technique is in the range of 80% to 90%.[11,12] Results of catheter stripping are summarized in Table 61-1.[7,11,13,14]

It should be noted that as a result of this procedure, there is invariably some amount of pulmonary embolization. Most patients will tolerate this well because the volume of thrombus is small. Some patients (e.g., those with pulmonary hypertension and those with right-to-left intracardiac shunts) should not be considered for catheter stripping. Patients with pulmonary hypertension may not have sufficient cardiac and pulmonary reserve to overcome the stress of the embolus. Patients with an intracardiac shunt are at risk for peripheral embolization and possible limb loss or stroke.[15]

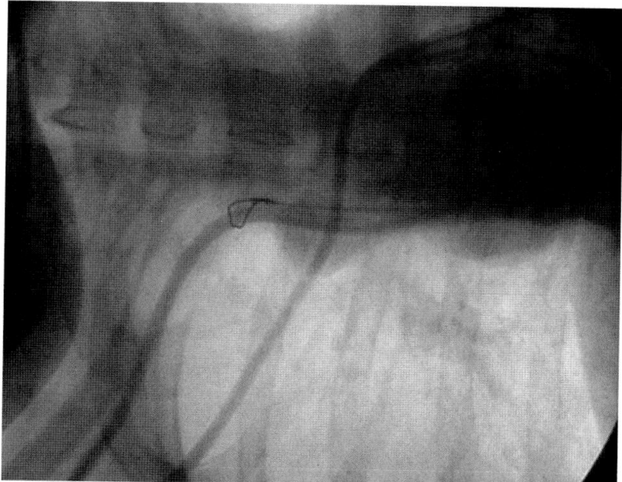

FIGURE 61-1 Catheter being stripped with snare.

In a comparison of balloon and stripping and lysis, Janne d'Othée et al[16] studied 66 patients who were treated with these techniques and found no significant difference in immediate success, complications, and durability of catheter function. The catheter patency at 6 months was between 28% and 35%. They concluded that, all techniques being similar, the choice of technique would be based on cost and preference of the patients and physicians.[16]

Central Vein Thrombosis

Thrombosis of a central vein usually occurs because of previous or current manipulation involving pacemaker wires or central venous catheters. The previous cannulation of the central veins results in inflammation, stricture, and thrombosis. This situation is properly referred to as secondary central vein thrombosis. The incidence of this phenomenon may be as high as 10% in patients with cancer.[5]

Spontaneous thrombosis of the central veins is a rare event, accounting for fewer than 15% of all cases of central venous thrombosis. The vast majority of cases of spontaneous central venous thrombosis (or Paget-Schroetter syndrome) are related to costoclavicular compression of the axillosubclavian vein as it crosses the thoracic outlet. Occasionally, Paget-Schroetter syndrome is due to a hypercoagulation disorder.[17]

Management

The differentiation between primary (spontaneous) and secondary venous thrombosis is based on the

TABLE 61-1 Results of Catheter Stripping

Author	Year	No.	Immediate success (%)	Median patency (days)
Brady et al.[12]	1999	131	95	89
Johnstone et al.[13]	1999	21	100	126
Rockall et al.[11]	1997	22	79	127
Haskal et al.[14]	1996	24	92	—
Crain et al.[7]	1996	40	98	84

patient history. Management of these two conditions is vastly different. Spontaneous thrombosis of the axillo-subclavian vein should be initially managed with anticoagulation and thrombolysis. This allows venography to determine the presence of compression at the costoclavicular margin. If the vein is compressed, rib resection and venolysis are needed to resolve the problem and to prevent recurrent thrombosis. If no compression is seen, the patient should be investigated for a hypercoagulation disorder and should be treated with anticoagulants.[18,19]

The management of secondary venous thrombosis is dependent on the degree of symptoms, the need for continued central venous access, and the estimated need for future central venous access. If the patient has severe symptoms and obtains no relief with heparin anticoagulation and arm elevation, lytic therapy should be considered.[20]

Thrombolytic infusion is used to clear a central vein of a moderately large occluding or partially occluding thrombus. There are several techniques that have been developed to clear a central venous thrombus. One of the principles of therapy is to probe the thrombus with a wire to estimate the firmness of the clot. Thrombus that has had time to organize and fibrose is unlikely to clear with thrombolytic infusion. If the guidewire passes readily through the clot, this indicates that the clot is relatively fresh and not firmly organized. In this instance, thrombolytic therapy has a good probability of succeeding.

The intravenous administration of a thrombolytic agent may be accomplished by means of peripheral, proximal, or direct infusion into the clot. Peripheral infusion is less specifically directed and often requires more time to succeed. For this reason, proximal or direct infusion of lytic agent is frequently favored. Proximal infusion requires puncture of the venous system at a location peripheral to the clot. The infusion catheter is then passed up to the clot, and the thrombolytic agent is infused into its margin. Direct infusion would involve passage of the catheter into the clot with direct injection of the lytic agent. This technique, frequently referred to as "lacing" the clot, is often followed by proximal infusion of the same agent. A further refinement of this method is the pulse-spray technique, in which a catheter with multiple side holes is passed into the clot and thrombolytic agent is force sprayed in pulses. The direct infusion accelerates the exposure of the thrombolytic agent to the clot and results in a more rapid dissolution.[21]

Once the clot is dissolved, venography is performed to image the vein and to identify the cause of thrombosis. In most instances, a stricture will be found in the central venous system. This is most likely the source of the clot. Correction of the stricture is important to prevent recurrence of the clot.

If the patient is not a candidate for thrombolytic therapy or if the patient's symptoms resolve with heparin anticoagulation, a prolonged course of anticoagulation should be instituted. Current recommendations indicate that the patient should be treated with warfarin for at least 3 months. Not doing so exposes the patient to the risks for rethrombosis, clot propagation, and pulmonary embolization.[22,23] The incidence of pulmonary embolism associated with secondary upper extremity central vein thrombosis has been estimated to be about 15%. Fatal pulmonary emboli are thought to occur with a frequency of approximately 1%.[24]

Pharmacomechanical Thrombectomy

Pharmacomechanical clot removal is an alternative to thrombolysis in management of central venous thrombosis. Devices such as the Arrow-Trerotola Percutaneous Thrombolytic Device (Arrow International, Redding, PA) have been reported in this application. This is a motor-driven fragmentation cage that is delivered on a 5F catheter (via a 6F sheath) into the graft lumen. The fragmentation cage self-expands as it rotates at 3000 to 4500 rpm. The mechanical disruption of the clot occurs as the fragmentation cage beats through the thrombus. It has the ability to dissolve fresh thrombus, as well as compacted white thrombus found at the arterial anastomosis.[25,26]

Another device that employs mechanical clot disruption is the AngioJet (Possis Medical, Minneapolis, MN). This device uses a pressurized stream of saline solution

TABLE 61-2 Percutaneous Transluminal Angioplasty Alone for Central Venous Lesions

Author	Year	No. of lesions	Primary patency, 12 mo (%)	Assisted patency, 12 mo (%)
Vesely et al.[29]	1997	20	25	47
Bhatia et al.[30]	1996	13	71	—
Quinn et al.[31]	1995	87	11	78
Gray et al.[32]	1995	29	20	33
Vorwerk et al.[33]	1995	27	57	—
Shoenfeld et al.[34]	1994	18	68	93
Criado et al.[35]	1994	13	62	69

injected via a multilumen catheter along with Venturi aspiration to clear clot. This has been found to be effective in clearing occlusion from central venous and arterial thrombosis.[27] The mechanical methods of clearing thrombus mechanically disrupt and liquefy the clot and in so doing may result in fewer episodes of bleeding and embolization. Removal of the clot may reduce febrile reactions. These devices are highly effective and are able to clear the clot within a vessel in a few minutes.

Central Venous Stenosis

Mechanism

Central venous stenosis is most commonly caused by inflammation associated with catheterization. The inflammation and the damage to the vein result in thrombosis and fibrous stricture. Stricture may be induced by the infusion of caustic agents into a central venous catheter. If the agents are not rapidly diluted by the central venous blood, they may cause damage to the endothelium and reactive fibrosis of the vein wall. This is more commonly associated with catheters that have been placed in a relatively peripheral position, such as the subclavian or the innominate veins. The incidence of this complication can be reduced by placing the catheter tips at the atrial-caval junction. When a catheter is positioned at this location, the chance that an infused agent will cause vein wall injury by either direct toxic interaction or osmolar effect is minimized.

Another mechanism resulting in central vein stenosis is catheter infection. Infected catheters may cause damage to adjacent endothelium, leading to a localized inflammatory process. The resolution of this inflammatory process may be a fibrous stricture that reduces the vein diameter or even occludes the vein entirely.

Central venous thrombosis may lead to subsequent central vein stricture. As the thrombus adheres to the vein wall, an inflammatory process develops. The resolution of the thrombus with dissolution of the clot and replacement of the organized thrombus with fibrous tissue may result in narrowing of the vein diameter.

Presentation

Many central venous strictures are asymptomatic. Based on a prospective screening program, one estimate places the incidence of unsuspected central venous strictures at 29% of a dialysis population.[28] Some such strictures come to light when a subsequent attempt is made to cannulate the central venous system. Difficulty with such cannulation may lead to investigations such as venography, which ultimately discover the central venous stricture.

Clinically silent central venous stenosis may present as the capacitance of the venous system becomes stressed. An example of such a stressful event is the placement of a new arteriovenous fistula for hemodialysis in a patient who has had multiple central venous cannulas. Some of these patients will have massive upper extremity swelling because the venous capacity is unable to manage the increased flow of the arteriovenous graft.

Some central venous strictures may present with dramatic, sudden onset of swelling of the upper extremities, the neck, the face, and the head. In such instances, it is likely that critical central venous stenosis has progressed to the point where the residual lumen has been compromised with thrombus and is now occluded.

Management

BALLOON ANGIOPLASTY

Once central venous thrombus has been dissolved, it is not uncommon to find a stricture of the vein in the area where the clot had formed. Frequently, this stenosis is the result of inflammation of the vein wall caused by the catheter itself. If the stricture exceeds 50% of the normal vein diameter, consideration should be given to angioplasty. Because venous strictures are fibrous, angioplasty must often be repeated to obtain a satisfactory result (Table 61-2).[29-35]

TABLE 61-3 Percutaneous Transluminal Angioplasty and Stenting for Venous Stenosis

Author	Year	No. of lesions	Primary patency, 12 mo (%)	Assisted patency, 12 mo (%)
Lumsden et al.[28]	1997	25	17	
Quinn et al.[31]	1995	87	12	100
Wisselink et al.[36]	1993	15	36	86

STENTING

Given the fibrous nature of these strictures, stenting is frequently required to maintain initial patency. With use of such an approach, initial technical success rates have been reported to be between 88% and 100% (Table 61-3).[28,31,36] Unfortunately, the long-term patency is not good, even with the addition of stenting. The reported long-term primary patency rate at 1 year is in the range of 17% to 33%.[28,31,36] The mean duration of primary patency with this procedure is only 5.7 months.[28] For those patients fortunate enough to present before reocclusion, the assisted primary patency rate at 1 year has been reported to be 47%; however, these patients are a minority. The cumulative 1-year patency rate is between 22% and 33%.[31,36] More recently Oderich and associates[37] have reported a 1-year primary patency of 27% and a secondary patency of 71%. After 2 years these numbers fall to 9% and 39%, respectively.[37]

In a recent review of stenting for central venous stenosis associated with hemodialysis access, Bakken and colleagues[38] report on 73 patients treated over an 8-year period. They compared those patients who underwent primary angioplasty with those who underwent primary stenting. They assessed the primary patency of the central vein, the assisted primary patency, and the survival of the ipsilateral dialysis access. They discovered that the results were essentially equivalent. There were no statistically significant advantages of primary stenting. They reported a 1-year primary patency of 21% and a 1-year assisted patency rate of 46%.[38]

COVERED STENTS

Given that bare metal stents have not solved the problem of central venous restenosis, and that a portion of the problem relates to the ingrowth of fibrous hyperplastic tissue through the stent interstices, the next logical step in treatment is the use of covered stents or stent grafts. Remarkably few reports are available that offer more than anecdotal accounts. No systematically recorded long-term results are available as of this time.

Quinn et al[39] have reported on use of covered grafts for both peripheral and central venous stenosis. In a series of 17 patients they reported that primary patency at 1 year was 32%. Their secondary patency at 1 year was 39%. They concluded that covered grafts do not prevent progressive dialysis access site failure.[39]

Ultimately, the role of vascular stents and stent grafts in the management of venous stricture is still uncertain. Although the stents do help maintain the initial angioplasty result, they are thrombogenic and may become the focus of more clot. Additionally, in dialysis-associated cases, recurrent aggressive fibrous ingrowth through the stent tends to limit the durability and the usefulness of this technique. Balloon angioplasty provides short-term benefit with some improvement in patency. The intermediate and the long-term results are far less than desired, but angioplasty is the only option in most cases. The role of central venous stent placement remains to be established.

SUMMARY

Central venous catheters have become an indispensable element in the modern care of patients. These devices, although clearly beneficial, do cause potential problems associated with malposition, thrombosis, and venous stricture. These conditions are rarely fatal, yet loss of catheter function and the associated disability mandate intervention. Endovascular therapy offers a wide range of opportunities to improve the condition of patients with a catheter-related complication. Although results are not perfect, the therapeutic interventions offered by endovascular therapy represent a significant advance in the care of these patients.

References

1. Lindsay RM, Rothera C, Blake PG: A comparison of methods for the measurement of hemodialysis access recirculation, *ASAIO J* 44:191–193, 1998.
2. Puel V, Caudry M, Le Métayer P, et al: Superior vena cava thrombosis related to catheter malposition in cancer chemotherapy given through implanted ports, *Cancer* 72(7):2248–2252, 1993.
3. Petersen J, Delaney JH, Brakstad MT, et al: Silicone venous access devices positioned with their tips high in the superior vena cava are more likely to malfunction, *Am J Surg* 178(1):38–41, 1999.
4. Schutz JC, Patel AA, Clark TW, et al: Relationship between chest port catheter tip position and port malfunction after interventional radiologic placement, *J Vasc Interv Radiol* 15(6):581–587, 2004.
5. Eastridge BM, Lefor A: Complications of indwelling venous access devices in cancer patients, *J Clin Oncol* 13:233–238, 1995.
6. Kowalski CM, Kaufman JA, Rivitz SM, et al: Migration of central venous catheters: implications for initial catheter tip positioning, *J Vasc Interv Radiol* 8(3):443–447, 1997.

7. Crain MR, Mewissen MW, Ostrowski GJ, et al: Fibrin sleeve stripping for salvage of failing hemodialysis catheters: technique and initial results, *Radiology* 198:41–44, 1996.
8. Meers C, Toffelmire EB: Urokinase efficacy in the restoration of hemodialysis catheter function, *J CANNT* 8:17–19, 1998.
9. Jean G: Haemopericardium associated with disruption of a clot using a flexible J-guide-wire in a haemodialysis catheter [letter], *Nephrol Dial Transplant* 13:1898, 1998.
10. Savader SJ, Haikal LC, Ehrman KO, et al: Hemodialysis catheter-associated fibrin sheaths: treatment with a low-dose rt-PA infusion, *J Vasc Interv Radiol* 11(9):1131–1136, 2000.
11. Rockall AG, Harris A, Wetton CW, et al: Stripping of failing haemodialysis catheters using the Amplatz gooseneck snare, *Clin Radiol* 52:616–620, 1997.
12. Brady PS, Spence LD, Levitin A, et al: Efficacy of percutaneous fibrin sheath stripping in restoring patency of tunneled hemodialysis catheters, *AJR Am J Roentgenol* 173:1023–1027, 1999.
13. Johnstone RD, Stewart GA, Akoh JA, et al: Percutaneous fibrin sleeve stripping of failing haemodialysis catheters, *Nephrol Dial Transplant* 14:688–691, 1999.
14. Haskal ZJ, Leen VH, Thomas-Hawkins C, et al: Transvenous removal of fibrin sheaths from tunneled hemodialysis catheters, *J Vasc Interv Radiol* 7:513–517, 1996.
15. Trerotola SO: Pulse-spray thrombolysis of hemodialysis grafts: not the final word, *AJR Am J Roentgenol* 164:1501–1503, 1995.
16. Janne d'Othée B: Tham JC, Sheiman RG. Restoration of patency in failing tunneled hemodialysis catheters: a comparison of catheter exchange, exchange and balloon disruption of the fibrin sheath, and femoral stripping, *J Vasc Interv Radiol* 17(6): 1011–1015, 2006.
17. Beygui RE, Olcott C, Dalman RL: Subclavian vein thrombosis: outcome analysis based on etiology and modality of treatment, *Ann Vasc Surg* 11:247–255, 1997.
18. Machleder HI: Evaluation of a new treatment strategy for Paget-Schroetter syndrome: spontaneous thrombosis of the axillary-subclavian vein, *J Vasc Surg* 17:305–317, 1993.
19. Urschel HC, Razzuk MA: Improved management of the Paget-Schroetter syndrome secondary to thoracic outlet compression, *Ann Thorac Surg* 52:1217–1221, 1991.
20. Machleder H: Veno-occlusive disorders of the upper extremity, *Curr Probl Surg* 25:44–67, 1988.
21. Valji K, Bookstein JJ, Roberts AC, et al: Pulse-spray pharmacomechanical thrombolysis of thrombosed hemodialysis access grafts: long-term experience and comparison of original and current techniques, *AJR Am J Roentgenol* 164:1495–1500, 1995.
22. DeWeese JA, Adams JT, Gaiser DI: Subclavian venous thrombectomy, *Circulation* 16(suppl 2):158–170, 1970.
23. Adams JT, DeWeese JA: Effort thrombosis of the axillary and subclavian veins, *J Trauma* 11:923–930, 1971.
24. Monreal M, Raventos A, Lerma R, et al: Pulmonary embolism in patients with upper extremity DVT associated to venous central lines: a prospective study, *Thromb Haemost* 72:548–550, 1994.
25. Trerotola SO, Johnson MS, Schauwecker DS, et al: Pulmonary emboli from pulse-spray and mechanical thrombolysis: evaluation with an animal dialysis-graft model, *Radiology* 200:169–176, 1996.
26. Trerotola SO, Vesely TM, Lund GB, et al: Treatment of thrombosed hemodialysis access grafts: Arrow-Trerotola percutaneous thrombolytic device versus pulse-spray thrombolysis. Arrow-Trerotola Percutaneous Thrombolytic Device Clinical Trial, *Radiology* 206:403–414, 1998.
27. Vesely TM, Williams D, Weiss M, et al: Comparison of the AngioJet Rheolytic catheter to surgical thrombectomy for the treatment of thrombosed hemodialysis grafts. Peripheral AngioJet Clinical Trial, *J Vasc Interv Radiol* 10:1195–1205, 1999.
28. Lumsden AB, MacDonald MJ, Isiklar H, et al: Central venous stenosis in the hemodialysis patient: incidence and efficacy of endovascular treatment, *Cardiovasc Surg* 5:504–509, 1997.
29. Vesely TM, Hovsepian DM, Pilgram TK, et al: Upper extremity central venous obstruction in hemodialysis patients: treatment with Wallstents, *Radiology* 204:343–348, 1997.
30. Bhatia DS, Money SR, Ochsner JL, et al: Comparison of surgical bypass and percutaneous balloon dilatation with primary stent placement in the treatment of central venous obstruction in the dialysis patient: one-year follow-up, *Ann Vasc Surg* 10:452–455, 1996.
31. Quinn SF, Schuman ES, Demlow TA, et al: Percutaneous transluminal angioplasty versus endovascular stent placement in the treatment of venous stenoses in patients undergoing hemodialysis: intermediate results, *J Vasc Interv Radiol* 6:851–855, 1995.
32. Gray RJ, Horton KM, Dolmatch BL, et al: Use of Wallstents for hemodialysis access-related venous stenoses and occlusions untreatable with balloon angioplasty, *Radiology* 195:479–484, 1995.
33. Vorwerk D, Guenther RW, Mann H, et al: Venous stenosis and occlusion in hemodialysis shunts: follow-up results of stent placement in 65 patients, *Radiology* 195:140–146, 1995.
34. Shoenfeld R, Hermans H, Novick A, et al: Stenting of proximal venous obstructions to maintain hemodialysis access, *J Vasc Surg* 19:532–539, 1994.
35. Criado E, Marston WA, Jaques PF, et al: Proximal venous outflow obstruction in patients with upper extremity arteriovenous dialysis access, *Ann Vasc Surg* 8:530–535, 1994.
36. Wisselink W, Money SR, Becker MO, et al: Comparison of operative reconstruction and percutaneous balloon dilatation for central venous obstruction, *Am J Surg* 166:200–205, 1993.
37. Oderich GS, Treiman GS, Schneider P, Bhirangi K: Stent placement for treatment of central and peripheral venous obstruction: a long-term multi-institutional experience, *J Vasc Surg* 32 (4):760–769, 2000.
38. Bakken AM, Protack CD, Saad WE, et al: Long-term outcomes of primary angioplasty and primary stenting of central venous stenosis in hemodialysis patients, *J Vasc Surg* 45(4):776–783, 2007.
39. Quinn SF, Kim J, Sheley RC: Transluminally placed endovascular grafts for venous lesions in patients on hemodialysis, *Cardiovasc Intervent Radiol* 26(4):365–369, 2003 Jul-Aug.

SECTION X

VENOUS DISEASE

CHAPTER

62

Catheter-Directed Thrombolysis for Lower-Extremity Acute Deep Venous Thrombosis

Anthony J. Comerota

Thrombolytic therapy for acute deep venous thrombosis (DVT) has been under investigation for decades.[1] The original studies evaluating systemic infusion of thrombolytic agents demonstrated improved clinical outcomes compared with anticoagulation.[2,3] Significantly better lysis, restoration of vein patency, and preservation of valve function were recorded. However, some patients failed to respond to systemic thrombolysis and some had minimal benefit, most likely because the systemically infused plasminogen activator could not come in contact with enough fibrin-bound plasminogen to produce enough plasmin necessary within the clot to effectively reduce the thrombus burden. Patients who received systemic thrombolysis had a higher risk of bleeding compared with patients treated with anticoagulation alone.[4] Therefore systemic thrombolysis for acute DVT fell into disfavor.

As alluded to earlier, the basic mechanism of thrombolytic therapy is activation of fibrin-bound plasminogen.[5] There is no better way to activate the fibrin-bound plasminogen within the thrombus than to deliver the plasminogen activator into the clot by a catheter. It is intuitive that the greater the admixture of plasminogen activator with thrombus, the more effective the treatment. This indeed seems to hold true with the observations of pharmacomechanical methods of thrombolytic therapy compared with catheter infusion techniques that do not incorporate mechanical means of plasminogen activator distribution.

This chapter focuses on patients receiving treatment for iliofemoral DVT with catheter-based thrombolytic techniques. This subset of patients is being solely addressed for two reasons: (1) patients with iliofemoral DVT represent a unique subset of patients with acute DVT, who are at highest risk for development of ongoing postthrombotic complications; and (2) the majority of the information available on catheter-directed techniques involves patients with iliofemoral DVT. However, a recently funded National Institutes of Health trial will address catheter-based thrombolysis in patients with both iliofemoral and proximal infrainguinal DVT.[6]

POSTTHROMBOTIC MORBIDITY

Iliofemoral DVT represents the most extensive form of acute DVT. Acute iliofemoral DVT is often associated with symptoms of lower-extremity pain, swelling, and cyanosis. This is frequently characterized as phlegmasia cerulea dolens. However, even in the absence of debilitating pain and cyanosis, edema that involves the entire lower extremity is frequently the clinical manifestation of thrombosis of the iliofemoral venous system.

The long-term postthrombotic sequelae of acute iliofemoral DVT are particularly morbid. Venous insufficiency occurs in more than 95%,[7] venous claudication is manifested in up to 45%,[8] and 15% of patients have venous ulceration within 5 years.[7]

The underlying pathophysiology of the postthrombotic syndrome is ambulatory venous hypertension. The two components producing ambulatory venous hypertension are residual venous obstruction and valvular incompetence. Although recanalization of the thrombosed venous segment may restore "patency," significant luminal obstruction remains in the vein because the recanalization channel is only a fraction of the diameter of the normal vein. Though this may not represent significant functional obstruction at rest, its physiologic importance is magnified during exercise. Shull et al.[9] demonstrated the additive effects of residual obstruction and valvular incompetence on ambulatory venous hypertension in patients after thrombosis. They found that patients with the highest ambulatory venous pressures had the most severe postthrombotic syndrome, resulting from the combination of both obstruction and valvular incompetence. Johnson et al.[10] followed patients with acute DVT treated with anticoagulation and confirmed these observations. They found that patients with the most severe postthrombotic syndrome were likely to have the combination of obstruction and valvular incompetence.

Studies have also demonstrated that valvular reflux is progressive from the time acute venous thrombosis is recognized. In a prospective observational study of patients receiving anticoagulation for acute DVT, Markel et al[11] showed that 17% of patients had valvular reflux by the end of the first week, 40% at 1 month, and 66% at 1 year. Valvular incompetence developed more commonly in patients presenting with occlusive thrombosis than in those with nonocclusive DVT. This study demonstrated that increasing amounts of time are required for some valves to become incompetent and that the more extensive the DVT, the more likely the patient is to have development of chronic venous insufficiency.

In a follow-up prospective study examining the natural history of patients receiving anticoagulation for acute DVT, Meissner et al.[12] found that early recanalization was important for the preservation of valvular function and that 85% to 90% of vein segments that did not develop reflux had complete lysis by 12 months. These studies indicate that persistent obstruction increases the severity of the postthrombotic syndrome and that early lysis preserves valve function. It is intuitive then that treatment specifically designed to eliminate thrombus should reduce the severity of postthrombotic symptomsby eliminating obstruction and preserving valvular function.

CURRENT RATIONALE FOR CATHETER-DIRECTED THROMBOLYTIC THERAPY

An understanding of the pathophysiology of the postthrombotic syndrome and the observations from carefully studied patients who received treatment with anticoagulation alone for acute DVT form an important part of the foundation of the recommendation for a strategy of thrombus removal. Familiarity of the results of series of venous thrombectomy and recognizing the outcomes of a large randomized trial of venous thrombectomy versus anticoagulation alone for acute iliofemoral DVT produce consistent observations. Patients who have patency restored to thrombosed veins have the lowest ambulatory venous pressure and the fewest postthrombotic symptoms.[13,14] Patients with persistent venous obstruction have the most severe postthrombotic symptoms because of their high ambulatory venous pressures. Therefore, it is apparent that the long-term benefits of any treatment designed to clear clot from the deep veins are directly related to its ability to achieve and maintain a patent deep venous system. Removing thrombus early in the course of acute DVT reverses the inflammatory and therefore the subsequent fibrotic consequences of thrombosis, thereby improving the likelihood that valve function will be preserved.

Early in the clinical course of the use of thrombolytic agents for acute DVT, 13 studies have been reported comparing anticoagulant therapy with thrombolytic therapy.[2,3,15-25] Two randomized studies reported results in patients treated with either anticoagulation or lytic therapy.[2,3] Follow-up ranged from 1.6 to 6.5 years. Long-term evaluation indicated that the majority of patients free of postthrombotic symptoms received thrombolytic therapy, whereas the majority of patients with severe postthrombotic morbidity received anticoagulation alone.

A persistently important question is whether lysis of acute DVT preserves valve function. In a long-term follow-up of a prospective randomized study, Jeffery et al.[23] showed significant functional benefit 5 to 10 years after successful lysis of acute DVT. The rate of early recanalization for streptokinase was 55% versus 5% for patients given treatment with heparin. This mirrors the overall observations of pooled results from randomized trials of systemic lytic therapy.[26] At follow-up, popliteal valve incompetence and venous insufficiency of the involved limb were evaluated with photoplethysmographic techniques, foot volumetry, and direct Doppler examination. The investigators compared those with initially successful lysis with lytic failures. Patients whose clot lysed demonstrated normal venous function compared with lytic failures ($p < .001$). Nine percent of patients in whom lysis was successful had an incompetent popliteal valve compared with 77% of those in whom lysis failed ($p < .001$). Therefore it appears that in patients without a contraindication to thrombolytic therapy, lysis of extensive DVT is preferred and indeed recommended. If successful, lytic therapy will preserve long-term venous function. Another important issue that has not yet been answered is whether lytic therapy for acute DVT reduces the incidence of recurrent DVT. I believe we are beginning to appreciate that the likelihood of recurrence is reduced when the bulk of acute thrombus is eliminated early.

The goals of treatment with catheter-directed thrombolysis for patients with iliofemoral DVT are (1) to prevent pulmonary embolism (PE), (2) to reduce or eliminate the acute symptoms of iliofemoral DVT, (3) to reduce or avoid the postthrombotic syndrome, and (4) to reduce the likelihood of recurrent venous thromboembolism. Patients who are successfully treated with catheter-directed thrombolysis will have patency restored to the venous segment treated. Efficient elimination of thrombus is likely to preserve valve function. Additionally, many patients who are treated, especially those with left-sided iliofemoral DVT, are likely to have an underlying iliac vein stenosis that will be identified after successful lysis. The underlying stenosis must be corrected to preserve long-term patency and to avoid recurrent thrombosis.

CATHETER-DIRECTED THROMBOLYSIS

During the generation of a clot, circulating Glu-plasminogen binds to fibrin, which converts the plasminogen molecule to Lys-plasminogen. This modification produces more binding sites for plasminogen activators and therefore more efficient production of plasmin after activation of Lys-plasminogen. The basic mechanism of thrombolysis is the activation of fibrin-bound plasminogen resulting in the production of plasmin.[5] It is intuitive that delivery of the plasminogen activator within the thrombus more effectively activates fibrin-bound plasminogen and is potentially safer than systemic infusion. In addition, intrathrombus delivery protects plasminogen activators from circulating plasminogen activator inhibitor and, more important, protects the active enzyme plasmin from neutralization by circulating antiplasmins (α_1-antiplasmin, (α_2-macroglobulin). If lysis can be accelerated, the overall dose and, subsequently, duration of lytic infusion should be reduced, thereby diminishing the risk of treatment-related complications.

Numerous authors have reported good outcomes of catheter-directed thrombolysis for acute DVT. Most of those reports are included in Table 62-1,[27-47] which also includes pharmacomechanical techniques used as adjuncts to catheter-directed lytic infusion. Generally, when patients with acute DVT are treated with catheter-based techniques, success rates in the 75% to 90% range can be anticipated. Bleeding complications typically occur in 5% to 11%. Bleeding complications are predominantly puncture-site bleedings with a few major distant bleedings. Fortunately, intracranial bleeding is a rarity. Symptomatic PE is uncommon, and fatal PE is rare.

An interesting report by Chang et al.[48] demonstrated the benefit of intrathrombus pulse-spray bolus dosing of recombinant tissue plasminogen activator (rt-PA) in a small group of patients. The pulse-spray technique infused 50 mg of rt-PA per treatment episode. After treatment, patients returned to their hospital rooms and were brought back the following day for repeated phlebographic evaluation and repeated treatment if necessary. Patients received treatment for a maximum of four sessions of pulse-spray thrombolysis. Significant or complete lysis was achieved in 11 of 12 extremities and 1 had 50% to 70% lysis. Although the average dose of rt-PA was 106 mg, bleeding complications were minor and no patient's hematocrit dropped more than 2%. This small observational study draws attention to the importance of high-pressure, pulse-spray infusion into the thrombus, demonstrating that lysis can continue in thrombus exposed to plasminogen activators long after the treatment session ends. These observations also have potential implications for the management of patients with acute arterial occlusions.

The National Venous Registry[31] is the largest single report to date of patients receiving lytic therapy for acute DVT. Seventy-one percent of these patients had iliofemoral DVT, and 25% had femoropopliteal DVT. Intrathrombus infusion of urokinase with catheter-directed thrombolysis was the preferred treatment. In the group of patients with acute first-time iliofemoral DVT, 65% had complete clot resolution.

There was a significant correlation ($p < .001$) of thrombus-free survival with the result of initial therapy. At 1 year, 78% of patients who initially had complete clot resolution had patent veins compared with only 37% of patients who had less than 50% lysis. In the group of patients with first-time iliofemoral DVT who had initially successful thrombolysis, 96% remained patent at 1 year. Initial lytic success also correlated with valve function at 6 months. Sixty-two percent of patients with less than 50% thrombolysis had venous valvular incompetence, whereas 72% of patients who had complete lysis had normal valve function ($p < .02$).

A quality-of-life (QoL) study was subsequently performed to determine whether lytic therapy altered the QoL in patients with iliofemoral DVT. Because all patients in the National Venous Registry were given treatment with catheter-directed thrombolysis, a cohort control of patients drawn from the institutions participating in the Registry was identified. Patients receiving treatment for iliofemoral DVT with anticoagulation from the same institutions were compared. All patients given treatment with anticoagulation were candidates for catheter-directed thrombolysis; however, they were given anticoagulation because of physician preference.[49] Patients were evaluated with a validated, disease-specific QoL questionnaire,[50] which was used to evaluate patients at 16 and 22 months after treatment. Ninety-eight patients were evaluated, with 68 receiving catheter-directed thrombolysis and 30 anticoagulation alone. Patient responses indicated that catheter-directed thrombolysis was associated with a better QoL than anticoagulation alone. QoL was directly related to initial treatment success. Successfully treated patients had a better Health Utilities Index, improved physical functioning, less stigma of chronic venous disease, less health distress, and fewer overall postthrombotic symptoms. Not surprisingly, patients in whom catheter-directed thrombolysis

TABLE 62-1 Review of Studies of Catheter-Directed Thrombolysis for Acute Deep Venous Thrombosis

			Results			Complications			
						Bleeding			
Author, year	Total no. of patients (limbs)	Intervention	Significant/ complete resolution, n (%)	Partial resolution, n (%)	No resolution, n (%)	Minor, n (%)	Major, n (%)	PE	Death caused by Rx (%)
Semba et al., 1994[27]	21 (27)	CDT with UK, angioplasty/stenting for residual stenosis	18 (72)	5 (25)	2 (8)	1 (4)	0 (0)	None	None
Semba et al., 1996[28]	32 (41)	CDT with UK, angioplasty/stenting for residual stenosis	21 (32)	9 (28)	2 (6)	0 (0)	0 (0)	None	None
Verhaeghe et al., 1997[29]	24	CDT with rt-PA, stenting for residual stenosis	19 (79)	5 (21)	0 (0)	0 (0)	6 (25)	None	None
Bjarnason et al., 1997[30]	77 (87)	CDT with UK, angioplasty, stenting, thrombectomy, bypass for residual stenosis	69 (793)	0 (0)	18 (21)	11 (14)	5 (6)	1	None
Mewissen et al., 1999[31]	287 (312)	CDT with UK, stenting for residual stenosis; systemic lysis (n = 6)	96 (31)	162 (52)	54 (17)	15 (28)	54 (11)	6	2 (<1)
Comerota and Kagan, 2000[32]	54	CDT with UK or rt-PA, thrombectomy for residual stenosis	14 (26)	28 (52)	6 (11)	8 (15)	4 (7)	1	None
Horne et al., 2000[33]	10	CDT with rt-PA	9 (90)	1 (10)	0 (0)	3 (30)	None	2 (20)	None
Kasirajan et al., 2001[34]	9	CDT with UK, rt-PA, or rPA	7 (78)	1 (11)	1 (11)	NA	NA	NA	NA
AbuRahma et al., 2001[35]	51	CDT with UK or rt-PA, stents/18	15 (83)	NR	NR	3 (17)	2 (11)	None	None
		Hep/33	1 (3)	NR	NR	3 (9)	2 (6)	2 (6)	None
Vedantham et al., 2002[36]	20 (28)	CDT with UK, rt-PA, or rPA, thrombectomy, stenting	23 (82)	NR	NR	None	3 (14)	None	None
Elsharawy and Elzayat, 2002[37]	35	CDT with SK, angioplasty, stent/18	13 (72)	5 (28)	0 (0)	None	None	None	None
		Hep/17	2 (12)	8 (47)	7 (41)	None	None	None	None

Castaneda et al., 2002[38]	15	CDT with rPA	15 (100)	NR	NR	None	None	None	None
Grunwald and Hofmann, 2004[39]	74 (82)	CDT with UK, t-PA, or rPA, angioplasty, stenting	54 (73)	26 (32)	NR	6 (8)	4 (5)	None	None
Laiho et al., 2004[40]	32	CDT with rt-PA/16	8 (50)	5 (31)	NR	4 (25)	2 (13)	2 (13)	None
		Systemic lysis with rt-PA/16	5 (31)	8 (50)	NR	6 (38)	1 (6)	5 (31)	None
Sillesen et al., 2005[41]	45	CDT with rt-PA, angioplasty, stenting	42 (93)	NR	NR	4 (8)	None	1 (2)	None
Jackson et al., 2005[42]	28	CDT with UK or rPA, stenting	5 (18)	20 (72)	NR	2 (7)	None	None	None
Ogawa et al., 2005[43]	24	CDT with UK/10	0 (0)	10 (100)	None	None	None	None	None
		CDT with UK + IPC/14	5 (36)	9 (64)	None	None	None	None	None
Kim et al., 2006[44]	37 (45)	CDT with UK/23	21 (81)	3 (11)	2 (8)	1 (4)	2 (7)	1 (4)	None
		CDT + PMT/14	16 (84)	3 (16)	None	None	1 (5)	1 (5)	None
Lin et al., 2006[45]	93 (98)	CDT with rPA, rt-PA, or UK, angioplasty, stenting/46	32 (70)	14 (30)	5 (11)	2 (4)	1 (2)	None	None
		PMT with rPA, rt-PA, or UK, angioplasty, stenting/52	39 (75)	13 (25)	4 (8)	2 (4)	None	None	None
Protack et al., 2007[46]	69	CDT with UK, t-PA, retavase, pulse-spray, mechanical thrombectomy, stenting, IVC filters	40 (63)	19 (30)	4 (6)	None	None	None	None
Goldenberg et al., 2007[47]	22	CDT and/or systemic lysis with mechanical thrombectomy/9	8 (89)	NR	NR	1	1	None	None
		Anticoagulation alone/13	5.5 (42)	NR	NR				

CDT, Catheter-directed thrombolysis; *Hep*, heparin; *IPC*, intermittent pneumatic compression; *IVC*, inferior vena cava; *NA*, not available; *NR*, not reported; *PE*, pulmonary embolism; *PMT*, pharmacomechanical thrombolysis; rPA, recombinant plasminogen activator; *rt-PA*, recombinant tissue plasminogen activator; *SK*, streptokinase; *t-PA*, tissue plasminogen activator; *UK*, urokinase.

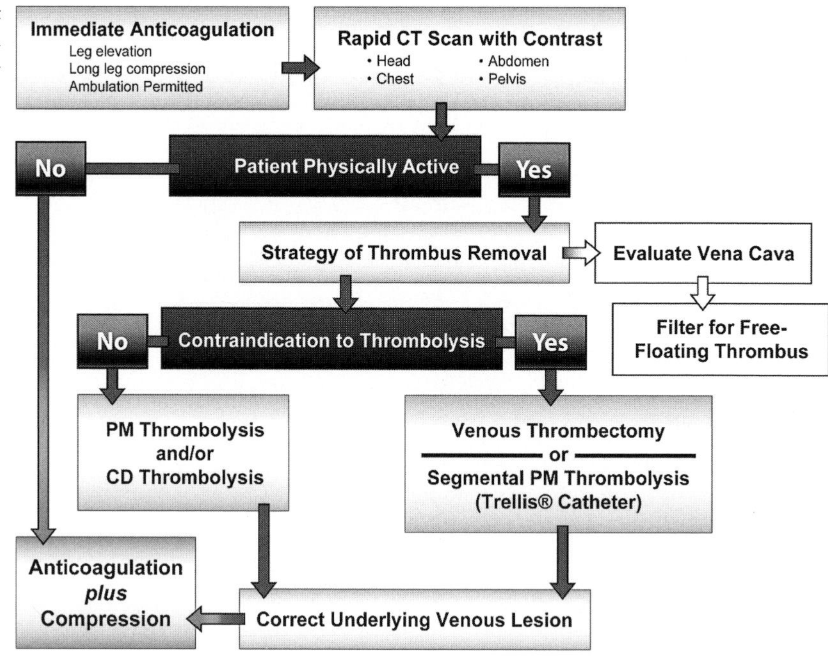

FIGURE 62-1 Algorithm illustrates our current treatment protocol for patients with iliofemoral DVT. *CD,* Catheter directed; *CT,* computed tomographic; *PM,* pharmacomechanical.

failed had outcomes similar to those treated with anticoagulation alone.

A small randomized trial performed by Elsharawy and Elzayat[37] compared catheter-directed thrombolysis with anticoagulation alone. Catheter-directed thrombolysis had considerably better outcomes at 6 months, demonstrating improved patency and vein valve function.

The above data are a compelling argument for catheter-directed thrombolysis. Larger randomized trials are required to establish definitive recommendations for care. Fortunately, two trials are underway, which will randomly assign patients with acute DVT to catheter-directed thrombolysis versus anticoagulation alone.[6,51]

PHARMACOMECHANICAL THROMBOLYSIS

Although good outcomes can be achieved with catheter-directed thrombolysis using the drip technique, treatment times are often unacceptably long and therefore bleeding risk and cost associated with therapy unacceptably high. This is evident by the recent report of Sillesen et al.[41] when they reported that 93% of their patients were successfully treated and discharged with patent veins, and more than 90% of patients discharged with patent veins had normal venous valve function at 1 year. However, the patients treated had a mean duration of symptoms of only 7 days, and patients with symptoms exceeding 14 days were excluded. Therefore, patients in this report would be expected to have the most acute thrombus, and one would anticipate that lysis would occur reasonably quickly. Treatment time for catheter-directed thrombolysis averaged 71 hours. This duration of acute care is logistically difficult if not impossible for many practitioners and many medical centers. The associated cost is high, especially considering that patients receiving lytic therapy are monitored in intensive care units (ICUs).

Mechanical techniques alone or in combination with thrombolysis have been developed to more rapidly clear the venous system. Vedantham et al.[36] evaluated the effectiveness of mechanical thrombectomy alone and in combination with pharmacologic thrombolysis in 28 limbs of patients with acute DVT. They evaluated multiple devices, including the Amplatz (ev3, Endovascular, Plymouth, MN), AngioJet (Possis Medical, Minneapolis, MN), Trerotola (Arrow International, Redding, PA), and Oasis (Boston Scientific/Meditech, Natick, MA) catheters. Venographic scoring was performed at each step of the procedure. Twenty-six percent of the thrombus was removed with mechanical thrombectomy alone, whereas adding a plasminogen activator solution to the mechanical technique (pharmacomechanical) removed 82% of the thrombus. These results include patients who had chronic occlusions that did not respond. Mechanical thrombectomy alone was highly successful for removing intraprocedural thrombus, which is generally gelatinous and does not contain cross-linked fibrin. Average infusion time was approximately 17 hours per limb, and 14% of patients had major bleeding complications.

Lin et al.[45] reported their 8-year experience of pharmacomechanical thrombolysis using a rheolytic catheter

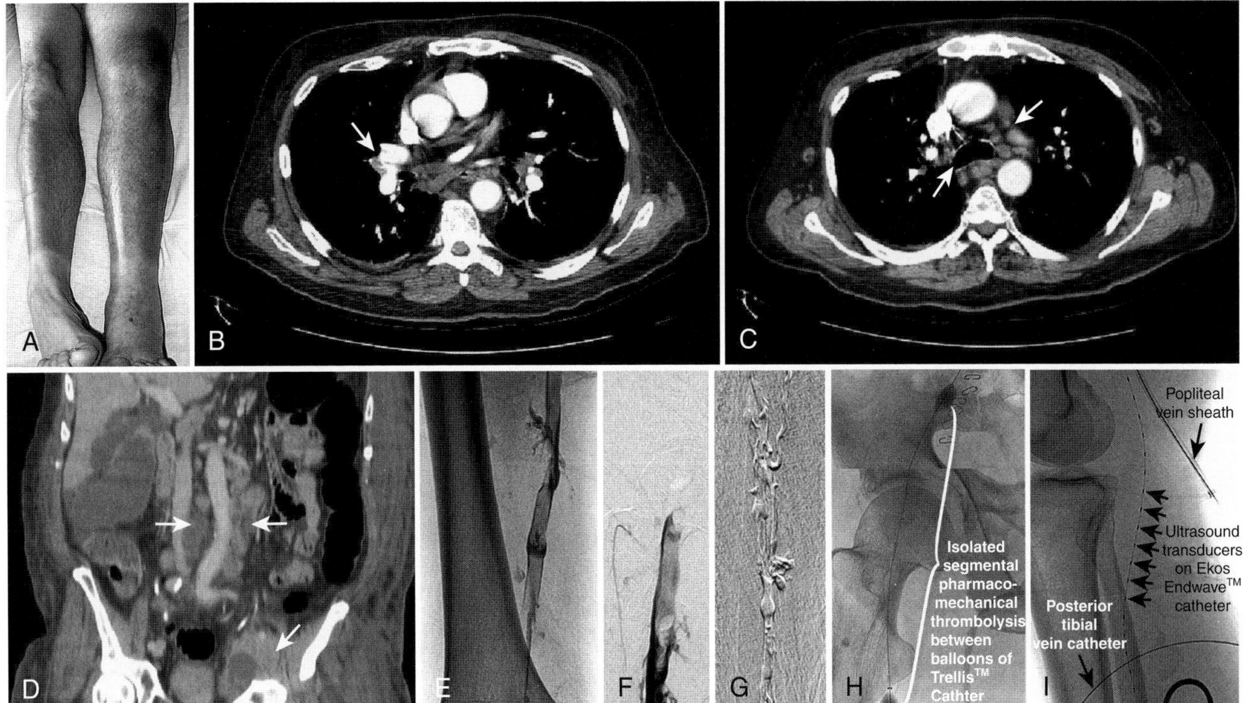

FIGURE 62-2 A 65-year-old white man was referred with phlegmasia cerulea dolens of his left leg. **(A)** 36 hours after a major abdominal laparotomy. Venous duplex demonstrated clot in the posterior tibial veins extending to the external iliac vein. A computed tomographic scan with contrast of the chest, abdomen, and pelvis was performed, which demonstrated asymptomatic pulmonary emboli **(B)** and mediastinal **(C)**, retroperitoneal *(arrows)*, and pelvic lymphadenopathy (**D**, *arrows*). The extensive thrombus is demonstrated by the catheter phlebogram of the femoral vein **(E, F)** and the silhouette of the calf thrombus **(G)** by the catheter in the posterior tibial vein at the ankle. The bulk of the thrombus from the proximal popliteal vein to the common iliac vein was treated with the Trellis catheter via an ultrasound-guided popliteal vein approach **(H)**. The clot in the posterior tibial and popliteal veins was treated with the EKOS EndoWave system **(I)**.

compared with catheter-directed lytic therapy with infusion alone. Of their 98 patients, 46 received catheter-directed thrombolysis alone and 52 received pharmacomechanical thrombolysis. Patients receiving the pharmacomechanical technique with the AngioJet catheter had significantly fewer phlebograms, shorter ICU stays, shorter hospital stays, and fewer blood transfusions. Bleeding complications were not different between the two groups. A smaller patient group treated with rheolytic thrombectomy was reported by Kasirajan et al.[34] and demonstrated that mechanical thrombectomy alone was less effective than combined pharmacomechanical thrombolysis.

The initial experience with ultrasound-accelerated thrombolysis was reported by Parikh et al.[52] Fifty-three patients were treated for acute DVT with use of the EKOS Endowave (EKOS, Bothell, WA) system. They included patients with both upper- and lower-extremity DVT in their report, and a variety of lytic agents were used. Complete lysis ($\geq$90%) was observed in 70% of the patients and overall lysis (complete and partial) observed in 91%. Mean infusion time was 22 hours, and 4% of patients had major complications, generally puncture-site hematomas. It was the authors' impression that, compared with historical controls (which is a weakness of this report), there was reduced treatment time and a reduced dose of lytic agents with ultrasound-accelerated thrombolysis.

An interesting new technique is isolated segmental pharmacomechanical thrombolysis (ISPMT), which is achieved with use of the Trellis catheter (Bacchus Vascular, Santa Clara, CA). This is a double-balloon infusion catheter that is inserted into the thrombosed venous segment, with the proximal balloon positioned just above the upper end (cephalic end) of the thrombus. When the balloons are inflated, the plasminogen activator is infused into the thrombosed segment isolated by the balloons. The intervening catheter assumes a spiral configuration and spins at 1500 rpm for 15 to 20 minutes. The liquefied and fragmented thrombus is aspirated and treatment success evaluated with repeated segmental phlebography. If successful, the catheter is repositioned, and additional thrombosed segments are treated. If residual thrombus persists, repeated treatment or other appropriate intervention (such as rheolytic thrombectomy, ultrasound-accelerated thrombolysis, balloon angioplasty, and/or stenting) is performed.

Martinez et al.[53] reported 52 consecutive limbs treated for iliofemoral DVT, the first 27 with catheter-directed thrombolysis and the following 25 with ISPMT

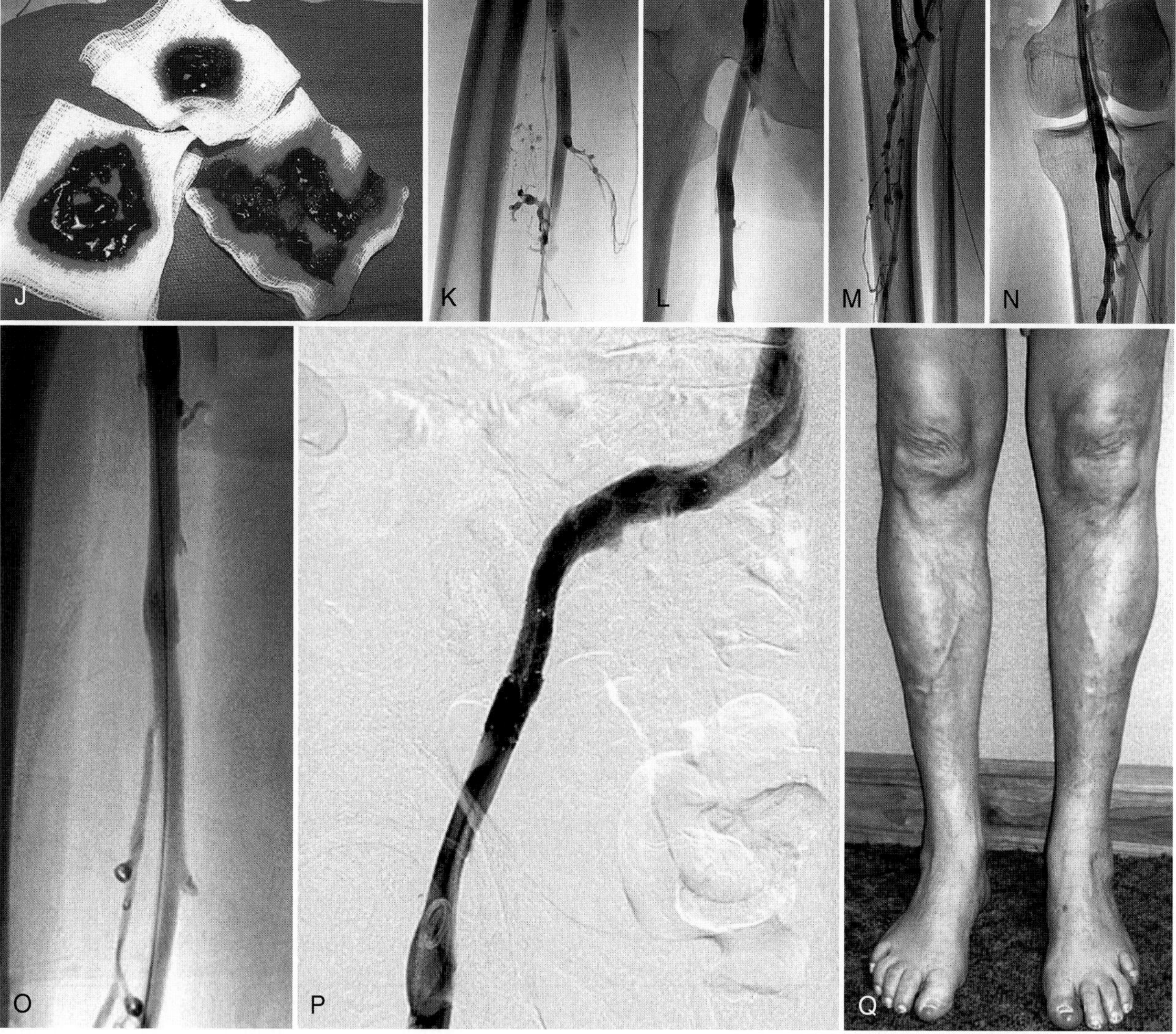

FIGURE 62-2 —*cont'd J-Q,* Liquefied and fragmented thrombus resulting from isolated segmental pharmacomechanical thrombolysis was aspirated via the Trellis catheter **(J)**. Segmental phlebography was performed to check the results of treatment before moving to an adjacent thrombosed segment **(K, L)**. Residual thrombus was removed with rheolytic thrombectomy with use of the AngioJet and iliac vein compression treated with a stent. A completion phlebogram shows patency of the calf, popliteal, femoral, and iliac veins, as well as supple valve cusps, suggesting that valve function persisted **(M-P)**. The patient received treatment with systemic chemotherapy for his underlying lymphoma. At 16 months **(Q)**, the patient was asymptomatic, had no postthrombotic symptoms, maintained lower-extremity venous patency with normal valve function, and fortunately had no evidence of lymphoma recurrence.

plus catheter-directed thrombolysis when necessary. Thrombus burden and treatment outcomes were quantified. Ninety-three percent of the patients were treated with rt-PA. Venoplasty and stenting were used to correct underlying stenoses in all patients, and all received long-term therapeutic anticoagulation. Sixteen of the 27 legs treated with catheter-directed thrombolysis required other adjunctive mechanical techniques to clear the thrombus, such as AngioJet, ultrasound-accelerated lysis, or pulse-spray techniques, whereas only 7 of the 25 limbs treated with ISPMT required additional adjunctive techniques. A larger percentage of the thrombus was removed with ISPMT compared with catheter-directed thrombolysis. Complete lysis ($\geq$90%) was achieved in 11% of limbs of patients with catheter-directed thrombolysis compared with 28% with ISPMT limbs ($p = .077$). Treatment time was shorter (23.4 vs. 55.4 hours, $p < .001$) and rt-PA dose was less (33.4 vs. 59.3 mg, $p = .009$) with ISPMT. Hospital and ICU length of stay were no different, which was believed to be due to the patients' underlying comorbidities rather than the treatment directed at their iliofemoral DVT. Eighteen percent of the limbs had complete lysis after use of the ISMPT catheter alone. This observation is consistent with that of O'Sullivan et al.[54] Bleeding complications occurred in 5% of patients undergoing catheter-directed thrombolysis alone and 5% of patients with ISPMT.

Our current approach to patients with iliofemoral DVT is to use ISPMT as an initial technique to remove the bulk of thrombus from the proximal venous system. Infrapopliteal and distal popliteal thrombus is treated with catheter-directed infusion and ultrasound-accelerated thrombolysis. Persistent segmental thrombus is treated with rheolytic thrombectomy techniques or balloon dilation, and persistent stenoses are treated with balloon dilation and stenting. This approach is summarized by the algorithm (Figure 62-1) and by the patient described in Figure 62-2.

SUMMARY

A strategy of thrombus removal should be offered to all patients with extensive DVT unless a compelling reason exists otherwise. This is recognized by the 2008 American College of Chest Physicians guidelines, which recommend both operative venous thrombectomy and catheter-directed thrombolysis for patients with iliofemoral DVT.[55] The potential advantage of pharmacomechanical techniques is also recognized in these guidelines.

Endovascular techniques are improving, as are the skill and judgment of the physicians caring for these patients. The net result is better patient outcomes with fewer complications. The importance of therapeutic long-term anticoagulation, which reduces the risk of recurrence, cannot be understated. Newer lytic agents, such as plasmin, and new antithrombotics, such as direct factor X_a inhibition and direct thrombin inhibitors, may improve efficacy and safety of anticoagulation as these agents are developed.

References

1. Comerota AJ: An overview of thrombolytic therapy for venous thromboembolism. In: Comerota AJ, editor: *Thrombolytic therapy,* Orlando, FL, 1988, Grune & Stratton, pp 65–89.
2. Arnesen H, Heilo A, Jakobsen E, et al: A prospective study of streptokinase and heparin in the treatment of deep vein thrombosis, *Acta Med Scand* 203:457–463, 1978.
3. Elliot MS, Immelman EJ, Jeffery P, et al: A comparative randomized trial of heparin versus streptokinase in the treatment of acute proximal venous thrombosis: an interim report of a prospective trial, *Br J Surg* 66:838–843, 1979.
4. Goldhaber SZ, Buring JE, Lipnick RJ, et al: Pooled analyses of randomized trials of streptokinase and heparin in phlebographically documented acute deep venous thrombosis, *Am J Med* 76:393–397, 1984.
5. Alkjaersig N, Fletcher AP, Sherry S: The mechanism of clot dissolution by plasmin, *J Clin Invest* 38:1086–1095, 1959.
6. Comerota AJ: The ATTRACT Trial: rationale for early intervention for illofemoral DVT, *Perspect Vasc Surg Endovasc Ther* 21(4): 221–224, 2009.
7. Akesson H, Brudin L, Dahlstrom JA, et al: Venous function assessed during a 5 year period after acute ilio-femoral venous thrombosis treated with anticoagulation, *Eur J Vasc Surg* 4:43–48, 1990.
8. Delis KT, Bountouroglou D, Mansfield AO: Venous claudication in iliofemoral thrombosis: long-term effects on venous hemodynamics, clinical status, and quality of life, *Ann Surg* 239:118–126, 2004.
9. Shull KC, Nicolaides AN, Fernandes e Fernandes J, et al: Significance of popliteal reflux in relation to ambulatory venous pressure and ulceration, *Arch Surg* 114:1304–1306, 1979.
10. Johnson BF, Manzo RA, Bergelin RO, et al: Relationship between changes in the deep venous system and the development of the postthrombotic syndrome after an acute episode of lower limb deep vein thrombosis: a one- to six-year follow-up, *J Vasc Surg* 21:307–312, 1995.
11. Markel A, Manzo RA, Bergelin RO, et al: Valvular reflux after deep vein thrombosis: incidence and time of occurrence, *J Vasc Surg* 15:377–382, 1992.
12. Meissner MH, Manzo RA, Bergelin RO, et al: Deep venous insufficiency: the relationship between lysis and subsequent reflux, *J Vasc Surg* 18:596–605, 1993.
13. Plate G, Akesson H, Einarsson E, et al: Long-term results of venous thrombectomy combined with a temporary arterio-venous fistula, *Eur J Vasc Surg* 4:483–489, 1990.
14. Plate G, Eklof B, Norgren L, et al: Venous thrombectomy for iliofemoral vein thrombosis: 10-year results of a prospective randomised study, *Eur J Vasc Endovasc Surg* 14:367–374, 1997.
15. Browse NL, Thomas ML, Pim HP: Streptokinase and deep vein thrombosis, *Br Med J* 3:717–720, 1968.
16. Robertson BR, Nilsson IM, Nylander G: Value of streptokinase and heparin in treatment of acute deep venous thrombosis. A coded investigation, *Acta Chir Scand* 134:203–208, 1968.
17. Kakkar VV, Flanc C, Howe CT, et al: Treatment of deep vein thrombosis. A trial of heparin, streptokinase, and arvin, *Br Med J* 1:806–810, 1969.
18. Tsapogas MJ, Peabody RA, Wu KT, et al: Controlled study of thrombolytic therapy in deep vein thrombosis, *Surgery* 74:973–984, 1973.
19. Duckert F, Muller G, Nyman D, et al: Treatment of deep vein thrombosis with streptokinase, *Br Med J* 1:479–481, 1975.
20. Porter JM, Moneta GL: Reporting standards in venous disease: an update. International Consensus Committee on Chronic Venous Disease, *J Vasc Surg* 21:635–645, 1995.
21. Marder VJ, Soulen RL, Atichartakarn V, et al: Quantitative venographic assessment of deep vein thrombosis in the evaluation of streptokinase and heparin therapy, *J Lab Clin Med* 89:1018–1029, 1977.
22. Watz R, Savidge GF: Rapid thrombolysis and preservation of valvular venous function in high deep vein thrombosis. A comparative study between streptokinase and heparin therapy, *Acta Med Scand* 205:293–298, 1979.
23. Jeffery P, Immelman EJ, Amoore J: Treatment of deep vein thrombosis with heparin or streptokinase: long-term venous function assessment (Abstract No. S20.3), *Proceedings of the Second International Vascular Symposium* London, September 11, 1986.
24. Turpie AG, Levine MN, Hirsh J, et al: Tissue plasminogen activator (rt-PA) vs heparin in deep vein thrombosis. Results of a randomized trial, *Chest* 97:172S–175S, 1990.
25. Goldhaber SZ, Meyerovitz MF, Green D, et al: Randomized controlled trial of tissue plasminogen activator in proximal deep venous thrombosis, *Am J Med* 88:235–240, 1990.

26. Comerota AJ, Aldridge SE: Thrombolytic therapy for acute deep vein thrombosis, *Semin Vasc Surg* 5:76–84, 1992.
27. Semba CP, Dake MD: Iliofemoral deep venous thrombosis: aggressive therapy with catheter-directed thrombolysis, *Radiology* 191:487–494, 1994.
28. Semba CP, Dake MD: Catheter-directed thrombolysis for iliofemoral venous thrombosis, *Semin Vasc Surg* 9:26–33, 1996.
29. Verhaeghe R, Stockx L, Lacroix H, et al: Catheter-directed lysis of iliofemoral vein thrombosis with use of rt-PA, *Eur Radiol* 7:996–1001, 1997.
30. Bjarnason H, Kruse JR, Asinger DA, et al: Iliofemoral deep venous thrombosis: safety and efficacy outcome during 5 years of catheter-directed thrombolytic therapy, *J Vasc Interv Radiol* 8:405–418, 1997.
31. Mewissen MW, Seabrook GR, Meissner MH, et al: Catheter-directed thrombolysis for lower extremity deep venous thrombosis: report of a national multicenter registry, *Radiology* 211:39–49, 1999.
32. Comerota AJ, Kagan SA: Catheter-directed thrombolysis for the treatment of acute iliofemoral deep venous thrombosis, *Phlebology* 15:149–155, 2000.
33. Horne MK III, Mayo DJ, Cannon RO III, et al: Intraclot recombinant tissue plasminogen activator in the treatment of deep venous thrombosis of the lower and upper extremities, *Am J Med* 108:251–255, 2000.
34. Kasirajan K, Gray B, Ouriel K: Percutaneous AngioJet thrombectomy in the management of extensive deep venous thrombosis, *J Vasc Interv Radiol* 12:179–185, 2001.
35. AbuRahma AF, Perkins SE, Wulu JT, et al: Iliofemoral deep vein thrombosis: conventional therapy versus lysis and percutaneous transluminal angioplasty and stenting, *Ann Surg* 233:752–760, 2001.
36. Vedantham S, Vesely TM, Parti N, et al: Lower extremity venous thrombolysis with adjunctive mechanical thrombectomy, *J Vasc Interv Radiol* 13:1001–1008, 2002.
37. Elsharawy M, Elzayat E: Early results of thrombolysis vs anticoagulation in iliofemoral venous thrombosis. A randomised clinical trial, *Eur J Vasc Endovasc Surg* 24:209–214, 2002.
38. Castaneda F, Li R, Young K, et al: Catheter-directed thrombolysis in deep venous thrombosis with use of reteplase: immediate results and complications from a pilot study, *J Vasc Interv Radiol* 13:577–580, 2002.
39. Grunwald MR, Hofmann LV: Comparison of urokinase, alteplase, and reteplase for catheter-directed thrombolysis of deep venous thrombosis, *J Vasc Interv Radiol* 15:347–352, 2004.
40. Laiho MK, Oinonen A, Sugano N, et al: Preservation of venous valve function after catheter-directed and systemic thrombolysis for deep venous thrombosis, *Eur J Vasc Endovasc Surg* 28:391–396, 2004.
41. Sillesen H, Just S, Jorgensen M, et al: Catheter-directed thrombolysis for treatment of ilio-femoral deep venous thrombosis is durable, preserves venous valve function and may prevent chronic venous insufficiency, *Eur J Vasc Endovasc Surg* 30: 556–562, 2005.
42. Jackson LS, Wang XJ, Dudrick SJ, et al: Catheter-directed thrombolysis and/or thrombectomy with selective endovascular stenting as alternatives to systemic anticoagulation for treatment of acute deep vein thrombosis, *Am J Surg* 190:864–868, 2005.
43. Ogawa T, Hoshino S, Midorikawa H, et al: Intermittent pneumatic compression of the foot and calf improves the outcome of catheter-directed thrombolysis using low-dose urokinase in patients with acute proximal venous thrombosis of the leg, *J Vasc Surg* 42:940–944, 2005.
44. Kim HS, Patra A, Paxton BE, et al: Adjunctive percutaneous mechanical thrombectomy for lower-extremity deep vein thrombosis: clinical and economic outcomes, *J Vasc Interv Radiol* 17:1099–1104, 2006.
45. Lin PH, Zhou W, Dardik A, et al: Catheter-direct thrombolysis versus pharmacomechanical thrombectomy for treatment of symptomatic lower extremity deep venous thrombosis, *Am J Surg* 192:782–788, 2006.
46. Protack CD, Bakken AM, Patel N, et al: Long-term outcomes of catheter directed thrombolysis for lower extremity deep venous thrombosis without prophylactic inferior vena cava filter placement, *J Vasc Surg* 45:992–997, 2007.
47. Goldenberg NA, Durham JD, Knapp-Clevenger R, et al: A thrombolytic regimen for high-risk deep venous thrombosis may substantially reduce the risk of postthrombotic syndrome in children, *Blood* 110:45–53, 2007.
48. Chang R, Cannon RO III, Chen CC, et al: Daily catheter-directed single dosing of t-PA in treatment of acute deep venous thrombosis of the lower extremity, *J Vasc Interv Radiol* 12:247–252, 2001.
49. Comerota AJ, Throm RC, Mathias SD, et al: Catheter-directed thrombolysis for iliofemoral deep venous thrombosis improves health-related quality of life, *J Vasc Surg* 32:130–137, 2000.
50. Mathias SD, Prebil LA, Putterman CG, et al: A health-related quality of life measure in patients with deep vein thrombosis: a validation study, *Drug Inf J* 33:1173–1187, 1999.
51. Enden T, Sandvik L, Klow NE, et al: Catheter-directed Venous Thrombolysis in acute iliofemoral vein thrombosis—the CaVenT study: rationale and design of a multicenter, randomized, controlled, clinical trial (NCT00251771), *Am Heart J* 154:808–814, 2007.
52. Parikh S, Motarjeme A, McNamara T, et al: Ultrasound-accelerated thrombolysis for the treatment of deep vein thrombosis: initial clinical experience, *J Vasc Interv Radiol* 19:521–528, 2008.
53. Martinez J, Comerota AJ, Kazanjian S, et al: The quantitative benefit of isolated, segmental, pharmacomechanical thrombolysis for iliofemoral DVT, *J Vasc Surg* 48:1532–1537, 2008.
54. O'Sullivan GJ, Lohan DG, Gough N, et al: Pharmacomechanical thrombectomy of acute deep vein thrombosis with the Trellis-8 isolated thrombolysis catheter, *J Vasc Interv Radiol* 18:715–724, 2007.
55. Kearon C, Kahn SR, Agnelli G, et al: Antithrombotic therapy for venous thromboembolic disease: American College of Chest Physicians Evidence-Based Clinical Practice Guidelines (8th edition), *Chest* 133:454S–545S, 2008.

CHAPTER

63

Inferior Vena Cava Filter Placement

Nirav Patel, Anil P. Hingorani, Enrico Ascher

Venous thromboembolism has been recognized to be a significant source of morbidity and mortality. The incidence of deep venous thrombosis is estimated to affect 48 per 100,000 persons annually, with an in-hospital case fatality rate resulting from complications of thromboembolism of 12%.[1] Pulmonary embolism (PE) occurs in as many as 630,000 patients annually, with an 11% first-hour mortality rate, which is more than 69,000 deaths.[2,3] Those surviving that first hour go on to have a 23.8% first-year mortality rate (150,000 deaths). What is even more startling is that the diagnosis of PE is being missed in 71% (400,000 patients).[4] There are 300,000 hospitalizations per year in the United States directly attributed to venous thrombotic disease, with studies reporting as many as 90% of patients admitted to the hospital.[5,6]

Lower-extremity deep venous thromboses (LEDVT) account for 88% to 96% of PEs. Upper-extremity deep venous thromboses (UEDVT) account for the remaining 4% to 12%.[7,8] It has also been shown that PE occurs in up to 30% to 50% of patients with LEDVT of iliac origin who are not anticoagulated. When comparing lower- and upper-extremity DVT, it has been shown that UEDVT is associated with higher morbidity and mortality rates.[9] PE from UEDVT is on the rise as a result of the increased use of central venous catheters.[10]

PRIMARY INDICATIONS FOR INFERIOR VENA CAVA FILTER

Anticoagulation has long been proved, and continues to be, the first-line therapy for prevention and treatment of PE. However, many occasions arise where this protocol is neither appropriate nor effective, and treatment must therefore be made available to those patients at risk for development of PE. In the presence of documented DVT or PE, a filtration device is indicated in patients for whom anticoagulation is contraindicated. Absolute indications are intracranial hemorrhage, massive hemoptysis, gross gastrointestinal bleeding, retroperitoneal hemorrhage, and thrombocytopenia. Another indication is development of PE while being therapeutically anticoagulated.

Relative indications for the placement of caval filters may include the presence of DVT/PE with cor pulmonale and metastatic disease in persons with a history of falling who may be at increased risk for intracranial hemorrhage with anticoagulation. Extension of existing DVT or new DVTs developing on anticoagulation are additional relative indications.

Furthermore, in those patients in whom there exists either a history or a high risk for the development of DVT, prophylactic implantations of filtration devices may be indicated.[11,12] This includes those patients who are deemed to be high risk for venous thromboembolism who will be undergoing hip or knee replacement surgery or gastric bypass for morbid obesity. Prophylactic placement of one or more vena cava filters is also indicated in situations of high-risk trauma, such as a spinal cord injury with an associated severe head injury, and complex pelvic fractures or multiple long-bone fractures.

THE EVOLUTION OF CAVAL INTERRUPTION

René-Théophile H. Laennec was the first to describe the phenomenon of PE in 1819.[13] It would not be until 1846 that Rudolph Virchow would postulate the pathogenesis of thromboembolism (endothelial damage, clotting tendency, and stasis)[13] and, later, the first postmortem observation of PE in 1856.[13] A newfound appreciation had been born for venous thrombosis and PE.

John Hunter in 1784 led the earliest efforts to prevent PE using the technique in which the femoral vein was ligated for thrombophlebitis. Others, such as Theodore E. Kocher and Theodor Billroth in 1883, Enrico Bottini in 1893, and Friedrich Trendelenburg in 1906, soon followed to build on John Hunter's principles. Trendelenburg made the first attempt in actually treating PE in 1908 when he conducted the first operation to surgically remove emboli from the pulmonary artery.[13] In his procedure the left side of the patient's chest was opened, exposing the common pulmonary artery. The proximal aorta and pulmonary artery were then encircled together through the transverse sinus of the pericardium and traction placed on that encircling band, thus occluding the vessels. The emboli were then extracted through a small pulmonary arteriotomy. Although the procedure was unsuccessful, he had thus set the stage for a new era—the possibility of a treatment for PE. A student of Trendelenburg, Martin Kirschner, would become the first surgeon to report the successful removal of a PE in 1924.[13] His adaptation of Trendelenburg's original operation, in which he obtained control of the proximal aorta and pulmonary artery by direct clamping of the vessels, was met with only minimal success—and few survivors. It would take four decades before significant changes in the surgical approach to pulmonary embolectomy would be realized when Edward H. Sharp developed his technique of pulmonary artery embolectomy by using cardiopulmonary bypass in 1961.[13]

Even as these pioneers were directing their attention toward the surgical correction of existing PE, other surgeons were developing techniques to prevent PE by obtaining partial extraluminal interruption of the inferior vena cava (IVC) that would limit the diameter of the IVC and trap emboli.[13] Their techniques included a variety of extraluminal clips, caval plication, and mattress suture patterns designed to trap emboli. The downfall of these techniques was that they all had a high incidence of IVC occlusion. These innovations, although timely in the evolution of the control of PE, would very soon be abandoned because of the nearly simultaneous introduction of more minimally invasive surgically implanted intraluminal filters that would revolutionarize the field. These new filters would permit those emboli that were trapped to be dissolved while maintaining IVC patency.

The modern era of limited surgical invasive prophylaxis of PE would begin when Bertram D. Cohn, at Maimonides Medical Center (Brooklyn, NY), applied for the first patent for an "Occlusive Device for the Inferior Vena Cava" on November 9, 1964. His device was constructed in a conical three-tier design with each tier deploying four expansion wings, which he implanted using endovascular technique in 12 dogs. At up to 8 months follow-up his results showed 5 animals with no IVC occlusion, 3 with early recanalization of caval occlusions, and 4 cavas remaining totally occluded. All of the animals survived without symptoms. The U.S. patent (number 3,334,629) for his device was awarded on August 8, 1967.

Later, at the 1967 Annual Clinical Congress of the American College of Surgeons, Kazi Mobin-Uddin would introduce his "umbrella" filter,[13] a silicone elastomer (Silastic)–covered umbrella-shaped device with six spokes radiating from the central hub with 18 3-mm perforations. This filter would be the first to gain wide acceptance in clinical use. Initially, the filter had a 23-mm diameter, but that was soon increased to 28 mm after evidence of its migration tendencies. Although the filter was effective in clot trapping, there was an 85% rate of IVC thrombosis, which led to its discontinuation.[13]

INTRALUMINAL FILTERS IN USE TODAY

Today, a number of successful devices are commercially available. Although there have been hundreds of published articles on the use of these vena cava filters, there has been no uniformity in how to accurately and consistently present the data obtained. This task is now being undertaken by a consensus committee of vascular surgeons.[13] Although all such intravenous filters have been effective in preventing PE in the majority of patients, each device has its own advantages, disadvantages, and complication rates. Which filtration device will be the right choice for the patient depends on the patency of the device, the luminal diameter of the vena cava, introducer sheath size of the device, site of venous access, anatomic variations affecting ease of placement, filter stability and migration, efficacy in clot trapping, PE recurrence rate, and any ferromagnetic properties that may affect future magnetic resonance imaging (MRI) examinations.

Greenfield Vena Cava Filters (Stainless Steel and Titanium)

The stainless steel Greenfield vena cava filter (SGF) was the first intraluminal filtration device to gain wide acceptance as an alternative to surgical ligation or partial extraluminal vena caval interruption.[14] Introduced in 1972, the SGF has survived the test of time and is the most widely studied intraluminal filtration device still in use today. The stainless steel Greenfield filter has a proved track record, with recurrence rates for PE to be as low as 3% to 5%. The thrombosis rate of the IVC is only 1% to 9%. The original device had a large 24F introducer sheath, which very often necessitated a venous cutdown for placement and subjected the patient to increased insertion site thrombosis.

As with any successful device, modifications were made to the Greenfield filter. Changes such as a modified hook design and a smaller introducer sheath were implemented in 1989 in the titanium Greenfield filter (TGF).[14] The new hook design significantly reduced the incidence of filter migration. The new 12F low profile made percutaneous placement successful in 97% of the patients. The TGF has no ferromagnetic properties, thus making it safe during MRI examination.

The design of the SGF and TGF permits thrombi to fill up to 80% of the filter capacity before a significant cross-sectional diameter reduction and caval occlusion occur. Drawbacks to the Greenfield filter are that it can only be placed in a maximum caval diameter limited to 28 mm. Also, its conical designs can cause tilting and leg asymmetry when incorrectly placed, thus making it ineffective in trapping emboli. The longstanding experience with the Greenfield vena cava filters and their results account for their dominance in the current cava filter market.

Bird's Nest Vena Cava Filter

Introduced in 1980, the Gianturco-Roehm Bird's Nest (BNF) Vena Cava Filter has the distinctive advantage of being able to be placed in large caval diameters of greater than 3 cm (4 cm maximum). It has a low-profile 14.5F introducer sheath, and its free-form configuration does not require centering in the IVC. When released from the carrier device the filter assumes a tangled "bird's nest" form—hence its name.

Disadvantages for this device are that it can be difficult to place in a short IVC. Seven centimeters is needed for proper placement. Another disadvantage is that the ferromagnetic properties of this filter make it susceptible to magnetic artifact during MRI examination. The BNF also has low IVC thrombosis rate of 2.9% to 7.6%, along with a recurrent PE rate of 1.1% to 2.7%.

Vena Tech—LGM Vena Cava Filter

The Vena Tech—LGM Vena Cava Filter was introduced by LGM (B. Braun Bethlehem, PA) in 1985 and received U.S. Food and Drug Administration approval in 1991.[13] It is unique in that it is constructed of a biocompatible metal known as Phynox, which is made up of cobalt, chromium, iron, nickel, and molybdenum. It has a six-leg conical design with six vertical stabilizing struts. The filter's self-centering design and low profile make it easy to place. The device has excellent clot-trapping efficiency and lacks ferromagnetic activity, thus producing only minimal MRI artifacts.

The Vena Tech—LGM Vena Cava Filter has a low PE recurrence rate of 0% to 2%. It has a high patency rate of 92% to 97%. A principal disadvantage of the device is its incomplete opening rates of 6% to 19%. This is most often seen when using the internal jugular approach, decreasing the filter's clot-trapping efficiency. The incomplete opening can be minimized, however, by rapid deployment from the carrier system. Another disadvantage of the filter is that incomplete opening leads to increased rates of migration with reported rates up to 12%. IVC thrombosis rates for this device have been reported at 8% in initial reports and 22% to 24% on subsequent reports (by ultrasound/MRI), with clinical symptoms present in 2% to 19% of patients.

Simon-Nitinol Vena Cava Filter

The Simon-Nitinol Vena Cava Filter was introduced in 1989[15] and is composed of a titanium and nickel thermal memory alloy. This allows the filter to be preoperatively formed for navigation at cool temperatures (less than 10° C), thus allowing it to assume its predetermined filter shape at body temperature when released at the selected location. This thermal memory alloy property gives the filter the advantage of being able to be navigated through tortuous vessels. Another advantage is its narrow introducer sheath (9F), which provides the vascular specialist with more options for access. Sites such as the brachial vein and left common femoral vein can now be approached with ease.

A disadvantage to this filter is the phenomenon of caudal drop that occurs when the filter is discharged from the carrier system, making the precise final filter location difficult to establish. Symptomatic occlusion rates (7% to 11%) are higher than have been reported with Greenfield or Bird's Nest filters, and caval penetration has been reported as high as 33%. The recurrent PE rate is up to 4.8%, with an IVC thrombosis rate ranging from 7% to 11%. The alloy produces only mild MRI artifacts and is considered safe for MRI examination.

TrapEase Inferior Vena Cava Filter

One of the most recent entrants into the field of IVC filters has been the TrapEase by Cordis (Bridgewater, NJ). Also made of nitinol, it uses a symmetric double-basket design. The principal advantages of this device relate to its 6F introducer sheath and the ability to deploy it without regard to puncture site. Its symmetric design allows for deployment from both the jugular and femoral approaches. Its small and flexible sheath allows puncture of relatively small-caliber veins such as the basilic vein.[16] This feature additionally limits the risk of local complications, such as hematomas.[17] Finally the design of the TrapEase helps to prevent tilting.

Despite the advantages of the TrapEase, there are some complications. The most common of these appears to be vena cava thrombosis.[18] This concern had been reflected in our series with an early 6.9% symptomatic thrombosis rate. With its symmetric design, the filter represents a two-tiered obstacle to flow. Although this may be advantageous in improving clot trapping, it may result in worsening flow disturbances. The TrapEase filter represents a promising addition to the filter armamentarium. Its advantages in terms of deployment are undeniable. Unfortunately, the long-term results are still unknown.

Retrievable Inferior Vena Cava Filters

The first removable vena cava filter for temporary protection from PE was proposed in 1967.[19] The availability of retrievable vena cava filters has stimulated considerable clinical interest and likely has contributed to the increased overall use of filters.[20] There are two types of nonpermanent filters—temporary and retrievable. A temporary IVC filter is usually attached to tethers for stabilization and/or removal without any other means for fixation to the wall of the IVC.[21] The tethers are guidewires or catheters that are usually externalized or buried subcutaneously at a venous access site.[21] Removal of the devices should be done within 2 to 6 weeks because the tethers can develop endothelial overgrowth, which makes them difficult to remove from the wall of the IVC.

Also there is a risk of infection with temporary tethered filters if left in too long. There are no approved temporary tethered filters in the United States, but devices are available elsewhere in the world.[21]

Retrievable IVC filters are designed similarly to conventional permanent filters but with modifications to the caval attachment sites that allow retrieval using a snare or specially designed filter grasper.[22] The potential advantage is that the filter can be retrieved or left in the patient to act as a permanent filter. In the United States, the Gunther Tulip (Cook Medical Eclipse, Bloomington, IN) and the Cordis OptEase (Cordis Endovascular) have labeling for percutaneous removal.[21] The (Bard Peripheral Vascular, [Bard, Murray Hill, NJ]) the Celect (Cook Medical, Bloomington, IN) and the Option filter (Angiotech, Vancouver, BC, Canada) are three retrievable filters that have recently entered the market.[21]

The ideal time to retrieve the IVC filter is still in question. A lot of it depends on the filter design and clinical indication for the filter placement. The process of caval filter retrieval is accomplished by using a snare or grasper to anchor the end of the retrieval filter and pull it into a guiding sheath. The main concern is endothelialization in the vena cava, which incorporates the filter into the wall of the endothelium, making retrieval impossible without injuring the native vessel.[22] Burbridge et al.[23] demonstrated that endothelialization can develop as soon as 2 weeks after IVC filter placement.

Currently Available Retrievable Inferior Vena Cava Filters

The Gunther Tulip Filter

The Gunther tulip filter is a nonmagnetic filter that can be inserted via either the femoral or jugular vein route. It has the shape of a half basket, with four centering wires extending outside the basket and a curvature designed to follow the IVC wall.[22] A retrieval hook is located at the apex of the filter. To retrieve this filter, a retrieval snare in an 11F sheath is used from the right jugular vein.[22] The filter should be removed within 14 days of placement. Studies have found a filter occlusion rate of 5%.[22]

The OptEase Filter

The OptEase filter is based on the permanent version of the TrapEase filter. It is made from a single nitinol metal tube and has a double-basket design with six straight struts connecting the proximal and distal baskets. In addition, the OptEase has a set of six fixation barbs to prevent cranial migration at the cranial end of the filter. There is a hook located at the caudal end to allow retrieval via a endovascular snare. The OptEase can be deployed via a femoral, jugular, and brachial approach through a 6F delivery system. It is the only retrievable filter that can be recovered from a femoral approach. The key advantage here is that recovery from the femoral approach avoids hemopneumothorax, myocardial injury, and arrhythmias.[22]

TECHNIQUE

Dependent on the suspected DVT origin, these filters may be placed in the IVC, superior vena cava (SVC), or the iliac veins. For most filters there are three basic options for venous access, the right internal jugular vein and the right and left common femoral veins. The choice of access depends on the site and extent of the DVT. The main advantages of the femoral approach over the jugular approach are (1) averting chances of pneumothorax or hemothorax caused by an attempt at catheterization of the jugular vein, (2) avoiding arrhythmia caused by manipulation of the guidewire into the right ventricle, and (3) potential dislodging of pacemaker electrodes. On this basis, some vascular specialists would prefer the approach via the right femoral vein. However, if this is not possible because of DVT or other local problems, the left femoral or right internal jugular vein may be considered, although this has become less of an issue with the new line of filters.

The preferred location for placement of a filter in the IVC is below the level of the renal veins, but indications do exist that call for a suprarenal filter placement option. In those circumstances where pathology has progressed to the level of the renal veins, such as malignancy or thrombus, it is acceptable to place a filter in the suprarenal IVC. Suprarenal filter placement should also be considered in patients who have had renal transplants and to preclude the potential complication of the gravid uterus compressing an infrarenally placed IVC filter in women who are still fertile or are pregnant.

The vascular specialist must also remain vigilant in an effort to identify those patients in whom anatomic variations exist. For those patients with dual IVCs, it is acceptable to place appropriately selected filters into the lumen of each cava using the techniques described below. Some patients will also have an IVC of greater than 4 cm diameter. Because there are currently no filters available appropriate for placement into megacava, the vascular specialist may elect to place bilateral iliac vein filters.

It is imperative to conduct a thorough preoperative examination of the proposed venous access site, navigated vessels, and point of release. Vessel diameters, anomalies, and potential obstructions are identified to assist in selecting the appropriate filter, access site, access route, and discharge location. The newer generation of noninvasive duplex ultrasound equipment has improved the available imaging quality of scanners, resulting in the increased application of duplex ultrasound in the diagnosis and management of vascular pathologies. The advantages of duplex ultrasound in preoperative examination of the filter candidate are manifold: the mobility of the duplex ultrasound equipment allows for performance of noninvasive examination of critically ill patients examined at their bedside, while reducing overall costs. In additional, recent investigators have reported the use of intravascular ultrasound for the use of placement of IVC filters.

Inferior Vena Cava Filter Placement

After noninvasive duplex examination to determine the patency of the venous access site, a percutaneous catheterization of either the jugular or the femoral vein is performed, with the patient under local anesthesia, with an 18-gauge hollow-bore needle. Ultrasound may also be used to direct the venous puncture, especially in obese patients.

After successful catheterization of the selected vein, a guidewire is threaded through the needle and into the IVC under continuous fluoroscopic visualization. The junction between L2 and L3 is then identified and marked with a radiopaque marker. Venacavogram is performed with a pigtail catheter and power injector. The renal veins are identified along with any venous anatomic anomalies. The dilator system with attached sheath is passed over the guidewire and positioned at the desired level under fluoroscopic guidance. The dilator and guidewire are then removed, leaving the sheath in place.

With use of fluoroscopic visualization, the carrier system is advanced through the sheath and positioned below the renal veins, and the filter is then discharged. In the IVC, the filter apex should be approximately 0.5 cm below the renal veins. Both the carrier and sheath are then removed together, and gentle manual compression is applied to the puncture site until hemostasis is obtained.

Superior Vena Cava Filter Placement

When considering UEDVT as a source of potential PE, the placement of a SVC filter must be considered. Placement of the SVC filter follows the same previously described steps for the IVC filter; however, a superior venacavogram must be performed to assess the length and diameter of the SVC before discharging the filter. The SVC is usually less than 3 cm in diameter and less than 7 cm length; therefore, all of the existing filtration devices, except for the Bird's Nest, may be considered suitable for intraluminal placement if no other contraindications are present. The ideal location for positioning the filter is in the SVC proximal to the innominate vein. It is important to understand that, when placing a filter in the SVC, a femoral kit must be used for the jugular approach and a jugular kit for a femoral approach. This will permit the filter apex to be properly oriented when it is released from the carrier device. Some filter manufacturers are now producing dual-purpose kits with delivery systems that may be used for either SVC or IVC filter implantation. To prevent the blockage of needed future access routes, special consideration must also be made if simultaneous IVC and SVC filters are to be deployed. If using a jugular approach the IVC filter is to be inserted first, followed by the SVC filter. For a femoral approach the SVC filter would be first deployed, followed by the IVC filter.

AFTER THE PROCEDURE

The patient should be confined to bed rest for the first hour after successful filter placement, primarily to reduce the incidence of bleeding at the access site. As with any permanently implanted device, long-term follow-up evaluations are required. Sequential x-ray examinations at 1 month, at 6 months for the first 2 years, and then annually thereafter should be conducted and compared with previous studies to determine whether any filter migration or any other pathology is present.

Additionally, clinical examinations should be conducted to evaluate the efficacy of the filter. Particularly, duplex sonography studies should be performed to establish the presence or absence of recurrent DVT or chronic venous insufficiency. A careful patient history must be elicited to determine the presence of symptoms consistent with caval thrombosis or PE. A positive review of systems will warrant the conduct of further, more specific, clinical studies. Finally, anticoagulation therapy should be continued unless otherwise contraindicated.

CONCLUSION

Experience with vena cava filters is extensive, and, when a vascular specialist with specialized training and considerable experience in filter placement performs the procedure, complications after vena caval filter placement are minimized. Local complications at the insertion site may include bleeding, infection, femoral or jugular vein thrombosis at the insertion site, traumatic arteriovenous fistula, and major hematoma requiring a return to the operating room for evacuation and control. Although infrequent, the vascular specialist must also remain vigilant for the presence of more serious complications after vena cava filter placement. Foremost is the possibility of postprocedural PE. Other reported complications have been misplacement of the filter, migration of the filter into the heart or pulmonary artery, and cardiac arrhythmia. Incomplete or asymmetric distribution of the filter struts in the vena cava may occur, as well as entanglement of the filter struts by ensnarement on the guidewire on its extraction. The cava itself may also become thrombosed or perforated—the perforation of a vena cava filter into the duodenum years after implantation of the filter has been reported. Perforation of the abdominal aorta by vena cava filter has also been reported.

Recent and exciting innovations in the development and use of vena cava filters include routine concomitant SVC and IVC filter insertions and the prophylactic placement of temporary filters in carcinoma, trauma, pregnancy, major orthopedic surgeries, and other situations where patients are predictably at high risk for thromboembolic events. The introducer catheters for these temporary filters remain indwelling, and the filters are then retrieved in 2 to 24 weeks, after the risk of PE has been either reduced or controlled. Several ongoing studies advocate the insertion of vena cava filters at the patient's bedside, and others are evaluating the placement of vena cava filters based on duplex ultrasound criteria alone, forgoing venacavogram.

The insertion of IVC and SVC filtration devices is a safe and effective therapy to prevent thromboembolism in those patients who are refractory to anticoagulation therapy or have contraindications to anticoagulation. The necessary endovascular technique for this procedure does require specialized training, and the best results are achieved by the vascular specialist with the most experience in placing these filters.

References

1. Anderson FA Jr, Wheeler HB, Goldberg RJ, et al: A population based perspective of the hospital incidence and case-fatality rates of deep vein thrombosis and pulmonary embolism. The Worcester DVT Study, *Arch Intern Med* 151:933–938, 1991.
2. Braverman SJ, Battey PM, Smith RB III: Vena caval interruption, *Am Surg* 58:188–192, 1992.
3. Alpert JS, Dalen JE: Epidemiology and natural history of venous thromboembolism, *Prog Cardiovasc Dis* 36:417–422, 1994.
4. Juni JE, Abass A: Lung scanning in the diagnosis of pulmonary embolism: The emperor redressed, *Semin Nucl Med* 21:282–29, 1991.
5. Arcelus JI, Caprini JA, Monreal M, et al: The management and outcome of acute venous thromboembolism: a prospective registry including 4011 patients, *J Vasc Surg* 38:916–922, 2003.
6. Wakefield TW, Greenfield LJ: Diagnostic approaches and surgical treatment of deep venous thrombosis and pulmonary embolism, *Hematol Oncol Clin N Am* 7:1251–1267, 1993.
7. Horattas MC, Wright DJ, Fenton AH, Evans DM, Oddi MA, Kamienski RW, Shields EF: Changing concepts of deep venous thrombosis of the upper extremity: report of a series and review of the literature, *Surgery* 104(3):561–567, 1988.
8. Gloviczki P, Kazmier FJ, Hollier LH: Axillary-subclavian venous occlusion: the morbidity of a nonlethal disease, *J Vasc Surg* 4(4):333–337, 1986.
9. Hingorani A, Ascher E, Hanson J, et al: Upper extremity versus lower extremity deep venous thrombosis, *Am J Surg* 174 (2):214–217, 1997.
10. Monreal M, Lafoz E, Ruiz J, Valls R, Alastrue A: Upper-extremity deep venous thrombosis and pulmonary embolism. A prospective study, *Chest* 99(2):280–283, 1991.
11. Langan EM III, Miller RS, Casey WJ III, et al: Prophylactic inferior vena cava filters in trauma patients at high risk: Follow-up examination and risk/benefit assessment, *J Vasc Surg* 30 (3):484–490, 1999.
12. Hingorani A, Ascher E, Ward M, Mazzariol F, Gunduz Y, Ramsey PJ, Yorkovich W: Combined upper and lower extremity deep venous thrombosis, *Cardiovasc Surg* 9(5):472–477, 2001.
13. Enrico Ascher MD, Anil P, Hingorani MD, William R: Yorkovich WR RPA; Inferior Vena Cava Filter Placement. In Moore WS, Ahn SS, editors: *Endovascular surgery*, ed 3, Philadelphia, 2001, WB Saunders Co.
14. Greenfield L, McCurdy J, Brown P, et al: A new intracaval filter permitting continued flow and resolution of emboli, *Surgery* 73:599–606, 1973.
15. Simon M, Athanasoulis C, Kim D, et al: Simon nitinol inferior vena cava filter: initial clinical experience, *Radiology* 172:99–103, 1989.
16. Davison B, Grassi C: TrapEase inferior vena cava filter placed via the basilic arm vein: a new antecubital access, *J Vasc Interv Radiol* 13:107–109, 2002.
17. Mewissen M, Erickson S, Foley W, et al: Thrombosis at venous insertion sites after inferior vena cava filter placement, *Radiology* 173:155–157, 1989.
18. Usoh F, Hingorani A, Ascher E, et al: Prospective randomized study comparing the clinical outcomes between inferior vena cava Greenfield and TrapEase filters, J Vasc Surg 52(2):394–399, 2010.
19. Williams R, Schenk W: A removable intracaval filter for prevention of pulmonary embolism: early experience with the use of the Eichelter catheter in patients, *Surgery* 68:999–1008, 1970.
20. Quirke TE, Ritota PC, Swan KG: Inferior vena caval filter use in U.S. trauma centers: a practitioner survey, *J Trauma* 43:333–337, 1997.
21. John Kaufman: Optional Vena Cava Filters: what, why, and when, *Vascular* 15(5):304–313, 2007.
22. Lin Peter H, Bush Ruth L, Lumsden Alan B: Vena cava filters in the treatment of acute DVT, *Endovasc Today* 40–50, 2005.
23. Burbridge BE, Walker DR, Millward SF: Incorporation of the Gunther temporary inferior vena cava filter into the caval wall, *J Vasc Interv Radiol* 7:289–290, 1996.

CHAPTER

64

Pulmonary Thrombolysis

Anthony J. Comerota, Subhash Thakur

Pulmonary embolism (PE) is unique among all cardiovascular diseases because its death rate has not declined since 1970.[1] This is likely because the standard treatment for PE, anticoagulation, has not changed in most medical centers in the United States. Relatively few patients are treated with a method designed to remove the embolic obstruction from the pulmonary arteries.

In 1959, Coon and Willis[2] estimated that PE caused 47,000 deaths each year in the United States. In 1970, Hume et al[3] estimated that 142,000 patients died of PEs and another 285,000 patients had nonfatal PEs on an annual basis. In 1975, the classic paper by Dalen and Alpert[4] studied the problem of venous thromboembolism by reviewing available data. These authors estimated that of the 200,000 patients in whom PEs developed, 10% would die within 1 hour. Of the remaining 90%, the majority (70%) did not have a correct diagnosis; in this group, the mortality rate was 30%. Among the 30% who survived for longer than 1 hour and whose condition was correctly diagnosed and treated, the mortality rate dropped to 8%. Carson et al[5] prospectively followed 399 patients with PEs and demonstrated a 9.5% in-hospital mortality rate, although only 2.5% died of PE. There was a 23% 1-year mortality rate. Clinically apparent recurrent PE was found in only 8.5% of patients; however, when present, it was associated with a 45% mortality rate. Most recently, Heit et al.[6] reported that PE was responsible for more than 300,000 deaths in the United States, positioning it as a more lethal condition than acute myocardial infarction or acute stroke.

NATURAL HISTORY OF PULMONARY EMBOLISM

To appreciate the importance of proper diagnosis and treatment of any disease, one must be aware of the natural history of the disease when it is not treated. The mortality rate of untreated PE is unacceptably high. In a randomized trial of anticoagulation versus no active treatment, Barritt and Jordan[7] found a 38% mortality rate in the group receiving no treatment compared with an 8% mortality rate in patients who were anticoagulated. This randomized study was terminated early by the Data and Safety Monitoring Committee because it was considered unethical to withhold treatment from subsequent patients with PE. Other retrospective studies have demonstrated a similarly high mortality rate ranging from 18% to 32%. It became evident that, when treatment was instituted, the mortality rate fell significantly to approximately 8%.[8]

Patients dying of PEs usually die within the first several hours of the acute embolic event, frequently before therapy is given. Those who survive longer have enough cardiorespiratory reserve to compensate for the pulmonary artery obstruction caused by the acute embolus. Alternatively, in many patients the initial PE is small enough that cardiorespiratory hemodynamics are not severely compromised, and these patients are not at risk of dying unless they sustain another embolic event.

Dalen and coworkers[9] studied the response of PEs to anticoagulant therapy. Fifteen patients had PEs confirmed arteriographically. Patients were treated with anticoagulation, and follow-up pulmonary arteriograms were obtained. Eighty-seven percent of patients had more than 25% obstruction of the pulmonary vasculature remaining on follow-up pulmonary arteriography. Ninety-three percent of patients had their vena cavas ligated, and 93% were anticoagulated with heparin. Therefore the follow-up pulmonary arteriogram indicated the natural resolution of the initial PE with anticoagulation, and any residual pulmonary vascular obstruction could not be due to recurrent PE. After a 2- to 3-week follow-up, 80% of the patients continued to have angiographically persistent PE, and, perhaps more important, 73% had elevated pulmonary artery pressures. These observations from 40 years ago are useful today in helping physicians adopt proper treatment strategies for PE.

More recently, Pengo et al.[10] studied the development of chronic thromboembolic pulmonary hypertension (CTPH) in patients presenting with a first episode of PE. Patients were treated only with anticoagulation. At 6 months and at 2 years, 1% and 3.8% of patients, respectively, had CTPH. It is intuitive that if only patients with acute right-sided heart strain were studied, the percentage with CTPH would be many-fold higher. They found that risk factors for development of long-term pulmonary hypertension were previous PE (odds ratio [OR], 19), younger age (OR, 1.79 per decade), large perfusion defect (OR, 2.22 per decile), and idiopathic PE (OR, 5.7).

EARLY CLINICAL TRIALS

Two large clinical trials sponsored by the National Institutes of Health (NIH) evaluated thrombolytic therapy versus standard anticoagulation for PEs. The Urokinase Pulmonary Embolism Trial (UPET) and the Urokinase-Streptokinase Pulmonary Embolism Trial (USPET) were important studies that evaluated arteriographic, lung scanning, and hemodynamic outcome of these two treatment modalities.[11,12] In these multicenter, arteriographically confirmed prospective clinical studies, patients were randomly assigned to receive lytic therapy (streptokinase [SK] or urokinase [UK]) or anticoagulation. All patients had follow-up pulmonary arteriograms and ventilation-perfusion scans. The results demonstrated that thrombolytic therapy rapidly improved arteriographic and lung scan findings during the resolution of PE ($p < .05$). Thrombolytic therapy significantly reduced pulmonary artery and right atrial pressure. Although there was a 42% rate of bleeding complications with lytic therapy, this was mostly due to the multiple invasive procedures performed as part of the protocol. A 27% rate of bleeding complications was observed in patients receiving standard anticoagulation.

These NIH-sponsored trials demonstrated that thrombolytic therapy rapidly improved resolution of PEs, as demonstrated by arteriography and lung scans. Perhaps more important, hemodynamic status improved after lytic therapy, with significantly reduced pulmonary artery and right atrial pressures. There was no difference in mortality rate between the two treatment groups; however, death was not considered a primary end point of either study during protocol design. In addition, all patients with PEs were randomly assigned, not just those who were at risk of dying or those with hemodynamic compromise. Therefore the absence of a survival benefit does not diminish the observed merits of lytic therapy for PE. If one were to propose a 50% reduction in mortality rate in patients given treatment with lytic therapy versus anticoagulation, and if all patients with PE were to be randomly assigned to either lytic therapy or anticoagulation, approximately 1000 patients would be required in each treatment arm of such a study designed to evaluate death as a primary end point (assuming an 8% mortality rate in patients given treatment with anticoagulation).[13]

LONG-TERM FOLLOW-UP

Long-term physiologic studies following patients in the NIH-sponsored trials subsequently evaluated the basic functional unit of the lung by measuring pulmonary capillary blood volume and oxygen-diffusing capacity.[14] At 1-year follow-up, significant benefit was observed in patients receiving lytic therapy who demonstrated greater pulmonary capillary blood volume and oxygen-diffusing capacity.

In a 7-year follow-up evaluation, surviving patients were studied with right-sided heart catheterization.[15] Pulmonary artery pressures and pulmonary vascular resistance were measured with the patient at rest and exercising. Patients treated with lytic therapy had significantly lower pulmonary artery pressures and pulmonary vascular resistance both at rest and after exercise. Additionally, when patients' functional status was assessed, 73% (8 of 11) of those who were given heparin were classified as having New York Heart Association functional class III or IV disease, compared with 25% (4 of 12) of those who were given a lytic agent, indicating the adverse long-term impact of CTPH and the benefit of early lysis of hemodynamically significant PE. These studies showed that early lysis of PEs rapidly improves cardiopulmonary hemodynamics, which translates into improved oxygenation, improving the basic functional unit of the lung, resulting in less long-term morbidity.

CONTEMPORARY TRIALS OF THROMBOLYTIC THERAPY FOR PULMONARY EMBOLISM

The historical NIH trials documented early improvement in lung scan results, arteriographic findings, and pulmonary hemodynamics in patients given treatment with thrombolytic agents compared with standard anticoagulation alone. The associated bleeding complications worried physicians, however, and lytic therapy was not widely accepted.

The clinical trials performed in the 1980s and the 1990s studied the hemodynamic effects of lytic therapy in patients with PE. These trials evaluated escalating doses of bolus infusions of plasminogen activators and compared those results with standard doses and with prolonged infusion of plasminogen activators.

The development of newer lytic agents, specifically recombinant tissue plasminogen activator (rt-PA)—which was not antigenic and caused minimal, if any, allergic reaction—generated an increased interest in the use of lytic agents for PE. Furthermore, dosage regimens were explored that would maximize lytic response and minimize bleeding complications. The mechanism of action, the suggested doses, the pharmacokinetics, and the side effects of heparin, SK, UK, and rt-PA are summarized in Table 64-1.

In 1984, Petitpretz et al.[16] reported on 14 patients with acute life-threatening PE who were treated with large-dose UK delivered directly into the right atrium. Patients were given 15,000 units/kg along with continuous anticoagulation with heparin. Compared with pretreatment observations, 12 of the 14 patients showed a significant decrease in pulmonary vascular obstruction and a significant reduction in total pulmonary vascular resistance. Despite these observations, there was no significant change in their cardiac index. Although there was a 40% reduction in fibrinogen and plasminogen levels, no serious bleeding complications were observed. The majority of the hemodynamic improvement in these patients occurred within 3 hours, demonstrating the rapidity of effect of lytic therapy.

In two patients, the clinical status and the hemodynamic variables did not change, and one of these patients died. Interestingly, neither fibrinogen nor plasminogen levels changed, indicating that these two patients did not have a lytic effect from the UK.

Effect of Lytic Therapy on Lung Scan and Arteriographic Resolution

Goldhaber et al.[17] evaluated 36 patients with arteriographic PEs to document whether rt-PA produced substantial clot lysis within 6 hours. The dose was 50 mg given intravenously over a 2-hour period, and, if necessary, an additional 40 mg was given over the next 4 hours. By 6 hours, arteriographic evidence of lysis was documented in 94% of patients, with marked lysis in 67%. The fibrinogen level dropped by 30% at 2 hours and by 36% at 6 hours, but only 2 of the 36 patients experienced major bleeding complications.

Verstraete et al[18] performed a multicenter European trial to evaluate whether intrapulmonary artery infusion of rt-PA was more effective than intravenous infusion. Patients were given a 10-mg bolus of rt-PA into the pulmonary artery, and this was compared with an intravenous infusion of rt-PA of 40 mg given over a 2-hour period. On repeated pulmonary arteriography, if the patient still had a massive PE, 50 mg of rt-PA was infused over the next 5 hours. The results indicated that intrapulmonary infusion of rt-PA does not offer significant benefit over the intravenous route. Furthermore, the authors suggested that a prolonged infusion of rt-PA of 50 mg over a 7-hour period (100 mg total) is superior to a single infusion of 50 mg over 2 hours.

It should be emphasized that although Verstraete infused the rt-PA into the pulmonary artery, it was not an intrathrombus infusion. Therefore it is not surprising that infusing the plasminogen activator above (proximal to) the embolus was not superior to standard intravenous infusion.

Goldhaber et al[19] compared rt-PA, 100 mg given intravenously over 2 hours, with the accepted standard dose of UK, 2000 units/lb bolus followed by 2000 units/lb per hour for 22 hours. Sixty-eight patients were studied; 45 were randomly assigned to receive rt-PA, and 23 were randomly assigned to receive UK. The end point chosen was improvement in the 2-hour pulmonary arteriogram and the 24-hour lung scan compared with baseline studies. All patients assigned to receive rt-PA received their intended infusion, but 9 of the 23 patients receiving UK had infusions terminated prematurely (because of a significant allergy in one and bleeding complications in eight). Early clot lysis was significantly better in patients given rt-PA, as documented by means of pulmonary arteriography. At 24 hours, however, there was no difference in lung scan results between the two treatment groups. Fibrinogen levels measured at 2 and 24 hours were no different between the two groups.

In 1990, Levine et al[20] demonstrated that a short course of rt-PA infused in a dose of 0.6 mg/kg over a 2-minute period showed significant early resolution of PE compared with a saline solution placebo. Thirty-four percent of patients given treatment with rt-PA showed a 50% or more resolution in their lung scans, compared with 12% in the placebo group ($p = .026$). By day 7, however, there was no difference between the two treatment groups. The authors concluded that a very short infusion of a high concentration of rt-PA accelerates thrombolysis of acute PEs with a minimal risk of bleeding.

Dalla-Volta et al.[21] demonstrated that a short course of a high dose of rt-PA showed significant arteriographic improvement in acute PEs compared with standard anticoagulation with heparin. The investigators in the second plasminogen activator Italian multicenter study randomly assigned 36 patients to receive either rt-PA as a 10-mg bolus followed by 90 mg infused over a 2-hour period or heparin at 1750 units/hr. Arteriographic improvement was significant in the group receiving rt-PA, but there was no change in patients receiving heparin. Mean pulmonary artery pressures were significantly reduced in the lytic group and rose somewhat in

TABLE 64-1 Characteristics of Agents Used in Treatment of Pulmonary Embolism

Agent	Nature	Mechanism	Dosage	Pharmacokinetics	Side effects	Comments
Unfractionated heparin	Anionic polysaccharide of alternating iduronate and glucosamine (—sulfated glycosaminoglycan)	Inhibition of antithrombin III, factor Xa, and factor IIa (thrombin)	5000-10,000 units IV bolus + 1000-2000 units/hr IV	Metabolized in reticuloendothelial system; excreted in urine, mainly as metabolites but also unchanged; half-life = 1-6 hr, average 1.5 hr	Hemorrhage, thrombocytopenia, allergy, ↑ aldosterone with ↑ K^+, alopecia, and osteoporosis on prolonged use	Concomitant antihemostatics, NSAIDs ↑ bleeding; check serum K^+ and PLT every second day
Low-molecular-weight heparin	Obtained by depolymerization of natural heparin from porcine intestinal mucosa	Inhibition of factor Xa and IIa via antithrombin	1 mg/kg subcutaneoulsy	Eliminated by kidney, half-life = 4.5 hr	Bleeding, anemia, thrombocytopenia, elevation of serum aminotransferase, diarrhea, nausea	Reduce dose in renal failure
SK	A protein from culture filtrate of *Streptococcus hemolyticus* group C	Complexes and activates plasma- and fibrin-bound plasminogen to plasmin	250,000 units IV/30 min + 100,000 units/hr for 24-72 hr	Cleared by both reticuloendothelial cells (initial) and SK-specific antibodies (later); half-life = 23 min	Hemorrhage, allergy, Guillain-Barré syndrome	Titrate dose with 2-4 times normal thrombin clotting time
UK	An enzyme initially from human urine, now cultured from human kidney cells	Directly converts plasminogen to plasmin	IV, 4400 units/kg per hour + 4400 units/kg per hour for 12 hr	Rapidly cleared by liver; half-life = 20 min	Hemorrhage; allergy less common than with SK	4400 units/kg = 2000 CTA units/lb (CTA units are obsolete)
rt-PA	Glycosylated protein of 527 residues with AA sequence of human t-PA	Activates fibrin-bound plasminogen to plasmin	100 mg IV in 2 hr	Metabolized by liver; half-life of rt-PA is 26.5-46 min; half-life of t-PA is 17-20 min	Hemorrhage; allergy less common than with SK and UK	t-PA will precipitate when diluted to <0.5 mg/dL in 5% dextrose in water; t-PA is incompatible with dopamine, dobutamine, or heparin
Reteplase	A nonglycosylated t-PA with 355 residues produced by *Escherichia coli*	Catalyzes cleavage of endogenous plasminogen to plasmin	Two 10-unit IV boluses, given 30 min apart	Metabolized by kidney and liver, half-life = 13-16 min	Bleeding, allergic reactions	Incomplete binding to fibrin leads to better clot penetration
Tenecteplase (Metalyse)	Glycosylated protein of 527 residues modified at three sites using Chinese hamster ovary cells	Activates fibrin-bound plasminogen to plasmin	Weight-based, 6000-10,000 unit single dose	Eliminated by liver, half-life = 65-132 min	Bleeding, nausea, vomiting, hypotension, anaphylaxis	Not compatible with dextrose solutions, resistant to inactivation by its endogenous inhibitor (PAI-1) compared to native t-PA

AA, Amino acid, *CTA*, Committee on Thrombolytic Agents; *IV*, intravenous; *K^+*, potassium; *NSAIDs*, nonsteroidal antiinflammatory drugs; *PLT*, platelet; *rt-PA*, recombinant tissue plasminogen activator; *SK*, streptokinase; *t-PA*, tissue plasminogen activator.

those patients given treatment with heparin. There was no difference in bleeding complications.

Meyer et al.[22] reported the results of the European study group for PEs, comparing the rt-PA regimen of a 10-mg bolus followed by 90 mg over the next 2 hours with UK given in a 4400 unit/kg bolus followed by 4400 units/kg over the next 12 hours. Sixty-three patients were randomly assigned, 29 to receive UK and 34 to receive rt-PA. The investigators found more rapid resolution at 2 hours in the patients receiving rt-PA; however, at the 12-hour point, arteriographic resolution and the decrease in pulmonary vascular resistance were equivalent in the two groups. Bleeding complications were also equivalent.

Goldhaber et al.[23] compared an equivalently high dose of UK with 100 mg of rt-PA given over the same time course. Ninety patients with PE were randomly allocated to receive either 100 mg of rt-PA given over a 2-hour period or UK, 3 million units given as a 1 million—unit bolus followed by 2 million units infused over the next 2 hours. Eighty-seven patients underwent repeated pulmonary arteriography after the 2-hour infusion. Arteriographic improvement was comparable in the two groups, with 79% of patients receiving rt-PA and 67% of patients receiving UK showing significant improvement. The mean change in the lung scans was similar in the two groups at 24 hours. Three patients had intracranial bleeding, two in the group receiving rt-PA and one in the group receiving UK.

Effect of Lytic Therapy on Cardiopulmonary Hemodynamics

As mentioned earlier, the NIH-sponsored trials demonstrated significantly reduced pulmonary artery and right atrial pressures in patients receiving lytic therapy versus anticoagulation. These early observations translated into long-term benefit when, after 1 year, lytic patients had improved pulmonary capillary blood volume and O_2 diffusion capacity and, after 7 years, had lower pulmonary artery pressures and pulmonary vascular resistance at rest and after exercise.

Goldhaber et al.[24] compared the effects of thrombolytic therapy on ventricular function and pulmonary perfusion with the effects of anticoagulation alone. One hundred one patients were randomly assigned to receive rt-PA infused at 100 mg over a 2-hour period, and 55 patients were given heparin. Thirty-nine percent of patients receiving rt-PA, compared with 17% of patients given heparin, had improvement in right ventricular wall motion (p=.005). There was significantly improved pulmonary perfusion in the group receiving rt-PA. Interestingly, in the heparin-treated group, two patients had subsequent fatal PE, and three had nonfatal PE.

European Multicenter Registry and Randomized Trial

The results of a multicenter registry for PE are helpful in placing thrombolytic therapy for PE into proper perspective. Konstantinides et al[25] evaluated the results of lytic therapy for PE in patients who were hemodynamically stable. The overall 30-day mortality rate was significantly lower in the 169 patients who received thrombolytic agents than in the 550 patients receiving anticoagulation alone (4.7% vs. 11.1%, p = .016). Primary thrombolysis was the only independent predictor of survival that reached statistical significance (p = .051) on multivariate analysis (OR, 0.46; 95% confidence interval, 0.21 to 1.00). The 30-day mortality rate after primary thrombolysis was also lower than for anticoagulation if patients were defined on the basis of presenting characteristics, such as age (younger than 65 years, 3.0% for primary thrombolysis vs. 9.2% for anticoagulation; older than 65 years, 7.1% for primary thrombolysis vs. 12.6% for anticoagulation), arterial hypotension (4.4% for primary thrombolysis vs. 14.9% for anticoagulation), arterial normotension (5.0% for primary thrombolysis vs. 8.1% for anticoagulation), syncope (4.4% for primary thrombolysis vs. 17.9% for anticoagulation), no syncope (4.9% for primary thrombolysis vs. 8.9% for anticoagulation), no recent major surgery (2.9% for primary thrombolysis vs. 12.3% for anticoagulation), and right ventricular enlargement on echocardiography (4.7% for primary thrombolysis vs. 11.1% for anticoagulation). The mortality rate was higher with thrombolytics than with heparin in patients after surgery (12.5% vs. 7.6%, respectively). The clinical factors that were associated with a higher mortality rate for both groups were the presence or the absence of syncope (14.4% vs. 7.8%; p = .12), arterial hypotension (12.6% vs. 3.7%; p = 0.021), congestive heart failure (13.9% vs. 7.7%; p = .013), and chronic pulmonary disease (17.1% vs. 8.8%; p = 0.032). Among the other adverse effects, the incidence of major bleeding was higher with thrombolytics than with heparin (21.9% vs. 7.8%, respectively), whereas the incidence of recurrent PE was lower (7.7% vs. 18.7%, respectively; p <.001). The latter was more common in patients with evidence of proximal deep vein thrombosis (17.2% vs. 11.4%, respectively; p = .06) and the echocardiographic presence of right-sided thrombi (26.7% vs. 15.7%, respectively; p = .09). Two cases of intracranial bleeding and one hemorrhagic death occurred in each group.

Konstantinides et al.[26] followed up with a randomized trial of patients with acute submassive PE who were hemodynamically stable. They randomly assigned their patients to heparin versus heparin plus 100 mg of alteplase infused over a 2-hour period. The primary end point was in-hospital death or clinical deterioration requiring an escalation of treatment, defined as the addition of pressors, secondary thrombolysis, endotracheal intubation, cardiopulmonary resuscitation, or emergency mechanical embolectomy, either catheter based or surgical. Two hundred fifty-six patients were randomly assigned, 118 to lytic therapy and 138 to anticoagulation alone. The anticoagulation-alone–treated patients had a significantly higher incidence of reaching the primary end point ($p = .006$). The 30-day event-free survival was significantly higher in the lytic therapy group ($p = .005$). Escalation of treatment was required in 25% of the anticoagulation-alone patients versus 10% in the lytic group ($p = .004$). Mortality was low in both groups (3.4%, anticoagulation alone; 2.2%, lytic therapy) and not different. No fatal bleeding or intracranial bleeding occurred in patients receiving lytic therapy.

The authors concluded that in patients with submassive PE, defined by right-ventricular dysfunction, right-ventricular enlargement, and evidence of elevated pulmonary artery pressures, lytic therapy significantly improved 30-day event-free survival. Long-term follow-up has not yet been reported from this patient sample.

Catheter-Based Pharmacomechanical Embolectomy

Most of the patients with PE can be treated effectively with systemic thrombolysis. However, some patients have major relative contraindications and others have absolute contraindications to systemic thrombolysis. Such patients with massive PE are at risk of hemodynamic deterioration and death if their cardiopulmonary hemodynamics are not improved.

Greenfield et al.[27] were the first to develop a catheter-based method to remove large PEs. This technique saved the lives of some; however, it was not widely accepted because of its cumbersome design.

Catheter-based fragmentation and aspiration were recently reported by Eid-Lidt et al.[28] when they reported results of 18 patients presenting with massive PE and right ventricular dysfunction. All patients underwent thrombus fragmentation with use of a pigtail catheter with subsequent thrombus aspiration in 13. They demonstrated that hemodynamic, arteriographic, and blood oxygen concentrations significantly improved after the procedure. The patients' systolic blood pressure improved, and there was a significant decrease in mean pulmonary artery pressure. In-hospital major complications were 11%; one patient died of refractory shock and one patient had an intracranial hemorrhage. However, the patient with intracranial hemorrhage had minor neurologic sequelae. Patients were not treated with thrombolytic therapy. There was no cardiovascular death or recurrent pulmonary thromboembolism during a mean follow-up of 12.3 months.

As technology advanced and our understanding of the use of plasminogen activators improved, it is clear that fragmentation of PEs after infusion of small doses of plasminogen activators can rapidly reduce pulmonary hypertension. Subsequent lysis of the fragmented thrombus further improves pulmonary perfusion and reduces pulmonary artery hypertension.

Twenty-five patients with hemodynamically important PEs were treated by Tajima et al.[29] with a modified rotational pigtail catheter. After embolic disruption, 13 mg of rt-PA was injected into the affected pulmonary arteries followed by manual clot aspiration. All patients survived, and their clinical status improved. After treatment, a pulmonary arteriography showed improved perfusion, resulting in a significant reduction in the mean pulmonary artery pressure and arteriographic score.

Zeni et al.[30] combined the infusion of plasminogen activators with rheolytic thrombectomy in 17 patients. Immediate angiographic improvement with relief of symptoms occurred in 16 of 17 patients. Fifteen patients survived the initial hospitalization, and 13 were alive 19 months later. Chauhan et al.[31] treated 14 patients with large PEs with rheolytic thrombectomy who had contraindications for systemic thrombolysis. Successful treatment occurred in 12 of the 14 patients. The 11 survivors reported significant improvement of symptoms.

Twenty-five patients with PEs were treated by Margheri et al.[32] with rheolytic thrombectomy. All patients were managed successfully with reduced pulmonary artery obstruction, improved perfusion, and improved arteriographic scores ($p < .001$). Four of the 25 patients died during their hospitalization. Twenty of the 21 remaining patients were alive after a mean follow-up of 61 months. Although mechanical pulmonary embolic fragmentation is possible in high-risk patients and reduces pulmonary artery pressure, clinical observation supports the contention that the combination of pulsed plasminogen activator solution into the thrombus during fragmentation is likely to yield better short-term and long-term results. Small doses (5-10 mg) of rt-PA diluted into a relatively large volume of saline solution and infused into the embolus are unlikely to cause bleeding complications yet offer the opportunity of clot dissolution after fragmentation as a result of the plasminogen activator penetrating the thrombus and binding to fibrin-bound plasminogen.

We have observed gratifying results in a small number of patients with massive PEs treated with rheolytic thrombectomy who had major contraindications to systemic thrombolysis (Figure 64-1). Pulse-spray fibrinolytic infusion during and/or after mechanical fragmentation of the thrombus rapidly restores cardiopulmonary hemodynamics and pulmonary perfusion and improves oxygenation.

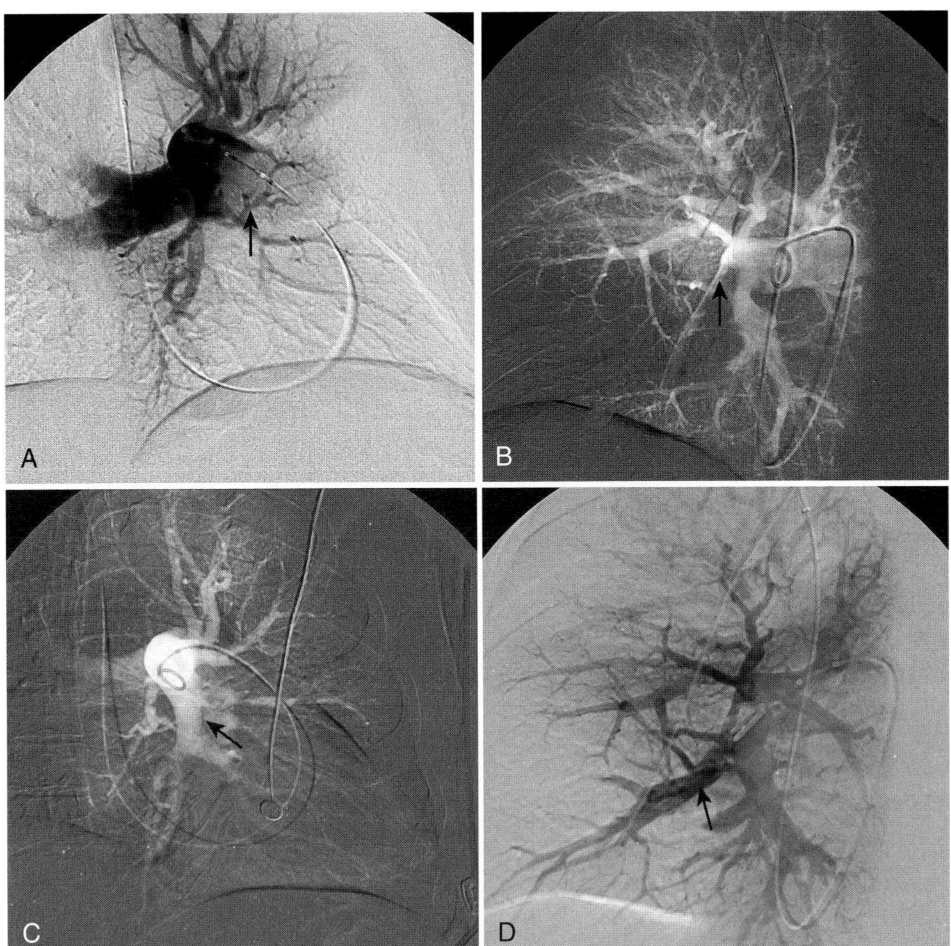

FIGURE 64-1 **A** and **B**, Marked dyspnea, hypoxia, tachycardia, and hypotension developed in a patient being treated for massive gastrointestinal bleeding, *(arrows)*. After treatment with rheolytic thrombectomy, (**C** and **D**) the patient had significantly improved pulmonary artery perfusion *(arrows)* improved oxygenation with resolution of dyspnea, and restored normal hemodynamics.

SUMMARY

Patients with PEs that raise pulmonary artery pressures to the points of affecting right-ventricular function have a substantially higher risk of hospital mortality and 1-year mortality. They also face a high risk of chronic thromboembolic pulmonary hypertension with its associated increased morbidity and mortality. As a result, all patients with PEs should be evaluated with a cardiac echocardiogram, assessing pulmonary artery pressure and right-ventricular function. Patients demonstrating abnormalities of the right side of the heart, such as right-ventricular dilation, deviation of the septum, tricuspid insufficiency, and documented pulmonary hypertension, should be considered for systemic thrombolytic therapy or catheter-based fragmentation with thrombolysis. Our treatment algorithm is summarized in Figure 64-2. This offers patients the best chance of restoration of cardiopulmonary hemodynamics with

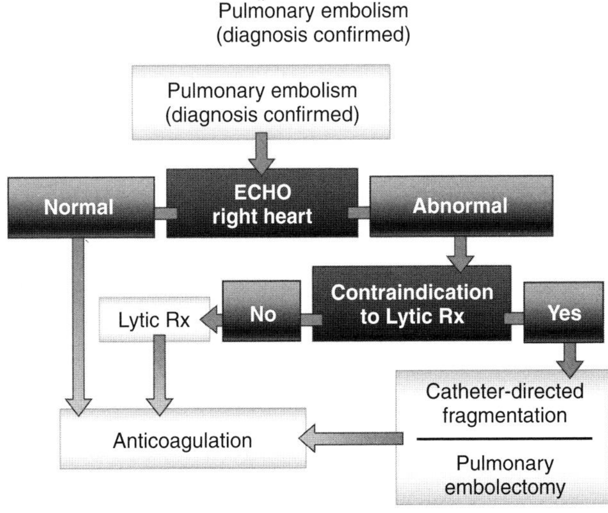

FIGURE 64-2 Treatment strategy for pulmonary embolism.

TABLE 64-2 Morbidity and Mortality at 0 to 24 Hours and 24 Hours to Follow-Up*

	ALL/Fe	Minor bleed		Major bleed		Vessel access bleed		IC bleed		Recurrent PE		Mortality		Survived		FU range
Drug	**24 hr**	**24 hr**	**FU**	**24 hr**	**FU**	**24 hr**	**FU**	**24 hr**	**FU**	**24 hr**	**FU**	**24 hr**	**FU**	**24 hr**	**FU**	**Days**
UK	7.6	37.1	18.0	12.3	2.6	34.2	13.3	0.7	0.3	2.6	8.9	1.6	8.8	97.9	90.4	8-365
SK	19.2	23.1	20.8	8.5	0.0	22.3	6.9	0.0	0.0	2.6	3.5	0.0	8.5	100	91.5	3-365
t-PA	1.7	30.0	6.8	8.8	0.9	10.8	0.0	0.9	0.0	0.6	3.6	1.4	4.0	98.6	95.3	2-365
Mean	6.8	31.2	16.2	10.1	1.2	20.4	6.3	0.6	0.1	1.5	5.9	1.3	6.9	98.6	92.7	–
Heparin	0.6	5.5	6.4	5.5	5.5	4.8	5.5	1.1	1.3	2.2	17.0	2.2	6.0	97.8	92.7	3-365
Total	0.6	5.5	6.4	5.5	5.5	4.8	5.5	1.1	1.3	2.2	17.0	2.2	6.0	97.8	92.7	–

Data from references 9, 10, 14, and 19-28.
*Six patients in UK group and five in heparin group were lost during the 1-year follow-up in the Urokinase Pulmonary Embolism Trial.
ALL, Allergy; *Fe*, fever; *FU*, follow-up; *IC*, intracranial; *PE*, pulmonary embolism; *SK*, streptokinase; *t-PA*, tissue plasminogen activator; *UK*, urokinase.

TABLE 64-3 Percentage Mortality by Cause 0 Hours to Follow-up*

Drug	Deaths	PE	Recurrent PE	Cancer	IC bleed	Others†	Follow-up, days
UK	10.0	2.7	0.5	0.5	0.5	3.7	1-365
SK	8.5	1.3	0.0	0.0	0.0	2.6	1-365
t-PA	4.8	1.1	0.6	0.9	0.3	2.0	1-365
Mean	7.8	1.6	0.6	0.7	0.4	2.8	–
Heparin	7.3	2.3	2.3	0.0	0.6	2.3	1-365
Mean	7.3	2.3	2.3	0.0	0.6	2.3	–

Data from references 9, 10, 14, and 19-28.
*Six patients in UK group and five in heparin group were lost during the 1-year follow-up in the Urokinase Pulmonary Embolism Trial.
†Others include deaths due to cardiac, cerebral thromboembolic, hemorrhagic, or investigatory complications.
IC, Intracranial; *PE*, pulmonary embolism; *SK*, streptokinase; *t-PA*, tissue plasminogen activator; *UK*, urokinase.

the lowest risk of complications and long-term chronic thromboembolic pulmonary hypertension.

Bleeding complications are the greatest concern, and, of the bleeding complications, intracranial hemorrhage is the most feared (Table 64-2). Evaluation of available data indicates that the true risk of intracranial bleeding is approximately 0.7% to 1.1%.

To treat significant bleeding complications, we would suggest infusing 8 to 10 units of cryoprecipitate followed by 2 units of fresh frozen plasma. Epsilon-aminocaproic acid in a dose of 5 mg can be given intravenously to neutralize any ongoing fibrinolytic effect. Overall mortality by cause (e.g., PE, complication of treatment, cancer, or other) is summarized in Table 64-3.

References

1. Anderson FA Jr, Wheeler HB, Goldberg RJ, et al: A population-based perspective of the hospital incidence and case-fatality rates of venous thrombosis and pulmonary embolism: the Worcester DVT Study, *Arch Intern Med* 151:933–938, 1991.
2. Coon WW, Willis PW: Deep venous thrombosis and pulmonary embolism: prediction, prevention and treatment, *Am J Cardiol* 4:611–616, 1959.
3. Hume M, Sevitt S, Thomas DP: *Venous Thrombosis and Pulmonary Embolism*, Cambridge, MA, 1970, Harvard University Press.
4. Dalen JE, Alpert JS: Natural history of pulmonary embolism, *Prog Cardiovasc Dis* 17:257–270, 1975.
5. Carson JL, Kelly MA, Duff A, et al: The clinical course of pulmonary embolism, *N Engl J Med* 326:1240–1244, 1992.
6. Heit JA, Cohen A, Anderson FJ: Estimated annual number of incident and recurrent, non-fatal and fatal venous thromboembolism (VTE) events in the US, *Blood* 106:267A, 2005.
7. Barritt DW, Jordan SC: Anticoagulant drugs in the treatment of pulmonary embolism: a controlled clinical trial, *Lancet* 1:1309–1313, 1960.
8. Alpert JS, Smith R, Carlson CJ, et al: Mortality in patients treated for pulmonary embolism, *JAMA* 236:1477–1480, 1976.
9. Dalen JE, Banas JS Jr, Brooks HL, et al: Resolution rate of acute pulmonary embolism in man, *N Engl J Med* 280:1194–1199, 1969.
10. Pengo V, Lensing AW, Prins MH, et al: Incidence of chronic thromboembolic pulmonary hypertension after pulmonary embolism, *N Engl J Med* 350:2257–2264, 2004.
11. Sasahara AA, Hyers TM: The Urokinase Pulmonary Embolism Trial. A national cooperative study, *Circulation* 39. SII-1, 1973.
12. Urokinase Pulmonary Embolism Trial Study Group: Urokinase-streptokinase embolism trial: Phase 2 results: a cooperative study, *JAMA* 229:1606–1613, 1974.
13. Anderson DR, Levine MN: Thrombolytic therapy for the treatment of acute pulmonary embolism, *Can Med Assoc J* 146: 1317–1325, 1992.

14. Sharma GVRK, Burleson VA, Sashara AA: Effect of thrombolytic therapy on pulmonary-capillary blood volume in patients with pulmonary embolism, *N Engl J Med* 303:842–845, 1980.
15. Sharma GVRK, Foland ED, McIntyre KM, et al: Longterm hemodynamic benefit of thrombolytic therapy in pulmonary embolic disease [abstract], *J Am Coll Cardiol* 15:65A, 1990.
16. Petitpretz P, Simmoneau G, Cerrina J, et al: Effects of a single bolus of urokinase in patients with life-threatening pulmonary emboli: a descriptive trial, *Circulation* 80:861–866, 1984.
17. Goldhaber SZ, Vaughn DE, Markis JE, et al: Acute pulmonary embolism treated with tissue plasminogen activator, *Lancet* 2:886–889, 1986.
18. Verstraete M, Miller GAH, Bounameaux H, et al: Intravenous and intrapulmonary recombinant tissue-type plasminogen activator in the treatment of acute massive pulmonary embolism, *Circulation* 77:353–360, 1988.
19. Goldhaber SZ, Kessler CM, Heit J, et al: Randomised controlled trial of recombinant tissue plasminogen activator versus urokinase in the treatment of acute pulmonary embolism, *Lancet* 2:293–298, 1988.
20. Levine MN, Hirsh J, Weitz J, et al: A randomized trial of a single bolus dosage regimen of recombinant tissue plasminogen activator in patients with acute pulmonary embolism, *Chest* 98:1473–1479, 1990.
21. Dalla-Volta S, Palla A, Santolicandro A, et al: PAIMS 2: alteplase combined with heparin versus heparin in the treatment of acute pulmonary embolism. Plasminogen activator Italian multicenter study 2, *J Am Coll Cardiol* 20:520–526, 1992.
22. Meyer G, Sors H, Charbonnier B, et al: Effects of intravenous urokinase versus alteplase on total pulmonary resistance in acute massive pulmonary embolism: a European multicenter doubleblind trial. The European Cooperative Study Group for Pulmonary Embolism, *J Am Coll Cardiol* 19: 239–245, 1992.
23. Goldhaber SZ, Kessler CM, Heit J, et al: Recombinant tissue-type plasminogen activator versus a novel dosing regimen of urokinase in acute pulmonary embolism: a randomized controlled multicenter trial, *J Am Coll Cardiol* 20:24–30, 1992.
24. Goldhaber SZ, Haire WD, Feldstein ML, et al: Alteplase versus heparin in acute pulmonary embolism: randomised trial assessing right-ventricular function and pulmonary perfusion, *Lancet* 341:507–511, 1993.
25. Konstantinides S, Geibel A, Olschewski M, et al: Association between thrombolytic treatment and the prognosis of hemodynamically stable patients with major pulmonary embolism: results of a multicenter registry, *Circulation* 96:882–888, 1997.
26. Konstantinides S, Geibel A, Heusel G, et al: Heparin plus alteplase compared with heparin alone in patients with submassive pulmonary embolism, *N Engl J Med* 347:1143–1150, 2002.
27. Greenfield LJ, Bruce TA, Nichols NB: Transvenous pulmonary embolectomy by catheter device, *Ann Surg* 174:881–886, 1971.
28. Eid-Lidt G, Gaspar J, Sandoval J, et al: Combined clot fragmentation and aspiration in patients with acute pulmonary embolism, *Chest* 134:54–60, 2008.
29. Tajima H, Murata S, Kumazaki T, et al: Hybrid treatment of acute massive pulmonary thromboembolism: mechanical fragmentation with a modified rotating pigtail catheter, local fibrinolytic therapy, and clot aspiration followed by systemic fibrinolytic therapy, *AJR Am J Roentgenol* 183:589–595, 2004.
30. Zeni PT, Blank BG, Peeler DW: Use of rheolytic thrombectomy in treatment of acute massive pulmonary embolism, *J Vasc Interv Radiol* 14:1511–1515, 2003.
31. Chauhan MS, Kawamura A: Percutaneous rheolytic thrombectomy for large pulmonary embolism: a promising treatment option, *Catheter Cardiovasc Interv* 70:121–128, 2007.
32. Margheri M, Vittori G, Vecchio S, et al: Early and long-term clinical results of AngioJet rheolytic thrombectomy in patients with acute pulmonary embolism, *Am J Cardiol* 101:252–258, 2008.

CHAPTER

65

Axillosubclavian Vein Thrombectomy, Thrombolysis, and Angioplasty

Samuel S. Ahn, Milton Conley, Justin S. Ahn

Compression at the thoracic outlet has both neurogenic and vascular components. The vast majority of compressive symptoms are neurogenic and are related to the brachial plexus. Only a minority of patients present with symptoms associated with the axillosubclavian artery and vein. The clinician must be aware that neurologic and vascular symptoms can coexist. The discussion in this chapter is limited to compressive problems of the axillosubclavian vein, as well as venous thrombosis of this segment caused by various catheters.

Axillosubclavian vein thrombosis (ASVT) can be divided into primary and secondary types. *Primary thrombosis* is due to external venous compression and trauma from a restrictive thoracic outlet. This is commonly known as Paget-Schroetter syndrome. Another often-used term is "effort thrombosis," which describes the frequent temporal relationship to upper-extremity exertion. Historically, Paget (in London) in 1875 and Von Schroetter (in Vienna) in 1884 independently described a syndrome of thrombosis involving the axillosubclavian vein.[1,2] In 1949, Hughes reviewed 320 cases of upper-extremity venous thrombosis that were collected from the medical literature.[3] Aware that this entity had been described previously, he named the condition Paget-Schroetter syndrome.

Secondary thrombosis is a relatively new phenomenon. Before 1950, almost all reports discussed primary thrombosis. With the advent and the common use of indwelling subclavian catheters, iatrogenically induced secondary ASVT has been known to occur. The cause is intimal injury by a foreign body, resulting in a localized area of increased thrombogenicity. Secondary venous thrombosis is associated with the presence of pacemakers, invasive monitoring with central lines and pulmonary artery catheters, and the presence of long-term indwelling venous catheters for dialysis and administration of hyperalimentation, antibiotics, and chemotherapeutic agents. Uncommon causes of ASVT include posttraumatic fibrosis, significant callus formation resulting from clavicular fracture, malignancies (breast, lung, and lymphoma) that result in extrinsic compression, radiation, and hypercoagulation states.

PAGET-SCHROETTER SYNDROME

Anatomy

Anatomically, the subclavian vein is the most anterior vascular structure of the thoracic outlet. It is bound anteriorly by the subclavius muscle and posteriorly by the anterior scalene muscle. The subclavian artery and the brachial plexus lie posteriorly between the anterior and the middle scalene muscles, which insert on the posterior-lateral aspect of the first rib. There may also be congenital bands and fibrous slips interdigitating with the neurovascular structures. Mechanical compression of the brachial plexus and the subclavian artery and vein between the first rib and the musculotendinous insertions is the principal cause of symptoms.

The primary abnormality of Paget-Schroetter syndrome involves the costoclavicular portion of the axillosubclavian vein. Compression occurs between the hypertrophied anterior scalene, the subclavius tendon, and the first rib. Venous thrombosis almost invariably occurs in this area. A less frequent, but recently discovered abnormality involves what researchers believe to be the subclavius posticus muscle, an aberrant muscle connecting the sternal end of the first rib and superior margin of the scapula. Found unilaterally in 11 out of 124 Japanese cadavers, the muscle runs along the anterior surface of the subclavian vein, crosses over the brachial plexus, and should be considered, particularly in cases of venous compression.[4]

History and Physical Examination

Paget-Schroetter syndrome is most commonly a result of excessive and unusual use of the arm. It occurs predominantly in the right upper extremity in males. It is noted that neurogenic thoracic outlet syndrome is more common in females. Frequently, patients are young and are engaged in athletic activities. Laborers performing strenuous work involving the upper extremities are also a significant patient group. A minority of patients are sedentary.

Patients note acute swelling, pain, and cyanosis, often after excessive use of the arm. Chronically, patients will complain of arm discomfort and the sensation of heaviness, which is made worse by activity and is relieved by rest.

Physical examination results vary according to the interval between the event and the initial evaluation. An acute presentation is frequently characterized by significant pain and edema. A chronic presentation may have few physical findings and may even show normal findings because of the development of venous collaterals. These collaterals can sometimes be appreciated on examination of the shoulder and the hemithorax. There may also be increased prominence of the veins of the hand and the forearm.

Patients with an unimpressive physical examination result may be requested to perform exacerbating exercises. The patient may complain of arm pain during these maneuvers, and the examiner may note a slight duskiness of the hand and the arm and increased venous prominence. Venous tenderness may be present. These signs and symptoms tend to resolve quite rapidly with cessation of the activity.

It is appropriate to note that, after more than half a century, Hughes' original description is still very accurate:

> Swelling is the usual initial complaint involving the whole arm from fingers to the shoulder, and frequently the lower neck or breast is involved. The swollen arm, while firm, rarely pits with finger pressure. The skin of the afflicted extremity is slightly cyanotic but may be mottled, and this coloration is more obvious in the hand and lower part of the forearm. Superficial veins are more prominent than usual as they act to form collateral circulation.[3]

Diagnosis

An initial noninvasive workup should be considered. The most common noninvasive modalities are duplex scanning, computed tomography, and magnetic resonance imaging.

Ultrasound imaging is fast, inexpensive, and safe, although its reliability has been questioned. Color duplex imaging is the most accurate study; however, its limitations must be understood. For example, visualization of part of the subclavian vein may be hampered by the overlying clavicle. Anatomically, the axillary vein, the distal subclavian vein, and sometimes the central subclavian vein may be visualized and may be amenable to compression. Noncompressible veins indicate that thrombus is present. The proximal subclavian and the innominate veins cannot be compressed because of their intrathoracic location. Sometimes echogenic thrombus may be visualized even when the venous segment is not accessible to compression. A nonobstructing thrombus is seen as a filling defect within a color-filled lumen. Complete obstruction shows an absence of color in the segment that is thrombosed. Absence of flow phases during respiration, abnormal waveforms, and prominent collaterals also suggest thrombosis.[5] The accuracy of this test depends on the skill and the familiarity of the operator and the radiologist.

The gold standard is venography, but this test carries the risk of renal contrast agent toxicity and allergic reactions. It is the most accurate modality in diagnosing short-segment stenoses and webs and can define the precise location and the extent of the occlusive process. Optimal visualization is obtained by injection of dye into the basilic vein, because contrast agent injected into the cephalic vein may bypass the axillary vein and flow into collaterals. Supine venography should be performed first with the arm at the side, followed by 90-degree abduction. It is common for thrombosis to extend from the jugular-subclavian junction centrally to the axillary and the brachial veins peripherally. Prominent venous collaterals are also often visualized.

Treatment

In Paget's original article, the patient was treated with a milk diet, leeches, mercury, and chalk with reportedly satisfactory results.[1] Since that time, improved methods have been developed.

Initial attempts to clear the venous obstruction included thrombectomy with patch angioplasty closure.[6] This had a high failure rate because of the thrombogenicity of the venous segment and the danger of maintaining anticoagulation in the immediate postoperative period. Surgical thrombectomy combined with thoracic outlet decompression was reported to have improved results.[7] In addition, the use of polytetrafluoroethylene bypass grafts from the axillary to the internal jugular veins has met with some success.[8] The jugular-subclavian vein bypass has been well described and is quite durable, especially with the addition of a radial artery-to-vein fistula.[9,10]

Currently, the majority of cases are best treated medically initially (e.g., via thrombolysis and anticoagulation), followed by surgical decompression of the thoracic outlet.[11-13] Endovascular intervention is performed if significant residual stenosis remains. Surgical bypass is reserved for refractory cases.

Anticoagulation

For many years, the accepted nonoperative method of treatment of ASVT was arm elevation in conjunction with heparin anticoagulation on a short-term basis, followed by long-term warfarin administration.[7,14] With this regimen, complete recovery was uncommon. Residual symptoms were reported in 40% to 85% of patients.[7,15,16] Disability can be significant, with chronic swelling, pain, and even ulceration. This is most likely because heparinization may prevent propagation of thrombus into the collateral circulation but will rarely result in clearing of the obstructive clot.

Thrombolytic Therapy

Catheter-directed thrombolytic therapy has become the treatment of choice for patients who are candidates for this procedure. These powerful lytic agents act by converting plasminogen to plasmin. Plasmin, a nonspecific serine protease, breaks down the fibrin in clots to soluble fibrin degradation products.

Urokinase was the most studied and most used thrombolytic agent for peripheral arterial and venous disease. Because of quality-control problems, however, it is no longer available in the United States, which has left a void in the thrombolytic armamentarium. Other thrombolytic drugs are available, and it is incumbent on the vascular surgeon to become familiar with these agents. Thrombolytic agents have been some of the most studied drugs in the history of medicine, but significant controversy still exists regarding their optimal method of administration. Most studies of venous disease involve treatment of deep venous thrombosis of the iliofemoral system. These dosage recommendations may be appropriate for upper-extremity venous thrombosis; however, consistent information from large studies is lacking. Therapy must be individualized, and the clinician must consult the most current pharmacologic data to determine the appropriate dosage protocol. A brief summary of available thrombolytic agents follows.

Streptokinase (SK) was the first thrombolytic agent to be developed. It is a single-chain nonenzymatic protein derived from β-hemolytic streptococci. Its pharmacokinetics are complex. SK initially binds with plasminogen, which then reacts with unbound plasminogen to cleave to plasmin. This can result in an unpredictable dose response. Pyrogenic and allergic reactions are common. SK is not as efficient in clot lysis as the newer agents; however, its one advantage is that it is relatively less expensive.

Tissue plasminogen activator (t-PA) is a naturally occurring enzyme thought to originate from vascular endothelium, although it is measurable in all human tissues. Pharmacologically, it is produced by recombinant DNA technology (rt-PA). It is a direct plasminogen activator and has more clot selectivity than SK. Its dose response is more predictable, and allergic reactions are rare. It is significantly more expensive than SK. Rt-PA and urokinase have been shown to be equally safe and effective for treating spontaneous axillosubclavian vein thrombosis.[17]

Reteplase is a deletion mutant of t-PA. It has slower clearance than t-PA, but its efficacy and its safety profile are similar.

There are few studies comparing the efficacy of these agents in the treatment of upper-extremity venous thrombosis. Therefore the clinician must exercise sound judgment and gain expertise in their use. The newer thrombolytic agents are probably preferable because of their better safety profile and more predictable dosing.

Technique of Thrombolytic Administration

Regional catheter-directed intravenous delivery of thrombolytic agents is preferable to systemic delivery. With the former procedure, the overall dose is reduced, and there is a lower risk of producing a systemic lytic state (which may precipitate bleeding). Thrombolytic efficacy is also improved.[18] All catheter-directed therapy is performed under radiographic guidance. The clinician should be familiar with basic endovascular techniques.

Venous access should be attained via percutaneous puncture of the basilic vein to ensure a more direct communication with the axillosubclavian vein. A guidewire is introduced to maintain venous access, the needle is removed, and a catheter is placed over the guidewire. A venogram is then obtained to delineate the anatomy. This image is retained for reference, and the guidewire is advanced across the thrombosis. An infusion catheter with multiple side holes is advanced over the guidewire and is placed within the clot. Next, the guidewire is removed, and the thrombolytic infusion may be started. An initial bolus or a lacing dose within the clot may improve lysis.

The patient should be assessed frequently for upper extremity changes as well as for complications. Repeated venography is performed within 24 hours to determine the degree of clot lysis, to check catheter position, and to adjust the dosage of the thrombolytic agent.

The incidence of bleeding complications increases with the length of infusion; thrombolysis that lasts longer than 72 hours is not recommended and has a significantly reduced chance of success. Postinfusion venography after the clot has been cleared will delineate the venous anatomy with respect to the site of occlusion and will provide information for future endovascular or vascular surgical options.

The clinician must be aware that venous thrombotic disease has two components: occlusion from the clot and valvular damage. Occlusive disease is cleared effectively in most instances; however, preservation of valvular function is less certain. The earlier thrombolytic therapy can be initiated, the greater its chance of success. There is no consensus regarding how long venous thrombus can be present before thrombolysis becomes of no value. Machleder[19] reported that when thrombolytic therapy was initiated within 8 days of the onset of symptoms, 82% of clots were lysed. When treatment was instituted after 10 days, however, there was no significant thrombolysis.

Bleeding complications are the greatest risk for patients receiving thrombolysis. The risk of bleeding is related more to the duration of therapy than to the dose. It has been difficult to correlate the risk of bleeding with specific coagulation parameters; however, it is known that a systemic lytic state (50% drop in fibrinogen, prolongation of thrombin time to two times normal) tends toward an increase in the incidence of hemorrhage.

Intracerebral hemorrhage is the most feared complication and occurs 1% to 2% of the time regardless of the thrombolytic agent used. Close neurologic monitoring is mandatory. Gastrointestinal hemorrhage usually represents an unsuspected ulcer or significant gastritis. The number of needle puncture sites should be kept to a minimum to avoid bleeding from these areas. A careful history and physical examination, as well as evaluation of laboratory parameters (complete blood cell count, kidney and liver panels, coagulation profile), are necessary. For a limited review of contraindications, see Box 65-1.

The concomitant use of heparin is controversial. Bleeding is increased with heparin use; however, clot formation along the catheter sheath is reduced. The relative risks and benefits must be weighed in each patient.

After the clot has been successfully lysed, the patient is maintained with therapeutic heparin while warfarin therapy is initiated to reduce the risk of rethrombosis.

Mechanical Thrombectomy

Shah and associates[20] recently reported on the successful use of power-pulse spray thrombectomy in three cases of Paget-Schroetter syndrome. This novel method involves the direct infusion of a thrombolytic agent into a clot via a catheter, followed by intravascular mechanical clot fracture and removal. Arko and associates[21] reported on the combination of mechanical thrombectomy with rapid low-dose thrombolysis. The group achieved widely patent veins with no residual stenosis in two patients, using Solera mechanical thrombectomy (Bacchus Vascular, Santa Clara, CA) followed by a 5-mg catheter-directed t-PA injection to remove any remaining thrombus. The low exposure time and dose prove advantageous in minimizing bleeding risks. Mechanical thrombectomy, combined with thrombolysis, offers a new potentially more effective approach for the treatment of axillosubclavian vein thrombosis; however, further investigative studies are needed.

Decompression of Thoracic Outlet

Decompression of the thoracic outlet is recommended if the following occur:

1. An apparent stricture is noted on venography.
2. A compressive abnormality is demonstrated by arm abduction during venography after vein patency has been restored.
3. Symptomatic patients with an occluded axillosubclavian vein demonstrate occluded collaterals when the arm is abducted during venography.

Transaxillary first rib resection is considered the procedure of choice and is based on an extensive body

BOX 65-1

CONTRAINDICATIONS TO THROMBOLYTIC THERAPY

Absolute

- Active internal bleeding
- Intracranial disease
- Recent hemorrhagic stroke (3 months)
- Recent eye operation (3 months)

Relative

- Uncontrolled hypertension
- Severe hepatic or renal disease
- Pregnancy
- Postpartum period (10 days)
- Recent history of bleeding peptic ulcer or gastritis
- Recent major surgery or organ biopsy (10-14 days)

of literature documenting its long-term effectiveness.[11,22-24] This procedure is generally performed after a 1- to 3-month period of warfarin anticoagulation. This has the advantage of avoiding surgical intervention at a time when the vein is most thrombogenic and when there may be a perivenous inflammatory reaction. Early surgical decompression has its advocates, but this approach is debated.[24-29] Angle et al.[30] found that early decompression was just as effective as the traditional staged decompression and did not result in increased perioperative morbidity or mortality. Some of the obvious benefits of early decompression include expedited treatment and a quicker return to normal physical activity. Lee et al.[31] suggest the potential effectiveness of nonoperative management; however, they also propose that younger patients (<28 years old) be offered early surgical decompression because of an increased tendency for long-term recurrent thrombosis. Various factors, such as patient preference, age, cost, and medical history should be considered when evaluating candidates for early surgical decompression.

Balloon Angioplasty

Balloon angioplasty (BA) is an effective method of treating residual stenosis after surgical decompression of the thoracic outlet. Recent evidence indicates that intraoperative BA combined with decompression surgery in one stage may significantly reduce the incidence of recurrent thrombosis.[32] Predecompressive BA is not recommended because it is largely ineffective as a result of unrelieved extrinsic compression.

Postoperative BA can be performed if a residual stricture of 50% or greater exists. It may also be considered if lesser stenosis is present with significant collaterals. There is a small subgroup of patients who may have a normal-appearing venogram but who still have symptoms. This group may have a thin web from fusion of valve leaflets, which is difficult to demonstrate on venography. A web generally occurs at the costoclavicular portion of the subclavian vein and may be appreciated on BA.

In another subgroup of patients who have undergone successful thrombolysis, very high-grade stenosis is demonstrated. This may reocclude despite warfarin therapy. BA with a small-diameter balloon is recommended to keep the vein open before surgical decompression. Leaving significant stenosis untreated in the face of improved symptoms and examination is unwise, because rethrombosis is the rule with unrelieved obstruction.

Technique

The technique of percutaneous guidewire access is the same as is described in the previous section. Venography is performed, which allows assessment of vein diameter and permits the selection of an appropriately sized standard arterial balloon. It is wise to undersize the balloon slightly for the first inflation to reduce the risk of rupture to the thin-walled vein. Larger balloon sizes can then be used as deemed appropriate. Full heparinization is recommended before BA because fractured intima will expose the thrombogenic subintimal layer. The balloon is passed over a guidewire and is advanced across the venographically delineated stenosis. The balloon is carefully inflated until a "waist" or a narrowing is seen as the balloon opposes the stenosis. Inflation pressure is increased until the waist disappears. Frequently, release of the balloon and follow-up venography demonstrate residual stenosis or elastic recoil. Repeating BA with higher inflation pressures or selecting the next-greater size of balloon is recommended. Clinical judgment and familiarity with endovascular techniques are mandatory.

Stenting

Stenting in the retroclavicular portion of the axillosubclavian vein should generally be avoided. The overriding clavicle or the underlying first rib (if not surgically resected) is a point of pressure during normal upper-extremity range of motion, which may cause stent deformity or fraying. In addition, placing a thrombogenic foreign body in a low-flow/low-pressure system may predispose to thrombotic occlusion.[33,34] A 22-patient case study in 2003 observed 100% reocclusion in all patients within 1 to 6 days after stent insertion, suggesting that intravenous stents are contraindicated in patients with Paget-Schroetter syndrome.[35]

Selective venous stenting does have its advocates, however. It has been recommended only after first rib removal to reduce the risk of venous trauma. The Wallstent is preferred over the rigid Palmaz (Johnson & Johnson, Warren, NJ) stent because of its greater deformability. Stent placement should be limited to patients who have at least 50% stenosis remaining after BA.[34] A 2001 case study that followed the aforementioned guidelines found good vein patency in 9 out of 14 patients after an average of 3.5 years following stent insertion in the axillosubclavian vein.[36] Patients with remaining strictures or stenosis after lysis, decompression surgery, and percutaneous transluminal angioplasty may benefit from intravenous stents.

Malignancy causing axillosubclavian vein compression and thrombosis is a difficult circumstance for which stent placement may be considered, especially in conjunction with radiation therapy.[37]

It must be kept in mind that there are few, if any, long-term studies to define the biologic reaction of stents in this venous system. Many of these patients are quite young and may be at risk for development of problems later. The timing, the complications, and the role of stenting in this disorder have yet to be clearly defined.

Surgery

If the previously mentioned techniques are unsuccessful in reestablishing venous patency and resolving symptoms, surgery may be considered. Various procedures have been described, but their efficacy remains to be established. A full description of these procedures is beyond the scope of this chapter, and the reader is encouraged to become familiar with the appropriate references.

Conclusion

The treatment of primary ASVT has evolved over the years since it was first described. Early treatment consisted of anticoagulation and, if anticoagulation was ineffective, direct venous surgery. At this time, thrombolytic agents, first rib resection, and endovascular techniques are recommended. The suggested method of treatment is as follows:

1. After anatomic delineation by means of venography, catheter-directed thrombolytic therapy is administered to reestablish patency.
2. Venography is used to define underlying venous compression or stenosis, and the patient is given warfarin for 4 to 12 weeks.
3. If stenosis or compression is found, first rib removal is performed to decompress the axillosubclavian vein.
4. After venous decompression, if repeated venography demonstrates significant remaining stenosis, BA is performed.
5. Remaining stenosis after BA warrants intravenous stent placement.

SECONDARY AXILLOSUBCLAVIAN VEIN THROMBOSIS

With the increasing use of indwelling venous catheters, secondary axillosubclavian vein thrombosis (SASVT) is quite common. Indwelling venous lines (e.g., central lines for monitoring and intravenous infusion, hemodialysis catheters, and pacemakers) are foreign bodies and cause localized areas of intimal injury, resulting in the potential for venous thrombosis.

The true incidence of SASVT is unknown because it is frequently silent and has a more benign course than primary ASVT; however, severely symptomatic cases are known to occur. The differences in presentation and outcome between the two are difficult to understand. Several studies have suggested that the incidence of SASVT is between 10% and 30%, although clearly it is much more common than is generally appreciated.[38-41]

Subclavian Hyperalimentation and Medication Delivery Catheters

Subclavian catheters used for hyperalimentation and medication delivery are extremely common. For these procedures, not only is there a foreign body within the subclavian vein, but also a hypertonic or an irritative solution is infused.

It is important to note three points with respect to the position and the diameter of the catheter, as well as the nature of the infusion time.

1. If the catheter tip is within the axillosubclavian vein instead of the superior vena cava, the risk for thrombosis increases from 21% to 60%.[42] The risk also increases from 2.3% to 10% if the catheter is placed in the subclavian vein as opposed to the internal jugular vein.[43]
2. A 16-gauge single-lumen catheter is much less likely to cause SASVT than a larger-bore multiple-lumen catheter.[44]
3. Intermittent infusions using the heparin lock system can reduce the incidence of thrombophlebitis.[45]

Transvenous Pacemakers

With the ubiquity of pacemakers, a significant incidence of symptomatic SASVT should be expected; however, clinical manifestations are extremely rare. In two studies of 125 and 212 patients, the incidence of symptomatic thrombosis was 2.4%.[46,47] Another study using venography noted that 44% of patients had severe luminal stenosis and 21% had total occlusion, but only one patient presented with arm edema.[48] Although venous thrombosis is quite common with transvenous pacemakers, it rarely presents a significant problem.

Subclavian Hemodialysis Catheters

Subclavian hemodialysis catheters were introduced in 1977. They provide immediate dialysis access until surgically placed arteriovenous fistulas or shunts have matured. SASVT with dialysis catheters is common and most often silent. Patients may suddenly have symptoms with significant arm swelling after placement of an arteriovenous fistula below a thrombosed axillosubclavian vein. Consideration should be given to performing duplex scanning or other diagnostic investigations before fistula placement when there has been an indwelling catheter in the ipsilateral subclavian vein. Chronically occluded axillosubclavian veins are probably not amenable to endovascular intervention, and a decision must be made whether a bypass around the occluded venous segment is indicated versus interruption of the fistula. Acute thrombosis is more difficult to document but may be amenable to lytic therapy and BA.[8,49] It is important to be aware of the potential for subclavian vein thrombosis before an arm arteriovenous fistula is placed so that the contralateral side can be used.

Recommended Treatment

Venous thrombosis related to the presence of an indwelling subclavian vein catheter is more common than is generally recognized. It is usually asymptomatic or minimally symptomatic. If practical, the inciting catheter should be removed, especially if the symptoms are not insignificant. This is usually possible with hyperalimentation and perhaps hemodialysis catheters but is more difficult and not advisable when pacemaker wires are present.

Anticoagulation with heparin followed by warfarin is appropriate for uncomplicated cases. Thrombolytic therapy should be reserved for complicated cases and significantly symptomatic patients.[50,51] The goal of anticoagulation is to reduce the extension of thrombosis and to preserve collaterals. Pulmonary embolism is also a risk and has been noted in up to 12% of patients.[52,53]

Catheter-directed thrombolytic therapy is appropriate in patients with severe arm edema.[54] Dissolution of the thrombus is faster and has fewer treatment failures than with anticoagulation alone. If significant underlying stenosis remains after lysis, BA must be considered. Stent placement has been reported, but the previously discussed concerns about extrinsic compression remain, particularly with the first rib intact.[55] Endovascular techniques appear to be comparable to surgical reconstruction, although repeated interventions may be required.

References

1. Paget J: *Clinical lectures and essays*, London, 1875, Longmans Green.
2. Von Schroetter L: Erkrankungen der Gefossl. In *Nathnogel: handbuch der pathologie und therapie*, Vienna, 1884, Holder, pp 421–433.
3. Hughes ESR: Venous obstruction in the upper extremity (Paget-Schroetter's syndrome), *Int Abstr Surg* 8:89–127, 1949.
4. Akita K, Ibukuro K, Yamaguchi K, Heima S, Sato T: The subclavius posticus muscle: a factor in arterial, venous or brachial plexus compression? *Surg Radiol Anat* 22:111–115, 2000.
5. Koksoy C, Kuzu A, Kutlay J, et al: The diagnostic value of colour doppler ultrasound in central venous catheter related thrombosis, *Clin Radiol* 50:687–689, 1995.
6. Campbell CB, Chandler JG, Tegtmeyer CJ, et al: Axillary, subclavian, and brachiocephalic vein obstruction, *Surgery* 82:816–826, 1977.
7. Adams JT, DeWeese JA: "Effort" thrombosis of the axillary and subclavian veins, *J Trauma* 11:923–930, 1971.
8. Currer CB Jr, Widder S, Ali A, et al: Surgical management of the subclavian and axillary vein thrombosis in patients with a functioning arteriovenous fistula, *Surgery* 100:25–28, 1986.
9. Hansen B, Feins R, Detmer DE: Simple extra-anatomic jugular vein bypass for subclavian vein thrombosis, *J Vasc Surg* 2:921–923, 1985.
10. Bell T, Stevens SL, Freeman MB, et al: Jugular venous bypass for subclavian vein obstruction, *Ann Vasc Surg* 8:390–393, 1994.
11. Adelman MA, Stone DH, Riles TS, et al: A multidisciplinary approach to the treatment of Paget-Schroetter syndrome, *Ann Vasc Surg* 11:149–154, 1997.
12. Schmacht DC, Back MR, Novotney ML, et al: Primary axillary-subclavian venous thrombosis: is aggressive surgical intervention justified, *Vasc Surg* 35:353–359, 2001.
13. Melby SJ, Vedantham S, Narra VR, et al: Comprehensive surgical management of the competitive athlete with effort thrombosis of the subclavian vein (Paget Schroetter syndrome), *J Vasc Surg* 47:809–820, 2008.
14. Coon WW, Willis PW III: Thrombosis of axillary and subclavian veins, *Arch Surg* 94:657–663, 1967.
15. Crowell LL: Effort thrombosis of the subclavian and axillary veins: review of the literature and case report with 2 year followup and venography, *Ann Intern Med* 52:1337–1343, 1960.
16. Tilney NL, Griffiths HJG, Edwards EA: Natural history of major venous thrombosis of the upper extremity, *Arch Surg* 101:792–796, 1970.
17. Gelabert HA, Jimenez JC, Rigberg DA: Comparison of retavase and urokinase for management of spontaneous subclavian vein thrombosis, *Ann Vasc Surg* 21:149–154, 2007.
18. Dake MD, Semba CP: Thrombolytic therapy in venous occlusive disease, *J Vasc Interv Radiol* 6(suppl):735–775, 1995.
19. Machleder HI: Evaluation of a new treatment strategy for Paget-Schroetter syndrome: spontaneous thrombosis of the axillary-subclavian vein, *J Vasc Surg* 17:305–317, 1993.
20. Shah AD, Bajakian DR, Olin JW, et al: Power-pulse spray thrombectomy for treatment of Paget-Schroetter syndrome, *AJR Am J Roentgenol* 188:1215–1217, 2007.
21. Arko FR, Cipriano P, Lee E, et al: Treatment of axillosubclavian vein thrombosis: a novel technique for rapid removal of clot using low-dose thrombolysis, *J Endovasc Ther* 10:773–778, 2003.
22. Roos DB, Edgar J: Poth lecture: thoracic outlet syndromes: update 1987, *Am J Surg* 154:568–573, 1987.
23. Feugier P, Aleksic I, Salari R, et al: Long-term results of venous revascularization for Paget-Schroetter syndrome in athletes, *Ann Vasc Surg* 15:212–218, 2001.
24. Urschel HC Jr, Patel AN: Surgery remains the most effective treatment for Paget-Schroetter syndrome: 50 years' experience, *Ann Thorac Surg* 86:254–260, 2008.
25. Pittam MR, Darke SG: The place of first rib resection in the management of axillary-subclavian vein thrombosis, *Eur J Vasc Surg* 1:5–10, 1987.
26. DeWeese JA: Results of surgical treatment of axillary-subclavian venous thrombosis. In Bergan JJ, Yao JST, editors: *Venous disorders*, Philadelphia, 1991, WB Saunders, pp 421–433.
27. Aziz S, Straehley CJ, Whelan TJ: Effort-related axillo-subclavian thrombosis. A new theory of pathogenesis and a plea for direct surgical intervention, *Am J Surg* 152:57–61, 1986.
28. Urschel HC, Razzuk MA: Improved management of Paget-Schroetter syndrome secondary to thoracic outlet compression, *Ann Thorac Surg* 52:1217–1221, 1991.
29. Caparrelli DJ, Freischlag J: A unified approach to axillosubclavian venous thrombosis in a single hospital admission, *Semin Vasc Surg* 18:153–157, 2005.

30. Angle N, Gelabert HA, Farooq MM, et al: Safety and efficacy of early surgical decompression of the thoracic outlet for Paget-Schroetter syndrome, *Ann Vasc Surg* 15:37–42, 2001.
31. Lee JT, Karwowski JK, Harris EJ, et al: 4th: Long-term thrombotic recurrence after nonoperative management of Paget-Schroetter syndrome, *J Vasc Surg* 43:1236–1243, 2006.
32. Schnieder DB, Dimuzio PJ, Martin ND, et al: Combination treatment of venous thoracic outlet syndrome: open surgical decompression and intraoperative angioplasty, *J Vasc Surg* 40:599–603, 2005.
33. Becker GJ, Holden RW, Mail JT, et al: Local thrombolytic therapy for thoracic outlet syndrome, *Semin Interv Radiol* 2:349–353, 1985.
34. Meier GH, Pollack JS, Rosenblatt M, et al: Initial experience with venous stents in exertional axillary-subclavian vein thrombosis, *J Vasc Surg* 24:974–983, 1996.
35. Urschel HC Jr, Patel AN: Paget-Schroetter syndrome therapy: failure of intravenous stents, *Ann Thorac Surg* 75:1693–1696, 2003.
36. Kreienberg PB, Chang BB, Darling RC III, et al: Long-term results in patients treated with thrombolysis, thoracic inlet decompression, and subclavian stenting for Paget-Schroetter syndrome, *J Vasc Surg* 33:S100–S105, 2001.
37. Beygui RE, Olcott CIV, Dalman RL: Subclavian vein thrombosis: outcome analysis based on etiology and modality of treatment, *Ann Vasc Surg* 11:247–255, 1997.
38. Horne MK III, Merryman PK, Mayo DJ, et al: Reductions in tissue plasminogen activator and thrombomodulin in blood draining veins damaged by venous access devices, *Thromb Res* 79:369–376, 1995.
39. Axelsson CK, Efsen F: Phlebography in long-term catheterization of the subclavian vein: a retrospective study in patients with severe gastrointestinal disorders, *Scand J Gastroenterol* 13: 933–938, 1978.
40. Smith VC, Hallett JW Jr: Subclavian vein thrombosis during prolonged catheterization for parenteral nutrition: early management and long-term follow-up, *South Med J* 76:603–606, 1983.
41. Feliciano DV, Mattox KL, Graham JM, et al: Major complications of percutaneous subclavian catheters, *Am J Surg* 138:869–874, 1979.
42. Clagett GP, Eberhart RL: Artificial devices in clinical practice. In Colman RW, editor: *Hemostasis and thrombosis: basic principles and clinical practice*, ed 3, Philadelphia, 1994, JB Lippincott, pp 421–433.
43. Kearns PJ, Coleman S, Wehner JH: Complications of long-term catheters: a randomized trial of central vs peripheral tip location, *J Parenter Enteral Nutr* 20:20–24, 1996.
44. Horattas MC, Wright DJ, Fenton AH, et al: Changing concepts of deep venous thrombosis of the upper extremity: report of a series and review of the literature, *Surgery* 104:561–567, 1988.
45. Weiss Y, Nissan S: A method for reducing the incidence of infusion phlebitis, *Surg Gynecol Obstet* 141:73–74, 1975.
46. Crook BRM, Gishen P, Robinson CR, Oram S: Occlusion of the subclavian vein associated with cephalic vein pacemaker electrodes, *Br J Surg* 64:329–331, 1977.
47. Williams EH, Tyers GFO, Shaffer CW: Symptomatic deep venous thrombosis of the arm associated with permanent transvenous pacing electrodes, *Chest* 73:613–615, 1978.
48. Stoney WS, Addlestone RB, Alford WC, et al: The incidence of venous thrombosis following long-term transvenous pacing, *Ann Thorac Surg* 22:166–170, 1976.
49. Wisselink W, Money SR, Becker MO, et al: Comparison of operative reconstruction and percutaneous balloon dilation for central venous obstruction, *Am J Surg* 166:200–205, 1994.
50. Jones JC, Balkcom IL, Worman RK: Pulmonary embolus after treatment for subclavian-axillary vein thrombosis, *Postgrad Med* 82:244–249, 1987.
51. Ameli FM, Minas T, Weiss M, Provan JL: Consequences of "conservative" conventional management of axillary vein thrombosis, *Can J Surg* 30:167–169, 1987.
52. Sassu GP, Chisholm CD, Howell JM, et al: A rare etiology for pulmonary embolism: basilic vein thrombosis, *J Emerg Med* 8:45–49, 1990.
53. Monreal M, Raventos A, Lerme R, et al: Pulmonary embolism in patients with upper extremity DVT associated with venous central lines: a prospective study, *Thromb Haemost* 72:548–550, 1994.
54. Chang R, Horne MK III, Mayo DJ, et al: Pulse-spray treatment of subclavian and jugular and venous thrombi with recombinant tissue plasminogen activator, *J Vasc Interv Radiol* 7:845–851, 1996.
55. Bhatia DS, Money SR, Ochsner JL, et al: Comparison of surgical bypass and percutaneous balloon dilatation with primary stent placement in the treatment of central venous obstruction in the dialysis patient: one-year follow-up, *Ann Vasc Surg* 10:452–455, 1996.

CHAPTER

66

Catheter-Directed Therapy of Superior Vena Cava Syndrome

Vikram S. Kashyap, Gregory Pierce

Superior vena cava (SVC) syndrome is caused by obstruction of venous flow in the SVC. This results in the classic findings of head and neck swelling, upper-torso venous engorgement and discomfort, and occasional respiratory embarrassment. SVC syndrome is rarely life threatening, but its clinical sequelae can cause serious morbidity.

SVC syndrome continues to be associated with a variety of benign and malignant diseases. In a majority of cases, SVC obstruction is due to malignant tumor or lymph node metastases in the thorax. Usually, the mediastinal process encroaches on or infiltrates the SVC, leading to progressive narrowing and causing secondary thrombosis. Lung cancer or lymphoma is the culprit in most cases, but other mediastinal tumors or metastatic disease can lead to SVC syndrome.[1] Of the benign conditions causing SVC syndrome, prolonged central venous catheterization with resultant thrombosis of the SVC is becoming a more frequent etiologic factor. Similarly, other long-term indwelling devices, including pacemaker electrodes, can lead to SVC thrombosis and occlusion. Rarer benign causes include mediastinal fibrosis, goiter, granulomatous disease, and radiation injury.[2]

SVC syndrome was first described by William Hunter in 1757. Interestingly, earlier in the twentieth century, a majority of cases of SVC obstruction had benign causes, usually infection. Currently, however, 60% to 80% of cases are due to thoracic or metastatic malignancies causing caval obstruction.[3] A similar change has occurred in the treatment of this syndrome. Technical advances and increased experience with endovascular therapies have led to wider use of catheter-directed modalities for SVC syndrome.

THERAPEUTIC OPTIONS FOR SUPERIOR VENA CAVA SYNDROME

SVC syndrome may develop in patients either acutely, because of sudden thrombosis, or gradually, because of external constriction leading to SVC stenosis. Regardless of the cause, patients may become extremely disabled. Usually, patients complain of facial, periorbital, neck, and bilateral arm swelling (Figure 66-1). Dilated superficial veins may develop over the upper chest, and eventually tortuous intrathoracic collaterals may develop based on the azygos and the hemiazygos venous systems (Figures 66-2 and 66-3). Respiratory symptoms are not uncommon, with patients complaining of dyspnea and occasionally associated dysphagia. A more difficult sequela of SVC syndrome to ascertain is the cognitive dysfunction that may result from cerebral venous hypertension. This cerebral venous edema can also cause headaches and sensory disturbances, including visual problems.

In cases where SVC syndrome is a result of malignant causes, multimodality treatment is needed. Traditional modalities for the treatment of SVC syndrome have included chemotherapy or radiation therapy in cases of external compression caused by a malignant process.[4,5] Clearly, these still remain the primary treatments for the underlying tumor. However, chemotherapy and/or radiation therapy provide limited symptomatic relief of SVC obstruction. These agents take a variable amount of time to affect the tumor, rarely improving the patient's condition until weeks have passed. Surgical revascularization of the SVC has been described, but prolonged patency of the surgical bypass is not ensured. Surgical bypass has been most successful with the use of spiral vein grafts; other allografts and prosthetic conduits have had less promising results, probably because of graft compression or thrombosis resulting from low-velocity flow.[6] These procedures require a median sternotomy and are often limited to selected patients with benign causes of SVC syndrome and a normal life expectancy.

A recent review at the Mayo Clinic identified 32 patients who had undergone SVC reconstruction over

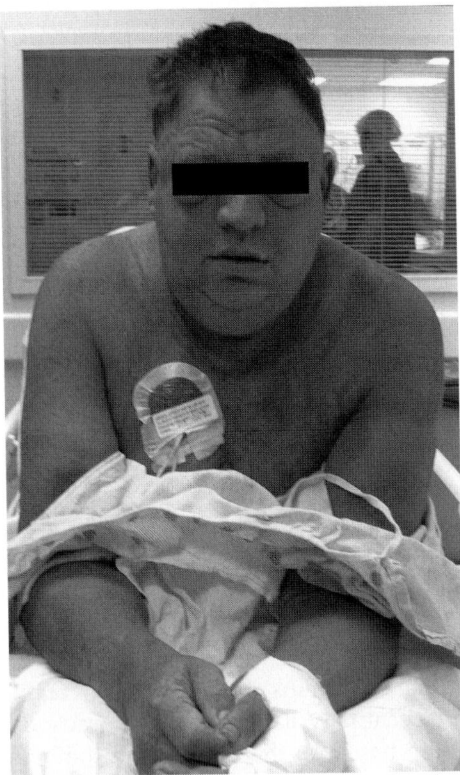

FIGURE 66-1 SVC syndrome in a male. Marked periorbital, facial, and upper-extremity edema is present.

an 18-year period.[7] All the procedures were done for nonmalignant disease, including mediastinal fibrosis in many of the cases. A majority of the reconstructions were done with use of the spiral saphenous vein graft technique. Primary patency rate of 53% and a secondary patency rate of 80% were achieved at 5 years. Of note, 17 additional secondary procedures (mostly endovascular) were needed in 8 patients to maintain patency. The authors concluded that the long-term secondary patency justified SVC grafting with spiral vein grafts for benign disease but that careful surveillance and occasional endovascular salvage were necessary.

Medical therapy is a reasonable alternative in patients with only minimal symptoms or in individuals with an extremely short life expectancy. This consists of bed rest, head elevation, and anticoagulation. Steroids and diuretic therapy may be added for laryngeal and peripheral edema, respectively. In an observational study of 107 patients, the rate of clinical improvement with use of steroids or diuretics was similar to that in patients receiving neither therapy.[8]

With the recent advent of endovascular techniques, increasing numbers of patients with SVC syndrome are being treated with catheter-based modalities. This can be regional thrombolysis, angioplasty, stent deployment, or a combination of the three. An algorithm for the treatment of SVC syndrome is based on the cause of the obstruction (Figure 66-4). Even though many modalities may be available, in general, the catheter-based interventions have received the most enthusiastic response in patients with malignant disease because of their efficacy and low morbidity.

RESULTS OF ENDOVASCULAR INTERVENTION

Endovascular treatment of SVC syndrome was first suggested in 1974 with the use of thrombolysis for SVC thrombosis.[9] Many investigators have documented the efficacy of thrombolytic treatment in SVC syndrome, but it has been most efficacious in the setting of central venous catheter–induced thrombosis. In most situations, the SVC occludes because of the presence of a discrete stenosis, and thrombolytic therapy alone leads to short-term resolution of the patient's symptoms. More often than not, however, the SVC reoccludes, and the patient's symptoms return. This realization has led to the use of venous angioplasty and stenting. Balloon angioplasty alone is associated with a very high recurrence rate, however.[10] This occurs because the chronic venous stenosis is elastic and exhibits substantial recoil. Thus the current status of endovascular treatment of SVC syndrome includes venous stent placement whenever a discrete lesion is found (Figure 66-5).

The early experience with SVC stenting involved Gianturco stents.[11] More recent series have used Wallstents or Palmaz stents in the SVC. Results from contemporary reports of the use of endovascular interventions for SVC syndrome are displayed in Table 66-1.[12-17] A majority of the patients in these series had SVC syndrome resulting from a malignant process in the thoracic cavity. Despite variations in the definition of success in these reports, some conclusions can be made. In a vast majority of cases, the endovascular intervention could be successfully performed. If this resulted in palliation of the obstructive symptoms, it was characterized as a technical success. The cumulative technical success rate approached 90%. Morbidity was also variably defined in these reports. Still, the rate of major complications from these procedures was small. Mortality could not be garnered accurately from these studies, because many did not report the traditional 30-day mortality rate. In a review of SVC stenting for malignant disease, Uberoi[18] found a high rate of technical success (95%-100%) and clinical success with resolution of symptoms (80%-95%). This was coupled with low rates of procedure-related complication or mortality. However, recurrence of symptoms occurred in up to 40% of cases with a mean recurrence rate of 13%.[18]

Despite these initial favorable results in series of limited patients, one must keep in mind that there are

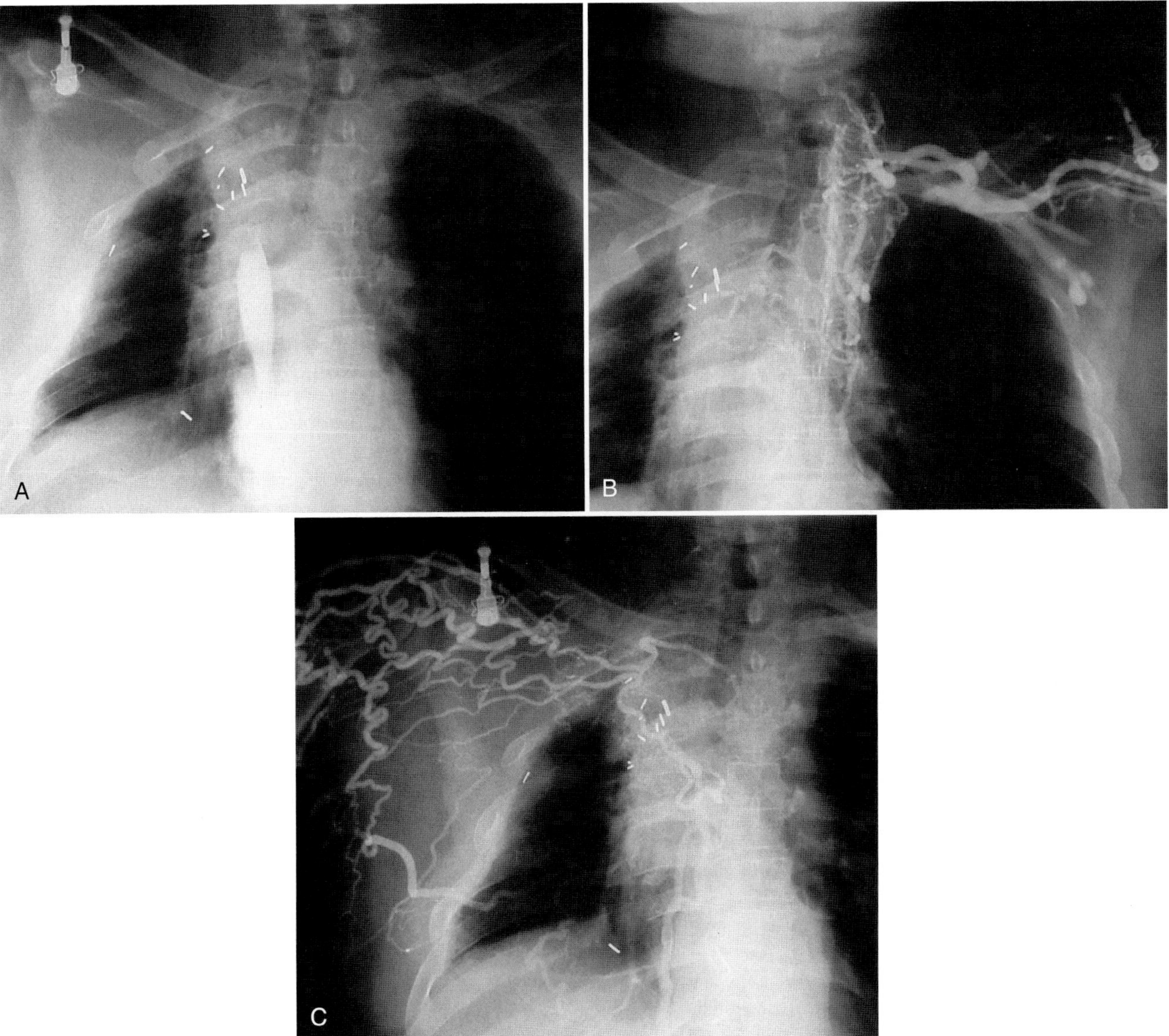

FIGURE 66-2 SVC syndrome in an elderly man with a mediastinal tumor. **A,** Venogram via the femoral route shows occlusion of the SVC. **B** and **C,** Left and right brachial venograms demonstrate extensive chronic occlusion in the brachiocephalic venous systems with multiple collaterals.

significant potential risks associated with intravascular stents. Perhaps of most concern is the potential for migration or embolization of the stent into the atrium or pulmonary circulation. The smooth concentric character of the underlying caval stenoses and the relatively short length of the SVC make stent selection critical in minimizing the likelihood of migration. Any intravascular prosthesis has the potential to become seeded with circulating bacteria and gross infection. Metallic stents are thrombogenic and prone to the effects of intimal hyperplasia; thus, multiple interventions with rethrombolysis or restenting may be required. More long-term data are clearly needed. That said, however, one must also keep in mind that most patients with SVC syndrome caused by malignancy have a grim prognosis, with a limited life expectancy.

TECHNICAL CONSIDERATIONS FOR ENDOVASCULAR THERAPY

The patient should be placed supine, but patients with SVC syndrome often cannot tolerate being completely flat for prolonged periods and need to be positioned semirecumbent for the procedure. One must prepare for multiple venous access sites for this procedure. Bilateral upper extremity venography through the basilic vein offers anatomic verification of SVC obstruction or stenosis. Also, the extent of the lesion and any collateral pathways can be documented (Figure 66-6). The upper-extremity approach is advantageous from multiple standpoints. First, and most important, it allows for the assessment of the patency of the upper-extremity and intrathoracic veins peripheral to the SVC occlusion. Thrombus frequently extends more peripherally to involve the brachiocephalic, subclavian, and even the axillary veins. These thrombosed or stenotic inflow channels will also require treatment, and antegrade access from the upper arms eases intervention on these vessels. Second, these patients who frequently have dyspnea can sit upright while undergoing thrombolysis, a comfort not permitted from a femoral approach. Femoral access is still required in most instances to allow for delivery of the inflexible large-diameter sheaths needed to deploy caval stents, but their introduction can be deferred until complete or near complete thrombolysis has been achieved. Finally, an upper-extremity approach avoids excessive use of contrast agents for visualization. Venography from the femoral route leads to significant loss of contrast agent through the right side of the heart and the pulmonary circulation.

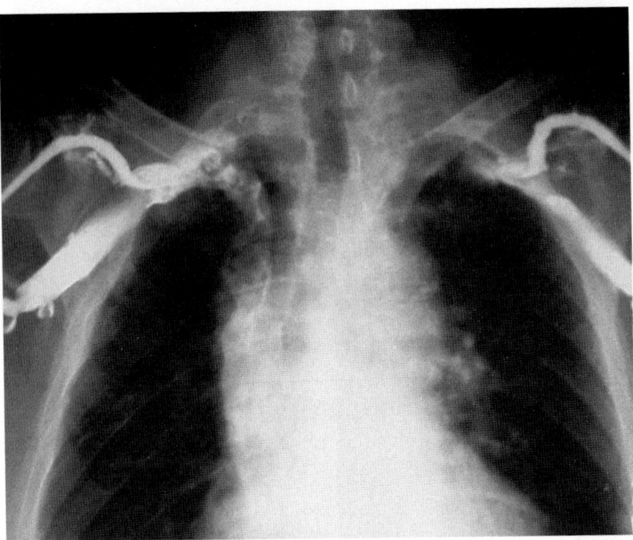

FIGURE 66-3 Bilateral simultaneous brachial vein injections demonstrate innominate vein and SVC occlusion, resulting in SVC syndrome. In this acute case, note the absence of significant collateralization, as seen in Figure 66-2.

For any intervention, the first step is an attempt to cross the thrombosed or the stenotic section with use of a hydrophilic guidewire. This can be challenging, and occasionally a wire must be placed from the arm access site and snared from the femoral catheter. If there is a documented thrombotic occlusion, catheter-directed thrombolysis is appropriate. This can be accomplished with use of a multi–side-hole catheter placed into the thrombus. Appropriate regional infusion doses of the thrombolytic agent (i.e., tissue plasminogen activator, urokinase) are used. During the infusion, heparin can be given systemically or through the catheter sheath to decrease the risk of pericatheter thrombosis. Fibrinogen levels should be checked every 6 hours during thrombolytic therapy, and thrombolysis should be discontinued if levels drop to less than 100 mg/dL or if there are any signs of uncontrollable bleeding. Repeated venography at 8- to 12-hour intervals allows visualization of the progression of thrombolysis. The procedure can be discontinued if successful recanalization has occurred. Thrombolysis should be terminated at 48 hours regardless of the outcome; continuing past this time adds little benefit and increases the bleeding risk significantly. If thrombolysis reveals an underlying stenotic lesion, angioplasty or preferably stenting of the SVC is performed. If no lesion is found, all catheters are removed, and the patient is given long-term warfarin anticoagulation therapy.

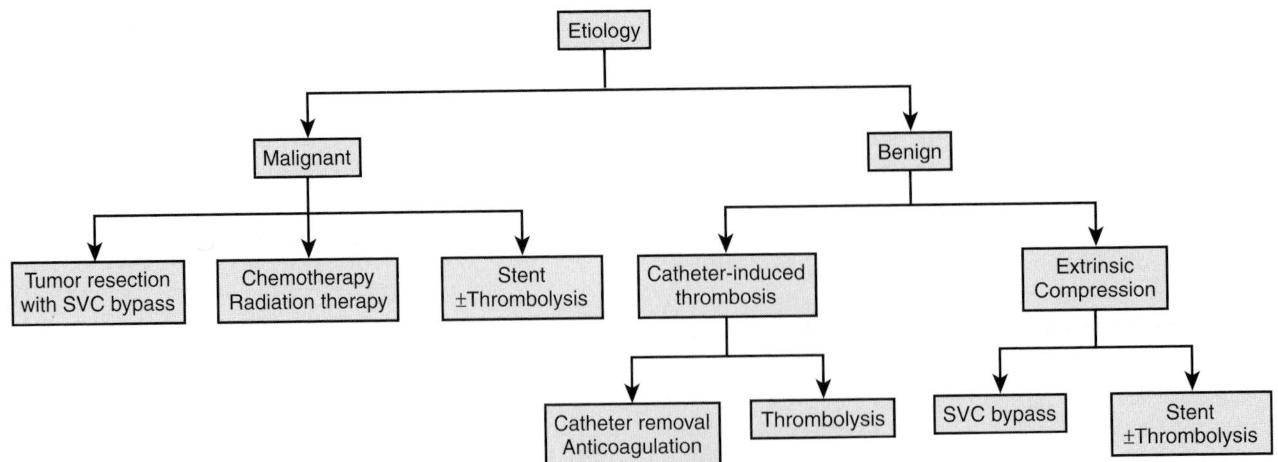

FIGURE 66-4 Algorithm for management of SVC syndrome based on cause.

For stenotic SVC lesions or stenoses revealed by means of thrombolysis, stenting of the SVC is a reasonable alternative. If no further intervention is performed, there is a high risk of rethrombosis. This may be acceptable in a patient with a very limited life expectancy or in the rare case of a possible surgical revascularization. Use of the Gianturco Z-stent (Cook, Medical, Bloomington, IN), Palmaz balloon-expandable stent, as well as the self-expanding Wallstent and nitinol SMART stents, has been described for SVC syndrome. The Gianturco Z-stent in 25-mm or 30-mm diameters may be preferable for stenting of isolated SVC stenoses. The Gianturco

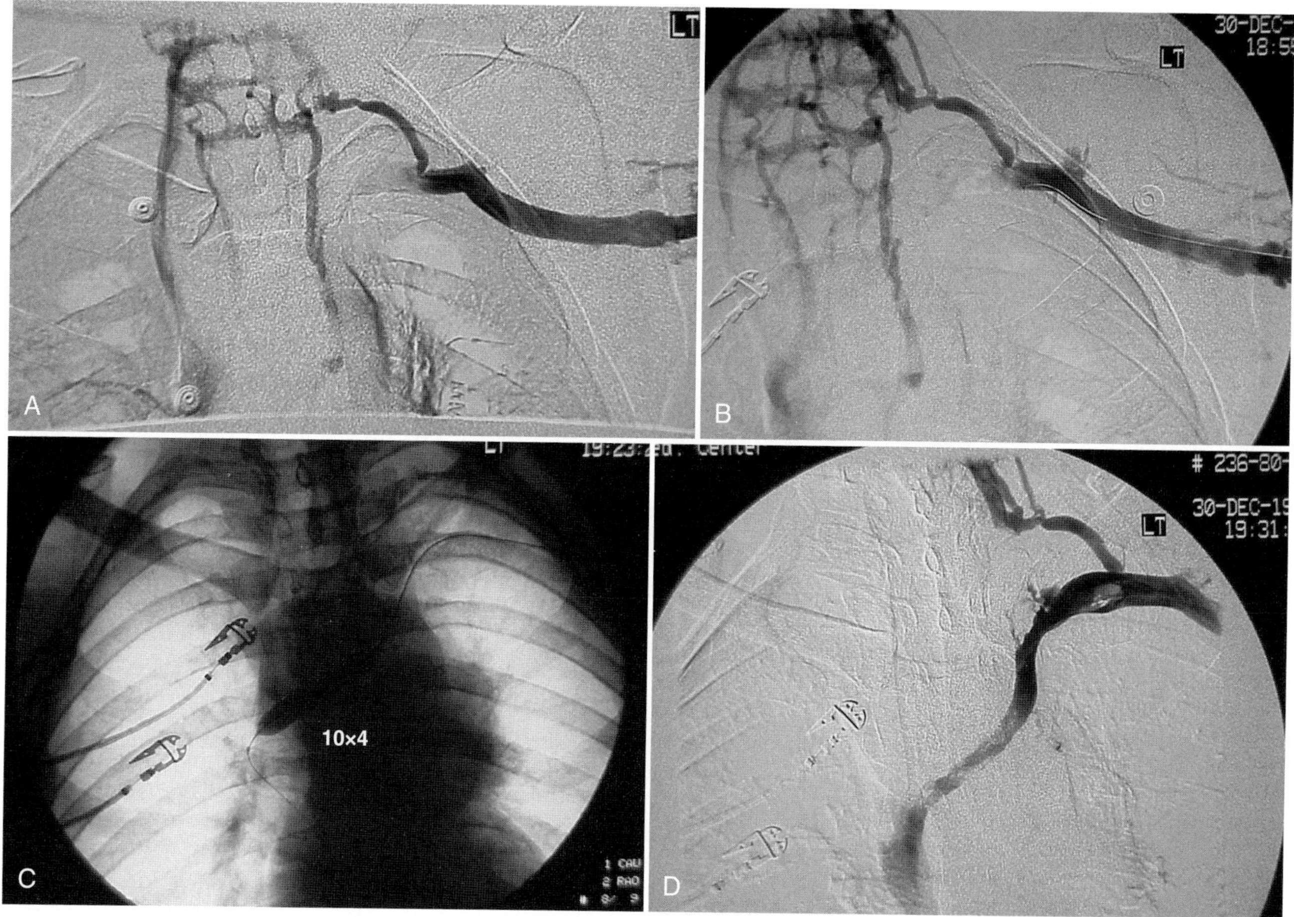

FIGURE 66-5 A 30-year-old man presented with the acute onset of significant left arm and neck edema. **A,** Venogram obtained through the left brachial vein demonstrates subclavian and innominate vein occlusion. **B,** Regional thrombolytic therapy was instituted through an infusion catheter placed via the left arm. **C,** After successful thrombolysis, a residual stenotic segment was treated with balloon angioplasty. **D,** Completion venogram demonstrates venous drainage in the SVC. The patient has remained symptom free for more than 6 months while continuing to receive treatment for malignancy.

TABLE 66-1 Selected Recent Experience With Endovascular Interventions for Superior Vena Cava Syndrome

Author	Year	Patients (n)	Malignant (%)	Morbidity/ mortality (%)	Follow-up (mean in months)	Durability
Shah et al.[12]	1996	13	100	NR	3.7	8% recurrence
Kee et al.[13]	1998	59	73	10/3	17	85% 1 yr secondary clinical patency
Smayra et al.[14]	2001	30	53	7/3	12	74% 1 yr secondary patency
Courtheoux et al.[15]	2003	20	100	0/5	2	94% symptom relief
Urruticoechea et al.[16]	2004	52	100	2/0	NR	17% reobstruction
Rizvi et al.[17]	2008	32	0	4/0	26	96% 3 yr secondary patency

NR, Not reported.

tracheobronchial Z-stent is available in large diameters and has small circumferential fixation hooks that prevent migration (Figure 66-7). Precise positioning is therefore possible. The Z-stents have relatively little metal in contact with the vessel wall, which may not inhibit tumor ingrowth to the same extent as other stents. The larger diameters achieved with use of these stents, as well as the relatively short life span of most patients with malignant occlusion, mitigate this disadvantage. A long, wide-bore angiographic sheath (up to 16F for the Gianturco Z-stent) is required for proper deployment of these stents. A systemic bolus dose of heparin is given before stent deployment. The Palmaz stent is another choice for SVC lesions. The Wallstent and SMART stent may be more suitable for the tortuous brachiocephalic veins, where stent flexibility is more of an issue. The confluence of the brachiocephalic veins and the SVC should not be encroached by the stents unless one plans a bilateral "kissing" technique. Often, these patients need further intervention, and stenting across an orifice can preclude that access site from future use. Given the low-flow state of the venous system and the presence of foreign material intraluminally, most authorities recommend postprocedure warfarin anticoagulation.

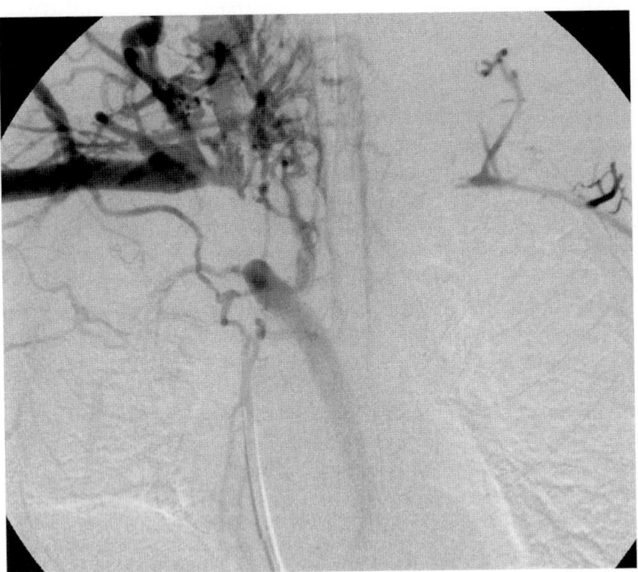

FIGURE 66-6 Brachial vein injections demonstrate SVC occlusion with collateral veins in the neck.

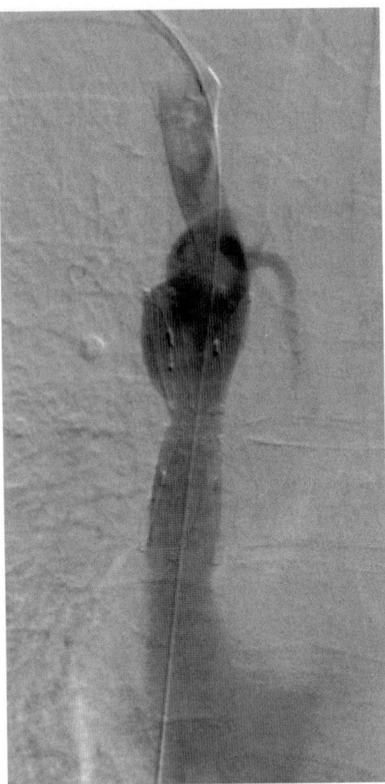

FIGURE 66-7 Successful treatment of SVC syndrome using a 25-mm × 5-cm Gianturco Z-stent with resolution of SVC occlusion and rapid emptying of contrast into the right atrium.

One must keep in mind several pitfalls when contemplating endovascular therapy for SVC syndrome. The use of thrombolytic therapy has the potential to cause bleeding in areas remote from the site where it is applied. Clearly, patients with contraindications such as recent intracranial hemorrhage or operation or pregnancy cannot be treated with thrombolysis. Additionally, exclusion of intracranial metastases before embarking on thrombolytic intervention is of paramount importance because of the high risk of intracranial bleeding. In cases where an intravascular stent is required, there is a potential for the prosthesis to become seeded with circulating bacteria and to incite thrombosis. Perhaps of most concern is the potential for migration or embolization of the stent into the atrium or pulmonary circulation. The Gianturco tracheobronchial Z-stent has several small barbs that permit precise deployment and prevent migration. Alternatively, if a self-expanding stent is going to be used, the largest device may need to be used (i.e., 14-mm diameter Wallstent, Palmaz 308) to prevent stent migration and to ensure embedding of the prosthesis into the vessel.

SUMMARY

SVC syndrome is a debilitating problem. It is usually found in patients with extensive mediastinal malignancy and limited life expectancy. The successful use of endovascular therapy to palliate SVC syndrome leads to dramatic improvement in the quality of life of patients who are terminally ill. Surgical therapy may still be useful in selected cases of SVC syndrome caused by benign disease or in cases of endovascular failure. Increasing endovascular experience and device improvement will lead to further application of endovascular therapy for this particularly debilitating syndrome.

References

1. Wilson LD, Detterbeck FC, Yahalom J: Clinical practice: superior vena cava syndrome with malignant causes, *N Engl J Med* 356 (18):1862–1869, 2007.
2. Rice TW, Rodriguez RM, Light RW: The superior vena cava syndrome: clinical characteristics and evolving etiology, *Medicine (Baltimore)* 85(1):37–42, 2006.
3. Chen JC, Bongard F, Klein SR: A contemporary perspective on superior vena cava syndrome, *Am J Surg* 160(2):207–211, 1990.
4. Armstrong BA, Perez CA, Simpson JR, et al: Role of irradiation in the management of superior vena cava syndrome, *Int J Radiat Oncol Biol Phys* 13(4):531–539, 1987.
5. Maddox AM, Valdivieso M, Lukeman J, et al: Superior vena cava obstruction in small cell bronchogenic carcinoma: clinical parameters and survival, *Cancer* 52(11):2165–2172, 1983.
6. Doty DB, Doty JR, Jones KW: Bypass of superior vena cava: fifteen years' experience with spiral vein graft for obstruction of superior vena cava caused by benign disease, *J Thorac Cardiovasc Surg* 99(5):889–895, 1990.
7. Kalra M, Gloviczki P, Andrews JC, et al: Open surgical and endovascular treatment of superior vena cava syndrome caused by nonmalignant disease, *J Vasc Surg* 38(2):215–223, 2003.
8. Schraufnagel DE, Hill R, Leech JA, et al: Superior vena caval obstruction: is it a medical emergency? *Am J Med* 70(6):1169–1174, 1981.
9. Williams DR, Demos NJ: Thrombosis of superior vena cava caused by pacemaker wire and managed with streptokinase, *J Thorac Cardiovasc Surg* 68(1):134–137, 1974.
10. Ali MK, Ewer MS, Balakrishnan PV, et al: Balloon angioplasty for superior vena cava obstruction, *Ann Intern Med* 107(6):856–857, 1987.
11. Irving JD, Dondelinger RF, Reidy JF, et al: Gianturco self-expanding stents: clinical experience in the vena cava and large veins, *Cardiovasc Intervent Radiol* 15(5):328–333, 1992.
12. Shah R, Sabanathan S, Lowe RA, et al: Stenting in malignant obstruction of superior vena cava, *J Thorac Cardiovasc Surg* 112 (2):335–340, 1996.
13. Kee ST, Kinoshita L, Razavi MK, et al: Superior vena cava syndrome: treatment with catheter-directed thrombolysis and endovascular stent placement, *Radiology* 206(1):187–193, 1998.
14. Smayra T, Otal P, Chabbert V, et al: Long-term results of endovascular stent placement in the superior caval venous system, *Cardiovasc Intervent Radiol* 24(6):388–394, 2001.
15. Courtheoux P, Alkofer B, Al RM, et al: Stent placement in superior vena cava syndrome, *Ann Thorac Surg* 75(1):158–161, 2003.
16. Urruticoechea A, Mesia R, Dominguez J, et al: Treatment of malignant superior vena cava syndrome by endovascular stent insertion: experience on 52 patients with lung cancer, *Lung Cancer* 43(2):209–214, 2004.
17. Rizvi AZ, Kalra M, Bjarnason H: Benign superior vena cava syndrome: stenting is now the first line of treatment, *J Vasc Surg* 47(2):372–380, 2008.
18. Uberoi R: Quality assurance guidelines for superior vena cava stenting in malignant disease, *Cardiovasc Intervent Radiol* 29 (3):319–322, 2006.

CHAPTER

67

Iliofemoral and Inferior Vena Cava Stenting in Chronic Venous Insufficiency

Seshadri Raju, Peter Neglen

Venous stenting has introduced a powerful yet minimally invasive outpatient technique in the management of chronic venous insufficiency (CVI) of the lower extremities. It is safe and efficacious and can replace traditional major open surgery in many patients for the correction of obstruction and, more surprisingly, to ameliorate symptoms associated with reflux as well. The technique is relatively simple in comparison with complex open venous surgery and is therefore likely to find greater application and benefit a larger set of patients with CVI. Later open surgery is not precluded, however, if the stent were to fail or occlude. For these reasons, this new technology is likely to have a profound impact on the management of CVI. Several unexpected clinical observations associated with venous stent experience also raise fundamental questions regarding the pathophysiology of CVI as currently understood, requiring a reappraisal.

The technique of venous balloon dilatation and stenting differs significantly from its arterial counterpart. Inattention to these details is a prescription for technical and clinical failure. Major technical points are shown in Box 67-1.

PATHOLOGY OF ILIAC VEIN OBSTRUCTION

Combined obstruction and reflux are now recognized as a major component of postthrombotic syndrome.[1] The importance of iliac vein obstruction in CVI had been underestimated in part because of diagnostic difficulties.[2] Venography lacks significant sensitivity in this area, and standard duplex technique has been unreliable as well. Intravenous ultrasound (IVUS), however, has proved to be a reliable diagnostic tool and has helped clarify iliac vein pathology.[3] A surprising IVUS finding in clinical cases has been the high prevalence of obstructive iliac vein lesions at arterial crossover points in nonthrombotic cases (Figure 67-1).[4] Stenting alone provides clinical relief in such cases, *even when associated reflux is left uncorrected*. In a group of 332 limbs that were stented for such lesions, outcome was compared at 2½ years in two subsets: one without associated reflux and the other with reflux that was left untreated. Cumulative relief of pain (77%, 82%), swelling (53%, 47%), and ulcer healing (76%, 67%) in the two subsets, respectively, were not different. In our own practice at the present time, iliac venous stenting is carried out as often for "primary" disease as for postthrombotic disease. Other rare etiologies, such as congenital anomalies, tumor compression, direct venous trauma, and retroperitoneal fibrosis, are occasionally (<1%) encountered.

Anatomically, the iliac vein is the terminal venous outflow pathway for the respective limb. Clinical experience indicates that this segment is hemodynamically important as well. Segmental obstructions of the femoral vein and the inferior vena cava (IVC) frequently tend to become clinically well compensated because of rich collateralization; these collaterals are parallel embryologic progenitors with normal forward flow.[5,6] In contrast, iliac vein collateralization is based on branch collaterals with reversal of normal flow pattern. The majority of symptomatic iliac vein obstructions tend to remain clinically uncompensated because of poor collateralization.[7] Collaterals that appear profuse on venography tend to be functionally inadequate. Venographic collaterals are present in only a third of cases with significant iliac vein stenosis whether primary or postthrombotic.[3] Part of this may be due to inadequate venographic opacification of altered flow patterns. A perivenous fibrous sheath frequently develops around postthrombotic iliac veins and retards collateral development as was observed by Rokitansky from autopsy studies in

BOX 67-1

MAJOR TECHNICAL POINTS IN VENOUS STENTING

The technique is different from arterial stenting in many respects.

- Femoral vein access can be obtained even at deep locations and is not restricted to compressible superficial sites. Access complications are rare with routine use of sealant devices.
- Large-size sheaths 10F or 11F are optimal.
- Stenting is *always* required in venous obstructions; balloon dilatation alone results in recoil and recurrence.
- "Kissing" balloon technique is not necessary in stenting common iliac vein.
- Iliac vein stents have to be extended 3-5 cm into IVC to avoid local migration of the stent and resultant recurrence of stenosis at iliocaval junction; contralateral flow is seldom affected.
- Large-caliber stents corresponding to normal native vein size should be used for adequate venous decompression of the limb. Undersized stents can malfunction or occlude.
- Avoid skip areas in the iliac vein even if it appears normal at the time of stenting. Skip areas tend to become stenotic with time.
- Long stent lengths are well tolerated and are seldom thrombogenic in and of themselves.
- Poor inflow or outflow into the stent and defects in the stent conduit itself result in stent malfunction or thrombosis. Use of IVUS is mandatory for optimal results. Venographic control alone is unsatisfactory.
- The stent assembly can and should be extended below the inguinal ligament if necessary to ensure adequate inflow into the stent. No instances of stent fracture or erosion caused by crossing the flexion crease have been observed. Risk of stent thrombosis is not increased.

IVC, Inferior vena cava; *IVUS,* intravenous ultrasound.

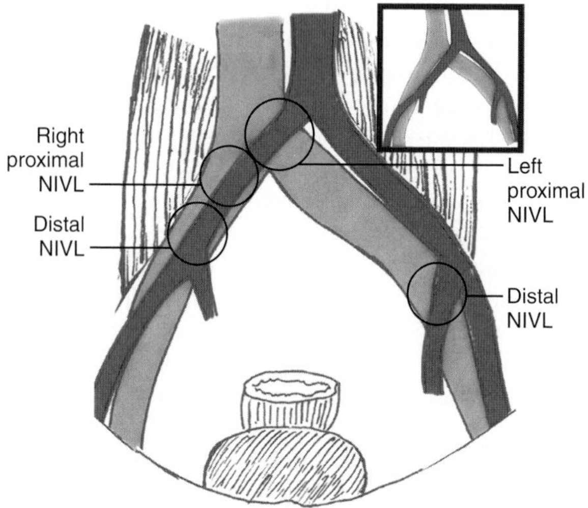

FIGURE 67-1 NIVLs occur at a number of arterial crossover points. There is considerable anatomic variation *(inset)* depending on the level of aortic bifurcation. Proximal lesions occur in relation to the common iliac artery on either side. Distal lesions are related to the iliac artery crossing of the vein on the right side and the hypogastric artery on the left side. Left-sided proximal lesions occur three to four times more commonly than on the right because the common iliac artery does not cross the vein in 75% of the population *(inset).* The incidence of distal lesions is roughly the same between the two sides.

1852. The process of iliac vein collateralization is not well understood. Thus iliac vein obstructions present a significant roadblock to venous outflow from the lower limb. In disseminated postthrombotic disease when multiple segments may have been involved, the iliac vein segment is often the main source of symptoms, and venous stenting of this segment alone may be sufficient to relieve symptoms. A thorough assessment of the iliac vein segment is therefore necessary in such cases, before concluding that symptoms are due to femoral vein pathology. Diffuse postthrombotic stenosis of the iliac vein may present no focal cues on venography and may be missed unless caliber changes are considered. IVUS is often required in such cases for definitive diagnosis.

Yet another curious feature of iliac vein pathology is the behavior of "primary" venous obstruction of nonthrombotic etiology. The term "nonthrombotic iliac vein lesion" (NIVL) is inclusive of both intrinsic lesions (webs and membranes) and extrinsic compression by the overlying artery. Although the lesion was originally described in some detail by McMurrich in 1906, there had been incomplete descriptions in the nineteenth century; many others have since added to its description. Controversy surrounds the exact etiology, whether it is ontogenic or results from traumatic pulsations of the overlying artery, but there is general agreement that the initial lesion is not postthrombotic. Eponymous nomenclature such as May-Thurner syndrome and Cockett's syndrome honor major contributors, but these designations are nondescriptive of the pathology. "Iliac vein compression syndrome" is misleading, because intrinsic lesions may be present as well. NIVL in asymptomatic form can be demonstrated in about 60% of the general population by modern imaging techniques.[8] Most will never have symptoms in their lifetime, whereas an estimated 3% eventually become symptomatic. The lesion is a common denominator in patients with CVI of nonthrombotic etiology. IVUS examination will reveal NIVLs in more than 90% of patients with class, etiology, anatomy, pathophysiology (CEAP) class 3 or higher with nonthrombotic disease.[4] In individual cases, an additional new stress factor such as trauma to the limb, cellulitis, venosclerosis of age, advancing arteriosclerosis of the overlying artery, congestive failure, or simply orthostasis and immobility of the limb can be identified as having precipitated symptoms in the context of previously silent NIVL. Contrary to the previous perception that the disease largely affects the left limb of young women, the median age in a recent series of 493 symptomatic limbs with IVUS-proved NIVL was 54 years, and both sexes and both limbs are now known to be involved, although there is predominance of women and the left side in disease cohorts. The preponderance of the left lower limb is curious and led Virchow to speculate that the lesion may explain the well-established observation that deep venous thrombosis (DVT) of the lower limb occurs several times more often on the left side. There are scores of well-documented reports in the literature of cases in which a preexisting silent NIVL appears to have led to the subsequent development of DVT and symptoms. Involvement of the left side is two to three times more frequent in other nonthrombotic CVI syndromes involving the superficial and/or the deep systems with reflux pathology. Therefore it is not unreasonable to speculate that the onset of reflux in the limb with a previously silent NIVL could play a precipitating role in symptom production as well. Moreover, stent correction of the NIVL alone leads to CVI symptom remission (pain, swelling, dermatitis, and even stasis ulceration) with the associated reflux remaining uncorrected, as detailed previously. These are features associated with *permissive* lesions, many of which occur in human pathology. A classic example is patent foramen ovale, which is present in about 25% of the general population and remains largely silent. In a small subset, however, symptoms will develop such as transient ischemic attacks or stroke from paradoxical embolus. Other examples of permissive lesions and associated secondary pathologies include ureteric reflux and pyelonephritis, obesity and diabetes, esophageal reflux and asthma, cricopharyngeal spasm and Zenker's diverticulum, and many others. The general therapeutic principle in all such complex pathologies is to correct the underlying permissive lesion, which alone is often curative without the need to address the secondary pathology that rendered the previously silent lesion symptomatic. Therapeutic response to stenting in NIVL is in accord with this experience.

INDICATIONS FOR INTRAVENOUS ULTRASOUND AND STENT PLACEMENT

All patients with CEAP clinical class 3 and higher should be considered for IVUS and possible stent placement if the symptoms are severe enough to warrant interventional treatment. Such patients would have had failure of conservative therapy with compression or were not candidates for such management in the first instance. In the latter category are patients who could not use compression because of either the local condition of the limb or other comorbid factors that preclude effective use of compression. This is a large subset. In many series, one third to one half of patients with advanced CVI have failure of compression for a variety of reasons. One subset not adequately covered by the CEAP classification is that of patients with recurrent cellulitis of the limb. An underlying iliac vein obstruction is commonly present in these patients.[9] Stasis dermatitis or ulcer is often present to offer a portal of entry for the infection, but a "spontaneous" variety of cellulitis without obvious skin breakdown is also known to occur.

Iliac vein obstruction should be suspected when severe symptoms are present in the absence of reflux on duplex examination. In other patients segmental reflux may be present but is insufficient to explain the severity of symptoms. For example, isolated popliteal reflux is a common finding in postthrombotic limbs but is generally asymptomatic unless associated with iliac vein pathology. Nontruncal varices, even if extensive, produce pain that is localized to the varices but is seldom of a nature that is so diffuse as to involve the calf or the entire extremity. These and other instances in which pain is disproportionate to duplex pathology should prompt consideration of iliac vein obstruction. Truncal reflux involving the great saphenous vein can by itself produce severe diffuse limb pain and, in some instances, stasis ulceration as well. It is nevertheless wise to investigate the iliac vein segment in such cases. Saphenous ablation alone may be ineffective or result in only partial relief of symptoms, particularly pain in the presence of a coincident iliac vein lesion. Significant leg swelling (beyond ankle edema) is not a feature of isolated saphenous reflux, and the presence of associated iliac outflow obstruction should be suspected when more extensive limb edema is present. In some instances, there is onset of new limb swelling after saphenous ablation because of the presence of an associated iliac vein lesion. When combined saphenous/iliac vein pathology is present, a stepwise treatment

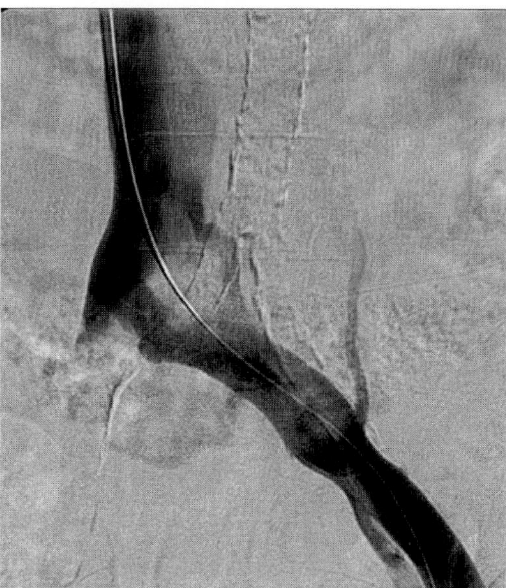

FIGURE 67-2 Arteriosclerosis of the overlying artery visible in this x-ray film may add compression to NIVL and precipitate symptoms.

algorithm can be devised on the basis of initial outcome after saphenous ablation. Some patients opt for total correction of both saphenous and iliac vein pathology in one sitting. Concurrent saphenous ablation by laser or microwave energy combined with iliac vein stenting is minimally invasive, safe, and effective.[10] Contrary to traditional teaching, saphenous ablation can be carried out safely without ill effects in the presence ("secondary" varix) of underlying chronic deep venous obstruction.[11]

Leg swelling is common in the elderly and constitutes an increasing subset with our aging population. Geriatric leg swelling can be disabling, particularly if significant pain is also present. Self-care and autonomous living are threatened and demand speedy resolution. Leg elevation and compressive therapy are often inapplicable or ineffective in this frail subset. Most are given diuretics with indifferent results. Ancillary factors such as increasing sedentary habitus, day-long orthostasis without calf exercise (sitting in a chair watching TV), congestive failure, or hormonal imbalance may be precipitating factors. Swelling may persist even after precipitating factors are corrected. Investigations may reveal a permissive NIVL augmented by venosclerosis or arteriosclerosis of the overlying artery (Figure 67-2). Iliac vein stenting may be appropriate in these cases.

Lymphedema cannot be differentiated clinically from venous obstruction. "Classic" clinical features of primary lymphedema such as early onset, bilaterality, family history, or long duration of painless leg swelling can be misleading, because venous leg swelling can present with similar features. A thorough venous investigation to rule out a correctible iliac vein lesion is warranted in all cases of leg swelling of uncertain etiology. Abnormal lymphoscintigraphy results alone are not indicative of primary lymphedema, because secondary lymphatic dysfunction is present in 30% of cases with deep venous obstruction. Secondary lymphatic dysfunction is thought to be the result of damage or exhaustion from overload.

CLINICAL ASSESSMENT

All patients who are potential candidates for iliac vein stent placement should undergo a thorough clinical evaluation including a detailed venous history and examination. The venous clinical severity scoring system (VCSS)[12] is useful in both initial assessment and gauging outcome. Assessment of limb swelling is imprecise at present. Plethysmographic techniques are cumbersome for routine clinical use. The VCSS system is based on patient history, which may be imprecise because patients tend to exaggerate or understate the degree of swelling based on the presence or absence of associated pain, respectively. Grading of swelling by physical examination (grade 0-3: none, pitting, ankle edema, and gross, respectively) is objective but crude; partial improvement within a single clinical grade cannot be precisely quantified. Such a partial improvement may have clinical bearing in some patients. For example if gross swelling involving the thigh and leg recedes to only leg swelling, or the degree of limb swelling appreciably diminishes in girth even if remaining gross, functional use of the limb may improve. In either case swelling will be marked as grade 3, allowing no accurate way of quantifying the improvement in swelling. Quality-of-life metrics specific for venous disease in clinically usable form are currently available.[13] Pain assessment is inadequately addressed in the CEAP and VCSS protocols at present. A visual analogue scale[14] is an easy and dependable metric of stent outcome in patients with CVI. About 20% of patients with other CVI features have no pain.

DIAGNOSIS

Venography is only about 50% sensitive to iliac vein stenosis even with transfemoral injection of contrast.[4,15] Venographic appearance of diagnostic interest may be variable in NIVL; in about a third of cases with NIVL, venographic appearance may be entirely normal (Figure 67-3). Postthrombotic lesions also have diverse venographic appearances (Figure 67-4). Because of the unreliability of venography, IVUS should be employed in symptomatic CEAP clinical class 3 and higher cases, even if venography is nonrevealing. IVUS has a

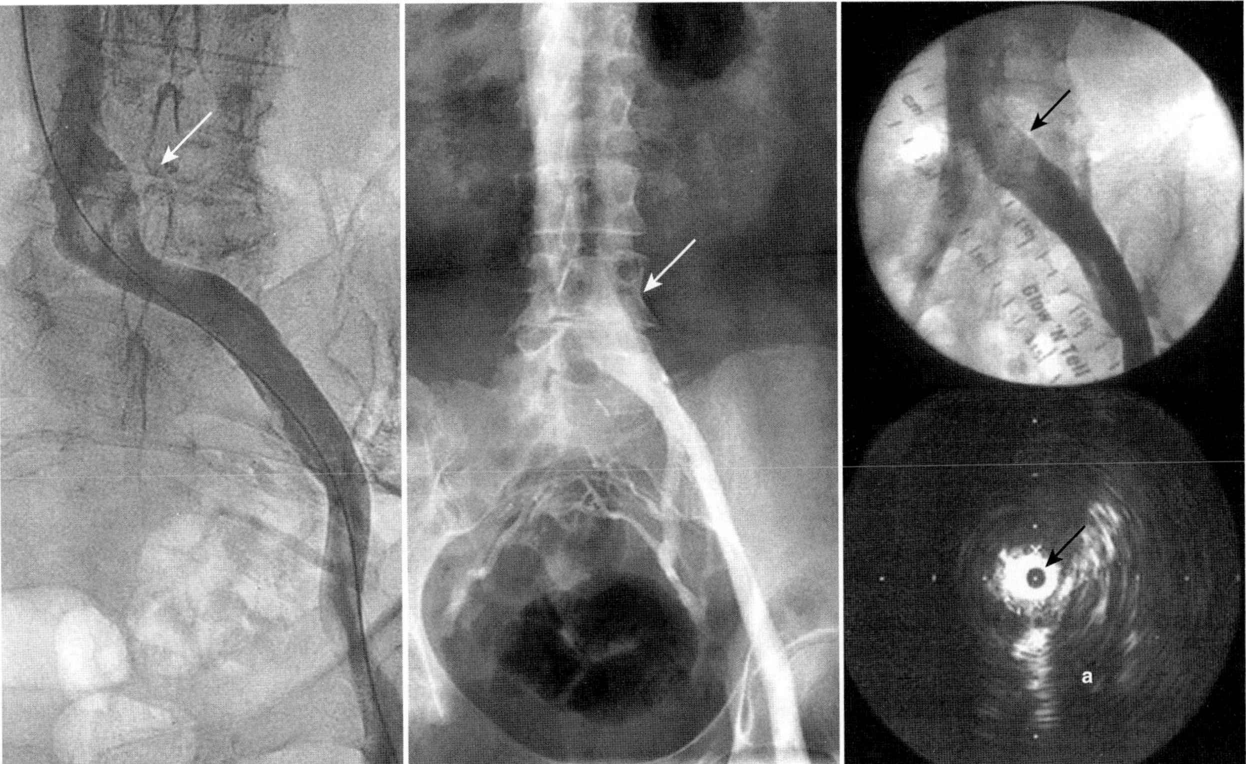

FIGURE 67-3 Venographic appearance of NIVL may be variable. "Classic" islandlike appearance *(left)* and broadening ("pancaking") of the terminal part of the common iliac vein *(center)* can be easily missed on cursory examination. Collaterals *(center)* are present in only a third of cases. The venogram may be entirely normal in frontal projections in about 30% of NIVL limbs. Lateral projections are helpful, but IVUS is more definitive. *Inset* shows a very tight lesion surrounding 6F IVUS catheter with normal venographic appearance *(right).*

diagnostic accuracy of more than 90% in iliac vein lesions.[4] With IVUS, iliac vein lesions can be definitively categorized as NIVLs, postthrombotic, or a combination. NIVLs are subsegmental, whereas postthrombotic lesions are segmental with wall fibrosis; trabeculae when present are easily visible (Figure 67-5). Diagnostic IVUS is best combined with concurrent iliac vein stenting, because IVUS is needed for stent placement as well. IVUS-positive NIVLs occur in proximal as well as distal locations in the iliac vein related to the overlying artery (see Figure 67-1). The crossover arterial segments and the location of the lesions differ somewhat between the right and left sides as is evident on IVUS examination. Conventional pressure measurements are positive in only a third of cases with symptomatic iliac vein obstruction.[3] Duplex technologies to identify iliac vein lesions are in development and have not been adequately validated for routine clinical use. High-resolution computed tomographic or magnetic resonance imaging can identify NIVL and other iliac vein lesions, but their sensitivity has not yet been determined.

A detailed thrombophilia investigation is helpful in making the decision on whether postoperative anticoagulation is needed and how long it should be continued.

TECHNIQUE OF ILIAC VEIN STENTING

General anesthesia is preferred for better pain control during balloon dilatation and recanalization maneuvers; in the elderly, superior cardiopulmonary control is afforded. Ipsilateral antegrade midthigh access through the femoral vein is used; the vein is deep in this location and carries a variable relationship (more often posterolateral) to the artery. With routine use of ultrasound guidance and employment of a sealant (VasoSeal) access complications are rare. Midthigh access has been found to be superior to others such as the popliteal entry or other remote locations in terms of maneuverability ("pushability") and use of shorter-length (150 to 180 cm) endovenous devices, while still allowing ample room for stent deployment below the inguinal ligament when needed without being constrained by the sheath. These advantages are particularly obvious when total iliofemoral occlusions have to be recanalized. A preliminary on-table venography is useful but not essential except in total occlusions. IVUS is the mainstay for assessment and stenting of the iliac vein and adjoining segments. In these roles it is superior to venography, in choice of optimal upper and lower landing sites for the stent assembly, assuring its proper deployment without

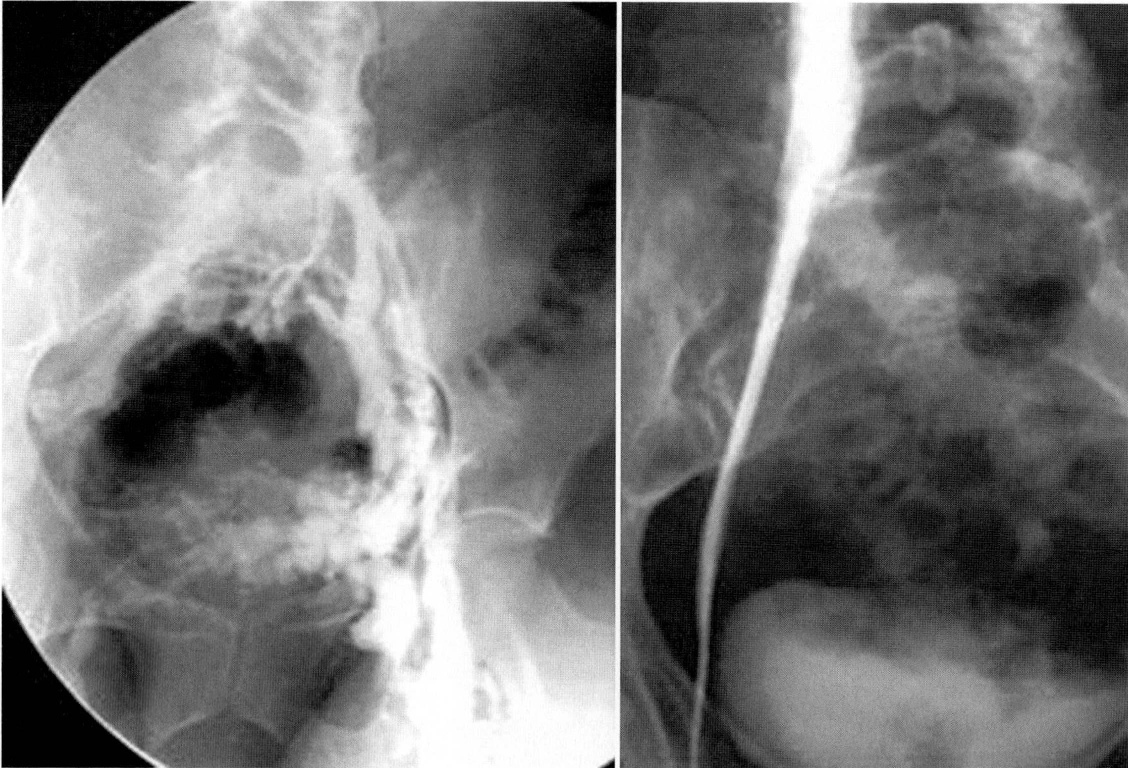

FIGURE 67-4 Variable appearance of postthrombotic stenosis. Lesion with profuse collaterals *(left)* and a diffuse lesion without collaterals *(right)*. A postthrombotic perivenous sheath that develops (see text) retards the development of collaterals. Less-obvious diffuse stenoses are often missed on venography. They are readily apparent on IVUS examination.

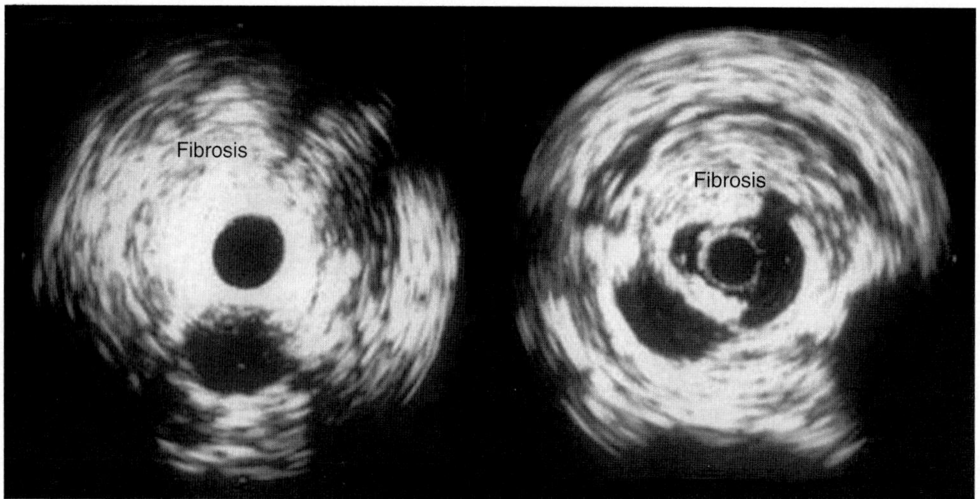

FIGURE 67-5 Wall fibrosis and trabeculae are obvious on IVUS examination. Wall fibrosis and many trabeculae are obscured on venography.

technical defects and minimizing radiation exposure. It can be used exclusively without contrast for stenting stenotic lesions in patients with renal dysfunction.

Successful outcome of venous stenting is dependent on adherence to basic principles of vascular surgery, ensuring adequate inflow and outflow into the reconstructed conduit and avoiding technical faults therein. This means that all lesions should be covered with stent(s) with no skip areas. Although the iliac vein appears mildly curvaceous on frontal projections, it in fact pursues a spiral course through the pelvis with sharp angulation at the pelvic brim. Successive stents should be significantly overlapped (3 to 4 cm) so as to avoid shelving at angulation points or stent separation.

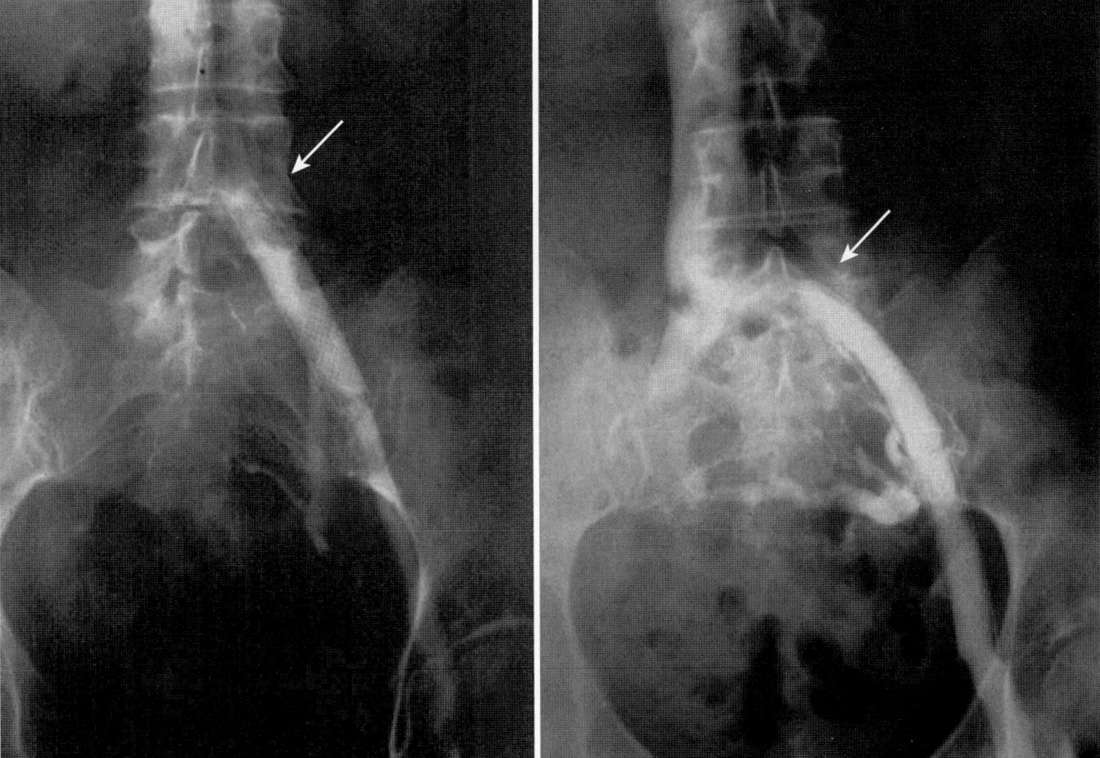

FIGURE 67-6 Recurrence of stenosis at iliac-IVC junction from local stent retraction/migration because of inadequate extension of the stent into the IVC *(left, center)*. The stent should be extended 3 to 5 cm into the IVC *(right)* to prevent such recurrence. Contralateral flow is seldom affected.

Stent separation occurs from local retraction or migration of individual braided stents at NIVL choke points and elsewhere because of dense fibrosis in postthrombotic disease. The iliocaval junction is a major choke point in NIVL, as well as postthrombotic cases. Extension of the stent for 3 to 5 cm into the IVC is necessary to avoid retrograde stent migration and recurrence of stent stenosis at this point (Figure 67-6). Contralateral flow is seldom affected by this practice. The femoral vein segment behind the inguinal ligament is another choke point requiring stent extension into the common femoral vein when retroinguinal stenosis is detected. Misguided compromise of these principles in an effort to minimize metal load may lead to poor clinical outcome from inadequate limb decompression or stent occlusion (Figure 67-7). Metal load per se does not appear to be thrombogenic, because extensive stent assemblies remain patent long term[6] provided all underlying lesions have been corrected (Figure 67-8). Stents can and should be extended below the inguinal crease in pursuit of these principles; stent compression, erosion, or fracture seldom occurs behind the inguinal ligament when braided self-expanding stents are used.[16] Stent malfunction caused by inadequate initial stenting can be salvaged by further iterant stenting to correct missed lesions.

RECANALIZATION OF OCCLUDED ILIOCAVAL VEINS

Many or most iliac vein occlusions, even including total occlusions of the IVC, can now be recanalized with modifications of the basic stent technique described earlier.[6,17] Access can frequently be obtained through the upper femoral vein even if it appears occluded on venography. Gradual dilatation of the fibrotic entry site in the postthrombotic vein to accommodate a size 10 or 11 sheath is usually necessary. If the common femoral vein is occluded at or below the inguinal ligament, a cutting balloon, Frontrunner device, atherectomy catheter, or laser-created channel may be selectively used to initiate guidewire entry into the occluded segment. Further progress of the Glidewire through the occluded vein segment(s) may be unexpectedly easy or variably difficult, testing patience and sometimes requiring further attempt(s) after a few weeks for eventual success. If guidewire progress is stalled, different guidewires of varying size, stiffness, and tip configurations are tried in sequence. Catheter support of the Glidewire is helpful in its passage. The Quickcross catheter is particularly useful in crossing several choke points in guidewire passage—behind the inguinal ligament, at the hypogastric and iliac

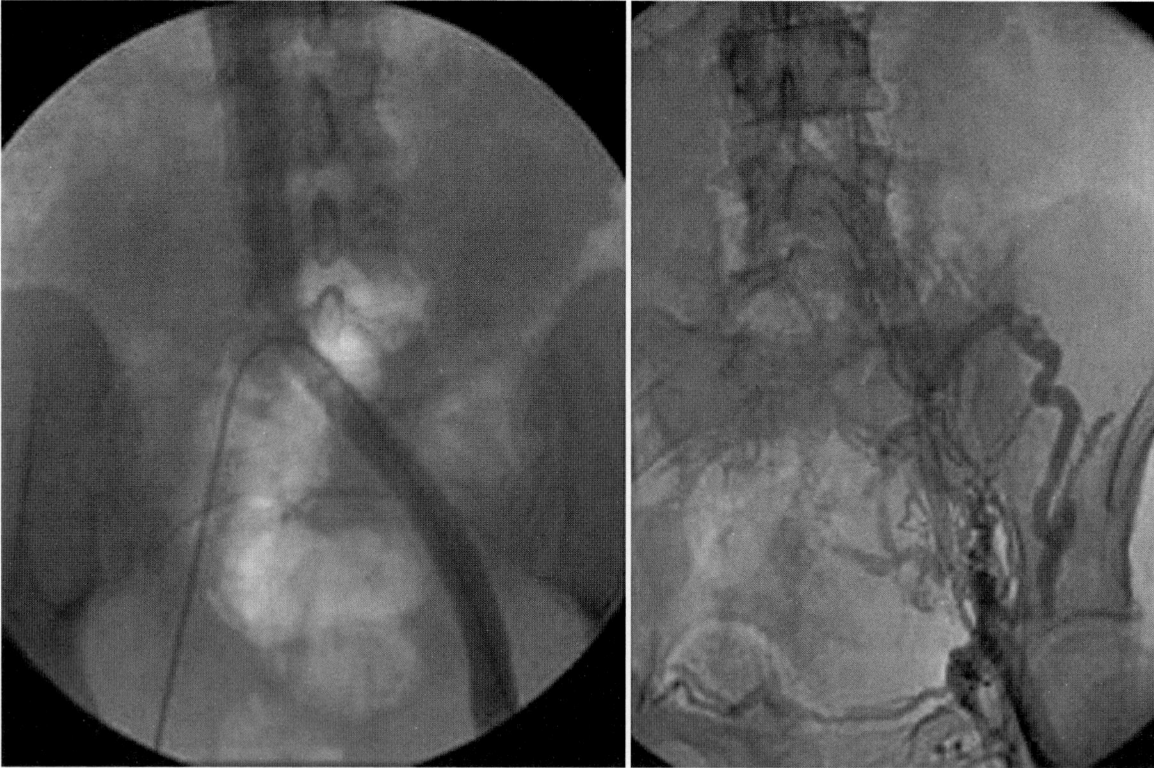

FIGURE 67-7 Deployed stent should approximate size of native vein being treated. Oversizing by one or two sizes (see text) is recommended. Undersizing can result in inadequate venous decompression of the limb *(left)* or stent thrombosis *(right)*.

artery crossover points through the iliac vein, and higher up at the renal and diaphragmatic levels in the IVC. Because collaterals are often present at these levels, proper direction of the guidewire with an angled-tip catheter is helpful. The process is "blind" and depends on feel and sense of anatomy because the occluded vein is invisible and venous occlusions generally involve the entire segment or segments in continuity. This procedure is enhanced by experience, but one is impressed by how the advancing guidewire invariably tends to track the occluded vein presumably because passage occurs through vascular channels in the organized thrombus not visible on venography. Off-course deviations of the guidewire through collaterals or otherwise are readily apparent and seldom pose a threat even if perforations were to occur. The guidewire can then be retracted and progress resumed in the proper direction without fear of clinical bleeding presumably because of the low prevailing pressure in the veins and restriction of local bleeding by perivenous tissues. Very rarely, the Glidewire can pass into the vertebral canal when traversing the pelvic brim through vertebral collaterals without being readily apparent in frontal projections. Vertical tracking of the guidewire at the center of the fourth and fifth lumbar vertebrae instead of to one side is a clue that should prompt lateral projection fluoroscopy for confirmation. No malsequelae resulted after withdrawal and redirection of the guidewire when this occurred. Entry of the guidewire into the open venous segment above the occlusion is indicated when it passes rapidly tracking the IVC into the right atrium. This can be confirmed by venography or preferably IVUS after minimal dilatation of the recanalized channel to allow passage of the IVUS catheter (6F). Once proper positioning of the guidewire has been confirmed, the occluded vein segments should be progressively dilated to native size (21 mm for the IVC, 16 mm for CIV, 14 mm for CIV, 12 mm for CFV). Because some recoil of the recanalized channel, particularly at the aforementioned choke points, occurs over time, overdilatation and oversized stenting by one or two sizes is recommended. This allows for aggressive postdilatation or later redilatation if recoil results in clinically significant restenosis. Such aggressive dilatation of a totally occluded venous cord may seem hazardous but appears to be entirely safe (Figure 67-9). Optimal proximal and distal landing sites for the stent assembly are chosen by IVUS examination.

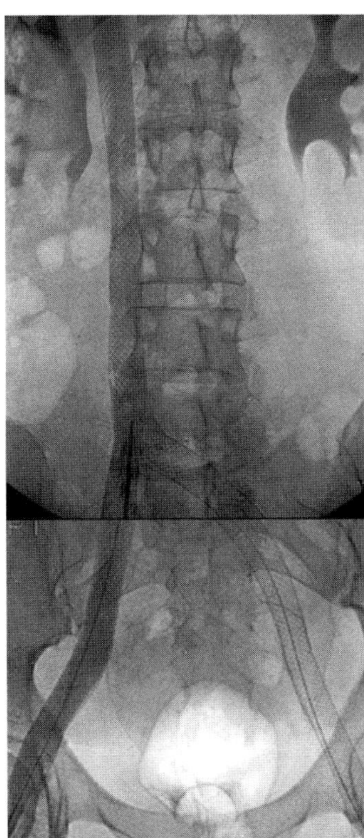

FIGURE 67-8 Extensive stenting of IVC and bilateral iliofemoral veins. Note crossing of the inguinal ligament to cover all stenotic lesions. Metal load per se does not seem to be thrombogenic. On the contrary, inadequate stenting to limit metal load may result in stent malfunction or even thrombosis (see text).

SPECIAL TECHNIQUES

Bilateral Stenting

Bilateral iliac vein stenting is necessary in about 20% of cases. Simultaneous bilateral iliac vein stenting can be accomplished by using the standard technique. In that event, the stents lie side by side in the vena cava ("double barrel"). This is not possible if staged bilateral stenting is performed because the older stent will tend to compress the newly placed contralateral stent. Such delayed contralateral stenting is desirable in many cases because the opposite limb tends to improve symptomatically after unilateral stenting. The mechanism is not clear but may be related to offloading from cessation of collateral circulation load. Staged delayed stenting requires fenestration of the existing stent in the vena caval segment. Often the Glidewire will pass through the interstices of the existing stent to initiate the fenestration process. If not, a TIPS needle may be used to penetrate the stent for guidewire passage (Figure 67-10).

Inferior Vena Cava Filters

When an IVC filter is present, IVUS should be used to determine whether a stenosis is present at the implantation site. The incidence of stenosis varies with the type of filter used. If a stenosis is present, the filter is moved away by repeated balloon dilatation[18] and the stent extended across. A variety of filters have been moved in this fashion without malsequelae (Figure 67-11).

POSTOPERATIVE ANTICOAGULATION AND STENT SURVEILLANCE

Aspirin has been found to be adequate in NIVL cases for stent maintenance. The risk of stent thrombosis is virtually nil in this subset. Aspirin may also be adequate in postthrombotic cases in which the thrombotic event was related to a transient thrombophilia in the past. Long-term warfarin anticoagulation is indicated in cases of recurrent thrombosis and in cases of specific thrombophilia. Perioperative low-molecular-weight heparin is standard in both NIVL and postthrombotic cases.

Routine stent surveillance by duplex or venography is carried out at 6 weeks and once a year in NIVL cases to detect features of stent malfunction (new or missed stenosis, inflow/outflow problems, intrastent abnormalities). Interval stent imaging will be required if symptoms recur. Seven percent of postthrombotic stents occlude, many of them in the recanalized subset. More intensive routine stent surveillance in the recanalized subset may be warranted.

OUTCOME

Iliocaval venous stenting is a safe and effective procedure. It is well tolerated even in the geriatric population. Thirty-day mortality has been zero in a consecutive series of 982 limbs.[19] There were no stent-related complications such as embolization, fracture, rupture of the vein, or infection. One instance of pelvic hematoma requiring transfusion recently occurred in a difficult recanalization procedure. The incidence of DVT (<30 day) was 1.5%.

There were no stent occlusions in 518 NIVL limbs and only 31 (7%) stent occlusions in 464 postthrombotic limbs followed long term. This results in impressive cumulative stent patency (Figure 67-12). Cumulative long-term improvement in pain and swelling was significant; *complete* relief of limb pain and swelling was achieved in a large fraction of these (Figure 67-13). Relief of swelling is somewhat inferior to that of pain partly because swelling is more recalcitrant than pain to relieve (curiously more often in early onset NIVL limbs) and partly because of metrics problems in quantifying pain (see earlier). Relief of pain associated with swelling often results in significant clinical benefit even if the latter is

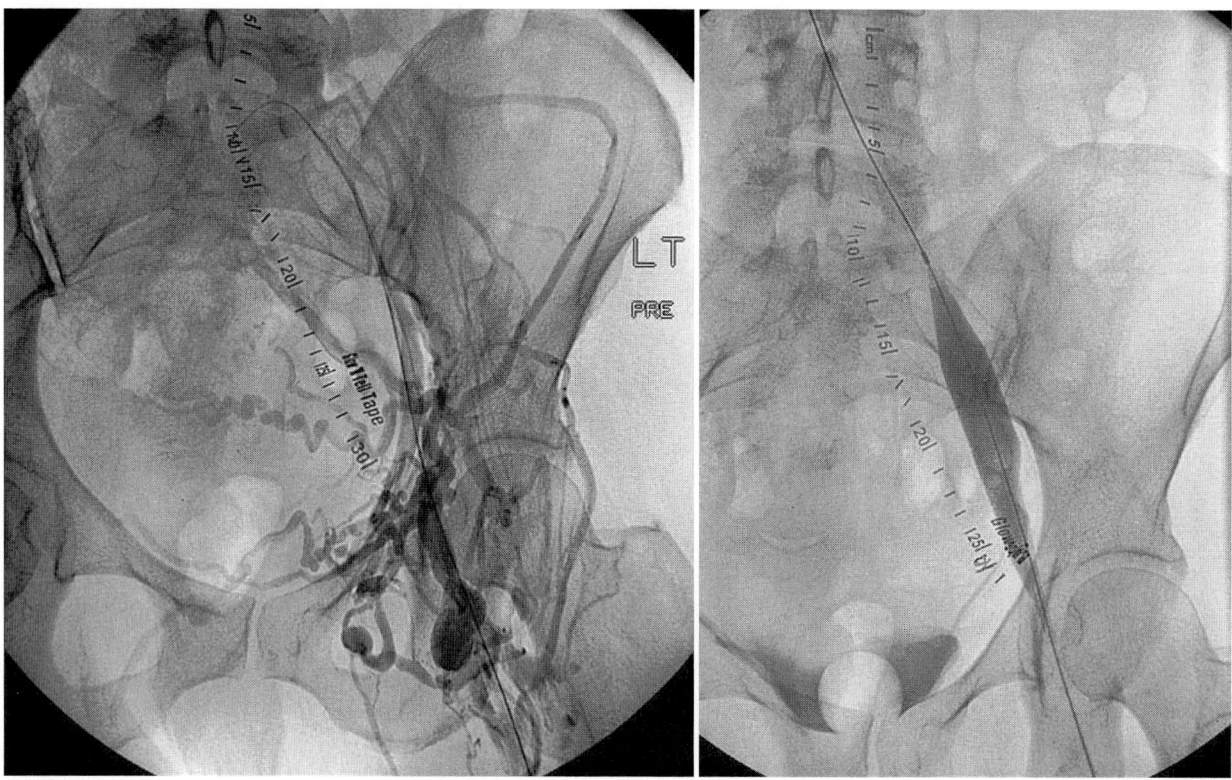

FIGURE 67-9 Aggressive dilatation of an occluded venous cord may seem hazardous but is necessary to accommodate a proper-sized stent. The practice seems to be safe (see text) presumably because any rupture that occurs is locally well contained by perivenous tissues aided by the low pressure prevailing in veins.

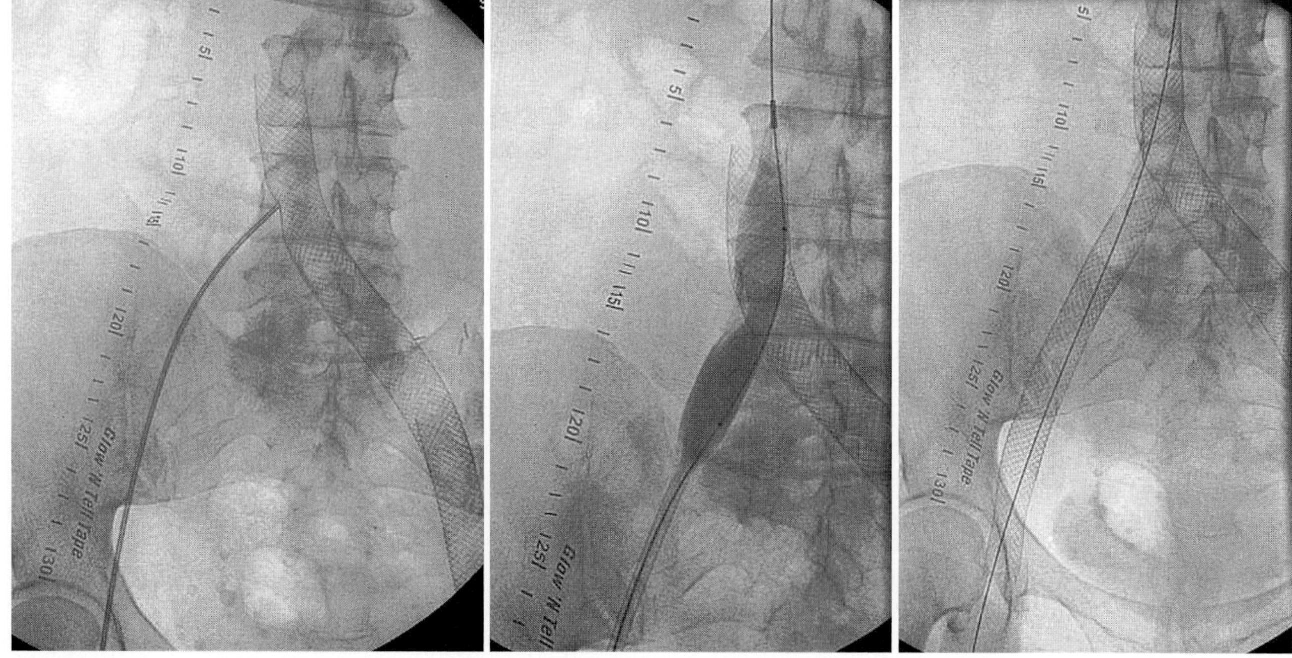

FIGURE 67-10 Use of TIPS needle to create a fenestrum in the resident stent in cases of staged bilateral stenting.

not completely or only partially relieved. Partial improvement in swelling can accrue clinical benefit, for example, enabling a previously wheelchair-bound patient to ambulate or discard assist devices for movement. Cumulative ulcer healing was 58% at 5 years (Figure 67-14) even though associated reflux when present was left uncorrected. Quality of life was significantly improved.

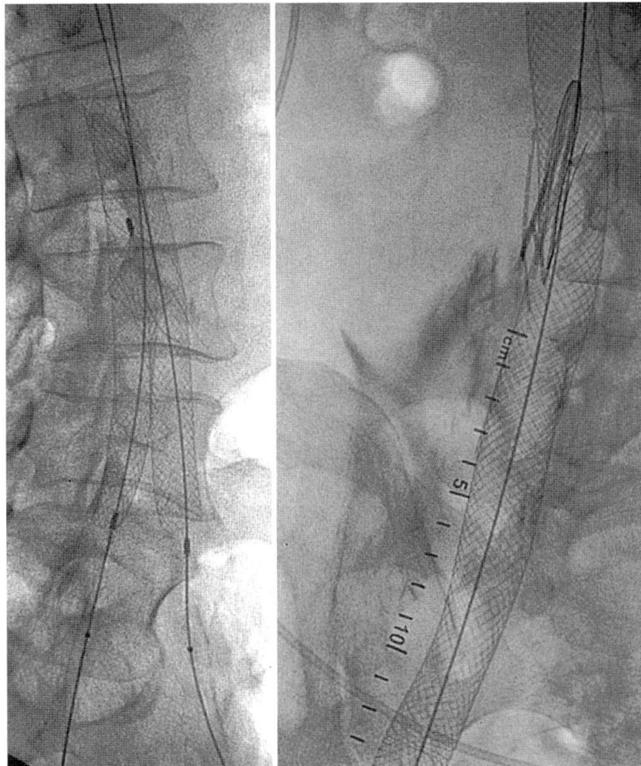

FIGURE 67-11 Filters are often encountered in iliocaval stenting and may be associated with significant stenosis at the implantation site (IVUS). They can be compacted by repeated balloon dilatation and stented across. All types of commercially available filters have been treated in this fashion without incident (see text). Note extension of the long stent below the groin crease. Risk of stent fracture, erosion, or propensity of increased thrombosis from this practice is very low in venous stenting.

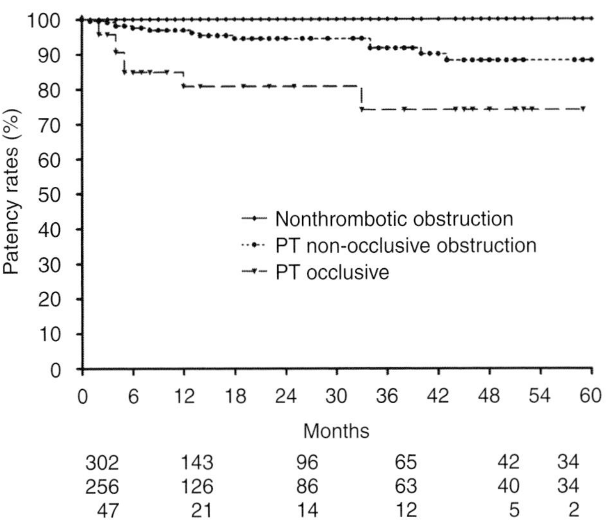

FIGURE 67-12 Long-term stent patency (cumulative) in NIVL and postthrombotic subsets. Stent occlusions virtually never occur in NIVL limbs (see text) and are restricted (7% incidence) to postthrombotic cases, particularly recanalized veins. Stent surveillance at planned regular intervals and timely correction of any stent abnormalities (inflow/outflow or intrastent) in the latter subset may further reduce stent thrombosis incidence.

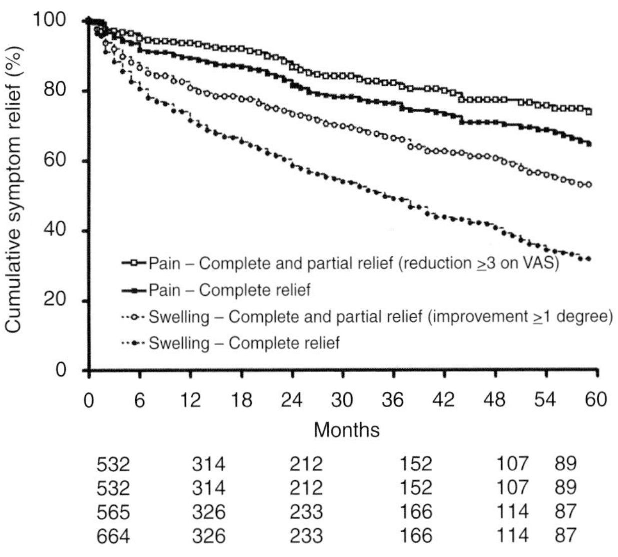

FIGURE 67-13 Cumulative improvement in pain (3/10 on visual analogue scale or greater) and swelling (grade 1 or greater; see text) after stenting. *Complete* relief of pain and swelling was noted in the majority with noted clinical benefit *(lower curves)*.

OBSTRUCTIONS OF THE INFERIOR VENA CAVA

IVC obstructions have many curious clinical features unexpected for lesions involving such a major venous pathway. This is related to the rich collaterals that develop in IVC obstructions, which have an embryonic basis (Figure 67-15). With the widespread use of imaging in clinical medicine many instances of incidental asymptomatic caval occlusions are now identified. Permanent anticoagulation is recommended in such instances to reduce the chances of DVT involving the distal venous tree and/or collaterals, which can precipitate symptoms in a previously asymptomatic patient. The iliac vein is the origin of most IVC collaterals, and its involvement in the thrombotic process invariably leads to symptom production. Successful catheter lysis of the thrombus can revert the patient to the previous asymptomatic state even though the vena cava occlusion itself remains unresolved.[6] Chronic disease in the iliac vein segment also appears to play a role in symptom development in IVC obstructions. In two thirds of patients with IVC obstructions, symptoms are unilateral involving the side with concurrent iliac vein disease.[6] Renal or hepatic dysfunction is rare in adults with IVC occlusions, presumably because of adequate collateral drainage. In Budd-Chiari syndrome the hepatic veins are often additionally involved in the occlusive process.

Stenosis and occlusions of the IVC are amenable to stent treatment.[6] Even total IVC occlusions involving the thoracic segment can be successfully recanalized with stents extending into the right atrium. Despite the long and extensive stenting required, patency appears to be excellent, similar to iliac vein stenting in postthrombotic disease. Outcome is also excellent. In a series of 99 cases that underwent stenting of the IVC, cumulative *complete* relief of pain and swelling at 3½ years was 74% and 51%, respectively.

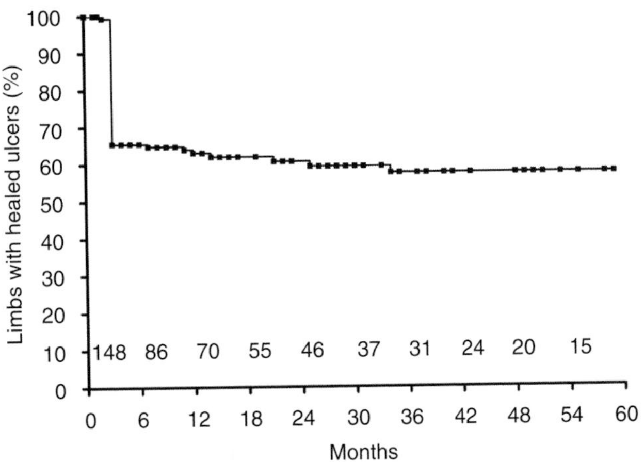

FIGURE 67-14 Cumulative complete ulcer healing after stenting. Ulcers that had not healed by 4 months after stenting were scored as unhealed and were not included if they healed later. After initial healing, very few ulcers recur, resulting in a flat curve. Many limbs had untreated residual reflux (see text), which raises fundamental questions regarding pathophysiology of venous stasis ulceration, which is commonly attributed to reflux, not obstruction.

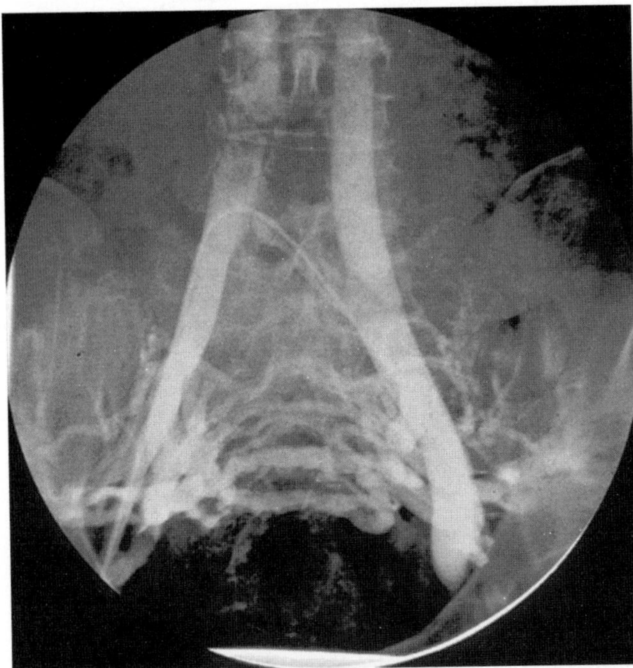

FIGURE 67-15 Extensive collateralization in a limb with IVC obstruction giving the appearance of double vena cava. Symptoms were minimal (vague limb pain) and transient in this instance. No specific treatment was offered, and long-term anticoagulation was recommended (see text). The collaterals arise from embryonic caval elements that are present in putative form. Most arise from the iliac vein, disease of which (acute or chronic) can precipitate symptoms.

References

1. Johnson BF, Manzo RA, Bergelin RO, et al: Relationship between changes in the deep venous system and the development of the postthrombotic syndrome after an acute episode of lower limb deep vein thrombosis: a one- to six-year follow-up, *J Vasc Surg* 21:307–312, 1995, discussion 13.
2. Neglen P, Thrasher TL, Raju S: Venous outflow obstruction: an underestimated contributor to chronic venous disease, *J Vasc Surg* 38:879–885, 2003.
3. Neglen P, Raju S: Intravascular ultrasound scan evaluation of the obstructed vein, *J Vasc Surg* 35:694–700, 2002.
4. Raju S, Neglen P: High prevalence of nonthrombotic iliac vein lesions in chronic venous disease: a permissive role in pathogenicity, *J Vasc Surg* 44:136–143, 2006, discussion 44.
5. Raju S, Fountain T, Neglen P, et al: Axial transformation of the profunda femoris vein, *J Vasc Surg* 27:651–659, 1998.
6. Raju S, Hollis K, Neglen P: Obstructive lesions of the inferior vena cava: clinical features and endovenous treatment, *J Vasc Surg* 44:820–827, 2006.
7. Raju S, Fredericks R: Venous obstruction: an analysis of one hundred thirty-seven cases with hemodynamic, venographic, and clinical correlations, *J Vasc Surg* 14:305–313, 1991.
8. Kibbe MR, Ujiki M, Goodwin AL, et al: Iliac vein compression in an asymptomatic patient population, *J Vasc Surg* 39:937–943, 2004.
9. Raju S, Tackett P Jr, Neglen P: Spontaneous onset of bacterial cellulitis in lower limbs with chronic obstructive venous disease, *Eur J Vasc Endovasc Surg*, 2008.
10. Neglen P, Hollis KC, Raju S: Combined saphenous ablation and iliac stent placement for complex severe chronic venous disease, *J Vasc Surg* 44:828–833, 2006.
11. Raju S, Easterwood L, Fountain T, et al: Saphenectomy in the presence of chronic venous obstruction, *Surgery* 123:637–644, 1998.
12. Rutherford RB, Padberg FTJ, Comerota AJ, et al: Venous severity scoring: an adjunct to venous outcome assessment, *J Vasc Surg* 31:1307–1312, 2000.
13. Launois R, Rebpi-Marty J, Henry B: Construction and validation of a quality of life questionnaire in chronic lower limb venous insufficiency (CIVIQ), *Qual Life Res* 5:539–554, 1996.
14. Scott J, Huskisson EC: Graphic representation of pain, *Pain* 2:175–184, 1976.
15. Negus D, Fletcher EW, Cockett FB, et al: Compression and band formation at the mouth of the left common iliac vein, *Br J Surg* 55:369–374, 1968.
16. Neglen P, Tacket P, Raju S: Venous stenting across the inguinal ligament, *J Vasc Surg*, 2008, Submitted.
17. Raju S, McAllister S, Neglen P: Recanalization of totally occluded iliac and adjacent venous segments, *J Vasc Surg* 36:903–911, 2002.
18. Vedantham S, Vesely TM, Parti N, et al: Endovascular recanalization of the thrombosed filter-bearing inferior vena cava, *J Vasc Interv Radiol* 14:893–903, 2003.
19. Neglen P, Hollis KC, Olivier J, et al: Stenting of the venous outflow in chronic venous disease: long-term stent-related outcome, clinical, and hemodynamic result, *J Vasc Surg* 46:979–990, 2007.

CHAPTER

68

Endovascular Ablation of Veins

Richard Brad Cook, David A. Rigberg

Varicose veins are a common condition, affecting an estimated 25% of women and 15% of men in the United States.[1] Aside from patients' concerns regarding cosmetics, varicosities themselves may be symptomatic and often manifestations of underlying venous insufficiency. Risk factors include female sex, advanced age, family history, and increased hydrostatic pressure, which can be brought on by a variety of factors. The majority (60%-80%) of varicose veins arise from incompetence of the saphenofemoral junction and associated great saphenous vein (GSV) reflux.[2,3] Left untreated, a subset of patients with significant superficial venous insufficiency will progress to the chronic phase characterized by lower-extremity edema, pigmentation, eczema, and ulceration.[4]

The gold standard treatment for saphenous vein reflux has been high ligation of the saphenous vein at the saphenofemoral junction with surgical removal of the distal vein and ligation of all tributary vessels. This procedure typically requires general anesthesia, although it can be performed with the patient under sedation with sufficient tumescent anesthetic administration. It is frequently accompanied by extensive postoperative bruising, pain, and scar formation. Complications include wound infections and saphenous nerve injury, and duplex-documented recurrence rates of 66% at 5 years have been reported for a variety of open venous procedures.[5] Alternatively, endovenous obliteration of the saphenous vein can be performed by using radiofrequency (RF) or laser energy.

RADIOFREQUENCY ABLATION

Endovenous radiofrequency ablation (RFA) has become the most common alternative approach to treating superficial and perforator venous reflux.[6] Indications for treatment are duplex-proved reflux of the GSV extending to the saphenofemoral junction or upper thigh along with concomitant symptoms of venous insufficiency. Reflux in the small saphenous vein can also be treated by either endovenous method. Indications for perforator treatment are reflux in the perforator vein, which can frequently be defined on a size basis (>3 mm) and usually the presence of an associated venous ulcer.

The VNUS Closure system (VNUS Medical Technologies, Sunnyvale, CA) uses an endovenous catheter (the Closure catheter) with bipolar electrodes at the tip to disperse energy generated from a RF generator. Energy delivered at high frequency (200-3000 kHz) heats tissue by a resistive mechanism whereby high-resistant tissues such as vein wall and valves are heated as the energy passes through, while lower-resistance fluids are not heated. A thermocouple device on the catheter provides constant evaluation of the impedance and temperature and automatically adjusts the power to maintain a constant temperature. The clinical effect is precise coagulation, vein shrinkage, closure, and ultimate obliteration of the vein with minimal thrombus formation. There are currently two types of catheters approved for treatment of saphenous veins and accessory branches. The ClosurePLUS catheter is available in 6F and 8F sizes. The 6F size can treat veins with diameters of up to 8 mm, and the 8F size can treat up to 12-mm vessels. Both are available in 60-cm and 100-cm lengths and can accommodate a 0.025-inch guidewire. The newer ClosureFAST catheter requires a 7F introducer sheath and also comes in 60-cm and 100-cm lengths. This catheter delivers energy simultaneously along a longer 7-cm length of vein and does not require a slow, continuous withdrawal of the catheter as is required when using the ClosurePLUS catheter. It also uses a higher temperature of 95° to 120° C compared with 85° to 90° C. With these changes, the average procedure time may be reduced from 15 to 20 minutes to 1.5 to 3 minutes.

RADIOFREQUENCY ABLATION OF THE GREAT SAPHENOUS VEIN

This procedure can be performed in either an office setting or an outpatient operative suite. Anesthetic can range from straight local to conscious sedation; in our practice, 5 mg of oral diazepam (Valium) is given after consent is obtained. All varicosities are marked with the patient in the standing position. Careful notation is then made as to the effect leg elevation has on the branches. Branches that disappear with leg elevation are generally not removed concomitant with saphenous ablation. However, those branches that persist with leg elevation are unlikely to resolve after saphenous treatment alone and are removed via the technique of microstab phlebectomy. Other practitioners never perform branch removal at the time of vein ablation, and there is literature supporting the idea that this allows for a reduction in the number of branches that must eventually be removed.[7] The patient is then positioned supine on a table with tilt capabilities. The course of the GSV is identified by duplex ultrasound from the saphenofemoral junction to the knee and marked. Careful evaluation is made for depth of the vein and tortuosity. Notation is also made of the caliber of the vein; if the pattern of saphenofemoral reflux is directed through alternative branches (such as an anterolateral thigh branch), access to the saphenous vein may be difficult. A relatively straight vein measuring at least 3 mm with the bed in Trendelenburg position is ideal.

The leg is then prepped in accordance with the planned procedure. If no adjunctive procedures are to be performed, a simple preparation of the groin and medial thigh to the level of the knee is undertaken. If more extensive work is planned, the leg may be prepped circumferentially. The skin above the access site is infiltrated with 1% buffered lidocaine without epinephrine. The vein is then percutaneously accessed either just below or above the knee under ultrasound guidance with use of a micropuncture kit (Figure 68-1). At this level, the venous course is linear, and there is a smaller risk of nerve injury. Applying topical nitroglycerin paste and using the reverse Trendelenburg position may help counteract any venospasm. Additionally, venospasm brought on by patient anxiety or a cold environment should be avoided. Great care is taken with the first puncture attempt, as this is usually the best opportunity for successful venous cannulation. A guidewire is then inserted, the needle is removed, a small skin incision is made, and the introducer sheath (6F-8F by 7 or 11 cm) is inserted with use of the Seldinger technique. An intraluminal position is confirmed by ultrasound examination and by aspirating dark, nonpulsatile blood from the side port (Figure 68-2). The appropriate catheter is then inserted and advanced under ultrasound guidance to 2 cm below the saphenofemoral junction. Ablation of the vein any closer to the saphenofemoral junction greatly increases the risk for development of deep venous thrombosis (DVT). The patient is then placed in Trendelenburg position to reduce lower-extremity venous pressure. Approximately 300 to 400 mL of a tumescent solution (0.1% lidocaine with epinephrine and bicarbonate in normal saline solution) is then injected via a 19-gauge spinal needle and either a high-pressure delivery system or a continuously filling hand-operated injector into the saphenous space surrounding the vein. The solution will compress the wall of the vein onto the catheter, aid in exsanguination of the vein, provide a thermal sink to shield adjacent tissues from radiant heat, and provide local anesthesia.

Once the catheter position is confirmed and tumescent solution is instilled, the positioning of the catheter tip is again confirmed in multiple planes via ultrasound examination (Figure 68-3). RF energy is delivered, and

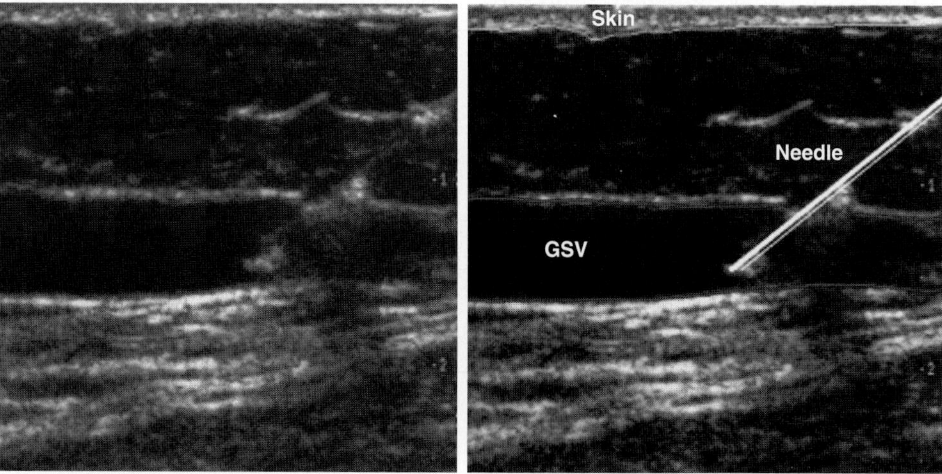

FIGURE 68-1 Longitudinal view demonstrating percutaneous access of the great saphenous vein (GSV). Great care must be taken while establishing venous access, as spasm of the vein can make subsequent attempts very difficult.

the vein wall is heated to the catheter's goal temperature. External pressure is applied by using the surgeon's hand or the ultrasound probe to assist in vein wall apposition to the catheter. Power will typically begin at 40 W and should drop to below 20 W within 10 seconds. Continued high power or inability to reach the set temperature usually indicates continued flow within the vessel that is cooling the treated segment or a catheter that is not in the vessel lumen. In this situation, catheter or patient repositioning or more forceful external pressure may be indicated. Energy is then delivered while the ClosurePLUS catheter is slowly withdrawn at a rate of 1 to 3 mm/s depending on the set temperature. The ClosureFAST catheter remains in position for 20 seconds and then is repositioned at roughly 7-cm segments, and the cycle is repeated. The segment closest to the saphenofemoral junction undergoes two cycles of treatment with the newer ClosureFAST system. The process continues until the introducer sheath is reached but should not continue while the treating element is inside the introducer. Contraction of the GSV with absence of flow is confirmed by ultrasound examination along with patency of the femoral vein and superior epigastric vein at the saphenofemoral junction (Figure 68-4). Although flow may be present, a characteristic white, thick-walled appearance of the treated vein should be noted. Residual varicosities may now be treated. At the conclusion, abdominal pads are positioned over the obliterated vein and secured with stockinette and pressure dressings. The patient is instructed to ambulate frequently but to avoid strenuous activities or heavy lifting for several days. Follow-up examination in 48 to 72 hours includes removal of dressings and repeated ultrasound scan to rule out thrombus extension into the femoral vein.

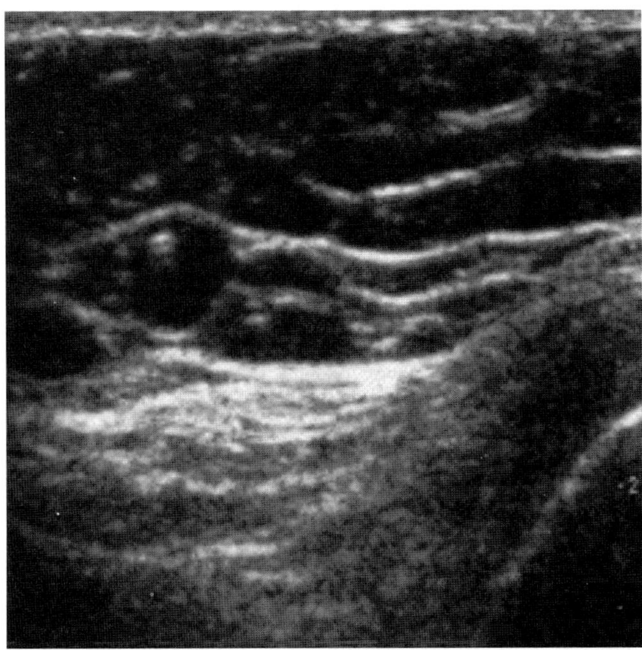

FIGURE 68-2 Pictured is a transverse view of the guidewire in the GSV. Confirmation should be obtained via ultrasound examination that the wire is within the vein and also that it is not in a branch before the sheath is placed.

RADIOFREQUENCY ABLATION OF THE LESSER SAPHENOUS AND PERFORATOR VEINS

Small saphenous vein treatment is performed similarly to GSV ablation with a few important differences. The patient is positioned prone. Great care must be taken in identifying the saphenopopliteal junction, because there is considerable variation in the location of this structure. Great care must also be taken in the placement of the tumescent anesthetic, because the vein is frequently quite superficial. Patients should be

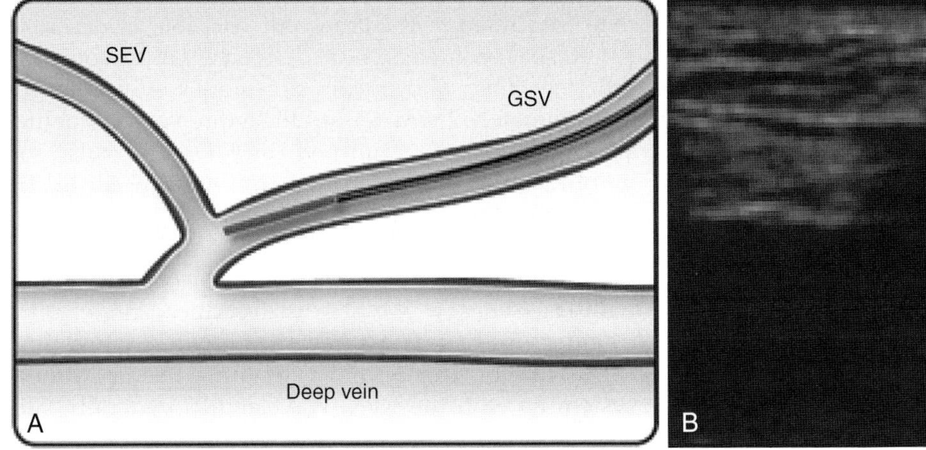

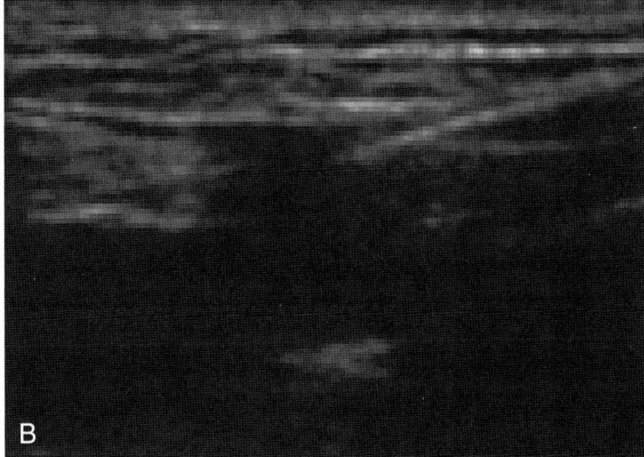

FIGURE 68-3 Schematic **(A)** and B-mode ultrasound scan **(B)** of laser fiber positioned at the superior epigastric vein (SEV) "before" the saphenofemoral junction. In addition to using the SEV as a guide, it is safest to position the catheter at least 2 cm from the deep system.

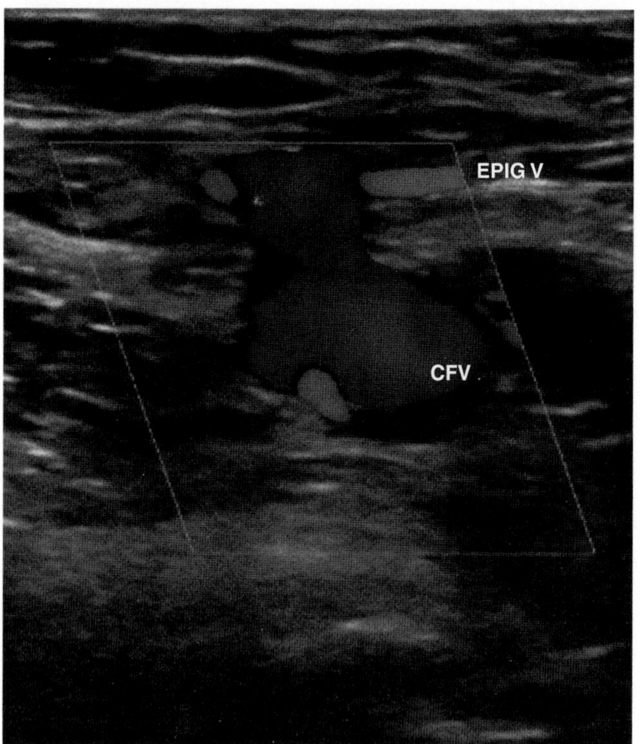

FIGURE 68-4 Ultrasound of saphenofemoral junction demonstrating closure of the saphenous vein and patency of the superior epigastric vein (EPIG V) and the common femoral vein (CFV). Both brightness and color-flow Doppler are used in the postprocedure evaluation.

carefully screened via ultrasound examination by the surgeon before selecting this technique over traditional open procedures for the small saphenous vein.

Perforator veins of the lower extremity are short and tend to be angulated, which makes the technique more challenging. Careful, thorough imaging and marking by ultrasound is necessary. Two catheters are currently available for RFA of perforator veins: the ClosurePLEX and the ClosureRFS. The confluence of the refluxing perforator vein with the deep venous system is identified, and the access site is marked by ultrasound. The perforator vein is accessed under ultrasound guidance with use of a flexible ClosurePLEX catheter or a more rigid ClosureRFS. The short catheter and needle are a single unit with the latter; when blood is aspirated from the vein, the needle is gently withdrawn. Tumescence is placed, and the treatment usually involves four quadrant positioning of the catheter by gently turning and leaning it. One of the great difficulties of perforator treatment is the difficulty in visualizing the vessel after the anesthetic has been injected. This makes it particularly troublesome when attempting to discern whether treatment has been effective. Patients are told to wait until their postprocedure ultrasound examination in 48 to 72 hours before we advise them on the status of the treated perforator vessel.

ENDOVENOUS LASER ABLATION

Lasers induce thermal reactions by using focused light energy. The light energy from a laser (*l*ight *a*mplification by *s*timulated *e*mission of *r*adiation) is monochromatic (one wavelength), and therefore the penetration into tissues can be adjusted depending on the wavelength chosen. Although the mechanism is not entirely clear, the direct and indirect thermal reactions caused by the laser induce vein wall coagulation, contraction, and obliteration of the vessel. In January 2002 the U.S. Food and Drug Administration approved endovenous laser treatment (EVLT). The 810-, 940-, 980-, and 1320-nm diode lasers have all been effective for EVLT, although two comparative studies have shown that patients treated with higher wavelengths reported less postoperative pain and were less likely to have ecchymosis.[8,9] In contrast to the RFA catheter, the temperature of the laser tip may reach 800° C, and the energy dissipates rapidly into surrounding tissue.

TECHNIQUE OF ENDOVENOUS LASER THERAPY

EVLT may also be performed in an outpatient setting. Anesthesia and patient positioning are identical to that for RFA. The GSV is accessed with an 18-gauge needle, a 0.035-inch guidewire is inserted and advanced to the common femoral vein, and a sheath is placed. The dilator and guidewire are removed, and the sheath is withdrawn to its starting position 1 cm distal to the saphenofemoral junction. The diode laser fiber is then inserted and advanced until the tip is flush with the end of the sheath. The sheath is then withdrawn to expose the distal 3 cm of the laser fiber. Positioning is confirmed by ultrasound examination and by direct visualization of the red aiming beam of the laser fiber through the skin. The tissue surrounding the vein is then infiltrated with tumescent solution as described for RFA. Laser energy is delivered continuously as the laser fiber and sheath are slowly withdrawn at approximately 2 mm/s until the entire vessel is obliterated. Results are confirmed, and DVT is ruled out by ultrasound at the conclusion of the procedure. The technique for small saphenous vein treatment is similar, again with the differences outlined for RFA treatment earlier. Perforator veins can also be treated with laser energy. The fiber is introduced under ultrasound guidance via a small sheath (16-18 gauge) into the perforator. There is not a combined needle/catheter system as with the RFA. Wavelengths generally cited in the literature are between 940 and 1320 nm. The procedure is otherwise performed similarly to the perforator RFA.

OUTCOMES OF ENDOLUMINAL THERAPY

In most studies, successful treatment is typically defined as an occluded vessel as demonstrated by the absence of flow on ultrasound examination. Traditional surgery results in recurrent venous reflux in approximately 15% and 20% of treated limbs at 1 and 5 years, respectively.[10] The primary cause of long-term recurrence is theorized to be neovascularization, although there are also patients with paired saphenous systems where the smaller retained vein becomes more prominent over time or even reflux from pelvic or abdominal veins.[11-13] With regard to RFA and EVLT of the saphenous vein, there is a body of literature documenting the safety and efficacy of these procedures. Ravi et al.[14] reported on one experience of 1091 consecutive limbs treated for GSV and small saphenous vein reflux with EVLT. Although 1 year follow-up was reported for only 200 limbs, there was a 96.7% and 91.0% rate of GSV and small saphenous vein occlusion for up to 1 year, and only one major complication (pulmonary embolus).[14] Agus et al.[15] reported on the Italian experience of 1076 limbs followed out to 3 years, which showed a success rate of 97%. With regard to multi-institutional studies, the Closure Group, with 31 sites participating, treated 31 limbs and reported varicose vein–free results of 88.2% and occlusion rates of 75% at 3 years, a rate of recurrence higher than many other series.[16] Most smaller case series have similar immediate results, with initial success rates approaching 100% and with a less than 10% recurrence on longer-term follow-up. Major complications, including saphenous nerve injury causing paresthesia, DVT, pulmonary embolism, and skin burns, were reported in less than 1% of treated limbs.[17]

ENDOLUMINAL VERSUS SURGICAL THERAPY

Studies have shown equivalent technical success and safety when comparing conventional surgery with endoluminal ablation. However, minimally invasive techniques are proving to be favorable when comparing perioperative morbidity and timing to full recovery. The EVOLVeS Study demonstrated a more rapid return to work for RFA versus high ligation and stripping (1.2 vs. 3.9 days), as well as improved quality of life (QoL) and global pain scores.[18] Cumulative 2-year recurrence was 14% in the RFA group and 21% with the open surgical cohort.[19]

EVLT has been compared with traditional high ligation and stripping in a paired analysis of 20 patients. Recurrence was observed in one patient after EVLT and none after conventional therapy. Swelling and bruising were less with EVLT with no difference in periprocedural pain.[20] Another nonrandomized controlled study compared early QoL outcomes of 132 patients undergoing EVLT and inverse stripping of the GSV.[21] The EVLT group had a better postoperative improvement in QoL, although the difference resolved by 12 weeks.

A randomized clinical trial that compared EVLT with ligation and stripping was completed in 2007. One hundred three consecutive patients were treated either by EVLT using continuous (29 patients) or stepwise (42 patients) laser withdrawal or ligation and GSV stripping (32 patients). Technical success was similar at 3 months, but the EVLT-treated patients had a quicker recovery as evidenced by earlier return to normal activity.[22]

COMPARING ENDOVENOUS LASER THERAPY AND RADIOFREQUENCY ABLATION

In a retrospective study, 77 limbs treated for saphenofemoral reflux by EVLT were compared with 53 limbs treated by RFA over a 3-year period. Both modalities were found to be equally effective, but three DVTs were reported after EVLT.[23] A prospective study of 499 limbs treated with EVLT for saphenofemoral reflux reported excellent results that were comparable to those of RFA. Initial treatment was 98.2% successful, and at 2-year follow-up 93.4% of limbs remained occluded. All recurrences occurred within 9 months. The most common adverse affects were tightness around the treated area, which was noted in 90% of patients, and bruising, which was noted in 24% of treated patients. No major complications occurred.[24]

Early results with endovenous small saphenous vein treatment are encouraging. The Leeds Vascular Institute reported its results using EVLT in small saphenous treatment, noting an initial 100% success rate in closing the veins and abolishing the reflux.[25] Another recent report noted that 94.4% of veins treated in this manner remained closed as of 1-year follow-up.[26] In addition, data are available regarding perforator ablation. In a series from 2005, 67 perforator veins were treated with EVLT, and an initial success rate of 98% was attained.[27]

With regard to QoL issues, anecdotal evidence and the two studies cited previously in this chapter suggest that endovenous ablation is an improvement over open venous surgery. However, this has been difficult to demonstrate in the literature. In a study comparing EVLT with high ligation and stripping, both postprocedural pain and bruising were decreased in the EVLT group.[28] In another trial comparing EVLT plus high ligation with traditional high ligation and stripping, swelling, bruising, and patient estimation of benefit of surgery were all greater in the EVLT group, although it is somewhat difficult to interpret these results given the unusual technique employed in the EVLT group.[20] This same criticism can be applied to a more recent study that demonstrated only minimal benefits to endovenous versus open treatment. Again, the endovenous group also had a high ligation performed.[29] With the rapid diffusion of endovenous ablation into the community, there are fewer patients undergoing traditional high ligation and stripping, and it seems unlikely that a larger prospective randomized trial focused on QoL issues can or will be conducted.

Comment must be made regarding DVT and endovenous ablation techniques. Hingorani et al.[30] published a series of saphenous vein RFAs in 2005 in which post-procedure duplex examination revealed a 16% incidence of DVT. These findings were contested, as other series did not report numbers of DVT approaching these. Nonetheless, it rather quickly became standard of care to ensure that all patients undergoing endovenous ablation must have an ultrasound examination, usually in the 48- to 72-hour time frame following the initial procedure. Ideally, the scan will demonstrate occlusion of the GSV, with patency of the superior epigastric vein maintained. Occasionally, the closure will extend beyond the epigastric vein and approach the saphenofemoral junction (Figure 68-5). There is no universally accepted algorithm for management in this situation. If there is clot protruding into the common femoral vein, most practitioners will treat this as a DVT, starting enoxaparin sodium (Lovenox) once the diagnosis is made. Follow-up ultrasonography can be performed 2 weeks later, and frequently the thrombus will have retracted out of the deep system.[23] Alternatively, one occasionally faces a situation where there appears to be clot flush with the common femoral vein. Therapy in this situation can range from formal anticoagulation to clopidogrel bisulfate (Plavix) or aspirin. The key is close patient follow-up with ultrasound as needed. In our series, we have seen this extension of clot in just over 1% of patients, and none has required more than a 2-week course of Lovenox before complete resolution of the thrombus away from the deep system.

CONCLUSION

The treatment of lower-extremity venous reflux disease via endovascular techniques has led to major

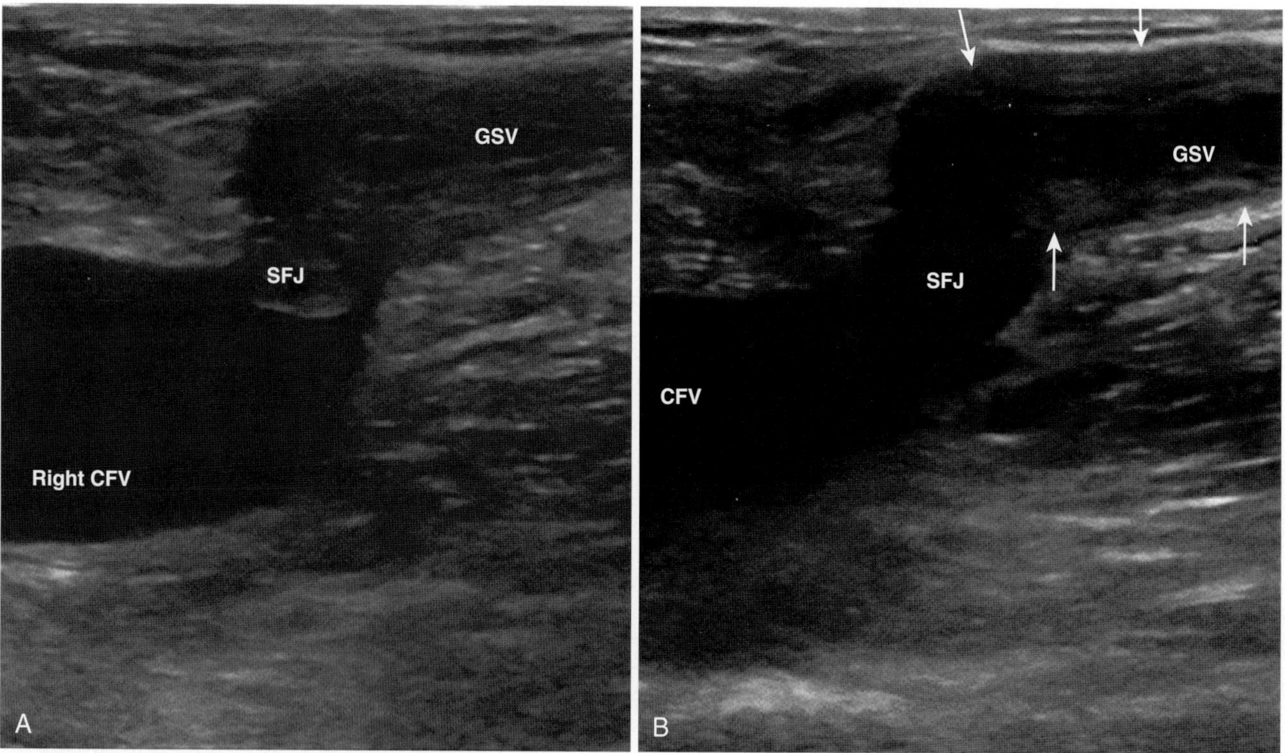

FIGURE 68-5 Extension of thrombus into the common femoral vein *(CFV)* is seen on this ultrasound scan. Follow-up ultrasonography performed 1 week later shows regression of the thrombus out of the saphenofemoral junction *(SFJ)* and safely back to the great saphenous vein *(GSV)*.

changes in the management of this constellation of disorders. What was once treated by a procedure requiring hospitalization and general anesthetic is now treated routinely in an office setting with rapid recuperation. Data regarding the longer-term outcomes from these procedures continue to accumulate, and it is likely that they will continue to be refined as technology improves. Like many new interventions, the keys to success are proper technique and appropriate patient selection. As the practitioner gains experience with GSV ablations, the more challenging short saphenous and perforator cases can also be approached. The availability of all these techniques should lead to patients receiving the appropriate treatment for a widely prevalent clinical problem.

References

1. Callam MJ: Epidemiology of varicose veins, *Br J Surg* 81:167–173, 1994.
2. Labropoulos N, Leon M, Nicolaides AN, et al: Superficial venous insufficiency: correlation of anatomic extent of reflux with clinical symptoms and signs, *J Vasc Surg* 20(6):953–958, 1994.
3. Cheatle T: The long saphenous vein: to strip or not to strip? *Semin Vasc Surg* 18:10–14, 2005.
4. Widmer LK, Mall TH, Martin H: Epidemiology and social medical importance of diseases of the veins, *Munch Med Wochenschr* 116:1421–1426, 1974.
5. Van Rij AM, Jiang P, Solomon C, et al: Recurrence after varicose vein surgery: a prospective long-term clinical study with duplex ultrasound scanning and air plethysmography, *J Vasc Surg* 38:935–943, 2003.
6. Bergan JJ: Endovenous saphenous vein obliteration. In Whittmore AD, Bandyk DF, editors: *Advances in vascular surgery*, vol 9, Chicago, 2001, Mosby, pp 123–132.
7. Welch HJ: Endovenous ablation of the great saphenous vein may avert phlebectomy for branch varicose veins, *J Vasc Surg* 44:601–605, 2006.
8. Proebstle TM, Moehler T, Gul D, et al: Endovenous treatment of the great saphenous vein using a 1,320 nm Nd:YAG laser causes fewer side effects than using a 940 nm diode laser, *Dermatol Surg* 31:1678–1683, 2005.
9. Kabnick LS: Outcome of different endovenous laser wavelengths for great saphenous vein ablation, *J Vasc Surg* 43:88–93, 2006.
10. Dwerryhouse S, Davies B, Harradine K, et al: Stripping the long saphenous vein reduces the rate of reoperation for recurrent varicose veins: five-year results of a randomized trial, *J Vasc Surg* 29:589–592, 1999.
11. Jones L, Braithwaite BD, Selwyn D, et al: Neovascularization is the principal cause of varicose vein recurrence: results of a randomized trial of stripping the long saphenous vein, *Eur J Vasc Endovasc Surg* 12:442–445, 1996.
12. Glass GM: Neovascularization in recurrent saphenofemoral incompetence of varicose veins: surgical anatomy and morphology, *Phlebology* 10:136–142, 1995.
13. Perrin M, Labropoulos N, Leon LR: Presentation of the patient with recurrent varices after surgery (REVAS), *J Vasc Surg* 43:27–34, 2006.
14. Ravi R, Rodriguez-Lopez JA, Trayler EA, et al: Endovenous ablation of incompetent saphenous veins: a large single-center experience, *J Endovasc Ther* 13:244–248, 2006.
15. Agus GB, Mancini S, Magi G: IEWG. The first 1000 cases of Italian Endovenous-laser Working Group (IEWG): rationale, and long-term outcomes for the 1999-2003 period, *Int Angiol* 25:209–215, 2006.
16. Nicolini P, Closure Group: Treatment of primary varicose veins by endovenous obliteration with the VNUS closure system: results of a prospective multicentre study, *Eur J Vasc Endovasc Surg* 29(4):433–439, 2005.
17. Van den Bos RR, Kockaert MA, et al: Technical review of endovenous laser therapy for varicose veins, *Eur J Vasc Endovasc Surg* 35:88–95, 2008.
18. Lurie F, Creton D, Eklof B, et al: Prospective randomized study of endovenous radiofrequency obliteration (closure procedure) versus ligation and stripping in a selected patient population (EVOLVeS Study), *J Vasc Surg* 38(2):207–214, 2003.
19. Lurie F, Creton D, Eklof B, et al: Prospective randomised study of endovenous radiofrequency obliteration (closure) versus ligation and vein stripping (EVOLVeS): two-year follow-up, *Eur J Vasc Endovasc Surg* 29(1):67–73, 2005.
20. De Medeiros CA, Luccas GC: Comparison of endovenous treatment with an 810 nm laser versus conventional stripping of the great saphenous vein in patients with primary varicose veins, *Dermatol Surg* 31:1685–1694, 2005.
21. Mekako AI, Hatfield J, Bryce J, et al: A nonrandomized controlled trial of endovenous laser therapy and surgery in the treatment of varicose veins, *Ann Vasc Surg* 20:451–457, 2006.
22. Darwood RJ, Theivacumar N, Dellagrammaticas D, et al: Randomized clinical trial comparing endovenous laser ablation with surgery for the treatment of primary great saphenous varicose veins, *Br J Surg* 95:294–301, 2008.
23. Puggioni A, Kalra M, Carmo M, et al: Endovenous laser therapy and radiofrequency ablation of the great saphenous vein: analysis of early efficacy and complications, *J Vasc Surg* 42:488–493, 2005.
24. Min RJ, Khilnani N, Zimmet S: Endovenous laser treatment of saphenous vein reflux: long-term results, *J Vasc Interv Radiol* 14:991–996, 2003.
25. Theivacumar NS, Beale RJ, Mavor AI, et al: Initial experience in endovenous laser ablation (EVLA) of varicose veins due to small saphenous vein reflux, *Eur J Vasc Endovasc Surg* 33(5):614–618, 2007.
26. Park SJ, Yim SB, Cha DW, et al: Endovenous laser treatment of the small saphenous vein with a 980-nm diode laser: early results, *Dermatol Surg* 34(4):517–524, 2008, discussion 524.
27. Proboebtle TM, Herdermann S: Early results and feasibility of incompetent perforator vein ablation by endovenous laser treatment, *Dermatol Surg* 33:162–168, 2007.
28. Rasmussen LH, Bjoern L, Lawaetz M, et al: Randomized trial comparing endovenous laser ablation of the great saphenous vein with high ligation and stripping in patients with varicose veins: short-term results, *J Vasc Surg* 46:308–315, 2007.
29. Kalteis M, Berger I, Messie-Werndl S, et al: High ligation combined with stripping and endovenous laser ablation of the great saphenous vein: early results of a randomized controlled study, *J Vasc Surg* 47(4):822–829, 2008, discussion 829.
30. Hingorani AP, Ascher E, Markevich N, et al: Deep venous thrombosis after radiofrequency ablation of greater saphenous vein: a word of caution, *J Vasc Surg* 40(3):500–504, 2004.

CHAPTER

69

Endoscopic and Percutaneous Techniques for Treatment of Incompetent Perforators

Peter Gloviczki, Alessandra Puggioni

Perforating veins of the leg drain blood from the superficial to the deep venous system of the leg. Unidirectional flow is assured by venous valves. Valves can be incompetent because of congenital absence or abnormal development *(congenital valvular incompetence)*, because of varicosity and dilation of the vein wall resulting in separation of the valve leaflets with leaky valves *(primary valvular incompetence)*, and because of post-thrombotic damage to the valves *(secondary valvular incompetence)*. Incompetent perforating veins have reversed venous flow, which in turn results in ambulatory venous hypertension. These hemodynamic changes contribute to development of varicose veins and ultimately lead to skin changes and venous ulcers because of extravasation of red cells and cytokines causing chronic inflammation of the subcutaneous tissue and the skin in the most sensitive area of the leg at and above the ankle.

The development of leg ulcers in patients who had varicose veins and incompetent perforating veins was observed as early as 1867 by John Gay.[1] Surgical interruption of incompetent perforating veins to decrease ambulatory venous hypertension and prevent venous ulcers was suggested by Linton in 1938.[2] The classic open Linton procedure to interrupt medial calf perforators through a long medial incision in the calf was further developed by Cockett[3] and Dodd[4]; the operation was ultimately abandoned because of high wound complication rates of the surgical incision, made frequently in an area of the leg close to an open or recently healed venous ulcer. In 1985 Hauer[5] first described the endoscopic approach for perforator vein ablation. Subfascial endoscopic perforator vein surgery (SEPS) became rapidly popular, with decrease of wound complications from 24% to less than 5%.[6-14] SEPS became the primary surgical technique for perforator ablation over the next two decades.

In the past few years, less-invasive office procedures, such as ultrasound-guided ablation of perforating veins, developed, using either small stab wounds for hook phlebectomy of perforators or performing completely percutaneous ablation of the perforators (PAPS) with heat (radiofrequency or laser)[14-16] or ultrasound-guided liquid or foam sclerotherapy.[17-20] The emergence of these techniques has led to increasing interest in minimally invasive therapy for the treatment of severe chronic venous insufficiency (CVI) and venous ulcers, and the number of procedures performed to treat incompetent perforators has increased significantly. However, the efficacy of perforator ablation, regardless of which technique is used, still remains intensely debated.

In this chapter we review surgical anatomy, rationale for treatment of incompetent perforating vein, and diagnostic evaluation of the patients. We describe the currently used endoscopic and minimally invasive percutaneous techniques of perforator vein ablations and discuss results of these interventions.

SURGICAL ANATOMY

Perforator veins connect the superficial to the deep veins, either directly to the main axial veins (direct perforators) or indirectly through muscular tributaries or soleal venous sinuses (indirect perforators). Perforating veins of the leg and thigh have one or two bicuspid valves that allow blood to flow from the superficial to the deep system (unidirectional flow); these valves usually are located beneath the fascia. Although the lower extremity has 80 to 140 perforating veins that are mostly small and not clinically significant, only a specific group has actual relevance and may contribute to the development of ambulatory venous hypertension. The lower-extremity perforators consist

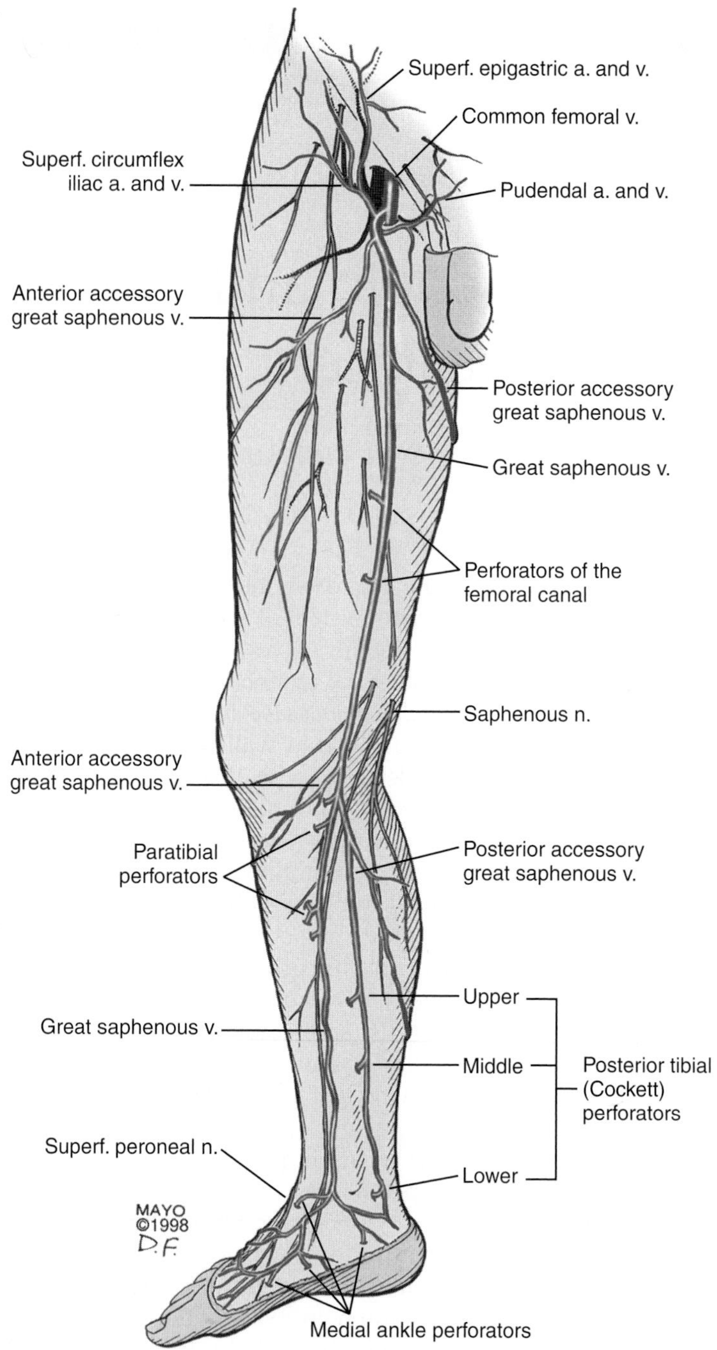

FIGURE 69-1 Superficial and perforating veins of the leg. *(Copyright Mayo Clinic.)*

of four main groups: foot, medial calf, lateral calf, and thigh perforators (Figure 69-1).

The most important perforators are the direct *medial calf perforators*, which cross the superficial posterior compartment. Among these, the posterior tibial perforating veins (Cockett perforators) connect the posterior accessory saphenous vein of the calf (posterior arch veins in the old terminology) to the paired posterior tibial veins (Figure 69-2). This is an important observation, because stripping or heat ablation of the great saphenous vein (GSV) will not affect flow through incompetent medial calf perforators. The most distal posterior tibial perforators (Cockett I) are located behind the medial malleolus, and the middle and upper posterior tibial perforators are located more proximally in the calf (at 7-9 cm and 10-12 cm from the medial malleolus, respectively) and about 2.5 cm medial to the tibia. More proximal direct perforating veins are saphenous vein perforators and include the paratibial direct perforators or 24-cm perforators, which are located closer to the tibia

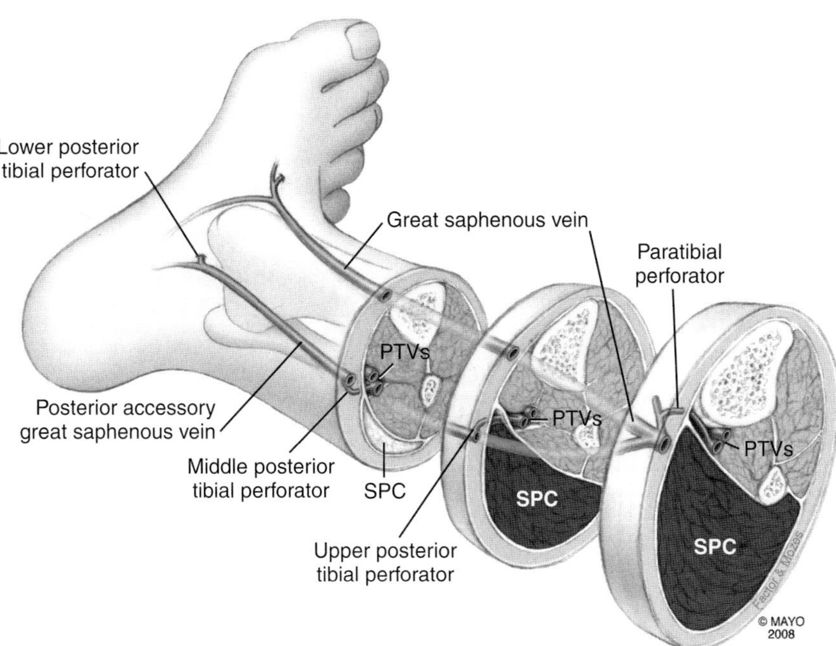

FIGURE 69-2 The topographic anatomy of medial calf perforators and the compartments of the calf. *(Copyright Mayo Clinic.)*

and 18 to 22 cm from the medial malleolus, and the so-called Boyd's perforators, which connect the GSV and its tributaries to the tibial or distal popliteal veins. Of probable clinical importance are also the posterolateral perforators, or peroneal perforators, which connect tributaries of the small saphenous vein to the peroneal veins. Thigh perforators are less developed than calf perforating veins; the main ones are the Dodd's perforators and the Hunterian perforators, which are located in the medial aspect of the thigh and connect the GSV to the popliteal or femoral veins.

Mozes et al.[21] found that only 63% of all medial calf perforators were directly accessible from the superficial posterior compartment. These comprise 32% of the mid posterior tibial, 84% of the upper posterior tibial, and 43% of lower paratibial perforating veins; the remaining traverse the intermuscular septum dividing the deep and superficial compartments or reside solely within the posterior deep compartment itself. To access these perforators during endoscopic dissections, a paratibial fasciotomy must be performed, incising the fascia of the posterior deep compartment (see Figure 69-2).

RATIONALE FOR TREATMENT

In CVI (clinical class 3-6, with use of the class, etiology, anatomy, pathophysiology [CEAP] classification)[22] skin changes and venous ulcers almost invariably develop in the gaiter area of the leg, the area between the distal edge of the soleus muscle and the ankle. This is where a large number of medial direct perforators are located. Although significant efforts have been made to elucidate the mechanism of skin ulcers, the pathophysiology of this process is still not well understood. Venous ulcers are thought to be the end result of high ambulatory pressures transmitted to the venous side of the capillary bed; this causes exudation of fluid and macromolecules out of the microcirculation of skin and subcutaneous tissues. Muscle contractions compress the intramuscular and intermuscular veins, and the blood from deep veins is returned to the heart. At the same time, it is redirected from the superficial to the deep veins via the perforating veins. During calf muscle contraction, incompetent perforating veins can raise pressures in the supramalleolar veins above 100 mm Hg.[23] Still, the hemodynamic significance of the incompetent perforating veins has been long debated. In 1988 Bjordal[24] suggested that incompetent perforating veins do not contribute to ambulatory venous hypertension, especially in limbs with superficial reflux alone. Burnand et al.[25] suggested that in patients with deep vein involvement ligation of perforating veins made no difference, and Stacey et al.[26] could not confirm improvement in calf muscle pump function after perforator ligation.

Incompetent perforating veins, however, have been observed in patients with CVI in 50% to 80% of the patients, with higher proportion in patients with ulcers than in those with skin changes only. In a study of Labropoulos et al.[27] that included 275 patients with CVI, 148 had incompetent perforators (54%); those with ulcers had perforators in 61% whereas those with skin changes only had incompetent perforators in 49%. In another study the same author found that the duration of outward flow in incompetent perforating veins in patients with ulcers was longer than in those without ulcers.[28] Perforator incompetence is usually associated with either superficial or deep venous incompetence or with both. Isolated perforator incompetence is rare; it occurs in fewer than 5%.

Another interesting observation is that the number and size of perforating veins also increases with the severity of the disease. The prevalence of incompetent perforating veins increased with the severity of the disease in a study by Delis et al.[29] Danielsson et al.[30] observed that limb volume, measured with air plethysmography in 36 patients with chronic venous disease, correlated with the diameter of the largest incompetent perforating vein of the calf. Patients with abnormally elevated venous volume resulting from severe valve incompetence had a median perforator diameter of 5.5 mm versus those with normal venous volume who had a median perforator diameter of 3.5 mm ($p = .001$, Mann-Whitney). Zukowski et al.[31] found that 70% of patients with venous ulcers had incompetent perforating veins of moderate to severe hemodynamic significance.

Several studies suggested that treatment of superficial reflux eliminates perforator vein incompetence. Although this may be true for patients with primary varicosity and C2 disease, it is certainly not the case in patients with more advanced CVI. The Edinburgh group found that in presence of deep venous reflux 72% of limbs will have persistent perforator vein incompetence after superficial venous surgery.[32]

PREOPERATIVE EVALUATION

Preoperative evaluation includes imaging studies to document superficial, deep, and/or perforator incompetence and to guide the operative intervention. The preferred test is duplex scanning that is considered the gold standard for evaluation of lower-extremity chronic venous disease. In patients with suspected iliac vein or inferior vena cava disease computed tomographic venography or magnetic resonance angiography needs to be performed.

Duplex scanning is suitable to establish deep vein obstruction or less-severe postthrombotic changes, and it determines the degree and distribution of valvular incompetence in segments of the superficial and deep veins and in the perforating veins. The test has 100% specificity and the highest sensitivity of all diagnostic tests to predict the sites of incompetent perforating veins.[10] Duplex scanning of the perforating veins is best performed on the non–weight-bearing limb while the patient is standing upright; manual compression/decompression maneuvers are performed above the identified perforator to detect reflux (Figure 69-3). In ultrasound flow analysis incompetent perforating veins have higher peak flow velocity and higher mean flow velocity and volume flow, longer time to peak reflux velocity, and greater reflux volume displaced outward. Perforator reflux duration cutoff value has been arbitrarily set at 0.5 second. All identified perforators are marked on the skin with a nonerasable marker.

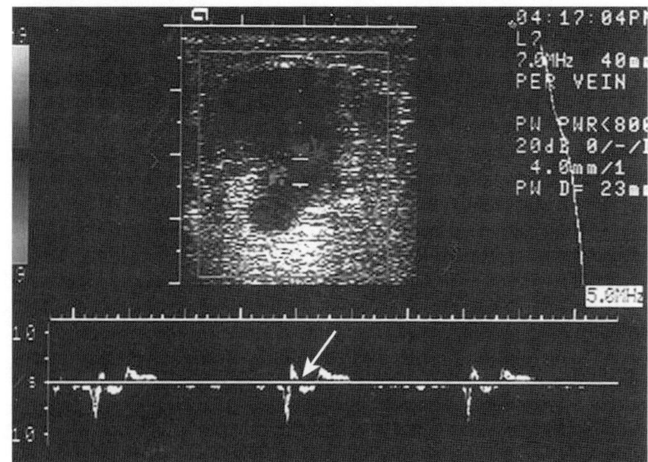

FIGURE 69-3 Duplex scan of an incompetent calf perforator. Bidirectional flow is confirmed with ultrasound scan.

Usually patients with CVI (C3-C6 disease) are candidates for selective perforator interruption. Patients with recurrent varicose veins may also need treatment of incompetent perforators that can be the sources of recurrence. Those with deep vein obstruction need perforating veins to assure venous return, and perforator interruption in these patients should not be performed.

TREATMENT OPTIONS

Endoscopic Subfascial Perforating Vein Surgery

Disappointments with the high wound complications of the open surgical perforator interruptions, pioneered by Robert Linton,[2] and later modified by Cockett[3] and Dodd,[4] opened the way for the much less invasive endoscopic techniques of perforator ligations. Hauer[5] described the first endoscopic subfascial interruption of incompetent perforating veins using a rigid scope. In 1991 O'Donnell[6] developed the first laparoscopic approach using a closed system and water irrigation to improve visualization in the subfascial plane. Conrad[7] and Gloviczki et al.,[8] working independently, modified the laparoscopic technique adding a tourniquet and CO_2 insufflation. This CO_2 technique expanded the operating space and allowed the surgeon to visualize, dissect, and clip the incompetent perforating veins.

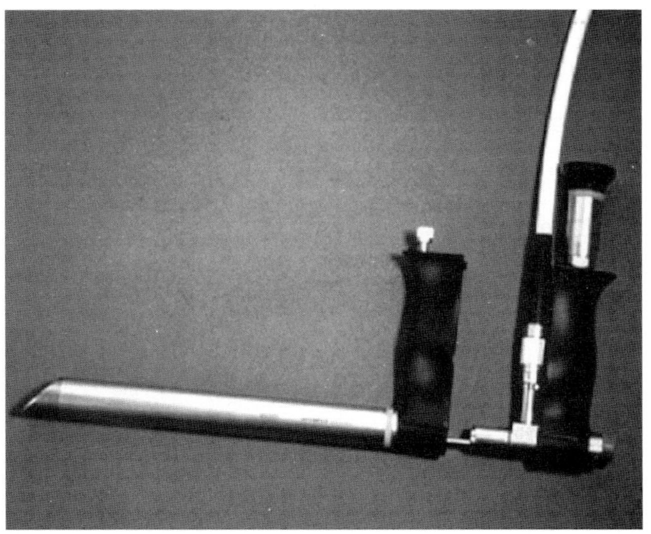

FIGURE 69-4 Rigid endoscope for the subfascial perforating vein interruption.

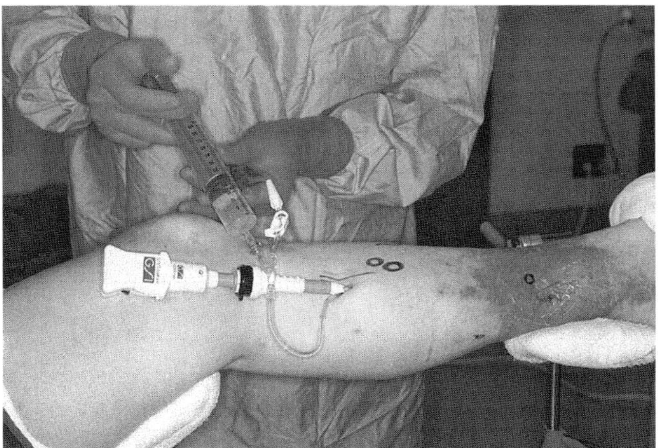

FIGURE 69-5 Dissection of the subfascial space by injecting 120 to 150 mL of saline solution into a plastic balloon, using the 10-mm port.

Bergan et al.[9] and Wittens with Pierik[10] used the single-scope technique (Figure 69-4), whereas the Mayo group perfected the two-scope technique with carbon dioxide insufflation and later with the use of a harmonic scalpel for division of perforating veins. Balloon dissection was also used to enlarge the subfascial plane (Figure 69-5). In the 1990s and early 2000s, SEPS soon replaced open surgery completely to treat incompetent perforating veins.[11,12,33-46]

Surgical Technique

The SEPS procedure is performed with the patient under general or regional anesthesia although some surgeons perform it with the patient under tumescent anesthesia.[33] The limb is first exsanguinated with an Esmarch bandage, and a bloodless field is provided by a pneumatic tourniquet placed on the proximal thigh inflated to 300 mm Hg.[13] One 10-mm endoscopic port is

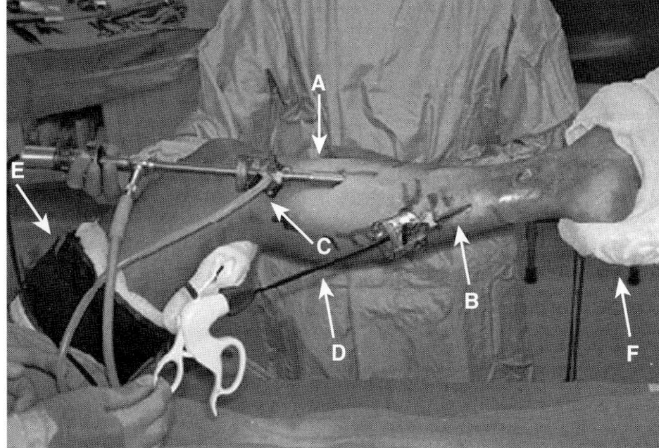

FIGURE 69-6 Two-port technique of the SEPS procedure. A 10-mm *(A)* and a 5-mm *(B)* port are used, CO_2 is insufflated into the subfascial space *(C)*, and a harmonic scalpel is used for perforator interruption *(D)*. *E,* Bloodless field is obtained with a thigh tourniquet. *F,* A leg holder is used to elevate the limb above the table for easy manipulation of the endoscopic instruments.

placed in the medial aspect of the calf 10 cm distal to the tibial tuberosity, proximal to the diseased skin (Figure 69-6). A 5-mm distal port is placed halfway between the first port and the ankle, about 5 cm more posteriorly, for easier dissection. To widen the subfascial space and facilitate access after port placement we routinely now use balloon dissection, popularized by Fogarty, Tawes, and Elias (see Figure 69-5). CO_2 is then insufflated into the subfascial space, and pressure is maintained around 30 mm Hg. The loose connective tissues between the calf muscles and the superficial fascia are sharply divided by using endoscopic scissors.

The subfascial space is widely explored from the medial border of the tibia to the posterior midline and down to the level of the ankle. All perforators encountered are divided with the harmonic scalpel. The perforators encountered during SEPS include the upper, middle, and lower posterior tibial perforators and the proximal *paratibial* perforators. A paratibial fasciotomy is next made by incising the fascia of the posterior deep compartment close to the tibia to avoid injury to the posterior tibial vessels and nerve. Although this can aid in distal exposure, reaching retromalleolar Cockett I perforators endoscopically is usually not possible and, if incompetent, may require a separate small incision over them to gain direct exposure.

After completion of the endoscopic portion of the procedure, stab avulsion of varicosities in addition to ablation or stripping of the GSV and/or small saphenous vein, if incompetent, is performed. The patient is discharged home the same day

Advantages of SEPS include avoidance of diseased or infected skin, visual control, complete division of mid and upper medial perforators, and low complication

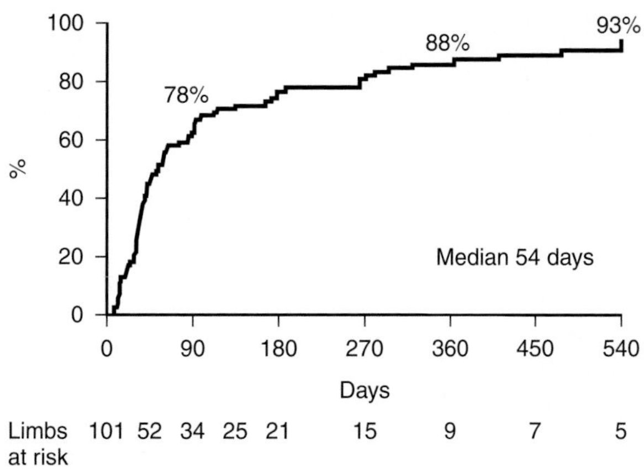

FIGURE 69-7 Ulcer healing after SEPS in 101 patients. *(From Gloviczki P, Bergan JJ, Rhodes JM, et al: Midterm results of endoscopic perforator vein interruption for chronic venous insufficiency: lessons learned from the North American subfascial endoscopic perforator surgery registry. The North American Study Group,* J Vasc Surg *29:489-502, 1999.)*

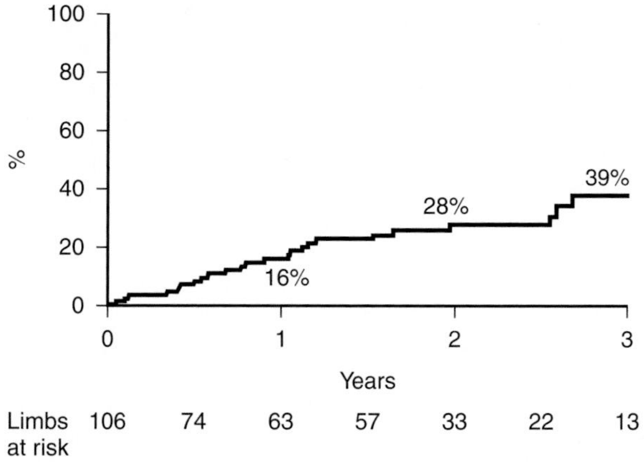

FIGURE 69-8 Ulcer recurrence after SEPS in 106 patients. *(From Gloviczki P, Bergan JJ, Rhodes JM, et al: Midterm results of endoscopic perforator vein interruption for chronic venous insufficiency: lessons learned from the North American subfascial endoscopic perforator surgery registry, The North American Study Group,* J Vasc Surg *29:489-502, 1999.)*

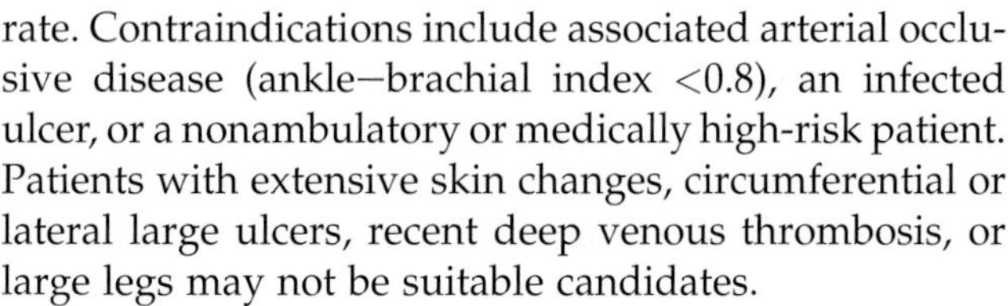
rate. Contraindications include associated arterial occlusive disease (ankle–brachial index <0.8), an infected ulcer, or a nonambulatory or medically high-risk patient. Patients with extensive skin changes, circumferential or lateral large ulcers, recent deep venous thrombosis, or large legs may not be suitable candidates.

Results

Retrospective data from the North American SEPS registry on 146 patients demonstrated an 88% ulcer healing rate at 1 year, with a median ulcer healing time of 54 days and a complication rate of 6% (Figure 69-7). Ulcer recurrence rate was 16% at 1 year and 28% at 2 years (Figure 69-8), significantly better than in most published series on nonoperative management.[11] In the Mayo Clinic experience 90-day ulcer healing rate was 80%, with a median time to ulcer healing of 35 days. The 1-, 3-, and 5-year cumulative ulcer recurrence rates were 4%, 20%, and 27%.[13] All ulcers in limbs with primary incompetence healed. Cumulative 5-year ulcer recurrence in post-thrombotic syndrome was 56% versus 15%, respectively, in limbs with primary valvular incompetence ($p = .001$) (Figure 69-9).

Similar results have been reported by several authors, so it is unclear whether or not SEPS is indicated in this subgroup of patients. Several other studies demonstrated a benefit of SEPS in early ulcer healing and decreased recurrence rates (Table 69-1).[13,38-46] Nonetheless, some studies did not prove the clinical efficacy of perforator vein reflux ablation, even in patients with ulcerated limbs. In a study by Scriven et al.,[34] combined perforator and superficial vein reflux ablation in ulcerated limbs with associated deep reflux did not result in clinical improvement compared to limbs treated with superficial reflux ablation alone. All these data

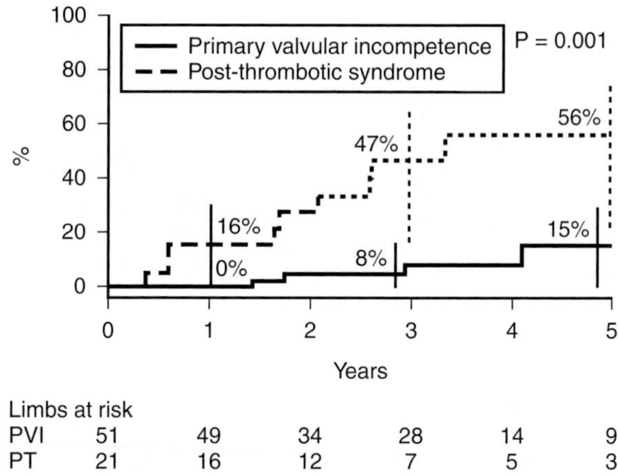

FIGURE 69-9 Ulcer recurrence after 103 SEPS procedures in limbs with primary valvular incompetence (n = 73) and postthrombotic syndrome (n = 30). *(From Kalra M, Gloviczki P, Noel, et al: Subfascial endoscopic perforator vein surgery in patients with post-thrombotic venous insufficiency: is it justified?* Vasc Endovascular Surg *36:41-50, 2002.)*

from perforator vein surgery trials came from nonrandomized cohorts that almost invariably lacked a comparison group. The Dutch SEPS trial was a randomized, prospective, multicenter study designed to compare SEPS versus conservative treatment for venous ulcers.[35] This study did not recognize an overall benefit of surgical treatment over compression alone except in selected cases of medial and/or recurrent ulceration and in patients who undergo the SEPS procedure in expert venous centers. Two thirds of the patients in this study underwent concomitant saphenous vein stripping and branch varicosity avulsion, making it difficult to ascertain how much clinical improvement can be attributed to SEPS alone.

TABLE 69-1 Results of 920 SEPS Procedures Published in 12 Series

First author, year	Limbs (n)	Limbs with history of ulcer (n)	Limbs with active ulcer (n)	Saphenous vein ablation (%)	Ulcer healing (%)	Limbs with ulcer recurrence (n)	Mean follow-up (mo)
Jugenheimer, 1992[38]	103	NR	17	NR	94	0	27
Pierik, 1995[39]	40	40	16	10	100	1	46
Bergan, 1996[9]	31	25	15	100	93	0	NR
Gloviczki, 1999[12]	146	122	101	60	84	26	24
Lee, 2001[40]	36	19	NR	92	89	2	14
Baron, 2001[41]	45	45	37	40	89	0	10
Iafrati, 2002[42]	51	51	29	55	74	7	38
Ciostek, 2002[38]	146	74	36	90	86	11	56
Kalra, 2002[13]	103	76	42	72	90	21	39
Bianchi, 2003[44]	74	74	58	77	91	4	44
Roka, 2006[45]	92	41	21	97	95	2	44
Ting, 2006[46]	53	15	34	100	100	3	31
TOTAL	920	582	406	72	90	77 (13%)	33

NR, Not reported; *SEPS*, subfascial endoscopic perforator vein surgery.

A meta-analysis by TenBrook at al.[36] analyzed data of 1140 SEPS procedures performed in 20 studies, 1 randomized trial, and 19 case series. The authors concluded that surgical management of venous ulcer including SEPS, with or without saphenous ablation, leads to an 88% chance of ulcer healing and a 13% chance of ulcer recurrence during a mean follow-up of 21 months. In an excellent recent review of the subject, O'Donnell[37] concluded that the role of incompetent perporator vein ablation alone or concomitant with ablation of the GSV awaits results of properly conducted randomized and controlled trials.

Percutanous Ablation of Perforators

Main limitations of endoscopic techniques such as SEPS include a steep learning curve, inability to treat perimalleolar and lateral perforators, and the need for general or regional anesthesia in most patients. To overcome these limitations of SEPS, a number of minimally invasive, percutaneous techniques of perforator ablation have been developed.

Duplex-Guided Sclerotherapy

Thibault from Australia described first in 1992 the injection of incompetent perforating veins using ultrasound guidance for recurrent varicose veins.[17] There are now many different sclerosing agents and techniques of performing this procedure; the most popular agents are sodium tetradecyl sulfate, sodium morrhuate, and polidocanol.[18,19] These solutions can be injected in liquid form or, alternatively, can be mixed with air within a close double-syringe system to create a foam.[20]

To perform sclerotherapy, 1 to 2 mL of sclerosing agent, liquid or foam, is injected into the perforating vein with use of ultrasound guidance, above the fascial opening. Complications are rare and may include hyperpigmentation, phlebitis, tibial vein thrombosis, skin necrosis, or allergy. Therefore patients with known allergic reactions or common contraindications to sclerotherapy agents cannot undergo treatment. Also the presence of arterial occlusive disease or vasculitis is a contraindication; accidental arterial injection may lead to significant tissue loss.

Early results of duplex-guided sclerotherapy of perforators reported by Guex[18] showed a 90% occlusion rate after three or fewer sessions. Masuda et al.[19] reported clinical results with ultrasound-guided sclerotherapy with sodium morrhuate in 80 limbs. Immediate obliteration of the perforators was obtained in 98% of cases. After treatment there was a significant improvement in venous severity scores and disability scores, and the authors observed an 86.5% ulcer healing rate with a mean healing time of 36 days. Skin complications with superficial skin necrosis occurred in 1.5%. Recurrence, defined as the presence of flow in a previously sclerosed perforating vein at duplex follow-up, was present in 23% of cases with a mean follow-up of 17 months. Ulcer recurrence rate was 32% at a mean of 20 months. Perforator recurrence was more common in limbs with ulcerations.

Cabrera et al.[47] reported on 116 patients with chronic venous disease who received treatment with foam sclerotherapy; ulcers healed in 83% of patients after 6 months. In the United States Bergan is the most enthusiastic proponent of foam sclerotherapy of perforating veins, and his early results have been promising.[48] Well-documented case series with long-term follow-up or randomized controlled studies on foam sclerotherapy of perforators are not available; concerns continue regarding frequencies of recanalization, any tibial vein thrombosis, and occasional systemic side effects of foam.

Duplex-Guided Laser Ablation

The procedure is technically much more demanding than saphenous laser ablation because of the short and often tortuous nature of these perforators.[14] Several different fibers and kits can be used for this procedure (Figure 69-10); however, none of them has been specifically designed for this purpose.[15,16]

The vein is punctured under duplex guidance, and an introducer and a sheath are advanced over a guidewire. The laser fiber is then inserted into the sheath with the tip positioned at least 0.5 to 1 cm from the deep veins. Two to three pulses are delivered for each perforating vein, one subfascially, one at the fascial level, and another suprafascially. Each segment should be treated either with 60 to 100 J using laser pulses or with 100 J/cm energy delivered with continuous pullback mode.

In the early experience reported by Proebstle and Herdemann,[14] a 940-nm diode laser and a neodymium: yttrium aluminum garnet laser with 1320 nm were used with laser fibers of 600-nm diameter; laser energy was delivered in a pulsed fashion using laser power in the range between 5 and 30 W. Of 67 perforators treated, 66 occluded. No major complications occurred. At 3-month follow-up all perforating veins remained occluded if 250 J or more was delivered at the time of treatment. Initial success with other wavelengths (980 nm) has also been reported. Long-term data are not available.

Duplex-Guided Radiofrequency Ablation

Radiofrequency ablation of incompetent perforating veins is performed with an ad-hoc rigid device, the ClosureRFS stylet (VNUS Medical Technologies Inc., Sunnyvale, CA). The stylet has two electrodes on the shaft and a removable needle trocar (Figure 69-11). The perforating vein is punctured with the stylet or with a needle followed by access over a guidewire, and tumescent anesthetic solution is injected around the vein. The segment of the vein that is treated should be the one immediately under the fascia and at least 0.5 cm away from the posterior tibial veins. For best results, the

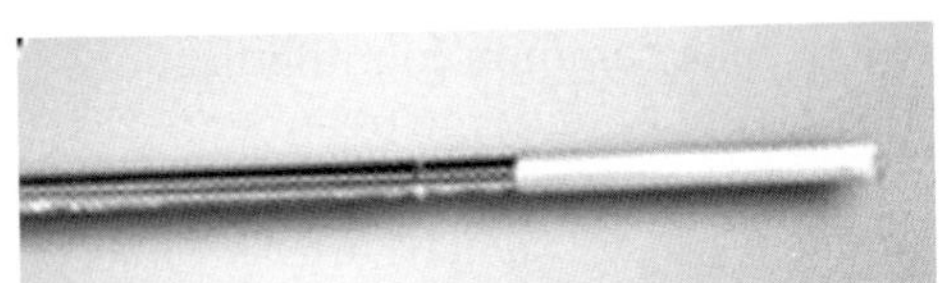

FIGURE 69-10 Vari-Lase Bright Tip (Vascular Solutions, Inc., Minneapolis, MN) for perforator laser ablation. *(Courtesy Vascular Solutions, Inc.)*

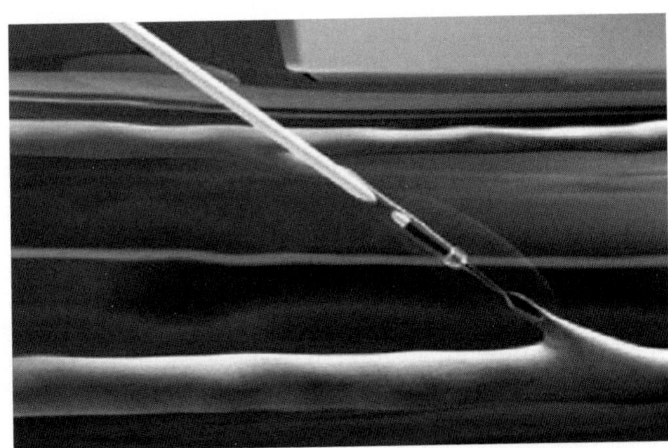

FIGURE 69-11 Radiofrequency ablation of the perforating vein (ClosureRFS stylet). *(Courtesy VNUS Medical Technologies Inc).*

TABLE 69-2 Comparison of the Clinical Efficacy of Endoscopic Versus Percutaneous Perforator Interruptions

		PAPS			
	SEPS	**Phlebectomy**	**RF**	**Laser**	**Sclerotherapy**
Proved efficacy	+++	+	+	+	+
Long-term data	++++	+	+	+	+
Invasive procedure	++++	+++	++	++	+
Treats all IPVs	+++	++	+++	+++	+++
Return to work	++	+++	++++	++++	++++
Repeatable	+	++	+++	+++	++++

IPV, Incompetent perforating vein; *PAPS,* percutaneous ablation of the perforators; *RF,* radiofrequency; *SEPS,* subfascial endoscopic perforator vein surgery.

device should be apposed against four different areas of the vein wall for a period of 1 minute each, and two or more segments of vein should be treated.[49]

The first report with this device came from Whiteley and colleagues[50]; these authors used the saphenous radiofrequency probe to treat perforating veins. Seven hundred seventy perforators were treated in 506 limbs, and 79% of the perforators remained occluded at 1 year.

Peden and Lumsden[49] presented initial data from a multicenter trial on treatment of 97 perforating veins in 55 limbs. Perforators were treated intravascularly or extravascularly. Occlusion rate after intravascular treatment was 91.2% at 3 weeks. Extravascular treatment had inferior results. Deep vein thrombosis developed in two patients. Long-term results with this treatment are not yet available.

CONCLUSION

Advanced CVI and venous ulcers are disabling conditions. The need for perforator interruption remains a subject of debate as the clinical significance of incompetent perforators, even though it seems evident, remains unconfirmed. The main question is of course whether incompetent perforating veins are the cause or the effect of the global venous incompetence in the limb. Ablation of the incompetent superficial system has been effective to reduce ulcer recurrence, but treatment of incompetent perforating veins, particularly in postthrombotic syndrome, remains elusive. Until additional well-designed, prospective, randomized studies become available to support grade 1A recommendation to treat incompetent perforators, it is up to the surgeon and the patient to select from the available treatment options. SEPS compared with PAPS has advantages and disadvantages (Table 69-2). Because minimally invasive perforator interruptions are now available at low risk and as an outpatient procedure, in most centers PAPS has become the first line of perforator treatment, even though midterm and long-term results with these techniques are not known. The procedure is, however, repeatable, with minimal morbidity. SEPS is reserved for recurrent or nonhealing ulcers for those patients in whom percutaneous techniques failed or are not possible.

References

1. Gay J: Lettsonian Lectures 1867, *Varicose disease of the lower extremities*, London, 1868, Churchill.
2. Linton RR: The operative treatment of varicose veins and ulcers, based upon a classification of these lesions, *Ann Surg* 107:582–593, 1938.
3. Cockett FB: The pathology and treatment of venous ulcers of the leg, *Br J Surg* 260–278, 1956.
4. Dodd H, Cockett FB: *The pathology and surgery of the veins of the lower limb*, E&S Livingstone, Ltd. Edinbugh and London 1956, pp344.
5. Hauer G: Endoscopic subfascial discussion of perforating veins: preliminary report [in German], *Vasa* 14(1):59–61, 1985.
6. O'Donnell TF: Surgical treatment of incompetent communicating veins. In *Atlas of venous surgery*, Philadelphia WB, Saunders. 111–124, 2000
7. Conrad P: Endoscopic exploration of the subfascial space of the lower leg with perforator interruption using laparoscopic equipment: a preliminary report, *Phlebology* 154–157, 1994.
8. Gloviczki P, Cambria RA, Rhee RY, et al: Surgical technique and preliminary results of endoscopic subfascial division of perforating veins, *J Vasc Surg* 23(3):517–523, 1996.
9. Bergan JJ, Murray J, Greason K: Subfascial endoscopic perforator vein surgery: a preliminary report, *Ann Vasc Surg* 10(3):211–219, 1996.
10. Pierik EG, van Urk H, Hop WC, et al: Endoscopic versus open subfascial division of incompetent perforating veins in the treatment of venous leg ulceration: a randomized trial, *J Vasc Surg* 26(6):1049–1054, 1997.
11. Gloviczki P, Bergan JJ, Menawat SS, et al: Safety, feasibility, and early efficacy of subfascial endoscopic perforator surgery: a preliminary report from the North American registry, *J Vasc Surg* 25:94–105, 1997.
12. Gloviczki P, Bergan JJ, Rhodes JM, et al: Midterm results of endoscopic perforator vein interruption for chronic venous insufficiency: lessons learned from the North American subfascial endoscopic perforator surgery registry. The North American Study Group, *J Vasc Surg* 29:489–502, 1999.
13. Kalra M, Gloviczki P, Noel AA, et al: Subfascial endoscopic perforator vein surgery in patients with post-thrombotic venous insufficiency: is it justified? *Vasc Endovasc Surg* 36(1):41–50, 2002.
14. Proebstle TM, Herdemann S: Early results and feasibility of incompetent perforator vein ablation by endovenous laser treatment, *Dermatol Surg* 33(2):162–168, 2007.
15. Black CM, Smilanich RP, Worth ER: Endovascular perforator ablation, *EV Today* October, 2007, pp63–70.
16. Elias S, Peden E: Ultrasound-guided percutaneous ablation for the treatment of perforating vein incompetence, *Vascular* 15 (5):281–289, 2007.
17. Thibault PK, Lewis WA: Recurrent varicose veins. II. Injection of incompetent perforating veins using ultrasound guidance, *J Dermatol Surg Oncol* 18(10):895–900, 1992.
18. Guex JJ: Ultrasound guided sclerotherapy (USGS) for perforating veins (PV), *Hawaii Med J* 59(6):261, 2000.
19. Masuda EM, Kessler DM, Lurie F, et al: The effect of ultrasound-guided sclerotherapy of incompetent perforator veins on venous clinical severity and disability scores, *J Vasc Surg* 43(3):551–556, 2006.
20. de Waard MM, der Kinderen DJ: Duplex ultrasonography-guided foam sclerotherapy of incompetent perforator veins in a patient with bilateral venous leg ulcers, *Dermatol Surg* 31 (5):580–583, 2005.
21. Mozes G, Gloviczki P, Menawat SS, et al: Surgical anatomy for endoscopic subfascial division of perforating veins, *J Vasc Surg* 24:800–808, 1996.
22. Eklöf B, Rutherford RB, Bergan JB, et al: The American Venous Forum International Ad Hoc Committee for Revision of the CEAP Classification: Revision of the CEAP classification for chronic venous disease: a consensus statement, *J Vasc Surg* 40:1248–1252, 2004.

23. Negus D, Friedgood A: The effective management of venous ulceration, *Br J Surg* 70(10):623–627, 1983.
24. Bjordal R: Flow and pressure studies in venous insufficiency, *Acta Chir Scand Suppl* 544:30–33, 1988.
25. Burnand KG, O'Donnell TF, Thomas ML: The relative importance of incompetent communicating veins in the production of varicose veins and venous ulcers, *Surgery* 82:9–14, 1977.
26. Stacey MC, Burnand KG, Layer GT, et al: Calf pump function in patients with healed venous ulcers is not improved by surgery to the communicating veins or by elastic stockings, *Br J Surg* 75:436–439, 1988.
27. Labropoulos N, Delis K, Nicolaides AN, et al: The role of the distribution and anatomic extent of reflux in the development of signs and symptoms in chronic venous insufficiency, *J Vasc Surg* 23:504–510, 1996.
28. Labropoulos N, Mansour MA, Kang SS, et al: New insights into perforator vein incompetence, *Eur J Vasc Endovasc Surg* 18:228–234, 1999.
29. Delis KT, Ibegbuna V, Nicolaides AN, et al: Prevalence and distribution of incompetent perforating veins in chronic venous insufficiency, *J Vasc Surg* 28:815–825, 1998.
30. Danielsson G, Eklof B, Kistner RL: Association of venous volume and diameter of incompetent perforator veins in the lower limb: implications for perforator vein surgery, *Eur J Vasc Endovasc Surg* 30:670–673, 2005.
31. Zukowski AJ, Nicolaides AN, Szendro G, et al: Haemodynamic significance of incompetent calf perforating veins, *Br J Surg* 78:625–629, 1991.
32. Stuart WP, Adam DJ, Allan PL, et al: Saphenous surgery does not correct perforator incompetence in the presence of deep venous reflux, *J Vasc Surg* 28(5):834–838, 1998.
33. Proebstle TM, Bethge S, Barnstedt S, et al: Subfascial endoscopic perforator surgery with tumescent local anesthesia, *Dermatol Surg* 28(8):689–693, 2002.
34. Scriven JM, Bianchi V, Hartshorne T, et al: A clinical and haemodynamic investigation into the role of calf perforating vein surgery in patients with venous ulceration and deep venous incompetence, *Eur J Vasc Endovasc Surg* 16:148–152, 1998.
35. van Gent WB, Hop WC, van Praag MC, et al: Conservative versus surgical treatment of venous leg ulcers: a prospective, randomized, multicenter trial, *J Vasc Surg* 44:563–571, 2006.
36. TenBrook JA Jr, Iafrati MD, O'Donnell TF Jr, et al: Systematic review of outcomes after surgical management of venous disease incorporating subfascial endoscopic perforator surgery, *J Vasc Surg* 39:583–589, 2004.
37. O'Donnell T Jr: The present status of surgery of the superficial venous system in the management of venous ulcer and the evidence for the role of perforator interruption, *J Vasc Surg* 48:1044–1052, 2008.
38. Jugenheimer M, Junginger T: Endoscopic subfascial sectioning of incompetent perforating veins in treatment of primary varicosis, *World J Surg* 16:971–975, 1992.
39. Pierik EG, Wittens CH, van Urk H: Subfascial endoscopic ligation in the treatment of incompetent perforating veins, *Eur J Vasc Endovasc Surg* 9:38–41, 1995.
40. Lee DW, Chan AC, Lam YH, et al: Early clinical outcomes after subfascial endoscopic perforator surgery (SEPS) and saphenous vein surgery in chronic venous insufficiency, *Surg Endosc* 15:737–740, 2001.
41. Baron HC, Saber AA, Wayne M: Endoscopic subfascial surgery for incompetent perforator veins in patients with active venous ulceration, *Surg Endosc* 15:38–40, 2001.
42. Iafrati MD, Pare GJ, O'Donnell TF, Estes J: Is the nihilistic approach to surgical reduction of superficial and perforator vein incompetence for venous ulcer justified? *J Vasc Surg* 36:1167–1174, 2002.
43. Ciostek P, Myrcha P, Noszczyk W: Ten years experience with subfascial endoscopic perforator vein surgery, *Ann Vasc Surg* 16:480–487, 2002.
44. Bianchi C, Ballard JL, Abou-Zamzam AM, et al: Subfascial endoscopic perforator vein surgery combined with saphenous vein ablation: results and critical analysis, *J Vasc Surg* 38:67–71, 2003.
45. Roka F, Binder M, Bohler-Sommeregger K: Mid-term recurrence rate of incompetent perforating veins after combined superficial vein surgery and subfascial endoscopic perforating vein surgery, *J Vasc Surg* 44:359–363, 2006.
46. Ting AC, Cheng SW, Ho P, et al: Clinical outcomes and changes in venous hemodynamics after subfascial endoscopic perforating vein surgery, *Surg Endosc* 17:1314–1318, 2003.
47. Cabrera J, Redondo P, Becerra A, et al: Ultrasound-guided injection of polidocanol microfoam in the management of venous leg ulcers, *Arch Dermatol* 140:667–673, 2004.
48. Bergan JJ, Pascarella L: Severe chronic venous insufficiency: primary treatment with sclerofoam, *Semin Vasc Surg* 18:49–56, 2005.
49. Peden E, Lumsden A: Radiofrequency ablation of incompetent perforator veins, *Perspect Vasc Surg Endovasc Ther* 19(1):73–77, 2007.
50. Whiteley MS, Price BA, Scott MJ, et al: Radiofrequency ablation of refluxing great saphenous systems, Giacomini veins, and incompetent perforating veins using VNUS closure and TRLOP technique, *Phlebology* 18:52, 2003.

SECTION XI

ENDOSCOPIC VASCULAR SURGERY

CHAPTER

70

Thoracoscopic Dorsal Sympathectomy

Samuel S. Ahn, Kyung M. Ro, Cecilia K. Wieslander

Since the end of the nineteenth century, cervicodorsal sympathectomy has been performed for numerous medical conditions, including several autonomically mediated vascular and neurologic disorders. Although it was first performed by Hughes in 1942,[1] Kux is best associated with thoracoscopic sympathectomy because of his publication of the results of more than 1400 procedures in 1951.[2] During the early 1950s, Kux performed his minimally invasive technique to visualize the sympathetic chain and the ganglia. The endoscopic approach provided the advantages of reduced morbidity and mortality without compromising the technical success rates seen with open sympathectomy. Variations of this endoscopic procedure have now been established as safe and effective treatments for palmar hyperhidrosis[3-22] (Ahn SS, unpublished data, 2000), Raynaud's syndrome,[7,15] Buerger's disease,[23] reflex sympathetic dystrophy/causalgia,[7,15,24,25] refractory cardiac arrhythmia,[7,26] and intractable visceral pain.[27,28] The predominant indication has been primary palmar hyperhidrosis, and widespread application of this technique in its treatment has been fueled by impressive technical and patient satisfaction rates. Morbidity and mortality are low, and further advances in minimally invasive endoscopic surgery may allow for widespread applicability and use.

PREOPERATIVE EVALUATION

A complete preoperative medical evaluation should exclude those patients with underlying or preexisting diseases of the lung and the thorax. Also, the evaluation should rule out hypermetabolic and hypercoagulable states. Potentially high-risk patients should be evaluated with a pulmonary function test to determine whether they will be able to tolerate single-lung ventilation during the operation.

Thoracoscopic sympathectomy has generally been contraindicated in patients with previous thoracic operations or pulmonary infections who may have dense adhesions that can impede thorough visualization of the sympathetic chain.[29] Yim et al.,[30] however, in a retrospective review of video-assisted thoracic surgery in patients with previous operations of the chest, found that reoperation using minimally invasive techniques did not incur greater morbidity or mortality; furthermore, fibrous adhesions complicated the procedure in only 5% of their cases.

Because of the positioning of the arms throughout the procedure, it is necessary to rule out thoracic outlet syndrome (TOS). The 90-degree angle of the airplane arm holder can potentially exacerbate symptoms associated with TOS by impinging on the brachial plexus and the vessels. If a patient has TOS diagnosed, the arm should be positioned to minimize compression of the thoracic outlet, and the upper extremity should be monitored for adequate peripheral pulses throughout the procedure.

SURGICAL TECHNIQUES

Anesthesia and Position

Thoracoscopic sympathectomy is performed with the patient under general endotracheal anesthesia with use of a double-lumen endotracheal tube with the lung deflated and nonventilated. Elia et al.[31] used local anesthesia and spontaneous breathing in a group of 15 patients and found it reduced costs and postoperative stays. The patient is placed in the lateral decubitus position with the ipsilateral arm abducted in an arm holder at a 90-degree angle (Figure 70-1, *A*). Good radial pulses should be palpable with positioning, and extreme care should be taken not to hyperextend the shoulder joint. The contralateral chest wall should be adequately extended to maximize expansion of the intercostal space and is then prepped and draped in the usual sterile fashion.

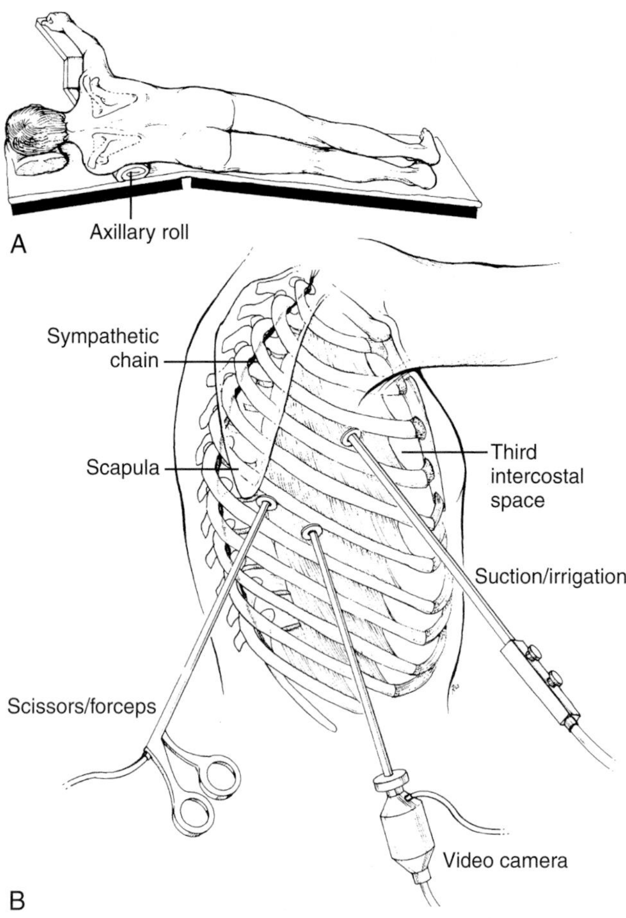

FIGURE 70-1 **A,** Patient in lateral decubitus position with ipsilateral arm abducted at a 90-degree angle. **B,** Port placement: one port in the third intercostal space, and two ports along the sixth intercostal space.

Ports and Instruments

Entrance into the chest cavity is through three separate 7-mm ports. Soft, flexible ports with blunted trocars and 5-mm endoscopic instruments (which include a suction/irrigator with an electrocautery hook apparatus, blunt-tipped scissors with electrocautery attachment, and a curved grasper) are preferred to avoid intercostal neuralgia. Bugmann et al.[32] reported using 5-mm ultrasonic coagulating shears, which eliminates the chance of injury to the distal nerve from electric current, with good results. Some investigators advocated the use of 2-mm instruments, reporting greater patient satisfaction rates, reduced operative time, and a decreased incidence of complications from compensatory hyperhidrosis and Homer's syndrome.[33,34] However, drawbacks are increased fragility of the instrument and limited visibility.[35] Because landmark identification is key in accident avoidance, an instrument with an adequate field of view is extremely important.[36]

The first port is placed in the sixth intercostal space in the posterior chest line, a second port is placed in the sixth intercostal space in the midchest line, and a third port is placed in the third intercostal space along the anterior chest line (see Figure 70-1, *B*). Note that the chest line is more posteriorly placed than the axillary line; this more posterior placement of the ports allows better visualization of the sympathetic nerves and eliminates the need to insert a fourth port to retract the lung.

Procedure

The endoscope is inserted through the port located along the sixth intercostal space in the posterior chest line to allow for optimal visualization of the upper thoracic cavity. All adhesions of the lung to the parietal pleura should be coagulated to allow for proper retraction of the lung. The ipsilateral lung is deflated mechanically and is retracted anteriorly and inferiorly. The superior aspect of the sympathetic chain and the extent of surgical dissection are identified through visualization of the subclavian artery. The azygos, the innominate, and the subclavian veins, along with the phrenic and the vagus nerves, should be promptly identified and preserved throughout the procedure. The phrenic and the vagus nerves run ventral to the vertebral bodies, in contrast to the sympathetic chain, which runs dorsal to the spine (Figure 70-2). Electrocautery is used solely to unroof the parietal pleura off the appropriate rib segments (first to fourth) to expose the sympathetic chain and should not be used in proximity of the nerve fibers (Figure 70-3, *A*).

The rami communicantes of the second and the third ganglion should be divided (and the fourth ganglion if the axilla is involved) while taking extreme precautions to avoid injury to the intercostal artery and vein (see Figure 70-3, *B*). If minor bleeding occurs, hemostasis can be controlled with pressure and suction. If major intercostal bleeding occurs, electrocautery can be used to control it; however, care should be taken to avoid injury to the intercostal nerves. The dissection proceeds in a rostral fashion and should be carried to the lower portion of the stellate ganglion. At this point, the nerve of Kuntz can be identified, which is a large branch of the T1 ramus that runs parallel and lateral to the trunk of the sympathetic chain at the inferior aspect of the superior stellate ganglion (Figure 70-4, *A*). The sympathetic chain is then resected inferiorly and caudally to the stellate ganglion at the level of the superior margin of the second rib (see Figure 70-4, *B*). The third ganglion and the chain just caudal to the end of the third ganglion are subsequently divided, corresponding to the level of the superior aspect of the fourth rib (see Figure 70-4, *C*). For palmar hyperhidrosis, only T2 and T3 should be resected to avoid the risk of Horner's syndrome; T4 can be included in the dissection if the axilla is severely affected. Sympathectomy for axillary hyperhidrosis has lower satisfaction levels than for palmar hyperhidrosis.[35,37]

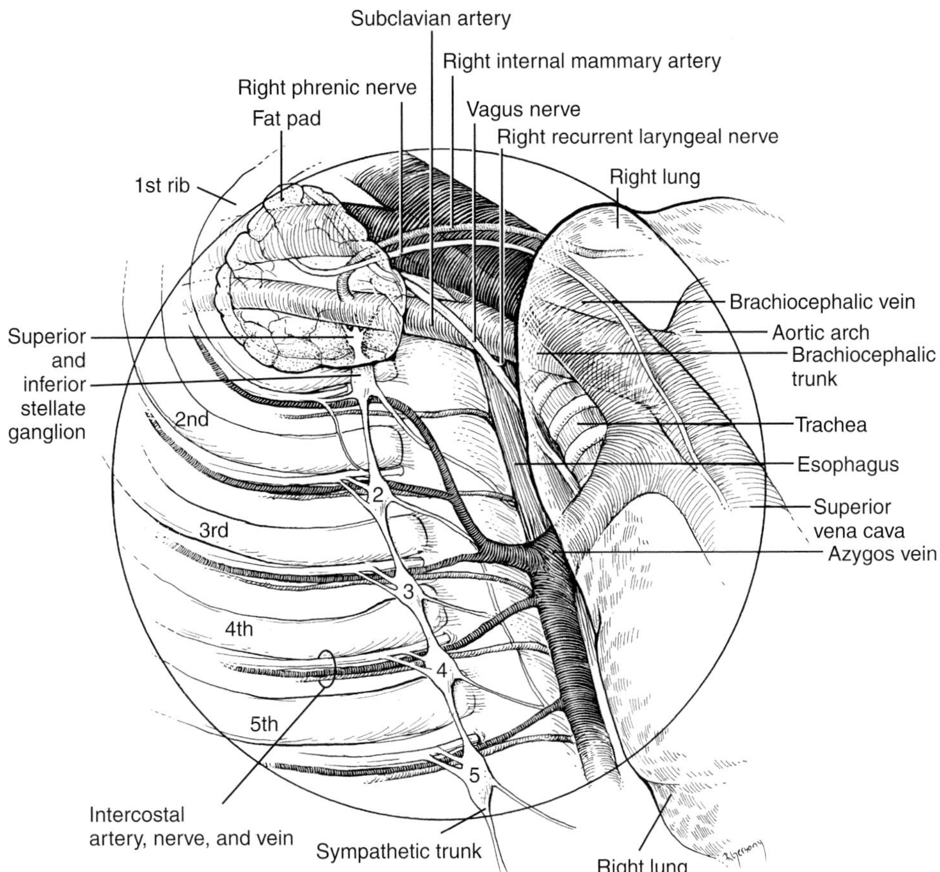

FIGURE 70-2 Sympathetic chain coursing over the neck of the ribs. Note the relationship to the azygos and the subclavian veins, as well as the phrenic and the vagus nerves.

The chain and the ganglia should be sent to the pathology department for intraoperative histologic confirmation. The wound should be inspected for good hemostasis, irrigated, and subsequently suctioned of all fluid. A 16F chest tube can be inserted through the middle port and placed under direct visualization. The lung is then reinflated with use of 30 to 40 mm Hg of positive pressure; adequate inflation should be confirmed with the endoscope. The incision is closed in two layers with use of heavy silk sutures, and the chest tube is secured in place. Steri-Strip (3M, St. Paul, MN) skin closures and OpSite dressings can be applied as needed.

If indicated and the patient is stable, the patient is repositioned to the contralateral side and is completely reprepped and draped, and the procedure is repeated on the other side.

POSTOPERATIVE CARE

Immediately after the operation, it is recommended that a chest x-ray film be obtained to rule out possible pneumothorax or pleural effusions. If no air leaks are present, the chest tube is removed in the recovery room. If air leaks do occur or there is a pneumothorax, the chest tube should not be removed until all air leaks have been completely sealed. Oral analgesics are adequate for most patients. Patients are discharged when there is adequate pain control and the chest tube is removed, usually the same day as surgery.

COMPLICATIONS

Possible short-term complications include pneumothorax, hemothorax, subcutaneous emphysema, pleural effusion, and segmental atelectasis.[38] Incomplete reinflation of the collapsed apical lobe results in postoperative complications from atelectasis and pneumothorax.[38] Rare complications, including false aneurysm of an intercostal artery and inferior brachial plexus injury, have been described in case reports.[39-41]

Long-term complications include intercostal neuralgia compensatory sweating in the trunk or the lower extremities, and Horner's syndrome. Compensatory hyperhidrosis is the most common and unpredictable side effect of thoracoscopic sympathectomy and is

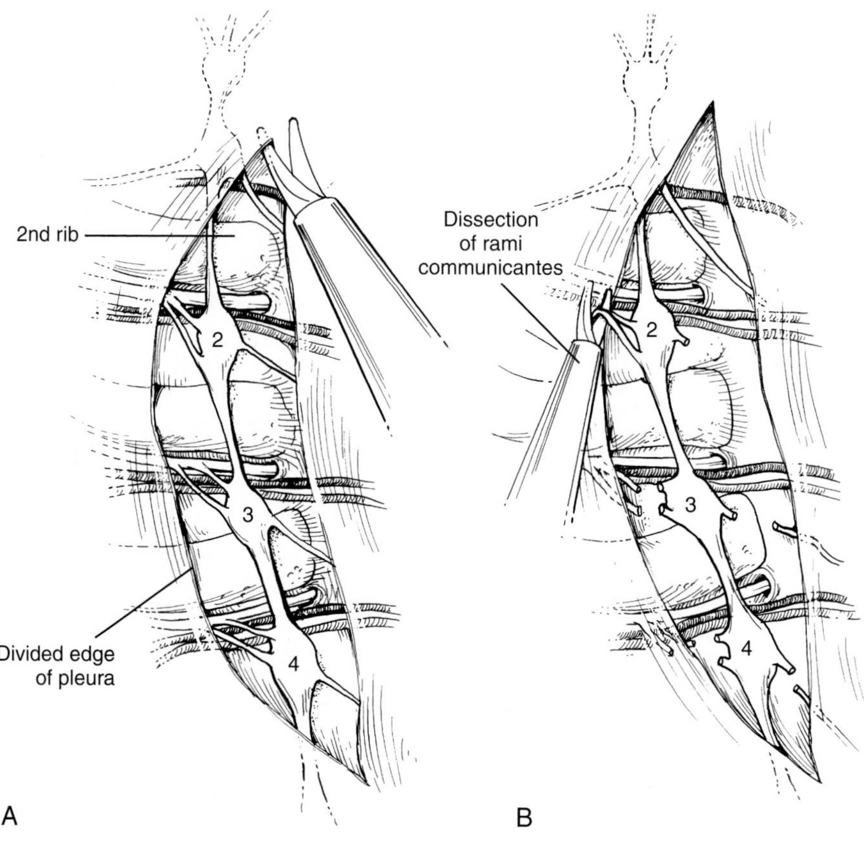

FIGURE 70-3 **A,** Pleural incision over sympathetic chain. **B,** Dissection of rami communicantes corresponding to T2-T3 (and T4 for axilla involvement).

reported to occur in 0% to 74.5% of cases (Table 70-1). The trunk and the lower extremities are primarily affected.* Most patients, however, find this less cumbersome than the original palmar hyperhidrosis.[12] In a previous study, fewer than 10% of those patients in whom compensatory hyperhidrosis developed believed the sweating to be severe, and anecdotal evidence suggests that the sweating often subsides over time.[6,38] Although the exact cause of compensatory hyperhidrosis is unclear, the extent of the sympathectomy and the postsurgical thermoregulatory response have been suggested.[6,14,15] In a separate study, however, Drott and Claes[42] could not confirm that an increase in the number of coagulated segments correlated with the degree of compensatory sweating. Nonetheless, surgeons should perform a minimal resection to reduce the risk of postoperative compensatory sweating. Resection of only the T3 ganglion for palmar hyperhidrosis has been shown to reduce the severity of compensatory sweating while still providing excellent results.[36,43,44] Atkinson and Fealey[45] reported good results for 10 patients who underwent sympathotomy, where the ganglia was preserved and the T2 and stellate ganglions were separated by a simple chain disconnection. None of their subjects reported moderate or severe compensatory hyperhidrosis when contacted for follow-up (average 5.6 months after surgery). Gustatory hyperhidrosis, albeit a less common postoperative complication, has also been reported to occur.[46,47]

Intercostal neuralgia may stem from a variety of factors, including thermal damage to the adjacent intercostal nerve during electroablation, unintentional dissection of the intercostal nerve, or compression injury while using large, rigid Thoracoports (Auto Suture, Norwalk, CT).[7] In an early series, Ahn et al.[7] reported two incidences of intercostal neuralgia while using rigid 12-mm Thoracoports; however, no additional complications of neuralgia were reported after the change to soft 7-mm ports.

Horner's syndrome, which results from damage to the stellate ganglion, is of most concern to patients. This condition can be either transient or permanent; transient Horner's syndrome is reported to occur in 0% to 23.5% of cases, with permanent symptoms occurring in 0% to 6%.[7,11] In a series of 17 patients with reflex sympathetic dystrophy treated with open sympathectomy of the entire stellate ganglion down to the third stellate ganglion, 91% of patients had favorable technical results; however, postoperative Horner's syndrome developed in all patients.[24] Interestingly, Horner's syndrome has been reported to occur with resection of only the second or the third ganglion using the

*References 6, 11, 14, 15, 17, 34, 38.

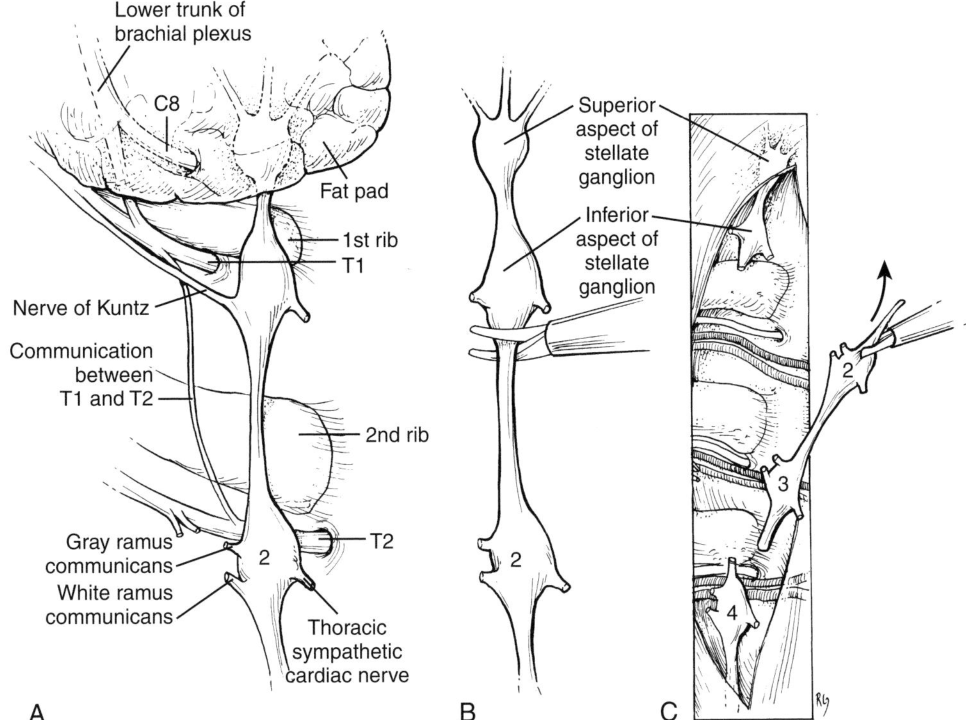

FIGURE 70-4 **A,** Inferior aspect of stellate ganglion, nerve of Kuntz, and T2. **B,** Area of dissection inferior to stellate ganglion. **C,** Resected portion of sympathetic chain, T2-T3.

supraclavicular technique.[48,49] To minimize the risk of permanent Horner's syndrome, the surgeon should take great care to visualize the multiple rami of the stellate ganglion, to identify the course of their direction, and to incise immediately caudal to it, above the level of the T2 ganglion. Transient Horner's syndrome may arise from traction of the stellate ganglion during partial resection of the sympathetic chain.[7] In addition, heat generation from electrocoagulation, misidentification of the second rib, and injury to the stellate ganglion from pulling on the sympathetic chain are potential causes of permanent Horner's syndrome.

The role of video assistance in thoracoscopic sympathectomy has been examined for its potential to help reduce complication rates. A study of 656 patients undergoing T1-T4 sympathectomy compared the results of thoracoscopic sympathectomy using video assistance versus direct visualization.[47] It suggested that video assistance may decrease the incidence of postoperative Horner's syndrome, as well as gustatory hyperhidrosis, while improving technical success rates (98% vs. 93%).[47]

RESULTS

Essentially an outpatient operation, thoracoscopic sympathectomy is usually performed as a simultaneous bilateral staged procedure.[50] Since 1990, several investigators using diverse techniques have reported their experiences with thoracoscopic sympathectomy, with undoubtedly varied results (see Table 70-1). For all indications, the failure of thoracoscopic sympathectomy has resulted primarily from inadequate ablation of the sympathetic nerves during electrocautery of the rami communicantes or regrowth of the nerve tissue.[7] To prevent failure, many investigators recommend obtaining intraoperative histologic confirmation of the resected portion of the sympathetic chain.[7,13,16] Although most surgeons limit their resection to T2-T3 to avoid the potential for Horner's syndrome, other investigators include the lower portion of the stellate ganglion, believing that fibers from this portion of the sympathetic chain supply regions of the upper extremity (see Table 70-1).

Claes et al.,[5] in an early series that included 130 patients, found that removal of the T2-T3 ganglion provided satisfactory results for the treatment of palmar hyperhidrosis, whereas resection of T4 was necessary to alleviate axillary hyperhidrosis. Resection limited to only the rami communicantes resulted in mixed conclusions, with investigators reporting success rates ranging from 71% to 100% and recurrence rates from 0% to 1.5%.[4,8,19,29] In a comparison of sympathetic chain versus rami communicantes resection, Gossot et al.[19] found that the occurrence rates for compensatory hyperhidrosis were equal; however, transection of the

TABLE 70-1 Thoracoscopic Sympathectomy: Summary of Literature

Year	Authors	Patients (n)	Ports (n)	Level of section	Ablation technique	Success (%)*	Follow-up (%)	Mean duration of follow-up (range)	Recurrence (%)	Horner's syndrome (%)	Compensatory sweating (%)
1990	Byrne et al.[3]	85 (PHH)	2	T2-T4; T5 if axilla involved	Electrocautery	95	100	43 mo (3-95 mo)	3	23.5 (T)	64
1993	Friedel et al.[4]	6 (PHH)	2	NS-T4; T5 if axilla severely involved; postganglionic rami only	Laser coagulation	100	100	18 mo	3	0	17
1993	Claes et al.[5]	130 (PHH)	1	Lower one third of stellate-T3; T4 if axilla involved	Electrocautery	98	99	6.5 mo (1-47 mo)	13	0.8 (P)	55
1994	Chen et al.[6]	180 (PHH)	1	T2-T4	Electrocautery	98	100	2.5 mo	0	0	70
1994	Ahn et al.[7]	9 (RSD)	3	Lower one third of stellate-T4	Resection + histology	100	100	11 mo (1-42 mo)	0	11 (T)	0
		6 (RS)				100	100				
		5 (PHH)				100	100				
		1 (RCA)				100	100				
1994	Herbst et al.[8]	270 (PHH)	1	T1/T2-T4 postganglionic rami only	Electrocautery	98	100	16.4 yr (9 mo-27.1 yr)	1.5	2.5 (P)	67
1995	Cohen et al.[9]	19 (PHH)	2	T2-T3	Resection	95	100	NS (1-13 mo)	0	0	11
1995	Ishibashi et al.[24]	4 (BD)	3	Lower one third of stellate-T3	Resection	100	NS	NS	NS	0	NS
1996	Wu et al.[10]	108 (PHH)	1	T2	Electrocautery	98	85	23.1 mo (2-35 mo)	0	0	36
1996	Kopelman et al.[11]	53 (PHH)	2	T2-T3	Electrocautery resection + removal	100	100	19.25 mo (11-26 mo)	0	11 (T) 6 (P)	67
1996	Graham et al.[12]	47 (PHH)	2	T2-T4	Diathermy	96	96	13 mo (3-36 mo)	4	0	56

1996	Lee and Hwang[13]	82 (PHH)	3	T2 (46%), T2-T3 (40%), T2-T4 (0.6%)	Resection + histology	100	100	6 mo	0	0	61
1996	Noppen et al.[14]	100 (PHH)	2	T2-T3	Electrocautery	98	100	>1 mo	0	1 (T)	45
1996	Bonjer et al.[15]	9 (RSD)	2	T2-T3	Resection	100	100	10 mo (1-24 mo)	62.5	0	22
		6 (PHH)		T3	Resection	100	100		0		
		4 (RS)		Between T2 and T3	Division	100	100		0		
1996	Josephs and Menzoian[16]	7 (RSD)	3	Lower one third of stellate-T4	Resection + histology	86	NS	NS	NS	0	NS
		2 (PHH)				100	NS	NS	NS	0	NS
1997	Cohen et al.[17]	84 (PHH)	1	T2-T3	Electrocautery	98	100	NS (1-23 mo)	0	0	25
1997	Dumont et al.[18]	20 (PHH)	2	T2 + T1-T4 ganglia and chains	Diathermy + resection	100	100	9.3 mo (2-19 mo)	100	5(T)	70
1997	Gossot et al.[19]	54 (PHH)	3	Lower one third of stellate-T4 or T5	Resection	100	100	11 mo	0	0	72
		62 (PHH)	3	T2-T4 or T5	Resection of rami only; electrocautery of rib 2-4 for 3-4	98	100	11 mo	5	0	71
1997	Lönroth et al.[27]	9 (TVP)	3	T4-T10 or T11	Electrocautery	100	100	3 mo	33	NS	NS
1998	Zacherl et al.[21]	352 (PHH)	NS	Below T1-T4	Electrocautery	93	83	16 yr	0	3.8 (P)	67
1998	Noppen et al.[28]	8 (TVP)	2	T5-T11 rami communicantes	Electrocautery	71	NS	NS	NS	NS	NS
1999	Hsia et al.[22]	47 (PHH)	1	T2	Electrocautery	100	100	12.8 mo (6-22 mo)	0	0	74.5
2000	Ahn (unpublished data)	59 (PHH)	3	T2-T3	Resection + histology	100	97	13.9 mo (1-79 mo)	0	3.8(T) 0.9(P)	1.9

*Success is defined as complete or partial improvement of symptoms. It is not defined as patient satisfaction with the result.
BD, Buerger's disease; *IVP*, intractable visceral pain; *NS*, not stated; *P*, permanent symptoms; *PHH*, primary hyperhidrosis; *RCA*, refractory cardiac arrhythmia; *RS*, Raynaud's syndrome; *RSD*, reflex sympathetic dystrophy; *T*, transient symptoms.

sympathetic chain conferred more severe compensatory hyperhidrosis.

Most reported studies of thoracoscopic sympathectomy relate to the treatment of primary palmar hyperhidrosis, with success rates ranging from 71% to 100% (see Table 70-1). Success and recurrence rates ranging from 93% to 100% and 0% to 13%, respectively, have been reported for the treatment of Raynaud's disease.[7,15] Survey of the literature reveals suboptimal results of thoracoscopic sympathectomy for the treatment of reflex sympathetic dystrophy, with initial success rates of 86% to 100% and recurrence rates as high as 62.5%.[15,16] As well, the results of thoracoscopic sympathectomy for the treatment of intractable visceral pain are mediocre, with initial success rates of 71% to 100% and a reported recurrence rate of 33% at 3-month follow-up.[27,28]

Although most investigators limit thoracoscopic sympathectomy to adults or to individuals with adequate physiologic development, several studies have reported on children and adolescents.[9,17,46,51] In their experience with pediatric and adolescent patients, Cohen et al. advocated performing sympathectomies during childhood to alleviate the social and the physical discomfort associated with palmar hyperhidrosis at an early stage of development. They concluded that the procedure was safe and effective at 4-year follow-up.[9,17,51] Lin,[46] in a larger series of 438 patients (875 procedures) with a mean age of 14.2 years, ablated the T2 or the T2 and T3 segments of the sympathetic chain along with the Kuntz fibers; he reported only one technical failure and a patient satisfaction rate of 93.2%. The rate of compensatory hyperhidrosis was a disappointing 86%, and the recurrence rates at 1-, 2-, and 3-year follow-up were 0.6%, 1.1%, and 1.7%, respectively. Additional reports, although based on smaller study populations, support the implementation of this procedure in children.[52,53] Despite these initial reports, the safety and the risk-benefit ratio in children should be evaluated further because thoracoscopic sympathectomy also affects the heart by causing a partial β-blocker effect.

SUMMARY

Because the volume of data continues to support the use of thoracoscopic sympathectomy for the treatment of palmar hyperhidrosis and other vascular disorders, we anticipate a growing acceptance of this endoscopic technique as the preferred treatment modality. Given its enormity and breadth, open surgical sympathectomy is rarely performed and has been replaced by a quick, safe, and minimally invasive alternative. Although the incidence of adverse side effects can be minimized if the procedure is performed properly, all patients must be adequately warned of potential complications, especially Horner's syndrome and compensatory hyperhidrosis. The benefits of this procedure, as defined by an increase in quality of life, are numerous and immeasurable and can potentially outweigh latent limitations.

References

1. Jonnesco T: Traitement chirurgical de l'angine de poitrine par la resection du sympathetique cervicothoracicque, *Press Med* 29:193–195, 1921.
2. Kux E: The endoscopic approach to the vegetative nervous system and its therapeutic possibilities, *Dis Chest* 20:139–147, 1951.
3. Byrne J, Walsh TN, Hederman WP: Endoscopic transthoracic electrocautery of the sympathetic chain for palmar and axillary hyperhidrosis, *Br J Surg* 77:1046–1049, 1990.
4. Friedel G, Linder A, Toomes H: Selective video-assisted thoracoscopic sympathectomy, *Thorac Cardiovasc Surg* 41:245–248, 1993.
5. Claes G, Drott C, Gothberg G: Endoscopic electrocautery of the thoracic sympathetic chain: a minimally invasive way to treat palmar hyperhidrosis, *Scand J Plast Reconstr Hand Surg* 27:29–33, 1993.
6. Chen HJ, Shih DY, Fung ST: Transthoracic endoscopic sympathectomy in the treatment of palmar hyperhidrosis, *Arch Surg* 129:630–633, 1994.
7. Ahn SS, Machleder HI, Concepcion B, Moore WS: Thoracoscopic cervicodorsal sympathectomy: preliminary results, *J Vasc Surg* 20:511–519, 1994.
8. Herbst F, Plas EG, Fugger R, Fritsch A: Endoscopic thoracic sympathectomy for primary hyperhidrosis of the upper limbs, *Ann Surg* 220:86–90, 1994.
9. Cohen Z, Shinar D, Levi I, Mares AJ: Thoracoscopic upper thoracic sympathectomy for primary palmar hyperhidrosis in children and adolescents, *J Pediatr Surg* 30:471–473, 1995.
10. Wu JJ, Hsu CC, Liao SY, et al: Contralateral temperature changes of the finger surface during video endoscopic sympathectomy for palmar hyperhidrosis, *J Auton Nerv Syst* 59:98–102, 1996.
11. Kopelman D, Hashmonai M, Ehrenreich M, et al: Upper dorsal thoracoscopic sympathectomy for palmar hyperhidrosis: improved intermediate-term results, *J Vasc Surg* 24:194–199, 1996.
12. Graham ANJ, Owens WA, McGuigan JA: Assessment of outcomes after thoracoscopic sympathectomy for hyperhidrosis in a specialized unit, *J R Coll Surg Edinb* 41:160–163, 1996.
13. Lee KH, Hwang PYK: Video endoscopic sympathectomy for palmar hyperhidrosis, *J Neurosurg* 84:484–486, 1996.
14. Noppen M, Herrgodts P, D'Haese, et al: A simplified T2-T3 thoracoscopic sympathicolysis technique for the treatment of essential hyperhidrosis: short-term results in 100 patients, *J Laparoendosc Surg* 6:151–159, 1996.
15. Bonjer HJ, Hamming JF, du Bois Najj, van Urk H: Advantages of limited thoracoscopic sympathectomy, *Surg Endosc* 10:721–723, 1996.
16. Josephs LG, Menzoian JO: Technical considerations in endoscopic cervicothoracic sympathectomy, *Arch Surg* 131:355–359, 1996.
17. Cohen Z, Shinar D, Kurtzbart E, et al: Laparoscopic and thoracoscopic surgery in children and adolescents: a 3-year experience, *Pediatr Surg Int* 12:356–359, 1997.
18. Dumont P, Hamm A, Skrobala D, et al: Bilateral thoracoscopy for sympathectomy in the treatment of hyperhidrosis, *Eur J Cardiothorac Surg* 64:975–978, 1997.
19. Gossot D, Toledo L, Fritsch S, Celerier M: Thoracoscopic sympathectomy for the upper limb hyperhidrosis: looking for the right operation, *Ann Thorac Surg* 64:975–978, 1997.

20. Lee LS, Lin CC, Ng SM, Au CF: The haemodynamic effects of thoracoscopic cardiac sympathectomy, *Eur J Surg* 580(suppl):37–38, 1998.
21. Zacherl J, Huber ER, Imhof M, et al: Long-term results of 630 thoracoscopic sympathecotomies for primary hyperhidrosis: the Vienna experience, *Eur J Surg* 580(suppl):43–46, 1998.
22. Hsia JY, Chen CY, Hsu CP, et al: Outpatient thoracoscopic limited sympathectomy for hyperhidrosis palmaris, *Ann Thorac Surg* 67:258–259, 1999.
23. Ishibashi H, Hayakawa N, Yamanoto H, et al: Thoracoscopic sympathectomy for Buerger's disease: a report on the successful treatment of four patients, *Surg Today* 25:180–183, 1995.
24. Olcott C, Eltherington LG, Wilcosky BR, et al: Reflex sympathetic dystrophy—the surgeon's role in management, *J Vasc Surg* 14:488–495, 1991.
25. Honjyo K, Hamasaki Y, Kita M, et al: An 11-year-old girl with reflex sympathetic dystrophy successfully treated by thoracoscopic sympathectomy, *Acta Paediatr* 86:903–905, 1997.
26. Ouriel K, Moss AJ: Long QT syndrome: an indication for cervicothoracic sympathectomy, *Cardiovasc Surg* 3:475–478, 1995.
27. Lönroth L, Hyltander A, Lundell L: Unilateral left-sided thoracoscopic sympathectomy for visceral pain control: a pilot study, *Eur J Surg* 163:97–100, 1997.
28. Noppen M, Meysman M, D'Haese J, Vincken W: Thoracoscopic splanchnicolysis for the relief of chronic pancreatitis pain: experience of a group of pneumologists, *Chest* 113:528–531, 1998.
29. Rutherford RB: Role of sympathectomy in the management of vascular disease. In: Moore WS, editor: *Vascular surgery: a comprehensive review*, Philadelphia, 1993, WB Saunders, pp 300–312.
30. Yim AP, Liu HP, Hazelrigg SR, et al: Thoracoscopic operations on reoperated chests, *Ann Thorac Surg* 65:328–330, 1998.
31. Elia S, Guggino G, Mineo D, et al: Awake one stage bilateral thoracoscopic sympathectomy for palmar hyperhidrosis: a safe outpatient procedure, *Eur J Cardiothorac Surg* 28:312–317, 2005.
32. Bugmann P, Robert J, Magistris M, Le Coultre C: Thoracoscopic sympathectomy using ultrasonic coagulating shears: a technical improvement in the treatment of palmar hyperhidrosis, *Pediatr Surg Int* 18:746–748, 2001.
33. Reardon PR, Preciado A, Scarborough T, et al: Outpatient endoscopic thoracic sympathectomy using 2-mm instruments, *Surg Endosc* 13:1139–1142, 1999.
34. Lee DY, Yoon HY, Shin HK, et al: Needle thoracic sympathectomy for essential hyperhidrosis: intermediate-term follow-up, *Ann Thorac Surg* 69:251–253, 2000.
35. Dumont P, Denoyer A, Robin P: Long-term results of thoracoscopic sympathectomy for hyperhidrosis, *Ann Thorac Surg* 78:1801–1807, 2004.
36. Dewey T, Herbert M, Hill S, et al: One-year follow-up after thoracoscopic sympathectomy for hyperhidrosis: outcomes and consequences, *Ann Thorac Surg* 81:1227–1233, 2006.
37. Doolabh N, Horswell S, Williams M, et al: Thoracoscopic sympathectomy for hyperhidrosis: indications and results, *Ann Thorac Surg* 77:410–414, 2004.
38. Ahn SS, Ro KM: Thoracoscopic sympathectomy: a case report, *Ann Vasc Surg* 12:509–514, 1998.
39. Atherton WG, Morgan WE: False aneurysm of an intercostal artery after thoracoscopic sympathectomy, *Ann R Coll Surg Engl* 79:229–230, 1991.
40. Lange JF: Inferior brachial plexus injury during thoracoscopic sympathectomy, *Surg Endosc* 9:830, 1995.
41. Hashmonai M, Kopelman D: Inferior brachial plexus injury during thoracoscopic sympathectomy [letter to the editor], *Surg Endosc* 10:459, 1996.
42. Drott C, Claes G: Hyperhidrosis treated by thoracoscopic sympathicotomy, *Cardiovasc Surg* 4:788–790, 1996.
43. Yazbek G, Wolosker N, Milanez de Campos J, et al: Palmar hyperhidrosis—which is the best level of denervation using video-assisted thoracoscopic sympathectomy: T2 or T3 ganglion? *J Vasc Surg* 42:281–285, 2005.
44. Van't Riet M, de Smet A, Kuilken H, et al: Prevention of compensatory hyperhidrois after thoracoscopic sympathectomy for hyperhidrosis, *Surg Endosc* 15:1159–1162, 2001.
45. Atkinson J, Fealey R: Sympathotomy instead of sympathectomy for palmar hyperhidrosis: minimizing postoperative compensatory hyperhidrosis, *Mayo Clin Proc* 78:167–172, 2003.
46. Lin TS: Transthoracic endoscopic sympathectomy for palmar and axillary hyperhidrosis in children and adolescents, *Pediatr Surg Int* 15:475–478, 1999.
47. Zacherl J, Imhof M, Huber ER, et al: Video assistance reduces complication rate of thoracoscopic sympathectomy for hyperidrosis, *Ann Thorac Surg* 68:1177–1181, 1999.
48. Adar R, Kurchin A, Zweig A, Mozes M: Palmar hyperhidrosis and its surgical treatment: a report of 100 cases, *Ann Surg* 186:34–41, 1977.
49. Keaveny TV, Fitzgerald PAM, Donnelly C, Shanik GD: Surgical management of hyperhidrosis, *Br J Surg* 64:570–571, 1977.
50. Yim AP: Simultaneous vs. staged bilateral video-assisted thoracoscopic sympathectomy [letter to the editor], *Surg Endosc* 10:459, 1996.
51. Cohen Z, Levi I, Pinsk I, Mares AJ: Thoracoscopic upper sympathectomy for primary palmar hyperhidrosis: the combined pediatric, adolescent and adult experience, *Eur J Surg* 580(suppl):5–8, 1998.
52. Rashid HI, Osman HS, McIrvine AJ: Thoracoscopic (upper thoracic) sympathectomy for primary palmar hyperhidrosis in children, *Int J Clin Pract* 52:537–538, 1998.
53. Imhof M, Zacherl J, Plas EG, et al: Long-term results of 45 thoracoscopic sympathectomies for primary hyperhidrosis in children, *J Pediatr Surg* 43:1839–1842, 1999.

CHAPTER

71

Laparoscopic Aortic Surgery

Willem Wisselink, Miguel Cuesta, Jeroen Diks, Hans M. E. Coveliers

Although not an endovascular technique, laparoscopic surgery merits discussion in this volume as a minimally invasive alternative for treatment of patients with aortoiliac occlusive or aneurysmal disease.

In 1993 Dion et al.[1] took the first step toward laparoscopic vascular surgery by performing a laparoscopy-assisted aortobifemoral bypass. Since then, various endoscopic vascular techniques and approaches have been developed, such as laparoscopic ligation of lumbar arteries, laparoscopy-assisted aortic surgery (laparoscopic dissection combined with a minilaparotomy to perform a conventional vascular anastomosis), hand-assisted laparoscopy, totally laparoscopic (both dissection and anastomosis carried out laparoscopically), robot-assisted laparoscopic techniques, endoscopic saphenous vein harvesting, endoscopic ligation of incompetent perforators, and hybrid procedures (laparoscopic techniques in simultaneous conjunction with endovascular methods).

To date, these laparoscopic techniques have been applied for treatment of vascular conditions such as endoleak after endovascular aneurysm repair (EVAR), aortoiliac occlusive disease, visceral artery occlusive disease, abdominal aortic aneurysm (AAA), and iliac aneurysm, all with the goal to improve the results of conventional, open surgery with presumed advantages such as decreased use of analgesics, shortened ileus, earlier ambulation, and shortened length of stay.

The objective of this chapter is to describe the most commonly performed laparoscopic vascular procedures, to evaluate the results of clinical studies on laparoscopic and robotic surgery, and to consider these against open and endovascular methods.

LAPAROSCOPIC LIGATION OF LUMBAR AND INFERIOR MESENTERIC ARTERIES AS A TREATMENT METHOD FOR TYPE II ENDOLEAK

Catheter embolization of patent lumbar arteries or IMAs, either alongside the limbs of the graft or via superior mesenteric or hypogastric arteries, has proved to be a valuable treatment option.[2] However, this method may not be technically feasible in all cases because of tortuosity of the collateral circulation or multiplicity of patent connections to the aneurysm sac. Efficacy of direct injection of thrombogenic material into the aneurysm sac is debated because pressure in the aneurysm may remain unaltered.[3,4] In 2000, our group first reported of a laparoscopic approach for treatment of a patient in whom treatment of persistent type II endoleak was deemed necessary and catheter embolization unlikely to succeed.[5]

Operative Technique

The patient is placed in a 60-degree right lateral decubitus position. The tip of the twelfth rib is palpated and an incision of 2-cm length made just anteriorly. A small retroperitoneal space is created in two directions, posteriorly by mobilizing the lower pole of the kidney and anteriorly toward the umbilicus. A dissecting balloon (Origin Medsystems, Menlo Park, CA) is introduced and the balloon insufflated to enlarge the created retroperitoneal space, thereby mobilizing the lower pole of the kidney anteriorly. The balloon is replaced by a 10-mm trocar and a 0-degree videoendoscope. Two additional 10-mm trocars are placed, one close to the iliac crest in the posterior axillary line, the other near the costal margin, in the anterior axillary line. After identification of the psoas muscle, the left ureter is being mobilized anteriorly and the infrarenal aorta exposed from the left renal artery to the iliac bifurcation. Intra-aneurysm pressure is measured by means of insertion of a laparoscopic needle attached to a pressure monitor. After dissection of the posterior aspect of the aneurysm, the left-sided lumbar arteries are controlled with surgical clips and divided. Subsequently, the right lumbar arteries are clipped and left undivided. If indicated, the anterior surface of the aneurysm is exposed and the inferior mesenteric artery (IMA) identified and clipped.

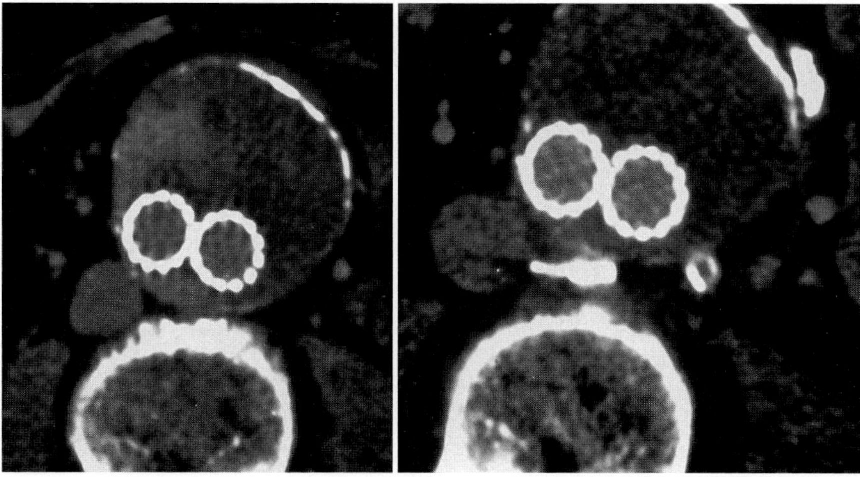

FIGURE 71-1 CT of type II endoleak before *(left)* and after *(right)* laparoendoscopic ligation of lumbar and inferior mesenteric arteries.

Spiral computed tomographic (CT) angiography is performed on the first postoperative day; at 3, 6, and 12 months; and semiannually thereafter.

Results

Between 1999 and 2002, 10 patients (9 men) presented with persistent type II endoleak more than 6 months (12 ± 5 months) after EVAR. The mean aneurysm diameter (6.5 ± 0.5 cm) had remained unchanged since the operation in 5 patients, slightly increased (2 and 5 mm, respectively) in 3, and significantly increased (11, 15, and 20 mm) in 3 others. Aneurysm volume in the latter 3 had increased with 15%, 25%, and 30%, respectively. Angiography revealed three (n = 1), four (n = 5), or six (n = 4) patent lumbar arteries, whereas the IMA was patent in six. Patent middle sacral arteries were found on two occasions. Vague abdominal and back pain had developed in 2 patients; the remaining had no symptoms. In 6 patients, prior catheter embolization had been attempted both via hypogastric collaterals and alongside the iliac limbs, and 1 patient had thrombin injected in the aneurysm sac, all without success.

There was one operative death because of venous bleeding in a Jehovah's Witness patient who had refused blood transfusion. In one other patient, a small retroperitoneal incision was made to facilitate difficult dissection of a large middle sacral artery. Mean operative time was 128 minutes (100-180 minutes); all patients had mechanical ventilation discontinued immediately after surgery without the need for admission to an intensive care unit (ICU). Regular diet was resumed 1 (n = 8) or 2 (n = 1) days after the operation, and all but one (5 days) patient left the hospital within 4 days after surgery. Postoperative spiral CT scan (n = 9) revealed, in one patient, a pair of unclipped, patent lumbar arteries. After immediate reoperation via the same approach with clipping of the remaining pair of lumbar arteries just at the aortic bifurcation, complete thrombosis of the aneurysm sac was radiographically confirmed (Figure 71-1).

Two other patients continued to have an endoleak in spite of absence of patent branch arteries. Subsequent angiography revealed a subtle, previously undiagnosed, type I endoleak. In the remaining patients (n = 7) complete exclusion of the aneurysm sac was demonstrated at the first postoperative scan. With a mean follow-up of 13 ± 7 months, seven patients have remained free from endoleak. In one patient with a remaining (type I) endoleak, the aneurysm diameter has increased; however, open repair to date has been refused. The other patient with a type I leak was converted to have open AAA repair shortly after the laparoscopic procedure. Aneurysm diameter has remained unchanged in four patients and decreased in three (by 2, 5, and 7 mm).

The role of endopressure as a means to judge completeness of lumbar ligation remains unclear. Continuous pressure registration revealed a straight line, without a pulse wave or other fluctuations in two cases, probably because the needle tip was embedded in thrombus. In two other cases, after injection of 0.5 mL of saline solution, a slightly dampened pressure curve was obtained with a mean pressure equal to systemic pressure. In both these patients, sac pressure decreased to approximately 30 mm Hg, nonpulsatile, after ligation of all branch arteries. This finding further indicates the need for safe and simple techniques to measure intrasac pressure. In two patients who continued to have an endoleak, a type I component probably had been present before the laparoscopic procedure but had not been recognized as such because of the multiple patent branch arteries. It is not inconceivable that the situation has actually been made worse by occluding the outflow of the aneurysm sac in the presence of a type I endoleak.

In conclusion, this procedure may be a less-invasive alternative to open repair in those patients in whom transcatheter embolization has been unsuccessful or is likely to fail. However, serious bleeding complications may arise because of periaortitis with dense adhesions between aortic wall and large venous structures, especially at the site of the aortic bifurcation. To validate this approach to therapy-resistant type II endoleak, long-term follow-up of a larger series is required.

LAPAROSCOPY-ASSISTED AORTOILIAC SURGERY

The purpose of these procedures is to limit the size of the abdominal wall incision by performing the surgical dissection and exposure of the aorta laparoscopically, followed by completion of the aortic anastomoses "by hand" via a minilaparotomy.

Alimi and coworkers[6] described their technique and reviewed its results in 2004. Between 1998 and 2003, they included 58 patients in a prospective study to undergo laparoscopy-assisted aortofemoral reconstruction with graft implantation through a 5-cm to 8-cm minilaparotomy. Fifty-one patients (88%) had claudication (category 2 or 3, Rutherford classification), and seven patients (12%) had tissue loss; at presentation they had TransAtlantic Inter-Society Consensus (TASC) C (n = 24, 41.4%) or D (n = 32, 55.2%) iliac lesions, and the last two patients (3.4%) had severe aortic lesions. Perioperative data for the first 29 patients, obtained during the first 34 months of the study (group 1), were compared with data for the last 29 patients, obtained during the last 32 months of the study (group 2). Follow-up consisted of clinical examination or duplex scanning, or both, at 1, 3, 6, and 12 months and yearly thereafter, and CT examination before discharge and then every 2 years. One intraoperative surgical conversion (1.7%) was necessary, and two other patients (3.4%) died in the immediate postoperative period. With experience, initial contraindications such as obesity or suprarenal artery aortic clamping were eliminated, making it possible to increase the percentage of patients included, from 53.7% during the first 34 months to 90.6% during the last 32 months (p = .003). The mean duration of the operative procedure decreased from 285 minutes in group 1 to 192 minutes in group 2 (p <.001), and the mean duration of aortic clamping decreased from 76.4 minutes in group 1 to 31.8 minutes in group 2 (p <.001). The number of early repeated interventions was reduced from three (10.3%) in group 1 to two (6.9%) in group 2 (p = not significant), and the clinical recovery period decreased from 7 days to 4.5 days (p = .05). During a mean follow-up of 26.7 months (range, 1-66 months) there were five repeated operations (9%) to treat late graft occlusion, establishing midterm primary and secondary patency rates of 89.3% and 91%, respectively. No aortic false aneurysms were detected, and no major amputations were performed. These authors concluded that their minimally invasive video-assisted technique was feasible and safe with a relatively short period of postoperative recovery and good midterm patency rate.

Another laparoscopy-assisted technique, hand-assisted laparoscopy (HALS), also has been applied to vascular disease.[7,8] With or without specifically designed "hand ports," a surgeon's hand is introduced in the abdominal cavity with maintenance of pneumoperitoneum and thus videoscopic exposure. Ferrari et al.[7] described 122 patients treated by HALS. Exclusion criteria were hostile abdomen (previous major abdominal or aortic surgery), bilateral diffuse common iliac and/or hypogastric aneurysms, massive aortoiliac calcifications, and severe cardiac insufficiency. Juxtarenal and proximal iliac aneurysms were not a contraindication, nor was obesity. In all patients, they performed a minilaparotomy (7-8 cm) both for laparoscopic hand-assisted dissection and for endoaneurysmorrhaphy. Mean laparoscopic and total operative times were respectively 64 ± 32 minutes and 257 ± 70 minutes, the mean aortic cross-clamping time was 76 ± 26 minutes, and the mean autotransfused blood volume was 1136 ± 711 mL. Overall mortality and morbidity were respectively 0% and 12.2%. Morbidity was surgery related in two cases (bleeding from an ipogastric artery lesion and a leg graft thrombosis). The mean ICU stay was 14.3 ± 13 hours. Oral food intake was resumed after 27.4 ± 15 hours, and patients were discharged after a mean of 4.4 ± 1.7 days. Operative times were not affected by obesity, suprarenal aortic cross-clamping, or aneurysm size. Both concomitant iliac aneurysms and bifurcated graft implantation (related to longer vascular reconstruction) involved significantly longer operative times. The learning curve of the procedure (comparing the first 30 patients with the last 92 patients) led to significantly shorter endoscopic, cross-clamping, and total operative times (p = .000). The mean follow-up was 28.6 ± 16 months. Three incisional hernias and one case of bowel occlusion were detected.

All these cases (3.4%) required laparoscopic treatment. The authors concluded that the HALS technique is a safe and minimally invasive treatment for AAA that could be considered as a bridge between open and total laparoscopic surgery.

TOTALLY LAPAROSCOPIC AORTOILIAC SURGERY

Obviously, the ultimate goal in laparoscopic vascular surgery is avoidance of abdominal incisions altogether, implicating the necessity for advanced laparoscopic skills to perform the aortic reconstruction.

Various techniques have been described to obtain surgical exposure of the aortoiliac trajectory and subsequently repair the diseased aorta.

To begin with, obtaining a stable and safe operative field is essential. Several methods have been developed, three of which are commonly used. First, a retroperitoneal approach toward the abdominal aorta can be used, as has been described earlier.[2] With use of a small flank incision, through digital dissection and subsequently with use of a dissection balloon, access to the aorta can be obtained. A problem in this approach, though, is the relatively small pneumoretroperitoneum that will easily collapse when suction is applied during surgery, thus leaving the surgeon without vision; therefore we use this approach for lumbar artery clipping only.

A second approach is creation of an "apron" from part of the peritoneum.[9] Through a transabdominal approach, a flap of the peritoneum is dissected and used to hang the bowels to the abdominal wall by means of transcutaneous stitches. This approach is time-consuming, and tearing of the thin retroperitoneal flap results in an immediate loss of the surgical field, and conversion to open surgery is necessary.

Finally, a method that uses extreme patient rotation (85-90 degrees)—as described by Coggia et al.[10]—can be used. This method uses an inflatable pillow positioned under the patient's left flank. After the operation table is tilted, the pillow is inflated and a maximum patient rotation is achieved. Subsequently, a transabdominal approach is performed in which the left colon can be dissected. By use of gravity, the left colon falls down and can be kept in place with a fan retractor, thus providing a stable operative field of the abdominal aorta.

Clinical Results

Recently, Coggia et al.[11] described their early and midterm results of total laparoscopic aortofemoral bypass (TLAFB). TLAFB was performed in 150 cases of severe aortoiliac occlusive disease. Aortic approaches included transperitoneal left retrocolic (n = 86), left retrorenal (n = 51), and direct (n = 4); the retroperitoneoscopic approach was used in nine cases. The procedure was totally laparoscopic in 145 patients (96.6%). Median operative and clamping times were 260 (120-450) and 81 (36-190) minutes, respectively. Thirty-day mortality was 2.7%. Nonlethal systemic, local vascular, and local nonvascular complications occurred in 21 (14.3%), 7 (4.8%), and 2 (1.3%) patients, respectively. Median return to general diet and ambulation was, respectively, days 2 and 3. Median hospital stay was 7 days. Follow-up was 25.2 ± 17.6 months (range, 1-60 months) with 3-year primary and secondary actuarial patency rates of 93% and 95.6%, respectively. They concluded that TLAFB gives early and midterm patency rates comparable with those of open direct repair but allows faster recovery and reduces operative trauma. A second problem of laparoscopic aortic surgery is creation of the aortic anastomosis. Because of the technical difficulty of this part, it seems to be reserved for a limited number of devoted specialists. With robotic assistance, however, the bar may be lowered, and this technique might be accessible to the more "common" vascular surgeon.

ROBOT-ASSISTED, TOTALLY LAPAROSCOPIC AORTOILIAC SURGERY

Even though laparoscopic training is a growing part of the surgical residency, major laparoscopic surgery is still restricted to devoted surgeons with extensive practice and expertise. Advanced laparoscopic surgery requires a great deal of skill and dexterity, mainly because of the technical difficulties emerging with this method.

These difficulties consist of unnatural eye-hand coordination, an unnatural working axis, two-dimensional vision, limited degrees of freedom, and the "fulcrum effect." The fulcrum effect is the unnatural movement of laparoscopic instruments; while moving the handle of the instrument to the right *outside* the patient, its tip moves leftward *inside* the patient.

Robotic assistance may help to overcome these difficulties. Recent surgical robots restore natural eye-hand coordination and a natural working axis. They use three-dimensional vision and have no fulcrum effect. Furthermore, 7 degrees of freedom are available, as opposed to the 5 degrees of freedom in conventional laparoscopic instruments. These conventional instruments use horizontal movement, vertical movement, depth movement, rotation, and opening and closing of the instrument. Robotic instruments however, use a "miniwrist" at the tip of the instrument. This wrist can articulate horizontally and vertically, thus adding 2 more degrees of freedom.

With overcoming the previously mentioned limitations of conventional laparoscopic surgery, robotic assistance may very well be of surplus value, especially in highly advanced laparoscopic procedures such as suturing a vascular anastomosis.

In 2001, the first robot-assisted TLAFB in the world was performed in our institution.[12]

Surgical Technique

Details of our method of aortic exposure have been described earlier.[12] After laparoscopic exposure of the infrarenal aorta (without use of the robot), two retroperitoneal tunnels are prepared from the groin incision toward the aorta by means of passing a blunt clamp, visualizing intra-abdominal passage with the endoscope.

The proximal aortic clamp is inserted through an separate stab incision in the abdominal wall, just below the xyphoid, and the distal clamp is inserted through an earlier placed trocar. Subsequently the robotic system, which is previously covered in sterile drapes, is introduced into the surgical field. The surgeon takes his or her place behind a remote console, from which the robotic arms are controlled. The endoscope is replaced by a 30-degree three-dimensional endoscope of the surgical system.

Under systemic heparinization, the aorta is clamped just distal to the renal arteries and below the IMA. An aortotomy is made with a pair of Potts scissors (EndoWrist Potts scissors; Intuitive Surgical, Sunnyvale, CA). A bifurcated polytetrafluoroethylene (W. L. Gore & Associates, Flagstaff, AZ) prosthesis is stained orange with rifampicin to prevent light reflections. An end-to-side anastomosis is made with a CV-4 polytetrafluoroethylene (W. L. Gore & Associates) running suture with two robotic needle drivers (EndoWrist Needle Drivers).

After completion of the aortic anastomosis the two graft limbs are tunneled to the groins where a conventional end-to-side anastomosis is performed to the common femoral artery.

Clinical Experience

Between 2004 and 2007, 24 patients underwent robot-assisted laparoscopic aortofemoral bypass in our institution.[13] This group was compared with a consecutive series (n = 30) treated with open surgical technique in the period just before our implementation of the robot-assisted technique.

Results

Both patient groups were similar as to ischemic symptoms, body mass index, cardiovascular risk factors, comorbidity, and extent of aortic disease. One patient in the robot group died 3 days after surgery of a massive myocardial infarction following uneventful early recovery. Operative times and aortic clamping times were significantly shorter in the "open" group (232.5 vs. 360 minutes, $p < .01$, and 50 vs. 71.5 minutes, $p = .02$), whereas postoperative data show a significant favor toward the "robot-assisted" group; ICU stay 1 versus 2 days ($p < .01$), resumption of normal diet 2 versus 5 days ($p < .01$), resumption of ambulation 3 versus 4 days ($p < .01$), and total hospital stay 6 versus 14.5 days ($p < .01$). We concluded that, in spite of longer operative and clamping times, robot-assisted laparoscopic aortic bypass was associated with a significantly quicker postoperative recovery compared with open surgical repair.

Stadler et al.,[14] between November 2005 and June 2006, performed 30 robot-assisted laparoscopic aortoiliac procedures (at the time of preparation of this chapter, their series had grown to well more than 100 patients, and a report of this largest series in the world will soon be published). Twenty-seven patients were prospectively evaluated for occlusive disease, two patients for AAA, and one for common iliac artery aneurysm. Dissections of the aorta and iliac arteries were performed laparoscopically by using the "modified Stadler method," a transperitoneal direct approach (Figure 71-2). The robotic system was used to construct anastomoses, to perform thromboendarterectomies, and, in most of the cases, for posterior peritoneal suturing. Robot-assisted procedures were successfully performed in all patients. The robot was used to perform both the AAA and common iliac artery aneurysm anastomoses and the aortoiliac reconstruction with patch and to complete the central, end-to-side anastomosis in another operation. Median operating time was 236 minutes (range, 180 to 360 minutes), with a median clamp time of 54 minutes (range, 40 to 120 minutes). Operative time is defined as the time elapsed from the initial incision to final skin closure. Median anastomosis time was 27 minutes (range, 20 to 60 minutes), and median blood loss was 320 mL (range, 100 to 1500 mL). No conversion was necessary, 30-day survival was 100%, median ICU stay was 1.8 days, and median hospital stay was 5.3 days. A regular

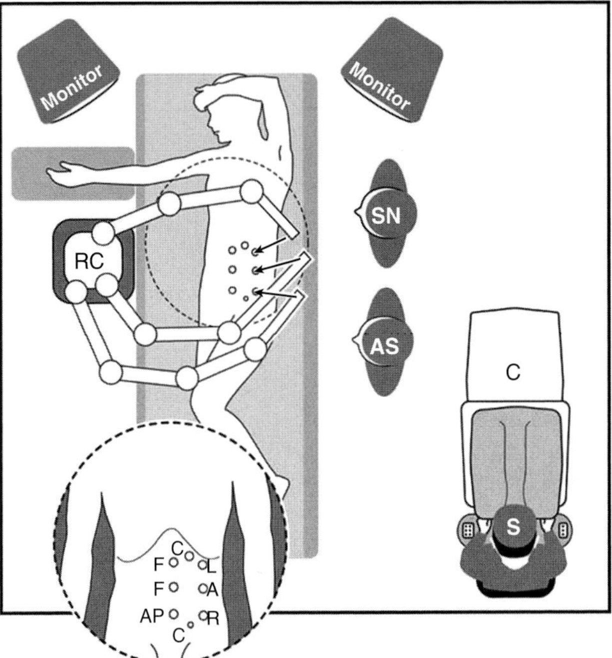

FIGURE 71-2 Setup in operating room and trocar positions. *AS*, Assistant; *C*, robot console; *RC*, robotic cart; *S*, surgeon; *SN*, scrub nurse. *Inset: A*, Surgical endoscope; *AP*, assistants' ports; *C*, aortic clamps; *F*, fan retractor; *L*, left robotic arm; *R*, right robotic arm.

oral diet was resumed after a mean time of 2.5 days. These authors concluded that robot-assisted laparoscopic surgery is a feasible technique for aortoiliac surgery. The da Vinci robotic system facilitated the creation of the aortic anastomosis and shortened aortic clamp time in comparison with our laparoscopic techniques.

To determine the current status of robot-assisted laparoscopic vascular surgery, we conducted a literature search.[15] Only five studies were identified describing a total number of 70 patients. In these studies, either the Zeus (Computer Motion, Santa Barbara, CA) (n = 15) or the da Vinci surgical system (Intuitive Surgical) (n = 55) was used to construct aortic anastomoses in surgery for aortoiliac occlusive or aneurysmal disease.

Study population and individual patient data were poorly described. Some of the studies described patient selection criteria for robot-assisted laparoscopic surgery. Patients with replacement of infected prostheses, with prior abdominal surgery, with redo surgery of occluded prostheses, and with class 4 American Society of Anesthesiologists were generally excluded.[13] Operative times varied from 188 to 480 minutes. ICU stay, reported only in some of the cases, varied from 1 to 2.1 days. Clamping time was reported from 54 to 95.9 minutes. Blood loss varied between 320 and 1000 mL. Anastomosis time is reported inconsistently, but when reported it varied from 27 to 40 minutes. The time to resume a normal diet varied between 1.3 and 3 days. Total hospital stay varied from 4 to 7.3 days. One of the 70 reported patients died after surgery. Seven of the 70 patients were converted to open surgery (10%). Reasons for conversion were either technical difficulties with the robotic system (n = 4) or an unstable operative field (n = 3). The technical difficulties with the robotic system consisted of failure of the robotic system and interference of the robotic arms outside the patient (Diks et al. Unpublished data, 2007).[16,17]

In summary, reported series show that robot-assisted laparoscopic aortic surgery is feasible and safe, with operative and clamping times similar and conversion rates smaller in comparison with series of totally laparoscopic aortoiliac surgery. However, the number of reported patients was small and the study quality of most series was low, preventing robust conclusions with respect to patient outcomes of robotic-assisted aortoiliac surgery compared with conventional laparoscopic surgery.

HYBRID PROCEDURES

Several authors have reported on laparoscopic techniques used to aid in endovascular vascular repair, so-called hybrid procedures. Kolvenbach's group[18] described different banding procedures and several ways to perform active graft fixation to improve the characteristics of the proximal aortic neck during EVAR. They also evacuated the thrombus to downsize the aneurysm and to prevent longitudinal shrinkage.

The same authors[19] performed totally laparoscopic aortohepatic bypass for aortic debranching during endovascular thoracoabdominal aneurysm repair, thereby extending the indications of EVAR. Laparoscopic techniques may also be used to obtain direct vascular access permitting insertion of a thoracic endograft directly into the aorta in patients with diseased iliac vessels.[20]

REVIEW OF CLINICAL STUDIES REPORTING ON LAPAROSCOPIC SURGERY PERFORMED FOR AORTOILIAC DISEASE

Recently, we performed a literature review including all articles that described original patient series.[21] Case reports and studies containing duplicate material were excluded. Data on operative, clamping, and anastomosis times; hospital stay; mortality; complications; and conversion were retrieved. Following strict criteria, 30 articles were deemed representative, including 8 articles on hand-assisted techniques (6 occlusive disease, 2 aneurysm), 6 laparoscopy assisted (3 occlusive disease, 3 aneurysm), 17 totally laparoscopic (11 occlusive disease and 6 aneurysm), and 2 robot-assisted series (1 occlusive disease and 1 aneurysm).

The total reported number of operated patients was 1044, 630 for occlusive disease and 414 for aneurysm repair.

Patient Selection

To identify which patients are potentially suitable candidates for laparoscopic vascular surgery, exclusion criteria were evaluated. The most frequently mentioned exclusion criteria were class 4 American Society of Anesthesiologists patients or those with severe nontreatable coronary disease, extensive aortic calcification, or associated visceral occlusive disease or who had undergone previous major abdominal surgery. In laparoscopic aneurysm repair, inflammatory and ruptured aneurysms were also mentioned as exclusion criteria. The more experienced authors did, however, operate in the presence of adiposity or concomitant visceral occlusive disease or if suprarenal clamping was necessary.

Conversion

In total, in 78 of 1044 patients (7%) laparoscopy was converted to open surgery. The rate of conversion varied, with the highest number of conversions occurring in the smaller series. In series of >50 patients conversion rates were less than 5% and in series of fewer than 20 patients up to 16%. In aneurysm repair the conversion rate was higher than in occlusive disease (39/630 vs. 39/414). Reasons for conversion were calcified aorta; bleeding from the cava, renal, or iliac veins or aorta; adhesions; the necessity of suprarenal clamping or inadequate exposure of the operative field because of collapse of the pneumoperitoneum or the pneumoretroperitoneum; or other technical difficulties. Self-imposed operative time limits (aortic cross-clamping time of more than 2 hours and total operative time of more than 4 hours) were sometimes a reason for conversion.

Clamping Time

Hand-assisted procedures had the shortest cross-clamping times, all less than 1 hour. Both laparoscopic-assisted and totally laparoscopic procedures reported clamping times varying from 54 to 146 minutes. Clamping times were a little shorter in operations for occlusive disease. Totally laparoscopic clamping times were at least 1.5 times longer than the comparative open series.

Anastomosis Time

Anastomosis time was reported only in some of the totally laparoscopic procedures and varied from 30 to 60 minutes for procedures without a robotic system and 41 to 74 minutes with a robotic system.

Operative Time

Operative time varied widely between both authors and laparoscopic techniques. Hand-assisted procedures had the shortest mean operative times, varying from approximately 2.5 to 4 hours. In laparoscopy-assisted techniques, both for aneurysm repair and occlusive disease, mean operative times of more than 4 hours were described, except for one study that reports less than 3 hours (occlusive disease).

In totally laparoscopic techniques the time varied from 4 to 6.5 hours. Operative times did not differ between aneurysm repair and occlusive disease. More recent studies report a shorter operative time than do the earlier studies.

The robot-assisted technique was used in 18 patients in two studies.[17,22] Reported mean operating times varied between 4 and 5.5 hours, certainly not shorter than those achieved without the use of a robotic system.

Morbidity

Reported complications included local wound problems (infection, seroma, dehiscence), respiratory and transient renal insufficiency, cardiac and mesenteric ischemia, splenic rupture, massive cholesterol embolization, graft thrombosis, and bleeding. Five injuries of the ureter are mentioned, and limb graft thrombosis is reported 11 times. Six instances of anastomotic bleeding were reported.

Mortality

Reported mortality rates, in total 26 of 1044 (2%), were in most series approximately 5% or less. Mortality in aneurysm repair was slightly higher than in occlusive disease (11/414 vs. 15/630). Mortality was mainly due to postoperative cardiac ischemic events, followed by mesenteric ischemia.

Hospital Stay

In all but six reports, mean hospital stay was 1 week or less, varying from 3 to 11 days, for both the total laparoscopic approach and the laparoscopic and hand-assisted approach regardless of the surgical procedure.

This systematic review shows that, since the introduction of laparoscopic surgery in 1993, only a small number of clinical studies on laparoscopic aortoiliac surgery have been published. A variety of laparoscopic techniques, approaches, and operative procedures were used, and most studies were of an observational character and contained a limited number of patients. In addition we assumed a considerable selection bias in all series because the publications do not adequately describe the characteristics of the whole cohort of consecutive patients under treatment. This limits the full evaluation of laparoscopic surgery in relation to open or endovascular techniques.

DISCUSSION

The potential benefits of laparoscopic aortoiliac surgery are found in the combination of its minimally invasive character (reduction of hospital stay and postoperative pain, earlier return to daily routines) and the durable results of conventional open surgery (less necessity for continuous follow-up and additional procedures).

For treatment of aortoiliac *occlusive* disease laparoscopic techniques appear safe and feasible with midterm patency rates identical to those of open surgery, (still) the gold standard for treatment of TASC C and D lesions. In good hands, therefore, laparoscopic aortobifemoral bypass may be considered a viable alternative, *if endovascular options are not indicated or failing.*

Few series have been published on laparoscopic *aneurysm* repair. These studies report longer operative times and higher conversion rates compared with laparoscopic surgery for occlusive disease, although mortality is comparable with that of open procedures. Laparoscopic aneurysm repair appears to be more difficult than bypass surgery and is routinely performed in a few centers only. This is in sharp contrast to the wide implementation of endovascular repair of aortic aneurysms, an even less invasive technique with a low mortality and a far shorter learning curve. Also, the anatomic requirements for an easy laparoscopic repair, a good infrarenal neck and normal iliac arteries, are identical to those favoring endovascular repair. Taking this into consideration, the results of laparoscopic aneurysm repair as of yet do not justify its broader implementation. With further advancements in laparoscopic technique, however, such as integration of preoperative imaging into the surgical field, smaller instruments, and better methods of exposure, the more "difficult" aneurysms that are not amenable to endovascular repair may very well be the future terrain of the laparoscopic surgeon. Obviously, wide availability and implication of branched endografts is a major counterforce to this development.

Therefore laparoscopic technique should become far less demanding to make wider implementation possible. Technical difficulties of the vascular anastomosis need to be addressed such as the development of vascular staplers or introduction of robotic equipment.

Only a few centers have reported on robotic laparoscopic aortoiliac surgery. Although the use of robots has not convincingly reduced operative time in the available series, experience is increasing rapidly, and the technique continues to evolve.

In conclusion, in spite of admirable efforts of dedicated pioneers, laparoscopic aortoiliac surgery is still in its infancy and is practiced on a modest scale worldwide. Although the technique appears safe and feasible, operative time is still long. Robotic assistance in laparoscopic aortic surgery holds promise for the future with rapidly evolving technical progress. The observational, noncomparative character and selection bias of most published series preclude strong statements on the broad value of laparoscopic vascular surgery in comparison with endovascular and open surgical techniques.

References

1. Dion YM, Kathouda N, Rouleau C, et al: Laparoscopy assisted aortobifemoral bypass, *Surg Laparosc Endosc* 3:425–429, 1993.
2. Amesur NB, Zajko AB, Orons PD, et al: Embolotherapy of persistent endoleaks after endovascular repair of abdominal aortic aneurysm with the ancure-endovascular technologies endograft system, *J Vasc Interv Radiol* 10(9):1175–1182, 1999.
3. Schurink GW, Aarts NJ, Van Baalen JM, et al: Experimental study of the influence of endoleak size on pressure in the aneurysm sac and the consequences of thrombosis, *Br J Surg* 87 (1):71–78, 2000.
4. Marty B, Sanchez LA, Ohki T, et al: Endoleak after endovascular graft repair of experimental aortic aneurysms: does coil embolization with angiographic "seal" lower intraaneurysmal pressure? *J Vasc Surg* 27(3):454–461, discussion 462, 1998.
5. Wisselink W, Cuesta MA, Berends FJ, et al: Retroperitoneal endoscopic ligation of lumbar and inferior mesenteric arteries as a treatment of persistent endoleak following endoluminal aortic aneurysm repair, *J Vasc Surg* 31:1240–1244, 2000.
6. Alimi YS, De Caridi G, Hartung O, et al: Laparoscopy-assisted reconstruction to treat severe aortoiliac occlusive disease: early and midterm results, *J Vasc Surg* 39:777–783, 2004.
7. Ferrari M, Adami D, Del Corso A, et al: Laparoscopy-assisted abdominal aortic aneurysm repair: early and middle-term results of a consecutive series of 122 cases, *J Vasc Surg* 43:695–700, 2006.
8. Fourneau I, Daenens K, Nevelsteen A: Hand-assisted laparoscopic aortobifemoral bypass for occlusive disease: early and mid-term results, *Eur J Vasc Endovasc Surg* 30:489–493, 2005.
9. Dion YM, Gracia CR, Estakhri M, et al: Total laparoscopic versus conventional abdominal aortic aneurysm repair: a case-control study, *J Vasc Surg* 42:906–910, 2005.
10. Coggia M, Javerliat I, Di Centa I, et al: Total laparoscopic versus conventional abdominal aortic aneurysm repair: a case-control study, *J Vasc Surg* 42:906–910, 2005.
11. Coggia M, Cerreau P, Di Centa I, et al: Total laparoscopic juxtarenal abdominal aortic aneurysm repair, *J Vasc Surg* 48 (1):37–42, 2008.
12. Wisselink W, Cuesta MA, Gracia C, et al: Robot-assisted laparoscopic aortobifemoral bypass for aortoiliac occlusive disease: a report of two cases, *J Vasc Surg* 36:1079–1082, 2002.
13. Diks J, Nio D, Jongkind V, et al: Robot-assisted laparoscopic surgery of the infrarenal aorta: the early learning curve, *Surg Endosc* 21:1760–1763, 2007.
14. Stadler P, Matous P, Vitasek P, et al: Robot-assisted aortoiliac reconstruction: a review of 30 cases, *J Vasc Surg* 5(Nov 2006):915–919. 44, 2006.
15. Diks J, Nio D, Wisselink W, et al: Robot assisted laparoscopic surgery for aortoiliac surgery: a systematic review. In *Medical robots*, Vienna, Austria, January 2008, I-Tech Education and Publishing.
16. Desgranges P, Bourriez A, Javerliat I, et al: Robotically assisted aorto-femoral bypass grafting: lessons learned from our initial experience, *Eur J Vasc Endovasc Surg* 27:507–511, 2004.
17. Kolvenbach R, Schwierz E, Wasilljew S, et al: Total laparoscopically and robotically assisted aortic aneurysm surgery: a critical evaluation, *J Vasc Surg* 39(4):771–776, 2004.
18. Kolvenbach R, Lin J: Combining laparoscopic and endovascular techniques to improve the outcome of aortic endografts. Hybrid techniques, *J Cardiovasc Surg (Torino)* 46(4):415–423, 2005.
19. Bakiovannis C, Cagiannos C, Wasilljew S, et al: Totally laparoscopic aortohepatic bypass for aortic debranching during endovascular thoracoabdominal aneurysm repair, *Eur J Vasc Endovasc Surg* 34(2):173–175, 2007.
20. Linsen MA, Jongkind V, Huisman L, et al: Direct videoscopic approach to the descending thoracic aorta for aortic arch endograft delivery: evaluation in a porcine model, *J Endovasc Therapy* 14(1):39–43, 2007.
21. Nio D, Diks J, Bemelman WA, et al: Laparoscopic vascular surgery: a systematic review, *Eur J Vasc Endovasc Surg* 263–271, 2007.
22. Nio D, Diks J, Linsen MAM, et al: Robot-assisted laparoscopic aortobifemoral bypass for aortoiliac occlusive disease: early clinical experience, *Eur J Vasc Endovasc Surg* 29:586–590, 2005.

CHAPTER

72

Endoscopic Vein Harvest

Juan Carlos Jimenez, Joshua C. Smith

Open saphenous vein harvest has traditionally been associated with long incisions and significant morbidity from postoperative wound complications (Figure 72-1). In patients with critical limb ischemia undergoing below-knee arterial bypass surgery, wound healing after open saphenectomy becomes an even greater challenge because of preexisting arterial occlusive disease. Lumsden et al.[1] first described video-assisted saphenous vein harvest in 1996. This technique allows for complete mobilization of the great saphenous vein (GSV) and other autogenous conduit sources with use of two or three skin incisions of 2 cm in length and use of carbon dioxide insufflation (Figure 72-2). Since then, endoscopic vein harvest (EVH) has been increasingly used for GSV and radial artery harvest during open coronary artery revascularizations. At our institution, more than 800 EVHs have been performed during cardiac surgery procedures. More recently, its use has been extended to minimally invasive harvest of autogenous conduits in peripheral vascular surgery. The development of newer endoscopic devices has allowed for a wider range of autogenous conduits to be harvested during minimally invasive distal bypass surgery with increased ease of use. These technologic advances, as well as development of technical operative modifications for EVH and minimally invasive distal bypass, have greatly expanded its role for vascular surgeons.

TECHNIQUES

Techniques for Endoscopic Harvest of the Great Saphenous Vein

Several endoscopic vein harvesting systems are currently available for mobilization and removal of the entire GSV from the groin to the ankle. At our institution, we use the Vasoview 7 Endoscopic Vein Harvesting system (Guidant, Indianapolis, IN). Before operation, vein mapping is performed to assess vein size, caliber, patency, and location of branch points. We also perform intraoperative ultrasonography to mark the course of the vein under sterile conditions before harvest and to maximize incision placement accuracy.

The initial incision is made three fingerbreadths posterior to the medial femoral or tibial condyles. A longitudinal 2-cm incision can be made either above or below the knee, and the vein is localized at this time with use of sharp dissection. A silicone elastomer (Silastic) vessel loop is then placed around the GSV. At this time, several more centimeters of vein can be bluntly dissected and mobilized from the surrounding subcutaneous tissue to ease placement of the blunt tip trocar (BTT) in the direction of the harvest. The BTT is placed into the subcutaneous space overlying the GSV, and approximately 25 cc of air is inflated into the port balloon to ensure a good seal with the adjacent skin. Leakage of carbon dioxide outside the harvest tunnel can lead to suboptimal visibility and bleeding during vein mobilization. A CO_2 cannula is then attached to a port on the BTT and continued at a flow rate of 3 to 5 L/min up to a maximal pressure of 10 to 15 mm Hg. Insufflation of the vein harvest tunnel facilitates placement of the 5-mm camera through the main port of the BTT and enhances visualization of the GSV within the subcutaneous space.

A conical tip is placed on the tip of the camera, and the vein is freed along its anterior and posterior surfaces with use of blunt dissection (Figure 72-3). Branches are skeletonized from surrounding soft tissue and exposed to maximal length before division with the bipolar dissector. The main goal before division of branches is to suspend the entire length of vein by its branches in the center of the harvest tunnel and allow maximal CO_2 insufflation for good visibility. Care must be taken at this time to avoid avulsion of large branches. Disruption of minor venous branches is not overly concerning, however, because the insufflation tends to control bleeding from these tributaries without the need for additional cauterization.

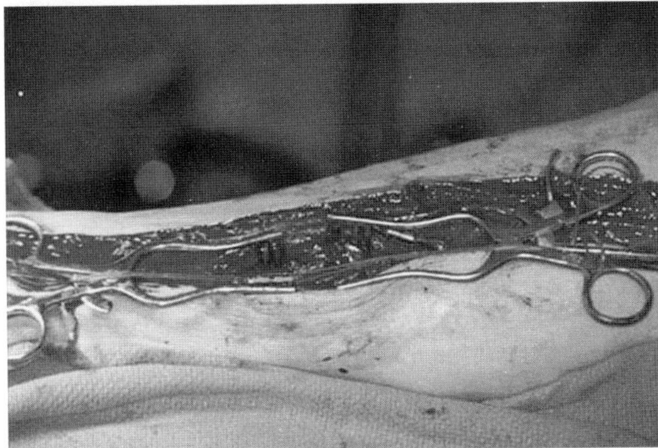

FIGURE 72-1 Traditional open saphenous vein harvest results in long incisions and significant patient morbidity.

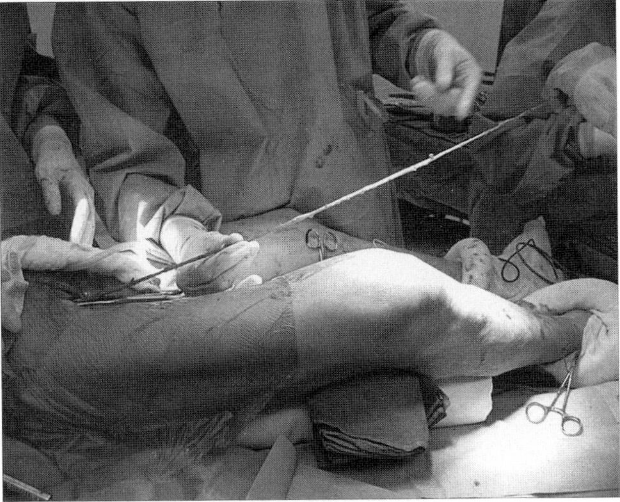

FIGURE 72-2 Harvesting long, continuous segments of greater and lesser saphenous vein is possible using endoscopic techniques.

After complete blunt dissection, the BTT is replaced with the vein harvesting cannula, which serves to retract, cauterize, and divide all branches. The Vasoview system provides a retractable C-ring, which is used in conjunction with the bipolar dissector to mobilize the main vein and provide countertension at each individual branch site. A retractable bipolar dissector is then used to cauterize and divide all branches at a setting of 15 to 25 W, while avoiding direct or collateral thermal injury to the vein wall. Care must be taken to avoid overaggressive retraction at this time, which may result in branch avulsion and bleeding within the tunnel. Once all branches are cauterized and divided, the vessel cradle (C-ring) is then run along the entire length of harvested vein to ensure that no branches remain. The vein can then be removed through a proximal and distal stab incision made directly at opposite ends of the harvest tunnel. We reinforce all cauterized side branches before limb salvage bypass with individual silk and Prolene sutures. Injured segments of vein must be repaired directly with Prolene suture, and, if luminal compromise is present, the affected segment of vein must be excised and venovenostomy performed. The vein is then prepared and flushed in usual fashion.

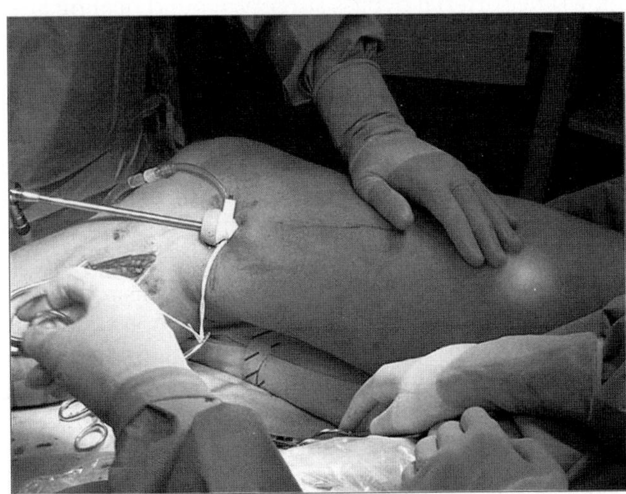

FIGURE 72-3 Harvesting long, continuous segments of greater and lesser saphenous vein is possible using endoscopic techniques.

Techniques for Endoscopic Harvest of the Small Saphenous Vein

EVH of the small saphenous vein is performed with the patient in the prone position. Preoperative vein mapping can be useful to determine length, diameter, and caliber of this vessel for use in lower-extremity limb salvage procedures. The small saphenous vein usually has more large branches than the GSV, and it lies deeper within the subfascial plane. Care must be taken to avoid injury to the sural nerve, which lies adjacent to the small saphenous vein in the leg. A 2-cm transverse incision is made in the upper leg below the knee joint distal to where the small saphenous vein dives deep and joins the popliteal vein. The vein is harvested and removed in similar fashion. A stab incision can then be made in the distal calf to remove the vein in its entirety. Minimally invasive popliteal–to–posterior tibial artery bypass can also be performed in this position with placement of the vein through the harvest tunnel in either reversed or nonreversed fashion (after treatment with a semiclosed valvulotome).

Modifications for Noncardiac Vascular Surgery and Limb Salvage

Despite its frequent use in the field of cardiac surgery for close to a decade, the use of EVH for minimally invasive distal limb salvage bypass has been validated more

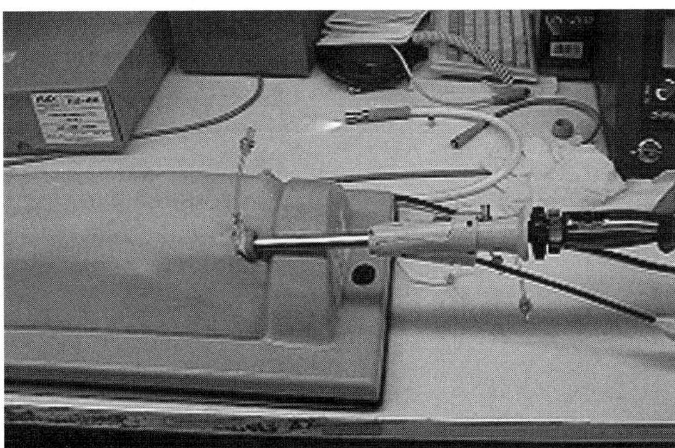

FIGURE 72-4 Simulator training equipment for learning endoscopic vein harvest techniques.

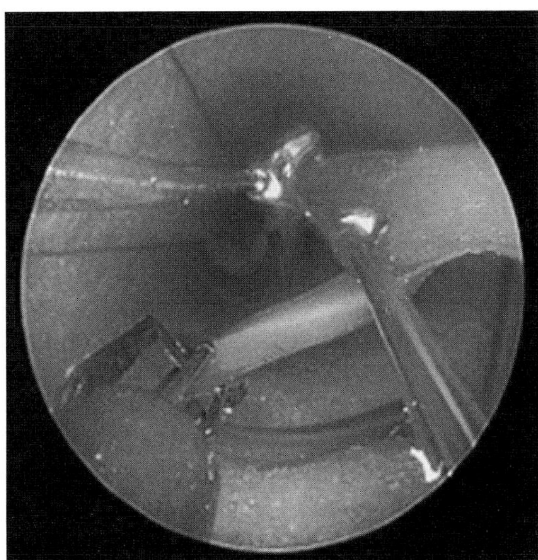

FIGURE 72-5 Simulator training for learning endoscopic vein harvest techniques.

recently by vascular surgeons.[2-7] At our institution, vascular surgeons and fellows underwent formal training on operative simulators before implementation in the operating room (Figures 72-4 and 72-5). This included familiarization with the different components of the device during formal training sessions with industry representatives and the review of video and other interactive materials during didactic sessions.[7]

Certain technical modifications have been implemented during EVH that facilitate use during lower-extremity limb salvage procedures. Longitudinal vein harvest incisions are preferred over the traditional transverse incisions, performed during cardiac surgery procedures, because they can be extended proximally and/or distally and used to simultaneously expose arterial targets for bypass. A medial EVH incision just above the knee at the level of the femoral condyle can be used to subsequently expose the above-knee popliteal artery

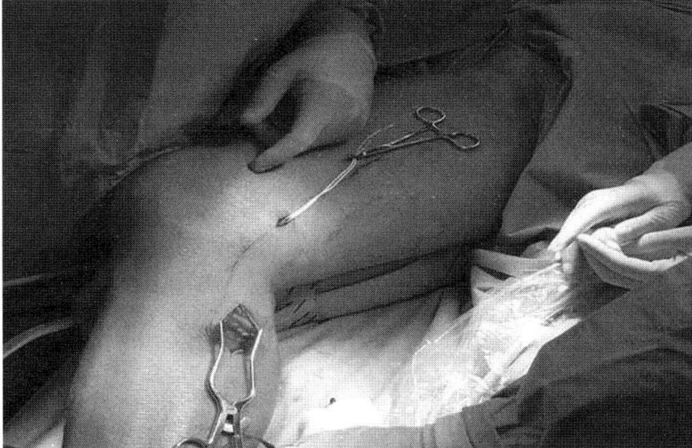

FIGURE 72-6 Typical incisions for below knee vein bypass using endoscopic vein harvest techniques.

after the GSV has been removed. A harvest incision just below the knee at the level of the tibial condyles can also be used for exposure of the below-knee popliteal artery, the tibioperoneal trunk, and the proximal peroneal and posterior tibial arteries. A longitudinal incision just proximal to the medial malleolus can be extended to expose the distal posterior tibial artery (Figure 72-6).

When ipsilateral GSV harvest is performed for limb salvage procedures, the harvest tunnel is frequently used for subcutaneous placement of the vein. It can be either reversed or placed in situ after valve lysis with the use of a semiclosed valvulotome. Meticulous hemostasis must be ensured within the harvest tunnel because bleeding and hematoma formation may jeopardize graft patency. We avoid the use of compression bandages when ipsilateral harvest is performed for limb salvage procedures, whereas this technique is frequently used after EVH for coronary artery bypass grafting. Patients are instructed to discontinue oral clopidogrel (Plavix) 7 days before the operation to minimize bleeding risk. We avoid the use of postoperative continuous intravenous heparin drips. Platelet antiaggregate therapy with aspirin or clopidogrel (Plavix) can usually be safely reinstated 24 to 48 hours after the operation.

RESULTS

EVH during coronary artery bypass surgery has demonstrated decreased wound complication rates and postoperative pain, improved cosmesis, similar graft patency rates, and increased patient satisfaction in several prospective randomized trials of open and minimally invasive techniques.[8-13] Although some early reports demonstrated increased operative times for EVH, the entire length of GSV from the groin to the ankle can be routinely harvested within 20 to 30 minutes.

TABLE 72-1 Results of Endoscopic Vein Harvest Used in Conjunction With Peripheral Arterial Bypass

Study	Year	Mean operative time (min)	Primary patency, %	Overall limb salvage (%)	Overall wound complication rate (%)
Jordan et al.[2]	2001	NA	69 (12 mo)	89	0.9
Suggs et al.[3]	2001	295	93 (12 mo)	92	4
Illig et al.[15]	2003	NA	60 (12 mo)	98	20.4
Erdoes and Milner[4]	2005	248	71.5 (18 mo)	91	7.5
Gazoni et al.[5]	2006	241.5	92.8 (21 mo)	96.5	13.8
Pulatt et al.[6]	2006	NA	30 (12 mo)	85	6
Jimenez et al.[7]	2007	410.4	78.5 (12 mo)	100	14

NA, Not available.

Griffith et al.[14] compared both open saphenectomy and EVH and studied the histologic findings of both techniques. There was no difference in endothelial, smooth muscle, and elastic lamina continuity. Medial and adventitial connective tissue uniformity was also not significantly altered.[14]

Several authors have demonstrated similar favorable results for EVH during distal limb bypasses, although no randomized controlled trials exist (Table 17-1).[2-7] Jordan et al.[2] endoscopically harvested 164 saphenous vein grafts for lower-extremity arterial reconstructive procedures over a 6-year period. With use of life table analysis, patency rates at 1, 3, and 5 years were 85%, 74%, and 68%, respectively. Fourteen (8.5%) patients had wound infections during the 30-day postoperative period, and two patients had harvest site hematomas. None of these wound complications led to either graft failure or limb loss.[2] The limb salvage rate was 89%.

A later study by Erdoes and Milner[4] yielded similar results. Infrainguinal bypass in 214 limbs was performed with use of endoscopically harvested saphenous vein over a 6-year period. The indication for bypass was limb salvage in 88.3%, claudication in 9.3%, and other in 2.4% (trauma and aneurysm). Assisted primary patency at 18 months was 77.2% by life table analysis. Wound complications occurred in 7.5% of patients with 2.5% of patients requiring readmission to the hospital. Only one patient early in the series required conversion to an open harvest.

Gazoni et al.[5] reviewed the results of patients who underwent femoral to below-knee arterial bypass grafting over a 27-month period. Fifty-nine patients underwent traditional open saphenectomy, and 29 had EVH. There was a trend toward improved patency rates in the EVH group compared with open harvest although no statistically significant difference was noted (92.8% vs. 80.6%). No significant differences were found between the two groups in postoperative complications, operative time, length of hospital stay, patency rates, limb salvage, and death. The incidence of wound complications was 3.4% in the EVH group and 15.3% in the open harvest group, although this difference also was not statistically significant.[5]

After implementation of technical modifications for limb salvage bypass, as well as formal systematic training by vascular surgeons at our institution, we noted 30-day primary and primary-assisted patency rates of 85.7% and 92.9%, respectively.[6] Actuarial primary assisted patency was 63.6%. The limb salvage rate at 19 months was 100%. One graft occluded within 30 days after tunnel hematoma in a patient who had a postoperative myocardial infarction and required a therapeutic heparin drip. One late hematoma was noted, and one patient demonstrated skin necrosis at the level of the ankle requiring prolonged hospitalization. Complete wound healing was achieved in 75% of patients with preoperative tissue loss because of critical limb ischemia.

Concerns regarding increased operative costs because of endoscopic equipment have prompted analysis of the financial impact of EVH and minimally invasive distal bypass.[15] Illig et al.[15] performed a cost analysis in patients undergoing both EVH and open saphenectomy for limb salvage procedures. Subset analysis revealed a significant reduction in total cost in the EVH group compared with the open group. Open saphenectomy proved more costly because of a significant increase in postoperative wound complications requiring readmission compared with patients who underwent EVH. EVH was also associated with a shortened length of stay, a decreased rate of major wound infections, and less need for early hospital readmissions.

COMPLICATIONS OF ENDOSCOPIC VEIN HARVEST

Despite several randomized trials demonstrating decreased wound complications with EVH, all wound complications associated with open saphenous vein harvest can occur with minimally invasive techniques. These include infection, dehiscence, hematoma, lymphocele, and limb swelling. A meta-analysis of 14 randomized studies performed by Athanasiou et al.[16] comparing minimally invasive versus conventional vein harvesting also found that EVH techniques were associated with a reduced risk of leg wound infections. However, infections occurring within the harvest tunnel after EVH usually require drainage of fluid collections contained in a closed space. Allen et al.[17] identified three closed-space tunnel infections out of 1,259 patients who underwent EVH. All three patients with closed-space infections also had early postoperative hematomas and had wound cultures positive for *Staphylococcus aureus*. Two patients were treated with unroofing the tunnel with an incision over its entire length. One patient was managed successfully by using closed-space irrigation with a Blake drain irrigated every 8 hours and gradually withdrawn over a 10-day period.

Carbon dioxide insufflation during EVH can result in hypercarbia,[18] pneumoperitoneum,[19] and CO_2 embolus.[20] Chiu et al.[21] randomly assigned 498 patients to high (15 mm Hg) and low (12 mm Hg) CO_2 insufflation groups for EVH during coronary artery bypass grafting. Transesophageal echocardiography with transgastric inferior vena cava views was used to monitor for the appearance of CO_2 bubbles. The incidence of CO_2 embolus was significantly elevated in the high-pressure insufflations group (13.3% vs. 6.5%, $p < .05$). Two patients in the high-pressure group required immediate cessation of insufflation. Although no patient exhibited hemodynamic alterations in either group in this study, massive CO_2 embolus with circulatory collapse has been noted in separate reports. All patients with visible CO_2 bubbles on transesophageal echocardiography were converted to open harvest, and these patients all exhibited subclinical injury to the vein wall.

When EVH is performed on the ipsilateral GSV during minimally invasive distal arterial bypass, care must be taken to avoid postoperative tunnel hematomas. Meticulous hemostasis in the subcutaneous tissue and reinforcement of all ligated branches must be ensured. Extension of existing incisions should be used in selected instances when significant bleeding is noted. Postoperative anticoagulation should be avoided. We also recommend avoidance of compression wraps when the ipsilateral GSV is used for graft tunneling because of possible compression of the vein within its subcutaneous position.

Although rare, skin necrosis has been reported after EVH, especially in the lower leg at the level of the ankle where minimal subcutaneous fat exists. Conversion to open harvest at this level should be performed if excessive resistance is noted during blunt dissection. At our institution, one patient exhibited full-thickness skin necrosis requiring flap coverage and ultimately leading to late graft failure. Early recognition and flap coverage is crucial, especially when the harvest tunnel is used for graft placement.

CONCLUSION

EVH has been used during coronary revascularization procedures for the past decade with decreased postoperative morbidity from wound complications, equivalent operative times, equal graft patency, and increased patient satisfaction. Vascular surgeons can (and should) learn to perform EVH for use with minimally invasive distal bypass procedures. EVH avoids long saphenous harvest incisions, which benefits patients with peripheral vascular disease undergoing limb salvage procedures. Additional technical modifications favor the use of EVH during minimally invasive distal arterial bypass.

References

1. Lumsden AB, Eaves III FF, Ofenloch JC, et al: Subcutaneous, video-assisted saphenous vein harvest: report of the first 30 cases, *Cardiovasc Surg* 4:771–776, 1996.
2. Jordan WD Jr, Alcocer F, Voellinger DC, et al: The durability of endoscopic saphenous vein grafts: a 5-year observational study, *J Vasc Surg* 34:434–439, 2001.
3. Suggs WD, Sanchez LA, Woo D, et al: Endoscopically assisted in situ lower extremity bypass graft: a preliminary report of a new minimally invasive technique, *J Vasc Surg* 34:668–672, 2001.
4. Erdoes LS, Milner TP: Encouraging results with endoscopic vein harvest for infrainguinal bypass, *J Vasc Surg* 42:442–448, 2005.
5. Gazoni LM, Carty R, Skinner J, et al: endoscopic versus open saphenous vein harvest for femoral to below the knee arterial bypass using saphenous vein graft, *J Vasc Surg* 44:282–288, 2006.
6. Pullatt R, Brothers TE, Robison JG, et al: Compromised bypass graft outcomes after minimal-incision vein harvest, *J Vasc Surg* 44 (2):289–294; discussion 294–295, 2006.
7. Jimenez JC, Lawrence PF, Rigberg DA, et al: Technical modifications in endoscopic vein harvest techniques facilitate their use in lower extremity limb salvage procedures, *J Vasc Surg* 45:549–553, 2007.
8. Allen KB, Griffith GL, Heimansohn DA, et al: Endoscopic versus traditional saphenous vein harvesting: a prospective, randomized trial, *Ann Thorac Surg* 66:26–32, 1998.
9. Puskas JD, Wright CE, Miller PK, et al: A randomized trial of endoscopic versus open saphenous vein harvest in coronary artery bypass surgery, *Ann Thorac Surg* 68:1509–1512, 1999.
10. Kiaii B, Moon BC, Massel D, et al: A prospective randomized trial of endoscopic versus conventional harvesting of the saphenous vein in coronary artery bypass surgery, *J Thorac Cardiovasc Surg* 123:204–212, 2002.
11. Schurr UP, Lahcat ML, Reuthebuch O, et al: Endoscopic saphenous vein harvesting for CABG: a randomized, prospective trial, *Thorac Cardiov Surg* 50:160–163, 2002.

12. Yun KL, Wu Y, Aharonian V, et al: Randomized trial of endoscopic versus open vein harvest for coronary artery bypass grafting: six-month patency rates, *J Thorac Cardiovasc Surg* 129:496–503, 2005.
13. Andreasen JJ, Nekrasas V, Dethlefsen C: Endoscopic vs open saphenous vein harvest for coronary artery bypass grafting: a prospective randomized trial, *Eur J Cardiothorac Surg* 34:384–389, 2008.
14. Griffith GL, Allen KB, Waller BF, et al: Endoscopic and traditional saphenous vein harvest: a histologic comparison, *Ann Thorac Surg* 69:520–523, 2000.
15. Illig KA, Rhodes JM, Sternbach Y, et al: Financial impact of endoscopic vein harvest for infrainguinal bypass, *J Vasc Surg* 37:323–330, 2003.
16. Athanasiou T, Aziz O, Skapinakis P, et al: Leg wound infection after coronary artery bypass grafting: a meta-analysis comparing minimally invasive versus conventional vein harvesting, *Ann Thorac Surg* 76:2141–2146, 2003.
17. Allen KB, Fitzgeral EB, Heimansohn DA, et al: Management of closed space infections associated with endoscopic vein harvest, *Ann Thorac Surg* 69:960–961.
18. Leissner KB, Woo A, Ortega R, et al: Endoscopic saphenous vein harvest: severe hypercarbia, *J Cardiothorac Vasc Anesth* 20:759–760, 2006.
19. Lehmann A, Lang J, Weisse U, et al: Pneumoperitoneum secondary to endoscopic harvest of saphenous vein graft, *Ann Thorac Surg* 69:1937–1938, 2000.
20. Tamim M, Omrani M, Tash A, et al: Carbon dioxide embolism during endoscopic vein harvesting, *Interact Cardiovasc Thorac Surg* 7:659–660, 2008.
21. Chiu KM, Lin TY, Wang MJ, et al: Reduction of carbon dioxide embolism for endoscopic saphenous vein harvesting, *Ann Thorac Surg* 81:1697–1699, 2006.

SECTION XII

MISCELLANEOUS ENDOVASCULAR TECHNIQUES

CHAPTER

73

The Transjugular Intrahepatic Portosystemic Shunt Procedure for Portal Hypertension

Jeffrey Jim, David Rigberg

The introduction of transjugular intrahepatic portosystemic shunt (TIPS) has given physicians an important tool in the treatment of patients with complications related to portal hypertension. The procedure was first described in 1971 by Rosch et al., and the first clinical TIPS was performed by Colapinto in 1983.[1,2] The use of a metallic stent was later reported by Palmaz et al. in 1985.[3] The first clinical TIPS in its current form was described in a patient in Germany in 1988.[4] Today, the TIPS procedure involves creation of a low-resistance channel between the portal system and the systemic circulation by placement of an expandable metal stent. It is a less-invasive alternative to surgery in patients with end-stage liver disease. It functions as a side-to-side portacaval shunt but obviates the associated morbidity and mortality of a surgically created shunt.

The Society of Interventional Radiology developed guidelines for the creation of a TIPS in 2001. A technically successful outcome was defined as the creation of a shunt that reduced the portal-systemic gradient to less than 12 mm Hg.[5] For procedures performed in experienced hands and at high-volume centers, the success rate approaches 100%, and procedure mortality should be less than 1%. If major complications occur in more than 3% of patients, then an internal quality review should be performed.[6]

Since its introduction, the TIPS procedure gained widespread acceptance as a viable method to treat ill patients with severe portal hypertension. However, as its use continued to expand, there was no consensus as to which patients should undergo placement of TIPS and the timing for this procedure compared with other medical and surgical therapies. In 1995, a National Institutes of Health–sponsored conference concluded that TIPS was effective in acute control and prevention of recurrent variceal bleeding.[7] Since then, numerous clinical trials have been performed, and new guidelines for the use of TIPS were published by the American Association for the Study of Liver Diseases in 2005.[8] Currently, the main indication for use of TIPS includes treatment and prevention for recurrent variceal bleeding and refractory ascites. However, its use in other selected clinical situations is also indicated.

INDICATIONS

Acute Esophageal Variceal Bleeding

The development of varices is common in portal hypertension, and variceal bleeding is a major cause of morbidity and mortality. Although most respond to pharmacologic or endoscopic interventions, a fraction of patients continue to bleed and will require portal decompression. TIPS has become the shunt procedure of choice because surgically created shunts are associated with a high mortality rate (31% to 71%).[9] In series of patients treated with TIPS after failure of medical therapy, hemostasis was achieved in more than 93% of patients and early rebleeding was seen in less than 13% of patients. Despite the success, there is still a high 6-week mortality rate of more than 35%.[10] This is because urgency of TIPS has been shown to be an independent predictor of mortality.[11] In addition, other preprocedural factors such as Model for End-stage Liver Disease (MELD) score, Acute Physiology, Age, and Chronic Health Evaluation (APACHE) II score, advanced liver disease, sepsis, and organ failure also predicted survival.[12] More recent work has suggested that TIPS be used in selective cases as primary treatment for acute variceal bleeding. In patients with a high portosystemic pressure gradient (>20 mm Hg), early TIPS placement led to less treatment failure and lower mortality rates compared with standard therapy.[13] Finally, although there is a defined role for TIPS in active and recurrent variceal bleeding, its use in primary prevention cannot be advocated. Studies have shown that pharmacologic therapy with β-blockade is considered the best approach to prevent initial bleeding from varices.[9] With its associated risks and complications, TIPS is thus not indicated for primary prophylaxis against variceal bleeding.

Variceal Rebleeding and Prevention

With the first episode of variceal bleeding, a patient is at risk for development of rebleeding. Multiple studies comparing TIPS with endoscopic therapy have demonstrated TIPS to be superior in prevention of rebleeding.[14] However, this benefit does not translate into improved patient survival and is associated with a higher incidence of hepatic encephalopathy.[15] Therefore TIPS should not be used as a first-line therapy to prevent rebleeding. It should be considered as a salvage therapy in situations where recurrent bleeding occurs despite maximal pharmacologic and endoscopic interventions.

Refractory Ascites and Hepatic Hydrothorax

Ascites is a common complication of cirrhosis, and its development carries a significant worsening of the prognosis. Approximately 90% of patients can be treated successfully with dietary sodium restriction and oral diuretics (furosemide and spironolactone). "Refractory ascites" has been defined as ascites that cannot be mobilized or the early recurrence of which cannot be satisfactorily prevented by medical therapy.[16] The first-line treatment for refractory ascites is repeated large-volume paracentesis. TIPS is considered if paracentesis is contraindicated or if the need for paracentesis is too frequent (generally considered as three times per month). Clinical improvement in ascites is seen in almost 75% of patients treated with TIPS.[17] A meta-analysis of 330 patients demonstrated that although TIPS was significantly better than paracentesis for control of refractory ascites (odds ratio = 0.14), it is associated with a higher rate of encephalopathy (odds ratio = 2.26) and had no statistically significant impact on patient survival.[18] Because of the drawbacks of TIPS, its use is therefore recommended only for those patients who are intolerant of repeated paracentesis. Hepatic hydrothorax develops in the setting of ascites if there is a communication between the thoracic and abdominal cavities. In small nonrandomized studies, TIPS has been shown to be effective in the management of symptomatic refractory hepatic hydrothorax with complete resolution or decreasing the frequency of thoracentesis.[19,20]

Budd-Chiari Syndrome

Budd-Chiari syndrome results from hepatic vein thrombosis leading to severe alterations in liver perfusion. Hepatic congestion leads to severe parenchymal injury, and the rationale for TIPS is to create an alternative venous outflow tract for the congested liver. Budd-Chiari can present in an acute fulminant form and a chronic ascitic presentation. Treatment of the acute form is usually with a surgical shunt or liver transplantation. However, there have been reports of successful treatment of the chronic form with TIPS. In a large series of 35 patients, the cumulative 1-year and 5-year survival rates without transplantation were 93% and 74%.[21]

Other Indications

Other potential application of TIPS include its use in hepatorenal syndrome. Small studies have demonstrated improvement in renal function in patients treated with TIPS.[22] In addition, there was a reduced incidence of hepatorenal syndrome in a study comparing TIPS with large-volume paracentesis for refractory ascites.[23] The use of TIPS in several other clinical conditions (hepatic veno-occlusive disease, portal hypertensive gastropathy, hepatopulmonary syndrome) has been described, but it is currently unclear whether there is a benefit, and therefore its use cannot be recommended.

CONTRAINDICATION

The absolute contraindications for a TIPS procedure include several clinical conditions, including congestive heart failure, severe pulmonary hypertension (mean pulmonary pressure >45 mm Hg), severe tricuspid regurgitation, severe liver failure, and presence of chronic recurrent portosystemic encephalopathy. Active systemic sepsis, infection, or severe coagulopathy will delay TIPS creation until the ongoing clinical condition is reversed. Multiple hepatic cysts, liver tumors, portal vein thrombosis, and obstruction of all hepatic veins are considered relative contraindications. Because of lack of supporting evidence, the use of TIPS in the primary prevention of variceal bleeding is also contraindicated.

PREPROCEDURE WORKUP

When a patient is referred, a comprehensive multidisciplinary approach should be undertaken to determine a patient's candidacy for TIPS. The patient should be under the care of a hepatologist (or gastroenterologist), and referral to a liver transplantation center should be considered. If a collective decision is made for the patient to undergo a TIPS procedure, a thorough preprocedure workup is undertaken. A thorough history should be elicited with additional focus on cardiopulmonary status and symptoms of encephalopathy. A physical examination is performed to evaluate for the presence of significant ascites or evidence of right-sided heart failure. Laboratory studies including complete blood cell count, metabolic panel, liver function studies, and coagulation parameters are obtained. A preoperative cardiac evaluation is warranted if there is a history of congestive heart failure, pulmonary hypertension, tricuspid regurgitation, or cardiomyopathy. This may include an echocardiogram or consultation with a cardiologist. Cross-sectional imaging of the liver (duplex ultrasound, computed tomography, or magnetic resonance imaging) should be obtained to evaluate liver anatomy and to document portal vein patency. If there is significant ascites, a pre-TIPS paracentesis should be performed to alleviate upward displacement of the liver. Coagulopathy should be treated with appropriate blood product transfusion before the procedure. A small liver is not a contraindication to TIPS; however, longer procedure time should be expected in these difficult cases.

TECHNIQUE FOR TRANSJUGULAR INTRAHEPATIC PORTOSYSTEMIC SHUNT

Although there are several commercially available catheter stent systems and each has its own proponents, it is our belief that no single system is better than the others. The technique of the TIPS procedure is fairly standard with minor variations depending on the practitioner and institution where the procedure is performed. Before the procedure, prophylactic broad-spectrum antibiotics should be administered and appropriate resuscitation completed. The procedure generally takes between 1 and 3 hours and is done in the angiography suite with use of conscious sedation. However, general anesthesia is used if the procedure is expected to be long or because of patient discomfort. The patient is positioned in the supine position and is prepped and draped in the usual sterile fashion. The internal jugular vein (usually right) is accessed under ultrasonic guidance with use of a micropuncture needle. The left internal jugular can also be used, and, although a femoral approach has been described, this latter technique is much more challenging. A guidewire is inserted, and a catheter is advanced past the right atrium into the inferior vena cava (Figure 73-1). The right hepatic vein is accessed, and wedged hepatic venography is obtained by either injection of contrast media or carbon dioxide. With use of the images as a guide, the cutting needle from the catheter stent system is advanced through the liver parenchyma in an anteroinferior direction to access the right portal vein. The needle is aspirated as it is withdrawn until portal venous blood is returned; correct positioning is confirmed with portal venography by injecting contrast, and a wire is advanced across the tract (Figure 73-2). Pressure measurements are obtained at this time from the portal vein, as well as the right atrium. The pressure difference between these two sites is the portosystemic gradient. Portal hypertension is defined as a pressure gradient greater than 12 mm Hg. If the pressure gradient is present, then the TIPS is placed. This is done by dilating the intrahepatic parenchymal tract with use of 8- to 10-mm balloon catheters, and an expandable metallic stent is deployed (Figure 73-3). Dilation of the

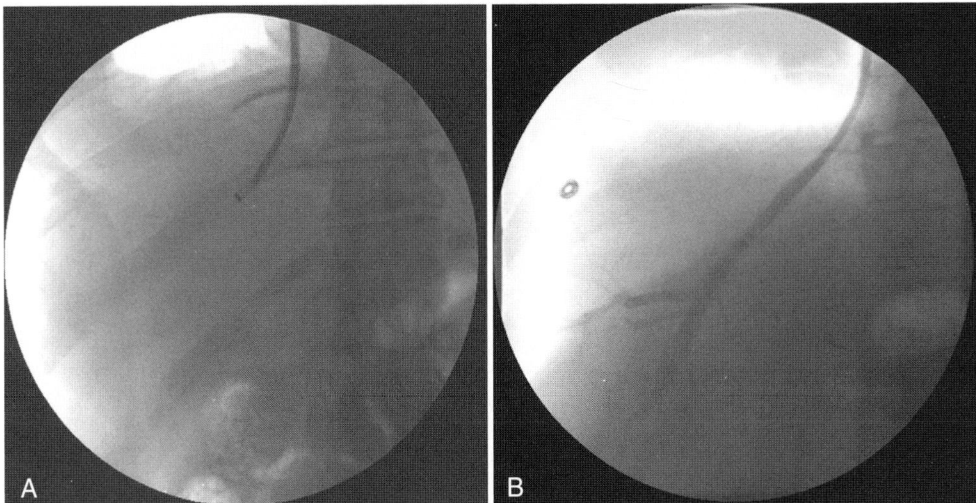

FIGURE 73-1 After cannulation of the right internal jugular vein, a guiding sheath has been positioned in the hepatic venous system **(A)**. An injection of contrast is performed **(B)** to confirm positioning before attempts are made with a Uchida needle to cross from the hepatic venous to portal venous circulation.

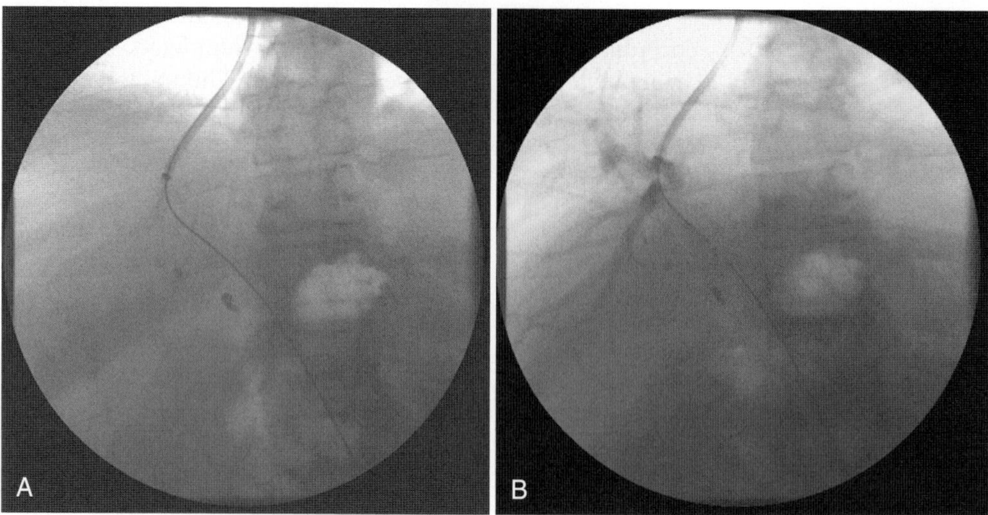

FIGURE 73-2 After successful crossing from the hepatic to portal venous beds, a wire has been positioned that will serve to preserve the tract and act as a guide for both the dilation of the tract and subsequent stent placement **(A).** The sheath allows for injection of contrast material with the wire in place **(B).**

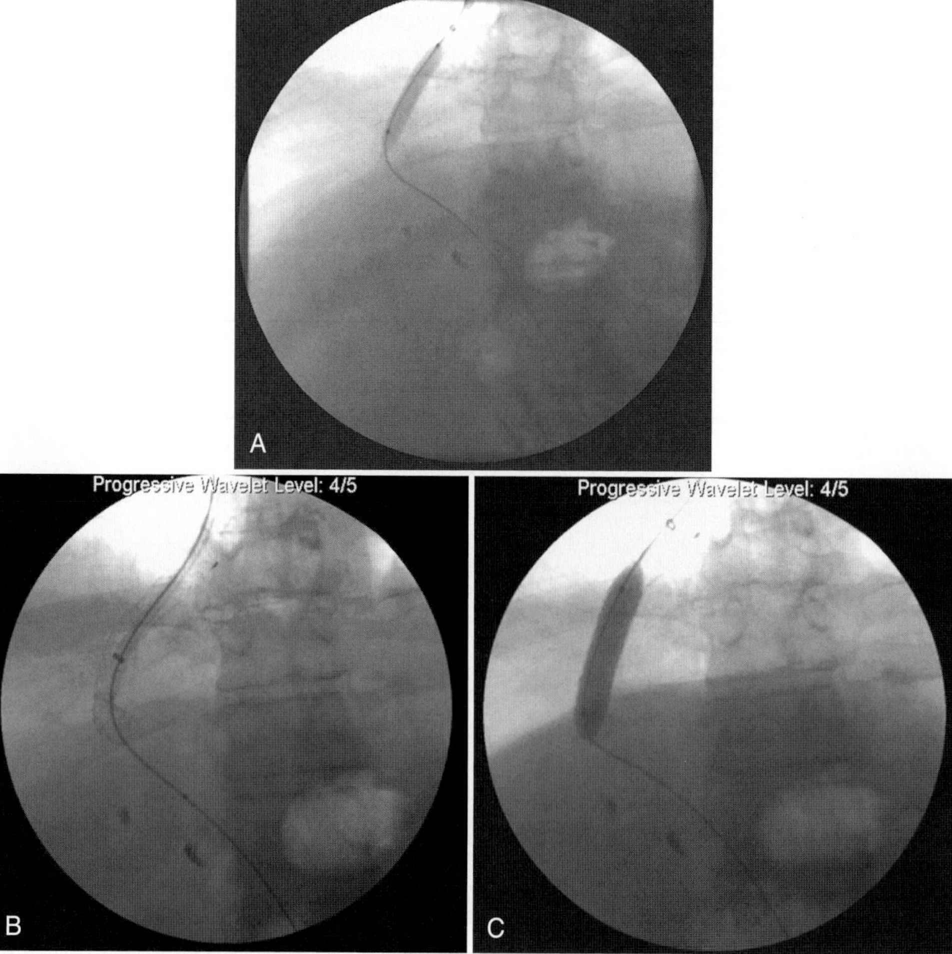

FIGURE 73-3 Initial balloon dilation of the tract is performed **(A),** followed by deployment of a stent **(B)** and postdeployment dilation **(C).** The pressure gradient from the portal to the hepatic sides is measured to help determine the final diameter of the TIPS.

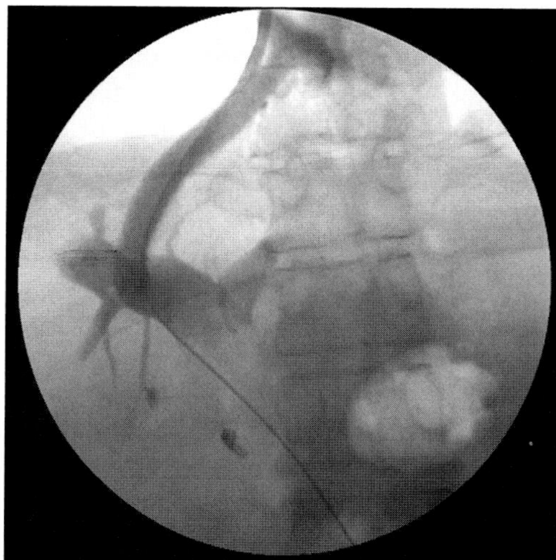

FIGURE 73-4 Completion image of TIPS after contrast injection shows a widely patent channel with flow directed from the portal venous circulation directly into the hepatic veins.

stent is then performed to the desired diameter (usually 10 mm). Poststent venography and pressure measurements again are performed to ensure adequacy of the procedure by documenting a decrease in the portosystemic gradient to less than 12 mm Hg (Figure 73-4). The catheter system is then withdrawn and hemostasis is achieved at the puncture site with manual compression.

POSTPROCEDURE CARE AND FOLLOW-UP

After the procedure, the patient is admitted to the hospital for observation for 1 to 2 days. A duplex ultrasound scan is obtained on the first postprocedure day to document patency of the TIPS. Serum electrolytes and liver function studies are obtained. After discharge, all patients with TIPS should undergo periodic follow-up according to a standard protocol. Routine surveillance ultrasound and laboratory studies should be obtained at least four times per year. Development of fever and bacteremia dictates admission and workup for stent infection. Finally, any recurrence of symptoms of portal hypertension necessitates workup for stent patency.

TRANSJUGULAR INTRAHEPATIC PORTOSYSTEMIC SHUNT STENOSIS/ THROMBOSIS

The major issue with TIPS is stenosis and thrombosis, which lead to return of the complications related to portal hypertension. Early thrombosis (<24 hours) is thought to be related to the thrombogenic potential of bile and is related to puncture of bile ducts during creation of the TIPS. Late stenosis (occurring in months) is caused by the development of a pseudointima and occurs in two patterns. Type 1 (diffuse stenosis) occurs along the entire length of the stent, whereas type 2 (focal narrow) usually occurs at the hepatic vein end of the stent. Although the primary patency rate at 1 year is approximately 40%, reintervention with balloon dilation and placement of additional stents have led to an acceptable secondary patency rate approaching 90%.[24] In addition, the use of covered stents has improved patency rates and decreased symptom recurrence. Recently published data using polytetrafluoroethylene-covered stent grafts for TIPS demonstrated 76% primary patency for the covered stents versus 36% for the bare stents at 2 years (actuarial data). Rates of encephalopathy were reduced as well.[25] Many institutions now routinely use covered stents for TIPS. Although duplex ultrasound can document patency of the TIPS, its use to establish degree of stenosis is limited. Velocity measurements may suggest flow limitation, but the degree of stenosis can only be determined with venography or pressure measurements. Thus, although duplex ultrasonography remains the noninvasive method to monitor shunt patency, some have advocated at least annual venography to evaluate for shunt stenosis and allow for secondary intervention.

COMPLICATIONS

Overall, the success rate for TIPS is high, and there is a low rate of morbidity and mortality. It has been reported that the direct procedure-related mortality ranges from 0% to 2% and the 30-day mortality rate ranges from 7% to 45%.[26-28] In addition to TIPS thrombosis, complications that arise can be divided into three categories: (1) those complications that arise directly from the technical aspects of the procedure, (2) those from creation of a portosystemic shunt, and finally (3) those that are specifically related to TIPS.

Complications From Technical Aspects of Procedure

Similar to other percutaneous procedures, puncture site morbidity and cardiac arrhythmia can occur. These can be reduced by cannulating the internal jugular vein with use of ultrasonic guidance and correcting electrolyte imbalances before the procedure. Although the reported incidence of liver capsule puncture is high (33%), the development of significant hemoperitoneum remains low.[26] This complication typically occurs in patients with a small, hard liver that is displaced superiorly by tense ascites or in those with a thrombosed portal vein. In the former situation, the procedure can be facilitated with a pre-TIPS paracentesis to smooth out the angle between the hepatic and portal veins. In the latter case, a preprocedure ultrasound scan should also be performed to document portal vein patency. Inadvertent creation of a fistula to the hepatic artery or biliary tree can also lead to various clinical consequences. A rare, but often fatal, complication is extrahepatic puncture of the portal vein resulting in exsanguinating hemorrhage. This is prevented by only using the branches for the portal vein for the placement of the stent. Extensive thrombosis of the TIPS, portal vein, and splenic vein has been reported in 10% of patients. Treatment include thrombolysis, suction thrombectomy, anticoagulation, or urgent liver transplantation.

Complications From Creation of Portosystemic Shunt

The primary complication is the development of portosystemic encephalopathy in 30% of patients after TIPS.[14,29] This rate is similar to that with surgically created shunts, and most can be treated medically. Post-TIPS encephalopathy usually develops 2 to 3 weeks after TIPS. Its treatment is similar to that of encephalopathy in other settings: reversing precipitating factors if present, minimizing dietary proteins, and medical therapy (e.g., lactulose, neomycin). For TIPS-related encephalopathy, occlusion of the shunt can resolve the encephalopathy but also reverse the therapeutic benefit of the TIPS.

Complications Specifically Related to TIPS

TIPS-related hemolytic anemia occurs in about 10% of patients.[30] The presenting sign of hyperbilirubinemia begins about 7 to 14 days after the TIPS procedure, and the hemolysis is thought to be caused by shear stress and trauma to red cells by the stent. Most cases are self-limited, but blood transfusions may be necessary. This process typically resolves spontaneously within 8 to 12 weeks. Severe hyperbilirubinemia without hemolysis can also occur in 5% of patients.[31] Although the cause of this condition is unknown, the development of this complication is associated with a markedly worse prognosis. Vegetative infection of the stent is rare but has been reported.[32] This will lead to bacteremia, fevers, and often occlusion of the stent with thrombus. TIPS infection can usually be treated with intravenous antibiotics.

CONCLUSION

Since its introduction approximately 20 years ago, TIPS is now a commonly used procedure to treat different processes related to portal hypertension. Although the shortcomings of poor primary patency and need for continued monitoring and repeated intervention exist, numerous studies have demonstrated the benefits of the TIPS procedure. With advances in stent technology, and continued investigation into portal hypertensive physiology, TIPS will likely have an even greater clinical applicability in the future.

References

1. Rosch J, Hanafee W, Snow H, et al: Transjugular intrahepatic portocaval shunt, *Am J Surg* 121:588, 1971.
2. Colapinto RF, Stronell RD, Gildiner M, et al: Formation of intrahepatic portosystemic shunts using a balloon dilatation catheter: preliminary clinical experience, *AJR Am J Roentgenol* 140:709, 1983.
3. Palmaz JC, Sibbitt RR, Reuter SR, et al: Expandable intrahepatic portacaval shunt stents: early experience in the dog, *AJR Am J Roentgenol* 145:821, 1985.
4. Rossle M, Richter GM, Noldge G, et al: Performance of an intrahepatic portacaval shunt (PCS) using a catheter technique: a case report, *Hepatology* 8:1348A, 1988.
5. Haskak ZJ, Martin L, Cardella JF, et al: Quality improvement guidelines for transjugular intrahepatic portosystemic shunts. SCVIR Standards of Practice Committee, *J Vasc Interv Radiol* 12:131, 2001.
6. Haskak ZJ, Martin L, Cardella JF, et al: Quality improvement guidelines for transjugular intrahepatic portosystemic shunts, *J Vasc Interv Radiol* 14:S231, 2003.
7. Shiffman ML, Jeffers L, Hoofnagle JH, et al: Role of transjugular intrahepatic portosystemic shunt treatment of portal hypertension and its complication: conference sponsored by the National Digestive Diseases Advisory Board, *Hepatology* 22:1591, 1995.
8. Boyer TD, Haskal ZJ: AASLD guideline: the role of transjugular intrahepatic portosystemic shunt in the management of portal hypertension, *Hepatology* 41:386, 2005.
9. D'Amico G, Pagliaro L, Bosch J: The treatment of portal hypertension: a meta-analytic review, *Hepatology* 22:332, 1995.
10. Vangeli M, Patch D, Burroughs AK: Salvage tips for uncontrolled variceal bleeding, *J Hepatol* 37:703, 2002.
11. Chalasani N, Clark WS, Martin LG, et al: Determinants of mortality in patients with advanced cirrhosis after transjugular intrahepatic portosystemic shunting, *Gastroenterology* 118:138, 2000.
12. Patch D, Nikolopoulou V, McCormick A, et al: Factors related to early mortality after transjugular intrahepatic portosystemic shunt for failed endoscopic therapy in acute variceal bleeding, *J Hepatol* 28:454, 1998.
13. Monescillo A, Martinez-Lagares F, Ruiz-del-Arbol L, et al: Influence of portal hypertension and its early decompression by TIPS placement on the outcome of variceal bleeding, *Hepatology* 40:793, 2004.
14. Mihas AA, Sanyal AJ: Recurrent variceal bleeding despite endoscopic and medical therapy, *Gastroenterology* 127:621, 2004.
15. Papatheodoridis GV, Goulis J, Leandro G, et al: Transjugular intrahepatic portosystemic shunt compared with endoscopic treatment for prevention of variceal rebleeding: a meta-analysis, *Hepatology* 30:612, 1999.
16. Arroyo V, Gines P, Gerbes AL, et al: Definition and diagnostic criteria of refractory ascites and hepatorenal syndromes in cirrhosis. International Ascites Club, *Hepatology* 23:164, 1996.
17. Somberg KA, Lake JR, Tomlanovich SJ, et al: Transjugular intrahepatic portosystemic shunts for refractory ascites: assessment of clinical and hormonal response and renal function, *Hepatology* 21:709, 1995.

18. D'Amico G, Luca A, Morabito A, et al: Uncovered transjugular intrahepatic portosystemic shunt for refractory ascites: a meta-analysis, *Gastroenterology* 129:1282, 2005.
19. Gordon FD, Anastopoulos HT, Crenshaw W, et al: The successful treatment of symptomatic, refractory hepatic hydrothorax with transjugular intrahepatic portosystemic shunt, *Hepatology* 25: 1366, 1997.
20. Siegerstetter V, Deibert P, Ochs A, et al: Treatment of refractory hepatic hydrothorax with transjugular intrahepatic portosystemic shunt: long-term results in 40 patients, *Eur J Gastroenterol Hepatol* 13:559, 2001.
21. Rossle M, Olschewski M, Siegerstetter V, et al: The Budd-Chiari syndrome: technical, hemodynamic, and clinical results of treatment with transjugular intrahepatic portosystemic shunt, *Surgery* 135:394, 2004.
22. Brensing KA, Textor J, Perz J, et al: Long term outcome after transjugular intrahepatic portosystemic shunt-stent in non-transplant cirrhotics with hepatorenal syndrome: a phase II study, *Gut* 47:288, 2000.
23. Sanyal A, Genning G, Reddy KR, et al: the NASTRA group: The North American Study for the Treatment of Refractory Ascites, *Gastroenterology* 124:634, 2003.
24. Saxon RS, Ross PL, Mendel-Hartvig J, et al: Transjugular intrahepatic portosystemic shunt patency and the importance of stenosis location in the development of recurrent symptoms, *Radiology* 207:683, 1998.
25. Bureau C, Pagan JC, Layrargues GP, et al: Patency of stents covered with polytetrafluoroethylene in patients treated by transjugular intrahepatic portosystemic shunts: long-term results of a randomized multicentre study, *Liver Int* 27(6): 742–747, 2007.
26. Freedman AM, Sanyal AJ, Tisnado J, et al: Complications of transjugular intrahepatic porto-systemic shunt (TIPS): a comprehensive review, *Radiographics* 13:1185, 1993.
27. LaBerge JM, Ring EJ, Gordon RL, et al: Creation of transjugular intrahepatic portosystemic shunts with the Wallstent endoprosthesis: results in 100 patients, *Radiology* 187:413, 1993.
28. Rossle M, Haag K, Ochs A, et al: The transjugular intrahepatic portosystemic stent-shunt procedure for variceal bleeding, *N Engl J Med* 330:165, 1994.
29. Riggio O, Merlli M, Pedretti G, et al: Hepatic encephalopathy after transjugular intrahepatic portosystemic shunt: incidence and risk factors, *Dig Dis Sci* 41:578, 1996.
30. Sanyal AJ, Freedman AM, Prudum PP, et al: The hematologic consequences of transjugular intrahepatic portosystemic shunts, *Hepatology* 23:32, 1996.
31. Rouillard SS, Bass NM, Roberts JP, et al: Severe hyperbilirubinemia after creation of transjugular intrahepatic portosystemic shunts: natural history and predictors of outcome, *Ann Intern Med* 128:374, 1998.
32. Sanyal AJ, Reddy KR: Vegetative infection of transjugular intrahepatic portosystemic shunts, *Gastroenterology* 115:110, 1998.

CHAPTER

74

Anesthetic Management for Endovascular Procedures

Kenneth Kuchta, Jordan D. Miller

The anesthesiology community has followed the development of endovascular surgery contributing to the research, as well as publishing periodic reviews of the implications for anesthesiologists. An early review article noted somewhat tepidly that the main advantage is that it is less invasive. The authors elaborate in that the technique allowed less anesthesia, an insignificant aortic occlusion time, less hemodynamic and metabolic stress, earlier ambulation and shorter hospital stays, and possibly less cost.[1] The most recent chapter in the American textbook *Miller's Anesthesia* is more exuberant, calling it "one of the most exciting developments in the treatment of peripheral vascular disease and has the potential to revolutionize current treatment modalities for aortic aneurysm, aortic dissection, and traumatic aortic injury."[2]

Very early on, anesthesiologists noted the remarkable stability offered by not clamping and unclamping the aorta. These observations have been borne out in published works along with the demonstration of a decreased stress response.[3-6] The most recent American College of Cardiology/American Heart Association (ACC/AHA) guidelines for perioperative cardiac risk classify endovascular procedures as intermediate risk versus the high risk of open repair of the aorta.[7] Nonetheless, there remains the concern about the possibility of conversion to open repair in essentially the same cohort of patients having significant cardiac, pulmonary, and other medical comorbidities now being managed in a high-risk procedure with increased severity because of the emergency setting.

Concerns with perioperative renal failure resulting from aortic clamping (even infrarenal) and hemodynamic instability have been supplanted by concerns with contrast-induced renal insufficiency. The less-invasive nature of the procedure has opened the opportunity to administer the anesthetic as a regional or even monitored anesthesia care (local with or without supplemental sedation) with the appropriate selection of cases for each anesthetic still being worked out. The less-invasive nature has also led to consideration of this technique for patients considered too high a risk for open procedures. Finally, the extension of this technique to the thoracic aorta, though the pathology is less prevalent, appears to offer even more dramatic advantages to the patient versus open repair because of the avoidance of a thoracotomy, high aortic clamp, and partial bypass. This has opened a number of additional concerns with the management of cord perfusion, as well as monitoring of cord function.

HEMODYNAMICS

Open repair of abdominal aneurysms has traditionally been challenging in anesthetics, primarily because of the requisite cross-clamping and unclamping of the aorta with consequent complex physiologic changes. Additionally, the need for transabdominal or even retroperitoneal incisions in patients who frequently have concomitant cardiac and/or pulmonary disease has added to the risks of these procedures. For open repair of the thoracic aorta, with the addition of thoracotomy, high aortic clamp and occasionally partial bypass further increase the anesthetic complexity. From even the early articles proposing endovascular repair, the less-invasive nature of the procedure was thought to offer significant benefit to the patient. Experience has demonstrated that the profound hemodynamic changes associated with aortic clamping are not reproduced in endovascular procedures. Several studies have borne out these observations indicating more stable hemodynamics (in association with aortic occlusion and reperfusion, as well as in an analysis of overall hemodynamic stability throughout the case) and evidence of less myocardial ischemia with endovascular repairs.[4,5,8,9] Of note, although open repairs seemed to have the most significant changes associated with aortic occlusion and reperfusion, in endovascular cases, changes occur with femoral artery clamping (not aortic occlusion) and subsequent limb reperfusion; nonetheless these changes were significantly less than seen with open procedures.[4] Undoubtedly these advantages are ultimately responsible for the classification of endovascular aortic repairs as intermediate-risk procedures versus the continued high-risk classification of open repairs in the most current ACC/AHA guidelines.[7]

CARDIAC

The most concerning perioperative morbidity and mortality among vascular patients are cardiac complications. With several centers reporting in the 1970s and 1980s approximately half of postoperative deaths after vascular surgery attributed to acute myocardial infarctions (MIs), interest in this area, in both screening and prevention, has continued in earnest since. Angiography data from the Cleveland Clinic at that time demonstrated significant coronary disease in 60% of vascular patients. Among those without symptoms, the rate was still 37%. Screening and preoperative intervention (coronary artery bypass grafting and subsequently percutaneous transluminal coronary angioplasty) were advocated on the basis of evidence of a protective effect during the subsequent vascular surgery with regard to cardiac complications. This was tempered with concerns about the perioperative/periprocedure morbidity and mortality of the cardiac intervention.[10] This debate has continued to the present. A very large Veterans Affairs study showed no difference in outcome in vascular patients with significant coronary disease if they were randomly assigned to revascularization (via coronary artery bypass grafting or percutaneous transluminal coronary angioplasty) versus merely proceeding with the proposed vascular surgery.[11] In this study patients with the most severe cardiac disease were excluded from the randomization, and one could argue that this is not an indication to forgo testing per se but that further cardiac intervention may not be beneficial. Nonetheless, detailed knowledge of the preoperative cardiac state of patients may significantly influence the perioperative management of the patient. Those with severe cardiac disease may be appropriately identified and treated before vascular surgery whereas those with less-severe disease may still receive perioperative care tailored to their degree of cardiac disease as the available therapeutic options are rapidly expanding.

Much of the early understanding of the pathophysiology of coronary artery disease was based on managing myocardial supply and demand. Thus coronary revascularization or percutaneous transluminal coronary angioplasty along with maintaining an adequate blood pressure and heart rate would improve supply. Hypertension and tachycardia were avoided to decrease demand. Invasive monitoring was seen as a way to fine-tune the hemodynamics. In fact early improvements in morbidity (at least in reinfarction rates) were attributed to newer drugs, as well as more invasive monitoring, that were becoming available at that time.[12]

Our current understanding of perioperative cardiac events is much more complex. An inflammatory and hypercoagulable state, hypoxia, and stress all probably play a role. It is important to note that stress itself seems to have a role beyond effects on heart rate and blood pressure and may involve stress and plaque rupture in the coronaries, increased free fatty acids, as well as other factors.[13] In fact, one study found that a majority of perioperative events were not associated with high-grade stenosis, suggesting that plaque rupture and acute thrombosis (not high-grade stenosis) may be more relevant in this setting.[14] Although the exact pathophysiology remains to be determined, this does open the opportunity for a number of other preventive measures beyond revascularization and tight hemodynamic control. This has led to several attempts to pharmacologically modify the perioperative responses to surgery and anesthesia to provide protection from adverse cardiac events.

Although the coronary vasodilator nitroglycerin would be an accepted treatment of perioperative ischemia, its prophylactic use has not been demonstrated to be efficacious.[15,16] Calcium channel blockers also appear to be attractive as coronary dilators, but a meta-analysis indicated significant reduction in ischemia but failed to showed a significant effect on MI or death unless the end points were combined.[17] This analysis has also been criticized for having very few events. Alpha$_2$-adrenergic agonists reduce the release of catecholamines, whereas statins may have beneficial effects beyond lowering cholesterol, but the evidence for each of these drugs with regard to beneficial effect in the perioperative period, although promising, probably needs further confirmation in large, well-designed studies. Aspirin via its antiplatelet effect has also been examined with conflicting results, as well as an increased risk for bleeding.[18]

Much of the modern discussion of the prevention of perioperative myocardial events has centered on the use of β-blockers. Two randomized controlled studies have largely driven this interest. In one, very-high-risk patients (having stress tests positive for ischemia) showed a decrease in MIs.[19] A second study in patients at risk for cardiac events demonstrated improved survival, but this difference started at 6 months after surgery.[20] Critiques of the studies have raised a number of concerns, and two subsequent studies failed to confirm the benefits of perioperative β-blockers. Of additional concern are two large studies; the first, a review of a large database (329 hospitals, 782,969 patients), indicated benefit for high-risk patients but no benefit and possible harm among low-risk patients.[21] A more recent large (8351 patients) randomized controlled study (the POISE trial) demonstrated a cardiac benefit from metoprolol (fewer cardiac deaths, nonfatal MIs, or cardiac arrests). There was, however, an increased incidence of death and stroke in the β-blocked group. Death of sepsis was also significantly higher in the metoprolol group. Of note, there was a significant increase in clinically significant hypotension and bradycardia among the metoprolol group.[22]

The 2007 ACC/AHA guidelines[7] attempt to provide some guidance in this matter especially when compared with those published in 2002. The guidelines continue their prior strategy of considering both the medical condition of the patient and the risk of the proposed surgical procedure to determine the cardiac recommendations. Of note, they consider endovascular procedures (and carotid endarterectomy) as intermediate-risk procedures versus major vascular procedures, which remain the "highest-risk procedures." They review the state of knowledge with respect to perioperative β-blocker therapy, noting recent studies failing to demonstrate efficacy in contrast to earlier positive trials. Thus the evidence seems to suggest benefit in high-risk patients or those with known coronary artery disease. Class I recommendation (that the therapy should be instituted barring contraindications) was thus limited to the patients with stress tests positive for ischemia and those already receiving β-blockers. The latter recommendation has been known for decades after early studies in which β-blockers were withdrawn with detrimental results. Other recommendations for vascular patients were less clear-cut. It is not uncommon for the typical patient having nonemergent vascular surgery to end up with the ACC/AHA recommendation to consider noninvasive testing "if it will change management." The guidelines apparently interpret changes in therapy to include a change in the planned surgery, the medical therapy, or the perioperative monitoring or delaying the surgery for further cardiac workup.[7] To this the authors would add changes in anesthetic management that go beyond the degree of monitoring. The anesthetic drugs used, the target hemodynamics, as well as the tradeoffs versus other medical conditions, may all be influenced by the specifics of the patient's cardiac disease. The guidelines seem to point to this with a rather lengthy description of goal of the consultation and need for communication among all the members of the preoperative team.[7] The need for effective communication is heightened with both the trend to offer this less-invasive alternative to the patient thought to be at too high a risk for open surgery and the constantly changing evidence with regard to the optimal perioperative cardiac management. (It should be noted that the 2007 ACC/AHA guidelines[7] predate the large POISE trial,[22] and it is unclear whether the guidelines will be modified on the basis of this trial's results, especially with respect to instituting perioperative β-blockers.) The relative chance for conversion to an open procedure with the increased risk involved (including the emergency nature of this conversion) further emphasizes the need for effective communication.

THORACIC

Surgical repair of the thoracic aorta has traditionally been a very demanding anesthetic case often involving thoracotomy with one-lung ventilation and high aortic cross-clamp usually in the typical vascular patient with cardiac, pulmonary, and other comorbidities. An additional concern with spinal cord ischemia may have further impact ranging from partial bypass (often with concomitant heparinization) to spinal cord drainage. If spinal cord monitoring were used, especially motor evoked potentials, this would usually dictate a major change in the anesthetic technique to minimize interference with this mode of monitoring.

Luckily, endovascular repair has eliminated the need for thoracotomy and high aortic cross-clamp. Although not extensively studied, the balloon aortic occlusion with the newer balloons that does not completely obliterate the lumen appears to have minimal effect on hemodynamics probably because of the short duration of inflation. All of this assumes that the case is not converted to an open procedure.

Barring an emergency conversion, by far the most troubling issue is the possibility of spinal cord ischemia. The anesthesia team is often closely involved with measures to minimize this complication. The team may be involved with placement of a lumbar drain either prophylactically or as part of the treatment. Because the patient could be taking antiplatelet therapy or require anticoagulation as part of the procedure, the concern with creating an epidural hematoma will of course be present. Although the guidelines for needle placement in the face of anticoagulation/antiplatelet therapy are evolving and not always straightforward, the anesthesiologist will probably rely heavily on the consensus statement for neuraxial anesthesia in the anticoagulated patient (the latest edition being available under consensus statements on the website of the American Society of Regional Anesthesia and Pain Medicine [http://www.asra.com]). For placement in an emergent situation (paraplegia after surgery in the absence of a preoperative lumbar drain) prior discussion among the teams involved would obviously be ideal. Likewise, the intraoperative goals for hemodynamics (especially mean blood pressure) and cerebrospinal fluid pressure should be delineated.

If spinal cord monitoring is to be used, the impact on the anesthetic choices should be realized by all teams involved. Motor evoked potentials are perhaps the most severe example, because they are the most influenced by anesthetics. The reader is referred to a review article on anesthetics and motor evoked potentials.[23] Even a cursory reading of this article leaves one with the impression that all anesthetics have some potential to interfere with motor evoked potential monitoring. A typical approach might include low-dose propofol 25 to 200 mcg/kg/min and remifentanil 0.125 to 0.375 mcg/kg/min.[24] It is not uncommon to avoid or minimize potent inhalation agents while the electrophysiologist monitoring the patient will often request discontinuation of muscle relaxants (after intubation). This is despite reported successful use of inhalation agents and even neuromuscular blockers while monitoring motor evoked potentials.[25-27] The goal of providing anesthesia while providing conditions of the reliable monitoring of the spinal cord is clearly a challenge often competing with the other objective of anesthesia (a motionless patient, with no recall of the procedure). Overall, a close collaboration among all the teams is essential with communication starting as early before surgery as possible.

RENAL

Perioperative renal dysfunction has long been a concern in open repairs of the aorta. This appears to be related to changes in renal hemodynamics with aortic clamping (decreased renal blood flow even with an infrarenal clamp, as well as redistribution of intrinsic perfusion to the renal cortex), hemodynamic instability, volume depletion, embolization of atheromatous material to the kidneys, and surgical trauma. Although a number of prophylactic techniques have been used including dopamine, loop diuretics, and mannitol, the maintenance of intravascular volume appears to be the most accepted practice to preserve renal function. With the elimination of the need for surgical clamping of the aorta with endovascular repair, the concerns regarding renal compromise from this etiology have been replaced with the specter of contrast-induced nephropathy (CIN).

With the increase in procedures using intravenous (IV) contrast, CIN ranks as the third leading cause of hospital-acquired renal failure. Its incidence ranges from 3.3% in those without preexisting renal disease to 26% for those with risk factors. Although it has been described as usually nonoliguric and transient with creatinine peaking at day 3 after contrast exposure, some patients require dialysis and have more significant morbidity and mortality. Risk factors include preexisting renal disease, diabetes, advanced age, congestive heart failure, the concomitant use of nephrotoxic agents, and intravascular volume depletion. The volume and type of contrast used are additional factors. Given the complex nature of renal physiology, it is not surprising that the pathophysiology of CIN is not completely understood. Changes in vasoconstriction, changes in renal hemodynamics, direct toxicity, and the generation of oxygen free radicals are among the most prominent causes postulated for CIN. Several prophylactic drugs have been suggested for the prevention of CIN including diuretics, mannitol, dopamine, fenoldopam, calcium channel blockers, and aminophylline with equivocal to negative benefits being demonstrated. The antioxidant/ renal vasodilator *N*-acetylcysteine has been studied with conflicting results.[28] Although a meta-analysis seems to suggest an overall benefit, a very small trial specifically in endovascular aortic repairs failed to show a benefit.[29]

Much of the interest has seemed to return to the mainstay of prophylactic therapy, hydration and clarification of the specific types of fluid that may be most beneficial. Normal saline solution may offer the best advantage. A small, randomized trial of Na bicarbonate produced favorable results and has spurred active interest in this area.[30] One large retrospective review, however, has cast some caution, finding detrimental renal effects with bicarbonate therapy.[31]

RESPIRATORY FUNCTION INCLUDING OBSTRUCTIVE SLEEP APNEA

A significant number of patients are at risk of complications in the immediate postoperative period because of obstructive sleep apnea (OSA).[32] OSA is the absence of air movement or a greater than 50% reduction in air movement for at least 10 seconds with a drop in oxygen saturation of greater than 4%. The more frequent the episodes the more severe the OSA. Severe OSA is more than 30 episodes per hour and moderate if more than 15 per hour. During the apnea the unsedated patient arouses and restores upper airway tone and resumes breathing. However, deep sleep is interfered with and the patient commonly has daytime somnolence. Repeated episodes of arousal lead to hypertension and may be responsible for middle-of-the-night acute MIs. The incidence of clinically significant OSA is 4% in men and 2% in women. This is probably a low estimate in the population needing endovascular therapy because it increases with age and obesity, both common in this group of patients. Those patients who come with a diagnosis and are receiving continuous positive airway pressure therapy should continue to use the device in the hospital. Changes in the settings, however, may be needed if the patient has a need for opiates or sedatives. Those patients who are suspected of having OSA on the basis of history of severe snoring, daytime somnolence, apnea episodes during sleep, and physical characteristics should be either studied in a sleep laboratory or assumed to have moderate sleep apnea. Continuous monitoring of pulse oximetry is warranted in the postoperative period until the patient's usual sleep pattern returns.

Pain medications suppress arousal and may lead to life-threatening apnea episodes. Typically, there is a decrease in rapid eye movement and deep non–rapid eye movement sleep after surgery followed by a rebound for several more days. These changes in sleep will increase the episodes of apnea and potentially can cause increased catecholamine release with an increased risk of arrhythmia, acute MI, hypertension, and negative-pressure pulmonary edema. The severity of the changes will be related to the amount, type, and duration of sedation given during and immediately after surgery.

The choice of anesthetic should be based on the usual criteria, but deep sedation to tolerate local or regional anesthesia is more likely to end with an obstructed airway, sudden arousal and movement, and unplanned general anesthesia. If emergent intubation is required, it may be difficult.

PRIOR ANESTHETICS

Frequently patients have had prior procedures. The records from those procedures if available will help in planning the anesthetic management. Difficulties encountered and possible causes are usually only available by reviewing the records themselves rather than summaries or surgical notes. Thus, if possible and time allows, these records should be obtained. The most useful information that these records provide are, for example, responses to sedatives, induction agents, ease of airway management, problems with intubation, and paradoxical effects of drugs.

ALLERGIES (PARTICULARLY CONTRAST-INDUCED)

Those patients who require contrast dye IV for their procedures who have a high likelihood for allergic reactions and those who are at risk because of previous reactions should receive the contrast agents with the lowest risk for allergic reaction. If the offending contrast agent that caused a reaction is known, it should be avoided. Nonionic agents have about one-tenth the risk for reaction as do ionic agents, though severe and life-threatening reactions do occur. The incidence of severe reactions is so low in the average patient that no attempt to decrease reactions is warranted. Overall risk may actually increase because agents used for prophylaxis carry their own risks. However, the use of prophylaxis in patients who are at high risk is more controversial. Those patients at increased risk of reaction are those with prior reaction to contrast agents, those with asthma, those with other drug allergies, and possibly those taking β-blockers. If prophylaxis is to be given then steroids are generally used. Steroids take hours to work; thus most tested regimens give two doses 1 day apart. Antihistamines do work for mild symptoms and possibly increase the efficacy of steroids; H_1 blockers are definitely used with possible improved efficacy if an H_2 blocker is also given. The time to peak effect and whether multiple doses need to be given are not clear. The most popular H_1 blocker, diphenhydramine (Benadryl), causes sedation and may cause a central anticholinergic reaction with excitement so does carry risks. Because no prophylactic regimen is fully protective, resuscitation measures must be available.[33] One must have a high index of suspicion for anaphylaxis to identify the reaction early to prevent serious complications. Because anaphylaxis may be biphasic in 20%, the length of time for observation must include the risk for recurrence.[34] However, most patients will not be discharged after endovascular procedures for the recommended 24 hours of observation.

PREOPERATIVE MEDICATIONS

Most anesthesiologists will suggest continuing all medications, though there are a few exceptions. Thus the patient is instructed to take all morning medications early on the morning of surgery with a sip of water. Those medications that have been controversial include the following.

- *β-Blocker therapy (see earlier discussion):* Maintaining patients with their routine β-blocker therapy is considered standard of care because acute β-blocker withdrawal can lead to overshoot of blood pressure and heart rate, and this is augmented by the stresses of the perioperative period.[35] Thus ACC/AHA concluded that patients already taking β-blockers should continue therapy through the perioperative period. Starting β-blocker therapy just for the surgery is controversial.[7,36]

- *Clonidine:* If patients are taking this drug before surgery, they should have it continued. Withdrawal symptoms occur frequently and may be difficult to treat.[37] Because some patients will be taking nothing by mouth (NPO) after surgery, switching such patients to Catapres-TTS before surgery may be warranted, but it takes 2 to 3 days to reach full replacement levels.
- *Angiotensin-converting enzyme inhibitors and angiotensin II receptor blockers:* Use of these medications, in particular if the patient is receiving diuretic therapy, increases the risk for hypotension during anesthesia.[38] Discontinuing the medication the morning of surgery may reduce the risk for hypotension,[39] but some patients will still have severe hypertension. Our suggestion is to continue these drugs unless the main concern is intraoperative hypotension.
- *Insulin, hypoglycemic agents:* These should be stopped when the patient is NPO.[40] Continue home glucose monitoring and respond to hypoglycemia and hyperglycemia as usual, taking into account NPO status. Tight glucose control may carry risks[41] for hypoglycemia and even poorer outcome. IV insulin may be preferable to subcutaneous insulin in the perioperative period because subcutaneous blood flow varies greatly during and immediately after surgery and anesthesia.
- *Metformin:* Stop before and do not give for 48 hours *after surgery.* Before restarting metformin renal function must be documented to have returned to baseline.[42]
- *Anticoagulants:* The use and whether to continue after surgery are at the discretion of the surgeon. From an anesthetic point of view, the guidelines of the American Society of Regional Anesthesia and Pain Medicine are used to determine the use of regional anesthesia (and placement of spinal drainage catheters) and its timing in patients receiving various anticoagulants (per the website at http://www.asra.com/consensus-statements/2.html).[43] In summary, some of the more commonly used drugs are as follows:
  - Nonsteroidal including aspirin low dose is OK for neuraxial block.
  - Antiplatelet agents: Clopidogrel (Plavix) or ticlopidine (Ticlid) precludes use of neuraxial block for 7 and 14 days, respectively.
  - Low-molecular-weight heparin: Enoxaparin (Lovenox) precludes use of neuraxial block for 1 day.
  - Warfarin (Coumadin) precludes use of neuraxial block until international normalized ratio is $\leq$1.3.
  - Heparin precludes use of neuraxial block until normal partial thromboplastin time and other test results.[43]

ANESTHETIC OPTIONS

Despite several studies showing the feasibility of endovascular procedures with the patient under regional or local anesthesia, a majority appear to be performed with the patient under general anesthesia.[44] Some investigators have suggested an advantage for regional or general anesthesia. Analyzing the large EUROSTAR database, Ruppert et al.[44] found benefit in cases not done with the patient under general anesthesia ranging from fewer intensive care unit admissions to shorter hospital stays and fewer systemic complications. When looking at the subset of higher-risk patients, defined as American Society of Anesthesiologists III and IV, a particular advantage was seen for cases not performed with use of general anesthesia including morbidity and mortality.[45] This analysis, however, suffers from its lack of randomization; in particular, the local anesthesia group was a very small segment of the study population coming from high-volume practices with one half coming from one center. Fewer additional procedures in the local anesthesia suggest simpler surgical problems with the inherent bias obvious. The conclusion could equally be that patients with more straightforward surgical problems did better especially when surgery was done in a particular high-volume center that does many of its cases with the patient under regional anesthesia.

In addition to these concerns, centers considering performing major endovascular procedures with the patient under predominantly local anesthesia should consider the attention to detail for administering the anesthesia and the modification of the surgical technique as described by Verhoeven et al.[46] that was tailored to maximize patient comfort and minimize the chance of patient movement during dissection, surgical manipulation, and limb ischemia.

Still practices that explore alternatives to general anesthesia offer opportunities for innovative ways to manage issues related to an awake patient. One such area is the common complaint of patients under local anesthesia with sedation, the discomfort of the urinary catheter used for bladder drainage. In many patients as the sedation is increased, they become restless, and when questioned it is not the radiologic procedure but the urinary drainage catheter that makes them feel as if they need to void. Multiple attempts to reduce the discomfort have been made. The use of lidocaine or other local anesthetics has been tried with variable success. More recently, tolterodine and oxybutynin have been given as prophylaxis for catheter-related discomfort. Although both have been shown to be partially effective they were used in patients who would continue to remain catheterized.[47] Patients with difficulty urinating might well have significant worsening of symptoms. Gabapentin has also been used prophylactically[48] and seems to work. Those institutions that do a large number of cases with the patients under local anesthesia seem to use urinary catheters less frequently.[46]

MENTAL FUNCTION

It has long been suspected that anesthesia and surgery cause cognitive changes. Whether these are related to anxiety, physical and emotional stress, or other factors is not clear. Recent studies using better controls and more sophisticated testing procedures continue. Postoperative delirium and postoperative cognitive dysfunction/decline (POCD) are the terms used to describe these problems. When studies are designed to look for these, both delirium (11%-43%) and POCD (15%-25%) are relatively common.[49] Delirium is unpleasant for the patient, family, and the medical staff, and it increases morbidity because patients may pull out IV lines or monitoring lines, cause injury, or prevent necessary procedures. There is a correlation with short-term and long-term mortality. Patients for endovascular surgery are at an increased risk because risk factors are age, severity of the surgery, preoperative cognitive deficits, level of education, and comorbidities. Available randomized controlled trials suggest that there is no significant difference in the incidence of delirium or POCD when general anesthesia and regional anesthesia are compared. Looking at these effects over time, the highest incidence is early with significant recovery at 3 months and 1 year. Although a small number of patients have residual effects at 3 months or later, most studies find the number to be similar to that in the control population.[50]

References

1. Kahn RA, Moskowitz DM, Marin M, et al: Anesthetic considerations for endovascular aortic repair, *Mt Sinai J Med* 69:57, 2002.
2. Miller RD: *Miller's anesthesia*, ed 6, Philadelphia, New York, 2005, Elsevier/Churchill Livingstone, p. 2089.
3. Huncke KW, Sopher MJ: Hemodynamic responses during repair of abdominal aortic aneurysms using endovascular grafts, *Anesth Analg* 84:SCA79, 1997.
4. Baxendale BR, Baker DM, Hutchinson A, et al: Haemodynamic and metabolic response to endovascular repair of infra-renal aortic aneurysms, *Br J Anaesth* 77:581, 1996.
5. Kahn RA, Moskowitz DM, Manspeizer HE, et al: Endovascular aortic repair is associated with greater hemodynamic stability compared with open aortic reconstruction, *J Cardiothorac Vasc Anesth* 13:42, 1999.
6. Salartash K, Sternbergh WC 3rd, York JW, et al: Comparison of open transabdominal AAA repair with endovascular AAA repair in reduction of postoperative stress response, *Ann Vasc Surg* 15:53, 2001.
7. Fleisher LA, Beckman JA, Brown KA, et al: ACC/AHA 2007 Guidelines on Perioperative Cardiovascular Evaluation and Care for Noncardiac Surgery: Executive Summary: A Report of the American College of Cardiology/American Heart Association Task Force on Practice Guidelines (Writing Committee to Revise the 2002 Guidelines on Perioperative Cardiovascular Evaluation for Noncardiac Surgery) Developed in Collaboration With the American Society of Echocardiography, American Society of Nuclear Cardiology, Heart Rhythm Society, Society of Cardiovascular Anesthesiologists, Society for Cardiovascular Angiography and Interventions, Society for Vascular Medicine and Biology, and Society for Vascular Surgery, *J Am Coll Cardiol* 50:1707, 2007.
8. Cuypers PW, Gardien M, Buth J, et al: Cardiac response and complications during endovascular repair of abdominal aortic aneurysms: a concurrent comparison with open surgery, *J Vasc Surg* 33:353, 2001.
9. Cuypers PW, Gardien M, Buth J, et al: Randomized study comparing cardiac response in endovascular and open abdominal aortic aneurysm repair, *Br J Surg* 88:1059, 2001.
10. Hertzer NR, Beven EG, Young JR, et al: Coronary artery disease in peripheral vascular patients: a classification of 1000 coronary angiograms and results of surgical management, *Ann Surg* 199:223, 1984.
11. McFalls EO, Ward HB, Moritz TE, et al: Coronary-artery revascularization before elective major vascular surgery, *N Engl J Med* 351:2795, 2004.
12. Rao TL, Jacobs KH, El-Etr AA: Reinfarction following anesthesia in patients with myocardial infarction, *Anesthesiology* 59:499, 1983.
13. Devereaux PJ, Goldman L, Cook DJ, et al: Perioperative cardiac events in patients undergoing noncardiac surgery: a review of the magnitude of the problem, the pathophysiology of the events and methods to estimate and communicate risk, *CMAJ* 173:627, 2005.
14. Ellis SG, Hertzer NR, Young JR, et al: Angiographic correlates of cardiac death and myocardial infarction complicating major nonthoracic vascular surgery, *Am J Cardiol* 77:1126, 1996.
15. Thomson IR, Mutch WA, Culligan JD: Failure of intravenous nitroglycerin to prevent intraoperative myocardial ischemia during fentanyl-pancuronium anesthesia, *Anesthesiology* 61:385, 1984.
16. Dodds TM, Stone JG, Coromilas J, et al: Prophylactic nitroglycerin infusion during noncardiac surgery does not reduce perioperative ischemia, *Anesth Analg* 76:705, 1993.
17. Wijeysundera DN, Beattie WS: Calcium channel blockers for reducing cardiac morbidity after noncardiac surgery: a meta-analysis, *Anesth Analg* 97:634, 2003.
18. Devereaux PJ, Goldman L, Yusuf S, et al: Surveillance and prevention of major perioperative ischemic cardiac events in patients undergoing noncardiac surgery: a review, *CMAJ* 173:779, 2005.
19. Poldermans D, Boersma E, Bax JJ, et al: The effect of bisoprolol on perioperative mortality and myocardial infarction in high-risk patients undergoing vascular surgery: Dutch Echocardiographic Cardiac Risk Evaluation Applying Stress Echocardiography Study Group, *N Engl J Med* 341:1789, 1999.
20. Mangano DT, Layug EL, Wallace A, et al: Effect of atenolol on mortality and cardiovascular morbidity after noncardiac surgery: Multicenter Study of Perioperative Ischemia Research Group, *N Engl J Med* 335:1713, 1996.
21. Lindenauer PK, Pekow P, Wang K, et al: Perioperative beta-blocker therapy and mortality after major noncardiac surgery, *N Engl J Med* 353:349, 2005.
22. Devereaux PJ, Yang H, Yusuf S, et al: Effects of extended-release metoprolol succinate in patients undergoing non-cardiac surgery (POISE trial): a randomised controlled trial, *Lancet* 371:2008, 1839.

23. Lotto ML, Banoub M, Schubert A: Effects of anesthetic agents and physiologic changes on intraoperative motor evoked potentials, *J Neurosurg Anesthesiol* 16:32, 2004.
24. Calancie B, Harris W, Brindle GF, et al: Threshold-level repetitive transcranial electrical stimulation for intraoperative monitoring of central motor conduction, *J Neurosurg* 95:161, 2001.
25. Bernard JM, Pereon Y, Fayet G, et al: Effects of isoflurane and desflurane on neurogenic motor- and somatosensory-evoked potential monitoring for scoliosis surgery, *Anesthesiology* 85:1013, 1996.
26. Kalkman CJ, Drummond JC, Kennelly NA, et al: Intraoperative monitoring of tibialis anterior muscle motor evoked responses to transcranial electrical stimulation during partial neuromuscular blockade, *Anesth Analg* 75:584, 1992.
27. Lang EW, Beutler AS, Chesnut RM, et al: Myogenic motor-evoked potential monitoring using partial neuromuscular blockade in surgery of the spine, *Spine* 21:1676, 1996.
28. Wong GT, Irwin MG: Contrast-induced nephropathy, *Br J Anaesth* 99:474, 2007.
29. Moore NN, Lapsley M, Norden AG, et al: Does N-acetylcysteine prevent contrast-induced nephropathy during endovascular AAA repair? A randomized controlled pilot study, *J Endovasc Ther* 13:660, 2006.
30. Merten GJ, Burgess WP, Gray LV, et al: Prevention of contrast-induced nephropathy with sodium bicarbonate: a randomized controlled trial, *JAMA* 291:2328, 2004.
31. From AM, Bartholmai BJ, Williams AW, et al: Sodium bicarbonate is associated with an increased incidence of contrast nephropathy: a retrospective cohort study of 7977 patients at Mayo Clinic, *Clin J Am Soc Nephrol* 3:10, 2008.
32. Gross JB, Bachenberg KL, Benumof JL, et al: Practice guidelines for the perioperative management of patients with obstructive sleep apnea: a report by the American Society of Anesthesiologists Task Force on Perioperative Management of patients with obstructive sleep apnea, *Anesthesiology* 104:1081, 2006.
33. Tramer MR, von Elm E, Loubeyre P, et al: Pharmacological prevention of serious anaphylactic reactions due to iodinated contrast media: systematic review, *BMJ* 333:675, 2006.
34. Ellis AK, Day JH: Incidence and characteristics of biphasic anaphylaxis: a prospective evaluation of 103 patients, *Ann Allergy Asthma Immunol* 98:64, 2007.
35. Miller RR, Olson HG, Amsterdam EA, et al: Propranolol-withdrawal rebound phenomenon. Exacerbation of coronary events after abrupt cessation of antianginal therapy, *N Engl J Med* 293:416, 1975.
36. Daumerie G, Fleisher LA: Perioperative beta-blocker and statin therapy, *Curr Opin Anaesthesiol* 21:60, 2008.
37. Geyskes GG, Boer P, Mees Dorhout: EJ: Clonidine withdrawal: mechanism and frequency of rebound hypertension, *Br J Clin Pharmacol* 7:55, 1979.
38. Kheterpal S, Khodaparast O, Shanks A, et al: Chronic angiotensin-converting enzyme inhibitor or angiotensin receptor blocker therapy combined with diuretic therapy is associated with increased episodes of hypotension in noncardiac surgery, *J Cardiothorac Vasc Anesth* 22:180, 2008.
39. Comfere T, Sprung J, Kumar MM, et al: Angiotensin system inhibitors in a general surgical population, *Anesth Analg* 100:636, 2005.
40. Walts LF, Miller J, Davidson MB, et al: Perioperative management of diabetes mellitus, *Anesthesiology* 55:104, 1981.
41. Gandhi GY, Nuttall GA, Abel MD, et al: Intensive intraoperative insulin therapy versus conventional glucose management during cardiac surgery: a randomized trial, *Ann Intern Med* 146:233, 2007.
42. Drug Information Sheet. http://packageinserts.bms.com/pi/pi_glucophage_xr.pdf. Bristol Myers Squib, 2006.
43. Horlocker TT, Wedel DJ, Benzon H, et al: Regional anesthesia in the anticoagulated patient: defining the risks (the second ASRA Consensus Conference on Neuraxial Anesthesia and Anticoagulation), *Reg Anesth Pain Med* 28:172, 2003.
44. Ruppert V, Leurs LJ, Steckmeier B, et al: Influence of anesthesia type on outcome after endovascular aortic aneurysm repair: an analysis based on EUROSTAR data, *J Vasc Surg* 44:16, 2006.
45. Ruppert V, Leurs LJ, Rieger J, et al: Risk-adapted outcome after endovascular aortic aneurysm repair: analysis of anesthesia types based on EUROSTAR data, *J Endovasc Ther* 14:12, 2007.
46. Verhoeven EL, Cina CS, Tielliu IF, et al: Local anesthesia for endovascular abdominal aortic aneurysm repair, *J Vasc Surg* 42:402, 2005.
47. Agarwal A, Dhiraaj S, Singhal V, et al: Comparison of efficacy of oxybutynin and tolterodine for prevention of catheter related bladder discomfort: a prospective, randomized, placebo-controlled, double-blind study, *Br J Anaesth* 96:377, 2006.
48. Agarwal A, Dhiraaj S, Pawar S, et al: An evaluation of the efficacy of gabapentin for prevention of catheter-related bladder discomfort: a prospective, randomized, placebo-controlled, double-blind study, *Anesth Analg* 105:1454, 2007.
49. Bryson GL, Wyand A: Evidence-based clinical update: general anesthesia and the risk of delirium and postoperative cognitive dysfunction, *Can J Anaesth* 53:669, 2006.
50. Newman S, Stygall J, Hirani S, et al: Postoperative cognitive dysfunction after noncardiac surgery: a systematic review, *Anesthesiology* 106:572, 2007.

CHAPTER

75

The Use of Embolization Techniques in Endovascular Surgery

Brian G. DeRubertis

Coincident with the technologic advances that have aided the development of endovascular approaches to arterial occlusive disease and aneurysm treatment has been the emergence of techniques of transcatheter arterial embolization. Embolization therapy describes the introduction of substances into the arterial system for the purpose of controlling hemorrhage, reducing blood flow to vascular lesions or malformations, excluding aneurysms or pseudoaneurysms, or interrupting blood flow to end organs. Catheters of increasing lower profile and microcoils of diameters as small as 0.018 inch have allowed interventionalists to perform transcatheter embolization throughout the vascular system. Common targets of embolic therapy now include aneurysms and malformations of the cerebral, pulmonary, visceral, and peripheral circulations.

EMBOLIC MATERIALS

Although this chapter primarily discusses the technical issues dealing with the use of thrombogenic coils, there are a number of materials that have been used for embolization of the peripheral vasculature, and advances in technology promise to bring further options for peripheral embolization. It is important for the surgeon to be familiar with the different materials used in embolization procedures, because each has its own distinct advantages and drawbacks, and different levels of expertise with endovascular interventions are required for effective results with the various materials. The following section briefly describes the embolic agents commonly used in the peripheral circulation.

Thrombogenic Coils

Among the most commonly used embolic materials are thrombogenic coils, often referred to as Gianturco or Guglielmi coils (Figure 75-1).[1,2] These are generally divided into macrocoils and microcoils. Macrocoils are coils typically delivered through 5F or 6F catheters (0.035-inch lumen diameter) to vessels of diameters ranging from 2 to 14 mm. Microcoils, on the other hand, are delivered through smaller 2F or 3F catheters (0.018-inch lumen diameter) to vessels ranging from 2 to 10 mm in diameter. Embolic coils are made of either stainless steel or platinum, and although both appear to be safe in patients undergoing magnetic resonance imaging subsequently, platinum coils are less likely to result in image artifact and distortion. Stainless steel coils have the advantage of superior radial strength, though secure placement is obtainable even for platinum coils with minimal vessel oversizing.

Coils are packaged in storage devices that keep them in their elongated uncoiled state, and on delivery into the target vessel the coil retains its preformed shape to result in obstruction of the vessel and ultimately vessel thrombosis (see Figure 75-1, *B*). Macrocoils retain shapes that include single-diameter coils, tapered coils, or other helical or irregular patterns. Microcoils are available in forms that remain straight (generally in diameters of 0.018 inch) or that reshape into coils. Although the coil itself has some thrombotic properties, the primary thrombogenicity of many coils comes from the small synthetic fibers that coat the coil. To deliver standard pushable (Gianturco) coils, an appropriately sized catheter is positioned in the target vessel to be embolized. The delivery system is then loaded into the catheter, and the coil is advanced with a guidewire until it exits the catheter and lodges in the vessel. Coils are used in a variety of settings, including endovascular repair of visceral and renal artery aneurysms, hypogastric artery embolizations (in conjunction with abdominal aortic aneurysm repair), treatment of arteriovenous malformations (AVMs), and exclusion of cerebral aneurysms.

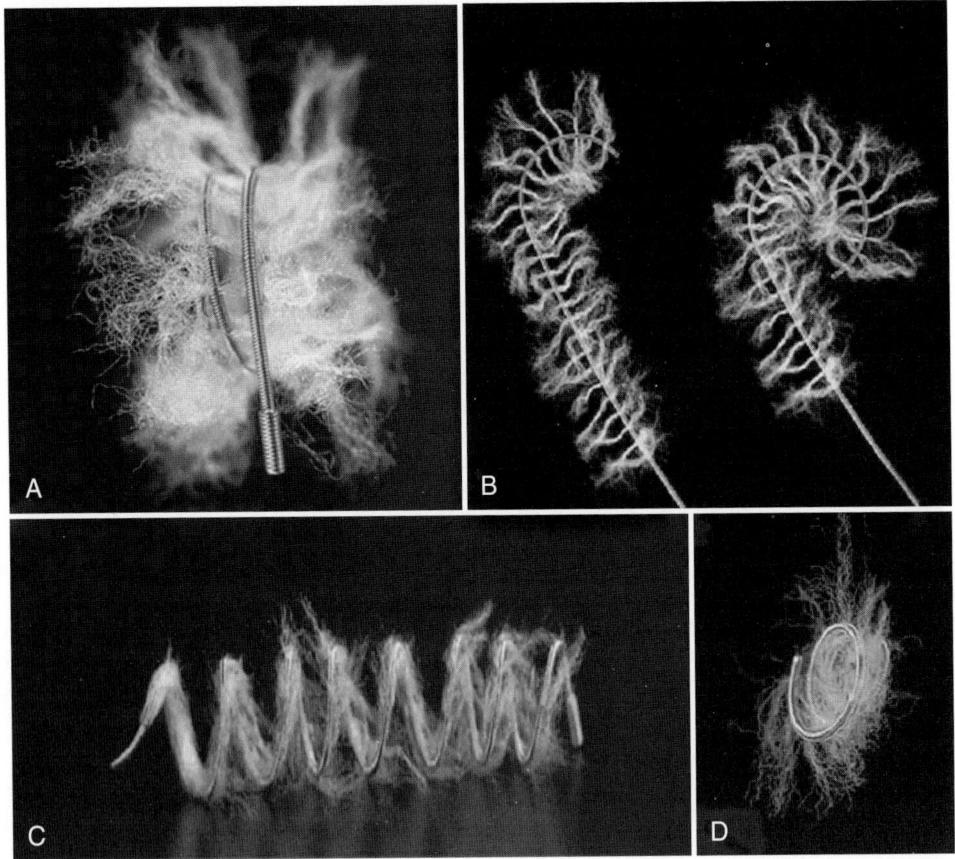

FIGURE 75-1 Thrombogenic coils range in size, shape, and deployment mechanism. They are generally constructed of stainless steel or nitinol alloy and coated with thrombogenic filaments. Although detachable coils **(A)** are becoming increasingly used because of their ability for precise deployment, pushable coils **(B-D)** are suitable for a wide range of peripheral applications. Nitinol coils are straightened in the deployment catheter, then retain their conformational shape on deployment **(B)**. Commonly used shapes include single-diameter coils **(C)** and tapered-diameter coils **(D)**.

Detachable (Guglielmi type) coils are similar to standard pushable coils except that they offer a more controlled delivery to a specific location (see Figure 75-1, *A*).[2,3] They are available in 0.018-inch and 0.035-inch platforms and are delivered with specially designed positioning catheters and push-wires. Generally, up to 95% of the coil can be delivered and still allow for retrieval and repositioning if placement is deemed suboptimal. When placement of the coil is satisfactory, the coil is released by either electromagnetic or mechanical properties. The use of detachable coils can be especially advantageous in areas where precise delivery and avoidance of thrombosis outside of the intended treatment region are crucial. For this reason, these coils have become very important adjuncts to coil embolization in the cerebral circulation for aneurysms and AVMs and in the peripheral circulation to avoid thrombosis in second- or third-order arterial bifurcations.

Polyvinyl Alcohol Foam Particles

Arterial occlusion can also be achieved by transcatheter delivery of embolic particles to the target vessel. Although a variety of particle types, such as Gelfoam and Avitene, have been used for embolization techniques, among the more commonly used agents are polyvinyl alcohol (PVA) foam particles (Cook Medical, Bloomington, IN). PVA foam particles are permanent embolic agents and are available in sizes that range from 90 to 2800 μm. They produce occlusion by causing an inflammatory reaction and thrombosis in the target vessel, and they have been demonstrated to have a low rate of recanalization. The particles are mixed in a suspension of contrast material before injection to allow visualization during fluoroscopy. An advantage of foam particles over coils is that the delivery catheter need not necessarily be positioned all the way to the target region. Instead, the surgeon can use particles of an appropriate size for target vessel occlusion and allow them to flow into position for occlusion. Although this strategy can be useful in embolization of certain vascular beds or vascular malformations, a drawback is that the particles can tend to aggregate after leaving the delivery catheter with the unintended consequence of occlusion more proximally than desired. Increasing the dilution ratio of the particles can decrease aggregation of particles and result in more distal embolization.

Gelatin Microspheres

Another type of occlusive particle that functions in a similar manner as PVA foam particles is the Embosphere gelatin microsphere (Biosphere Medical, Rockland, MA). These particles are spherical microporous beads composed of an acrylic polymer (trisacryl) linked to gelatin. The microspheres are hydrophilic and compressible, allowing relatively large particles (up to 700 μm) to be delivered through 3F microcatheters (0.019- to 0.023-inch inner lumen diameter). Like PVA foam particles, they must be mixed with a contrast agent to allow for visualization during fluoroscopy. Because microspheres are less prone to aggregation than PVA foam particles, they have the theoretic advantage of increased accuracy of delivery and fewer proximal occlusion events. Gelatin microspheres have been demonstrated to be useful in the embolization of benign and malignant tumors, vascular malformations, and sources of acute hemorrhage.

Liquid Embolics

Liquid embolic agents include cyanoacrylate and ethylene vinyl alcohol. Cyanoacrylate is a liquid adhesive agent that hardens on contact with blood after extrusion from the catheter. The polymerization process that occurs when it contacts blood results in an exothermic reaction that causes vessel wall injury and coagulative occlusion of the vessel. Cyanoacrylate is often used for AVMs and is delivered through a microcatheter positioned at the nidus of the malformation to achieve occlusion of the outflow vessels, as well as the arterial inflow. After deployment of the embolic through a microcatheter placed in a coaxial fashion through a larger guiding catheter, the microcatheter is removed to prevent adherence to the solidifying material.

Onyx (ev3 Inc., Plymouth, MN) is a commercially available liquid embolic composed of ethylene vinyl alcohol copolymer dissolved in dimethyl sulfoxide, the nonadhesive properties of which reduce the chance of adherence of the catheter to the embolic material on polymerization. It is indicated for the presurgical embolization of brain AVMs, though it has been used for embolization of vascular lesions in the peripheral circulation as well. Onyx is generally delivered through a coaxial technique, with use of a dimethyl sulfoxide–compatible microcatheter positioned at the primary target location. It is radiopaque and thus does not require mixing with a contrast agent for visualization.

Vascular Plugs

The Amplatzer Vascular Plug (AGA Medical Corporation, Plymouth, MN) is an occlusion device composed of a cylindrical nitinol wire mesh that is delivered through an appropriately sized guiding catheter positioned at the desired site of occlusion. This device is prepackaged in a loading device that aids in easy introduction of the device into a guiding catheter and also contains a delivery cable that allows for recapture and repositioning of the plug before the cable is removed. The nitinol mesh allows visualization of the device under fluoroscopy during and after deployment. The device comes in diameters that range from 2 to 22 mm (delivered through 5F to 9F guiding catheters), and the manufacturer recommends oversizing of approximately 30% to 50% of vessel diameter. The availability of large-diameter plugs and the precise deployment of the device make it an attractive option for use in occlusion of large vessels, such as in embolization of hypogastric arteries before endograft placement for iliac aneurysms.

TECHNICAL ISSUES IN EMBOLIZATION PROCEDURES

Access and Sheath Support

Important principles for vascular embolization include thorough preembolization and postembolization angiography, catheter placement in the desired region of occlusion, and stable coaxial sheath or guide catheter support. Standard arterial access via puncture with an 18-gauge followed by guidewire and sheath placement is typical. Next, unselected aortography in the area of interest is performed. At this point, the patient is systemically anticoagulated with 100 units/kg of intravenous heparin before selective catheterization of the target vessel is attempted to prevent unintended thrombosis of adjacent vessels or main arterial trunks proximal to the area of interest. Although systemic anticoagulation can prolong the time to thrombosis of the desired vessel, complete target vessel thrombosis generally occurs after the activated clotting time returns to normal, and the placement of large guide catheters or sheaths into second- or third-order branch vessels without systemic anticoagulation puts the patient at risk for thrombotic complications. After anticoagulation, selective or superselective catheterization is performed to acquire a full angiographic road map of the vessel or lesion (i.e., aneurysm, AVM) requiring embolization. Attention must be given to identifying all inflow and outflow vessels leading to lesions such as aneurysms or to identifying nidus points in lesions such as AVMs. Obtaining complete views of the lesion or target vessel usually requires angiography performed in multiple obliquities. Once adequate imaging has been performed, an embolization strategy is developed and coaxial sheath support is established. A supportive exchange wire such as a Stiff Angled Glidewire (Terumo, Somerset, NJ) or a Rosen wire (Cook Medical) allows placement of a long sheath or guiding catheter into the target vessel. Next, additional support can be provided by establishing a "triaxial" system in which a smaller microcatheter (Renegade; Boston Scientific, Natick, MA, or RapidTransit; Cordis, Warren, NJ) is housed within a 0.035-inch catheter (Figure 75-2). For example, in coiling a distal splenic artery aneurysm, a Rosen exchange wire can be placed in the distal splenic artery after angiography to track a 65-cm Super Arrow Flex 6F sheath (Arrow International, Reading, PA) through the celiac trunk and into the midsplenic artery. Next, a 90-cm 6F Angled Glide Catheter (Terumo) is advanced over the Rosen wire into the aneurysm sac. The 0.035-inch Rosen wire is then removed, and a 0.021-inch catheter (2.8F 155-cm length RapidTransit; Cordis) over a 0.014-inch wire (300 cm Asahi Grand Slam; Abbott Vascular, Abbott Park, IL) is advanced to select individual outflow vessels off the aneurysm sac. Using a steerable 0.014-inch wire/0.021-inch microcatheter through the 0.035-inch catheter system can give additional maneuverability and torque to enable superselective access of outflow vessels and can allow for additional support when delivering coils.

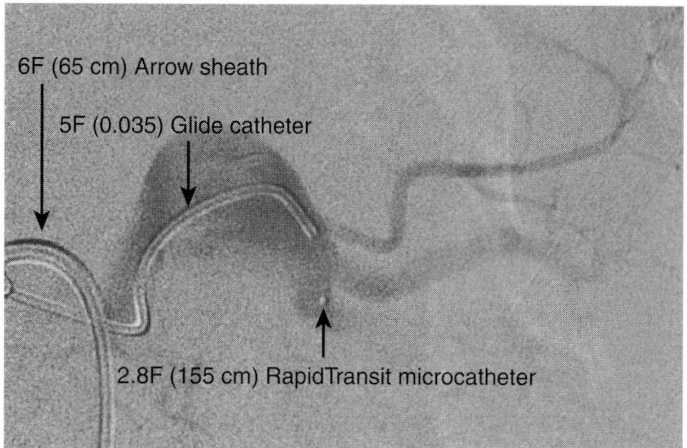

FIGURE 75-2 Selective catheterization of individual outflow branches of this splenic artery aneurysm is facilitated by use of a triaxial system. A 6F sheath houses a 5F Glide catheter, which in turn supports a 2.8F microcatheter through which 0.018-inch coils can be delivered. The placement of the microcatheter within the larger 5F catheter provides additional support during coil delivery and enables easier catheterization of outflow vessels by "absorbing" some of the tortuosity within the system.

Techniques for Coil Delivery

Once stable and supportive access has been established, delivery of embolic agents can be performed. There are several commonly used techniques for delivery of thrombogenic coils. A scaffolding technique describes the nesting of several smaller coils within a larger coil that acts as an anchoring framework. First, coil of high radial force appropriately sized to the vessel diameter is delivered over a 1- to 2-cm segment of the artery requiring embolization. Next, the guidewire and microcatheter are advanced into the region of the artery containing this coil, and smaller-diameter filament-coated thrombogenic coils are delivered in a nested fashion within this larger well-secured coil by weaving the microcatheter proximally and distally during deployment (Figure 75-3, *A*). Deployment location of the coil can also be secured by anchoring the initial portion of the coil in a side branch off the target vessel and then weaving the microcatheter proximally and distally while supporting the system with the 0.035-inch catheter and sheath (see Figure 75-3, *B*). For the embolization of broad-necked aneurysms, stent- or balloon-supported modeling and embolization can be performed. This requires a sheath sufficiently large to house the microcatheter used for coil delivery alongside a noncompliant angioplasty balloon or stent delivery system. First, the microcatheter is advanced over a guidewire until it is situated in the aneurysm. Next, a second guidewire is advanced intraluminally in a buddy-wire fashion past the aneurysm and is used to guide an angioplasty balloon into position over the neck of the aneurysm. The balloon is then subjected to a low-pressure (2-3 atm) inflation to isolate the aneurysm from the lumen of the vessel, and coils are delivered into the aneurysm sac (see Figure 75-3, *C*). This technique allows coiling of a wide-necked structure while minimizing the risk that the coils will spill into the vessel lumen. Alternatively, an appropriately sized stent can be deployed across the neck of the aneurysm with the microcatheter positioned in the sac. After stent deployment, coils can be delivered through the microcatheter into the sac. After coil delivery, the microcatheter is withdrawn.

EMBOLIZATION OF SPECIFIC LESIONS IN THE PERIPHERAL VASCULATURE

Arteriovenous Malformations

AVMs can be difficult to treat surgically because of their hypervascularity, and complete surgical resection can be difficult because of the associated blood loss. Percutaneous embolization now plays an important role in the treatment of AVMs that require intervention, both before surgery and as an isolated treatment modality. Unfortunately, the large number of arterial inflow vessels, as well as the multiple outflow vessels, can make embolization of these structures challenging, and multiple embolizations are usually required over a number of sessions. The management of these lesions

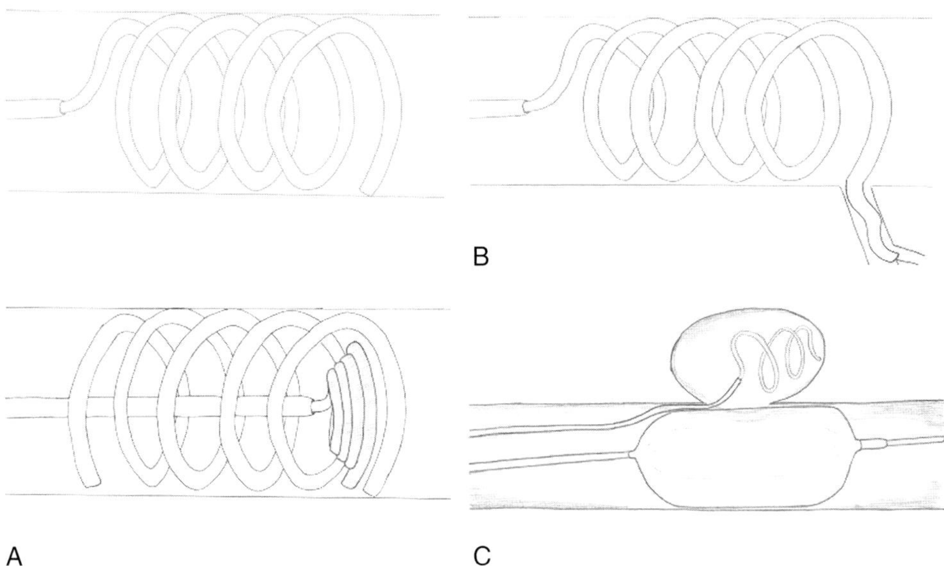

FIGURE 75-3 Delivery of coils or other embolics always requires stable sheath placement into the target vessel, followed by deployment through 5F (0.035-inch platform) or 2.8F (0.018-inch platform) catheters. Deployment methods include a "nesting" technique **(A)** in which smaller-diameter coils are deployed into a larger-diameter coil that is slightly oversized for the vessel and deployed first. A vessel branch **(B)** can also be used to anchor the coil during delivery. Broad-necked aneurysms can be embolized with a "balloon-assisted" technique **(C)** in which a microcatheter positioned into the aneurysm sac is used for coil delivery while a balloon is inflated across the neck of the aneurysm to prevent escape of coils into the vessel.

requires careful consideration of the advantages and difficulties posed by open surgical resection, percutaneous sclerosant injections, and intra-arterial embolization. Because these are benign lesions, both the patient and the physician should understand that intervention is used to control symptoms and not necessarily achieve cure in most circumstances and that many patients requiring intervention are best managed with a combination of surgery and percutaneous intervention.[4] Enthusiasm for intervention should be tempered against the realization that a long-term treatment strategy is essential to control the lesion without causing undue morbidity.[5]

The role of intra-arterial embolization therapy has increased as low-profile microcatheters and an increasing range of embolic agents have become available. The primary goal of intra-arterial embolization is identification and occlusion of the nidus of the malformation where the inflow and outflow vessels communicate. After initial angiography, superselective catheterization of the inflow vessels is required to access the nidus. Embolization of proximal feeding vessels should not be performed as collaterals quickly develop to perfuse the nidus, and subsequent access to the nidus becomes more difficult on subsequent procedures.

The choice of embolic material depends largely on the size of the arteriovenous connection and the volume of flow through the lesion. Fistula-like high-output lesions can be seen in renal or pulmonary AVMs, and these lesions may be amenable to coil embolization using 0.035-inch delivery catheters supported by 6F to 8F guiding catheters.[6-9] Alternatively, extremity AVMs typically have multiple nidus points supplied by numerous small feeding vessels that are too small for the use of thrombogenic coils. Embolization of these lesions has been performed most successfully with the use of liquid embolics or PVA foam particles delivered through tapered microcatheters (2.4F/1.9F Echelon or 2.7F/1.5F Marathon; ev3).[4,10,11] The low profile of the distal end of the microcatheter allows for greater access to the nidus of the malformation through the small feeding vessels. The microcatheter can be supported in a triaxial configuration with a 0.035-inch catheter and 6F to 8F guiding catheter.

Postembolization angiography should demonstrate reduced vascularity of the lesion although complete disruption of flow through the lesion AVM is uncommon. The need to sufficiently reduce flow through the lesion to control symptoms should be balanced against the potential compromise in perfusion to the normal tissues.

Published results for extremity AVM embolization demonstrate the complexity of the decision regarding initiation of treatment and chronic nature of this condition. Tan et al.[10] reported the outcome of 30 patients referred by evaluation and treatment of extremity AVM over a 15-year period. These patients included equal numbers of both upper- and lower-extremity lesions. Of this group, 11 patients had symptoms deemed insufficient to warrant surgical or percutaneous intervention, and, of these, only 1 had progression of symptoms over the study period. Of those with symptoms sufficient to warrant endovascular intervention, 6 were determined to be unsuitable for intervention because of anatomy considered to be unsafe for embolization. The remaining 13 patients underwent 27 embolization procedures with cyanoacrylate or PVA, averaging 2.1 sessions per patient (range of one to five per patient). In these 13 patients, 3 had complete angiographic and clinical resolution of the AVM, 5 had clinical symptom control despite persistence of the AVM on angiography, and 5 had no significant improvement in symptoms. White et al.[4] reported the results of 20 patients undergoing intervention for extremity AVM. Seventy-five percent of these had symptom control with either embolization alone (11 patients) or embolization and resection (4 patients), with follow-up as long as 16 years. The remaining 5 patients required amputation, and all of these patients were found to have extensive AVMs involving all three tibial vessels.

Hypogastric Artery Embolization

Hypogastric artery embolization is commonly performed by vascular surgeons in conjunction with endovascular repair of iliac artery aneurysms.[12,13] In patients with common iliac aneurysm or combined aortoiliac aneurysm, endovascular repair with currently available bifurcated endografts must extend past the hypogastric artery to achieve a distal fixation and seal in the external iliac artery. In these patients, embolization of the ipsilateral hypogastric artery is required to prevent retrograde type II endoleak through the pelvic circulation (Figures 75-4 and 75-5).

Although this procedure can be performed coincidently with the placement of the endograft, some prefer to stage the procedures to reduce contrast load to the kidneys in a single procedure and allow the patient to recover from the embolization procedure before aneurysm repair. The hypogastric artery is usually approached most easily from the contralateral side (see Figure 75-4, *A*). The procedure begins with contralateral common femoral artery access followed by unselected arch aortography. After crossing the aortic bifurcation and placing a stiff exchange wire in the external iliac artery, a 45-cm 6F Balkan sheath (Cook Medical) is positioned at the origin of the hypogastric. Selective catheterization of the hypogastric is easily accomplished at this point with a Cobra 2 catheter; then placing an exchange wire into the hypogastric will allow the sheath to be advanced over its obturator into the orifice of the hypogastric artery. Positioning of the sheath within the origin of the hypogastric artery allows for angiography during coil deployment and provides firm support during delivery to ensure that the delivery catheter does not back out of the artery during coil delivery, thus allowing coils to migrate into the lower-extremity circulation.

Coil selection is based on the vessel diameter, and significant oversizing should be avoided as it prevents the coils from assuming their preformed shape. The coil should be positioned in the main trunk of the vessel to preserve distal collateral pelvic blood flow and reduce the likelihood of buttock claudication (see Figure 75-4, *B*). For hypogastric artery embolization, coils ranging in diameter from 6 to 10 mm are initially used as a scaffold, and additional tapered coils (Tornado; Cook Medical) of smaller diameter can then be nested within the scaffolding for complete occlusion.

Some groups have reported successful use of the Amplatzer Vascular Plug (AGA Medical Corporation) as an alternative to coils for embolization of the hypogastric artery.[14-16] Vandy et al.[14] compared 23 consecutive patients undergoing endovascular aneurysm repair with Amplatzer Vascular Plug embolization of the hypogastric artery with 19 patients whose adjunctive hypogastric embolization used coils. They found that the plug was effective in all cases, whereas one patient who received coil embolization required a secondary embolization procedure. Furthermore, there were no episodes of plug migration and two episodes of coil migration. Incidence of buttock claudication was significantly lower in the vascular plug group compared with the coil group (9% vs. 35% respectively, $p < .027$). Patients undergoing vascular plug embolization required an average of 1.35 devices (at an average cost of $470 per patient), compared with 7.53 devices (at a cost of $1496 per patient).

Splenic Artery Aneurysm

Endovascular management of visceral artery aneurysms is becoming increasingly common. The most prevalent visceral artery aneurysms are those of the splenic artery,[17] and treatment options for these lesions include open or laparoscopic splenectomy, laparoscopic splenic artery ligation, or endovascular repair with coil embolization.[18-20] The decision between these treatment options depends on the patient's medical comorbidities, anatomic considerations regarding the splenic artery and the aneurysm, and the risk of treatment-related splenic infarction. Although spleen preservation is preferable, intraparenchymal or distal hilar aneurysms generally require splenectomy to prevent the postembolization syndrome associated with splenic infarction. Aneurysms of the proximal section or midsection of the splenic artery can be treated by interruption of blood flow through the main trunk of the artery, thus relying on collateral flow from the short gastric arteries to maintain splenic perfusion. The primary goal in endovascular

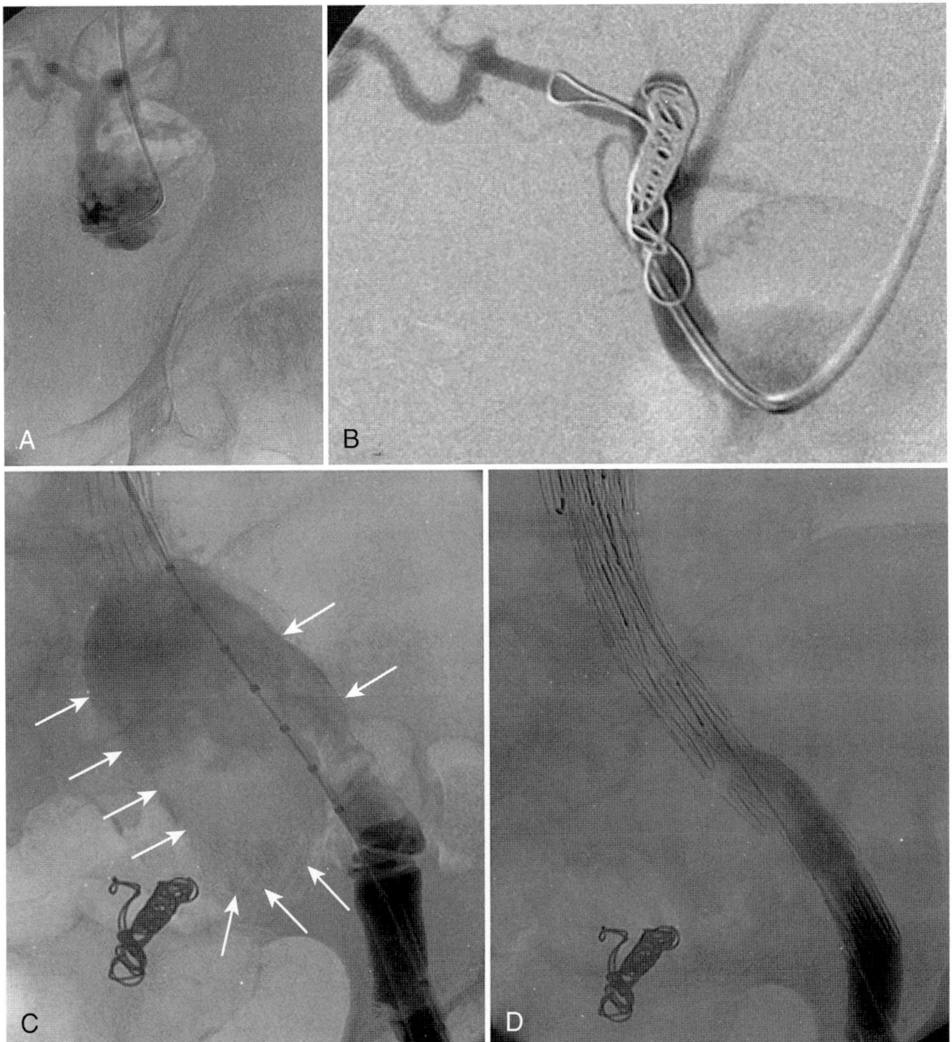

FIGURE 75-4 Coil embolization of the hypogastric artery in association with endovascular aneurysm repair. The hypogastric artery is usually best approached from contralateral access **(A)**. After placement of a sheath in the target region of the vessel, coils are delivered. The coils should be targeted for the origin of the vessel to preserve distal collateral flow, although the presence of a concomitant hypogastric artery aneurysm sometimes requires placement of coils into the distal aspect of the main trunk of the artery **(B)**. Flow through the hypogastric artery **(C)** and the common iliac artery aneurysm **(D)** is excluded after extension of the endograft component into the external iliac artery.

management of these aneurysms is placement of thrombotic coils in normal-appearing artery proximal and distal to the aneurysm, thus completely excluding the aneurysm, while preventing extension of the coil or thrombus into the splenic hilum.

Splenic artery embolization begins with unselected aortography at the T12-L1 interspace in the later projection to identify the origin of the mesenteric vessels. Next, an SOS Omni catheter (AngioDynamics, Queensbury, NY) or Cobra 2 catheter is used to selectively catheterize and image the celiac trunk and splenic artery. After confirming that the aneurysm has appropriate anatomy for endovascular therapy, the catheter is advanced over a 0.035-inch guidewire into the distal splenic artery. Next, this guidewire is changed to a stiff exchange wire, which is then used to position a long sheath or guiding catheter well into the splenic artery. Because of the oftentimes extreme tortuosity of the splenic artery (Figure 75-6), the exchange wire must be positioned quite distally in the main trunk of the splenic artery. The patient should be systemically anticoagulated at this point to prevent thrombotic complications caused by the presence of a large sheath in the mesenteric vessels. If the aneurysm is located in the main trunk of the splenic artery (Figure 75-7) without additional side branches or hilar vessels emanating from it, then 0.035-inch coils can generally be placed safely through a 5F or 6F end-hole delivery catheter distally and proximally to exclude the aneurysm. If the aneurysm approaches the hilum or there are additional branches off the aneurysm that require selective catheterization and embolization (Figure 75-8), then the use of 0.018-inch coils

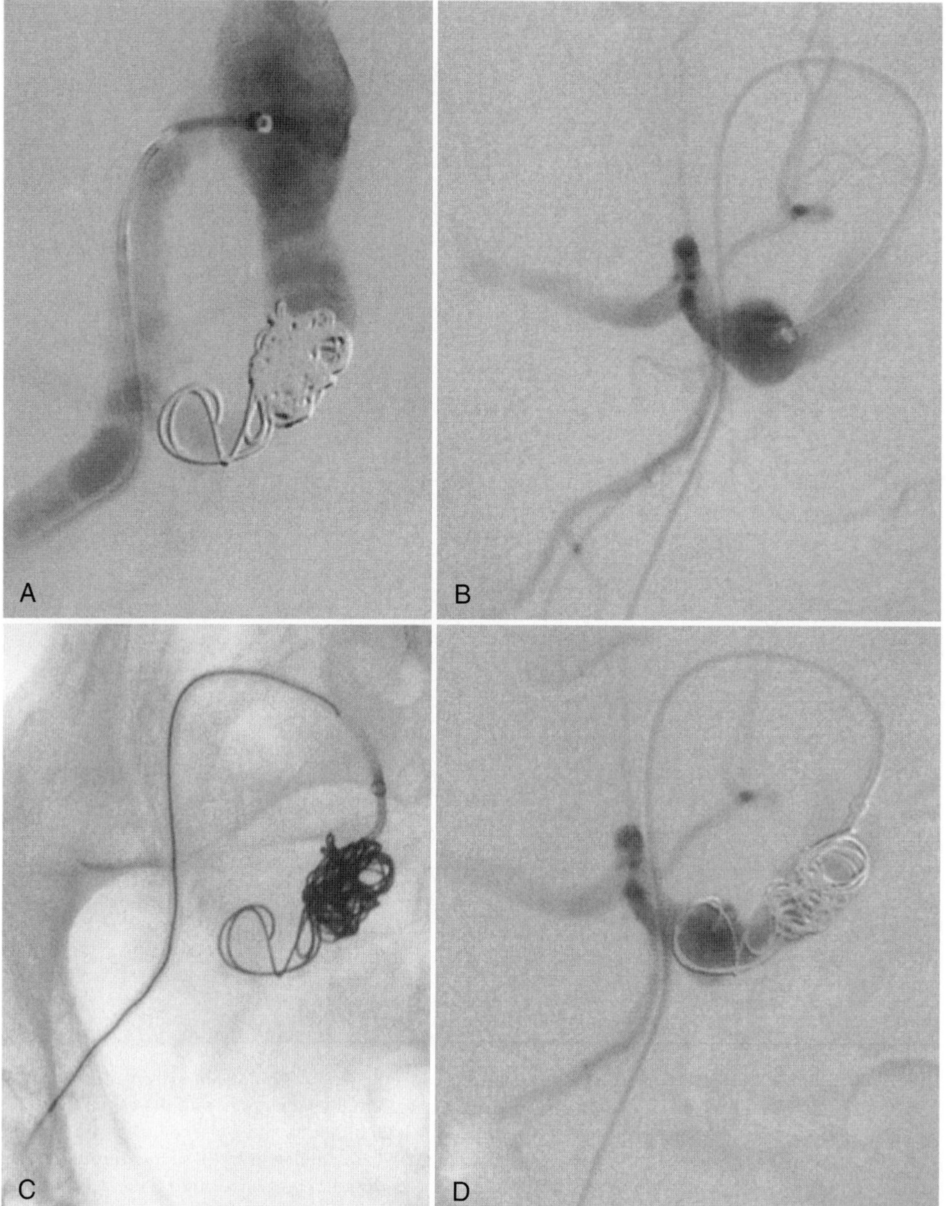

FIGURE 75-5 Coil embolization of a hypogastric artery aneurysm in conjunction with endograft extension into the external iliac for a common iliac artery aneurysm 5 years after initial aortic aneurysm repair. Coils were placed in the distal aspect of the main trunk of the hypogastric artery to prevent back-bleeding into the hypogastric aneurysm **(A).** This was accomplished by placing a 6F sheath into the target region of the hypogastric artery **(B),** then advancing a 5F delivery catheter **(C)** to precisely position the coil and provide additional support in a coaxial fashion. Note position of coils proximal to the main bifurcation point to preserve distal collateral flow **(D).**

through a microcatheter may be preferable. Use of a triaxial system in this case allows the 0.023-inch or 0.019-inch microcatheter to be supported by both the 0.035-inch catheter and the sheath/guide catheter, thus offering increased torque and handling of the catheter during catheterization of the branch vessels, as well as additional safety and stability during coil deployment. Detachable coils may be helpful in this setting to ensure precise deployment of the coil without extension into the distal hilar branches.

Although most splenic artery aneurysms have a fusiform morphology, an alternative strategy for saccular aneurysm includes packing of the aneurysm with coils without occlusion of the main trunk of the artery. This has been described in conjunction with balloon-assisted neck remodeling to prevent the coils from entering the main splenic artery in aneurysms with a wide-based neck.[21] This maneuver is performed as described above, with inflation of an angioplasty balloon across the neck of the aneurysm as coils are deployed through

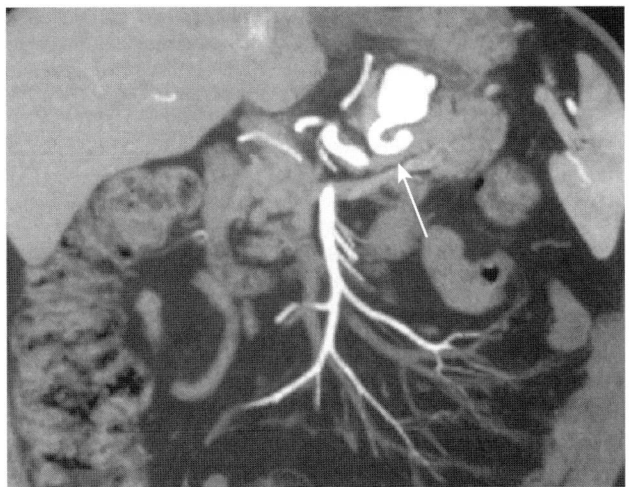

FIGURE 75-6 Splenic artery aneurysms located in the midportion of the main trunk of the splenic artery are ideally suited for endovascular exclusion. Although this aneurysm is situated in an appropriate position for endovascular intervention, the tortuosity often found in the proximal splenic artery *(arrow)* can make sheath placement and catheter navigation difficult.

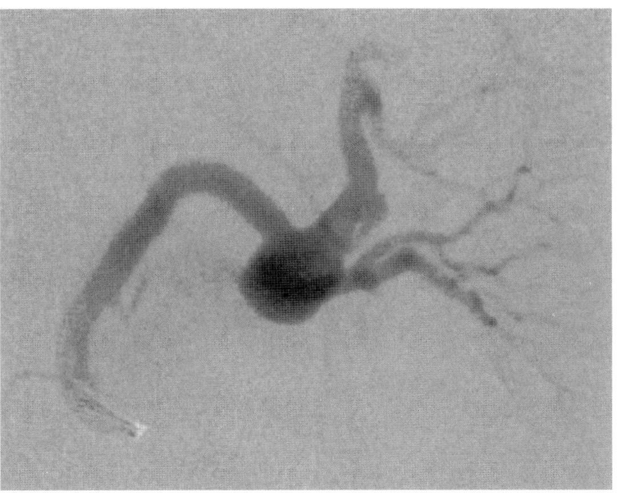

FIGURE 75-8 Splenic artery aneurysms approaching the hilum of the spleen are difficult to approach through interventional techniques because of the increased risk of thrombosis extending into the hilar branches and development of postinfarction syndrome. Treatment of aneurysms in this location can be facilitated by superselective catheterization of branch vessels and precise deployment of detachable coils.

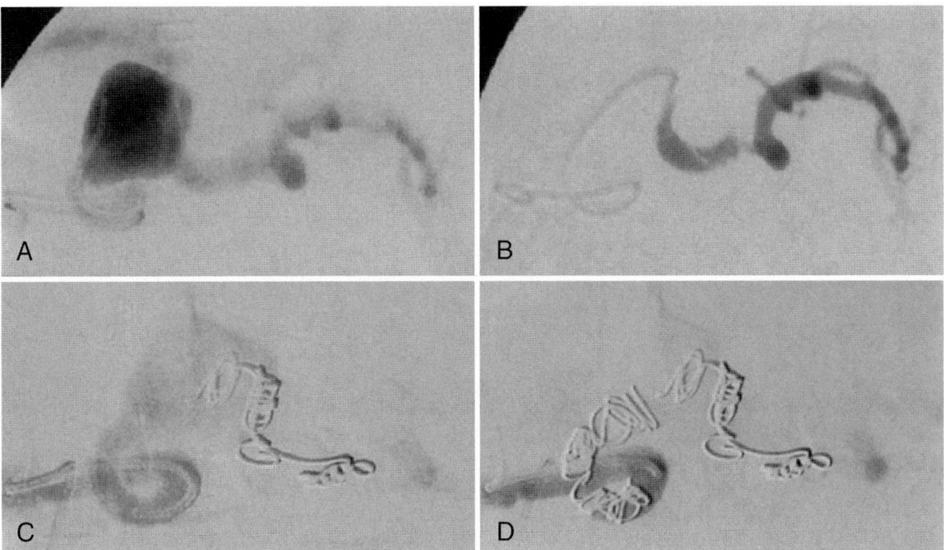

FIGURE 75-7 Splenic artery aneurysms situated in the midportion of the main splenic artery are ideally suited for endovascular intervention **(A).** Selective catheterization of the outflow branch of the vessel is required **(B),** followed by deployment of coils distal to the aneurysm but proximal to the hilar branches **(C).** This allows collateral flow from the short gastric vessels to provide continued splenic perfusion but prevents back-bleeding into the aneurysm. Next, the catheter is withdrawn to allow coil delivery into the proximal splenic artery **(D).**

a microcatheter positioned into the aneurysm sac. A theoretical disadvantage of embolization of the sac alone (and not the undilated main artery) is that systemic pressure may still be transmitted through the thrombosed neck into the aneurysm, thus leaving some continued risk of rupture. There are currently insufficient long-term data to determine whether this method will prove less durable than coil embolization of the main splenic artery, or whether either endovascular approach will result in long-term outcomes equivalent to open repair or splenectomy.

The high technical success rate with endovascular management of splenic artery aneurysms has made it the first-line therapy for these lesions in some centers. Loffroy et al.[18] achieved a 94.1% success rate in 17 patients undergoing attempted coil embolization of splenic artery aneurysms. The single failure was a result of inability to cannulate the distal outflow of an intraparenchymal aneurysm. These authors reported a 23% postembolization syndrome caused by microinfarcts seen on computed tomographic scan. Similar results were described by Piffaretti et al.,[22] who treated 15 patients with a technical success rate of 93% and a postembolization syndrome rate of 30% with no episodes of pancreatitis, splenic abscess, or surgical conversion. Patients were followed by magnetic resonance imaging with a mean follow-up of 36 months. One patient had reperfusion of the sac in the follow-up period, which was treated with repeated embolization.

CONCLUSION

Advances in technology and increased endovascular abilities have allowed surgeons to use embolization techniques for a variety of applications throughout the peripheral vascular system. Multiple options exist in terms of embolic materials, and each has its own advantages and required level of expertise for effective use. A thorough knowledge of the different materials is essential for selecting the proper embolic for a specific purpose. The placement of supportive sheaths or guiding catheters and the use of coaxial systems to deliver embolic materials further increases the safe and effective delivery of embolic materials. Long-term outcome data are necessary before firm conclusions can be drawn regarding the durability of intravascular embolization procedures relative to open surgical techniques.

References

1. Wallace S, Gianturco C, Anderson JH, et al: Therapeutic vascular occlusion utilizing steel coil technique: clinical applications, *AJR Am J Roentgenol* 127(3):381–387, 1976.
2. Guglielmi G, Viñuela F, Duckwiler G, et al: Endovascular treatment of posterior circulation aneurysms by electrothrombosis using electrically detachable coils, *J Neurosurg* 77(4):515–524, 1992.
3. Coley SC, Jackson JE: Endovascular occlusion with a new mechanical detachable coil, *AJR Am J Roentgenol* 171(4): 1075–1079, 1998.
4. White RI Jr, Pollak J, Persing J, et al: Long-term outcome of embolotherapy and surgery for high-flow extremity arteriovenous malformations, *J Vasc Interv Radiol* 11(10):1285–1295, 2000.
5. Flye MW, Jordan BP, Schwartz MZ: Management of congenital arteriovenous malformations, *Surgery* 94(5):740–747, 1983.
6. Huppert PE, Duda SH, Erley CM, et al: Embolization of renal vascular lesions: clinical experience with microcoils and tracker catheters, *Cardiovasc Intervent Radiol* 16(6):361–367, 1993.
7. Mori T, Sugimoto K, Taniguchi T, et al: Renal arteriovenous fistula with rapid blood flow successfully treated by transcatheter arterial embolization: application of interlocking detachable coil as coil anchor, *Cardiovasc Intervent Radiol* 27(4): 374–376, 2004.
8. Remy-Jardin M, Dumont P, Brillet PY, et al: Pulmonary arteriovenous malformations treated with embolotherapy: helical CT evaluation of long-term effectiveness after 2–21-year follow-up, *Radiology* 239(2):576–585, 2006.
9. Mager JJ, Overtoom TT, Blauw H, et al: Embolotherapy of pulmonary arteriovenous malformations: long-term results in 112 patients, *J Vasc Interv Radiol* 15(5):451–456, 2004.
10. Tan KT, Simons ME, Rajan DK, et al: Peripheral high-flow arteriovenous vascular malformations: a single-center experience, *J Vasc Interv Radiol* 15(10):1071–1080, 2004.
11. Osuga K, Hori S, Kitayoshi H, et al: Embolization of high flow arteriovenous malformations: experience with use of superabsorbent polymer microspheres, *J Vasc Interv Radiol* 13(11): 1125–1133, 2002.
12. Mehta M, Veith FJ, Ohki T, et al: Unilateral and bilateral hypogastric artery interruption during aortoiliac aneurysm repair in 154 patients: a relatively innocuous procedure, *J Vasc Surg* 33(2 suppl):S27–S32, 2001.
13. Lee CW, Kaufman JA, Fan CM, et al: Clinical outcome of internal iliac artery occlusions during endovascular treatment of aortoiliac aneurysmal diseases, *J Vasc Interv Radiol* 11(5): 567–571, 2000.
14. Vandy F, Criado E, Upchurch GR Jr, et al: Transluminal hypogastric artery occlusion with a nitinol vascular plug during endovascular aortic aneurysm repair, *J Vasc Surg* 48(5):1121–1124, 2008.
15. Resnick SA, Eskandari MK: Outcomes of Amplatzer Vascular Plugs for Occlusion of Internal Iliacs during Aortoiliac Aneurysm Stent Grafting, *Ann Vasc Surg* [Epub ahead of print], 2008 Jul 9.
16. Pellerin O, Caruba T, Kandounakis Y, et al: Embolization of the internal iliac artery: cost-effectiveness of two different techniques, *Cardiovasc Intervent Radiol* 31(6):1088–1093, 2008.
17. Pulli R, Dorigo W, Troisi N, et al: Surgical treatment of visceral artery aneurysms: a 25-year experience, *J Vasc Surg* 48(2): 334–342, 2008 Aug.
18. Loffroy R, Guiu B, Cercueil JP, et al: Transcatheter Arterial Embolization of Splenic Artery Aneurysms and Pseudoaneurysms: Short- and Long-Term Results, *Ann Vasc Surg* 22 (5):618–626, 2008.
19. Ikeda O, Tamura Y, Nakasone Y, et al: Nonoperative management of unruptured visceral artery aneurysms: treatment by transcatheter coil embolization, *J Vasc Surg* 47(6):1212–1219. Epub 2008 Apr 28, 2008.
20. Tulsyan N, Kashyap VS, Greenberg RK, et al: The endovascular management of visceral artery aneurysms and pseudoaneurysms, *J Vasc Surg* 45(2):276–283, 2007.
21. Uchiyama D, Koganemaru M, Abe T, et al: Coil embolization of splenic artery aneurysm with preservation of the parent artery using a neck remodeling technique, *J Vasc Interv Radiol* 18 (3):447–450, 2007.
22. Piffaretti G, Tozzi M, Lomazzi C, et al: Splenic artery aneurysms: postembolization syndrome and surgical complications, *Am J Surg* 193(2):166–170, 2007.

CHAPTER

76

Cell Therapy Strategies to Treat Chronic Limb-Threatening Ischemia

Darwin Eton MD FACS

Biologic revascularization offers the promise of a durable low-risk, inexpensive modality to treat chronic severe limb ischemia. Its only theoretical drawback is that efficacy is not immediate compared with surgery or catheter-based intervention.

Research in cell biology is creating opportunities for imitating, amplifying, and inhibiting biologic processes to treat disease. Research into the mechanisms of vascularization has been evolving on two fronts. On the one hand, physicians who treat the dysvascular patient are striving to harness and enhance this natural process. On the other hand, oncologists are seeking to involute tumors by attacking vessel formation.

Neovascularization is a natural process that occurs throughout our lives. Any surgeon reoperating on a patient within a month of a previous procedure in the same operative field readily witnesses the neovascularization that accompanies wound healing in the form of increased bleeding. The focus of this chapter is to summarize nascent attempts to orchestrate the revascularization of ischemic tissue using cell therapy approaches.

THE PROGENITOR CELL

Following union of the sperm with the ovum, a totipotent embryonic stem cell is produced encoding the information that yields all human tissue. This information is completely passed on with each division until the morula phase (16 cells). Until then, each cell is totipotent; that is, it can generate an entire human being. Differentiation begins to occur at the 16-cell stage and is when the mature (more differentiated) progenitor stem cell originates.

Adult progenitor cells are specialized stem cells that respond to specific protein signals to divide asymmetrically to create an exact copy of themselves, as well as a sister cell that can go on to become specific tissue (e.g., endothelium). Niches of progenitor cells are located throughout our body, with sizeable populations located in the bone marrow (BM). They are present throughout our lives and respond to protein signals to divide and enter the peripheral blood (PB) stream to home to tissue in need of repair. Adult progenitor cells are readily isolated from the mononuclear cell (MNC) fraction of the BM and PB.

Many components of the MNC fraction (monocytes, macrophages, lymphocytes) contribute to neovascularization. MNC secrete proangiogenic factors such as vascular endothelial growth factor (VEGF), basic fibroblast growth factor (b-FGF), monocyte chemotactic protein (MCP-1), platelet-derived growth factor (PDGF) and angiopoietin-1, to name a few. The leukocyte fraction of the MNC secretes enzymes needed to restructure the vascular network (e.g., membrane metalloproteinases, elastase, tissue plasminogen activator, and collagenase). In addition, cells that are not part of the MNC fraction (aggregating platelets, polymorphonuclear leukocytes) also release proangiogenic and antiangiogenic proteins.

Endothelial progenitor cells (EPC) come from the MNC fraction and have been reported to promote angiogenesis following injection into ischemic muscle.[1-5] EPC express a number of endothelial-specific cell-surface markers and exhibit numerous endothelial properties.[1-3,6]

NEOVASCULARIZATION

Angiogenesis starts with local proteolysis within the vessel wall. New conduit begins to form at these weakened areas as neighboring endothelial cells (EC) and vascular smooth muscle cells (SMC) proliferate and migrate out of the vessel into the periadventitial soft tissue. The nascent vasculature is strengthened by the migration of pericytes around it, effectively blocking transmural seepage. All of this is orchestrated by proteins released locally. Angiogenesis per se is seen on angiography as a blush or as increased flow. Arteriogenesis is the formation of medium-sized vessels. Their larger diameter supports a higher volume rate of flow, which is proportional to their radius to the fourth power. Another name is collateral-genesis. These are visible on angiography.

THE INFLUENCE OF AGE AND DISEASE

The kinetics of neovascularization changes as we age. A child who occludes the superficial femoral artery can grow up with such good collateralization as to not manifest any disability except under the most strenuous activity. This is not true in the elderly,[7-14] and other atherosclerotic risk factors are reported to reduce progenitor cell availability and function, thus limiting their therapeutic usefulness in these dysvascular patients. The concentration of circulating EPC appears to be a better predictor of vascular disease than the combined Framingham risk factor score.[15,16] In patients with severe coronary artery disease, the colony-forming capacity and migratory activity of BM-derived CD34+/CD133+ MNCs (EPC cytokines) are markedly reduced.[17] Reduced neovascularization was observed after xenogeneic transplantation of these older MNCs into the ischemic hind limb of nude rats. Specific subsets of circulating CD34+ cells are decreased in patients with atherosclerosis.[18] A subset of BM Lin−/cKit−/Sca-1− cells that may be EPC-rich are profoundly affected by aging and hyperlipidemia.[14] The EPC (CD133+/VEGFR2+) count appears inversely related to the severity of congestive heart failure.[19] A senescent environment significantly affects progenitor cells. The aging milieu includes reduced levels of angiogenic cytokines, defects in the BM stem cell niche, altered hemostatic cascade, altered neurochemical pathways, altered growth factors, and their receptors. Moreover, at least in a murine model, the neovascularization capacity of transplanted BM-MNCs (discussed later as a clinical strategy) is reported to be impaired with aging.[20] However, aging does not hamper the revitalization of neovascularization in old mice in response to transplantation of young BM-MNCs.[20]

Ischemic tissues express signaling proteins (e.g., stroma-derived factor-1α, and hypoxia inducible factor-4) that enter the circulation and travel to the marrow and other progenitor cell niches. These proteins bind receptors on reparative progenitor cells and promote their proliferation and migration into the circulation, where they home to the site of ischemia/injury by following the protein concentration gradient. These signaling proteins thus orchestrate recruitment of these reparative progenitor cells from their niches to the tissues in need. Responsiveness to these proteins is impaired in the elderly because of decreased cell surface receptor presentation (e.g., CXCR4) and diminished receptor effectiveness following binding with the signaling protein. The reduced signals for mobilization and homing limit the ability of EPC to even initiate repair. For instance, the EPC from diabetic patients have a reduced capacity to induce angiogenesis in vitro.[21,22] Thus dysvascular patients in dire need of neovascularization are at a severe disadvantage compared to a young healthy patient. Hence, approaches to restore or enhance precursor function are needed to promote angiogenesis more effectively.

Further complicating this problem is the presence of severe arterial disease. Blood flows preferentially around occlusive vascular beds. This not only slows delivery of the signaling protein out of the ischemic tissue on the venous side but also detours mobilized progenitor cells away from the ischemic tissue on the arterial side.

ANGIOGENESIS STRATEGIES

Efforts to address these problems form the basis of the clinical research described below. Strategies include the following:

1. Direct protein injection (VEGF, FGF,...) into ischemic tissue
2. Direct MNC injection into the ischemic muscle
   - A. MNCs are extracted from the patient's bone marrow (BM-MNC)
   - B. MNCs are extracted from the patient's peripheral blood (PB-MNC)
3. MNC arterial embolization into the ischemic limb
4. Boosting the BM and PB MNC count with granulocyte−colony stimulating factor (G-CSF)
5. Combination of a programmed pneumatic compression pump and G-CSF

Strategy 1: Direct Protein Injection Into Ischemic Tissue

Experimental and clinical efficacies were reported early on regarding single factor injection. However, further research is elucidating the complexity of angiogenesis, and single factor stimulus is now regarded as insufficient. For instance, VEGF promotes endothelial tube formation. This alone is insufficient to support meaningful blood flow because of tube fragility. Adding PDGF promotes pericyte migration, strengthening the endothelial tube. Observations such as this are what led to the advancement of cell therapy strategies. MNC infusion into ischemic tissue provides not only EPCs, but also the signaling proteins and structural enzymes enabling the angiogenesis process. Nevertheless, there is a role for pharmacologic enhancement. For example, angiotensin II receptor blockade has been reported to improve EPC proliferation and function.[23]

Strategy 2: Direct Mononuclear Cell Injection Into Ischemic Muscle

In this strategy MNCs are harvested from the bone marrow (BM-MNC) or peripheral blood (PB-MNC) and injected directly into ischemic muscle with a 25- or 27-gauge needle. The 0.75 mL injections are usually 2.5 cm apart, requiring about 50 injections and requiring sedation and analgesia. Patients report increasing warmth and decreasing ischemic pain as early as 1 week later. In our early experience, we harvested 500 mL of marrow from each iliac crest in the operating room. The process is slow (3-5 mL was harvested at a time) to reduce contamination by circulating red blood cells. Many trocar entries at different depths into the iliac crest were required and were done under general anesthesia. A unit of packed red blood cells was usually given to the patient. The marrow was then filtered in the operating room through a 500-micron then a 200-micron filter to remove bone and fat. The effluent was then processed in the stem cell laboratory by differential centrifugation using a CS3000-Plus blood-cell separator (Baxter, Deerfield, IL) to 95% purity over 4 hours and then delivered in a final volume of 40 to 60 mL containing 2 to 3 $\times$ 10^9 MNC. The MNC differential obtained in our patients was lymphocytes 66 $\pm$ 17%, monocytes 22 $\pm$ 11%, and polymorphonuclear leukocytes 10 $\pm$ 8%. The platelet count was 395 $\pm$ 41 $\times$ $10^3/\mu L$. There were 5 $\times$ 3 10^7 CD34$-$ cells (marker for EPC). Thus there was some contamination with platelets, red cells, and neutrophils. Polymorphonuclear leukocyte esterase from neutrophils adversely affects angiogenesis. New cell separators now yield MNC at 30 minutes, although perhaps at a lower purity. They can be used in the operating room right after cell harvest. G-CSF has been used to reduce the volume of marrow to be harvested tenfold (see later discussion),[24] reducing the volume of marrow harvest substantially and permitting the procedure to be done under local anesthesia in a minor operating room environment without transfusion.

Progenitor cell composition influences outcome. For example, the presence of hematopoietic progenitors (erythroblasts and myeloblasts) and lymphocytes favors angiogenesis.[25] In mice, CXCR4(+) BM cells exhibit an increased therapeutic potential for blood flow recovery after acute ischemia. Mechanistically, CXCR4(+) BM cells' higher migratory capacity and their increased release of paracrine factors may contribute to enhanced tissue repair. Supernatants of CXCR4(+) BMCs were reported to be enriched with the proangiogenic cytokines hepatocyte growth factor (HGF) and PDGF-BB.[26] Angiographic evidence of neovascularization in one of our patients is illustrated in Figure 76-1, which shows a foot angiogram just before midfoot amputation for gangrene, and a follow-up angiogram 20 months after MNC injection. MNC injection was *not* the sole therapy applied to this patient, though. This patient also wore a programmable pneumatic compression pump on his leg for 1 hour at a time three times per day for several months, which may have contributed to the excellent angiographic results (see later discussion).

When EPCs are injected into ischemic muscle, incorporation into sites of neovascularization has been reported,[1,5,27-32] though at a much lower rate than initially thought. In fact the survival of the injected cells in the ischemic muscle may in fact be brief (hours to a couple of days) and the observed angiogenesis actually a result of the chemical release of a battery of proangiogenic cytokines. Nevertheless, MNC implantation in ischemic limbs is hypothesized to enhance angiogenesis by supplying the needed reparative progenitor cells in high concentration directly into the ischemic tissue, replete with proangiogenic cytokines. Collateral vessel formation, with incorporation of EPC into new capillaries has been reported in ischemic skeletal muscle and myocardium in animals and in humans. The local concentrations of angiogenic factors (beta-FGF, VEGF, angiopoietin-1), and of angiogenic cytokines (interleukin 10, tumor necrosis factor 10) indeed elevate in the implanted tissues. Differentiation into other lineage cells, such as osteoblasts or fibroblasts, has not been reported.

Since early clinical reports of BM-MNC and PB-MNC intramuscular injection in chronically ischemic limbs, many supportive, albeit often anecdotal reports of limb salvage, ischemic wound healing, diminished ischemic pain, increased exercise tolerance, increased warmth have been presented. These have been corroborated with evidence of improved hemodynamics, increased tissue oxymetry, and even angiographic collateral development.[33-44]

Although PB-MNCs are easier to obtain (phlebotomy) than BM-MNC (bone marrow aspiration), data on equivalent effectiveness are mixed. Only recently have reports been published showing PB-MNC may be as effective as BM-MNC implantation[45-48] One particular cell type, the human PB-MNC CD 31+ cell has been reported to have robust angiogenic and vasculogenic properties.[49]

One of the earliest clinical trials in which BM-MNCs were harvested and injected into ischemic muscle is the Therapeutic Angiogenesis Using Cell Transplantation (TACT) Study.[33] In Group A, saline was injected

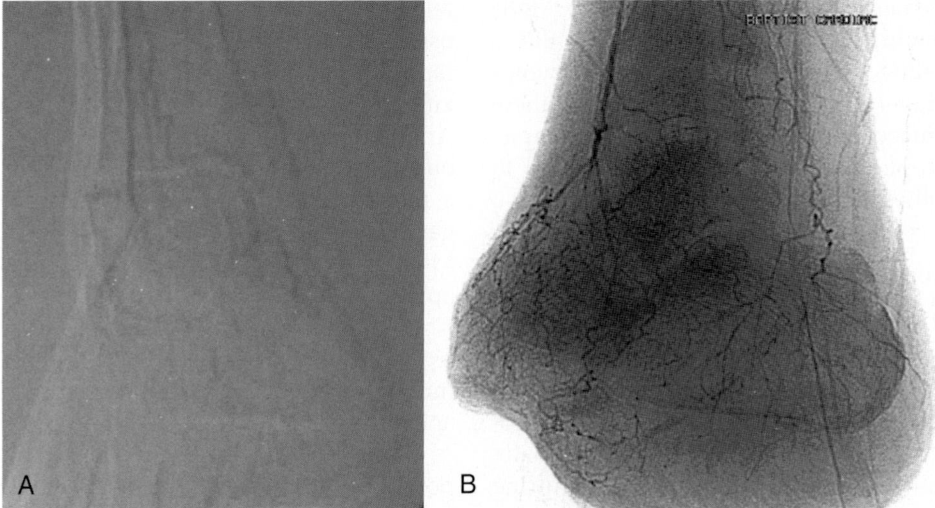

FIGURE 76-1 Angiogram of a foot of a 76-year-old diabetic renal transplant recipient who initially presented with severe rest pain and gangrene of his forefoot. **A,** Pre-MNC injection and preamputation; note the paucity of collateral vessels. **B,** Twenty months after midfoot amputation and injection of BM-MNC into the calf, ankle, and foot, along with use of the Art Assist Device. Neovasculature corresponded with improved hemodynamics, improved $TcPO_2$, and complete healing of an open amputation

into the contralateral limb as a control. The ankle–brachial index (ABI) in legs injected with BM-MNC increased from 0.34 (95% CI 0.27–0.40) at baseline to 0.47 (0.41–0.52) at week 4 in 17 of 25 limbs. No changes in ABI were seen in legs injected with saline. Another 20 patients (group B) with bilateral leg ischemia were randomly injected with BM-MNC in one leg and PB-MNC in the other to assess differences in clinical response. As in Group A, the ABI and the transcutaneous oxygen tension ($TcPO_2$) increased, though less so in the limbs injected with PB-MNC, compared to those injected with BM-MNC. The ischemic rest pain in legs treated with BM-MNC resolved in 16 of 20 patients, but in only 3 of the PB-MNC–treated limbs. Improvements were sustained at 24 weeks for both groups of patients.

This study as well as others performed in Asia and Europe report at least 80% of patients benefit following direct BM-MNC injection into ischemic tissue, without major adverse effects.[5,32] Review articles analyze the use of MNC for the treatment of critical limb ischemia.[50]

We and others have observed that patients with thromboangitis obliterans (Buerger disease) have had a particularly good response to BM-MNC injection in the severely ischemic limb. We attributed part of this benefit to the known benefit of tobacco cessation. However, changes in serum levels of angiogenesis related factors after BM cell infusion are beginning to be reported in these patients.[51] Soluble vascular cell adhesion molecule-1 (sVCAM-1), C-reactive protein (CRP), and adrenomedulin serum levels 24 hours after BM cell infusion were significantly ($p < 0.05$) increased compared with those before treatment. VEGF serum levels significantly increased between 1 week and 3 months after treatment ($p < 0.05$). Adrenomedulin receptor stimulation increases the cellular production of nitric oxide. Nitric oxide serum levels after BMI treatment increased significantly 2 weeks after treatment ($p < 0.05$). Nitric oxide synthase has been shown to have an essential role in mobilizing stem and progenitor cells.[52]

Increasing cellular diversity may be advantageous. In a phase I clinical trial, patients with limb ischemia were infused with a cell product consisting of BM-MNC and mesenchymal stem cells (a source of pericyte progenitors and angiogenic regulators). At 10 months, improvements in walking time, ankle–brachial pressure, and quality of life were reported. Angiographic and 99mTc-TF perfusion scintigraphy scores confirmed increased perfusion in the treated limbs.[41]

Strategy 3: Mononuclear Cell Arterial Embolization Into the Ischemic Limb

It is not clear whether single session intra-arterial catheter injection of MNC into the ischemic limb offers a therapeutic advantage over intramuscular injection. The theoretical advantage of intra-arterial injection is a more uniform distribution of cells in the ischemic limb. The disadvantage is the pass through of a substantial number of cells into the systemic circulation, with trapping in organs. Nevertheless, efficacy in promoting angiogenesis is reported[53] following intra-arterial infusion. Intra-arterial catheter BM cell injection with or without autologous intramuscular BM cell injection was compared.[38] No adverse reactions were reported. Significant and sustained improvement in pain-free walking distance, ABI, and pain score were reported using both regimens. Although a lower rate of amputation was observed in the combination group, this did not reach statistical significance. These data were supported by the Transplantation of Autologous BM-MNC in Patients with Peripheral Arterial Disease Study.[44] A larger study in China found similar improvement of ischemia symptoms following single session intra-arterial and single session intramuscular BM-MNC delivery.[54]

Strategy 4: Boosting the Circulating Progenitor Cell Population

Boosting the circulating progenitor cell count to promote angiogenesis has been investigated as a means to offset the decreased number and function of these cells in the elderly dysvascular patient. G-CSF is a lineage specific colony-stimulating factor produced by monocytes, fibroblasts, and endothelial cells (ECs). G-CSF is not species specific and has been shown to have minimal direct in vivo or in vitro effects on the production of hematopoietic cell types other than the neutrophil and monocyte lineage. G-CSF is indicated for the mobilization of hematopoietic progenitor cells into the peripheral blood for collection by leukapheresis (Food and Drug Administration [FDA] approved), to be used for bone marrow rescue following chemotherapy. Following G-GSF administration, the circulating number of these progenitor cells is increased dramatically. Granulocyte-macrophage colony-stimulating factor (GM-CSF) has also been used clinically and experimentally for the mobilization of increased numbers of progenitor cells capable of engraftment.

Until the late 1980s GM-CSF and G-CSF were only considered to be hematopoietic growth and differentiation factors. Bussolino et al.[55] reported that endothelial cells (EC) respond to these cytokines too. Both induce EC to proliferate and migrate and stimulate repair of mechanically wounded endothelial monolayers.[55,56] Bussolino et al went on to study the angiogenic activity of human G-CSF in the rabbit cornea. G-CSF had definite proangiogenic activity without any sign of inflammatory reaction. They concluded that G-CSF and GM-CSF induce EC to express an activation and differentiation program (including proliferation and migration) related to angiogenesis.

BOOSTING THE CIRCULATING PROGENITOR CELL POPULATION: ISCHEMIC LIMB ANIMAL DATA

Takagi et al.[57] reported that 100 mg/kg per day of G-CSF augments neovascularization following BM-MNC (1×10^7 cells) transplantation (BMT) in rat hind limb ischemia. One week after unilateral hind limb ischemia was surgically induced in Lewis rats, the laser Doppler blood perfusion index (LDBPI), the number of angiographically detectable collateral vessels, and the capillary density determined by alkaline phosphatase staining increased significantly in the BMT/G-CSF group versus the BMT alone group. G-CSF significantly increased VEGF mRNA and FGF-2 mRNA in the hind limb muscle.

Grundmann et al[58] hypothesized that intra-arterial cytokine application using implantable infusion pumps may stimulate arteriogenesis in a large-species model of peripheral vascular disease. They also compared continuous and intermittent infusion. Twenty-four pigs underwent unilateral occlusion of the right femoral artery and received either GM-CSF continuously, GM-CSF intermittently, or phosphate-buffered saline (PBS). After 1 week, collateral conductance was determined under maximal vasodilatation with adenosine and by using a pump-driven extracorporal shunt system. Conductance showed a significant stimulatory effect of GM-CSF on arteriogenesis. Flow measurements under reactive hyperemia were consistent with these results. Measurements of ankle–brachial indices were not sensitive enough to detect the differences in collateral growth between the three groups. These results demonstrated the proarteriogenic properties of GM-CSF in a pig model, revealing comparable efficacy of continuous and intermittent intra-arterial infusion using an implantable pump. They also showed that ABI is an insensitive measure to determine angiogenesis compared with flow or combined flow-pressure measurements.

Ohki et al.[59] demonstrated that local G-CSF administration into ischemic tissue increased capillary density. VEGF induces EPC mobilization. Blockade of the VEGF pathway blocked G-CSF-induced angiogenesis. Blocking the VEGF/VEGFR1, but to a much lesser extent, the VEGF/VEGFR2 pathway in G-CSF-treated animals delayed tissue revascularization in a hind limb model. G-CSF modulates angiogenesis by increasing myelomonocytic cells (VEGFR1+ neutrophils) and their release of VEGF. G-CSF augmented the number of circulating VEGF receptor-2 (VEGFR2) EPCs compared with untreated controls. Ohki et al.[59] concluded that G-CSF injection into ischemic tissue provides a novel and safe therapeutic strategy to improve neovascularization.

Zhang et al.[60] investigated BM-MNC and PB-MNC for therapeutic angiogenesis in the ischemic hind limb of mice. One month after injection of BM-MNC into the ischemic limb muscle, laser Doppler analysis showed that the blood flow ratio was significantly increased (0.67 ± 0.02 vs. 0.44 ± 0.02). Alkaline phosphatase and immunohistochemical analyses showed that capillary density increased significantly ($95.25 \pm 0.07\%$ vs. $39.6 \pm 0.04\%$). Zhang et al.[60] then treated 15 patients with nonhealing arterial ulceration with subcutaneous injections of G-CSF to mobilize progenitor cells. PB-MNC were harvested and transplanted directly into the ischemic limb. Six ulcers healed. Two months after PB-MNC implantation, ankle–brachial index, walking distance, pain scale, and $TcPO_2$ were significantly improved ($p < 0.005$).

Jeon et al.[61] hypothesized that combined angiogenic therapies may be superior to monotherapy for the treatment of limb ischemia. One day after the surgical induction of hind limb ischemia, mice were randomized to receive no treatment, EPC mobilization with G-CSF administration, BM-MNC transplantation using a fibrin matrix, or a combination of EPC mobilization with BM-MNC transplantation using a fibrin matrix. Microvessel density and β-FGF and VEGF expression were all significantly increased except in the nontreatment group and were highest in the combined EPC mobilization and BM-MNC transplantation group. This study demonstrated that the combination of BM-MNC transplantation and EPC mobilization potentiates the angiogenic efficacy of either therapy alone in the mouse hind limb ischemia model.

Ieda et al.[62] investigated whether 10 days of subcutaneous G-CSF by itself or in combination with intra–ischemic muscular injection of HGF plasmid can promote vasculogenesis and angiogenesis. Hind limb ischemia was induced in BALB/c nude or C57/BL6 mice that received BM transplantation from green fluorescent protein (GFP)-transgenic mice. The G-CSF+HGF group had a higher laser Doppler blood perfusion index, higher microvessel density, and a lower incidence of hind limb necrosis than the other groups. Confocal laser microscopy revealed that GFP-positive cells were visible in the vasculature of the ischemic area. Some of the GFP positive cells were clearly co-immunostained with α smooth muscle actin as well as von Willebrand factor. G-CSF–mobilized stem cells coexpressed CD49d and CD34, which would have promoted their adhesion to cells in the ischemic muscle that expressed HGF-induced VCAM-1. The combination of G-CSF and HGF had a significant synergistic effect, suggesting that the combination of mobilization of BM stem cells to the peripheral circulation, and their recruitment to the ischemic area potentiate angiogenesis and vasculogenesis.

We reported our results using a murine model to study the effect of stroma-derived factor 1 (SDF-1) on promoting angiogenesis. This is an important signaling protein that is produced from distressed tissue and helps recruit reparative cells from their niches throughout the body. Hind limb ischemia was created by femoral artery and vein resection in BL6 mice.[63,64] NIH 3T3/SDF-1 cells (NIH 3T3 mouse fibroblasts retrovirally transduced with the SDF-1 gene) were injected into the ischemic hind limb musculature to increase production of SDF-1. G-CSF (Neupogen, 25 mcg/kg/day) was injected intraperitioneally daily for 3 days after surgery to stimulate progenitor cell mobilization into the circulation. Angiogenesis was measured as the recovery of blood flow using laser Doppler blood perfusion imaging (LDBPI) (Figure 76-2, *A*). The LDPI perfusion ratio was significantly higher in the SDF-1 alone group and the G-CSF alone group compared to the saline injected control group 3 weeks after surgery. Combined treatment with both SDF-1 and G-CSF resulted in an even better perfusion ratio versus the single treatment groups. Mice were sacrificed 21 days after surgery. More CD34− cells, increased capillary density, and less apoptotic muscle cells were found in both G-CSF and SDF-1 treated groups ($p < 0.05$ vs. other groups) (Figure 76-2, *B*). These data support the notion that the combination of G-CSF–mediated progenitor cell mobilization and SDF-1–mediated homing of EPC promotes neovascularization in the ischemic limb and increases the recovery of blood perfusion. To demonstrate the source of the progenitor cells that participate in neovascularization in the ischemic limb, mice whose BM had been replaced with BM from GFP mice underwent femoral vessel resection. Green fluorescent cells present in the ischemic muscle were observed at the ischemic site (Figure 76-3, *A*). GFP+ cells were confirmed by immunostaining using anti-GFP Ab (Figure 3, *C*). GFP+ cells co-localized with CD34+ marker using either immunofluorescence staining (Figure 76-3, *B*) or immunochemical staining (Figure 76-3, *D*), suggesting that at least some of the BM-derived progenitor cells participate directly in angiogenesis in the ischemic mouse limb. To further characterize the fate of engrafted cells, BM cells from Tie2-lacZ transgenic mice were transplanted into wild-type mice intravenously after femoral vessel ligation. Significantly more X-gal–positive cells were detected in the ischemic muscles (Figure 76-4, *A*) than in the nonischemic muscles (Figure 76-4, **C**) 1 week after surgery. Because the lacZ gene in the injected BM cells is controlled by the EC specific Tie2 promoter, the X-gal positive cells are EC cells. This was further confirmed by alkaline phosphatase staining on the same slide (Figure 76-4, *B*). These data indicate that BM cells can home to the ischemic site, and that some differentiate into EC in mice.

BOOSTING THE CIRCULATING PROGENITOR CELL POPULATION: ISCHEMIC LIMB CLINICAL TRIALS

Kudo et al.[65] injected PB-EPCs into both ischemic limbs of two patients (1.0×10^5 and 1.6×10^5 CD34+ cells/mL) pretreated with G-CSF in whom reconstruction was not possible.[65] $TcPO_2$ in each limb increased

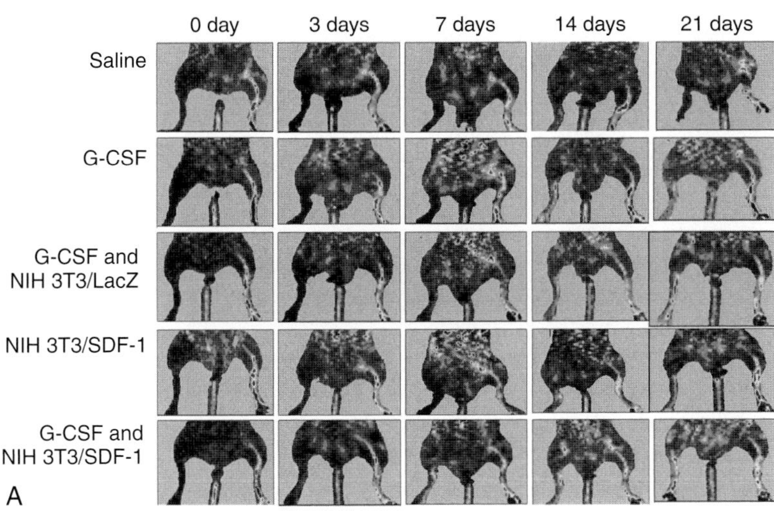

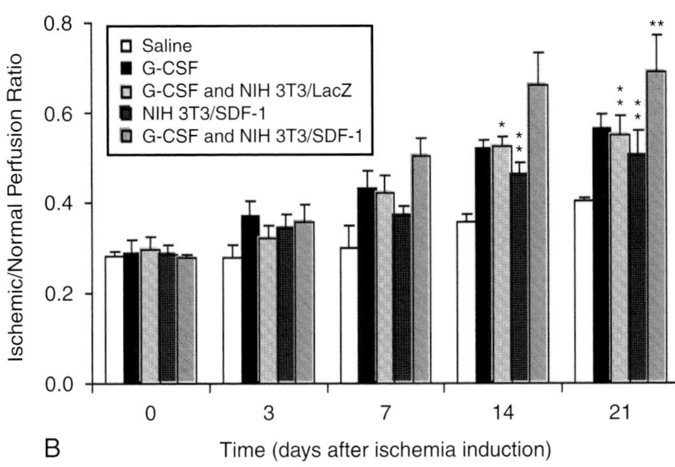

FIGURE 76-2 Effect of G-CSF and SDF-1 on reperfusion in ischemic hind limb of mice. The blood flow of the lower limbs was measured using an LDPI analyzer, followed by calculation of the perfusion ratio of the ischemic limbs (right) to normal limbs (left). **A,** Representative LDPI images at indicated time points. **B,** Quantitative measurement of perfusion ratio of ischemic limbs to that of normal limbs (n = 6). $*p < 0.05$ versus saline group. $**p < 0.05$ versus G-CSF–treated and SDF-1– treated groups.

and clinical symptoms improved. Newly visible collateral blood vessels were seen on angiogram.

Kawamura et al.[66] treated 92 patients with critical limb ischemia with approximately 4.0×10^7 CD34+ PB-MNCs. The PB-MNCs were mobilized into the circulation by G-CSF, collected by apheresis, and centrifuged. The cell suspension was injected into the ischemic muscle of limbs at 50 to 70 sites (0.5-1 mL at each site). At 6 weeks, CD34+ and factor VIII staining were strong and correlated with capillary formation. The mean serum VEGF level increased 176%. Of 11 nondiabetic patients (DM(−)) who were not receiving hemodialysis (HD(−)), there were no amputees. Of 19 patients in the HD(+)DM(−) category, there were no amputations in Fontaine stage I, II, and III patients, whereas three limbs and one toe were amputated in Fontaine stage IV patients. Of 13 patients in the HD(−)DM(+) category, none of the Fontaine stage I, II, or III patients underwent amputation, but 6 Fontaine stage IV patients underwent amputation. Of 49 patients in the HD(+) DM(+) category, 38 (78%) were Fontaine stage IV, 71% (27/38) of whom had a toe or a limb amputation. In 9 patients older than 80 years of age, one toe and one limb were amputated. Kawamura et al.[66] concluded that diabetes and/or renal failure adversely affect limb salvage of Fontaine class IV patients using stem cell transplantation.

Van Royen et al.[67] evaluated the effects of GM-CSF in patients with peripheral artery disease in a double-blinded, randomized, placebo-controlled study in 40 patients with moderate or severe intermittent claudication. No benefit was observed. However, for optimal angiogenesis, severe ischemia resulting in continual release of signaling proteins would seem necessary. Patients with claudication are significantly ischemic only on exertion. Moreover, the level of ischemia typically falls off within minutes of cessation of exercise. Therefore claudicants may not be optimal patients for this strategy. Patients with chronic critical limb ischemia (forefoot rest pain, tissue loss) have ischemia all day long, and are the most optimal candidates.

Huang et al.[68] assessed safety, efficacy, and feasibility of autologous transplantation of G-CSF–mobilized PB-MNC in the treatment of critical limb ischemia in 28

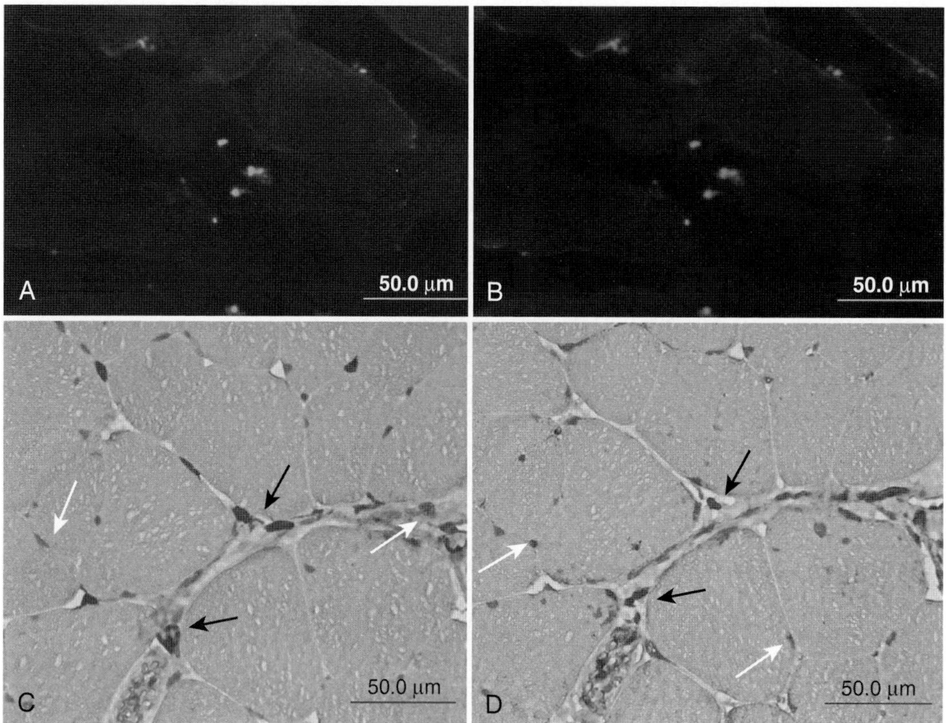

FIGURE 76-3 Identification of BM cells in ischemic muscle. GFP cells from BM were detected in ischemic muscle by direct fluorescent microscopy **(A)** and immunochemical staining **(C)**. GFP cells are co-localized with CD34 marker by immunofluorescence staining **(B)** and immunochemical staining **(D)** on a continuous section of **(C)**. *Black arrows* point to cells that are positive for both GFP and CD34. Brown: positively stained for GFP **(C)** or CD34 **(D)**, purple: negative cell *(white arrow)*.

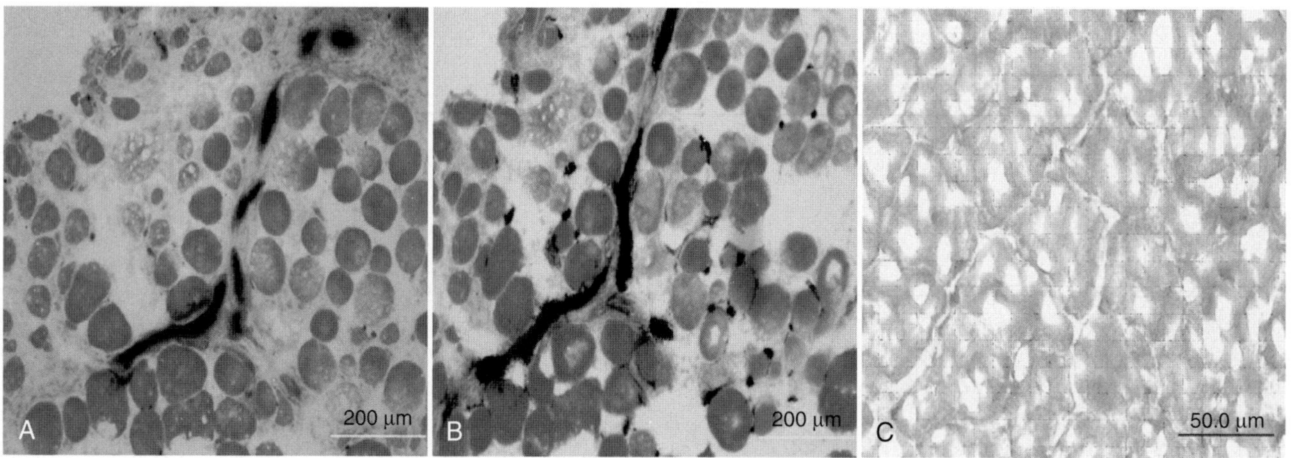

FIGURE 76-4 BM cell differentiation into EC after engrafted into ischemic muscle. BM cells from Tie2-lacZ transgenic mouse were IV injected into WT mouse after ischemic surgery. X-gal staining of ischemic **(A)** and nonischemic **(C)** muscle recovered one week after surgery. The ischemic sample **(A)** was further stained for alkaline phosphatase **(B)**.

diabetic patients. Half were randomized to receive recombinant human G-CSF (600 mcg/day) subcutaneously for 5 days. Their PB-MNCs were collected and transplanted by multiple intramuscular injections into the ischemic limbs. At the end of 3 months, lower limb pain and ulceration were significantly improved in the patients in the transplant group. The laser Doppler blood perfusion of lower limbs increased from 0.44 ± 0.11 to 0.57 ± 0.14 perfusion units (p <0.001). Mean ABI increased from 0.50 ± 0.21 to 0.63 ± 0.25 (p <0.001). A total of 14 of 18 limb ulcers (77.8%) of transplanted patients were completely healed after cell transplantation, whereas only 38.9% of limb ulcers (7/18) were healed in the control patients ($p < 0.016$ vs. the transplant group). No adverse effects from cell transplantation were observed, and no lower limb amputation occurred in the patients who underwent transplant procedures. In contrast, five control patients had lower limb amputation ($p < 0.007$, transplant vs. control group). Angiographic scores were significantly improved in the transplant group compared with the control group ($p < 0.003$).

Gu et al.[24] reported a large series of 145 ischemic limbs treated in 129 patients with BM-MNC. Group 1 patients (N = 35, 43 limbs) were pretreated with G-CSF 300 mcg/day for 2 days. Group 2 patients were not (N = 94, 102 limbs). Presenting limb symptoms were gangrene (Gp1 N = 7 limbs, Gp2 N = 22), ischemic ulcer (Gp1 N = 12, Gp2 N = 23), ischemic rest pain (Gp1 N = 19, Gp2 N = 41), claudication (Gp1 N = 5, Gp2 N = 13). MNCs were isolated by gradient density centrifugation from BM aspirated from the iliac crest (196 ± 17 mL in Gp1, 377 ± 39 mL in Gp2). They were returned to the patient either by intra-arterial infusion in the popliteal artery or intramuscularly in the ischemic calf. The patients were reevaluated 2 months later. G-CSF boosted the MNC yield ($p < 0.001$) to $5.6 \pm 2.1 \times 10^9$/L cells in Gp1 (range 1–9 $\times 10^9$/L) from $1.0 \pm 0.9 \times 10^9$/L in Gp2 (range 0.6–6.7 $\times 10^9$/L). This represents a 10.8-fold increase in MNC per milliliter of BM harvested. $TcPO_2$ increased equally in both groups. The ABI also improved more than 0.15 in 44% of Gp1 versus 33% of Gp2 limbs ($\xi^2 = 1.36$, $p = 0.215$), as did the walking distance. Symptom resolution in Gp1 versus Gp 2 was complete in 39% versus 35% and partial in 56% versus 49% of limbs. The authors concluded that autologous BM-MNC implantation has a therapeutic effect in the treatment of lower limb ischemia. G-CSF increases the yield of BM-MNC in the harvested BM 10.8 fold, reducing the amount of BM needed to be harvested significantly.

Long-term data regarding the clinical effect of treating critical limb ischemia with G-CSF mobilized autologous PB-MNC are becoming available.[47] During a 5-year period (2001–2006), 50 of 162 patients so treated died. The median follow-up time for surviving patients was 26.4 months. The 2-year survival rate was 65% for the 140 patients with arteriosclerosis (ASO) and 100% for the 11, 4, and 7 patients with thromboangiitis obliterans (TAO), diabetic gangrene (DG), and connective tissue disease (CTD), respectively. The 1-year amputation-free rates for ASO, TAO, DG and CTD were 70%, 79%, 75%, and 83%, respectively. Common serious adverse events included heart failure (15 cases), myocardial infarction (15 cases), serious infection (13 cases), stroke (10 cases), and malignant tumor (9 cases). Significant negative prognostic factors associated with overall survival were ischemic heart disease and collection of a small number of CD34+ cells. Factors associated with time to amputation and amputation-free survival were a combination of Fontaine classification and lower limb gangrene and history of dialysis.

Strategy 5: G-CSF and the Programmed Pneumatic Compression Device

In our latest effort to address the diminished number and function of circulating reparative progenitor cells in the elderly dysvascular patient, and to overcome the impaired rate of presentation of these cells to the ischemic tissue as a result of arterial disease, we treated patients with severe limb threatening ischemia with an intermittent programmable pneumatic compression device (PPCD) during a prolonged period of exposure to G-CSF.[69] This is the least invasive and potentially least expensive approach to arteriogensesis and can be accomplished at home. It is the only approach that addresses both the biologic problem and the hemodynamic problem at the same time.

The ArtAssist Device (ACI Medical, Inc., San Marcos, CA) is a PPCD used to increase arterial blood flow in patients with severe limb ischemia patients.[70-73] Sequential venous emptying under calf, ankle, and foot pneumatic compression cuffs increases the arteriovenous gradient locally, which lowers the resistance across the capillary network and increases blood flow into the ischemic tissue. Additionally, the rapid cuff inflation is believed to cause the endothelium to release nitric oxide, a powerful vasodilator[74,75] and stimulator of arteriogenesis (the formation and widening of medium-sized blood vessels).[76] The patient must be seated during use. The duration of each treatment is 1 hour at a time, for a minimum of 3 hours daily. Use continues until the ischemic wounds heal, and pain is relieved.

External counter pulsation therapy has been used clinically to relieve angina and improve myocardial ischemia in patients with refractory angina pectoris. Efficacy has been associated with increased number and colony forming units of circulating EPCs.[77] Whether this happens with PPCD use for limb ischemia is in the process of being determined. The association of PPCD use with arteriogenesis has been inferred from angiography,[78] sustained improved arterial hemodynamics, and increased skin perfusion.[79] However, PPCD use is associated with variable outcomes, particularly in elderly patients with diabetes, renal failure, and/or congestive heart failure (CHF). We believe this in part may be attributed to the reduced number and function of circulating reparative progenitor cells in these populations, and as discussed earlier, could in part be offset by the administration of G-CSF. We used Filgrastim (Amgen, Thousand Oaks, CA) administered subcutaneously at a dose of 10 mcg/kg once every 3 days for a total of 10 doses. This differs from the FDA-approved dose

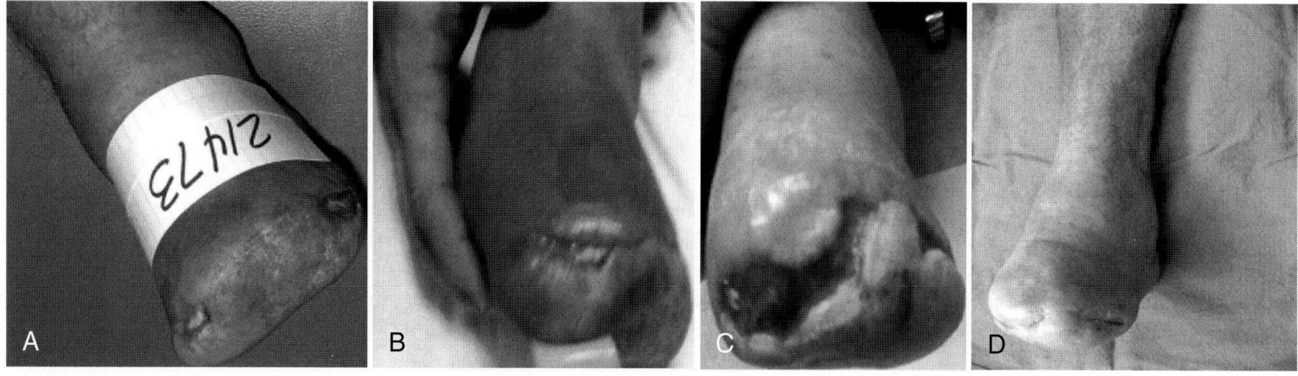

FIGURE 76-5 *Patient 1:* Serial images of transmetatarsal wound. **A,** 1 month after femoral peroneal graft occlusion and outflow embolization following balloon angioplasty of a graft stenosis. **B,** 2 weeks after A: Amputation wound necrosis continues. **C,** 6 weeks after A: Granulation tissue beginning to form after wound completely opened. **D,** Wound healed after 5 months using the ArtAssist device and 10 G-CSF injections in the first month.

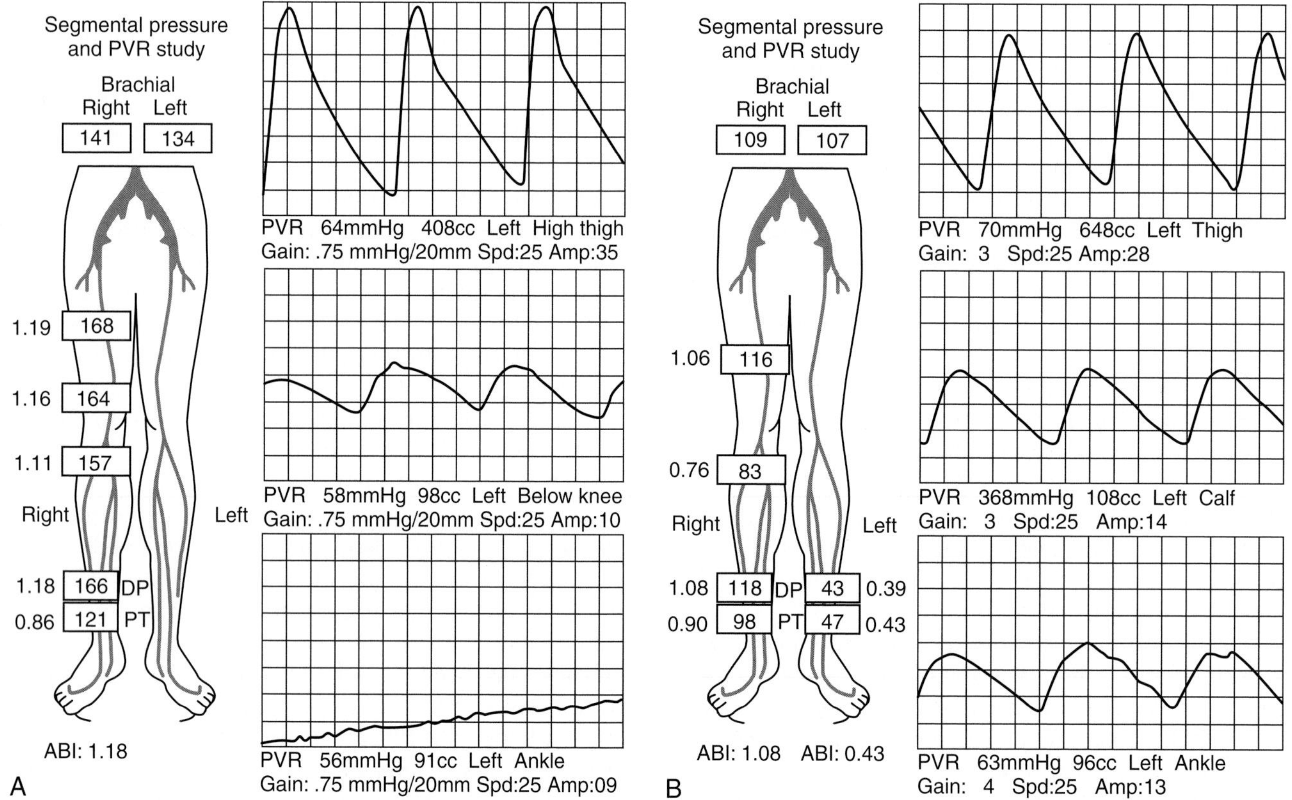

FIGURE 76-6 *Patient 1:* Pulse volume recordings. **A,** Ankle–brachial Index (ABI) was 0 (9/25/2009), and there was no pulsatility at the ankle level before enrollment. **B,** ABI = 0.43 on 4/8/2009, and pulsatility returned at the left ankle. **C,** ABI = 0.64 on 6/3/2009.

for stem cell mobilization in oncology applications: 10 mcg/kg daily, followed by plasmapheresis on day 5. The reason is that our protocol does not require plasmapheresis. We expect the concentration of reparative progenitor cells to increase dramatically following G-CSF dosing, followed by homing of a significant number of these cells to the ischemic tissues elaborating the appropriate signaling proteins (e.g., SDF-1). The PPCD helps drive the circulation through the ischemic bed, increasing progenitor cell presentation there. In our experience, the white blood cell count rose 4 to 7 fold the first day after a dose (28–50 $\times$ 10^3 cells per mL) and dropped to 2 to 4 fold the second day. We administer the G-CSF every third day. By giving 10 doses, the effect was extended throughout the first month of PPCD use. Our 72-hour dosing interval may also reduce the rare

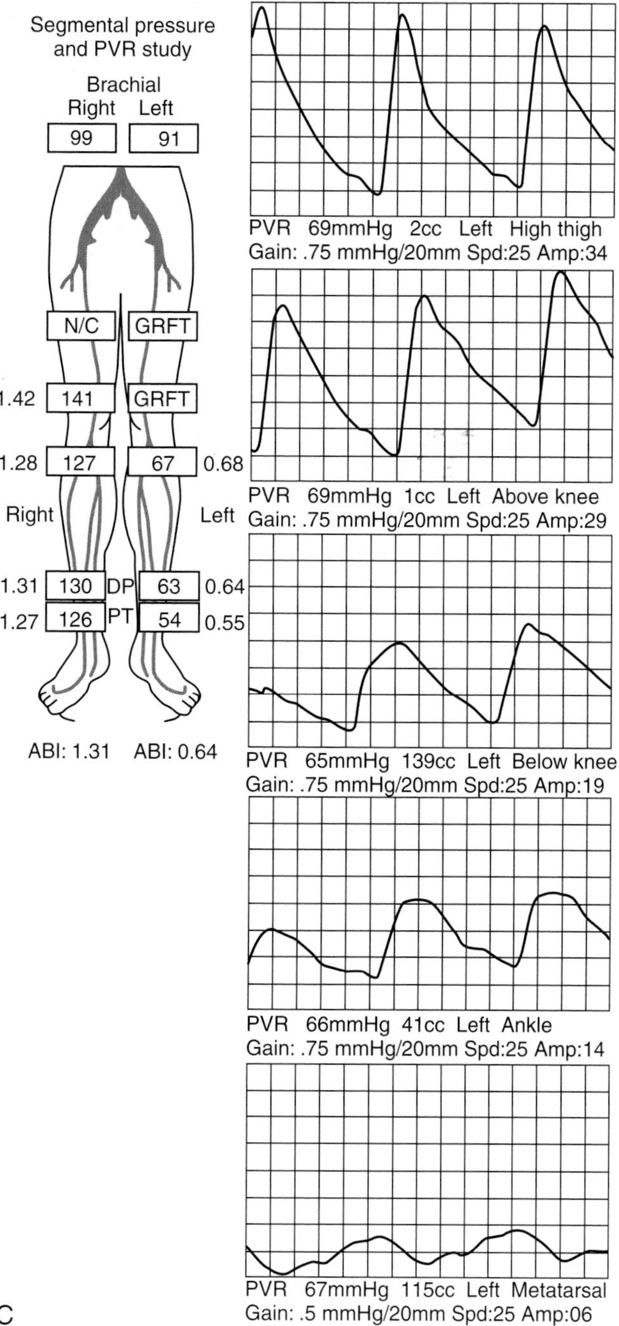

FIGURE 76-6—cont'd

incidence of myocardial infarction and splenic rupture reported with G-CSF. Two patient clinical courses are summarized in the following section.

Patient 1 is an active 56-year-old white man who developed necrosis of a previously healed transmetatarsal amputation (TMA). His history includes bilateral carotid endarterectomy, coronary artery revascularization (CABG), and femoral-peroneal bypass with TMA for forefoot gangrene. He is human immunodeficiency virus (HIV) positive and is on antiretroviral therapy. His viral counts were undetectable. During surveillance of the graft, progressive stenosis of the conduit led to catheter angioplasty 6 months after surgery. This was complicated by distal graft occlusion and outflow embolization. His healed TMA wound completely dehisced. In lieu of BKA, he consented to the combined strategy of G-CSF and use of the PPCD, with approval from his HIV physician. Enrollment started October 17, 2008. The open TMA wound (Figure 76-5) was managed with Silvercel (Johnson & Johnson, Warren, NJ), and

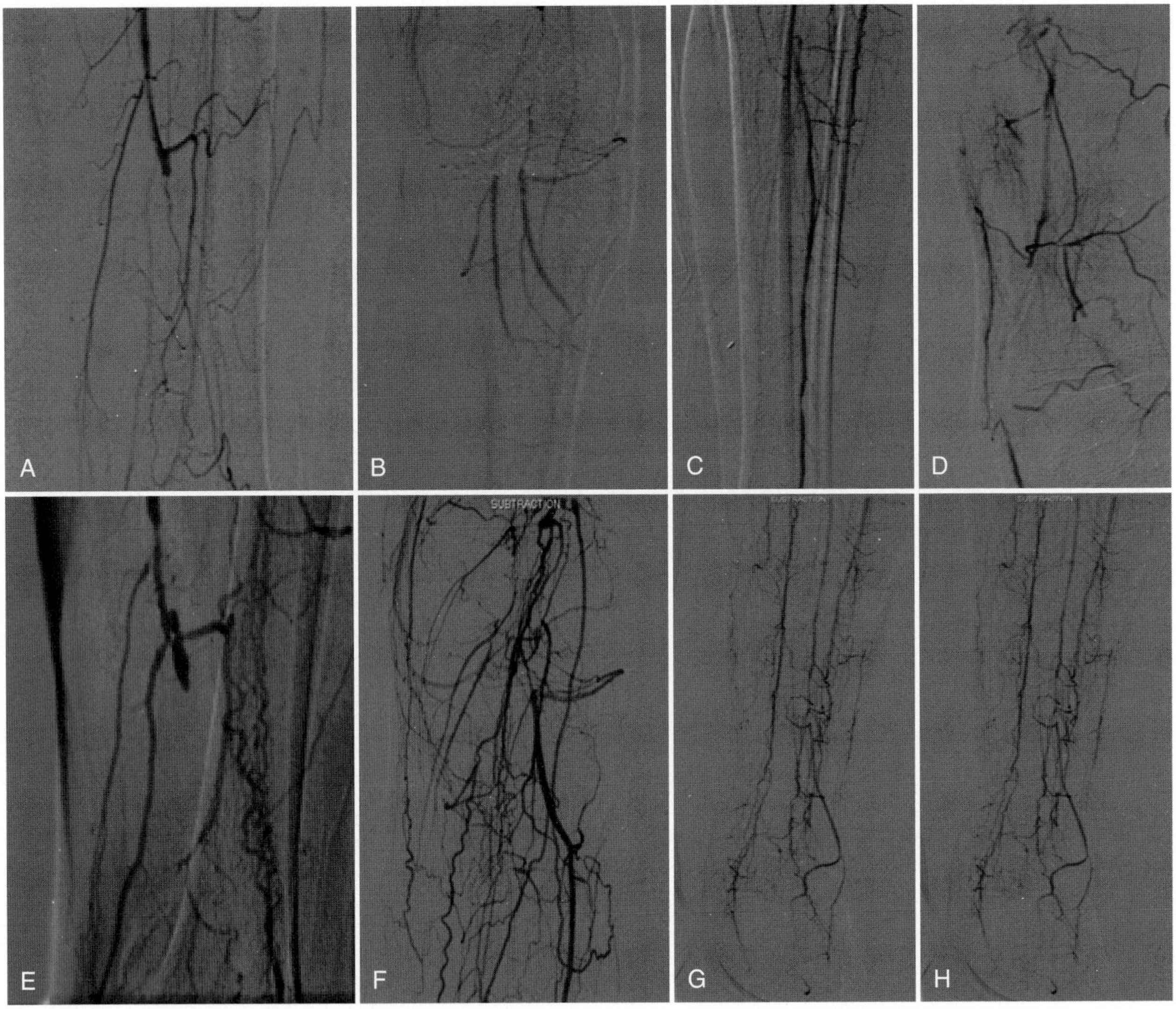

FIGURE 76-7 *Patient 1:* Angiography. **A** to **D** were obtained on initial referral. **E** to **H** were obtained at 6-month follow-up. Note increased collateral vessels at all levels from above knee (**E** vs. **A**), below knee (**F** vs. **B**), calf (**G** vs. **C**), and ankle (**H** vs. **D**).

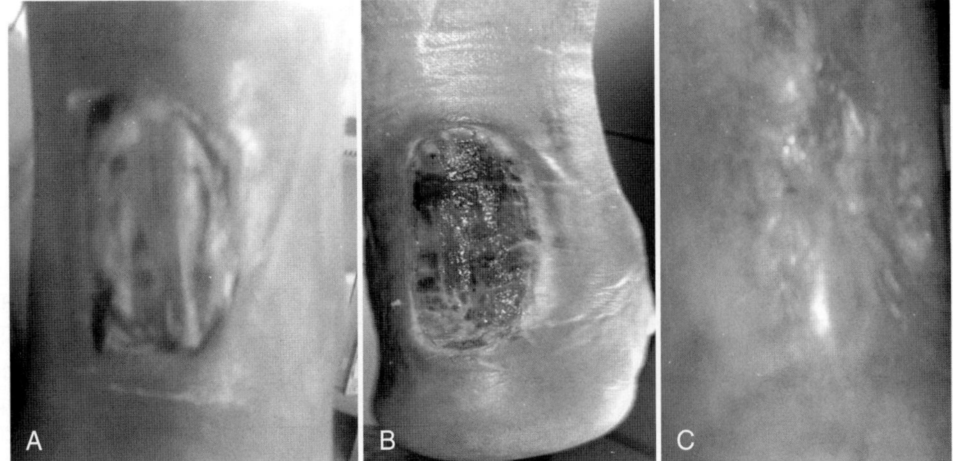

FIGURE 76-8 *Patient 2:* Exposed Achilles tendon. **A,** On presentation. **B,** 5 months later. **C,** 1 year later.

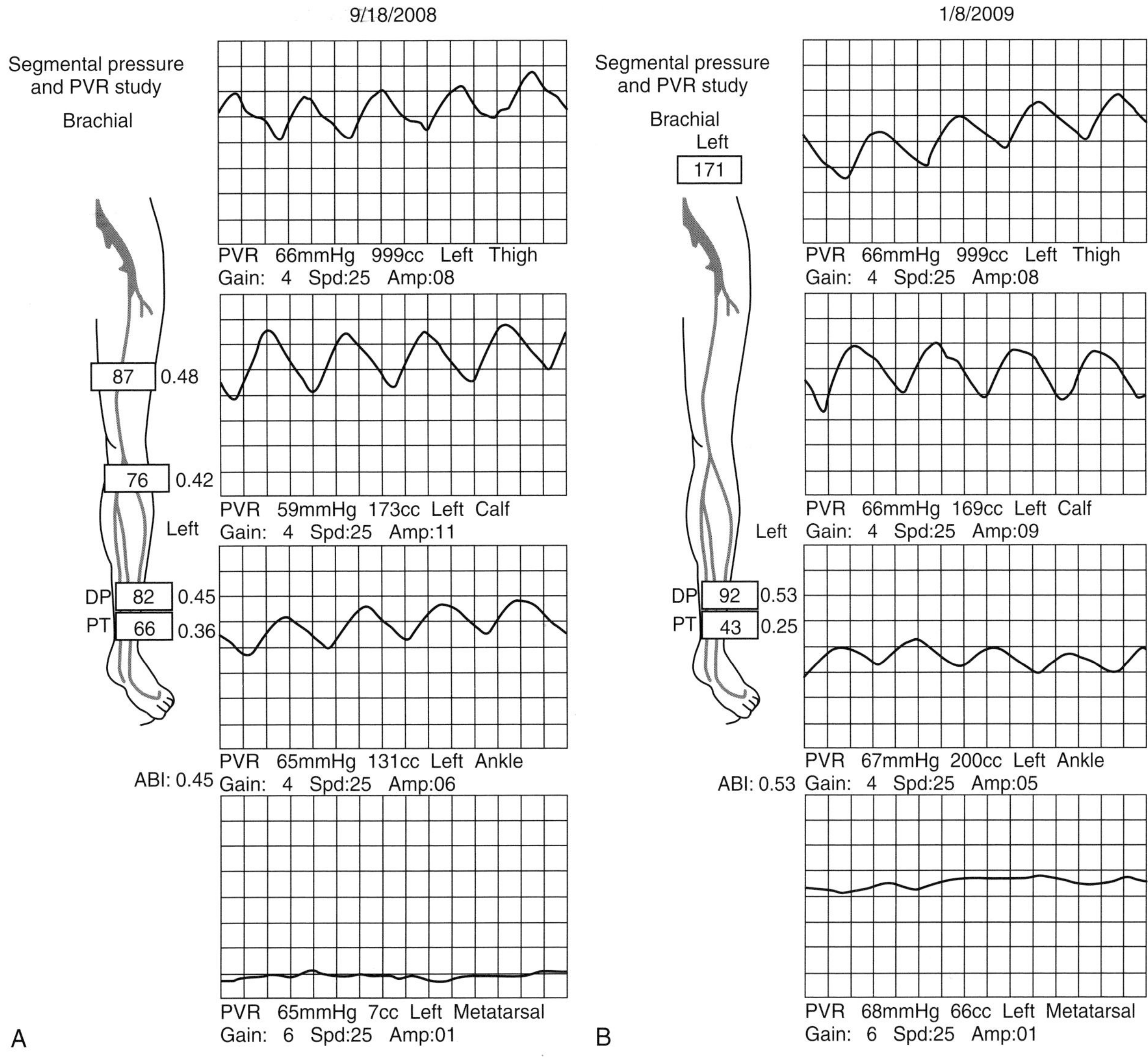

FIGURE 76-9 *Patient 2:* Pulse volume recordings. **A,** Before enrollment: No pulsatility at the transmetatarsal level on the left (9/18/2008), ABI = 0.43. **B,** ABI = 0.53 on 1/8/2009. It rose to 0.58 on 4/8/2009 (not shown). **C,** ABI = 0.67 on 11/18/2009. **D,** ABI = 1.05 on 6/15/2010.

eventually healed. The $TcPO_2$ on the foot dorsum rose from 3 mm Hg preenrollment to 24 mm Hg (April 8, 2009). The ABI rose from 0 (September 25, 2008) to 0.43 (April 8, 2009) to 0.64 (June 3, 2009). Ankle pulsatility was absent on enrollment, but was observed on the April 8, 2009 and June 3, 2009 pulse volume recording (PVR, Figure 76-6). Figure 76-7 shows the remarkable neovascularization by angiography.

Patient 2 is a 44-year-old morbidly obese woman with insulin-dependent diabetes and a history of CABG, renal insufficiency, and CHF, who was referred after her second failed left leg bypass. She had exposed Achilles tendon, a dorsal ankle ulcer, and ischemic rest pain. Superficial femoral, popliteal, and tibial artery occlusive disease reduced her ABI to 0.4. Previous iliac stents had been placed for ipsilateral external iliac artery stenoses. She was enrolled October 7, 2008. An equine pericardium (Pegassus, Irvine, CA) was applied for 5 weeks, then removed. AlloDerm (LifeCell, Branchburg, NJ) was applied after a 1-month hiatus and removed 4 weeks later. Silvercel was applied when there was no biologic dressing. Figure 76-8 shows the healing progression of the large ulcer over her exposed Achilles tendon. The preenrollment $TcPO_2$ measured from the skin overlying the medial calcaneous and on the foot dorsum was 23 mm Hg (September 18, 2008) and 1 mm Hg (October 7, 2008), respectively. These rose to 46 and 35 mm Hg (September 22, 2009). No pulsatility was recorded on her preenrollment PVR at the metatarsal level (September 18, 2008), at which time her ABI was 0.43. Pulsatility was seen at this level on August 17, 2009, at which time her ABI was 0.64 (Figure 76-9). By

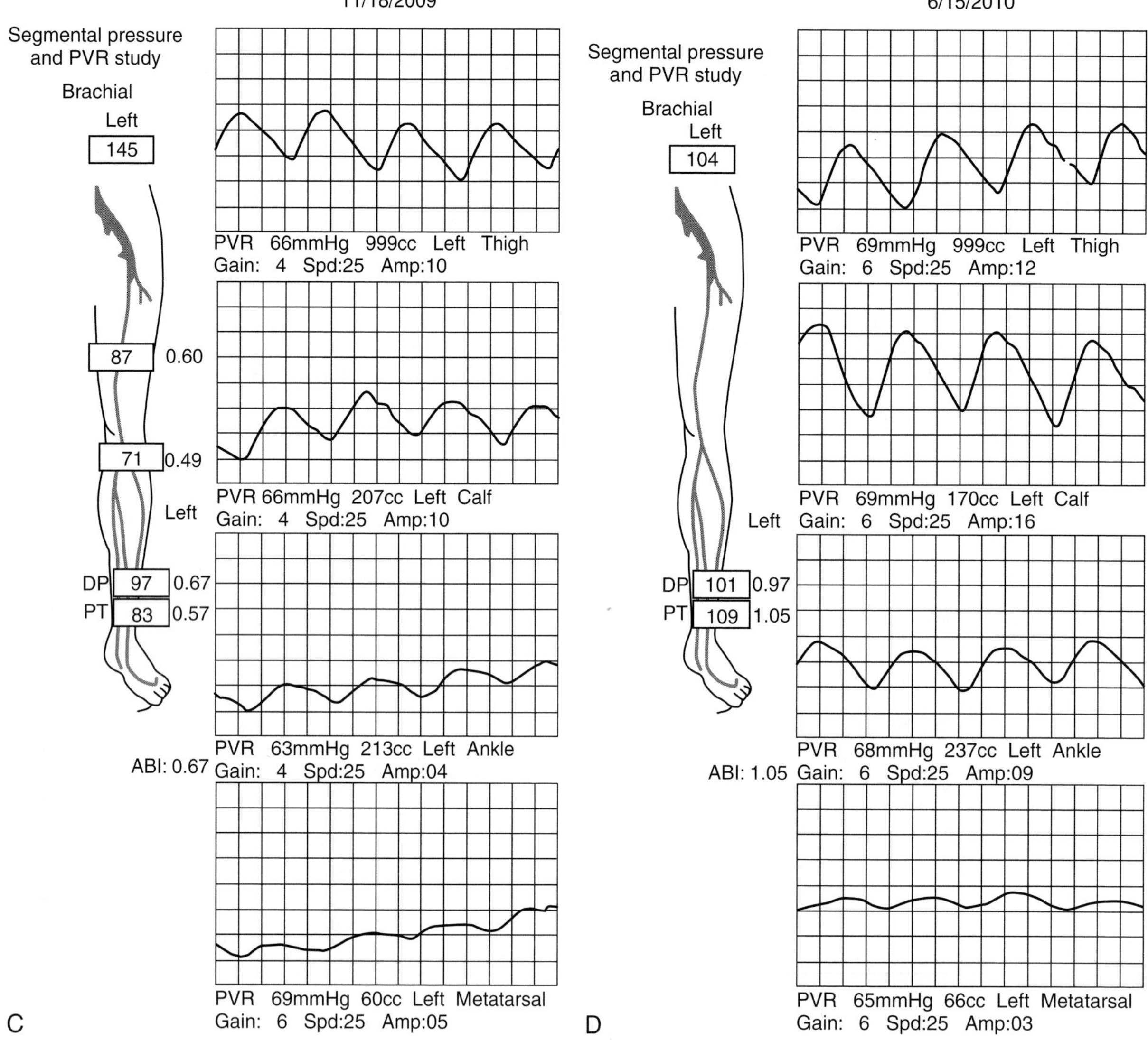

FIGURE 76-9—cont'd

November 18, 2009, her ABI rose to 0.67, and on June 15, 2010 her ABI rose to 1.05. Most important, her digital photoplethysmography tracings (Figure 76-10) were nearly flat in all five toes of her left foot until November 18, 2009, at which time pulsatility is observed in digit 1, and by June 15, 2010 she has perceptible pulsatility in all five toes. Figure 76-11 shows the neovascularization by angiography.

Healing of a dehisced TMA wound (Patient 1) or an ankle wound with exposed Achilles tendon (Patient 2) would be challenging even in the setting of good arterial perfusion. That healing occurred in the setting of severe ischemia suggests efficacy. Healing correlated with hemodynamic and angiographic evidence of neovascularization. This occurred despite severe comorbidities in both patients—coronary artery disease in both, and renal insufficiency, diabetes and congestive heart failure in Patient 2. Nevertheless, our experience is limited, and a control group was not part of this compassionate use evaluation. Moreover, the preoperative angiograms were provided by the referring institutions, using different equipment and contrast injection protocols than the final angiograms.

Nevertheless, this technique has many advantages. As discussed earlier in this chapter, investigators have attempted to promote neovascularization by delivering large numbers of progenitor cells directly into ischemic tissue in a single session, either by multiple intramuscsular injections or by arterial embolization. Our approach avoids the associated costly and invasive hospital-based BM harvest, ex vivo cell processing, and cell reinjection required in these neovascularization strategies. Moreover, our approach overcomes the problems of nonuniform progenitor cell distribution

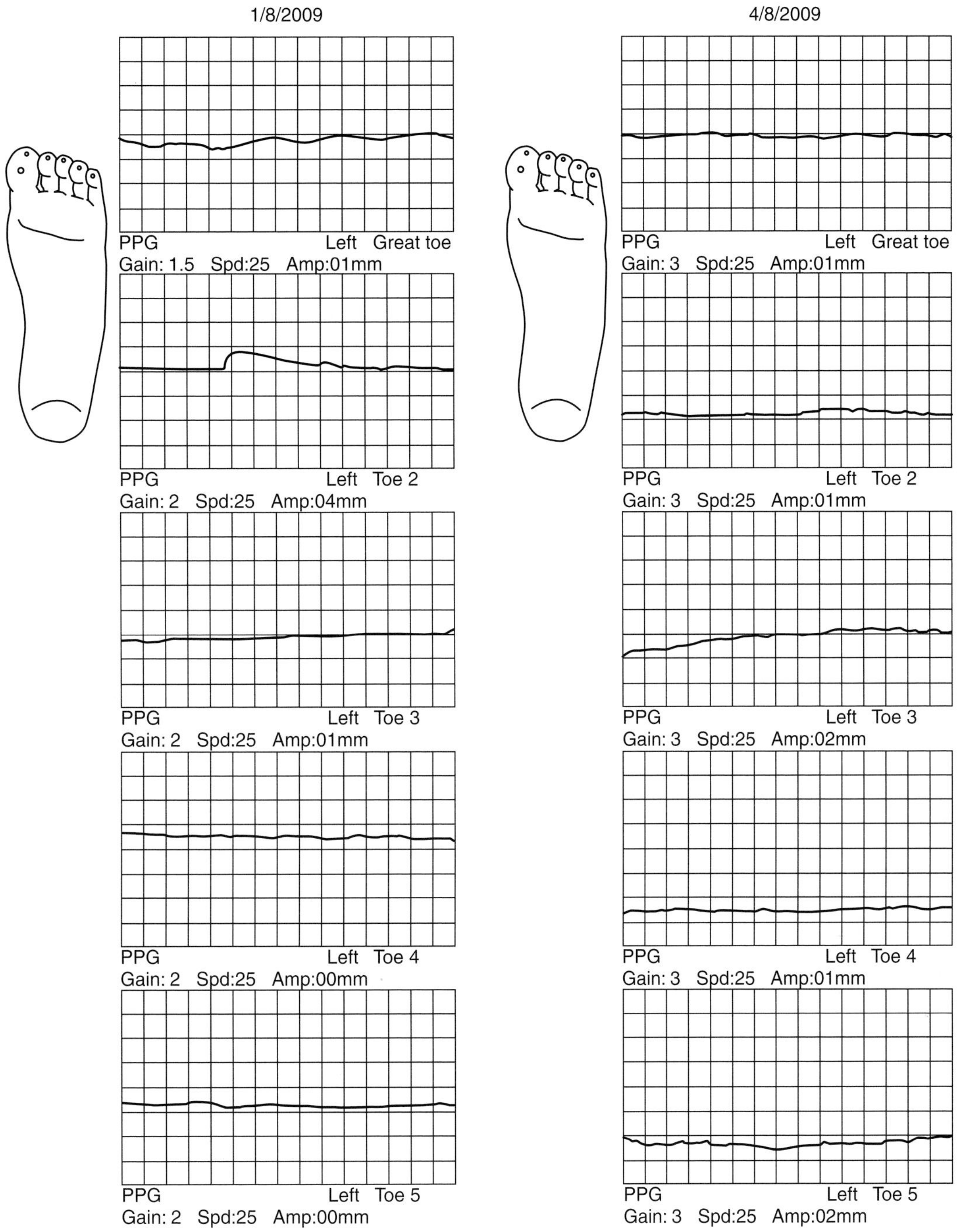

FIGURE 76-10 *Patient 2:* Toe photoplethysmography. Note gradual return of pulsatility in all five toes by 6/15/2010 from little to no pulsatility on 1/8/2009.

following direct injection into the ischemic calf musculature, along with the limited survival of these cells. Although single session intra-arterial injection has the potential to provide a more uniform progenitor cell distribution, significant pass-through results in cell sequestration in other organs.

Finally, unlike the immediate revascularization benefit provided by catheter or surgical interventions, this strategy took many months to achieve wound healing. Whether healing can be further accelerated by alternate G-CSF dosimetry, increasing the frequency of daily PPCD sessions, or both remains to be seen. Stem cell mobilization strategies are evolving. A prospective randomized study comparing use of the PPCD alone with PPCD plus G-CSF is being planned by us to confirm synergy.

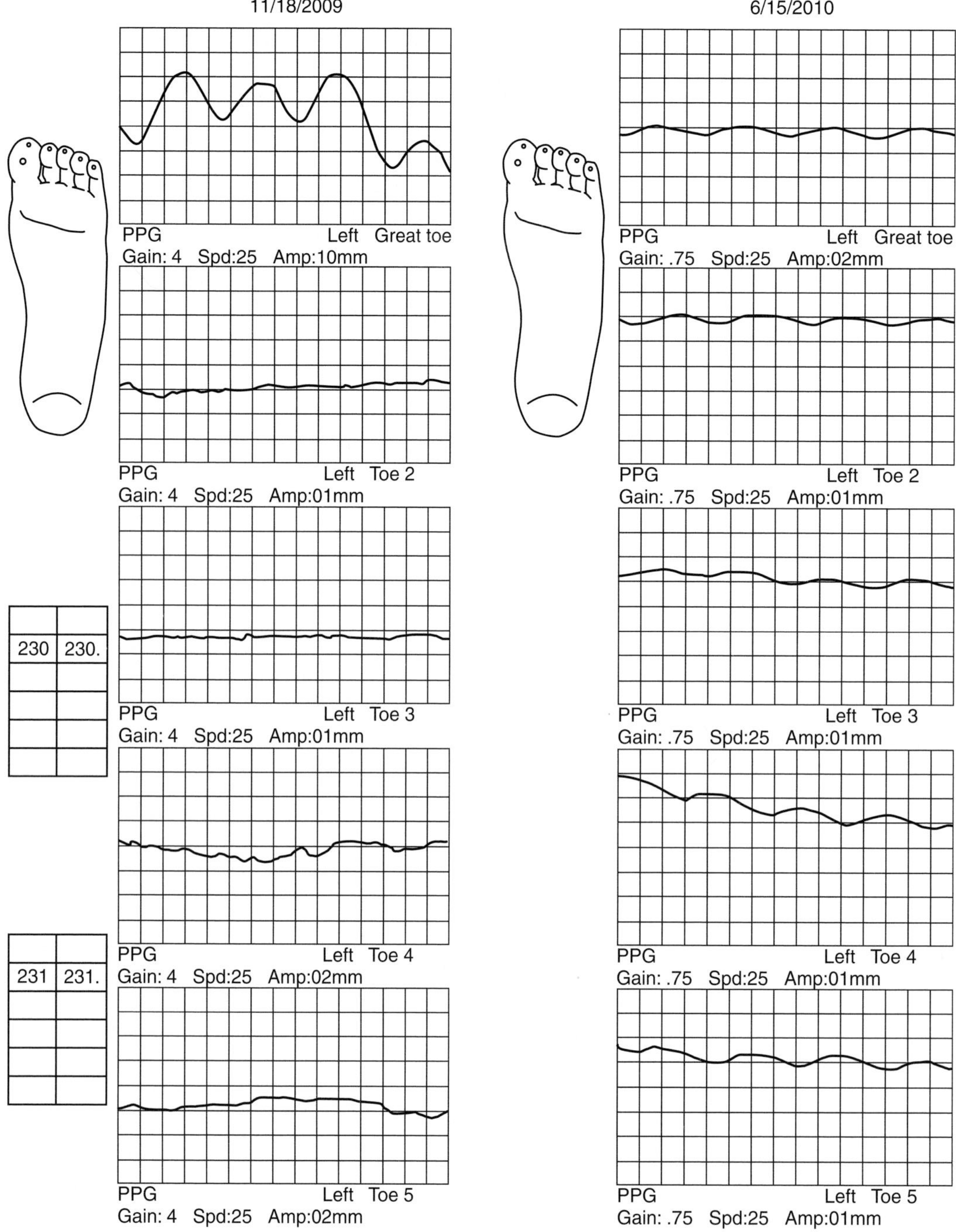

FIGURE 76-10—cont'd

CONCLUSION

Can cell-based therapies solve our medical challenges today? Unlike most research in which seeing the forest through the trees is challenging, research in cell therapy is quite the opposite. The forest is obvious—two cells make a human being. Progenitor cells within each of us are probably the closest we will get to a fountain of youth. Understanding how these cells communicate, as well as what happens to them with age and exposure to atherosclerotic risk factors, will offer insight into reparative biology. Today the experimental techniques are in place to answer questions about cytokine expression, apoptosis, and gene regulation. In addition techniques are evolving to up-regulate or down-regulate gene expression, providing an opportunity to restore progenitor cell function in the diseased sate. Finally, therapeutic angiogenesis by transplantation of induced

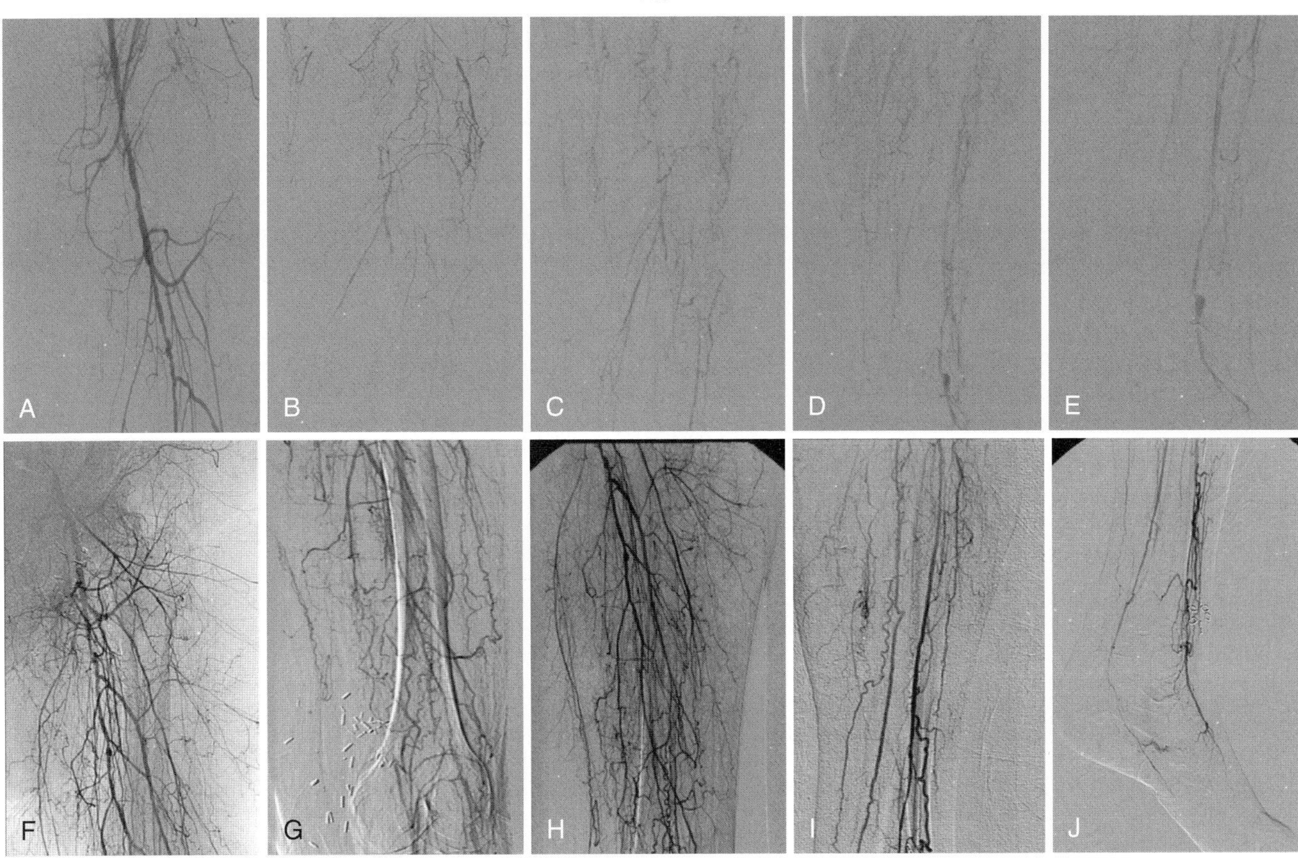

FIGURE 76-11 *Patient 2:* Angiography. **A** to **E** were obtained on initial referral. **A,** Iliofemoral. **B,** Above-knee popliteal. **C,** Below-knee popliteal. **D,** Calf. **E,** Ankle. **F** to **J** were obtained at 1-year follow-up. The 1-year angiogram was not obtained earlier because of renal insufficiency. Note increased collateral vessels at all levels.

pluripotent stem cells (novel stem cells induced from somatic cells) is just beginning to be reported.[80] Cell therapy to achieve angiogenesis should be achievable.

REFERENCES

1. Asahara T, Masuda H, Takahashi T, et al: Bone marrow origin of endothelial progenitor cells responsible for postnatal vasculogenesis in physiological and pathological neovascularization, *Circ Res* 85:221–228, 1999.
2. Lin Y, Weisdorf DJ, Solovey A, Hebbel RP: Origins of circulating endothelial cells and endothelial outgrowth from blood, *J Clin Invest* 105:71–77, 2000.
3. Peichev M, Naiyer AJ, Pereira D, et al: Expression of VEGFR-2 and AC133 by circulating human CD34(+) cells identifies a population of functional endothelial precursors, *Blood* 95:952–958, 2000.
4. Reyes M, Dudek A, Jahagirdar B, et al: Origin of endothelial progenitors in human postnatal bone marrow, *J Clin Invest* 109:337–346, 2002.
5. Murohara T, Ikeda H, Duan J, et al: Transplanted cord blood-derived endothelial progenitor cells augment postnatal neovascularization, *J Clin Invest* 105:1527–1536, 2000.
6. Tongers J, Roncalli JG, Losordo DW: Role of endothelial progenitor cells during ischemia-induced vasculogenesis and collateral formation, *Microvasc Res* 79(3):200–206, 2010.
7. Rivard A, Fabre JE, Silver M, et al: Age-dependent impairment of angiogenesis, *Circulation* 99:111–120, 1999.
8. Gennaro G, Menard C, Michaud SE, et al: Age-dependent impairment of reendothelialization after arterial injury: role of vascular endothelial growth factor, *Circulation* 107:230–233, 2003.
9. Bach MH, Sadoun E, Reed MJ: Defects in activation of nitric oxide synthases occur during delayed angiogenesis in aging, *Mech Aging Dev* 126:467–473, 2005.
10. Swift ME, Kleinman HK, DiPietro LA: Impaired wound repair and delayed angiogenesis in aged mice, *Lab Invest* 79:1479–1487, 1999.
11. Wang H, Keiser JA, Olszewski B, et al: Delayed angiogenesis in aging rats and therapeutic effect of adenoviral gene transfer of VEGF, *Int J Mol Med* 13:581–587, 2004.
12. Rauscher FM, Goldschmidt-Clermont PJ, Davis BH, et al: Aging, progenitor cell exhaustion, and atherosclerosis, *Circulation* 108:457–463, 2003.
13. Heiss C, Keymel S, Niesler U, et al: Impaired progenitor cell activity in age-related endothelial dysfunction, *J AmColl Cardiol* 45:1441–1448, 2005.
14. Zhu S, Liu X, Li Y, et al: Aging in the atherosclerosis milieu may accelerate the consumption of bone marrow endothelial progenitor cells, *Arterioscler Thromb Vasc Biol* 27:113–119, 2007.

15. Hill JM, Zalos G, Halcox JP, et al: Circulating endothelial progenitor cells, vascular function, and cardiovascular risk, *N Engl J Med* 348:593–600, 2003.
16. Vasa M, Fichtlscherer S, Aicher A, et al: Number and migratory activity of circulating endothelial progenitor cells inversely correlate with risk factors for coronary artery disease, *Circ Res* 89:E1–E7, 2001.
17. Heeschen C, Lehmann R, Honold J, et al: Profoundly reduced neovascularization capacity of bone marrow mononuclear cells derived from patients with chronic ischemic heart disease, *Circulation* 109:1615–1622, 2004.
18. Boilson BA, Kiernan TJ, Harbuzariu A, et al: Circulating CD34+ cell subsets in patients with coronary endothelial dysfunction, *Nat Clin Pract Cardiovasc Med* 5:489–496, 2008.
19. Valgimigli M, Rigolin GM, Fucili A, et al: CD34+ and endothelial progenitor cells in patients with various degrees of congestive heart failure, *Circulation* 110:1209–1212, 2004.
20. Sugihara S, Matsura T, Yamamoto Y: Age related BM-MNC dysfunction hampers neovascularization, *Mech Ageing Dev* 128(9):511–516, 2007.
21. Loomans CJ, de Koning EJ, Staal FJ, et al: Endothelial progenitor cell dysfunction: a novel concept in the pathogenesis of vascular complications of type 1 diabetes, *Diabetes* 53:195–199, 2004.
22. Tepper OM, Galiano RD, Capla JM, et al: Human endothelial progenitor cells from type II diabetics exhibit impaired proliferation, adhesion, and incorporation into vascular structures, *Circulation* 106:2781–2786, 2002.
23. Kobayashi N, Fukushima H, Takeshima H, et al: Effect of eplerenone on endothelial progenitor cells and oxidative stress in ischemic hindlimb, *Am J Hypertens* 23(9):1007–1013, 2010.
24. Gu YQ, Guo LR, Zhang J, et al: *Enhanced mobilization of mononuclear cells by G-CSF reduces the volume of bone marrow needed to induce angiogenesis in lower limb ischemia [abstract]*, Naples, FL, January, 2008, Annual Meeting of the Southern Association of Vascular Surgery.
25. Iso Y, Soda T, Sato T, et al: Impact of implanted bone marrow progenitor cell composition on limb salvage after cell implantation in patients with critical limb ischemia, *Atherosclerosis* 209(1):167–172, 2010.
26. Seeger FH, Rasper T, Koyanagi M, et al: CXCR4 expression determines functional activity of bone marrow-derived mononuclear cells for therapeutic neovascularization in acute ischemia, *Arterioscler Thromb Vasc Biol* 29(11):1802–1809, 2009.
27. Takahashi T, Kalka C, Masuda H, et al: Ischemia- and cytokine-induced mobilization of bone marrow-derived endothelial progenitor cells for neovascularization, *Nat Med* 5:434–438, 1999.
28. Asahara T, Masuda H, Takahashi T, et al: Bone marrow origin of endothelial progenitor cells responsible for postnatal vasculogenesis in physiological and pathological neovascularization, *Circ Res* 85:221–228, 1999.
29. Asahara T, Takahashi T, Masuda H, et al: VEGF contributes to postnatal neovascularization by mobilizing bone marrow-derived endothelial progenitor cells, *EMBO J* 18:3964–3972, 1999.
30. Kocher AA, Schuster MD, Szabolcs MJ, et al: Neovascularization of ischemic myocardium by human bone-marrow-derived angioblasts prevents cardiomyocyte apoptosis, reduces remodeling and improves cardiac function, *Nat Med* 7:430–436, 2001.
31. Grant MB, May WS, Caballero S, et al: Adult hematopoietic stem cells provide functional hemangioblast activity during retinal neovascularization, *Nat Med* 8:607–612, 2002.
32. Luttun A, Carmeliet G, Carmeliet P: Vascular progenitors: from biology to treatment, *Trends Cardiovasc Med* 12:88–96, 2002.
33. Tateishi-Yuyama E, Matsubara H, Murohara T, et al: Therapeutic angiogenesis for patients with limb ischaemia by autologous transplantation of bone-marrow cells: a pilot study and a randomised controlled trial, *Lancet* 360:427–435, 2002.
34. Miyamoto M, Yasutake M, Takano H, et al: Therapeutic angiogenesis by autologous bone marrow cell implantation for refractory chronic peripheral arterial disease using assessment of neovascularization by 99mtc-tetrofosmin (tf) perfusion scintigraphy, *Cell Transplant* 13:429–437, 2004.
35. Higashi Y, Kimura M, Hara K, et al: Autologous bone-marrow mononuclear cell implantation improves endothelium-dependent vasodilation in patients with limb ischemia, *Circulation* 109:1215–1218, 2004.
36. Shintani S, Murohara T, Ikeda H, et al: Augmentation of postnatal neovascularization with autologous bone marrow transplantation, *Circulation* 103:897–903, 2001.
37. Huang PP, Li SZ, Han MZ, et al: Autologous transplantation of peripheral blood stem cells as an effective therapeutic approach for severe arteriosclerosis obliterans of lower extremities, *Thromb Haemost* 91:606–609, 2004.
38. Van Tongeren RB, Hamming JF, Fibbe WE, et al: Intramuscular or combined intramuscular/intra-arterial administration of bone marrow mononuclear cells: a clinical trial in patients with advanced limb ischemia, *J Cardiovasc Surg (Torino)* 49(1):51–58, 2008.
39. Franz RW, Parks A, Shah KJ, et al: Use of autologous bone marrow mononuclear cell implantation therapy as a limb salvage procedure in patients with severe peripheral arterial disease, *J Vasc Surg* 50(6):1378–1390, 2009.
40. Lara-Hernandez R, Lozano-Vilardell P, et al: Safety and efficacy of therapeutic angiogenesis as a novel treatment in patients with critical limb ischemia, *Ann Vasc Surg* 24(2):287–294, 2010.
41. Lasala GP, Silva JA, Gardner PA, et al: Combination stem cell therapy for the treatment of severe limb ischemia: safety and efficacy analysis, *Angiology* 61(6):551–556, 2010.
42. Cobellis G, Silvestroni A, Lillo S, et al: Long-term effects of repeated autologous transplantation of bone marrow cells in patients affected by peripheral arterial disease, *Bone Marrow Transplant* 42(10):667–672, 2008.
43. Duong Van Huyen JP, Smadja DM, et al: Bone marrow-derived mononuclear cell therapy induces distal angiogenesis after local injection in critical leg ischemia, *Mod Pathol* 21(7):837–846, 2008.
44. Bartsch T, Brehm M, Zeus T, et al: Transplantation of autologous mononuclear bone marrow stem cells in patients with peripheral arterial disease (the TAM-PAD Study), *Clin Res Cardiol* 96(12):891–899, 2007.
45. Huang PP, Yang XF, Li SZ, et al: Randomized comparison of G-CSF-mobilized peripheral blood mononnuclear cells versus bone marrow-mononuclear cells for the treatment of patients with lower limb arteriosclerosis obliterans, *Thromb Haemost* 98(6):1335–1342, 2007.
46. Moriya J, Minamino T, Tateno K, et al: Long-term outcome of therapeutic neovascularization using peripheral blood mononuclear cells for limb ischemia, *Circ Cardiovasc Interv* 2(3): 245–254, 2009.
47. Horie T, Onodera R, Akamastu M, et al: Long-term clinical outcomes for patients with lower limb ischemia implanted with G-CSF-mobilized autologous peripheral blood mononuclear cells, *Atherosclerosis* 208(2):461–466, 2010.
48. Onodera R, Teramukai S, Tanaka S, et al: Bone marrow mononuclear cells versus G-CSF-mobilized peripheral blood mononuclear cells for treatment of lower limb ASO: pooled analysis for long-term prognosis, *Bone Marrow transplant* 17. EPub ahead of print, 2010.

49. Kim SW, Kim H, Cho HJ, Lee JU, Levit R, Yoon YS: Human peripheral blood-derived CD31+ cells have robust angiogenic and vasculogenic properties and are effective for treating ischemic vascular disease, *J Am Coll Cardiol* 56(7):593–607, 2010.
50. Sprengers RW, Lips DJ, Moll FL, et al: Progenitor cell therapy in patients with critical limb ischemia without surgical options, *Ann Surg* 247(3):411–420, 2008.
51. Tachi Y, Fukui D, Wada Y, et al: Changes in angiogenesis-related factors in serum following autologous bone marrow cell implantation for severe limb ischemia, *Expert Opin Biol Ther* 8 (6):705–712, 2008.
52. Aicher A, Heeschen C, Mildner-Rihm C, et al: Essential role of endothelial nitric oxide synthase for mobilization of stem and progenitor cells, *Nat Med* 9:1370–1376, 2003.
53. Chochola M, Pytlík R, Kobylka P, et al: Autologous intra-arterial infusion of bone marrow mononuclear cells in patients with critical leg ischemia, *Int Angiol* 27(4):281–290, 2008.
54. Gu YQ, Zhang J, Guo LR, et al: Transplantation of autologous bone marrow mononuclear cells for patients with lower limb ischemia, *Chin Med J (Engl)* 12(11):963–967, 2008.
55. Bussolino F, Ziche M, Wang JM, et al: In vitro and in vivo activation of endothelial cells by colony-stimulating factors, *J Clin Invest* 87(3):986–995, 1991.
56. Bussolino F, Colotta F, Bocchietto E, et al: Recent developments in the cell biology of granulocyte-macrophage colony-stimulating factor and granulocyte colony-stimulating factor: activities on endothelial cells, *Int J Clin Lab Res* 23(1):8–12, 1993.
57. Takagi Y, Omura T, Yoshiyama M, et al: Granulocyte-colony stimulating factor augments neovascularization induced by bone marrow transplantation in rat hindlimb ischemia, *J Pharmacol Sci* 99(1):45–51, 2005.
58. Grundmann S, Hoefer I, Ulusans S, et al: Granulocyte-macrophage colony-stimulating factor stimulates arteriogenesis in a pig model of peripheral artery disease using clinically applicable infusion pumps, *J Vasc Surg* 43(6):1263–1269, 2006.
59. Ohki Y, Heissig B, Sato Y, et al: Granulocyte colony-stimulating factor promotes neovascularization by releasing vascular endothelial growth factor from neutrophils, *FASEB J* 19(14):2005–2007, 2005.
60. Zhang H, Zhang N, Li M, et al: Therapeutic angiogenesis of bone marrow mononuclear cells (MNCs) and peripheral blood MNCs: transplantation for ischemic hindlimb, *Ann Vasc Surg* 22 (2):238–247, 2008.
61. Jeon O, Song SJ, Bhang SH, et al: Additive effect of endothelial progenitor cell mobilization and bone marrow mononuclear cell transplantation on angiogenesis in mouse ischemic limbs, *J Biomed Sci* 14(3):323–330, 2007.
62. Ieda Y, Fujita J, Ieda M, et al: G-CSF and HGF: combination of vasculogenesis and angiogenesis synergistically improves recovery in murine hind limb ischemia, *J Mol Cell Cardiol* 42 (3):540–548, 2007.
63. Tan Y, Shao H, Eton D, et al: Stromal cell-derived factor-1 enhances pro-angiogenic effect of granulocyte colony stimulating factor, *Cardiovasc Res* 73:823–832, 2007.
64. Shao H, Tan Y, Eton D, et al: Statin and stromal cell derived factor-1 additively promote angiogenesis by enhancement of progenitor cells incorporation into new vessels, *Stem Cells* 26 (5):1376–1384, 2008.
65. Kudo FA, Nishibe T, Nishibe M, et al: Autologous transplantation of peripheral blood endothelial progenitor cells (CD34+) for therapeutic angiogenesis in patients with critical limb ischemia, *Int Angiol* 22(4):344–348, 2003.
66. Kawamura A, Horie T, Tsuda I, et al: Clinical study of therapeutic angiogenesis by autologous peripheral blood stem cell (PBSC) transplantation in 92 patients with critically ischemic limbs, *J Artif Organs* 9(4):226–233, 2006.
67. van Royen N, Schirmer SH, Atasever B, et al: START Trial: a pilot study on STimulation of ARTeriogenesis using subcutaneous application of granulocyte-macrophage colony-stimulating factor as a new treatment for peripheral vascular disease, *Circulation* 112(7):1040–1046, 2005.
68. Ping Ping H, Shangzhu L, Mingzhe H, et al: Autologous transplantation of granulocyte colony–stimulating factor–mobilized peripheral blood mononuclear cells improves critical limb ischemia in diabetes, *Diabetes Care* 28:2155–2160, 2005.
69. Eton D, Yu H: Enhanced cell therapy strategy to treat chronic limb-threatening ischemia, *J Vasc Surg* 52(1):199–204, 2010.
70. Louridas G, Saadi R, Spelay J, et al: The ArtAssist device in chronic limb ischemia: a pilot study, *Int Angiol* 21:28–35, 2002.
71. Van Bemmelen P, Gitlitz DB, Faruqi RM, et al: Limb salvage using high- pressure intermittent compression arterial assist device in cases unsuitable for surgical revascularization, *Arch Surg* 136:1280–1285, 2001.
72. Montori VM, Kavros SJ, Walsh EE, et al: Intermittent compression pump for nonhealing wounds in patients with limb ischemia: the Mayo Clinic experience (1998-2000), *Int Angiol* 21:360–366, 2002.
73. Kavros SJ, Delis KT, Turner NS, et al: Improving limb salvage in critical ischemia with intermittent pneumatic compression: a controlled study with 18-month follow-up, *J Vasc Surg* 47(3): 543–549, 2008.
74. Liu K, Chen L, Seaver AV, et al: Influences of inflation rate and duration on vasodilatory effect by intermittent pneumatic compression in distant skeletal muscle, *J Orthop Res* 17:415–420, 1999.
75. Guzman RJ, Abe K, Zarins CK: Flow-induced arterial enlargement is inhibited by suppression of nitric oxide synthase activity in vivo, *Surgery* 122(22):273–280, 1997.
76. Untank JL, Fath SW, Burkhart HM, et al: Wall remodeling during luminal expansion of mesenteric arterial collaterals in the rat, *Circ Res* 79:1015–1023, 1996.
77. Barsheshet A, Hod H, Shechter M, et al: The effects of external counter pulsation therapy on circulating endothelial progenitor cells in patients with angina pectoris, *Cardiology* 110(3):160–166, 2008.
78. Van Bemmelen P, Char D, Giron F, et al: Angiographic improvement after rapid intermittent compression treatment (ArtAssist®) for small vessel obstruction, *Ann Vasc Surg* 17:224–228, 2003.
79. Eze AR, Comerota AJ, Cisek PL, et al: Intermittent calf and foot compression increases lower extremity blood flow, *Am J Surg* 172:130–135, 1996.
80. Suzuki H, Shibata R, Kito T, et al: Therapeutic angiogenesis by transplantation of induced pluripotent stem cell-derived Flk-1 positive cells, *BMC Cell Biol* 11(1):72, 2010.

CHAPTER

77

Billing and Coding in an Endovascular Practice

Sean P. Roddy

The major focus in most vascular surgical practices is patient care and quality outcomes. While holding these goals primary, one can also evaluate the process by which care is rendered to optimize billing, coding, and, ultimately, reimbursement. Everything done in medicine that involves a patient can be described with a diagnosis and a procedure. This includes patient assessment, operative intervention, and diagnostic evaluation. When one takes a diagnosis code, links it to a procedure code, and adds up to three modifiers, a claim is generated. That claim is usually submitted to an insurance carrier by electronic methods. The appropriateness of the coding involved leads to both timely reimbursement by the insurance carrier and minimal risk of "fraudulent" billing. Each time a claim is rejected for any reason, the chance of that claim ever being paid to the physician decreases significantly. Therefore all efforts should be centered on generating a "clean" claim that is without error, is medically appropriate, and describes the intervention correctly. This chapter is only a guideline for the physician because each insurance payer has its own rules and regulations. Please consult your local carriers for specific details on claim submission.

DIAGNOSIS CODING

The World Health Organization (WHO) created the ninth edition of the *International Classification of Diseases* (ICD-9) in 1977 to track diseases worldwide. The National Center for Health Statistics altered this manual for use in the United States, and therefore "clinical modification" has been added to the title. The concept for this categorization evolved originally from the London Bills of Mortality in the 1600s, which described the reasons for death in the citizens of England. In 1937, the concept left Great Britain and was renamed the International List of Causes of Death. Finally, the WHO developed the first edition of the *International Classification of Diseases* tracking both mortality and, for the first time, morbidity in 1948. The current edition is updated annually, effective October 1 each year, and is divided into two sections.[1] The first section is a numerical list of diseases presented as code numbers in a tabular form, and the second section is an alphabetical index of the disease entries with corresponding diagnostic code numbers. Each ICD-9 code is composed of a three-, four-, or five-digit number. With increasing specificity, there are more digits. A common error is the use of a probable or a suspected diagnosis. A patient has the diagnosis of right lower quadrant abdominal pain and not appendicitis while in the emergency department. Only after laparotomy, if significant inflammation and/or infection is identified, does the patient officially have the diagnosis of appendicitis. If the patient has a normal appendix, no bill should ever be generated that includes a diagnosis of appendicitis. It is also important to use the most clinically suitable description listed in the ICD-9 manual for a patient's given condition whenever possible. That said, there are instances where several diagnoses will all be medically appropriate.

PROCEDURAL CODING

Procedure codes are taken from the *Current Procedural Terminology* (CPT) book.[2] This is currently in its fourth edition and is sometimes abbreviated CPT-4. This manual is created, maintained, and copyrighted by the American Medical Association (AMA), which updates it annually effective January 1 each year. It is used by physicians, researchers, and managed care as a systematic listing of all procedures that are currently performed. CPT descriptors are always a five-digit number and broken down into standard codes and add-on codes. Standard codes are those that can be submitted by themselves. Add-on codes cannot and must be accompanied by other specific code(s) as well. An example of an add-on code is CPT 35700 (reoperation, femoral-popliteal or femoral-tibial, more than 1 month after original procedure). This code provides value for the added difficulty in performing reoperative leg bypass surgery. Therefore payment for CPT code 35700 would require that one of the nine standard lower-extremity revascularization codes be submitted as well.

CPT codes for physician reimbursement are also designated as either category I or category III. Category I codes are the typical five-digit number codes with which most people are familiar. On the other hand, category III codes are four digits followed by a "T." These are referred to as temporary or emerging technology codes. They usually describe the use of a device not approved by the Food and Drug Administration or an investigational procedure. Most category III codes are not reimbursed by insurers unless converted at some point to a category I code but are in place to help with data collection by Medicare, private insurers, and other interest groups. An example is CPT code 0075T, which describes transcatheter placement of extracranial vertebral or intrathoracic carotid artery stents. Category III codes are limited in duration with a maximum of 5 years.

More than one procedure on the same date, in the same session, or within a global period may require use of an appropriate modifier. Modifiers are two-digit numbers that can be added to a claim that describes circumstances allowing for full or partial payment in situations that would otherwise be denied by the insurer. Additionally, the National Correct Coding Initiative (or NCCI) reviews codes quarterly to decide what can and cannot be billed together routinely based on current practice, billing patterns, and trends. For example, the -59 modifier can be used to notate distinct procedural services or an exception to the NCCI. The modifiers are listed both in the front of the CPT manual each year and in their own section in the Appendix.

It is also important to understand that when more than one CPT code is billed on the same session, the highest valued code is paid in its entirety. All subsequent nonradiologic codes are paid at 50% of their independent value. This decrease is termed the "multiple procedure discount" taking into account the overlap in work before, during, and after multiple procedures done on the same date of service. Imaging codes (i.e., the radiology codes that begin with the number 7) or vascular laboratory codes are not subject to this discount. Additionally, add-on codes are exempt from this fee reduction because they are created solely for use with other codes.

Two specific modifiers important in billing radiologic codes include the -TC (or technical component) modifier as well as the -26 (or professional component) modifier. When the equipment is owned by a practice in an office setting, that practice would bill with no modifier; this is termed "billing global." That includes both the technical component and the professional component for a given test. If a test is performed in the hospital where the hospital owns the equipment, a physician would typically bill with a -26 modifier. This signifies that the physician is performing and interpreting the test but does not own the equipment, purchase the catheters/stents/balloons/contrast, manage the facility, and employ the staff required to perform the procedure.

CPT codes can be grouped into three general categories. These include evaluation and management codes, surgical procedure codes, and radiologic codes. Evaluation and management codes are typically patient and practitioner interaction such as office visits, consultations, and hospital evaluations. Patient encounter billing is a separate topic and will not be discussed further in this chapter. Surgical procedure codes involve the work and care around the time of an operation. This is best described by a "global surgical package." This package includes all preoperative care, intraprocedural care, and postoperative care for a given time period. In most instances, that global period extends from the day before surgery to 90 days after the procedure. Minor surgery, however, may have a 0-day global period (just the actual date of the procedure) or a 10-day global period associated with it that extends from the day of surgery to 10 days after the procedure. Global packages also include discussion with the patient about the procedure, alternatives, risks, benefits and consent issues, and documentation of preoperative notes.

All radiologic codes in CPT are further classified in one of three categories: catheter manipulations, imaging studies, and interventions. Endovascular billing uses all three and is termed "component coding." Catheter manipulations occur when vessels are traversed and selected most commonly via a femoral or brachial artery puncture. Imaging includes the interpretation of angiography in various vascular beds. Interventions include things such as embolization, angioplasty, stent placement, atherectomy, thrombolysis, intravascular foreign body retrieval, or endograft deployment. In the coding world, there are five interventional systems. These include arterial, venous, lymphatic, portal, and pulmonary. The remainder of this chapter will be dedicated to endovascular treatments on the arterial side.

CATHETER MANIPULATION

Catheterization coding requires description in an operative record of the arterial entry site, vessels traversed within the body, and final resting point for the end of the catheter at the time of imaging. Any movement of the catheter should be noted including the subsequent imaging and/or intervention. An important topic in endovascular coding is selective and nonselective catheterization with regard to a vascular family. Nonselective implies that the puncture vessel itself is cannulated for imaging or a catheter is advanced along the artery retrograde from the puncture into the aorta. It does not matter whether the access site is the brachial artery or the femoral artery. If a catheter is advanced from either extremity vessel into the aorta, a nonselective aortic catheterization has occurred. This is described by CPT code 36200.

Selective catheterization occurs when cannulation of a vessel is performed at a branch point. In most circumstances, this will be a named vessel coming off the aorta itself. A vascular family is a network of vessels that originate from an arterial branch point off a nonselective vessel. This initial vessel is termed first order. As further branching occurs within that family, the arteries are designated second order and third order. There is work involved manipulating the catheter to access the desired vessel. Branch point negotiation beyond third order is not recognized in component coding. When selective catheterizations occur below the diaphragm, CPT codes 36245, 36246, and 36247 describe first-, second-, and third-order catheterizations, respectively. When selective catheters are placed within vascular families above the diaphragm, CPT codes 36215, 36216, and 36217 again describe first-, second-, and third-order catheterizations, respectively. Every vascular family that is selected during an angiogram for imaging and/or intervention purposes will generate a separate and distinct catheter CPT code. Also, the same vessel can be different based on the puncture site or anatomic variation (e.g., the left common carotid artery [CCA] is a first-order catheterization in standard arch anatomy but is a second-order vessel in bovine aortic arch anatomy as a branch off the innominate artery). Therefore when describing catheter manipulations in an operative report, it is important to note all branch entry points in a given examination for billing purposes. This was set up to describe the quantity of physician work dedicated to placing a catheter into a given artery. Advancing a catheter farther into a vessel has a different amount of work associated with it compared with pulling that catheter back from a branch into the aorta and placing the catheter in a separate and distinct vessel. If the catheter is brought back into a nonselective position and a separate vascular family is catheterized, this will necessitate an additional catheter code. For example, if the right common femoral artery (CFA) is punctured, this would generate the nonselective CPT catheterization code 36140. This describes retrograde femoral artery access. If the catheter is advanced into the aorta, the nonselective catheterization code, 36200, would be recorded, and this would nullify the 36140 code. The 36200 code contains the work described within the 36140 code, as well as the additional work required to advance the catheter into the aorta. Similarly, if the left renal artery is cannulated as a first-order catheterization, the code 36245 would take the place of the 36200 code; 36245 contains the relative value associated with the work required not only to get the catheter into the aorta but also to select the left renal artery. If the catheter is pulled back into the aorta and then placed in the right renal artery, which is an entirely different vascular family, a separate and distinct 36245 code would be appropriate. Bilateral renal artery selective catheterization would allow for billing the CPT code 36245 twice. If a catheter is further advanced within a given vascular family, branch points will need to be negotiated. A selective catheterization of the celiac artery would be termed "first order" similar to the renal artery cannulation described above and billed at 36245. However, if the catheter is advanced into the common hepatic artery past the left gastric and splenic artery branch points, the catheter is now in a "second-order" vessel. Second-order catheterization below the diaphragm is CPT code 36246 and includes the work of 36245 plus the work to enter the second-order vessel. Further advancement of the catheter into the proper hepatic artery past the gastroduodenal artery branch point is a "third-order" catheterization. Third-order catheterization is billed as a 36247 and, following the previous examples, voids and replaces the prior 36246 code.

If one enters a vascular family and proceeds to second- or third-order catheterization, there are times when the catheter is pulled back within that family (but not back into the aorta) and a separate second- or third-order branch is selected for further angiography. An example is selective catheterization through the innominate artery into the right CCA for carotid imaging. This is a second-order catheterization above the diaphragm (36216). The catheter is pulled back into the innominate artery and then into the right subclavian artery for further imaging. Placement of the catheter into the right subclavian artery is a "subsequent second- or third-order" catheterization and is billed with the add-on CPT code 36218. Similarly, if this occurred below the diaphragm, 36248 would be used.

IMAGING

Imaging includes image intensifier manipulation, table positioning, contrast injection, and interpretation of the angiography in a specific vascular bed. All hospital-based imaging necessitates use of the -26 modifier to designate only the professional component of the imaging

CPT code. As a general rule, when a catheter is repositioned and imaging occurs, another code is generated. Some imaging requires a selective catheter placement. Therefore nonselective catheterizations such as 36200 could never be used at the same time as any of these imaging codes. Examples include renal, visceral, spinal, adrenal, and pelvic arteriography. Coding these types of imaging with a nonselective catheterization would be a red flag to insurance carriers for inappropriate billing practices.

To start, the basic examination is coded first followed by subsequent examinations. Abdominal aortography (75625) and bilateral lower-extremity arterial runoff (75716) are standard basic imaging codes for vascular surgeons. However, some subsequent examinations include the basic examination. An example for this includes a renal artery selective arteriogram. Both the unilateral (75722) and bilateral (75724) renal arteriogram codes include selective renal angiography, as well as flush aortography. Therefore a basic abdominal aortogram (75625) would never be coded at the same time as a selective renal arteriogram (75722) because the renal study includes the work for interpreting the aortogram, as well as the selective renal images. Visceral angiography (75726) is similar and also includes flush aortography.

In previous years, many practices did a diagnostic angiogram and identified a lesion that could be treated with an endovascular therapy. Anywhere from 1 day to several days later, the same angiogram was repeated at the time of percutaneous intervention. This allowed for payment on the angiography twice for the same clinical condition. To discourage this practice and to ensure that Medicare would pay only once for angiography, version 10.3 of the NCCI created an edit on October 1, 2004, in the policy manual that bundled imaging with intervention except if the -59 modifier was added to the imaging CPT code.[4] Therefore one must dictate into the operative report if no prior angiography was done in a given clinical situation, which then allows addition of the -59 modifier to the imaging codes for reimbursement.

ENDOVASCULAR INTERVENTION

The last component of endovascular billing is the concept of interventions. These include embolization, transluminal angioplasty, stent placement, atherectomy, thrombolysis, transcatheter foreign body retrieval, or endograft deployment. Most of these procedures are described through two CPT codes: one code that begins with a 3 (what you did in the angiography suite) and another code that begins with a 7 (what you saw on the monitor in the angiogram). The latter code is the radiology supervision and interpretation code submitted with a -26 modifier to signify professional fee billing.

Multiple interventions are often performed on the same vessel in the same session. The AMA CPT correct coding guidelines would allow for reporting all the endovascular techniques required to percutaneously treat an occluded vessel provided each was done with appropriate intent. There has been a recent change in Medicare policy effective October 1, 2007, as described in version 13.3 of the NCCI *Coding Policy Manual for Medicare Services.*[3] Previously, one could perform an angioplasty and have an inadequate result such that a stent was required. Both the angioplasty and stent were billed. The angioplasty required appending a -59 modifier in the claim to certify that an attempt at percutaneous transluminal angioplasty (PTA) was pursued, but the result was inadequate requiring stent salvage. As of 2008, Medicare will only pay for the final endovascular procedure that is considered successful. Therefore a patient could have an atherectomy that required angioplasty with subsequent stenting. Only the stenting procedure would be reimbursable. This is in line with the overall Medicare policy that unsuccessful procedures are not reportable. However, endovascular interventions are usually considered additive rather than alternative to each other. Therefore an appeal has been submitted at this time by the Society for Vascular Surgery and the Society of Interventional Radiology but is pending.

INTERVENTIONAL CODING DESCRIPTIONS

PTA involves inflation of a balloon within a stenotic or occluded vessel. The procedure is coded per vessel treated and grouped into "renal or other visceral," "aortic," "iliac," "femoral-popliteal," "brachiocephalic trunk or branches," "tibioperoneal trunk and branches," and "venous" for coding purposes. An additional radiology supervision and interpretation code is added for each vessel (CPT 75962-75968, 75978) treated. The first peripheral artery PTA includes use of 75962 whereas all subsequent peripheral vessels treated with PTA allow for the add-on code 75964. Similarly, the initial renal and visceral PTA permits billing 75966 whereas all subsequent renal or visceral PTA require the add-on code 75968. If several inflations are performed at varying locations along a given vessel, only one intervention can be submitted for reimbursement. There is one set of codes that describes open angioplasty (CPT 35450-35460) and another set that covers a percutaneous approach (CPT 35470-35476) to the same vessel. It is important to differentiate between the two. For example, iliac PTA done at the time of a leg bypass through a contralateral percutaneous groin puncture would be billed differently than an iliac PTA approached retrograde through the exposed ("open") CFA. A hard copy image of the inflation must be preserved for documentation purposes in all cases.

Atherectomy follows the same rules as PTA. There are similar groupings as listed above (except there is no venous category) and a likewise division between open (CPT 35480-35485) and percutaneous (35490-35495) approaches. The radiology supervision and interpretation codes (75992-75996) mirror PTA for each vessel subject to plaque excision.

Endovascular stent placement is based on a different convention. There are actually only four stent codes for all vessels (excluding carotid and vertebral arteries). CPT code 37205 describes percutaneous deployment of the first stent, and 37206 is an add-on code used to describe each additional *vessel* treated. Similarly, CPT code 37207 and the add-on code 37208 are used in the open setting. All four codes require use of the same radiology supervision and interpretation code (75960). If four vessels are treated with stents through percutaneous access, four 75960 codes, three 37206 codes, and one 37205 code can be submitted for reimbursement. It is important to remember that stents are coded per vessel and not per stent. There is no difference in superficial femoral artery (SFA) or renal artery stent placement as far as billing is concerned for deployment of the device. The ICD-9 diagnosis will differ on the claim, but the stent CPT coding is identical. Also, if three individual stents are placed in the SFA, component coding guidelines would treat the intervention as if only one stent were placed for that endovascular therapy. However, *CPT Assistant* (an update published by the AMA) states that lesions in the SFA that are distinct from those in the popliteal artery are separately reportable.[5] Also, when both an external iliac artery and an ipsilateral CFA stenosis are treated, each therapy is reportable provided the lesions are not contiguous.[6]

Only the carotid and vertebral artery have different codes for stenting. Cervical carotid artery stenting with (37215) or without (37216) distal protection is special in that this represents a divergence from component coding. The work associated with catheter placement, selective imaging of the carotid arteries, placement of the stent, and use of a protection device are all bundled into one code. The inclusion of multiple procedures in one CPT code is termed bundling. Arch angiography, which is typically performed before selective carotid catheterization, is not bundled into these codes and may be reported separately. A similar situation exists with regard to intrathoracic carotid and extrathoracic vertebral artery stenting. Bundling for this intervention is described by CPT code 0075T, a category III code, for the initial vessel and 0076T, an add-on code, for each subsequent vessel treated at the same session.

Embolization (37204, 75894) implies percutaneous placement of a thrombogenic material through a selective catheter in an attempt to occlude an aneurysm, arteriovenous malformation, or bleeding site. Glue and coils are typical agents employed in the process. Additionally, most embolization procedures are followed by contrast angiography to evaluate the adequacy of the thrombosis. This follow-up study is reportable (75898) for each operative field treated. In 2007, a bundled CPT code (37210) was introduced to describe all work associated with uterine fibroid embolization. This includes all catheters, imaging, and techniques for vessel occlusion. There is no associated radiology supervision and interpretation code. As is usually the case, creation of an all-encompassing procedure unfortunately lowered the total relative value of this intervention compared with the prior component coding descriptions.

Thrombolysis is the administration of a clot-dissolving agent through a catheter that may open a clotted artery or vein. It is important to note that there is a difference between injection and infusion in the CPT manual. The CPT codes for thrombolysis (37201, 75896) necessitate an actual prolonged infusion by pump of the agent in an area outside the angiography suite. Instilling a thrombolytic drug through a catheter as a bolus by hand is termed "injection" and therefore not reimbursable. Thrombolysis is usually administered in a hospital setting, and a follow-up study is performed to evaluate the effectiveness of the treatment. Follow-up angiography through an existing catheter when the patient returns to the angiography suite is coded 75898. It is inappropriate to rebill the thrombolytic codes because they are only for the initiation of therapy and not for continued use on subsequent dates of service. Additionally, the infusion catheter may be exchanged to continue thrombolysis and reposition the catheter for optimal drug delivery. The removal and replacement of this catheter is described by CPT codes 37209 and 75900.

Primary arterial mechanical thrombectomy (37184) includes both clot disruption by an endoluminal device and instilling thrombolytic agent while in the angiography area. This code is reported per vessel. Each additional vessel treated in the same setting on the same date of service can be described by the add-on CPT code 37185. This is in direct contrast to secondary arterial mechanical thrombectomy (37186) for salvage after an embolic event is identified from arterial manipulation, PTA, or stent deployment. This add-on CPT code describes the work associated with extracting debris from a distal vessel by all endovascular methods. *Primary* means the patient went to the angiography for the purpose of mechanical thrombectomy, and *secondary* implies salvage after an untoward event has occurred.

Both thoracic (TEVAR) and infrarenal (EVAR) aortic aneurysm repair by endograft follow similar conventions. In a stepwise fashion, report the main device deployment first. This is based on the type of endograft implanted. EVAR is reported based on the main body graft configuration: aorta to aorta tube graft (34800), modular with one docking limb (34802), modular with two docking limbs (34803), bifurcated unibody graft (34804), or aorto-uniiliac graft (34805). The radiology supervision and interpretation code for all of the above listed EVAR possibilities includes 75952. Placement of the initial docking limb(s) is bundled into the main body code. When a modular bifurcated graft is transformed into an aorto-uniiliac prosthesis with either a formal graft converter or an aortic cuff placed proximally, the two devices are collectively reported with CPT code 34805. Additional extensions both proximally and distally per vessel treated are reported separately. The first extension is described by CPT codes 34825 and 75953. Each additional vessel treated by endograft extension is represented by 34826 and 75953. The radiology supervision and interpretation CPT code 75953 is the same for the first as well as the subsequent extensions such that subsequent submissions would require the use of a -59 modifier to identify that the replication of an identical code is not an accidental duplicate bill. TEVAR reporting is somewhat different. The initial graft placement is predicated on coverage of the left subclavian artery (LSA). If the graft occludes the orifice of the LSA, CPT codes 33880 and 75956 are appropriate. If the graft is placed caudad to that artery, CPT codes 33881 and 75957 are correct. Any additional distal endograft extensions at the time of the initial TEVAR are not separately reportable. However, proximal endograft extensions done at the time of initial TEVAR are appropriate. The first proximal extension is described by 33883 and 75958. Any additional proximal extensions are codes with 33884 and 75958. If a proximal extension(s) causes coverage of the LSA, the 33881, 33883, and 33884, as well as their radiology supervision and interpretation codes, are voided and are replaced by 33880 with 75956. Distal extensions are only reportable when done at a separate setting from the initial graft placement. Codes 33886 and 75959 describe placement of as many distal TEVAR extensions as necessary at a date subsequent to the main body deployment.

Next, the arterial catheter placements are considered. Most patients will have two nonselective catheters (36200 × 2): one in each femoral artery that extends into the aorta. If selective catheterization is performed, appropriate component coding rules apply. Any open arterial exposure is described. Usually femoral artery exposure and simple repair is coded with 34812, but complex primary repair (35226), prosthetic patch angioplasty (35286), and common femoral endarterectomy (35371) may supersede an exposure code. CPT code 34820 denotes iliac artery exposure as necessary, and 34833 conveys iliac artery exposure with the additional creation of a prosthetic graft conduit to assist in sheath insertion when small or heavily diseased external iliac arteries are encountered. When a brachial artery exposure (and repair) is warranted, CPT code 34834 is appropriate. All radiologic supervision and interpretation is then summarized. Any separately reportable services are then added such as stenting or PTA outside of the endograft landing zone (e.g., left renal stent placement), embolization of arteries that do not contain an endograft (e.g., internal iliac artery or inferior mesenteric artery), or deployment of an aneurysm pressure sensor (34806). Cross-femoral bypass with prosthetic conduit at the time of EVAR is described by the add-on code 34813. With regard to TEVAR, left arm revascularization may be required. Open subclavian to carotid artery transposition at the time of TEVAR is coded 33889. Carotid to subclavian artery bypass with prosthetic, an alternative to transposition, is reported with the traditional coding, 35606. If the LSA and the left CCA are both occluded and a carotid-to-carotid artery bypass with prosthetic is placed in a retropharyngeal tunnel, a specially designed CPT code for use at the time of TEVAR is appropriate (33891).

ADDITIONAL BILLING ISSUES

Central to all reimbursement in a physician practice is some type of billing, scheduling, and registration information technology system. These software packages must be user friendly for support staff and organize the large volume of demographic data required in claim submission. They also allow for reasonable office schedule templates and maximal use of clinic time. Many systems have interfaces with most insurance companies including Medicare, United Healthcare, Aetna, and Blue Cross/Blue Shield that provide immediate eligibility verification. They also employ scrubbing programs that identify global periods, medical necessity policies, and NCCI edits. Use of these computer models promotes efficiency in patient check-in and scheduling, higher clean claim creation rates, and improved throughput for charge entry. Electronic medical records in both the office and the vascular laboratory are also beneficial on many levels. Physicians can have access to them after hours, which can help in immediate patient care issues. Electronic medical records can include all the necessary information for billing at a given encounter level and allow for templating with future follow-up visits as well. There are immediate fax options, which may improve communication in a timely fashion with referring physicians and therefore may increase referrals.

The largest income source in a vascular surgery practice is typically reimbursement for procedures performed. There must be a system of checks and balances in regard to this procedure billing. Procedures (both open and endovascular) should be tracked from booking to charge entry. Having all procedure reports faxed to one central number for review to ensure none are misplaced is an added fail-safe mechanism. Missing even one procedure per month can lead to thousands of lost cash revenue per year for a practice.

Review rejection reports for trends on a routine basis. Insurers will periodically upgrade the scrubbing software, and this may lead to denial of claims that were previously paid. Only by systematic evaluation can changes be identified and remedied. Be aware of medical necessity edits or local coverage determinations. These may limit payments on procedures such as vascular laboratory studies, debridements, or Unna boot placement.

SUMMARY

Vascular surgery open coding and endovascular component coding are complex and difficult. Physicians must be involved in this process. Operative notes and angiography reports are also "billing receipts." Treat them as such and include an appropriate diagnosis for medical necessity, a list of all imaging, catheterizations, and interventions for endovascular work, and individual procedures for open surgery. The physician must have a general understanding of what is billed in a given procedure so that he or she can dictate a description that is clear and not disputable for each CPT code involved.[7] Computer software eases the burden significantly.

References

1. *2008 Physicians' Professional ICD-9-CM International Classification of Diseases Volumes 1&2*, Salt Lake City, 2007, The Medical Management Institute.
2. *Current Procedural Terminology CPT 2008 Professional Edition*, Chicago, 2007, American Medical Association.
3. *The National Correct Coding Sourcebook, Version 13.3*, Salt Lake City, 2007, The Medical Management Institute.
4. *The National Correct Coding Sourcebook, Version 10.3*, Salt Lake City, 2004, The Medical Management Institute.
5. Surgery: Cardiovascular System, 35474 (Q&A), *CPT Assistant* 16(8):10, 2006.
6. Bonus Feature: Surgery: Cardiovascular System, *CPT Assistant* 17:12, 2007.
7. *The 2008 SIR Interventional Radiology Coding CD*, Fairfax, VA, 2008, Society of Interventional Radiology.

CHAPTER

78

Pharmacologic Adjuncts to Endovascular Procedures

Peter F. Lawrence

For patients who undergo endovascular procedures, pharmacologic adjuncts play a critical role, because antiplatelet drugs, anticoagulants, and vasodilators are used in most endovascular procedures and thrombolytic agents are used in those patients with a thrombosed graft, artery, or vein.[1] In addition, patients who need these procedures often have coexisting cardiovascular disease and are receiving either antiplatelet drugs or anticoagulation before the procedure; they will also need to be given antiplatelet drugs or anticoagulation after the procedure to optimize the outcome. During the procedure, anticoagulation is required while catheters are in the vessels, while there is interruption of blood flow, or as a stent or graft is being placed in a vessel, to maintain vessel patency. Although there may be rare instances when anticoagulation is not used in endovascular procedures, such as when a patient has concomitant head trauma with a high risk for bleeding, pharmacologic agents are universally used during endovascular procedures, unless specifically contraindicated. It is therefore incumbent on the endovascular surgeon to be familiar with alternative antiplatelet, anticoagulant, vasodilator, and thrombolytic drugs.[2] This includes the indications for the agents, knowledge about when to start and/or stop them at appropriate intervals, and familiarity with the effects of each agent on arterial and venous patency. However, it must also be recognized that there are very few prospective data on the use of these agents in endovascular procedures, and therefore the use of most pharmacologic adjuncts is empiric and based on experience and/or traditions acquired during training.

ANTIPLATELET DRUGS

Antiplatelet drugs alter platelet activation at the site of vascular injury, which is usually necessary for the development of arterial thrombosis.[3] Antiplatelet drugs work by decreasing platelet aggregation and inhibiting thrombus formation. They are particularly effective in the arterial circulation, where anticoagulants have little effect. They are widely used not only in the primary and secondary prevention of thrombotic cerebrovascular or cardiovascular disease but also when arterial interventions are being performed and after they have been performed to maintain patency of the artery.[4] Antiplatelet drugs increase the risk of bleeding; low-dose aspirin increases the risk of major bleeding twice that of placebo, but the annual frequency of major bleeding is only 1.3 patients per thousand higher than bleeding from placebo.

The most important antiplatelet drugs are cyclooxygenase inhibitors (aspirin); adenosine diphosphate (ADP) receptor inhibitors (clopidogrel [Plavix]); phosphodiesterase inhibitors (cilostazol [Pletal]); adenosine reuptake inhibitors (dipyridamole [Persantine]); and glycoprotein IIB/IIIA inhibitors (abciximab [ReoPro], eptifibatide [Integrilin], and tirofiban [Aggrastat]), the last three of which are only used intravenously.

Aspirin

Aspirin, also known as acetylsalicylic acid, irreversibly inhibits the enzyme cyclooxygenase, resulting in reduced platelet production of thromboxane A_2, a powerful vasoconstrictor that lowers cyclic adenosine monophosphate (AMP) and initiates platelet release. Recent studies show that acetylsalicylic acid modulates signaling through nuclear factor κB, a transcription factor that plays a major role in many biologic functions. For some people, aspirin does not have a significant effect on platelets, and these patients are known to have aspirin resistance. Women are more likely to have resistance than men. In one study, 28% of patients were resistant, although other studies have found that only 5% are truly resistant and that the others are noncompliant in using aspirin.

Salicylic acid is a weak acid that is poorly soluble in the stomach, which can delay absorption for 8 to 24 hours. Most salicylate is bound by protein whereas the rest remains in the active, ionized state. Up to 80% of salicylic acid is metabolized in the liver. Salicylates are excreted mainly by the kidneys, with first-order kinetics, and a half-life of about 2 to 4.5 hours. The usual dose of aspirin is 81 mg/day to 325 mg/day. Increasing aspirin doses do not result in a greater antiaggregate effect.

The main side effects of aspirin are gastrointestinal (GI) ulcers, gastric bleeding, and tinnitus, especially in higher doses. Although enteric-coated aspirin is promoted to reduce GI symptoms, in one study enteric coating did not reduce this risk. Aspirin in combination with clopidogrel or warfarin also increases the risk of upper GI tract bleeding. Aspirin can cause prolonged bleeding after operations for up to 10 days. In one study, diffuse bleeding was associated with aspirin alone or in combination with another nonsteroidal antiinflammatory drug in 19 out of the 20 who had to have a second operation. There is still an increased risk of gastric bleeding when aspirin is taken with alcohol or warfarin. Aspirin is also known to cause hemolytic anemia in patients who have glucose-6-phosphate dehydrogenase deficiency, depending on the severity of the disease. People with kidney disease, hyperuricemia, or gout should not take aspirin because it inhibits the kidneys' ability to excrete uric acid.

Clopidogrel

Clopidogrel is an oral antiplatelet agent used to inhibit platelet-initiated thrombosis in coronary artery disease, peripheral vascular disease, and cerebrovascular disease. Clopidogrel's actions are related to the ADP receptor on platelet cell membranes; the specific ADP receptor that clopidogrel irreversibly inhibits is $P2Y_{12}$, which is important in platelet aggregation and the cross-linking of platelets by fibrin.[5] The blockade of this receptor inhibits platelet aggregation by blocking activation of the glycoprotein IIb/IIIa pathway. Activation of this receptor complex is the "final common pathway" for platelet aggregation, the cross-linking of platelets by fibrin. Platelet inhibition can be seen 2 hours after a single dose of clopidogrel.

Clopidogrel is indicated for prevention of vascular ischemic events in patients with symptomatic atherosclerosis, including acute coronary syndrome without ST-segment elevation and ST elevation myocardial infarction (MI), and is also used, along with aspirin, for the prevention of thrombosis after placement of intracoronary and peripheral angioplasties and stents.

Clopidogrel is rapidly absorbed after oral administration, with peak plasma levels of the circulating metabolite occurring approximately 1 hour after dosing. This metabolite has an elimination half-life of about 8 hours. After an oral dose of clopidogrel, approximately 50% is excreted in the urine and approximately 45% in the feces in the 5 days after dosing.

Serious adverse drug reactions associated with clopidogrel therapy include severe neutropenia (incidence: 1/2000), thrombotic thrombocytopenic purpura (incidence: 4/1,000,000), and hemorrhage. The incidence of hemorrhage may be increased by the concomitant administration of aspirin. GI hemorrhage occurs in 2.0% of users, and cerebral hemorrhage occurs with an incidence of approximately 0.2%. Nonsteroidal antiinflammatory drugs should not be used in those taking clopidogrel, because of increased risk of GI hemorrhage

Glycoprotein IIb/IIIa Receptor Antagonists

Glycoprotein IIb/IIIa receptor antagonists block receptors on the platelet for fibrinogen and von Willebrand factor. They are currently available only in intravenous form.

Abciximab is a platelet aggregation inhibitor primarily used during and after coronary artery procedures such as angioplasty but also may be used during peripheral angioplasty procedures. It prevents platelets from adhering to either themselves or the vessel wall. Abciximab is made from the Fab fragments of an immunoglobulin that targets the glycoprotein IIb/IIIa receptor on the platelet membrane. Its mechanism of action is inhibition of glycoprotein IIb/IIIa. Abciximab has a plasma half-life of about 10 minutes; however, platelet aggregation usually takes 24 to 48 hours to recover.

Abciximab is indicated for use in individuals undergoing percutaneous coronary and peripheral angioplasty with or without stent placement. The use of abciximab in this setting is associated with a decreased incidence of ischemic complications and a decreased need for repeated revascularization in the first month after the procedure. It is not an appropriate drug for patients undergoing emergency surgery because the bleeding time may take 12 to 24 hours to recover. The drug can be used for patients with diabetes and chronic renal insufficiency.

Most adverse effects of abciximab are due to its antiplatelet effects, including an increased risk of bleeding; the most common type of bleeding is GI hemorrhage. Thrombocytopenia, a rare but serious complication of abciximab, can last for up to 5 days after initial drug administration. Platelet transfusion is the treatment but may have limited effectiveness, because the drug will also bind to the new platelets.

Dipyridamole

Dipyridamole inhibits platelet phosphodiesterase, causing an increase in cyclic AMP with potentiation of the action of prostaglandin I_2—it opposes the action of thromboxane A_2. It is rarely used today because there are better agents with fewer side effects and lower cost.

ANTICOAGULANT DRUGS

An anticoagulant is defined as any substance that prevents coagulation or stops thrombosis; it is useful in primary and secondary prevention of deep vein thrombosis (DVT), pulmonary embolism, and MI and in some cases of stroke.[6] Consequently, many patients who undergo endovascular procedures are taking anticoagulants to treat their coexisting cardiovascular disease. Anticoagulants are routinely used during endovascular procedures and after endovascular procedures to prevent catheter, device, or vessel thrombosis during the implantation and manipulation of the blood vessel and after treatment to increase the patency of the vessel.

Heparin

Heparin is a naturally occurring anticoagulant, produced by basophils and mast cells, which are composed of a highly sulfated glycosaminoglycan biologic substance. It has the highest negative charge density of any known biologic molecule. It is usually made from pig intestine and bovine lung. It activates antithrombin (AT) III, which blocks thrombin from clotting blood. Low-molecular-weight heparin (LMWH) is a more highly processed form of heparin that has more predictable plasma levels with fewer side effects, so it does not require close monitoring of coagulation.

Although heparin is used primarily for anticoagulation, its normal physiologic role in the body remains unclear, because normal in vivo anticoagulation is achieved mostly by endothelial cell–derived heparan sulfate proteoglycans. Heparin is stored in the secretory granules of basophils and mast cells and released only during tissue injury. It has been proposed that the main purpose of heparin is to prevent bacterial invasion at sites of tissue injury.

Heparin, a member of the glycosaminoglycan family of carbohydrates, is a polymer with a molecular weight ranging from 3 to 50 kDa, although most commercial heparin preparations are in the range of 12 to 15 kDa because of the mixtures of polymers of different weights. One unit of heparin is the quantity required to keep 1 mL of cat's blood fluid for 24 hours at 0° C. The effects of heparin are measured in the laboratory by the partial thromboplastin time (aPTT).

Heparin binds to the enzyme inhibitor AT, causing a conformational change that results in activation of AT, which then inactivates thrombin and other proteases involved in blood clotting, such as factor Xa. The formation of a complex between AT, thrombin, and heparin results in the inactivation of thrombin.[7]

LMWHs and fondaparinux, which are more uniform in molecular weight, are increasingly used in preference to heparin. They target anti–factor Xa activity rather than AT. With LMWH and fondaparinux, there is a reduced risk of heparin-induced thrombocytopenia (HIT), and monitoring of the aPTT is also not required, because the aPTT is insensitive to alterations in factor Xa.

Heparin is given parenterally, because it is degraded when taken by mouth. It can be injected intravenously or subcutaneously, but intramuscular injections may cause hematomas and therefore are contraindicated. Because of its short half-life of approximately 1 hour, heparin must be given frequently or as a continuous infusion; however, LMWH, which has a longer half-life and more predictable anticoagulant effect, is given once or twice daily. If long-term anticoagulation is required, heparin is often used primarily to start anticoagulation therapy until the oral anticoagulant warfarin (Coumadin) takes effect. In rare situations, such as pregnant patients who require anticoagulation, LMWH may be injected for up to 9 months, because warfarin passes the placental barrier and is contraindicated in pregnancy.

Adverse reactions include HIT, which is an immunologic reaction to heparin, resulting in the destruction of platelets.[8] This condition is usually reversed by discontinuing the heparin and can generally be avoided with the use of LMWH. There is also a mild form of thrombocytopenia associated with early heparin use, which resolves without stopping heparin. In addition heparin can cause an elevation of serum aminotransferase levels, which has been reported in as many as 80% of patients receiving heparin. It disappears with discontinuation of the drug. Hyperkalemia also occurs with heparin use in 5% of patients receiving heparin and is due to heparin-induced aldosterone suppression. Rare side effects include alopecia and osteoporosis when heparin is used for long periods of time.

Low-Molecular-Weight Heparin

LMWH consists of only short chains of the polysaccharide, with an average molecular weight of less than 8000 Da. LMWH is obtained by fractionation of polymeric heparin. LMWH differs from unfractionated heparin in a number of ways, including the average molecular weight; the need for only once or twice daily dosing; the absence of monitoring the aPTT; and the lower risk of bleeding, osteoporosis, and HIT. In addition, the anticoagulant effect of heparin is reversible with protamine sulfate, whereas its effect on LMWH is limited.

Because LMWH does not require aPTT monitoring and can be given subcutaneously, outpatient treatment is possible in patients who are transitioning from warfarin to LMWH or vice versa. LMWH also does need to be monitored in patients with renal dysfunction, because LMWH has renal clearance.

The usual dose of LMWH (Lovenox) for therapeutic anticoagulation is 1 mg/kg given every 12 hours, although another option is 1.5 mg/kg given once daily.

Fondaparinux

Fondaparinux is a synthetic inhibitor of factor Xa, composed of five sugars (pentasaccharide) that bind to AT. It is a smaller molecule than LMWH.

Direct Thrombin Inhibitors

Direct thrombin inhibitors, such as argatroban, lepirudin, bivalirudin, and dabigatran, are used primarily in patients who require heparinization but who have HIT and are at risk for vascular thrombosis.[9] Although used during endovascular procedures, the drug is costly and there is limited experience with monitoring anticoagulation during an endovascular procedure.

Oral Anticoagulants

Oral anticoagulants, such as warfarin, are a class of drugs that act by antagonizing the effects of vitamin K. Warfarin is the most widely prescribed anticoagulant drug in North America.[10] It was approved for use as an anticoagulant in 1954. Despite its advantages, warfarin has many disadvantages, including interaction with many medications, a requirement for regular blood testing by the international normalized ratio (INR) to ensure that the anticoagulation is within the therapeutic range, and a significant risk of bleeding. Patients aged 80 years or more may be especially susceptible to bleeding complications with a rate of 13 per 100 person-years. Because it takes up to 72 hours for the oral anticoagulant effect to reach therapeutic levels, in cases in which an immediate effect is required heparin must be given concomitantly

Warfarin is a synthetic derivative of coumarin, a chemical found naturally in many plants. Warfarin and related coumarins decrease blood coagulation by inhibiting vitamin K epoxide reductase, an enzyme that recycles oxidated vitamin K to its reduced form after it has participated in the carboxylation of several blood coagulation proteins, mainly prothrombin and factor VII.[11] For this reason, drugs in this class are also referred to as vitamin K antagonists.

Warfarin is prescribed for patients with a high risk of thrombosis, such as those with atrial fibrillation, prosthetic heart valves, DVT, pulmonary embolism, and antiphospholipid syndrome and after MI. Because it takes up to 72 hours for the oral anticoagulant effect to reach therapeutic levels, in cases where an immediate effect is required, heparin must be given concomitantly.

The target INR varies by disease state but is usually in the 2 to 3 range for most conditions, whereas an INR of 3 to 4 may be recommended for patients with mechanical heart valves.[12] Loading regimens vary by institution and physician but are useful in getting patients to full anticoagulation without overshooting on their INR. Warfarin interacts with many medications and some foods—these interactions may enhance or negate warfarin's anticoagulation effect. Consequently, monitoring of the INR and a stable diet will facilitate a consistent level of anticoagulation. During the initial prescription of the drug, blood tests are needed regularly, with the interval between tests lengthened as a stable INR level is achieved.

The most common complication of warfarin is hemorrhage.[13] The annual risk of bleeding is estimated at 1% to 3%, and the risk of bleeding is higher if the INR is elevated above therapeutic levels. The risk of bleeding is also increased when warfarin is combined with antiplatelet drugs such as clopidogrel or aspirin, and bleeding is increased in the elderly and in those receiving hemodialysis.

The most dreaded complication of warfarin is skin necrosis, which occurs more frequently after initiating treatment in patients with a deficiency of protein C.[14] Warfarin initially decreases protein C levels faster than coagulation factors, so the initial effect of warfarin is to promote thrombosis. The system becomes temporarily tilted toward thrombus formation, leading to a prothrombotic state. Administering heparin before warfarin acts on AT and helps reduce the risk of thrombosis. Patients who are given heparin first will have a reduced risk of skin necrosis related to the transient hypercoagulable state.

Warfarin is contraindicated in pregnancy, because it passes through the placental barrier and may cause bleeding in the fetus. Warfarin use during pregnancy is associated with spontaneous abortion, death, and preterm birth.

The effects of warfarin can be reversed with vitamin K or fresh frozen plasma. For patients with an INR between 4.5 and 10.0, a small dose of oral vitamin K is usually sufficient.

Warfarin interacts with many drugs, and protein-bound drugs can displace warfarin from serum albumin, with an increase in INR. Many antibiotics, such as metronidazole, will increase the effect of warfarin, whereas other broad-spectrum antibiotics reduce the normal bacterial flora in the bowel, which make significant quantities of vitamin K. Food also may contain large quantities of vitamin K and may reduce the warfarin effect. Thyroid activity also influences warfarin requirements, and hypothyroidism makes patients less responsive to warfarin treatment.

VASODILATOR THERAPY

During endovascular procedures, vasodilators are often used to help visualize arteries during angiography; to differentiate between spasm, stenosis, and thrombosis and to break spasm that may reduce patency after an endovascular procedure; and to ascertain the success of the endovascular procedure.

Nitroglycerin

Nitroglycerin or glyceryl trinitrate is a vasodilator that has been in medical use since the 1870s and is frequently used in endovascular procedures for rapid arterial dilation. It dilates veins more than arteries but will dilate both rapidly, particularly when placed directly into an artery through a catheter.

Mitochondrial aldehyde dehydrogenase converts nitroglycerin into nitric oxide, which is a potent naturally occurring vasodilator.

Nitroglycerin can cause severe hypotension, and in some cases bradycardia.

Doses for intra-arterial use range from 1 to 2 mcg/kg, or 100- to 200-mcg boluses can be repeated as necessary, with close monitoring of the blood pressure and discontinuation if hypotension occurs.

Papaverine

Papaverine, an opium alkaloid, is a direct smooth muscle relaxant used in the treatment of vasospasm during endovascular procedures. It can also be applied directly to blood vessels during open surgery.[15] It originates in the poppy plant but differs in pharmacologic action from the other opiates.

The mechanism of action appears to be due to inhibition of the enzyme phosphodiesterase, causing an elevation of cyclic AMP levels.

Side effects of papaverine treatment include arterial hypotension, ventricular tachycardia, flushing of the face, tachycardia, and paradoxical aggravation of cerebral vasospasm.

Doses of 15 to 30 mg of intra-arterial papaverine, up to a maximum of 60 mg/hr, can be given intra-arterially to improve visualization of the artery. Close monitoring for hypotension is mandatory.

THROMBOLYTIC THERAPY

Thrombolysis is the dissolution of blood clot by pharmacologic means. It works by stimulating the body's normal fibrinolytic system through the infusion of analogs of tissue plasminogen activator (t-PA), the protein that normally activates plasmin, the major enzyme responsible for thrombus dissolution. T-PA is a serine protease, found on endothelial cells, and is the enzyme that catalyzes the conversion of plasminogen to plasmin. Thrombolysis is used to open thrombosed arteries and veins, prosthetic and autogenous grafts, and thrombosed stents and endografts.[16,17] It is also used in MI, ischemic stroke, DVT, acute angioaccess occlusion, and pulmonary embolism.[18,19] Thrombolysis is also indicated to clear occluded catheters that are placed in central or peripheral veins.

Thrombolytic drugs are made through recombinant technology, where activators of plasminogen are manufactured by bacteria. Commonly used thrombolytic drugs include alteplase (recombinant t-PA; Activase), reteplase (Retavase), tenecteplase (TNKase), and urokinase (Abbokinase). They are usually delivered in combination with intravenous heparin or LMWH.[20]

T-PA catalyzes the conversion of plasminogen into plasmin by cleaving the single-chained plasminogen into two chains, linked by a disulfide bond, and called plasmin. Plasmin works by clearing the cross-linked fibrin mesh, breaking the backbone of the thrombus, and making the clot soluble and subject to further proteolysis by other enzymes.

Because the major risk of thrombolysis is bleeding, it should not be used in patients who have had recent bleeding, uncontrolled hypertension, hemorrhagic stroke, or surgery or other invasive procedures within the previous 10 days. Other relative contraindications include bleeding disorders, diabetic retinopathy, and untreated hypertension.

MANAGEMENT OF PATIENTS RECEIVING ANTIPLATELET DRUGS AND/OR ANTICOAGULATION BEFORE AN ENDOVASCULAR PROCEDURE

Many patients are receiving antiplatelet medications or anticoagulation before a procedure, often for underlying cardiovascular disease, as either prevention or therapy. The endovascular surgeon must decide how critical it is to continue the antiplatelet/anticoagulation and whether the same or another regimen will be required after the procedure to maintain success of the procedure. The usual approach is to determine the risk of being without antiplatelet drugs or anticoagulation for the period of treatment and, if it is not high, to continue antiplatelet drugs and discontinue anticoagulation before the procedure, because anticoagulant alternatives are usually used during the procedure. Optimally, anticoagulation during a procedure that has a risk of bleeding should be reversible and specifically designed for the procedure.

Warfarin (Coumadin)

Warfarin has a number of chronic indications, including use for atrial fibrillation, DVT, and after prosthetic aortic and mitral valve replacement. In each indication, the endovascular surgeon must assess the risk of a thrombotic complication if the anticoagulation is stopped. If the risk is low for a thrombotic event when the warfarin is stopped, discontinuing it during the periprocedural time is recommended, and bridging with a shorter half-life anticoagulant such as heparin or LMWH is recommended (Table 78-1).

For patients with prosthetic heart valves or subacute bacterial endocarditis, where the risk of a thrombotic event is high when anticoagulation is discontinued for even a few days, bridging with heparin is the optimal approach. The use of LMWH or unfractionated heparin allows them to be discontinued during or after the procedure if there are bleeding complications and yet protects the patient from a thrombotic event during the procedure, because the heparin need only be discontinued for a short period of time during the procedure and can be restarted immediately when the risk of bleeding has diminished. Table 78-2 shows one commonly used method of bridging when patients require anticoagulation during the periprocedural period.

For patients who are receiving anticoagulation for embolic prophylaxis from conditions such as atrial fibrillation, and who have not had a prior event, warfarin may be discontinued for 4 to 5 days before the procedure and the prothrombin time and INR measured immediately before the procedure to determine the extent of residual anticoagulation and the subsequent risk of bleeding. Most endovascular surgeons will proceed with the procedure if the INR is 1.8 or less, but if a procedure with a higher risk of bleeding is being performed, such as thrombolysis, the INR should be less than 1.5. Table 78-2 demonstrates a typical order set for a patient who is receiving treatment with long-term warfarin and needs to have it discontinued before the procedure.

For most patients who require postprocedural warfarin, it should be resumed as soon as the bleeding risk is low. For many patients, this occurs at the end of the procedure, and warfarin can be restarted on the evening of

TABLE 78-1 Antithrombotics

Antiplatelet	**COX inhibitors**	e.g., Acetylsalicylic acid (Aspirin)
	ADP receptor/P2Y$_{12}$ inhibitors	e.g., Clopidogrel, Ticlopidine
	Glycoprotein IIb/IIIa inhibitors	e.g., Abciximab
	Other	e.g., Dipyridamole
Anticoagulants	**Vitamin K antagonists** (inhibit II, VII, IX, X)	e.g., Warfarin
	Heparin group	e.g., Low-molecular-weight heparin (Dalteparin, Enoxaparin)
	Factor Xa inhibitors (with some II inhibition)	e.g., Oligosaccharides (Fondaparinux)
	Direct factor Xa inhibitors	e.g., Xabans (Apixaban)
	Direct thrombin inhibitors	e.g., Hirudin, Argatroban
Thrombolytic	**Plasminogen activators**	e.g., tPA (Alteplase, Reteplase, Tenecteplase) e.g., UPA (Urokinase)
	Other serine endopeptidases	e.g., Ancrod

TABLE 78-2 Protocol for Bridging From Warfarin to Heparin

Preop day 1	Hold warfarin (Coumadin).
Preop day 2	Hold Coumadin. Give Lovenox 1 mg/kg every 12 hr.
Preop day 3	Hold Coumadin. Give Lovenox 1 mg/kg every 12 hr.
Preop day 4	Hold Coumadin. Give Lovenox 1 mg/kg every 12 hr.
Preop day 5	Hold Coumadin. Hold Lovenox.
Day of procedure	Depending on bleeding risk, restart Coumadin (loading dose) and Lovenox 1 mg/kg in the evening.
Postop day 1	Coumadin loading dose and Lovenox 1 mg/kg every 12 hr.
Postop day 2 and 3	Coumadin normal dose and Lovenox 1 mg/kg every 12 hr.
Postop day 4	Give Lovenox in the AM and check an INR.INR goal = 2-3.

INR, International normalized ratio; *Postop*, postoperative; *Preop*, preoperative.
NOTE: One successful protocol for converting a patient from Coumadin to heparin while maintaining anticoagulation. Conversion to heparin should be considered in patients who require continuous anticoagulation and who are undergoing a procedure with a risk of bleeding, such as thrombolysis, open surgery, or certain endovascular procedures.

the procedure. Patients who have warfarin discontinued for a short period of time do not require an overlap with heparin unless they have protein C deficiency. Patients who have warfarin stopped for a longer period of time (>1 week) need to have heparin used initially for several days before the institution of warfarin to avoid the hypercoagulable state associated with the initiation of warfarin alone.

Antiplatelet Therapy

Patients receiving antiplatelet therapy before an endovascular procedure rarely need to have the drug discontinued. Exceptions to this principle are patients who are taking clopidogrel and require a hybrid, or combined endovascular and open, procedure. In this case, discontinuation of the clopidogrel for 5 to 7 days is recommended. The most challenging dilemma is a patient who undergoes coronary angioplasty with stenting and is the early (<6 months) period, when clopidogrel use is mandatory to prevent stent thrombosis and early death. Because these patients cannot have their clopidogrel stopped, open procedures should be avoided. If an open procedure is required, exogenous platelets should be available before starting the procedure and techniques used in the operating room to limit bleeding.

POSTPROCEDURE OPTIONS FOR ANTIPLATELET DRUGS AND ANTICOAGULATION

Every endovascular procedure requires some form of antiplatelet drug or anticoagulant after the procedure. Although the decision for specific drug use may seem arbitrary, the principle of using some antiplatelet drug after an endovascular procedure is rational, because virtually all patients have either underlying cardiovascular disease, an injured endothelium where the procedure was performed, or an uncovered device. When the intervention has been in the artery, then antiplatelet drugs should suffice. When the intervention has been in the veins, such as with iliac vein stenting for May-Thurner syndrome, then warfarin anticoagulation is required for the first few months after the procedure.

References

1. Norgren L, Hiatt WR, Dormandy JA, et al: FGR, on behalf of the TASC II Working Group. Inter-Society Consensus for the Management of Peripheral Arterial Disease (TASC II), *J Vasc Surg* 45(1):S5–S67, 2007.
2. Donayre CE: Current use of low molecular weight heparins, *Semin Vascul Surg* 9:362–371, 1996.
3. Tsu EC: Antiplatelet drugs in arterial thrombosis: a review, *Am J Hosp Pharm* 35(12):1507–1515, 2005.
4. Robless P, Mikhailidis DP, Stansby G: Systematic review of antiplatelet therapy for the prevention of myocardial infarction, stroke or vascular death in patients with peripheral vascular disease, *Br J Surg* Volume 88(14):787–800, 2001, Number 6.
5. Arepally GM, Ortel TL: Heparin-induced thrombocytopenia, *N Engl J Med* 8:809–817, 2006, 355.
6. Dayal R, Bernheim J, Clair DG, et al: Multimodal percutaneous intervention for critical venous occlusive disease, *Ann Vasc Surg* 19(2):235–240, 2005.
7. Bjork I, Lindahl U: Mechanism of the anticoagulant action of heparin, *Mol. Cell. Biochem* 48:161–182, 1982.
8. Junqueira D: Unfractionated heparin versus low molecular weight heparin for avoiding heparin-induced thrombocytopenia in postoperative patients, *Cochrane Reviews*, www.cochrane.org/reviews, November 2008.
9. Hirsh J, O'Donnell M, Eikelboom JW: Beyond unfractionated heparin and warfarin: current and future advances, *Circulation* 116(5):552–560, 2007.
10. Holbrook AM, Pereira JA, Labiris R, et al: Systematic overview of warfarin and its drug and food interactions, *Arch. Intern. Med* 165 (10):1095–1106, 2005.
11. Ansell J, Hirsh J, Poller L, et al: The pharmacology and management of the vitamin K antagonists: the Seventh ACCP Conference on Antithrombotic and Thrombolytic Therapy, *Chest* 126(suppl 3):204S–233S, 2004.
12. Baglin TP, Keeling DM, Watson HG: Guidelines on oral anticoagulation (warfarin): third edition—2005 update, *Br J Haematol* 132(3):277–285, 2006.
13. Hylek EM, Evans-Molina C, Shea C: Major hemorrhage and tolerability of warfarin in the first year of therapy among elderly patients with atrial fibrillation, *Circulation* 115(21):2689–2696, 2007.
14. Chan YC, Valenti D, Mansfield AO: Warfarin induced skin necrosis, *Br J Surg* 87(3):266–272, 2000.
15. Takeuchi K, Sakamoto S, Nagayoshi Y, et al: Reactivity of the human internal thoracic artery to vasodilators in coronary artery bypass grafting, *Eur J Cardiothorac Surg* 26(5):956–959, 2004.
16. Semba CP, Murphy TP, Bakal CW, et al: Thrombolytic therapy with use of alteplase (rt-PA) in peripheral arterial occlusive disease: review of the clinical literature. The Advisory Panel, *J Vasc Interv Radiol* 11(2):149–161, 2000.
17. Kent KC: Thrombolytic therapy for peripheral vascular disease, *J Vasc Surg* 22(1):126, 1995.
18. Comerota AJ, Gravett MH: Iliofemoral venous thrombosis, *J Vasc Surg* 46(5):1065–1076, 2007.
19. Sugimoto K, Hofmann LV, Razavi MK, et al: The safety, efficacy, and pharmacoeconomics of low-dose alteplase compared with urokinase for catheter-directed thrombolysis of arterial and venous occlusions, *J Vasc Surg* 37(3):512–517, 2003.
20. Kessel DO, Berridge DC, Robertson, et al: Infusion techniques for peripheral arterial thrombolysis, *Cochrane Database Syst Rev* (1):CD000985, 2004.

Index

The letter t indicates a table, b indicates a box, and f indicates a figure.

C

D

F

G

H

I

M

N

O

P

S

T

U

V

W

X

Y

Z